McGRAW-HILL REVIEW FOR THE NCLEX-RN® EXAMINATION

Edited by

Frances D. Monahan, PhD, RN, ANEF
Professor
Department of Nursing
SUNY Rockland Community College
Suffern, New York

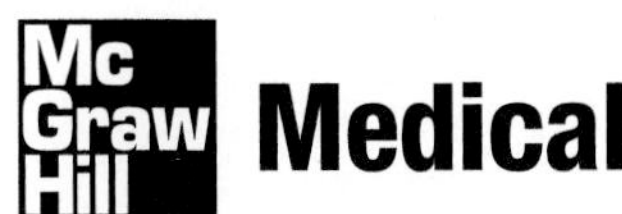

New York Chicago San Francisco Lisbon London Madrid Mexico City
Milan New Delhi San Juan Seoul Singapore Sydney Toronto

The McGraw-Hill Companies

McGraw-Hill Review for the NCLEX-RN® Examination

1 2 3 4 5 6 7 8 9 0 0 9 8

Set ISBN 978-0-07-146077-4
Set MHID 0-07-146077-2
Book ISBN 978-0-07-154710-9
Book MHID 0-07-154710-X
CD ISBN 978-0-07-154711-6
CD MHID 0-07-154711-8

Notice

Medicine is an ever-changing science. As new research and clinical experience broaden our knowledge, changes in treatment and drug therapy are required. The authors and the publisher of this work have checked with sources believed to be reliable in their efforts to provide information that is complete and generally in accord with the standards accepted at the time of publication. However, in view of the possibility of human error or changes in medical sciences, neither the authors nor the publisher nor any other party who has been involved in the preparation or publication of this work warrants that the information contained herein is in every respect accurate or complete, and they disclaim all responsibility for any errors or omissions or for the results obtained from use of the information contained in this work. Readers are encouraged to confirm the information contained herein with other sources. For example and in particular, readers are advised to check the product information sheet included in the package of each drug they plan to administer to be certain that the information contained in this work is accurate and that changes have not been made in the recommended dose or in the contraindications for administration. This recommendation is of particular importance in connection with new or infrequently used drugs.

This book was set in Berkeley Book by Aptara, Inc.
The editors were Quincy McDonald and Christie Naglieri.
The production supervisor was Sherri Souffrance.
Project management was provided by Aptara, Inc.
The designer was Eve Siegel; the cover designer was Kelly Parr.
Quebecor World Dubuque was printer and binder.

This book is printed on acid-free paper.

Library of Congress Cataloging-in-Publication Data

Monahan, Frances Donovan.
McGraw-Hill review for the NCLEX-RN examination / Frances D. Monahan. — 1st ed.
p. ; cm.
Includes index.
ISBN-13: 978-0-07-146077-4 (pbk. : alk. paper)
ISBN-10: 0-07-146077-2 (pbk. : alk. paper)
1. Practical nursing—Examinations, questions, etc. 2. National Council Licensure Examination for Practical/Vocational Nurses—Study guides. I. Title. II. Title: Review for the NCLEX-RN examination.

[DNLM: 1. Nursing Care—Examination Questions. WY 18.2 M734m 2008]
RT62.M58 2008
610.73076—dc22

2007029498

DEDICATION

Dedicated with all my love—first and foremost to the memory of my husband, William T. Monahan, also to my family and friends who support and tolerate me while I work and bring meaning and happiness to my days:

- Michael M. Monahan, my son;
- Kerryane T. Monahan, my daughter, and Robson Diniz, my son-in-law;
- John Donovan, my brother;
- Gerard Donovan, my brother, and Anita Donovan, my sister-in-law;
- Claire T. Torpey, my aunt;
- Suzanne M. Reynolds;
- Mary Ellen Wyllie;
- Josephine and James Hammer.

Many thanks to all of them.

CONTENTS

CONTRIBUTORS

FEATURED EDITORS

Charlotte E. Blackwell, RN, BSN, MSEd
Pharmacology
Instructor, Department of Nursing
Wake Technical Community College
Raleigh, North Carolina

Judy E. White, RNC, MA, MSN
Maternal-Child Health and Sample Test Question
Faculty, Southern Union State Community College
Opelika, Alabama

CONTRIBUTORS

Susan E. Abbe, PhD, RN
Nursing Curriculum Specialist
Connecticut Community-Technical Colleges
Hartford, Connecticut

Sharon A. Aronovitch, PhD, APRN, BC, CWOCN
Faculty, School of Nursing
Excelsior College
Albany, New York

Mary Sharon Boni, PhD, RN, CCRN
Professor & Dean
School of Nursing and Allied Health Administration
Fairmont State University
Fairmont, West Virginia

Susan R. Bulecza, RN, MSN, CNS, APRN, BC
Florida Department of Health
Office of Public Health Preparedness
Tallahassee, Florida

Patricia D. Coyne, RNC, MSN, MPA
Maternal-Newborn Instructor
Cochran School of Nursing
Yonkers, New York
Adjunct Professor, Maternal-Newborn Nursing
Rockland Community College
Suffern, New York

Paula M. Crawford, RN, MSN
Assistant Professor
Nursing Department
Orange County Community College
Middletown, New York

Dale A. Lange Crispell, RN, BSN, MA
Instructor, Department of Nursing
SUNY Rockland Community College
Suffern, New York

Mary Rose Driggers, RN, MSN
LPN-ADN Online Program Director and Nursing Instructor
Health Technology Division
Davidson Country Community College
Lexington, North Carolina

Miriam Freud, RN, MSN
Director, Adult Day Care Center
Friedwald Center for Rehabilitation & Nursing
New City, New York

Anne Hussey, BS, MSEd, RN (Retired)
Education Specialist School Nurse
Portsmouth Middle School
Portsmouth, New Hampshire

Laima M. Karosas, PhD, APRN
Associate Professor of Nursing
Quinnipiac University
Hamden, Connecticut

Dorothea Lever, RN, MS, CDE, CCRN
Associate Professor and Coordinator
Department of Nursing
SUNY Rockland Community College
Suffern, New York

Lisa L. Lombard, MD
Diplomat American Board of Anesthesiology
Boston, Massachusetts

Jana Henson Lyner, MSN, RN
Faculty, Department of Nursing
Pensacola Junior College
Pensacola Florida

M. Bridget Nettleton, PhD, RN,
Dean, School of Nursing
Excelsior College
Albany, New York

Tina Peer, MS, RN
Assistant Professor of Nursing
Associate Degree Nursing Program
College of Southern Idaho
Twin Falls, Idaho

Patricia Sue Ragsdale, MSN, RN
Assistant Professor of Nursing
University of Arkansas at Little Rock
Little Rock, Arkansas

Joyce Grant Scott, MSN, BSN, ASN, CLNC, RN
Associate Professor of Nursing
University of Arkansas at Little Rock
Little Rock, Arkansas

Lovely Varghese, MSN, FNP, BC, CNOR
Educator, Department of Nursing Education
Columbia Presbyterian Medical Center
New York, New York

Susan M. Wicks, RNc, BS, MS
Advanced Medical-Surgical Nursing Faculty
Cochran School of Nursing
St. John's Riverside Health Care System
Yonkers, New York
NCLEX-RN Presenter
Pace University
Pleasantville, New York

Denise D. Wilson, PhD, APN, FNP, ANP
Associate Professor
Mennonite College of Nursing
Illinois State University
Normal, Illinois
Family Nurse Practitioner
Medical Hills Internists & Pediatrics
Bloomington, Illinois

PREFACE

Dear **Soon-to-be Registered Nurse**,

The purpose of this book is to help you be successful on the NCLEX-RN® examination so that you can obtain your license as a registered nurse. You have worked long and hard to successfully complete your basic nursing program. Now the one thing between you and your license is the NCLEX-RN examination.

This book is designed to guide your review study. There is a vast amount of nursing knowledge and it can be organized and focused upon in different ways. This book is designed to review the content most likely to appear on the examination and approach it from the perspective of the examination. Thus, the book begins with a discussion of the test itself to direct your focus. Because time is a limited and valuable commodity for all of you as you begin life after nursing school, strategies for studying in the most effective, time-efficient manner also are discussed.

A unique feature of this text is a preparatory chapter on language. Despite advanced study, you may often have a few words whose meanings were never clearly mastered. Encountering one of these words in a test question can result in a wrong answer. Hence, some of the words that are often used in nursing but are prone to being misunderstood are identified, defined, and their use illustrated in sentences reflective of nursing practice. There is also a chapter on test-taking strategies. You may have already used many of these, but reviewing them as a unit helps to ensure that you are approaching the NCLEX-RN with the sharpest test-taking skills possible. The chapter even provides exercises to allow you to practice key skills.

The next 30 chapters of the book present the review of nursing content. The title of each chapter consists of one of the major NCLEX-RN test plan categories followed by the subcategories and topics from the plan to be covered in that chapter. Precise headings found on the NCLEX-RN test plan have been used to help you think about the content in the same way that the test is organized and the questions are designed. There are separate sections in the text dealing with the child-bearing client and with gerontology just as there are in the test plan. Care of the pediatric client is incorporated throughout the text. *Icons in the margin are alerts that the information applies specifically to a pediatric client or a child-bearing client.*

To help you recognize and learn critical points of content, the following alerts, which highlight key pieces of information, have been included in the chapters:

Assessment Alerts are key considerations related to assessing a particular type of client. These are factors with potential for significant impact on the client's health status if they not recognized and usually represent variations from the norm.

Nursing Intervention Alerts are dos and don'ts of practice that have significant import for the client's well being and that apply to a specific client problem not to all clients.

Clinical Alerts are specific items of information unique to a health problem, treatment, or test, which if not known can lead to incorrect interpretation of a clinical situation and an incorrect nursing action.

Practice Alerts are critical guidelines such as legal requirements or standards, which relate to the practice of nursing in general.

In addition to the alerts, complications and client teaching are highlighted areas because each is a separate section on the NCLEX-RN test plan. A complications heading follows the Rx heading in the presentation of health problems, surgery, treatments, and diagnostic tests whenever there are significant complications that should be known. In addition, there is a table summarizing complications related to major disorders. A section on client teaching, which lists specific information that needs to be taught to the client, is part of the presentation of virtually every health problem and major diagnostic or treatment modality.

Think Smart—Test Smart boxes found throughout the book are designed to make you stop and think about the differences between similar or frequently confused words or concepts, the different ways the information could be worded, how questions could be asked in different ways to test the same content, or to identify a memory trick related to content to be learned.

Also unique to this book are worksheets at the end of each chapter. These worksheets allow you to actively engage with the content; help to further "cement" content into memory; and provide a check of your understanding of basic facts and concepts. This is important because NCLEX-RN is primarily a test of application of knowledge and one cannot apply what one does not know.

Of course, the book also contains hundreds of practice questions. Practice questions are given at the end of each chapter as well as in the last chapter of the book, which consists of 198 pages of questions. Questions are both in the form of NCLEX-RN questions with multiple choice and as alternative types of questions. For all questions, the correct answer is explained; for multiple-choice questions, reasons why options are incorrect are also given. In many cases, these explanations are "mini lectures," which serve to synthesize and or highlight an area of information. Thus the content review chapters and the final question chapter work together to present key concepts for review.

I believe that this book will help you be successful on the NCLEX-RN. It is based on more than 25 years of teaching nursing students and giving NCLEX-RN review classes. I wish you success on the examination and hope that you find nursing a fulfilling and rewarding profession.

Sincerely,

Fran Monahan, PhD, RN, ANEF

Part I

TESTING SMART

CHAPTER 1

Preparing for NCLEX-RN®

PART 1: THE TEST

Purpose of NCLEX-RN®

The purpose of this examination is to protect the safety of the public. The examination is designed to determine whether candidates for licensure as registered nurses have the minimum level of knowledge needed to practice competently, knowledgeably, and safely at an entry level.

In preparing for the examination, key words from the stated purpose of the examination that you should think about are minimum level, safely, and entry level. These words can help focus your preparation and ease your mind. What they tell you is that the examination questions will test general principles and commonly encountered patient care situations. The focus will not be on testing obscure pieces of knowledge applicable only rarely in practice. Neither will the test focus on situations that demand a complexity of judgment, which can be expected only with time and experience. What can be expected to be stressed are nursing assessments and actions that protect patients from harm. This means that in preparing, you must give special attention to facts and procedures that promote physical safety, emotional safety, and protection from, or early identification of, disease complications or iatrogenic problems.

Development of the NCLEX-RN®

Knowing the basic process by which the examination is developed will further help direct your preparation. It will reinforce the fact that the questions focus on critical information regularly used by new graduates in daily practice.

NCLEX-RN® has been developed by the National Council of State Boards of Nursing (NCSBN) and is updated on the basis of a work-study analysis of what new graduates do in the workplace. All aspects of nursing practice are observed and then classified into categories and subcategories. These categories and subcategories then form the basis of the test plan, which specifies the content to be covered and the number of questions to be asked related to each area. Job analyses are done periodically and the test plan is changed, if required, according to the results. This ensures that the test remains accurate and consistent with current practice. Content of the examination is matched to the scope of practice.

In selecting the content to be tested, there are two major considerations: the frequency with which the information is needed in day-to-day practice and the criticality of the information to the patient.

The test questions are written by nurses who practice in a setting where they work with new graduates. The questions are carefully edited for any type of bias. They are also reviewed for clarity and correctness of the key by other practitioners. This ensures that the questions and answers represent accepted principles of safe practice and not a regional practice or opinion.

The Test Plan Content

The content is organized around four categories of human needs, which have been identified by the NCSBN. The four categories and their related subcategories are as follows:

- Safe, effective care environment
  —Management of care
  —Safety and infection control
- Health promotion and maintenance
  —Growth and development through the lifespan
  —Prevention and early detection of disease
- Psychosocial integrity
  —Coping and adaptation
  —Psychosocial adaptation
- Physiological integrity
  —Basic care and comfort
  —Pharmacological and parenteral therapies
  —Reduction of risk potential
  —Physiological adaptation

Each of these subcategories constitutes 5–13% of the test except for Reduction of Risk Potential and Physiological Adaptation each of which accounts for 12–18% of the total questions.

Integrated throughout each of the client needs categories are the steps of the nursing process, caring, communication and documentation, and teaching and learning.

NCLEX-RN® Style

In preparing for any examination, it is always helpful to have some idea of what to expect in terms of style. This helps prevent surprises, which can be distracting and can create anxiety. Knowing about the examination style in advance, helps free your mind to focus on the content of the questions. Some key points about the style of the NCLEX-RN® are that it

- uses the term "client," not "patient," to refer to the recipient of care.
- is an integrated examination, that is, it covers clients of all ages, backgrounds, and levels of health or illness.
- is gender neutral.
- is reviewed to remove any culturally biased terms.
- has primarily a multiple-choice format: stem and four options only one of which is the answer to the question.
- includes some other types of questions, for example,

—those that require the test taker to fill in the blanks with numerals or words rather than selecting an answer from a list of four options.

Example:

What is the normal heart rate in a newborn?

_____beats per minute.

—those that contain pictures/diagrams and ask the test taker to identify a particular site by touching the correct area on the diagram.

Example:

Where would the nurse auscultate for the apical pulse?

The test taker has to touch an area on a diagram of the chest. If the test taker touches the correct area or "hot spot," the answer is correct.

—those that present a list of assessment findings or nursing actions, etc., and ask the test taker to identify all those that are appropriate for a particular type of patient.

Example:

Which of the following are risk factors for cancer of the breast?

Mark all that apply.

- Family history
- Nulliparity
- Age over 50 years
- Late menopause
- Breast-feeding
- Cigarette smoking
- Provides a drop-down calculator as needed.

Administration of the NCLEX-RN®

To be admitted to the NCLEX-RN®, you need

- an Authorization to Text letter (This is sent to you upon receipt of application and fees and verification of eligibility.)
- two forms of ID—one of which must be a photograph ID and both of which must be signed

NCLEX-RN® is administered by computer. Taking the test on the computer is not complicated; it only requires use of the SPACE bar, the ENTER key, and for fill-in-the-blank answers, the keyboard. For multiple-choice and other similar questions, the cursor is moved to highlight the option selected as the answer by pressing the SPACE bar. When the option(s) selected is highlighted, the ENTER button is pressed. Then there is an opportunity to check your answer selection. If the option(s) highlighted is not the answer you want to give, you may change to another. If the answer you wish to give is highlighted, you press the ENTER key a second time to register your answer. Some very important points for you to remember about taking the examination are that

- after the ENTER key is pressed a second time to register your answer, there is no returning to the question or changing the answer.
- every question must be answered; you cannot skip a question.
- there is no penalty for guessing.

Number of Questions on the NCLEX-RN®

As a test taker, you of course, would like to know as part of your mental preparation and planning for the examination, how many questions you will be asked. For the NCLEX-RN®, there is no precise answer to this question because it is a computer adaptive test (CAT). This means that the computer selects the next question based on whether your answer to the previous question was right or wrong. If the previous answer was correct, the computer will select a slightly more difficult question for the next one; if the answer was incorrect, the computer will present a slightly easier question. Thus, each person takes a unique test. The maximum number of questions a candidate can have is 265. However, the computer is programmed to make a decision of competent or incompetent based on the level of difficulty of questions answered correctly or incorrectly so relatively few candidates receive 265 questions. The minimum number of questions a candidate can receive is 75. Of these 75, 15 pretest items, i.e., items that are being tested for future use, are interspersed. These pretest items do not influence your passing or failing.

Examination Time

In preparing for an examination, it is also important to know how much time you will be allowed to complete it. The total time allowed for the NCLEX-RN® is 6 hours. If at the end of 6 hours, you have not answered enough questions for the computer to determine whether you are competent, you fail by default. Based on the maximum of 265 questions and the maximum time of 6 hours (360 minutes), there is slightly more than one and a third minutes allowed per question. However, since few candidates receive the maximum allowable number of questions, the time available is generally more. Nonetheless, time is not unlimited so you should not spend excessive time on any one question.

Report of Pass—Fail

Forty-eight hours after you take the test, the Board of Nursing in the state where you are applying for licensure gets the pass/fail result. The Board then checks that all other requirements for licensure are met, and then sends out your results. Results are only reported in writing and never by telephone.

If you have failed the examination, it may be taken again in 3 months. How many times the test may be repeated depends on the State Board of Nursing.

NCLEX Myths

The NCLEX-RN® is one of the most important examinations that nurses ever take. To reach the point of taking the examination, much time, energy, and money have been invested and many sacrifices have been made. Because of these facts, you will hear many stories about the examination and receive much advice. This type of impromptu shared information often contributes to "myths" about the NCLEX-RN®, which serve as sources of undue anxiety. Some of the more common myths, and the corrections to them, are presented below.

The number of questions one receives indicates pass or fail.—This is not true. Candidates can answer the minimum number of questions, all of which are difficult, correctly and pass. Other candidates can answer the minimum number of questions, all of which are easy, and fail. It is not the number of items but the difficulty of the items that determines pass or fail.

Extra long tests are given randomly to selected test takers.—This is not true. The number of questions is determined by the difficulty of questions you answer correctly or incorrectly.

One needs to memorize everything.—This is not true. The test is looking at determining safe, entry-level practice based on the job analysis of what new graduates actually do in the work place. It is also testing generally accepted standards/methods of care. It is not testing rare, regionally variable information.

How good you are with the computer determines how well you do on the examination.—The Educational Testing Service has done research on the question as to whether computer skill influences examination performance. The results show that the test-taker's computer skill does not influence the score on the examination.

For more information about NCLEX, see the NCLEX Candidate Bulletin which can be accessed at the NCSBN Web site www.ncsbn.org.

PART 2: STUDYING FOR THE TEST

Study smart and study well! Remember, this is your future. It represents short-term sacrifice for a long-term gain.

Identify Areas for Intensive Review

Evaluate your own strengths and weaknesses. Often, it is a temptation to spend most of your study time reviewing material you already know quite well. This is because what you know best is most often material that you like, find easy, and are interested in (that is why you learned it well in the beginning). It is comfortable material and makes you feel good about taking the examination. *Avoid this pitfall. Spend most of the time on what you do not know so well.*

Begin identifying what you do not know so well by thinking about what areas you did least well on in nursing school or had the least experience with—write them down. These may be broad areas of practice, for example, pediatrics or mental health/psychiatric nursing or specific topics such as acid—base balance, burns, or problems of the nervous system. If you are not a recent graduate, also identify those things that you did well in nursing school but have not had any recent experience with; these areas will need review but not as much time as those areas you did not know really well in the beginning. Be careful about assuming that since you have a lot of experience in a practice area you do not need to review. Remember NCLEX is a theory/textbook-oriented examination. The questions and answers are based on what "should be" in practice, not on the shortcuts and improvisations that "are." Whether you are a new or a not-so-new graduate, review the list of topics in the NCLEX-RN® test plan found in this book and judge your level of comfort with each, referring of course to the list you made as the first part of this exercise. Mark with two checks those topics you feel you really do not know; make one check by those that you probably do not know really well. This will serve as a guide to make sure you review the areas most important to you.

Select Backup Review Materials

This book, like all review books, is written in an abbreviated format that assumes basic understanding and focuses on key points. If you never mastered an area well or you encounter content in this book that you do not understand the basis of, it is important to go to a basic classroom text for clarification and additional discussion.

NCLEX-RN® utilizes selected texts as references. Lists of text books are sent to schools of nursing with directions to indicate those which are used in the curriculum and to add any that are used but do not appear on the list. Reference texts are selected based on the extent of use in schools of nursing. Questions are designed to address basic principles of practice about which all texts agree, not to test about uncommon pieces of information, which are debatable. The current list can be accessed at the NCSBN Web site.

Develop a Realistic Schedule for Review

Dividing up material into achievable goals is smart. Each time you meet a goal, you feel more positive about yourself and your ability to deal with the material and the examination. This reduces stress and hence supports your ability to be successful. There are different ways to develop a realistic schedule. One way is to determine the number of days until you are scheduled to take the NCLEX-RN®. Also, determine how many hours on how many of these days can you realistically study. Be sure to allow for down time. After all, no one can study without a break and everyone must eat, sleep, bathe, etc. Tally total available study times/hours. Now assign study times/hours to the topics for review. Working from the test plan topics that you have marked according to how well you feel you know them, assign hours first to the topics needing in-depth review. These are the most important topics to review because you have already acknowledged that you do not feel you know them. Next, assign study times to those topics, which you decided you probably do not know well, and then to those needing a less-detailed review. Finally, place the topics in the order you will study them. Alternate hard and easy topics and topics you like with those you do not like—this will help keep you from shortening your scheduled study time.

To have enough time to study well you may need to make some temporary changes in your lifestyle. You may need to take time off from work, negotiate sharing of household tasks with others in the house, delay some projects or activities, and limit your social life. Only you can determine what is the best approach to ensure the time you need for study but as you consider your options remember—cramming is not one of them. It will not work. There is way too much material.

Select a Study Place That Works for You

Your study place should be quiet and convenient. A place you will be undisturbed but with space for your study materials. It should have good light to facilitate reading without developing eyestrain and/or a headache, a comfortable seat, and an ambient temperature that is not so warm that it makes you sleepy and not so cold that it distracts you from studying. Lying in bed or on a couch to study is not a good idea as it is at best relaxing, and at worst, sleep-inducing. A certain level of awake alertness is necessary for successful studying.

Select a Study Time That Works for You

Different people are most alert at different times of the day. Some people are "morning people" and concentrate best on first getting up; others are night people and concentrate best in the evening. Some people have periods of best function at two different times of the day. Analyze yourself to determine when your most productive intellectual periods are and then plan to study the most challenging material during these times. Plan to review material that needs less intense study at other times. If you have family responsibilities around which you must organize study time, involve family members in planning how to make your best study times available for working on your NCLEX-RN® review.

Make Use of All Available Time for Study

You can learn a great deal, relatively painlessly, by making good use of small amounts of available time throughout the day. You may have done this during nursing school. If so, recall some of your strategies. If not, begin to develop time-effective study techniques now.

Examples of how you can capitalize on bits of unused time:

- Review a brief set of laboratory values, the principles of a nursing procedure, or assessment parameters for a specific disease in the 5 minutes before you take a shower, then use the time in the shower to repeat them to yourself.
- Write information to be learned on an index card(s) and study when standing in line at the grocery store or when waiting to pick children up at the school bus, etc.

Prepare Yourself for Studying

Collect your notes, books, pens, highlighters, etc.

Eliminate potential distractions: Shut off the cell phone; get out of range of the land phone; shut off the TV, CD player, and radio.

Go to the bathroom.

Refresh yourself: Wash your face and hands. Brush your teeth.

Get something to drink.

Do whatever you need to do so that you will not feel uncomfortable or have to interrupt your studying.

Study Effectively

When you study, engage yourself with the content; mechanical reading of notes is useless. Research shows that the more actively you engage with the content, the better you learn. So take notes, underline or highlight, repeat content out loud; walk back and forth while you memorize; try to think what questions could be asked about the subject being reviewed.

Use a sequence of study—rest/reward—review. For example, study for 50 minutes. Take a 10-minute break. Reward yourself. Have a cup of tea or take a shower. Do not get involved in a mentally demanding activity that will cause you to lose your focus on the examination material. Take 10 minutes to review the material you just studied. As you review, mark any areas for which you think, "I don't really know that" or "I had forgotten about that." Go back and review the marked areas at the beginning of your next day's study.

To keep up your motivation, you can also do things like putting signs on your wall that say "You can do it." or "This will be over in__days." You can plan to go out to eat or buy a new dress if you meet your goal. Again, think about what motivational tricks work for you and use them.

Know When to Stop

When scheduling study, it is also important to recognize when you have studied to your capacity. Your time is valuable and you do not want to waste it by trying to study when you are beyond your ability to concentrate. It is better to take a break or accomplish something else that needs to get done and then return to studying with refreshed concentration. You will learn more in the end. So, again analyze yourself. You did a lot of studying in nursing school. What is the length of time you can usually concentrate? What are the telltale signs of when you are no longer learning effectively? Take these factors into consideration as you schedule study.

WORKSHEET

QUESTIONS

Do you have key facts from this chapter on your NCLEX-RN® knowledge ring? Complete the worksheet below to help you check.

1. Why is passing the NCLEX-RN® a requirement for being licensed as a registered nurse?
2. At what level of practice is the NCLEX-RN® designed to measure competence?
3. What are the two major considerations in the selection of content to be tested on the NCLEX-RN®?
4. Who are the writers of NCLEX-RN® test questions?
5. What is the predominant type of question found on the NCLEX-RN®?
6. How many questions does one have to get right in order to pass the NCLEX-RN®?
7. What is the maximum length of time that one can take to complete the NCLEX-RN®?
8. Do you need to be proficient in use of a computer in order to do well on NCLEX-RN®?
9. Can you skip a question on NCLEX-RN® and go back to it if you are not sure of the answer?
10. Does having the test stop when only 75 questions have been answered mean that you have failed?

ANSWERS & RATIONALES

WORKSHEET ANSWERS

1. Why is passing the NCLEX-RN® a requirement for being licensed as a registered nurse?

Answer
To protect the safety of the public by limiting the practice of Registered Nursing to those individuals who have passed an examination, which documents ability to practice competently, knowledgeably, and safely.

2. At what level of practice is the NCLEX-RN® designed to measure competence?

Answer
Entry-level Registered Nurse Practice.

3. What are the two major considerations in the selection of content to be tested on the NCLEX-RN®?

Answer
Frequency with which the information is needed in day-to-day practice and the criticality of the information to the patient.

4. Who are the writers of NCLEX-RN® test questions?

Answer
Registered nurses who work with new graduates in their practice.

5. What is the predominant type of question found on the NCLEX-RN®?

Answer
Multiple-choice question.

6. How many questions does one have to get right in order to pass the NCLEX-RN®?

Answer
It varies because NCLEX-RN® is a computer adaptive test and the decision on whether a test taker passes or fails is based on the difficulty of the questions answered and not on the absolute number.

7. What is the maximum length of time that one can take to complete the NCLEX-RN®?

Answer
6 hours.

8. Do you need to be proficient in use of a computer in order to do well on NCLEX-RN®?

Answer
No, studies have shown that computer proficiency has no effect on passing or failing.

9. Can you skip a question on NCLEX-RN® and go back to it if you are not sure of the answer?

Answer
No, a question cannot be skipped and once a question has been answered and the ENTER key has been hit the second time to register the answer, one cannot go back to the question.

10. Does having the test stop when only 75 questions have been answered mean that you have failed?

Answer
When the test stops after the minimum of 75 questions have been answered can mean one either passed or failed. The pass/fail decision is based on the difficulty of the questions answered correctly or incorrectly, not on the number.

CHAPTER 2

Test and Language Basics

To answer an examination question correctly, knowing the subject content is not enough. You have to clearly understand each part of the question in the context of nursing and correctly interpret the meaning of the question itself. Because nursing is a practice profession and the NCLEX-RN is measuring basic practice competencies, questions typically contain a clinical scenario followed by the question stem. In the case of multiple-choice questions, options follow.

When taking an examination, it is important for you to recognize each of these question parts, so read the following definitions and look at the example carefully.

- *Clinical scenario*: This part of the question tells you about the clinical situation.
- *Stem*: This part of the question contains the actual problem/question to be answered.
- *Options*: These are the answer choices provided. Options are also called alternatives and in the case of traditional multiple-choice questions, consist of one correct answer (the key) and three distracters or incorrect answers.

It is important that you read and understand each of these parts correctly for a lot of reasons.

- Facts provided in the scenario are often critical to selecting the best answer to the question. If these facts are not correctly understood, it is difficult to select the best answer.
- If the question being asked is not correctly understood, distracters, which sometimes answer a different question than the one asked in the stem or assume information not provided in the stem or in the scenario, are more likely to be perceived as the correct answer.
- Most questions also contain key words. These are words that direct the answer; hence, attention to them along with clear understanding of their meaning is essential.

KEY WORDS

Because key words are so important in determining the correct answer to a question, a list of frequently used key words is presented below for your review. Note that some of the words are negative.

First
Priority
Next
Best
Most
Least
Appropriate
Inappropriate
Last
Suitable
Not
Early
Late
Immediately
Initial
Only
After
Every
Expected
Contraindicated
Partial
Unexpected
Independently
Common
Uncommon

The following question illustrates the use and importance of a key word:

When giving medications to a client, what should the nurse do first?

1. Position the client
2. Check the client's identity
3. Explain what he/she is going to do
4. Ask how the client is feeling

In this example, all options are correct nursing actions when giving medications but which one is the correct answer is determined by the qualifying word "first." The first action is to check the client's identity.

Practice identifying key words by completing the following exercise:

WORKSHEET 1: IDENTIFICATION OF KEY WORDS

Directions: Read each of the following questions. If the question contains a key word, underline it.

1. Which clinical manifestation would the nurse expect when assessing a client admitted with a diagnosis of bacterial pneumonia?
2. Which sign should alert the nurse to a potential problem in a client with a history of a CVA?
3. What is the primary goal for the hospice care of a client with lung cancer?
4. Which nursing intervention should be given priority in the plan of care for a teenager with sickle cell anemia?
5. The nurse is assessing the nutritional status of a client who is 3 months pregnant. Which information is most important for the nurse to obtain?
6. The nurse is obtaining a health history of a debilitated client with sacral pressure ulcers. Which question should the nurse ask to elicit information effectively about the client's dietary intake?
7. Which behavior by a client with a newly created colostomy should alert the nurse to the need for teaching regarding skin care?
8. What is the best way to assess for shortness of breath in a 3-year-old client with congenital heart disease?
9. The nurse is assessing a family's ability to provide emotional support to a family member diagnosed with cancer. Which observation is most essential?
10. In analyzing a teenage primipara's need for teaching, the clinic nurse should ask which question?
11. Which finding should the nurse expect when checking urinary output of a client with SIADH?
12. Which information would be most helpful when preparing to do a home assessment prior to discharge of a low birth weight newborn?
13. Why is it important to monitor pulse rate in a client on digoxin?
14. A 25-year-old woman comes to the clinic complaining of lower left abdominal pain. Which additional information should the nurse obtain initially?
15. Which assessment question should receive priority?

FREQUENTLY MISUNDERSTOOD/MISREAD ENGLISH WORDS

Almost everyone has one or more words that he/she somehow learned incorrectly and as a result misunderstands its precise meaning. These can be very common, simple words and often the person is unaware of the error. This can be a particular problem when English is a person's second language, or is not the language of the household. Words that are similar in spelling and in pronunciation are particularly at risk of being misread, misused, or misunderstood. Because errors of this type can cause an NCLEX-RN question to be answered incorrectly, a list of potentially misleading, common English words follows. Each word is followed by its definition and a sentence illustrating its use in nursing practice. You should read each one carefully and ask yourself if you were clear about the use of the word and its meaning. If your answer is Yes—great! If the answer is No, mark the word to be reviewed again.

Accept—to agree or receive.

Examples:
The client accepted the diagnosis of breast cancer with surprising calm.

The client accepted the nurse's recommendation that all his drugs be ordered at the same pharmacy.

Except—indicates something is to be omitted or left out.

Example: All the assessment findings except the rash are consistent with a lower respiratory infection.

Advice—suggestion, guidance, or counsel.

Example: The client asked the nurse for advice on the best way to apply the ileostomy bag.

Advise—to give a suggestion, guidance, or counsel.

Example: The nurse advised the new mother to nap in the afternoon when the baby is sleeping.

Assent—to agree to.

Example: The nurse assented to a change in unit assignment for the day.

Ascent—to rise or to climb.

Example: The ascent of carbon monoxide levels in an enclosed area when a car is left running is rapid and can result in fatality.

Breath—air pulled into the lungs in one inhalation.

Example: Take a deep breath and hold it while I listen with the stethoscope over your lungs.

Breathe—the act of inhaling and exhaling air from the lungs.
Example: Breathe in slowly and deeply through your mouth.

Caster—wheel on a swivel.
Example: Many pieces of hospital equipment such as IV pumps and over-the-bed tables are on casters for ease of transport.

Castor—oil from castor beans, used as a laxative.
Example: A single dose of castor oil was ordered as part of the prep for the client's upcoming bowel surgery.

Charted (Not chartered)—entered in the client record.
Example: The nurse charted the appearance of the wound in the client's record.

Sight (Not site or cite)—vision.
Example: Eyesight typically declines with age.

Site (not cite)—location.
Example: The planned donor site for the skin graft was the left, upper, outer thigh.

Coarse (not course)—rough, uneven.
Example: The skin of clients with hypofunction of the thyroid is often coarse in texture.

Course—progression, order, direction.
Example: The course of the disease is characterized by exacerbations and remissions.

Compliment—praise.
Example: The supervisor complimented the nurse on her efficient handling of the multiple emergency admissions, which occurred during her shift.

Complement—add to or mix well.
Example: Participation in a support group can complement individual counseling.

Complaint—expression of something wrong.
Example: The client's chief complaint was a sharp pain in the left chest.

Compliant—willing to follow requirements or directions.
Example: The client verbalized a desire to be compliant with the medication regimen but stated he could not be because he could not afford to buy the medications ordered.

Continuous—going on without stopping.
Example: The client was receiving continuous feedings via a nasogastric tube.

Continually—happening at regular intervals or again and again.
Example: The client continually complained of nausea while receiving the antibiotic.

Defective—faulty or abnormal.
Example: The neonate was diagnosed with a defective mitral valve.

Deficient—lack of.
Example: Genetic syndromes characterized by deficient chromosomal material are more often fatal than those characterized by excess chromosomal material.

Dessert (not desert)—sweet foods served at the end of a meal.
Example: The nurse advised the client to eliminate desserts as a step in controlling weight.

Uninterested (not disinterested)—not caring.
Example: The client appeared markedly uninterested in learning about the prescribed diet.

Elicit—draw out information.
Example: The nurse's questions while obtaining the client history are designed to elicit complete, accurate information on which to base a nursing diagnosis.

Illicit—illegal.
Example: When obtaining a history, questions should be asked about the use of prescription drugs, over-the-counter drugs, herbal preparations, nutritional supplements, and illicit drugs.

Imminent (not Eminent)—about to happen.
Example: An aura, unique to the individual, is often the sign of an imminent seizure.

Farther—greater distance.
Example: The client should be ambulating farther than the bathroom.

Further—more.
Example: Before discharging the client, the physician decided further discussion with the family concerning plans for home care was necessary.

Former—the first of two. (Latter refers to the second of two.)
Example: Nausea and vomiting are common side effects to some medications.The former is a symptom because it cannot be seen, felt, or heard by an external observer; the latter is a sign because it can be observed.

Healthy—not ill, well.
Example: The child appeared healthy.

Healthful—promoting wellness.
Example: Adequate daily intake of calcium is healthful.

Lose—misplace, be deprived of.
Example: Clients lose central vision with macular degeneration; they lose peripheral vision with glaucoma.

Loose—opposite of tight.

Example: Loose bowel movements can be a problem for clients following an intestinal resection.

Nauseous—inducing a feeling of nausea.

Example: The nauseous smell of the drainage made the dressing difficult to change.

Nauseated—experiencing nausea.

Example: The client became nauseated 2 hours after the chemotherapy was administered.

Past—time gone by, ago.

Example: The time is past that medications could have helped; now surgery is the only option.

Passed—moved along, went away, departed, succeeded on a test.

Examples:

The suppository passed the rectal sphincter without difficulty.

The client passed a renal calculus last evening.

Patient—recipient of care.

Example: The patient thanked the nurse for making her comfortable.

Patience—tolerance or understanding.

Example: Patience is often needed when dealing with sick children.

Peace—calmness, tranquility.

Example: Helping the client achieve peace of mind is a goal of the hospice nurse.

Piece—part or section.

Example: The piece of the Foley catheter that inflates to hold the catheter in the urinary bladder is called the balloon.

Personal—private.

Example: Use of personal information about clients is governed by the HIPAA regulations.

Personnel—employees.

Example: Nurses are licensed health care personnel.

Prescribe—order for.

Example: The nurse practitioner prescribed the antibiotic Cipro for the client with a urinary tract infection.

Proscribe—prohibit.

Example: Leaving the unit with the narcotics key is proscribed.

Principal—of major importance.

Example: A principal use of digitalis is to strengthen the contraction of the myocardium in cases of heart failure.

Principle—a truth.

Example: The principle underlying use of a fan for cooling is that one of the ways heat is lost from the body is by convection.

Proceed—go on, continue.

Example: The nurse proceeded with the dressing change after the client had stopped coughing.

Precede—go before.

Example: Mild signs of an upper respiratory infection preceded the development of the rash.

Quite—a great deal.

Example: The client was quite verbal regarding his opinion of his care.

Quit—leave or stop.

Example: The client stated he wished he could quit smoking.

Rise—get oneself up.

Example: The client who had a CVA said to the nurse "I look forward to the day I can rise out of the bed in the morning without assistance."

Raise—lift or elevate an object or person.

Example: During a breast examination, the client needs to raise her arms over her head so the contours of the breast can be inspected.

Stationary—not moving.

Example: The brake on the wheelchair should be set when the client is being moved in or out of the chair in order to keep the chair stationary and help prevent the client from falling.

Stationery—paper.

Example: Official letters should be written on stationery imprinted with the agency letterhead.

Statute—legal restriction.

Example: The statute of limitation for malpractice cases differs state to state.

Stature—person's size.

Example: The client's stature was consistent with a diagnosis of hypopituitary dwarfism.

Adequate—sufficient.

Example: It is the nurse's responsibility to determine if the client's 24-hour fluid intake and output is adequate.

Aggravate—make worse.

Example: Straining at stool will aggravate hemorrhoids.

Allay—put at rest or cause to subside.

Example: Providing the client with information about a procedure to be done can allay anxiety.

Anticipate—take up or use ahead of time.

Example: Prior to entering an isolation room, it is important that the nurse anticipate client needs so that she is prepared with knowledge and equipment to provide the needed care."

Avoid—keep away from.

Example: Immunosuppressed clients need to avoid crowds because of the risk of exposure to infection.

Competitive—contest between rivals.

Example: In competitive inhibition of enzyme activity, the inhibitor competes with the substrate for binding on the enzyme.

Compromised—to endanger.

Example: Circulation to the lower extremities is compromised when the client is in lithotomy position.

Assume—take for granted.

Example: The nurse should never assume the client has understood instructions; validation of understanding by repeating the instructions or by return demonstration is always necessary.

At least—the very minimum.

Example: If the client refuses to lie in the prone position, at least have him lie on his side."

Confer—consult or to bestow.

Example: The Client Care team conferred to determine the best approach to manage the bladder retraining program of a newly admitted client.

Deny—declare not to be true.

Example: Clients sometimes deny use of illegal drugs because they fear the reaction of the health care provider.

Determine—to come to a decision or to obtain first hand knowledge.

Example: To determine the causative organism of a wound infection, a culture is done.

Differentiate—discriminate or identify differences.

Example: When examining the chest, it is important to differentiate between crackles and wheezes.

Exacerbate—worsen.

Example: Exposure to cold and damp can exacerbate the symptoms of a sinus infection.

Enhance—augment.

Example: Comfort measures such as clean linen, a back rub, and pleasant music can enhance the action of pain medications.

Excessive—more than acceptable, exorbitant.

Example: The bleeding was excessive following the surgery.

Expectorate—cough up and spit out mucus.

Example: To prevent spread of infection, the nurse instructed the client to expectorate into a tissue and dispose of it in the provided plastic bag.

Flushed—any tinge of red.

Example: The client's face was flushed and he was warm to the touch.

Flaccid—without resistance.

Example: A flaccid muscle is one with less than normal tone.

Tense—rigid, feeling nervous.

Examples:

A sign of increased intracranial pressure in a neonate is a tense fontanelle.

The client complained of feeling extremely tense whenever an interview with the psychiatrist was scheduled.

Hoarseness—grating sounds.

Example: Hoarseness is a characteristic symptom of laryngitis.

Impinge—come into close contact.

Example: The CAT scan showed that the tumor was impinging on the recurrent laryngeal nerve thus accounting for the hoarseness.

Inept—not apt, unable to do well.

Example: The client remained inept at handling the insulin syringe, so additional teaching was planned.

Insulation—prevent transfer of electricity, heat, or sound.

The insulation in the walls of hospital rooms helps clients to rest by decreasing nose heard from other areas of the unit.

Intact—without injury.

Example: The client's skin remained intact despite the long period of bed rest.

Isolation—loneliness, separation.

Examples:

Clients having intracavitary radiation treatments are at risk for feelings of isolation.

Clients presenting with active, drug resistant tuberculosis are placed in isolation.

Lead to—results in.

Example: An untreated streptococcal sore throat can lead to glomerulonephritis in susceptible children.

Least likely—in the smallest degree, lowest chance.

Example: The client least likely to develop constipation is the one with a liberal fluid and roughage intake, who exercises regularly, and obeys the urge to defecate.

Most likely—to the greatest degree, highest chance.

Example: Of antibiotics, diuretics, or calcium channel blockers, the drugs most likely to cause allergic reactions are the antibiotics.

Liberally—freely, unchecked.

Example: The client should be encouraged to use the Calamine lotion liberally to control the itch of the poison ivy.

Predispose—create a tendency to.

Example: Use of immunosuppressant drugs predisposes the client to infection.

Permit—let.

Example: Elevating a Foley catheter drainage bag above the level of the client's pelvis permits backflow of urine into the bladder.

Profuse—pouring forth.

Example: Vaginal drainage was yellow, profuse, and malodorous.

Refrain—keep oneself from doing.

Example: The client was instructed to refrain from lifting anything over 5 lbs following repair of his hernia.

Sparingly—frugally.

Example: It is important to apply the skin preparation sparingly in accordance with the directions.

Spasm—involuntary contracture.

Example: The client complained of repeated leg spasms during the night.

Sedentary—physically inactive.

Example: A sedentary lifestyle predisposes to obesity.

Check your basic test vocabulary by completing the following vocabulary exercise.

WORKSHEET 2: VOCABULARY

Directions: Match the definitions in column B with the words in column A.

Column A

1. _____Site
2. _____Coarse
3. _____Imminent
4. _____Deficient
5. _____Former
6. _____Enhance
7. _____Impinge
8. _____Tense
9. _____Predispose
10. _____Sedentary
11. _____Except
12. _____Principal
13. _____Loose
14. _____Exacerbate
15. _____Profuse

Column B

a. something to be left out
b. progress
c. without intending to
d. rough
e. create a tendency to
f. saturate
g. location
h. a truth
i. at any time
j. unable to do well
k. inactive
l. shaky
m. opposite of tight
n. eliminate
o. pouring forth
p. easy going
q. of major importance
r. cause discomfort
s. rigid
t. worsen
u. about to happen
v. first of two
w. misplace
x. augment
y. lack of
z. come into close contact

WORKSHEET 3

QUESTIONS

Do you have key facts from this chapter on your NCLEX-RN knowledge ring? Complete the worksheet below to help you check.
Directions: For items 1 to 5, read each question. If the question contains a key word, underline it.

1. Which nursing intervention should be given priority in the plan of care for a client with newly diagnosed tuberculosis?
2. In formulating a teaching plan for home care of a client with lung cancer, which information is most essential to include about the use of oxygen?
3. In caring for a client receiving outpatient chemotherapy for metastatic breast cancer, which instruction should the nurse include about the care of the central line?
4. When administering an IM medication using Z-track technique, what is the next step the nurse should take after injecting the medication into the muscle?
5. When assessing a client's response to Toprol XL, which finding would be unexpected?

Directions: For items 6 through 10, read each sentence carefully and decide if the underlined word is used correctly or incorrectly in the sentence. Write Correct or Incorrect at end of each sentence.

6. The client's nutritional status was <u>compromised</u> when he eliminated almost all sources of protein from his diet.
7. The nurse reported that the client was <u>inept</u> after reviewing laboratory reports that showed immunosuppression.
8. The medication <u>allayed</u> the pain as indicated by the client's statement that her pain was almost gone.
9. On first encountering a client, <u>statute</u> should be noted as part of the general assessment survey.
10. After the client drew up the incorrect amount of insulin and then contaminated the needle, the nurse concluded that the client needed <u>farther</u> teaching.

ANSWERS & RATIONALES

ANSWERS FOR WORKSHEET 1: IDENTIFICATION OF KEY WORDS

Directions: Read each of the following questions. If the question contains a key word, underline it.

1. Which clinical manifestation would the nurse expect when assessing a client admitted with a diagnosis of bacterial pneumonia?

Answer
Which clinical manifestation would the nurse <u>expect</u> when assessing a client admitted with a diagnosis of bacterial pneumonia?

(continued)

2. Which sign should alert the nurse to a potential problem in a client with a history of a CVA?

Answer

Which sign should alert the nurse to a <u>potential</u> problem in a client with a history of a CVA?

3. What is the primary goal for the hospice care of a client with lung cancer?

Answer

What is the <u>primary</u> goal for the hospice care of a client with lung cancer?

4. Which nursing intervention should be given priority in the plan of care for a teenager with sickle cell anemia?

Answer

Which nursing intervention should be given <u>priority</u> in the plan of care for a teenager with sickle cell anemia?

5. The nurse is assessing the nutritional status of a client who is 3 months pregnant. Which information is most important for the nurse to obtain?

Answer

The nurse is assessing the nutritional status of a client who is 3 months pregnant. Which information is <u>most</u> important for the nurse to obtain?

6. The nurse is obtaining a health history of a debilitated client with sacral pressure ulcers. Which question should the nurse ask to elicit information effectively about the client's dietary intake?

Answer

The nurse is obtaining a health history of a debilitated client with sacral pressure ulcers. Which question should the nurse ask to elicit information <u>effectively</u> about the client's dietary intake?

7. Which behavior by a client with a newly created colostomy should alert the nurse to the need for teaching regarding skin care?

Answer

Which behavior by a client with a newly created colostomy should alert the nurse to the need for teaching regarding skin care? <u>No keyword.</u>

8. What is the best way to assess for shortness of breath in a 3-year–old client with congenital heart disease?

Answer

What is the <u>best</u> way to assess for shortness of breath in a 3-year–old client with congenital heart disease?

9. The nurse is assessing a family's ability to provide emotional support to a family member diagnosed with cancer. Which observation is most essential?

Answer

The nurse is assessing a family's ability to provide emotional support to a family member diagnosed with cancer. Which observation is <u>most</u> essential?

10. In analyzing the need for teaching a teenage primipara, the clinic nurse should ask which question?

Answer

In analyzing the need for teaching a teenage primipara, the clinic nurse should ask which question? <u>No keyword.</u>

11. Which finding should the nurse <u>expect</u> when checking urinary output of a client with SIADH?

Answer

Which finding should the nurse expect when checking urinary output of a client with SIADH?

12. Which information would be most helpful when preparing to do a home assessment prior to discharge of a low birth weight newborn?

Answer

Which information would be <u>most</u> helpful when preparing to do a home assessment prior to discharge of a low birth weight newborn?

13. Why is it important to monitor pulse rate in a client on digoxin?

Answer

Why is it important to monitor pulse rate in a client on digoxin? No keyword.

14. A 25-year–old woman comes to the clinic complaining of lower left abdominal pain. Which additional information should the nurse obtain initially?

Answer

A 25-year–old woman comes to the clinic complaining of lower left abdominal pain. Which additional information should the nurse obtain initially?

15. Which assessment question should receive priority?

Answer

Which assessment question should receive priority?

ANSWERS FOR WORKSHEET 2: VOCABULARY

Column A	Column B
1. _g__Site	a. something to be left out
2. _d__Coarse	b. progress
3. _u__Imminent	c. without intending to
4. _y__Deficient	d. rough
5. _v__Former	e. create a tendency to
6. _x__Enhance	f. saturate
7. _z__Impinge	g. location
8. _s__Tense	h. a truth
9. _e__Predispose	i. at any time
10. _k__Sedentary	j. unable to do well
11. _a__Except	k. inactive
12. _q__Principal	l. shaky
13. _m__Loose	m. opposite of tight
14. _t__Exacerbate	n. eliminate
15. _o__Profuse	o. pouring forth
	p. easy going
	q. of major importance
	r. cause discomfort
	s. rigid
	t. worsen
	u. about to happen
	v. first of two
	w. misplace
	x. augment
	y. lack of
	z. come into close contact

ANSWERS FOR WORKSHEET 3

Do you have key facts from this chapter on your NCLEX-RN knowledge ring? Complete the worksheet below to help you check.

Directions: For items 1 to 5, read each of the following questions. If the question contains a key word, underline it.

1. Which nursing intervention should be given priority in the plan of care for a client with newly diagnosed tuberculosis?

Answer

Which nursing intervention should be given priority in the plan of care for a client with newly diagnosed tuberculosis?

2. In formulating a teaching plan for home care of a client with lung cancer, which information is most essential to include about the use of oxygen?

Answer

In formulating a teaching plan for home care of a client with lung cancer, which information is most essential to include about the use of oxygen?

3. In caring for a client receiving outpatient chemotherapy for metastatic breast cancer, which instruction should the nurse include about the care of the central line?

Answer

No keyword.

4. When administering an IM medication using Z-track technique, what is the next step the nurse should take after injecting the medication into the muscle?

Answer

When administering an IM medication using Z-track technique, what is the next step the nurse should take after injecting the medication into the muscle?

5. When assessing a client's response to Toprol XL, which finding would be unexpected?

Answer

When assessing a client's response to Toprol XL, which finding would be unexpected?

Directions: For items 6 through 10, read each sentence carefully and decide if the underlined word is used correctly or incorrectly in the sentence. Write Correct or Incorrect at end of each sentence.

6. The client's nutritional status was compromised when he eliminated almost all sources of protein from his diet. *Correct*

7. The nurse reported that the client was inept after reviewing laboratory reports that showed immunosuppression.

   Incorrect, inept means unable to do well. The client was inept at changing his dressing is a correct use of the term.

8. The medication allayed the pain as indicated by the client's statement that her pain was almost gone. *Correct*

9. On first encountering a client, statute should be noted as part of the general assessment survey.

   Incorrect, the word should be stature.

10. After the client drew up the incorrect amount of insulin and then contaminated the needle, the nurse concluded that the client needed farther teaching.

    Incorrect, the word should be further.

CHAPTER 3

Sharpening Your Test-Taking Skills

To be as sharp as possible when answering test questions, follow these steps:

- Identify the parts of a question
  - —the scenario which tells you about the situation
  - —the stem which contains the actual problem/question to be answered
  - —for multiple choice questions, the options or alternatives, which consist of one correct answer (the key) and three distracters or incorrect answers. Distracters sometimes answer a different question than the one asked in the stem or they may assume information not provided in the stem. As a result, they can seem like a good choice and hence are good distracters. Remember that if any part of an option is incorrect, the whole answer is wrong.
- Read the words in the question carefully. Identify "tricky" English words and think about their meaning. Jot down the meaning over each such word and then reread using the definition.
- Determine what the question is asking—read twice and try rephrasing it in easier terms. Once you identify the specific question and its subject, then you can focus on what you know about it.
- Identify what facts provided in the stem or scenario are relevant to the question.
- Ask if the option makes sense for this client—eliminate the option from consideration if the answer is No—even if under other circumstances it is a high-priority action.
- Look for key words—those that direct the answer—when you read the question. Take special note of a negative key word.
- As you read the question, think of your answer and then see if it is among the choices. Do not select the first answer that looks right; however, read all the options carefully.
- Always select an answer within the RN scope of practice.

  Example:
  Which of the following is a basic nursing responsibility related to drug administration?

  1. Monitoring the client's response to the administration of the drug *Correct*
  2. Determining the appropriate drug dosage
  3. Selecting the best route of administration of the drug
  4. Ordering the drug from the pharmacy

- When not certain of an answer, select the most complete option.

  Example:
  Which is the best definition of a medication?

  1. Chemical that treats symptoms of disease
  2. Drug used for a therapeutic effect *Correct*
  3. Pharmacological preparation used to reverse disease
  4. Plant, animal, or mineral substance which prevents disease

- Do not change your answer unless you are certain it is incorrect.

APPROACHES TO SPECIFIC TYPES OF QUESTIONS

Questions That Require Priority Setting

Guidelines for establishing priorities are as follows:

- The nurse should always assess (gather pertinent data) before deciding on and taking an action. This is reflected in the steps of the Nursing Process: assess, diagnose, plan, intervene, and evaluate.
- Physiological needs must be met first. The client must be kept alive for anything else to be important. Next in importance are safety needs and then come psychological needs. This is outlined in Maslow's hierarchy.
- When prioritizing physiological needs remember your ABCs: airway, breathing, and circulation.
- Which answer will keep the client safe/prevent client harm? It is especially relevant when the question deals with laboratory values, drug administration, and nursing procedures.
- Assessment of equipment never takes precedence over assessment of the client.

Communication Questions

Therapeutic communication promotes expression of feelings and ideas and also conveys acceptance and respect. Like any communication, it involves both verbal and nonverbal components. Major techniques to facilitate therapeutic communication are as follows:

- Communicate in an accepting and respectful manner. Address (refer to) the client by his/her given name—not by a nickname, a room number, or "sweetie." Names other than the given name should only be used upon the client's request or permission. Clients should be asked, not told, whenever appropriate. This allows for client decision making and hence communicates respect for the client as an able, intelligent individual.

  Examples:
  What would you like to do first?
  What would you like to talk about?

- Use open-ended questions. These are questions that cannot be answered with a Yes or a No.

  Examples:
  What do you think about this plan?
  What questions do you have?
  How do you feel about going home tomorrow?
  Tell me about your headaches.

- Reflect feelings expressed by the client. Remember that feelings are expressed verbally and nonverbally. These may be contradictory but feelings expressed nonverbally are usually true because nonverbal communication is harder to control. Reflection indicates empathy, allows validation of the perceived feelings, and allows the client to "look at" his/her feelings. Words used in reflection should be neutral unless the client uses an emotionally charged word.

  Examples:
  You seem sad.
  You seem unsure.
  You must feel lonely sometimes.
  I get the feeling you are upset.

  Do not say:
  You are depressed.
  You can't make a decision.
  It must be awful being alone all the time.
  You must be really mad at your neighbor.

- Focus the conversation on important areas.

  Examples:
  Let's talk a little more about . . .
  You were talking about the problem you had with changing your dressing, let's go back and explore that further.

- Paraphrase or restate what the client has said in your own words. This allows the client to validate the message or correct misunderstanding.

  Examples:
  What you are saying is . . .
  Let me make sure I understand . . .
  What I hear you saying is . . .

- Summarize the communication.

Therapeutic communication also involves (a) active listening, (b) stating observations made about the client but never any that would embarrass or anger the client ("You look rested" or "You seem quiet today." Not "You look terrible."), (c) reflecting empathy or an understanding of the importance of a situation to the client in a neutral, nonjudgmental manner ("It must be very disheartening . . ."), (d) sharing hope, humor, and feelings, (e) using touch and silence, (f) asking pertinent questions, and (g) giving information.

Nontherapeutic (blocking) communication techniques hinder further communication and expression of feelings and may induce negative responses. Some examples of nontherapeutic communication techniques are:

- Asking unnecessary personal questions: "Why are you just living with Mary rather than marrying her?" "Why are you still living at home?" "How come you haven't bought a house?"
- Giving personal advice or opinions: "If I were you I would make my son move out." "I think you should stop cooking for the whole family."
- Flip or automatic responses, use of cliches: "Everything will work out." "Don't worry." "It happens all the time but it doesn't mean anything."

Redirecting the conversation or changing the subject, expressing sympathy, asking "why," verbalizing approval or disapproval, responding defensively, passively or aggressively, and arguing also block therapeutic communication.

When answering a communication question, begin by reviewing the above principles. Then determine what the question is asking. If the question is asking what is the nurse's best response, what is the most appropriate response, what is the most therapeutic response, or what response will best support a therapeutic relationship, eliminate nontherapeutic options. Do this by identifying options that involve nontherapeutic responses: options that give opinions, options that brush off the client's concerns; options that contain emotionally charged, defensive, accusatory, or otherwise upsetting or offensive wording, and options that contain judgmental wording.

Example:
A client who has been hospitalized for 2 weeks says to the nurse "I can't stay here anymore, I have to get back to my family." Which is the most appropriate response for the nurse to make?

a. "Don't worry. Your family will be fine."

b. "If I were you, I'd take advantage of the rest you're getting while away from the family."

c. "Would you like to talk about how you feel?" *Correct*

d. "Is your family unable to get along without you?"

In some cases, the question may be asking you to identify the nontherapeutic or inappropriate response. Be alert for this when reading questions and then select the option containing a response that would be incorrect for the nurse to make as the answer.

Example:
A client states "My family doesn't seem to understand my illness." Which response on the part of the nurse would most likely block further discussion?

a. "They may not seem to, but I'm sure they do." *Correct*

b. "In what way do they react to give you that feeling?"

c. "Your family doesn't seem to understand."

d. "What makes you think that?"

Client-Teaching Questions

There are different types of client-teaching questions. Some are very straightforward simply asking what should the nurse teach. This type of question addresses the planning or implementation phase of the nursing process.

Example:
Which instruction/information should the nurse include in the teaching plan for a client with genital herpes?

Which instruction/information should the nurse give to a client with genital herpes?

A variation on this type of question asks you to identify not what needs to be taught but *when* or *by whom*, teaching is needed.

Example:
Which client should be taught about the need for potassium in the daily diet?

a. Client taking daily NSAIDS for arthritis

b. Client taking Toprol XL daily for hypertension

c. Client taking Fosamax weekly for osteoporosis

d. Client taking Hydrodiuril daily for fluid retention *Correct*

Other client-teaching questions ask not what should be taught but how does the nurse know the teaching was understood. These are client-teaching questions that address the evaluation phase of the nursing process. Was the teaching effective? Did the client learn? These questions may be phrased in a positive or negative way.

Positive questions ask you to select an answer that is a correct statement or activity—something that should be done or said.

Examples of positively phrased questions:

Which statement made by a client with hepatitis B following discharge teaching indicates that instruction was effective?

Which statement made by a client with hepatitis B indicates that discharge instructions were understood?

Negatively phrased questions ask you to identify the answer that indicates the client does not know, has misunderstood, or has not learned. It requires that you identify an incorrect statement—not a correct one. Negative questions require that you choose from the options the one that is incorrect or should not be said or done. Note that negative questions do not necessarily have a negative word (not, no, incorrect, etc.) in the stem.

Examples of negatively phrased questions:

Which statement made by a client taking Fosamax once a week for the treatment of osteoporosis indicates that the directions for taking the medication were not understood?

Which action taken by a client who has been taught to self-administer insulin indicates that further teaching/instruction is necessary?

Which statement made by the mother of a child diagnosed with bronchiolitis indicates a need for teaching?

A client's daughter is assisting her to the bathroom. Which observation by the nurse suggests that teaching is needed?

Delegation Questions

These typically ask what duties can be assigned to a nurse aide or an LPN/LVN and when a physician, social worker, respiratory therapist, or other member of the health-care team should be notified or consulted.

WORKSHEET

IDENTIFYING FACILITATING AND BLOCKING RESPONSES

Directions: Read each statement or set of statements and decide if therapeutic communication is being facilitated or blocked. Write your decision at the end of each.

1. Client: "I'm so worried about my surgery."
   Nurse: "We do 10 of these procedures every week and they all come out fine."
2. Client: "I keep thinking about my husband and how he is managing at home by himself."
   Nurse: "You just have to put him out of your mind and concentrate on getting better."
3. Client: "I don't know how I am going to cope with all the bills from being in the hospital."
   Nurse: "I'll have a social worker stop by to go over your insurance."
4. Client's daughter: "I don't know how I am going to arrange care for my mother at home while I work."
   Nurse: "If it were me I would put her in a nursing home where she would have round-the-clock care."
5. Client: "I am such a burden on everybody since I had the stroke."
   Nurse: "What makes you say that?"
6. Client: "I'll never learn how to give myself this injection."
   Nurse: "Of course you will."
7. Infant client's mother: "I'm afraid that I will forget how to correctly prepare the baby's formula when I get home."
   Nurse: "Would you like me to go over the procedure with you one more time?"
8. Client: "Having that test was the worst experience I've had in my whole life."
   Nurse: "Tell me what happened."
9. Client: "I have to begin to have my husband help with the housework when I get home."
   Nurse: "Do you have a plan in mind as to how you are going to do this?"
10. Client: "I can't use a diaphragm anymore; it's just too messy and inconvenient."
    Nurse: "Would you like information on other forms of birth control?"
11. Client: "My son doesn't want to visit me anymore. He says I am always complaining."
    Nurse: "Children expect their parents to be perfect. He'll get over it."
12. Client: "I can't do anything right."
    Nurse: "You shouldn't feel that way. Things will be different when you're better."
13. Client: "I am so upset about my roommate's visitor tripping over my slippers yesterday."
    Nurse: "My advice to you is to forget it—she didn't get hurt."
14. Client: "My son-in-law refused to bring my granddaughter to visit me."
    Nurse: "That's mean; it must make you angry."
15. Client: "I don't think I am going to make it out of here. I am just so weak."
    Nurse: "You are very depressed."

ANSWERS & RATIONALES

IDENTIFYING FACILITATING AND BLOCKING RESPONSES

Directions: Read each statement or set of statements and decide if therapeutic communication is being facilitated or blocked. Write your decision at the end of each.

1. Client: "I'm so worried about my surgery."
   Nurse: "We do ten of these procedures every week and they all come out fine."

Blocked. This response provides false reassurance and may even be interpreted as flip. It does not acknowledge the client's concern nor encourage further sharing.

2. Client: "I keep thinking about my husband and how he is managing at home by himself."
   Nurse: "You just have to put him out of your mind and concentrate on getting better."

Blocked. This response does not acknowledge the client's concern and is a form of personal advice. It effectively shuts off further discussion.

3. Client: "I don't know how I am going to cope with all the bills from being in the hospital."
   Nurse: "I'll have a social worker stop by to go over your insurance."

Blocked. This response indicates that the topic of the client's concern has been heard but it offers a solution which may or may not be acceptable to the client. It does not offer the client a choice or the opportunity to further specify or discuss concerns or feelings.

4. Client's daughter: "I don't know how I am going to arrange care for my mother at home while I work."
   Nurse: "If it were me I would put her in a Nursing Home where she would have round the clock care."

Blocked. This response gives advice and shuts down further discussion of the problem.

5. Client: "I am such a burden on everybody since I had the stroke."
   Nurse: "What makes you say that?"

Facilitated. This is an open ended question that encourages the client is to explore his or her feelings.

6. Client: "I'll never learn how to give myself this injection."
   Nurse: "Of course you will."

Blocked. This response gives false reassurance and constitutes a cliché.

7. Infant Client's Mother: "I'm afraid that I will forget how to correctly prepare the baby's formula when I get home."
   Nurse: "Would you like me to go over the procedure with you one more time?"

Facilitated. This response recognizes the mother's concern and offers, not dictates, an appropriate option.

8. Client: "Having that test was the worst experience I've had in my whole life."
   Nurse: "Tell me what happened."

Facilitated. This response indicates willingness to hear the client and encourages exploration of feelings and events.

9. Client: "I have to begin to have my husband help with the housework when I get home."
   Nurse: "Do you have a plan in mind as to how you are going to do this?"

Facilitated. This question can be answered yes or no but it opens the for the nurse to guide the client in the discussion and evaluation/revision/development of a plan.

10. Client: "I can't use a diaphragm anymore; its just too messy and inconvenient."
    Nurse: "Would you like information on other forms of birth control?"

Facilitated. This response recognizes the client's concern and offers an appropriate option in response.

11. Client: "My son doesn't want to visit me anymore. He says I am always complaining."
    Nurse: "Children expect their parents to be perfect. He'll get over it."

Blocked. This response is cliché in nature and does not recognize the validity of the client's concern.

12. Client: "I can't do anything right."
    Nurse: "You shouldn't feel that way. Things will be different when you're better."

Blocked. This response although somewhat "gentle" in its wording, offers false reassurance, may be construed as judgmental, and does not allow the client to further explain his or her feelings and concerns. It also contains an element of cliché.

13. Client: "I am so upset about my roommate's visitor tripping over my slippers yesterday."
    Nurse: "My advice to you is to forget it - she didn't get hurt."

Blocked. This response offers advice and trivializes the client's concern.

14. Client: "My son in law refused to bring my grand daughter to visit me."
    Nurse: "That's mean; it must make you angry."

Blocked. This response is judgmental and presumes to know what the client is feeling.

15. Client: "I don't think I am going to make it out of here. I am just so weak."
    Nurse: "You are very depressed."

Blocked. This response makes a judgment about the client. It does not encourage the client to discuss feelings not does it seek to validate interpretation of the client's communication.

Part II

CONTENT REVIEW

CHAPTER 4

Test Plan Category:

Safe, Effective Care Environment

Sub-category: Management of Care

Topics:
- Legal Rights and Responsibilities
- Client Rights
- Information Technology
- Confidentiality/Information Security
- Informed Consent
- Advance Directives
- Ethical Practice
- Concepts of Management
- Delegation
- Establishing Priorities
- Supervision
- Continuity of Care
- Resource Management
- Collaboration with the Multidisciplinary Team
- Advocacy
- Referrals
- Case Management
- Consultation
- Performance Improvement/Quality Improvement
- Staff Education

LEGAL RIGHTS AND RESPONSIBILITIES

PROFESSIONAL LEGAL ISSUES

Legal controls on the practice of nursing are to protect the public. Law provides a framework for

- identifying what nursing actions are legal,
- differentiating the nurses' responsibilities from those of other health care professionals,
- establishing the boundaries of independent nursing actions, and
- assisting in maintenance of a standard of nursing practice.

Nurse Practice Act

- This is a set of laws defining the scope of nursing practice.
- Each state has its own Nurse Practice Act usually administered by the State Board of Nursing.
- Most Nurse Practice Acts address performing services for compensation, specialized knowledge bases, use of the nursing process, and components of nursing practice.

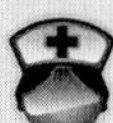

Practice Alert

The nurse needs to obtain and read the Nurse Practice Act for the state that she/he intends to practice in.

Licensure

- License is a legal credential conferred by a state granting permission to an individual to practice a given profession.
- It is commonly required for professions requiring direct contact with clients.
- Licensure requires that a level of competency be demonstrated by the individual seeking a license; for an RN license this is done by passing the NCLEX-RN.
- Mandatory licensure for registered nursing is the standard in the United States—one must have a valid nursing license to work in any state, territory, or province.
- RN Nurse Licensure Compact (NLC) is a mutual recognition licensure model which allows a nurse to be licensed in his or her state of residence but to practice physically or electronically in other ccompact states. Practice in compact states is subject to each state's practice law and regulation.
- Each state or jurisdiction establishes its own licensing laws, which usually require graduation from an approved nursing educational program, passing score on the NCLEX-RN, a good moral character, good physical and mental health, and disclosure of criminal convictions.

Standards of Care

- Standards of care are authoritative statements that define an acceptable level of patient care (professional practice).
- These are used to evaluate the quality of care provided by the nurse and, therefore, become legal guidelines for nursing practice.
- American Nurses Association (ANA) has developed general standards and guidelines for more than 20 specialty nursing practice areas.
- State Nurse Practice Acts describe standards of practice that apply to a nurse in the particular state.
- Individual health care agencies may have developed standards of care for selected patient problems, e.g., critical pathways, clinical pathways.

Malpractice

- Malpractice is the term used when a nurse while performing her/his responsibilities commits an act of negligence resulting in harm to the patient.
- Harm must be based on the failure to act in a *prudent professional* manner and within professional standards.
- Nurse must have had a professional duty toward the person receiving the care for malpractice to have occurred.

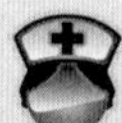

Practice Alerts

Regulation of the practice of nursing serves two purposes: protection of the public and accountability of the individual practitioner's actions.

Malpractice is present only if a breach of duty was the cause of the injury.

LEGAL ISSUES AFFECTING PATIENTS

Legal issues affecting patients are those that occur when a wrong has been committed against a patient or a patient's property.

Defamation of Character

- Defamation of character occurs when information about an individual is detrimental to his/her reputation.
- The communication, which is considered to be malicious and false, may be spoken (slander) or written (libel) and may be about patients or other health care providers.

- The nurse must
  - —document only objective information in the medical record,
  - —use professional terms,
  - —avoid discussing patients and other health care providers in public places where there is the possibility of being overheard, and
  - —use only acceptable avenues to confidentially report behavior of patients or other health care providers.

Privileged Communication

- Privileged communication is the information shared by an individual with certain professionals and that does not need to be revealed in a court of law.
- The nurse needs to know what the state she/he is practicing in says about privileged communications.

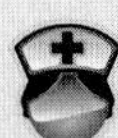

Practice Alert

All states do not recognize the nurse–patient relationship as one of privileged communication. States that do recognize the relationship as privileged may not recognize all communications between patient and nurse as privileged.

Emergency Care

- Certain actions provided by a health care professional may be legal in emergency situations and not legal in nonemergency situations.
- During a true emergency, *consent* is implied as the court considers that a reasonable person in a life-threatening situation would give permission for treatment.
- "Good Samaritan Acts" protect the nurse against negligence when she/he provides voluntary assistance to an individual in an emergency situation.
- Within a health care agency, the emergency policies and procedures of the institution govern what the nurse can do, and so a nurse must know these. The courts have held that a nurse can do things immediately necessary, even if the activity is normally considered a medical function, provided she/he has the expertise to carry out the act. The nurse is protected from a charge of practicing outside the scope of practice if the *protocols* established by the institution's medical staff are followed.

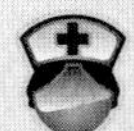

Practice Alert

Hospitals and health care agencies are expected to have policies and protocols to be followed during an emergency situation, e.g., "code." The standard of "reasonable care" is used when emergency care is given in a *noninstitutional* setting.

Refusing Treatment

- This issue arises out of the belief in and respect for the autonomy of the patient.
- The two forms of refusing treatment are when the patient discharges himself/herself from the hospital against medical advice *or* when he/she refuses certain treatment when in the hospital.

CLIENT RIGHTS

Patients have the right to expect they will be treated in a certain way, receive adequate information, and have their confidentiality maintained when they are interacting with the health care system.

DIGNITY

- Dignity is the right to receive compassionate nursing care.
- It is an essential professional nursing value.
- The nurse demonstrates respect for the worth and uniqueness of individuals—patients and colleagues.
- The nurse advocates for the respect and dignity of human beings.

AUTONOMY

- Autonomy is the right of self-determination.
- The nurse must respect the patient's right to make decisions about and for himself/herself.
- Examples of respect for an individual's autonomy are obtaining informed consent, facilitating patient choice for treatment, allowing patient to refuse treatment, and maintaining confidentiality.
- Individuals may lose autonomy when they fall ill; family interactions may leave the patient out of the decision-making process.

PATIENT'S BILL OF RIGHTS

- This document was developed by the American Hospital Association (AHA) in 1972 and was revised in 1992.
- It outlines an individual's right to inspect his/her medical record and to receive information about the medical care received during a hospital stay. In addition, the Bill speaks for the right to respectful care, relevant and understandable information, advance directive, consideration of privacy, consent or decline participation in research, continuity of care, and information of hospital policies and practices.
- In 2001, the McCain-Edwards-Kennedy/Ganske-Dingell Patients' Bill of Rights was passed. The Bill addresses such additional issues as shared decision making, the right to be informed of all medical options, and the right to refuse treatment.

ACCESS TO MEDICAL RECORD

The medical record

- contains medical information as well as personal information about the patient.
- is considered the property of the health care agency, but the patient has a legal interest and right to the information.
- can be accessed by those with a legitimate interest, which is generally accepted as referring to patient care, professional education, administrative functions, auditing functions, research, public health reporting, and criminal law requirements.

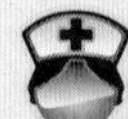

Practice Alert

Information may be shared between health care providers who are responsible for patient care within a health care facility. Health care agencies have a responsibility to establish policies and procedures to protect patient confidentiality as well as falsification or alteration of the medical record. Nurses are held accountable for upholding the Patient's Bill of Rights. Under conditions of danger to another human being, autonomy would not be absolute.

CONFIDENTIALITY/INFORMATION SECURITY

A patient's privacy will be respected and information that is shared about a patient to a health care provider will not be made public without the patient's consent.

HEALTH INSURANCE PORTABILITY AND ACCOUNTABILITY ACT (HIPAA)

- The Act is a federal privacy standard that protects the patient's medical records and other identifiable health information whether maintained on paper, computer, or orally communicated.
- It requires the maintenance of confidentiality and ensures the privacy of patients.
- Patients can obtain copies of their medical records.
- Providers must provide patients with written notice of practices and patients' rights.
- Limitations are placed on information shared: what, where, and with whom.

COMPUTERIZED MEDICAL DATABASE

- Serious concern arises around patient privacy and confidentiality as health care information becomes more and more electronically accessible.
- ANA supports nine principles in keeping with patient advocacy and trust in regard to advances in technology and patient's health information.

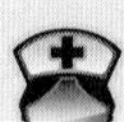

Practice Alert

Health care agencies need to have policies and procedures in place to ensure privacy and confidentiality of computerized patient information. Ultimately, patients will have increased control over their own information and there will be significant penalties in place if the policies are violated.

INFORMED CONSENT

- An individual has the right to understand the choices being offered around medical treatment and the right to voluntarily agree or refuse treatment.
- The client must receive a description of the procedure, alternatives for treatment, risks involved in treatment, and probable results. The law holds obtaining *consent for medical treatment* to be the responsibility of the physician, **but** the nurse has a responsibility of notifying the physician if she/he determines that the client does not seem to understand.
- Consent can be oral or written, although a written consent is usually preferred.
- A blanket consent for "any procedure deemed necessary" is not usually considered adequate for specific procedures.
- *Consent for nursing care* is implied when the nurse asks the client to do something and the client does not refuse the care.
- To give consent, a person must be competent, i.e., able to make judgments based on rational understanding.
- Clients have the right to change their mind and can *withdraw consent*; if this occurs, the nurse must notify the physician.
- *Consent for a minor* to receive treatment is usually provided by a parent or legal guardian.

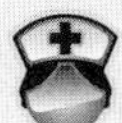

Practice Alerts

The nurse may witness the signing of the consent form for medical treatment.

The client has the right to refuse any aspect of care offered.

ADVANCED DIRECTIVES

These are the wishes of an individual expressed in a legal document when the individual is no longer capable of giving his/her own consent in certain health care situations. The document is prepared in *advance* of the situation and *directs* others how to act on behalf of the individual.

LIVING WILL

- Provides preferences around end-of-life care.
- "*If–Then*" plan: "If" something happens, then "I want X done." "If" must be a diagnosis made by a physician.
- States vary in their requirements—originally, living wills were advisory for families and physicians, but now some states have laws that require the physician to honor the living-will stipulation. If a physician does not agree with the patient's decision, then she/he must withdraw from the case and refer the patient to another physician.

DURABLE POWER OF ATTORNEY

- This is a legal document that designates a substitute decision maker for general or specific health care and medical decisions should the individuals not be able to decide for themselves.
- Durable power of attorney can be combined with a living will. This document is considered the most flexible as the individual who has been assigned the durable power of attorney can make decisions as the situation changes.

PATIENT SELF-DETERMINATION ACT

- Effective as of 1992, the Act requires health care facilities receiving Medicare and Medicaid reimbursement to recognize advance directives.
- Patients on admission to a health care agency must be given the opportunity to determine what lifesaving or life-prolonging actions they want to have carried out. The health care agency must follow the patient's advance directives. The agency is required to provide the individual with enough information to make an informed decision.
- Issues that are usually addressed in an advanced directive are specific treatment to be refused or desired, when the directive is to take effect, and specific hospitals and physicians to be consulted. As a clinical advocate, the nurse helps the family members determine a course of action.
- Frequently, it is the nurse who has to assess a client's level of understanding and provide the education as well as obtain the client's signature. ANA has come out with a statement that the nurse should have a primary role in education, research, patient care, and advocacy.

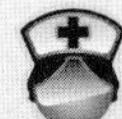

Practice Alert

Nurses are expected to learn the law regarding advance directives in the state in which they are practicing as well as the policies and procedures of the health care agency in which they are working.

ETHICAL PRACTICE

- It involves reasoning that is rational, systematic, and based on ethical principles and codes rather than on emotions or intuition.
- Ethical decision making has the patient's well-being at the center of it.
- Nurses have a responsibility for ethical considerations to patients, employing agency, and physicians.

PROFESSIONAL ETHICAL CODES

- Ethical codes are guidelines that provide a framework for ethical behavior, which in turn provides direction to moral reasoning and action. Nursing ethics focus on the practice of nursing.
- Codes provide direction; however, they do not eliminate moral dilemmas.
- The individual health care professional must be motivated to act morally.

ANA Code of Ethics

- The ANA Code of Ethics was adopted in 1950 and its last revision was in 2001.
- It contains general moral standards for nurses to follow.
- It is considered to be nonnegotiable with regard to nursing practice.
- It is patient focused, whether the patient is an individual, family, group, or community.

ICN Code of Nursing Ethics

- The ICN Code of Nursing Ethics was adopted in 1953.
- It contains four principal elements: standards for nurses and people, practice, profession, and coworkers.
- These elements provide a framework for standards of conduct.

The Codes use the word "patient" versus "client" in identifying the recipient of nursing care. Patients are the center of nurses' practice.

RELATIONSHIPS

Nurses need to be concerned about their relationships with colleagues (nurses and physicians) as well as patients in order to provide compassionate care. All the nurses' relationships ultimately affect the patient.

Nurse–Patient–Family Relationship

- When patients enter the health care system, they have no option but to trust the nurse when they need care—unavoidable trust. An uneven power structure is created between patients and nurses, and patients and nurses and families. Nurses promise to be the best nurses they can be. They promise to be candid, sensitive, attentive, and never to abandon the patient.
- A second component of the nurse–patient–family relationship is patient advocacy. The nurse identifies unmet needs and follows up to address the needs appropriately. When advocating for a patient, the nurse moves from the patient to the health care system to address the health care needs of the patient.

Nurse–Nurse Relationship

- Nurses are a community that works together for a common good using professional traditions to guide its practice.
- When a nurse has reason to believe a colleague is placing a client in jeopardy or another colleague in harm, she/he has a responsibility to deal with the offending coworker.

Nurse–Physician Relationship

Physicians and nurses are members of the health care community working together for the health and well-being of the patient.

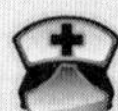

Practice Alert

Nurses can never take for granted the fragility of a client's trust. The best interests of the client are not served if the nurse and physician do not view themselves as members of a common community.

BIOETHICAL ISSUES

Bioethics is the domain of ethics that focuses on moral issues in the field of health care.

Acquired Immune Deficiency Syndrome

- AIDS bears a social stigma due to its association with sexual behavior and drug use.

- The primary ethical issues are testing for the presence of HIV and maintaining privacy, which include questions of whether health care providers and patients should undergo required or voluntary testing and how much information should be released to others.
- Statutory laws provide direction to the duty to warn sexual partners of individuals with HIV.
- There are only a few situations in which a nurse could ethically refuse to care for a patient with HIV; one example might be if the nurse was pregnant.

Abortion—Pro-Choice/Pro-Life

- The central ethical dilemma is the right to life of the fetus or the women's right to control her own body by choosing whether or not to have a baby. The question is—is the fetus a person a or nonperson?
- Abortion is legal during the first trimester. The US Supreme Court in *Roe v. Wade* ruled that states cannot ban abortion in the first and second trimester, except for certain reasons during the second trimester.

Child Abuse

- Physical, sexual, emotional abuse, and neglect are actions considered to be forms of family violence.
- Neglect is the most common form of child abuse.
- The nurse must be alert for the signs of abuse and is required to report possible abuse. The responsibility to maintain confidentiality is waived when child abuse is suspected.
- All states have mandatory child abuse reporting laws. Abuse does not need to be confirmed in order to be reported. There is legal protection for nurses in most states who report suspected cases in good faith.
- There are legal sanctions for health care providers who fail to report suspected abuse cases.

End of Life—Right to Die

Technology and the increased elderly population have raised many ethical dilemmas. Nurses are involved in ethical decision making around such things as euthanasia, assisted suicide, and termination of life-sustaining treatment.

Genetic Screening

- Genetic screening involves the professional counseling of individuals or couples about their risk for genetically linked diseases.
- Information obtained from genetic screening may be useful for individuals and couples; however, it can create a situation where the individuals involved do not know what to do with the information.
- Stem cell research offers hope for correction of genetic diseases.

Organ Transplant

- Organs may come from living donors or from donors who have just died.
- Ethical issues include such concerns as allocation of organs, selling of body parts, children as potential donors, and clear definition of death. Two major twenty-first century issues are (a) societal pressure for organ harvesting due to global demand for organs and (b) individuals questioning their own moral beliefs about death and the legal definition of death as it relates to organ donation.
- Bioethicists continue to search for answers to philosophical questions about life and death.

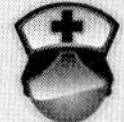

Practice Alert

Nurses need to learn the laws around bioethical issues in the state where they are practicing as well as the institution's policies where they are employed.

CONCEPTS OF MANAGEMENT

- Management is a process to achieve organizational goals.
- Nursing management is the process of getting nursing staff to provide care to patients.
- The nurse manager plans, organizes, directs, and controls financial, material, and human resources in order to provide the most effective care possible to groups of patients and their families.

PLANNING

Planning is the determination of what needs to be done. Its essential elements are

- objectives,
- strategic planning,

- budget, and
- setting priorities.

Objectives

- Objectives are the specific measurable statements that flow from the philosophy and mission of the institution that identify what needs to be achieved by the nursing unit.
- When the statement refers to the institution, it is called a goal.

Strategic Planning

- Strategic planning refers to the long-range planning by a health care organization; it provides the direction that the organization will go in over the next 3–5 years.
- It is based on the values, philosophy, and mission of the health care organization and the vision of its leaders.

Budget

- Budget is the allocation of resources on the basis of forecasted needs.
- It is a numerical expression of expected revenues and expenditures of the nursing service department.
- The objective for making a budget is to ensure the attainment of desired goals in the most cost-effective manner.
- There are two types of budgets: operating budget and capital budget. The operating budget includes manpower resources, supplies, minor equipment, overhead expenses, salaries, and benefits while the capital budget includes items of considerable expense, such as major pieces of equipment.

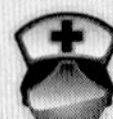

Practice Alert

The nurse manager is accountable for maintaining the nursing service department budget and needs to monitor the department budget reports.

Setting Priorities

The nurse leader determines the importance of activities and establishes the order in which the activities will be carried out. Setting priorities involves decision making.

ORGANIZING

Organization involves determination of how the planning is to be accomplished, how the parts are to be arranged into a functioning whole, and how the activities are to be coordinated to achieve a goal. Hence it is a means to an end, not an end in itself. Its essential elements are

- organizational structure
- position/job descriptions
- team building
- staffing

Organizational Structure

The formal organizational structure is the official arrangement of positions (organizational chart) and should be based upon goals of the institution and philosophy and objectives of the department.

The informal organizational structure is the unofficial personal relationship among workers, which influences their working effectiveness.

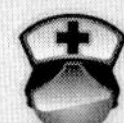

Practice Alert

The nurse manager needs to be able to use both the formal and the informal structure.

Organizational principles

- Unity of Command—an employee should be responsible to only one supervisor.
- Requisite Authority—when responsibility is delegated to a subordinate, the subordinate must also be given authority over the resources needed to accomplish the task.
- Continuing Responsibility—when a superior delegates responsibility to a subordinate, it does not diminish the superior's responsibility for the function.
- Organizational Centrality—an individual has more information available when she/he interacts directly with more individuals in the organization and becomes more powerful.

Position/Job Description

- Position/job description is a formal written document that describes the principal duties and scope of responsibilities for a particular position.
- It facilitates wage and salary administration, manpower planning, and assists with recruitment, selection, placement, orientation, and evaluation of employees.

Team Building

- Team building focuses on both task and relationship aspects of a group's functioning and is intended to increase efficiency and productivity.

- Team building involves data gathering about the team and its functioning, diagnosing strengths and areas needing development, and addressing team problems.
- Successful teams reflect open and effective communications, members that are committed to the team, clearly identified roles and responsibilities of the members, and trust and collegiality.

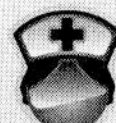

Practice Alert

The most important activities in team building are data gathering and diagnosing.

Staffing

- The purpose of staffing is to provide the nursing unit with the appropriate number and type of persons to perform the tasks required for patient care.
- Assignment methods are functional, team, primary, and modular.

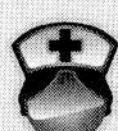

Practice Alert

There needs to be a uniform staffing pattern for the nursing service department versus a different one for each individual nursing unit.

LEADING

Leading is the process of getting the organization's work done. Its essential elements are

- leadership,
- supervision,
- decision making,
- shared governance,
- change agent,
- managing conflict,
- power—authority, and
- time management.

Leadership

- Leadership is the ability to influence other people. A nurse leader can inspire the nursing staff to work together to accomplish the nursing unit's goals.
- Formal leadership is when the nurse has legitimate authority as defined by the health care organization.
- Informal leadership is when a staff member exercises leadership without the management role.
- Present-day theories of leadership evolve from the principles of quantum mechanics and reflect a fusion of the earlier theories of leadership: trait, behavior, and contingency theories.
- Six perspectives of quantum leadership are charismatic, transactional, transformational, connective, shared, and servant leadership.

Supervision

- Supervision refers to the guidance, oversight, and evaluation of a member of the nursing team to whom the nurse leader has delegated an activity. It is an opportunity for the nurse to encourage the development of team members.
- Effective supervision utilizes the skills of communication, human relations, and teaching.
- Supervision is a mutual effort on the part of the individual being supervised and the person supervising.

Decision Making

- The decision-making process involves a series of steps that the nurse manager goes through to make a logical, well-informed, rational choice.
- Decision making always involves evaluating several possible solutions and making a choice.

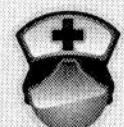

Practice Alert

A decision not to do something is still a decision.

Shared Governance

- Shared governance is based on a philosophy that nursing practice is best determined by nurses.
- It involves a network of nurses making nursing practice decisions in a decentralized environment.
- The outcome is that nurses participate in an accountable forum to control their own practice.
- Such forums can be in the form of councils or advisory boards.

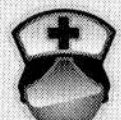

Practice Alert

Shared governance allows staff nurses significant control over major decisions affecting nursing practice.

Change Agent

- Change is a continual unfolding process.
- This process begins with the present state, moves through a transition state, and comes to the desired state. Having once arrived at the desired state, the process starts again.
- Change agent is the individual who helps to achieve the results during the dynamic process.
- Planned change has four steps: designing the change, planning the implementation, implementing the change, and integrating the change. Choosing change strategies depends on the amount of resistance anticipated and the degree of power the change agent has over the situation.
- Resistance to change occurs for a variety of reasons and comes from three major sources: technical concerns—concern about the change being a good idea, psychosocial needs—Maslow's hierarchy of needs, and threats to a person's position and power.

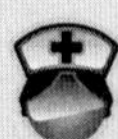

Practice Alert

A leader uses interpersonal skills to influence others to accomplish the specific objectives.

Managing Conflict

- Conflict management begins with a decision of "if and when" to intervene.
- It deals with conflict of issues, not personalities.
- Participants are responsible for working toward solutions and an open and full discussion of the problem is required.

Strategies

- Maintain equity in each party's presentation of their information.
- Establish an environment where positive as well as negative feelings can be expressed.
- Engage in active listening of all parties.
- Restate key themes and encourage both parties to provide feedback.
- Develop alternative solutions and a plan to carry them out. Follow up on the plan.
- Provide positive feedback.
- Never blame.

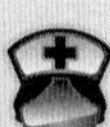

Practice Alert

Failure to intervene during a conflict can escalate the situation. Conflict management is a difficult process that consumes time and energy.

Power—Authority

- Power is the ability to influence other people even when there is resistance on the part of the other person.
- There are four types of power: authority—the power granted to a nurse or a group of nurses by virtue of position; reward—the promise (by the nurse manager) of money, goods, services, recognition, or other benefits; expertise—the special knowledge an individual (nurse) is believed to have; coercion—-the threat (by the nurse manager) of physical, economic, or psychological pain or harm.

Time Management

- In time management, what is really being managed is not time but how time is being used.
- An important aspect of time management is establishing one's own goals and time frames.
- There are seven principles of time management: goal setting, time analysis, priority determination, daily planning, delegation, interruption control, and evaluation.
- Assignment sheets that reflect the patient care assignments for each staff member as well as staff member's individual worksheets are tools to assist one in organizing time.

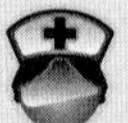

Practice Alert

Establish a "to-do" list to assist in organizing your time. Learn to say no to low-priority demands on your time.

CONTROL

Control is the process of establishing standards of performance, measuring performance, and evaluating performance and providing feedback.

Information Systems

- Information systems are complex automated systems that are integrated through networked computers to process data.
- The common information systems are management information system, hospital information system, and nursing information system.
- Automated systems offer efficient organization, management, and storage and retrieval of information.

Total Quality Management

- Total quality management is the framework for the nurse manager to manage both costs and quality of patient care.

- It is a management philosophy that emphasizes a commitment to excellence.
- Total quality management is the umbrella philosophy that supports the process of continuous quality improvement.
- Continuous quality improvement is the process that systematically determines ways to improve patient care.
- Joint Commission on the Accreditation of Healthcare Organizations (The Joint Commission) provides standards that help health care institutions focus on the quality improvement efforts.
- Components of quality management are developing a comprehensive plan, setting standards and benchmarks, carrying out performance appraisals, and focusing on intradisciplinary and interdisciplinary assessment and improvement.

Performance Appraisal

- Performance appraisal is the formal evaluation of an employee by a nurse manager.
- The employee's behavior is evaluated against a standard that identifies what the employee is expected to perform.
- The position description is the basis for the performance behaviors.
- The main reason for conducting a performance appraisal is to provide constructive feedback to the employee.
- Performance appraisals are frequently used in the decisions for salary increases and promotions.

Appraisals need to be in writing, done once a year, and shared with the employee. Employees should have the opportunity to respond and have an avenue for appeal.The manager needs to have adequate opportunity to observe the employee and should keep anecdotal notes as well as the staff nurse's self-assessment.

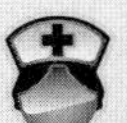

Practice Alert

The performance appraisal focuses on behaviors *not* personality traits or characteristics. Performance appraisals are part of the employee's permanent record.

DELEGATION

- Delegation is the process where responsibility and authority are transferred to another individual who accepts the responsibility and authority.
  —Responsibility is an obligation to accomplish a task.
  —Accountability refers to accepting ownership for the results.
  —Authority is the right to act. By transferring authority, the delegator is empowering the delegate to accomplish the task. When the delegator retains the authority, the delegate cannot accomplish the task and sets the delegate up for failure.
- Delegation empowers others and builds trust, enhances communication and leadership skills, and develops teamwork.
- Effective delegation enables the delegator to accomplish more and be more productive.

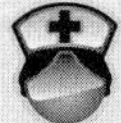

Practice Alert

The nurse can delegate only those tasks for which she/he is responsible. Along with responsibility, she/he must transfer authority.

DELEGATION PROCESS

The delegation process involves five steps:

- Define the complexity of the task and its components.
- Determine to whom to delegate; ask such questions as: Are specific qualifications necessary? Is performance restricted by practice acts, standards, or position description? Is training or education required? Match the task to the individuals' abilities and who is available to perform the task.
- Provide clear communications about expectations: describe the task, provide a reason for the task, identify on what standards the task will be evaluated, and identify any constraints for completing the task.
- Reach mutual agreement about the task, validate understanding.
- Monitor and evaluate the results; the leader/manager needs to remain accessible. If problems develop, handle privately. Give praise when it is due.

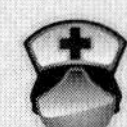

Practice Alert

When defining the task and expectations clearly establish where, when, and how. Analyze performance with respect to the established goals.

ACCEPTING DELEGATION

- Determine if you have the skills required and if not is the delegator willing to educate/train you.
- Make sure you are clear on the time frame, feedback mechanisms, and other expectations.
- Keep the delegator informed on a continual basis.

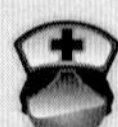

Practice Alert

Accepting delegation means you accept full responsibility for the outcome and its benefits or liabilities.

OBSTACLES TO DELEGATION

- Potential barriers to delegation can be environmental or the delegator's beliefs.
  —Environmental barriers include organizational culture, poor communication and interpersonal skills, and human and fiscal resources.
  —Majority of barriers to delegation arise from the delegator herself/himself and involve three conflicts: trust versus control, approval versus affiliation, and democratic ideal versus classic.

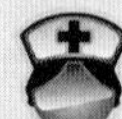

Practice Alert

Delegation takes time but a failure to delegate wastes time.

ESTABLISHING PRIORITIES

- Establishing priorities is the process of determining a preferential sequencing of activities.
- Classifications:
  —High, moderate, or low.
  —Urgent and important, important but not urgent, urgent but not important, busy work or wasted time.
- The nurse needs to have a rationale for priority setting and must use knowledge of the biological and behavioral sciences in deciding how activities will be prioritized.
- Two theories most commonly utilized are
  —Maslow's Hierarchy of Needs, which centers on five needs: physiological, safety, belonging, esteem, and self-actualization. Needs are organized hierarchically and the focus is on meeting lower-level needs before higher-level needs can be met.
  —Levine's Conservation Principles, which stresses four components necessary for a meaningful existence: conservation of energy, structural integrity, personal integrity, and social integrity.

FACTORS AFFECTING PRIORITY SETTING

- *Time management*: When time is managed effectively, the level of productivity will increase. Knowing how long an activity will take will influence the planning process.
- *Policies and procedures:* Provide a framework for the nurse to know what to do in a given situation.
- *Experience*: Past experiences of the nurse will influence the way she/he sets priorities.
- *Patient preferences*: Patient's likes and dislikes, as well as wishes, can influence priority setting.

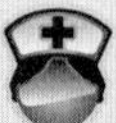

Practice Alert

Because the nurse is responsible for a large number of activities in the course of a day, she/he needs to write down the priorities.

CONTINUITY OF CARE

- Continuity of care refers to the coordination of health care services for patients when they move from one health care setting to another as well as among different health care providers.
- Continuity of care enables uninterrupted care.

DISCHARGE PLANNING

- Getting discharged is the process of leaving one level of health care for another, such as leaving the hospital for home, or leaving the hospital for another health care facility.
- Effective discharge planning involves ongoing, comprehensive assessment of the patient, development of nursing diagnoses, and establishment of individualized plans of care.
- Client, family or significant other, and health professional are included in the planning.

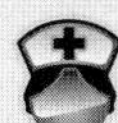

Practice Alert

Discharge planning begins on admission to a health care facility. Discharge planning includes the client and family or significant other in the planning process. Discharge planning includes all health professionals involved in the care of the individual.

RESOURCES

- Preparing referrals is a systematic problem-solving approach to identify community resources needed in the care of patients.
- As much information as possible about the patient should be provided in the process of making a referral: personal and health data, activities of daily living, disabilities/limitations, financial resources, and community supports.
- When making a referral, a nurse uses problem-solving, priority-setting, coordinating, and collaborating skills.

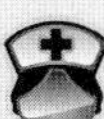

Practice Alert

When making a referral, instructions must be written clearly and be easily understood by the client and family members.

CONSULTATION

- Consultation is a method for obtaining information about the client.
- The nurse discusses client needs with other health care providers.
- Nurses also consult with client's family members to obtain information.

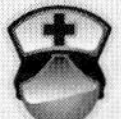

Practice Alert

Community-based nursing involves nursing care that extends beyond institutional boundaries and involves a network of services.

COMMUNITY-BASED HEALTH CARE

- Community-based health care is a system that provides health-related services within the context of where people spend their time.
- It is holistic in nature designed to provide services that focus on restoring and promoting health and preventing illness.
- *Integrated health care system* is one type of community-based framework whose goal is to facilitate care across health care settings.

INFORMATION TECHNOLOGY

- It replaces or supplements the written medical record.
- Computerized Medical Record provides for the retrieval of patient data by individuals who require the information.
- Data about the individual is constantly available, quality is monitored, and individuals can share activities influencing their health status.

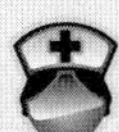

Practice Alert

Nurses need to assume accountability as they collaborate with other health care professionals.

RESOURCE MANAGEMENT

- Resource management is the process used to determine fiscal, human, and material needs of the nursing service department and nursing unit.
- Effectiveness of resource management depends on the ability of the nurse leader to make decisions.
- Decentralization model requires the nurse leader to be knowledgable about resources.

BUDGET

- It is a plan for the acquiring, distributing, and using the money necessary to run the organization.
- Budgets provide a foundation for managing and evaluating fiscal performance of the organization and each nursing unit receives a portion of the total organization budget.
- The nurse leader sets goals and objectives for the nursing unit in order to plan effectively for the fiscal needs of the unit and be able to submit an appropriate budget.
- The budgeting process consists of the operating budget (revenues and expenses for the upcoming year) and the capital budget (equipment and renovations to meet long-term goals).

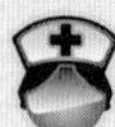

Practice Alert

To be fiscally responsible, the nurse is required to become familiar with the language of budgeting.

STAFFING

- It is the process of determining the appropriate number and type of nursing staff needed to deliver quality nursing care and meet the nursing unit's objectives.
- Staffing needs are determined by nurse–patient ratios, nurse–shift ratios, and staff mix ratios.
- Recruitment and retention of nurses are important components of the staffing process.
- Patient classification systems are used for determining workload requirements and staffing needs.
- A component of staffing is scheduling, i.e., determination of which staff member works which shift and on which days of the week.

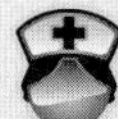

Practice Alert

Staffing and scheduling involve planning to meet the needs of the nursing unit.

SUPPLIES AND EQUIPMENT

- Supplies are the materials related to client care needed to operate the nursing unit.
- The nurse leader needs to determine the amount of materials necessary to carry out the activities of the nursing unit without having excess materials.
- Nurse leaders also are being asked to be involved in product selection.

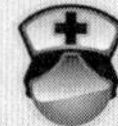

Practice Alert

Nurses need to educate themselves about the particular products being used within their nursing unit.

CASE MANAGEMENT

- This involves management of the type of nursing care delivery system that provides for the assessment, planning, implementing, coordinating, monitoring, and evaluating services received by clients provided by the entire health care team.
- It advances multidisciplinary collaboration.
- It emphasizes quality and cost-effective care.

Case Manager—Nurses often assume the role of case manager. A nurse carries a client caseload from admission to discharge and may also oversee clients in the outpatient setting following discharge. The case manager's key role is to assess, plan, facilitate, and advocate for patients. The case manager may have a client load but more frequently supervises and collaborates with the primary caregiver assigned to the clients. Case managers act as client advocates.

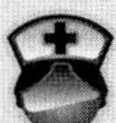

Practice Alert

Critical thinking, communication, planning, and evaluation are skills needed by the case manager.

CRITICAL PATHWAYS

- Critical pathways are the guidelines that provide direction for optimum daily patient care.
- They standardize care and reduce variation in patient care.
- They outline care activities as well as expected outcomes all of which are developed by a multidisciplinary team.
- Based on nursing diagnosis and critical pathways, the case manager immediately knows if expected outcomes are being met.

MULTIDISCIPLINARY TEAM

- Each member of the team is equal and respected for his/her unique contribution(s).
- Collaboration, which involves sharing information and knowledge, is critical to team function.
- Nurses often play key roles in multidisciplinary teams as team leader and team member.

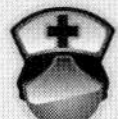

Practice Alert

Collaboration requires nurses to understand what other health professionals have to offer and what they bring to the situation.

PERFORMANCE IMPROVEMENT (QUALITY IMPROVEMENT)

Performance improvement is a model that represents actions and processes used by a health care organization to reduce costs and improve quality of health care.

QUALITY ASSURANCE (QUALITY ASSESSMENT AND IMPROVEMENT)

Quality assurance is a systematic process used to assure excellence in the health care provided to clients. Three components of evaluation are involved: structure, process, and outcome evaluation. Structure evaluation focuses on the setting where care was provided. Process evaluation looks at how the care was given. Outcome evaluation focuses on demonstrating the changes that have occurred as a result of the nursing care provided.

TOTAL QUALITY MANAGEMENT/ CONTINUOUS QUALITY IMPROVEMENT

Total quality management involves a systematic process focusing on improving the quality of care. Individuals from a variety of departments determine how care needs to be provided. They decide what outcomes are desired.

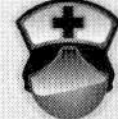

Practice Alert

TQM/CQI are focused on establishing procedures for improving the quality of care and not on identifying mistakes.

NURSING AUDIT

- Nursing audit is a review of client records to determine if specific criteria have been met.
- The audit is either *retrospective*—evaluation of a client's chart after discharge—or *concurrent*—evaluation of the patient's care while the individual is still receiving it.
- Nursing audit reflects the performance of a group of individuals versus a single individual.

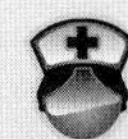

Practice Alert

Quality is everyone's responsibility.

STAFF EDUCATION

Staff education is the process of enhancing staff performance.

ORIENTATION

- Orientation involves acquainting the new graduate or employee with the workplace to socialize and reduce anxiety.
- It usually is a shared responsibility between the Staff Education Department, which focuses on organization-wide information, and the nursing manager or delegate who focuses on the particular nursing unit.
- It can last for several weeks to several months.
- Preceptorship or mentorship are two methods that are used to orient new employees. Preceptors are selected from experienced staff nurses to assist new graduates to obtain the necessary knowledge and skills structured to their particular needs. Mentors are experienced nurses who support, guide, and nurture a person over a much longer period of time than just orientation. A mentor instills a sense of self-confidence and self-esteem in the mentee.

IN-SERVICE EDUCATION (ALSO REFERRED TO AS "ON-THE-JOB TRAINING")

- In-service training consists of programs offered by the institution to keep staff members current with the protocol that has changed and new equipment used within the organization.
- It can be a cost-effective method for assuring that the staff is maintaining current levels of expertise.

CONTINUING EDUCATION

- Educational programs offered outside the health care agency which nurses attend to maintain expertise throughout their professional careers.
- They can be workshops, seminars, conferences, short courses, or online courses.
- Contact hour is the system for recognizing participation in a nonacademic credit offering.

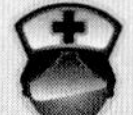

Practice Alert

Mandatory continuing education is related to renewing of a nurse's professional licensure and a predetermined number of contact hours are required by many states. Voluntary continuing education is not related to relicensure.

WORKSHEET

TRUE & FALSE QUESTIONS

Mark each of the following statements True or False. Correct all False statements in the space provided.

1. Case management, a type of nursing care delivery model, advances multidisciplinary collaboration. ___ T ___ F

2. Critical pathways are guidelines that delineate patient care activities as well as outcomes, and standardize and reduce variation in patient care. ___ T ___ F

3. Information shared by an individual with certain professionals that does not need to be revealed in a court of law is called privileged communication. ___ T ___ F

	T	F
4. The standard of "reasonable care" is used when emergency care is given in a health care setting.	___	___
5. Nursing audit is when patient records are reviewed to determine if specific criteria or standards have been met.	___	___
6. The process used to determine fiscal, human, and material needs of the nursing unit is called resource management.	___	___
7. Staffing needs are determined by nurse–patient ratios, nurse–shift ratios, and staff mix ratios.	___	___
8. The budgeting process consists of the operating budget, which includes equipment and renovations to meet long-term unit goals, and the capital budget, which focuses on revenues and expenses of the nursing unit for the upcoming year.	___	___
9. Ethical decision making has the patient's well-being at the center of it.	___	___
10. Neglect is the most common form of child abuse.	___	___
11. The professional counseling of individuals or couples about their risk for genetically linked diseases is called genetic screening.	___	___
12. AIDS bears a social stigma due its association with the right to life of the fetus and organ harvesting.	___	___
13. When a patient is undergoing a medical procedure, she/he needs to receive a description of the medical procedure, alternatives for treatment, risks involved in the treatment, and probable results.	___	___
14. Discharge planning begins on admission to a health care facility.	___	___
15. A computerized medical record replaces or supplements the traditional written medical record.	___	___
16. The process of determining a preferential sequencing of activities is called delegation.	___	___

MATCHING QUESTIONS

Match the following

17. ___ CEU	a. Defines the scope of nursing practice
18. ___ Accountability	b. Employee is responsible to only one supervisor
19. ___ In-Service Education	c. Philosophy that emphasizes a commitment to quality of patient care
20. ___ Patient's Bill of Rights	d. Determination of what needs to be done
21. ___ Nurse Practice Act	e. Continuing Education Unit
22. ___ Standards of Care	f. Document that describes the duties and responsibilities for a particular position
23. ___ Strategic Planning	g. Formal evaluation of an employee by a nurse manager

(continued)

24. ___ Planning	h. Individual's right to inspect his/her medical record and to receive information about medical care
25. ___ Position Description	i. Statements that define an acceptable level of care
26. ___ Unity of Command	j. Accepting ownership for the result
27. ___ Leadership	k. Individual that helps achieve the results during the dynamic process of change
28. ___ Change Agent	l. Ability to influence other people
29. ___ Total Quality Management	m. Programs offered by the health care facility to keep staff current
30. ___ Performance Appraisal	n. Long-range planning

APPLICATION QUESTIONS

1. An advance directive is a legal document that allows an individual to express his/her wishes prior to the health care situation occurring. The two most common advance directives are:
   a. living will and durable power of attorney
   b. informed consent and confidentiality
   c. Nurse Practice Act and licensure
   d. Patient's Bill of Rights and standards of care

2. Case management is a type of nursing care delivery system. It consists of the client, case manager, and support services and resources. The circles reflect the organization of the case management delivery system. Place an X in the circle indicating where the case manager would be, a Y in the circle indicating where the client would be, and a Z in the circle indicating where the support services and resources would be.

Figure 4–1.

3. Which of the following are advantages of the case management nursing care delivery system? (Select all that apply.)
   a. promotes multidisciplinary team collaboration
   b. is cost effective
   c. increases quality of care
   d. is time consuming

4. Case management is a type of nursing care delivery model that incorporates assessment, planning, implementation, coordinating, monitoring, and evaluation into the services received by clients by means of which primary concept?
   a. multidisciplinary team collaboration
   b. patient-focused care
   c. managed care
   d. differentiated practice

5. Four broad management functions that a nurse manager uses to achieve nursing organizational goals are:
   a. planning, organizing, directing, and controlling.
   b. strategic planning, team building, leadership, and performance evaluation.
   c. situational, interactional, transformational, and contingency processes.
   d. autocratic, democratic, and laissez-faire behaviors.

6. A staff nurse has the responsibility for the care of five clients. She is working with a nursing assistant in the care of the clients. The staff nurse will assign specific

care for clients to the nursing assistant. The nursing assistant will carry out the necessary care on the assigned clients and report back to the staff nurse. This is an example of how the nursing assistant does what? (Select all that apply.)
a. assumes responsibility
b. is accountable
c. makes decisions
d. delegates to another individual

7. The ability to influence other people is called:
a. leadership
b. management
c. decision making
d. supervision

8. The following organizational chart depicts which management principle?
a. chain of command
b. division of labor
c. staff organization
d. case method

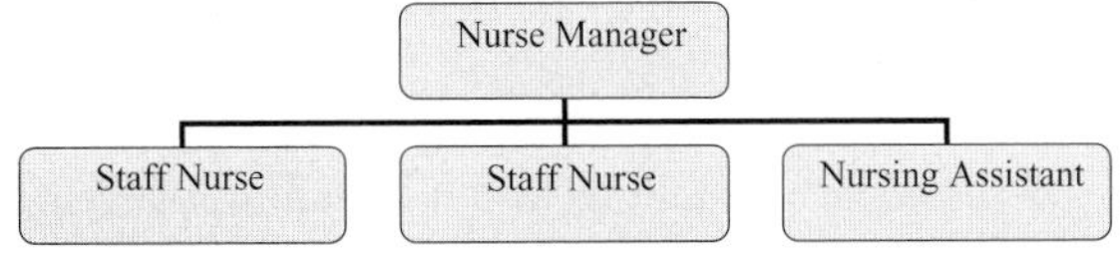

Figure 4–2.

9. The first thing a nurse does when planning for effective use of time is to:
a. assess his/her actual use of time
b. establish goals and priorities
c. consider what activities can be delegated
d. write down his/her client care assignment

10. The potential effectiveness of a decision depends on which of the following? (Select all that apply.)
a. personal value system of the decision maker
b. kind of data used in making the decision
c. defensibility of the decision
d. selling the decision

11. Some decisions are best made by a group rather than by the nurse alone. What is an advantage of group decision making?
a. promotes ownership of decision
b. individual opinions are influenced by others
c. dependency is fostered
d. formal and informal role and status positions evolve

12. The Health Insurance Portability and Accountability Act (HIPAA) protects the
a. patient's medical and health information
b. patient's right to refuse treatment
c. patient from third-party payers
d. patient's need to have liability insurance

13. The coordination of health care services for patients when they move from one health care setting to another is called:
a. continuity of care
b. discharge planning
c. consultation
d. integrated health care system

14. Delegation is the process where one individual can accomplish the necessary tasks with and through another. Place the five steps of delegation in the correct order.
a. communicate the expectations
b. define the task
c. determine to whom to delegate
d. supervise and evaluate the result
e. reach agreement about the task

15. The American Nurses Association (ANA) Code of Ethics addresses moral standards for nurses to adhere to and is patient focused. The phrase "patient focused" means it encompasses the:
a. patient, family, and group or community
b. patient only
c. patient and family
d. patient and nurse

16. A nurse's relationships center on three specific types: nurse–patient–family relationship, nurse–nurse relationship, and nurse–physician relationship. Which phrase best describes the nurse–nurse relationship?
a. Working together for a common good through respect.
b. Working together as members of a common community.
c. Working together to meet unmet needs and to address them.
d. Working together.

17. Mandatory continuing education is a/an:
a. requirement for renewal of a nurse's professional license in some states.
b. component of the Nurse Practice Act.
c. system for receiving nonacademic credit for attendance.

(continued)

d. institutional offering to keep professional staff current.

18. The concept of decentralized decision making is often associated with which of the following?
    a. shared governance
    b. team nursing
    c. interdisciplinary practice model
    d. primary nursing

19. When a nurse delegates, she/he gets the legal authority for the delegation from:
    a. Nurse Practice Act
    b. American Nurses Association Standards of Practice
    c. American Nurses Association Code of Ethics
    d. Public Health Act

20. As a nurse manager, you have been asked to delegate the preparation of the daily staffing assignment to your assistant. The task has been determined to be one that could be delegated to someone else and free you up for other responsibilities. You recognize the experience your assistant has working on the nursing unit; you also recognize that the individual is able to handle the new responsibility. However, you find that you are unwilling to delegate the daily staffing assignment. Which answer might explain your reluctance to delegate? (Select all that apply.)
    a. You question if this is a good use of your assistant nurse manager's time and skill.
    b. You feel that your assistant nurse manager is already overloaded and this new assignment would just add to an already difficult situation.
    c. You fear that your assistant may not know all the specifics that go into developing a staffing assignment and that staff members who are used to certain patients will no longer be assigned them.
    d. You know that this would be an opportunity for your assistant to develop in the role of nurse manager.

21. The legal credential conferred by a state that allows the nurse to practice nursing is called:
    a. license
    b. certification
    c. advanced practice
    d. Nursing Practice Act

22. What do the initials CEU stand for?
    a. Continuing Education Unit
    b. Chief Executive for Urbanization
    c. Code of Ethics for the Uninsured
    d. Collective Education Union

23. A sound planning process is important to the success of any health care organization. One type of planning is called strategic planning. Which statement best describes the process of strategic planning?
    a. Strategic planning is the effort by a hospital to plan the direction the organization will go in, taking into consideration the hospital's mission, philosophy, values, and stakeholders. It is a proactive process. It looks at future goals and strategies to meet the opportunities and threats of the external and internal environment.
    b. Strategic planning is when a group of people with a common purpose and common goals come together to discuss an idea that needs to be accomplished. A communication pattern is established to ensure that information is disseminated. All members of the group are encouraged to actively participate.
    c. Strategic planning is when resources to manage patient care are determined and monitored.
    d. Strategic planning is when a staffing pattern is developed that considers the availability of qualified staff and the acuity levels of the patients. The planning often utilizes patient-classification systems, benchmarking data, and regulatory requirements for decision making.

24. When a nurse in performing her/his responsibilities commits an act of negligence it is called
    a. malpractice
    b. tort
    c. misdemeanor
    d. criminal negligence

25. Critical pathways can be defined as
    a. guidelines that provide direction for optimum daily patient care.
    b. collaboration where nurses are equal team members.
    c. acting as a patient advocate.
    d. information shared by professionals that does not have to be revealed in a court of law.

ANSWERS & RATIONALES

TRUE & FALSE ANSWERS

Mark each of the following statements True or False. Correct all False statements in the space provided.

1. Case management, a type of nursing care delivery model, advances multidisciplinary collaboration. *True*
2. Critical pathways are guidelines that delineate patient care activities as well as outcomes, and standardize and reduce variation in patient care. *True*
3. Information shared by an individual with certain professionals that does not need to be revealed in a court of law is called privileged communication. *True*
4. The standard of "reasonable care" is used when emergency care is given in a health care setting. *False*

   "Reasonable care" standard is used in emergency situations that occur outside a health care institution.
5. Nursing audit is when patient records are reviewed to determine if specific criteria or standards have been met. *True*
6. The process used to determine fiscal, human, and material needs of the nursing unit is called resource management. *True*
7. Staffing needs are determined by nurse–patient ratios, nurse–shift ratios, and staff mix ratios. *True*
8. The budgeting process consists of the operating budget, which includes equipment and renovations to meet long-term unit goals, and the capital budget, which focuses on revenues and expenses of the nursing unit for the upcoming year. *False*

   The operating budget is the component that focuses on revenues and expenses of the nursing unit and the capital budget is the component that focuses on long-term unit goals.
9. Ethical decision making has the patient's well-being at the center of it. *True*
10. Neglect is the most common form of child abuse. *True*
11. The professional counseling of individuals or couples about their risk for genetically linked diseases is called genetic screening. *True*
12. AIDS bears a social stigma due its association with the right to life of the fetus and organ harvesting. *False*

    The social stigma of AIDS is due to its association with sexual behavior and drug use.
13. When a patient is undergoing a medical procedure, she/he needs to receive a description of the medical procedure, alternatives for treatment, risks involved in the treatment, and probable results. *True*
14. Discharge planning begins on admission to a health care facility. *True*
15. A computerized medical record replaces or supplements the traditional written medical record. *True*
16. The process of determining a preferential sequencing of activities is called delegation. *False*

    Setting priorities is the process of determining a sequencing of activities

MATCHING ANSWERS

Match the following:

17. __e__ CEU	a. Defines the scope of nursing practice
18. __j__ Accountability	b. Employee is responsible to only one supervisor
19. __m__ In-Service Education	c. Philosophy that emphasizes a commitment to quality of patient care
20. __h__ Patient's Bill of Rights	d. Determination of what needs to be done
21. __a__ Nurse Practice Act	e. Continuing Education Unit
22. __i__ Standards of Care	f. Document that describes the duties and responsibilities for a particular position
23. __n__ Strategic Planning	g. Formal evaluation of an employee by a nurse manager
24. __d__ Planning	h. Individual's right to inspect his/her medical record and to receive information about medical care
25. __f__ Position Description	i. Statements that define an acceptable level of care
26. __b__ Unity of Command	j. Accepting ownership for the result
27. __l__ Leadership	k. Individual that helps achieve the results during the dynamic process of change
28. __k__ Change Agent	l. Ability to influence other people
29. __c__ Total Quality Management	m. Programs offered by the health care facility to keep staff current
30. __g__ Performance Appraisal	n. Long-range planning

APPLICATION ANSWERS

1. An advance directive is a legal document that allows an individual to express his/her wishes prior to the health care situation occurring. The two most common advance directives are:
   a. living will and durable power of attorney
   b. informed consent and confidentiality
   c. Nurse Practice Act and licensure
   d. Patient's Bill of Rights and standards of care

Rationale

Correct answer: a.

a. A living will provides for an individual's preferences around end-of-life care; durable power of attorney designates a substitute decision maker for health care and medical decisions should the individual not be able to decide.

Incorrect answers: b, c, and d.

b. Informed consent is the right of an individual to understand the choices being offered around medical treatment and the right to agree or disagree; confidentiality is when the patient's privacy will be respected and information about the patient will not be made public.

c. Nurse Practice Act is a set of laws defining the scope of nursing practice; licensure is a legal credential conferred by a state that grants permission to an individual to practice a given profession.

d. Patient's Bill of Rights outlines the individual's right to inspect his/her medical record and to receive information about medical care; standards of care are statements that define an acceptable level of professional practice.

2. Case management is a type of nursing care delivery system. It consists of the client, case manager, and support services and resources. The circles reflect the organization of the case management delivery system. Place an X in the circle indicating where the case manager would be, a Y in the circle indicating where the client would be, and a Z in the circle indicating where the support services and resources would be.

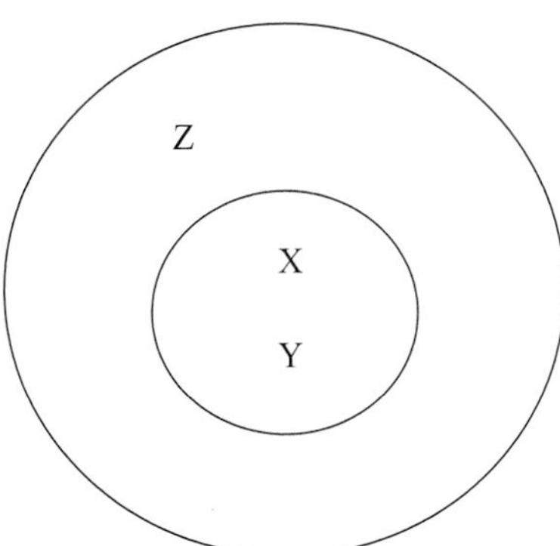

Figure 4–3.

Rationale

Correct answer: X and Y in the center circle and Z in the outside circle.

X—The case manager is the individual in the center, along with the patient, of the nursing care delivery system. She/he is responsible for the assessment, planning, implementing, coordinating, monitoring, containing costs, and evaluating services received by clients.

Y—The client is the other individual in the center of the nursing care delivery system because the primary focus of case management is the client.

Z—Support services and resources surround the core, they represent all the client's needs.

3. Which of the following are advantages of the case management nursing care delivery system? (Select all that apply.)

a. promotes multidisciplinary team collaboration

b. is cost effective

c. increases quality of care

d. is time consuming

Rationale

Correct answers: a, b, and c.

a. An advantage of the case management model is that it promotes a collaborative process for quality cost-effective outcomes; it is a process of interactions within health care network, which enables a client to receive needed services.

b. An advantage of the case management model is that outcomes result in more effective use of services and lessen costs.

c. A principal advantage of the case management model is the client receives more services and has fewer unmet needs.

Incorrect answer: d.

d. A disadvantage of the case management model is that the nurse case manager is responsible for coordinating a broad range of services for a client and managing the individual from admission through discharge and possibly after discharge making the model rewarding but also time consuming.

4. Case management is a type of nursing care delivery model that incorporates assessment planning, implementation, coordinating, monitoring, and evaluation into the services received by clients by means of which primary concept?

a. multidisciplinary team collaboration

b. patient-focused care

c. managed care

d. differentiated practice

Rationale

Correct answer: a.

a. The focus of case management is having the entire health team work together to provide the best care possible to the client.

Incorrect answers: b, c, and d.

b. Patient-focused care is what all models of nursing care delivery are concerned about.

c. Managed care refers to a system in which the use of health care services are controlled and monitored to ensure that policies are followed and that costs are minimized.

d. Differentiated practice is the practice of making a distinction between nursing roles based on education, experience, and competencies.

(continued)

5. Four broad management functions that a nurse manager uses to achieve nursing organizational goals are
   a. planning, organizing, directing, and controlling.
   b. strategic planning, team building, leadership, and performance evaluation.
   c. situational, interactional, transformational, and contingency processes.
   d. autocratic, democratic, and laissez-faire behaviors.

Rationale

Correct answer: a.

   a. The nurse manager plans, organizes, directs, and controls in order to provide the most effective care to groups of patients and their families.

Incorrect answers: b, c, and d.

   b. Strategic planning, team building, and leadership, performance evaluation are all essential elements of the management process.
   c. Situational, interactional, transformational, and contingency are names of leadership theories.
   d. Autocratic, democratic, and laissez-faire are names of leadership styles.

6. A staff nurse has the responsibility for the care of five clients. She is working with a nursing assistant in the care of the clients. The staff nurse will assign specific care for clients to the nursing assistant. The nursing assistant will carry out the necessary care on the assigned clients and report back to the staff nurse. This is an example of how the nursing assistant does what? (Select all that apply.)
   a. assumes responsibility
   b. is accountable
   c. makes decisions
   d. delegates to another individual

Rationale

Correct answers: a and b.

   a. The nursing assistant accepts the responsibility to carry out the necessary care on the assigned patients.
   b. By reporting back to the staff nurse the nursing assistant demonstrates accountability for her/his actions; the nursing assistant by accepting the assignment has an obligation to periodically report back to the delegator.

Incorrect answers: c and d.

   c. The staff nurse is the individual using decision making to determine which nursing staff member would be best to delegate the particular patient assignment.
   d. The nursing assistant is the person being delegated to rather than being the person doing the delegation; the staff nurse is the delegator.

7. The ability to influence other people is called
   a. leadership
   b. management
   c. decision making
   d. supervision.

Rationale

Correct answer: a.

   a. Leadership is when a nurse leader can inspire the nursing staff to work together to accomplish the nursing unit's goals.

Incorrect answers: b, c, and d.

   b. Management is the process of achieving organizational goals.
   c. Decision making is the process that a nurse goes through to make a logical, well-informed choice.
   d. Supervision is the process where an individual provides direction to assure that activities are being carried out properly.

8. The following organizational chart depicts which management principle
   a. chain of command
   b. division of labor
   c. staff organization
   d. case method

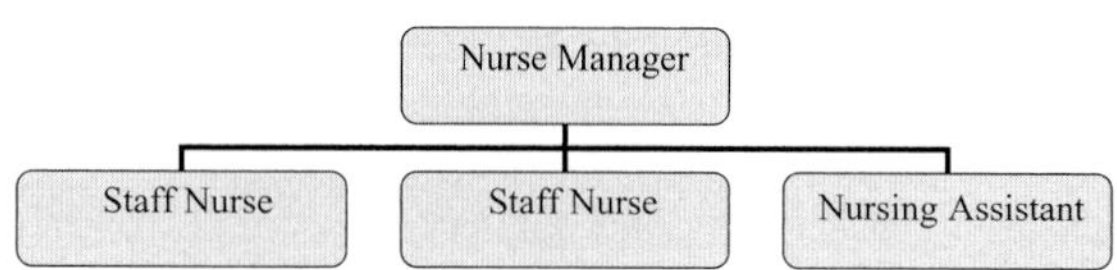

Figure 4–4.

Rationale

Correct answer: a.

   a. Chain of command represents the path of authority and accountability for decision making; the nurse manager gives direction to the nursing staff; the size of the chain of command will vary depending on the size of the nursing unit.

Incorrect answers: b, c, and d.

   b. Work that is divided into specific tasks and assigned to individuals or groups.
   c. Staff assists the line organization to carry out its function; the above diagram depicts the line organization.
   d. Case method is a nursing delivery system where

a nurse works with only one patient and meets all the individual's needs; today called private duty nursing.

9. The first thing a nurse does when planning for effective use of time is to
   a. assess his/her actual use of time.
   b. establish goals and priorities.
   c. consider what activities can be delegated.
   d. write down his/her client care assignment.

Rationale

Correct answer: a.

a. The nurse can only control how time is used; time is a resource that can be managed; it is important to first think about how you go about utilizing time before considering other principles of time management.

Incorrect answers: b, c, and d.

b. It is appropriate to determine what activities are important and establish outcomes; although important it is not the first thing the nurse thinks about.

c. At times, delegation is an effective activity of time management; although important to consider it is not the first thing the nurse thinks about.

d. Writing assignments down is a tool used by the nurse to help organize one's time.

10. The potential effectiveness of a decision depends on which of the following? (Select all that apply.)
    a. personal value system of the decision maker
    b. kind of data used in making the decision
    c. defensibility of the decision
    d. selling the decision

Rationale

Correct answers: a, b, c, and d.

a. Many factors enter into the ability for problem identification; one factor that can influence problem identification is the decision maker's personal value system.

b. The generation of alternatives; if good alternatives are not generated, a good decision cannot be made.

c. Can the decision maker support the outcome(s) and explain why the particular alternative was chosen if she/he had to support the decision to colleagues and nursing administration.

d. Acceptance of the decision by those who will be affected by it is a key component to not having the decision fail.

11. Some decisions are best made by a group rather than by the nurse alone. What is an advantage of group decision making?
    a. promotes ownership of decision
    b. individual opinions are influenced by others
    c. dependency is fostered
    d. formal and informal role and status positions evolve

Rationale

Correct answer: a.

a. There is greater likelihood of supporting the decision that the members of the group have contributed to.

Incorrect answers: b, c, and d.

b. Individual opinions influencing others in the group is a disadvantage of group decision making.

c. Dependency on the group by an individual member is a disadvantage of group decision making.

d. Role and position hierarchy may occur within the group and influence the decision making process; this possibility is considered a disadvantage to group decision making.

12. The Health Insurance Portability and Accountability Act (HIPAA) protects the
    a. patient's medical and health information
    b. patient's right to refuse treatment
    c. patient from third-party payers
    d. patient's need to have liability insurance

Rationale

Correct answer: a.

a. The Act is a federal privacy standard that protects the patient's medical records and other identifiable health information. The Act requires confidentiality and ensures the privacy of patients.

Incorrect answers: b, c, and d.

b. The right of the patient to refuse treatment is based on belief in the autonomy of the patient; it is not an Act.

c. Third-party payers are insurance companies and government programs that pay providers for health services provided to individuals.

d. Liability insurance is purchased by the nurse from an insurance company that accepts the risk of being sued.

13. The coordination of health care services for patients when they move from one health care setting to another is called

(continued)

a. continuity of care
b. discharge planning
c. consultation
d. integrated health care system

Rationale

Correct answer: a.

a. Continuity of care enables uninterrupted care when a patient leaves one facility and moves to another.

Incorrect answers: b, c, and d.

b. Discharge planning is a type of continuity of care where ongoing and comprehensive planning takes place prior to a patient leaving a health care facility.
c. Consultation is a method for obtaining information about the patient.
d. Integrated health care system is a type of community-based framework that facilitates care across health care settings.

14. Delegation is the process where one individual can accomplish the necessary tasks with and through another. Place the five steps of delegation in the correct order.
a. communicate the expectations
b. define the task
c. determine to whom to delegate
d. supervise and evaluate the result
e. reach agreement about the task

Rationale

Correct answers: b, c, a, e, and d.

b. Define the complexity of the task and its components.
c. Match the task to the individual's ability and who is able to perform the task.
a. Describe the task and provide a reason for the task; identify what standards the task will be evaluated on.
e. The nurse leader needs to validate that the task and expectations have been understood by the person being asked to carry out the task.
d. The nurse leader needs to remain accessible and evaluate performance based on the established goals.

15. The American Nurses Association (ANA) Code of Ethics addresses moral standards for nurses to adhere to and is patient focused. The phrase "patient focused" means it encompasses the
a. patient, family, and group or community
b. patient only
c. patient and family
d. patient and nurse

Rationale

Correct answer: a.

a. The nurse values and is committed to the uniqueness of the individual patient. When addressing the uniqueness of the patient the nurse must also recognize the patient's place in the family, in a group, or in the community.

Incorrect answers: b, c, and d.

b. The patient is more than just an individual; the patient can also be a family, a group, or a community.
c. The phrase "patient focused" includes not only the patient and family but it also encompasses the community in which the patient lives.
d. The nurse has the commitment to the recipient of nursing and health care.

16. A nurse's relationships center on three specific types: nurse–patient–family relationship, nurse–nurse relationship, and nurse–physician relationship. Which phrase best describes the nurse–nurse relationship?
a. Working together for a common good through respect.
b. Working together as members of a common community.
c. Working together to meet unmet needs and to address them.
d. Working together.

Rationale

Correct answer: a.

a. The nurse–nurse relationship requires active listening, acceptance and nonjudgmentalism, feedback, flexibility, and respect

Incorrect answers: b, c, and d.

b. The nurse and the physician work together as members of a common community.
c. The nurse identifies unmet needs and follows up to address the needs appropriate in the nurse–patient–family relationship.
d. Working together is a phrase that speaks to any relationship not specifically to the nurse and his/her relationships.

17. Mandatory continuing education is a/an
a. requirement for renewal of a nurse's professional license in some states.
b. component of the Nurse Practice Act.
c. system for receiving nonacademic credit for attendance.
d. institutional offering to keep professional staff current.

Rationale

Correct answer: a.

a. Some State Boards of Nursing regulations require that a certain number of continuing education contact hours be obtained before a nurse's license can be renewed.

Incorrect answers: b, c, and d.

b. The Nurse Practice Act defines the scope of nursing practice.

c. Frequently at the end of a continuing education program a certificate will be provided to the attendee that states the number of Continuing Education Units the program has been granted.

d. In-service programs provided by the institution.

18. The concept of decentralized decision making is often associated with which of the following?
    a. shared governance
    b. team nursing
    c. interdisciplinary practice model
    d. primary nursing

Rationale

Correct answer: a.

a. Shared governance is when staff members are involved in the decision-making process.

Incorrect answers: b, c, and d.

b. In team nursing, the team leader assumes a centralized decision-making role.

c. In this model team, members function independently and make independent decisions.

d. In primary nursing, decision making is centralized with the primary nurse.

19. When a nurse delegates, she/he gets the legal authority for the delegation from
    a. Nurse Practice Act
    b. American Nurses Association Standards of Practice
    c. American Nurses Association Code of Ethics
    d. Public Health Act

Rationale

Correct answer: a.

a. State laws and regulations are set forth through individual state's Nurse Practice Act that define the scope of nursing practice.

Incorrect answers: b, c, and d.

b. ANA Standards of Practice is not a legal documents; it is a document that provides general standards and guidelines for the practice of nursing.

c. ANA Code of Ethics contains general moral standards that nurses are expected to follow in their professional practice.

d. The Public Health Act is a component of federal legislation that focuses on the public safety.

20. As a nurse manager, you have been asked to delegate the preparation of the daily staffing assignment to your assistant. The task has been determined to be one that could be delegated to someone else and free you up for other responsibilities. You recognize the experience your assistant has working on the nursing unit; you also recognize that the individual is able to handle the new responsibility. However, you find that you are unwilling to delegate the daily staffing assignment. Which answer might explain your reluctance to delegate? (Select all that apply.)
    a. You question if this is a good use of your assistant nurse manager's time and skill.
    b. You feel that your assistant nurse manager is already overloaded and this new assignment would just add to an already difficult situation.
    c. You fear that your assistant may not know all the specifics that go into developing a staffing assignment and that staff members who are used to certain patients will no longer be assigned them.
    d. You know that this would be an opportunity for your assistant to develop in the role of nurse manager.

Rationale

Correct answers: a, b, and c.

a. As a nurse manager, you are expressing the feeling "I would rather do it myself"; this is a barrier to delegation.

b. As a nurse manager, you have not assessed the ability of the individual to do the job or the time needed for the individual to do the activity; this is a barrier to delegation.

c. The nurse manager fears the loss of control; this is a barrier to delegation.

Incorrect answer: d.

d. This is an example of effective delegation not a barrier to delegation.

21. The legal credential conferred by a state that allows the nurse to practice nursing is called
    a. license
    b. certification
    c. advanced practice
    d. Nursing Practice Act

Rationale

Correct answer: a.

a. A license is the legal credential that allows an individual to practice nursing.

(continued)

Incorrect answers: b, c, and d.

b. Certification is the process that grants recognition that an individual has met predetermined criteria specified for practice in his/her area of specialization.

c. Advanced practice is recognition of advanced education, usually a masters degree, in a specialty area.

d. Nurse Practice Act is a set of laws that defines the scope of nursing practice.

22. What do the initials CEU stand for?
   a. Continuing Education Unit
   b. Chief Executive for Urbanization
   c. Code of Ethics for the Uninsured
   d. Collective Education Union

Rationale

Correct answer: a.

a. Continuing Education Unit is the term used to describe the contact hour(s) received for a continuing education program.

Incorrect answers: b, c, and d.

Names do not stand for anything.

23. A sound planning process is important to the success of any health care organization. One type of planning is called strategic planning. Which statement best describes the process of strategic planning?
   a. Strategic planning is the effort by a hospital to plan the direction the organization will go in, taking into consideration the hospital's mission, philosophy, values, and stakeholders. It is a proactive process. It looks at future goals and strategies to meet the opportunities and threats of the external and internal environment.
   b. Strategic planning is when a group of people with a common purpose and common goals come together to discuss an idea that needs to be accomplished. A communication pattern is established to ensure that information is disseminated. All members of the group are encouraged to actively participate.
   c. Strategic planning is when resources to manage patient care are determined and monitored.
   d. Strategic planning is when a staffing pattern is developed that considers the availability of qualified staff and the acuity levels of the patients. The planning often utilizes patient-classification systems, benchmarking data, and regulatory requirements for decision making.

Rationale

Correct answer: a.

a. Strategic planning is long-range planning that provides the direction the organization will go in, over several years.

Incorrect answers: b, c, and d.

b. The statement describes team building.

c. The statement describes the budget process.

d. The statement describes the staffing process.

24. When a nurse in performing her/his responsibilities commits an act of negligence it is called
   a. malpractice
   b. tort
   c. misdemeanor
   d. criminal negligence

Rationale

Correct answer: a.

a. Malpractice is the term used to describe negligence by a nurse; malpractice is professional negligence.

Incorrect answers: b, c, and d.

b. Tort is a civil wrong committed by one person against another.

c. Misdemeanor is a crime of lesser infraction of the law and is punished by imprisonment of less than a year or a fine.

d. Criminal negligence is when the crime falls outside the boundaries of a simple error and reflects a serious lack of concern to the safety of the patient.

25. Critical pathways can be defined as
   a. guidelines that provide direction for optimum daily patient care.
   b. collaboration where nurses are equal team members.
   c. acting as a patient advocate.
   d. information shared by professionals that does not have to be revealed in a court of law.

Rationale

Correct answer: a.

a. Critical pathways outline care activities as well as outcomes in providing direction for patient care.

Incorrect answers: b, c, and d.

b. This type of collaboration takes place when the nurse is a member of a multidisciplinary team.

c. Acting as a patient advocate is associated with the role of the nurse in case management.

d. The information is considered privileged communication.

CHAPTER 5

Test Plan Client Needs Category:

Safe, Effective Care Environment

Sub-category: Safety and Infection Control

Topics: Accident Prevention
Disaster Planning
Emergency Response Plan
Error Prevention
Handling Hazardous and Infectious Materials
Home Safety
Ergonomic Principles
Injury Prevention
Medical and Surgical Asepsis
Reporting of Incident/Event/Irregular Occurrence/Variance
Safe Use of Equipment
Security Plan
Standard/Transmission-Based/Other Precautions
Use of Restraints/Safety Devices

ACCIDENT PREVENTION

- The main causes of accidental death in order of frequency are motor vehicle accidents, falls, poisoning, drowning, fires, and burns.
- The type of accident for which an individual is at the greatest risk is related to his/her normal growth and development.
- Most falls occur at home and are the number one cause of hospital admission for trauma among older adults; illness, medications, alcohol use as well as environmental factors cause these falls.
- Over the age of 65, hip fractures account for most admissions for trauma.
- Accident prevention requires client teaching and removal of dangers.

Client Teaching for Self-Care

AGE-RELATED ISSUES

School-age children

- Children must stay away from strangers.
- They must use protective equipment when participating in sports.
- Bicycles and scooter safety: Children should wear helmets, ride proper size bicycles, and know rules of road.

Adolescents (risk takers)

- Car safety: Adolescents are involved in more accidents than any other age group. They should wear seat belts, comply with driving rules, never drive when drunk, and never ride with anyone who is impaired.
- They are likely to experiment with drugs and this increases risk of all other types of accidents.

Adults

- Adults should adopt healthy lifestyle habits, techniques of stress management, and dangers of alcohol and other abuses.

Older adult

- Older adults have an increased risk for falls, burns, and car accidents.
- The risk factors are confusion, sensory deficit (peripheral vision loss, decreased lens accommodation, decreased night vision, cataracts, increased threshold for hot and cold, decreased hearing), impaired judgment, impaired mobility (limited ROM, kyphosis with change in center of gravity, and decreased muscle strength), slow reflexes, uncooperative, incontinence/urgency, anxiety/emotional lability, CV disease with impaired perfusion, respiratory disease with impaired oxygenation, medications affecting level of consciousness or BP, postural hypotension, new to unit, attached equipment.
- Measures to decrease the risk:
  —adequate lighting on outdoor walkways and in halls, stairways, and rooms; nightlights in children's, older adult, and guest rooms.
  —use of nonglare lights.
  —elimination of obstacles such as clutter, doormats, small rugs.
  —control of bathroom hazards through use of grab bars, nonslip strips or tub mat, and raised toilet seat.
  —childproof caps on medications.
  —discard of unused or outdated medications by flushing down the toilet.
  —installation of smoke detectors and fire extinguishers in the home.

DISASTER PLANNING

- Disaster Preparedness
  —Proactive planning is designed to structure the disaster response prior to its occurrence.
  —Effective planning focuses on the problems that have the potential of occurring.
- There are two types of disasters: natural and man-made.
  —Natural disasters are the "result of an ecological disruption or threat that exceeds the adjustment capacity of the affected community"(World Health Organization), for example, earthquakes, floods, hurricanes, and tornadoes.
  —Man-made disasters are emergency situations caused by human beings, for example, biological and biochemical terrorism, chemical spills, and nuclear events.
- Health care facilities may also identify disasters as external or internal.
  —External disasters occur outside the hospital, involve a large number of injured persons who will be sent to the hospital, do not affect health care facilities' infrastructure but do place a strain on their resources.
  —Internal disasters cause disruption of routine services and result in a large number of persons getting injured.
- The two types of disaster planning are "agent-specific approach" and "all-hazards approach."

—Agent-specific approach focuses on preparing for disasters that are most likely to occur in a community due to such factors as geographic locations (e.g., hurricane).

—All-hazard approach is a conceptual model that incorporates components of disaster management that are consistent across all types of disaster events, as many disasters have similarities.

MAJOR CHALLENGES IN DISASTER PLANNING

- Communication is a major priority in any disaster plan. Planning for ways that health care workers and the public can receive accurate information is critical.
- Leadership responsibilities and the distribution of all types of resources need to be determined in advance.
- Advance warning and evacuation procedures need to be included in the planning.
- Use of mass media to disseminate information to the public, particularly regarding health problems such as water safety or food contamination is important.
- Triage and distribution of patients to health care facilities is crucial at the time of a disaster.
- Patient tracking during a disaster is extremely important.

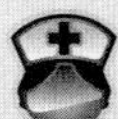

Practice Alert

Disaster planning cannot take place in a vacuum. It requires the involvement of the hospital, community agencies, and local government officials.

NURSING ROLE

- Nurses should actively participate in the development of the disaster plan.
- They should define their roles across the disaster continuum.
- They should initiate disaster prevention measures such as removal of hazards, establish early warning systems, or develop public awareness campaigns.
- Nurse managers should identify educational needs of the nursing staff and other members of the health care community.
- The nursing department needs to maintain a nursing database to be able to rapidly mobilize nurse resources.

EMERGENCY RESPONSE PLAN

- Purpose: An emergency response plan is needed to have an organizational structure and procedures in place to respond to major emergencies.
- Such a plan addresses all types of emergencies in a systematic and coordinated manner.
- It should identify information systems and protocols necessary to handle all types of disasters.
- It must be comprehensive, simple, and flexible to be effective.
- Agency employees must be educated about the plan.
- Disaster drills need to be carried out to test the plan.

SECURITY PLAN

- A security plan ensures the security of the buildings and grounds of the hospital for the safety and welfare of the clients, employees, and visitors.
- Measures that come within the domain of a security plan include traffic control, employee identification, client, visitor, and vendor identification, security policies and procedures, and liaison with local law enforcement.

TRIAGE

Triage is a process used for prioritizing which patients are to be treated first.Categories of triage are disaster triage, daily triage, and special condition triage.

- Disaster triage is when the decisions are based on doing the greatest good for the greatest number. The goal is to treat the needs of the largest number of individuals by delaying care to people who will not survive or will consume too many resources. The disaster triage nurse determines which patients need care, in what order they should receive care, and which patients will not receive care.
- Daily triage is when decisions are based on identifying and treating the sickest individuals first. This model of triage is used routinely in emergency departments.
- Special condition triage involves weapons of mass destruction and requires the wearing of special protective equipment by the health care personnel.

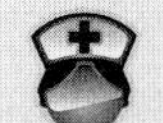

Practice Alert

The first priority in a disaster is human safety.

ERROR PREVENTION

- An error is the failure to complete a planned action or the use of a wrong plan to achieve a goal. Prevention of error focuses on improving the delivery of care and not on placing blame.
- Medical errors are the result of a complex interaction of multiple factors.
- Most medical errors are preventable.
- Frequent types of errors involve the client receiving the wrong medication, incorrect diagnosis leading to an incorrect choice of treatment, equipment failure, infections, blood transfusion-related injuries, and failure to check client identification.

INJURY PREVENTION

Nursing strategies need to be aimed at health promotion. Prevention often involves a lifestyle change for the individual. Falls, burns, poisons, and electrical hazards are common injuries that individuals sustain. The nurse is often the primary person overseeing the environmental factors.

USE OF SAFE EQUIPMENT

- Equipment-related accidents occur when a piece of equipment malfunctions, needs repair(s), is used incorrectly or inappropriately, or when an electrical hazard occurs.
- Regular checks of all equipment are requirements for safety prevention.
- Nurses must be alert for signs of faulty equipment (frayed cords, unusual sounds, etc.) and remove it from use and initiate a follow-up check.

ERGONOMIC PRINCIPLES

- Ergonomics is concerned with designing the job to fit the worker as opposed to forcing the worker to fit the job.
- In ergonomic principles, the focus is on the worker's joints, muscles, nerves, tendons, and bones.
- The goal of application of these principles is to reduce human error, fatigue, discomfort, and stress, and positively impact overall performance.

Following are its essential elements:

- principles of body mechanics
- posture
- lifting techniques
- positioning
- transfer
- assistive devices

PRINCIPLES OF BODY MECHANICS

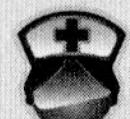

Practice Alert

Use of good body mechanics reduces fatigue and the risk of injury.

- Maximize stability by using a wide base of support and keeping the center of gravity low.
- Prevent abnormal twisting of the spinal column by facing in the direction of the movement.
- Use both the arms and the legs to balance activity.
- Save work by rolling, turning, or pivoting rather than lifting.
- Use large muscles, for example, muscles of thigh, buttock, and shoulders rather than small muscles, for example, muscles of the spine and arms, which are more susceptible to injury.
- Obtain the assistance of other individuals as necessary.

LIFTING TECHNIQUE

- Begin by assessing the weight to be lifted to determine if additional assistance (human or mechanical) is needed.
- Tighten stomach muscles.
- Bend the knees.
- Keep weight to be lifted close to body.
- Maintain trunk erect and knees bent.
- Avoid twisting the body.

POSTURE

- When the body is in correct body alignment, it is considered to be balanced.
- The center of gravity is the point at which the mass is centered.
- When in a standing position, the center of gravity in humans is located at the center of the pelvis. The wider the base of support and the lower the center of gravity an individual maintains, the greater the stability.

POSITIONING

- Maintenance of proper body alignment while in bed or sitting is important for reducing the risk of injury to the musculoskeletal system.
- Correct body alignment also contributes to a client's psychological and physical well-being.
- Devices used to properly position clients include pillows, sandbags, splints, and bed boards.
- Five common positions are
  —Fowler's position in which head of the bed is elevated by 45—60 degrees and knees are slightly elevated without pressure,
  —supine position, which involves resting on the back with legs extended such that feet are in plantar flexion and heels are touching the bed surface,
  —side-lying position in which (lateral position) body rests on side with weight on the dependent hip and shoulder,
  —Sims' position in which weight is placed on the anterior ilium, humerus, and clavicle; upper shoulder and arm are internally rotated; and upper leg and thigh are adducted and internally rotated, and
  —prone position in which the individual lies flat on the abdomen with the head turned to the side; shoulders, head, and neck are in an erect position; and feet are in plantar flexion.

TRANSFER

- Transfer involves assisting a client to move between bed and chair or wheelchair or between bed and stretcher. Principles to consider are center of gravity, base of support, and maintaining balance.

ASSISTIVE DEVICES

Assistive devices include

- aids for transferring, repositioning, and lifting clients. Some commonly used aids are
  —gait belts,
  —friction-reducing sheets, and
  —mechanical chairs and lifts.
- aids for walking: These enhance the client's balance and ability to bear weight. Some commonly used aids are
  —walkers
    - They need to extend from the floor to the client's hip joint.
    - Elbows need to be flexed about 30 degrees.

  —canes
    - They need to extend from the floor to the client's thigh joint.
    - Elbow needs to be flexed about 30 degrees.
    - Tip of cane should be placed 4 inches to the side of the foot.

  —crutches
    - Length of the crutches as well as the placement of the hand bars needs to be measured.
    - Crutches need to be three fingerbreadths below the axilla for length.
    - Elbow needs to be flexed at a 30-degree angle for the correct positioning of the hand bars.
    - Crutch gait is the gait a person assumes when using crutches.
    - The five crutch gaits are four-point gait, three-point gait, two-point gait, swing-to gait, and swing-through gait.

Nursing Process Elements

- Apply the principles of body mechanics correctly at all times to prevent injury
- Allow the client some control over mobility even when using an assistive device because it is not uncommon for older clients to view the use of assistive devices, particularly walking devices, as a weakness and loss of independence
- Teach the client using a cane to hold the cane in the opposite hand from the leg with the defect. This allows weight to be supported on the stronger leg and the cane

- When transferring a client, be sure that the procedure has been explained to both the client and any person assisting with the transfer

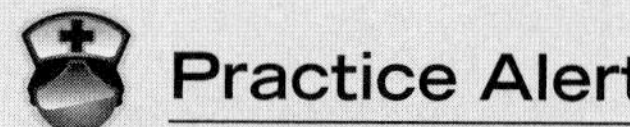

The nurse should serve as a role model in the practice and teaching of sound body mechanics.

HOME SAFETY

Home environmental assessment checks are often carried out by the nurse.

- The key areas inspected are
  - —exterior of the home for hazards such as lighting, broken steps or pavement, nonsturdy handrails, etc.
  - —interior with special attention to kitchen, bath, and stairways for inadequate lighting or glare, clutter, small rugs, or mats that can slip. If there are young children in home, are electrical outlets covered, are there window guards, are there safety locks on cabinets where cleaning supplies, etc., are stored, and are they stored in original containers? Can all doors be opened from inside without a key, are telephone emergency numbers accessible, are there batteries in detectors, are extension cords in good repair and used appropriately, are outlets overloaded, is a flashlight available, is water temperature in normal range, are dials on stove readable, and are combustible materials properly stored (not under stairwells)? Is there lead paint in use and are Radon levels in acceptable range?
- Actual and potential risks related to client safety need to be identified, therefore, the client's developmental stage as well as the client's daily routines must be identified.
- Home safety must be planned with the client, family members, or caregiver.
- Family members or caregivers may need to be taught how to implement a safe environment.

HANDLING HAZARDOUS AND INFECTIOUS MATERIALS

- A hazardous material is a material capable of causing a harmful physical or health effect. Hazardous wastes can be liquids, solids, contained gases, or sludges.
- Resource Conservation and Recovery Act (RCRA) identifies a hazardous waste as one that exhibits at least one of the four characteristics—ignitability, corrosivity, reactivity, or toxicity.
- Federal, state, and local agencies oversee the handling of hazardous materials to protect the public from harm.

HANDLING AND STORAGE

- Hazardous materials need to be stored correctly to prevent spills and uncontrolled reactions, and to minimize employee exposure.
- Three principles form the basis of the plan for safe handling of hazardous materials:
  - —minimize exposure to harmful materials through product substitution and keeping limited quantities on hand.
  - —assume all chemicals are hazardous and handle accordingly.
  - —use proper control measures, such as, written policies and procedures, education, and protective equipment.
- Hazardous materials need to be stored based on their compatibility and not necessarily in the alphabetical order. Substances need to be stored in their original containers.
- To decrease individual exposure to hazardous materials, common engineering controls, such as, local exhaust and general ventilation can be used. Other protective items that could be employed are safety glasses, gloves, and/or hearing protection.
- Development of a plan for safe handling of the hazardous or infectious material needs to include five elements.
  - —Element one requires maintenance of a current hazardous-waste inventory listing, which should include the full chemical name, storage location, quantities, and information regarding the hazard.
  - —Element two speaks of the labeling of all containers.
  - —Element three addresses maintaining a Material Safety Data Sheet(s).

- —Element four plans for employee education and training.
- —Element five provides for regular review and updating of the plan.

MATERIALS

Biological Agents

- Agents of concern are highly pathogenic bacteria and viruses.
- The Center for Disease Control (CDC) has classified specific agents as category A, B, or C.
  - —Category A agents are the most dangerous (anthrax, botulism, plague, smallpox, tularemia, viral hemorrhagic fever viruses, etc.). These agents are given the highest priority in disaster planning as they pose the most potential threat to the public.
  - —Category B agents are the second most dangerous agents (brucellosis, salmonella, melioidosis, psittacosis, Q fever, typhus fever, viral encephalitis, etc.).
  - —Category C represents "emerging" agents (Nipah fever, Hantavirus, etc.).
- Client history and physical condition are key tools in assessing the client's exposure to a biological agent, when making a diagnosis.
- Principles of infection control, beginning with universal precautions, are essential to managing the client.

Radiation

- Radiation is "energy emitted by atoms that are unstable."
- Radioactive contamination is the "presence of radiation-emitting substances in a place where it is not desired."
- Radiological incident is when people or the environment is exposed to radiation or radioactivity through accident or misuse. The exposure may lead to death but more commonly, exposure only requires decontamination and monitoring of the client.
- Nurses need to limit the time spent with radioactive clients, to remain at a distance whenever possible, and to wear protective devices.

OCCUPATIONAL SAFETY AND HEALTH ADMINISTRATION (OSHA)

- OSHA aims to ensure worker safety and health in the United States by working with employers and employees to create better working environments thereby preventing work-related injuries, illnesses, and deaths.
- Since its inception in 1970, OSHA has helped to cut workplace fatalities by more than 60% and occupational injury and illness rates by 40%.
- Guidelines have been developed that require the agency to identify, evaluate, and control safety and health hazards, and provide for emergency response for hazardous-waste operations.
- The agency is also responsible to see that employers develop and implement a written safety and health program for their employees involved in hazardous-waste operations.

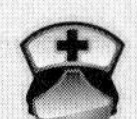

Practice Alert

Nurses need to be familiar with established procedures and protocols of the agency for handling hazardous and infectious materials.

MEDICAL AND SURGICAL ASEPSIS

- Asepsis is the absence of disease-causing microorganisms.
- There are two types of asepsis: medical asepsis and surgical asepsis.

MEDICAL ASEPSIS

Medical asepsis requires infection control practices that reduce and prevent the spread of microorganisms. Objects are considered "clean," which means the absence of almost all microorganisms.

- Hand washing in medical asepsis
  - —It is done to remove soil and transient organisms from hands in order to reduce microorganism count.
  - —It requires use of a vigorous, rubbing motion of about 10 seconds on all areas of the hands with a soap followed by rinsing under running water.
  - —Hands are pointed downward when washing to prevent contamination of arms with dirty water from the hands.

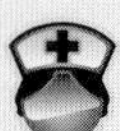

Practice Alert

Hand washing is the single most basic technique in preventing the spread of microorganisms. Contaminated hands are a prime cause of cross infection

- Isolation precautions: standard precautions
  - —Standard precautions are considered tier one precautions by the Center for Disease Control and Prevention (CDCP).
  - —These precautions apply to blood, fluids, secretions, excretions (except sweat), nonintact skin, and mucous membranes of all clients.
  - —Hand washing, wearing of gloves, care of equipment and linens, and disposal of sharp instruments and needles are precautions considered under this heading.
  - —A private room is not necessary.

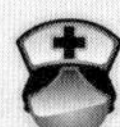

Practice Alert

Standard precautions are required to be used for all hospitalized individuals.

- Isolation precautions: transmission-based precautions
  - —Transmission-based precautions are used in addition to standard precautions.
  - —The three categories of these precautions are "airborne", "droplet", and "contact" precautions.
  - —A private room is required for airborne precautions and a private room or cohort group for droplet or contact precautions.
  - —Depending on the disease and type of precautions, a mask, gown, and gloves may also be needed.
    - ▪ Negative-pressure airflow of at least six exchanges per hour plus a mask or respiratory protection device is needed for airborne precautions (pulmonary TB, SARS, measles, etc.).
    - ▪ Mask is needed for droplet precautions (pneumonia, streptococcal pharyngitis, rubella, etc.).
    - ▪ Gloves and gowns are needed for contact precautions (colonization or infection with multidrug-resistant organisms, enteric pathogens, and major wound infections).

SURGICAL ASEPSIS

- Surgical asepsis is the elimination of all microorganisms, including pathogens and spores, from an area to render the area sterile.
- Sterile technique is implemented to maintain the sterility of the area.
- It is used in the operating room, for special procedures, and also for many procedures carried out at the bedside.
- A nurse must consider seven principles when maintaining sterile technique:
  - —Sterile objects remain sterile only as long as only sterile items touch them.
  - —All objects used in a sterile field must be sterile.
  - —Sterile objects or a sterile field is considered contaminated if they are out of the nurse's vision or below the nurse's waist.
  - —Exposure to prolonged airborne microorganisms will contaminate a sterile object or field.
  - —Fluid flows in the direction of gravity.
  - —Sterile surfaces coming in contact with moisture are considered contaminated due to capillary action.
  - —Edges of the sterile field are considered to be contaminated.

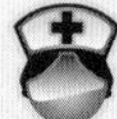

Practice Alert

Assemble all equipment that will be needed prior to beginning the procedure. If an object becomes contaminated during the procedure, discard it immediately.

REPORTING OF INCIDENT/EVENT/IRREGULAR OCCURRENCE/VARIANCE

INCIDENT REPORT

An incident (irregular occurrence, event, or variance) report is

- an organization's tool used in risk management for reporting and recording accidents and unusual occurrences that could potentially affect a client, a family member, or an employee.

- a comprehensive presentation of the occurrence that should be thorough, accurate, and done in a timely manner.
- used to provide information about the incident for statistical data and for future prevention.
- made out by the person who identifies the accident or unusual occurrence; this may not be the person who was actually involved in the incident. Names of any witnesses to the incident are included in the report.

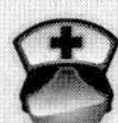

Practice Alert

The incident report must be completed as soon as possible in order to assure the most accurate information.

Risk Management

- Risk management is a system of identifying potential hazards and eliminating them before harm occurs.
- It is a planned program of loss prevention and liability control whose purpose is to identify sources of risks, analyze, classify, and prioritize risks, develop a plan to manage and reduce frequency of risks, and evaluate and develop risk-reduction programs.
- For it to be successful, all departments within the organization must be involved in the risk-management program and commitment from top management as well as the board of directors is needed.
- High risk areas are
  —medication errors,
  —falls,
  —complications following diagnostic procedures,
  —faulty electronic monitoring devices,
  —dissatisfaction with care, and
  —refusal of treatment or refusal to sign for consent of treatment.

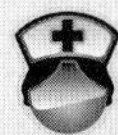

Practice Alert

Since nurses are involved with clients 24 hours a day, the nursing department is critical to the success of a risk-management program.

Sentinel Events

The Joint Commission on Accreditation of Healthcare Organization (The Joint Commission) includes a review of organizational activities in relation to a sentinel event, in order to improve quality of health care. A sentinel event is defined by The Joint Commission as an unexpected occurrence involving death or serious physical or psychological injury or any process variation for which a recurrence would carry a significant change of a serious adverse outcome.
The health care agency must

- develop mechanisms for identifying, reporting, and managing these events.
- conduct a timely analysis of the cause of the event, implement steps to reduce the risk, and monitor the effectiveness of the improvements.

USE OF RESTRAINTS/SAFETY DEVICES

- Regulatory guidelines for use:
  —Reason for use must be clearly stated
  —Use must be part of the client's medical treatment
  —All less restrictive interventions must be tried first
  —Other disciplines must be consulted
  —There must be supporting documentation
- Physician's order is required for the use of restraints.
  —The order must be based on an in-person assessment of the client. In case of an emergency, the assessment must be done within 1 hour.
  —The order must state the type of restraint, location, client behaviors for which restraint is to be used, and a specified time frame. It is never ordered PRN. Least restrictive type must be used.
- Risks associated with restraints are
  —they compress and interfere with function of devices or tubes,
  —they damage skin and underlying tissues from friction and pressure,
  —suffocation or choking may occur with improperly applied jacket restraint,
  —impaired ventilation may occur with too tight belt restraint, and
  —neurovascular compromise may occur with extremity restraint.

Nursing Process Elements

- Do a baseline assessment of the condition of area where restraint is to be placed, follow with ongoing and PRN assessment

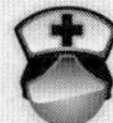

Practice Alert

Assess proper placement of restraint, skin condition, temperature, color, and sensation of restrained area at least once every hour. When an extremity restraint is used, if extremity distal to restraint is cold, pale, cyanotic, numb, tingling, or painful, remove restraint stat, notify physician, and stay with the client to protect extremity from further injury.

- Pad skin and bony prominences.
- Use quick release tie.

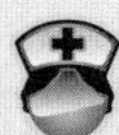

Practice Alert

Attach restraints to bed frame, which moves when height of head or foot of bed is changed, and never to side rails.

- Periodically release restraints to check condition of restrained parts.
- Determine if restraint is still needed at least q 24 hours.
- Document behavior requiring restraint, type of restraint, time applied, procedure used in applying, condition of body part restrained, response to the restraint, time of releases and assessments with findings, and family understanding of restraint.

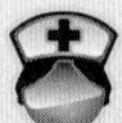

Practice Alert

Application of restraint may be delegated but RN is responsible for assessment of need, selection of alternative interventions, evaluation of effectiveness, and assessment for complications.

Alternatives to Restraints

- Repeated orientation to surroundings, activities, and treatments.
- Use of orientation cues such as family pictures, clocks, and calendars.
- Provision of appropriate amounts of sensory stimulation.
- Use of relaxation techniques.
- Assessment of the effectiveness of medications and initiate change PRN.
- Elimination of uncomfortable treatments.
- Scheduled toileting, exercise, and ambulation.

Think Smart–Test Smart

This chapter contained a lot of information about safety issues and the prevention of different types of injuries. Remember that regardless of the type of threat to safety, the nurse's first priority and therefore first intervention is to remove the client from immediate danger.

WORKSHEET

TRUE & FALSE QUESTIONS

Mark each of the following statements True or False. Correct all false statements in the space provided.

1. A tool used in risk management to report an accident or unusual happening is called an incident report. ___ T ___ F
2. Risk management is a system of identifying potential hazards and eliminating them before harm occurs. ___ T ___ F

3. Only the nursing department is involved in risk-management programs. ____ T ____ F

4. The abbreviation The Joint Commission stands for the "Joint Commission on Accreditation of Healthcare Organizations. ____ T ____ F

5. A sentinel event is defined as an unexpected occurrence involving death or serious physical or psychological injury or risk of injury. ____ T ____ F

6. The purpose of hand washing is to remove all microorganisms from the hands. ____ T ____ F

7. Standard precautions are classified as tier one precautions and require the person to be in a private room. ____ T ____ F

8. A client diagnosed with active tuberculosis would be placed on airborne precautions in conjunction with standard precautions. ____ T ____ F

9. Contaminated hands are a prime cause of cross infection. ____ T ____ F

10. The procedure used to eliminate all microorganisms, including pathogens and spores, is called surgical asepsis. ____ T ____ F

11. One principle of surgical asepsis states that "edges of a sterile field or container are considered to be contaminated." ____ T ____ F

12. A sterile field is an area free from microorganisms that is able to receive sterile and nonsterile items. ____ T ____ F

13. Most medical errors are considered to be preventable. ____ T ____ F

14. The nurse uses critical thinking in the assessment of actual and potential environmental risks to client safety. ____ T ____ F

15. When assessing actual and potential environmental risks it is helpful for the nurse to get a sense of the client's daily routines at home. ____ T ____ F

16. According to the National Fire Prevention Association, home fires are a major cause of death and injury. ____ T ____ F

17. The risk of motor vehicle accidents is highest among teen drivers than any other age group.

18. The Joint Commission for Accreditation of Healthcare Organization sets standards to address the nurse's responsibility for maintaining client safety. ____ T ____ F

19. One of the first questions the nurse would ask when doing a "fall assessment" on a client would be "Does the client have a history of falling?" ____ T ____ F

20. There are two types of disasters: man-made and natural.

21. An earthquake is classified as a man-made disaster. ____ T ____ F

22. "Agent-specific" approach to disaster planning focuses on preparing for disasters that are most likely to occur in a community.

23. Communication is a major priority in disaster planning. ____ T ____ F

(continued)

24. The purpose of an Emergency Response Plan is to have an organizational structure and procedures in place to respond to major emergencies. ___ T ___ F

25. Triage is the process for prioritizing which patients are to be treated first. ___ T ___ F

26. Disaster triage is when decisions are based on identifying and treating the sickest individuals first.

27. The first priority in a disaster is human safety. ___ T ___ F

28. A hazardous material is a material capable of causing a harmful physical or health effect. ___ T ___ F

29. Hazardous materials are removed from their original containers and placed in agency-specific containers for storage. ___ T ___ F

30. The Center for Disease Control (CDC) has classified hazardous agents as Category A, B, or C. Category A is the most dangerous agent. ___ T ___ F

31. The standard of "reasonable care" is used when emergency care is given in a health care setting. ___ T ___ F

APPLICATION QUESTIONS

1. Which of the following events would be considered a "natural disaster?" (Select all that apply.)
   a. Flood
   b. Meteorological phenomena
   c. Fire
   d. Nuclear event

2. When does a communicable, infectious disease outbreak management become disaster management?
   a. Once public health officials determine that the outbreak exceeds the capability and resources available to handle it
   b. At the beginning of the outbreak as communicable diseases are a serious threat to the population
   c. The disaster plan would need to be implemented only if the outbreak was a Category A biological agent
   d. When it is determined that the outbreak is an internal disaster

3. In handling a chemical, you accidentally spilled a small amount of the contents on your hand. What would be the best course of action for you to take?
   a. Immediately wash the affected hand and remove any clothing that the chemical might have come in contact with
   b. Call the Poison Control Center to determine what medication needs to be applied to the area to counteract the chemical
   c. Wrap your hand in a towel to protect it from exposure to the air
   d. Do nothing

4. While making rounds, the nurse finds that a client's IV of Ringer Lactate was running at 75 ml/hr. The kardex stated that the IV ordered was D5W. The nurse's notes in the chart stated that the IV had been changed 2 hours ago and the drip rate had been set. The first thing the nurse would do is
   a. change the IV solution
   b. inform the person who hung the incorrect IV about the occurrence
   c. make out an incident report
   d. report the incident to the nurse in charge

5. A planned program of loss prevention and liability control is called
   a. risk management
   b. critical pathways
   c. peer review
   d. quality assurance

6. A client is admitted to the nursing unit with a diagnosis of mycoplasma pneumonia. The admitting physician did not order the client to be placed on any form of precautions. Which isolation precautions would be best for the client to be on?

a. Transmission-based precautions
b. Universal precautions
c. Sterile precautions
d. Standard precautions

7. Mr. Smith is one of the 10 clients on your team. You are making out the team assignment and must decide whom to assign Mr. Smith. The CNA is new to the unit and you have not worked with her that much; RN1 has been caring for two postoperative patients; RN2 will be attending a continuing education program for about 1 hour during the shift. Select the most appropriate staff member to take care of Mr. Smith.
a. RN2
b. CNA
c. RN1
d. Request a float nurse

8. Which of the following activities would be an example of implementing medical asepsis? (Select all that apply.)
a. Mopping the floor
b. Hand washing
c. Covering hair with a cap
d. Wearing sterile gloves

9. Disinfection and sterilization processes are two methods of eliminating microorganisms. Place a "D" in front of the methods that are examples of disinfection and an "S' in front of methods that are examples of sterilization.
a. ___alcohol
b. ___moist heat
c. ___ethylene oxide gas
d. ___boiling water

10. A nurse would use surgical asepsis at the client's bedside in the following situations. (Select all that apply.)
a. Inserting an IV
b. Applying a sterile dressing
c. Inserting a urinary catheter
d. Suctioning the oropharynx and trachea

11. A nurse fills out an incident report in situations when someone could have been or did get hurt. The incident report needs to maintain the same qualities as all other types of documentation. Important guidelines the nurse needs to follow are (select all that apply):
a. Document an objective description of the incident
b. Document accurate information about the incident
c. Document the incident in a timely manner
d. Document the information in an organized manner

12. A "sentinel event" is defined as
a. an unexpected occurrence involving death or serious physical or psychological injury or risk of injury
b. an emergency treatment that is provided to a client without his/her consent
c. a situation where a client's behavior requires the use of restraints
d. a system of identifying potential hazards and eliminating them before harm occurs

13. A safe environment is an environment that includes which of the following factors? (Select all that apply.)
a. Basic needs are met
b. Physical hazards are reduced
c. Sanitation is maintained
d. Nursing standards of care are implemented

14. Falls are one of the leading environmental hazards reported in hospitals. One of the most common occurrences that precipitates a client fall is
a. getting out of bed to go to the bathroom
b. leaving the side rails down
c. experiencing stress, anxiety, and fatigue
d. slipping on a wet floor

15. If a client falls, the nurse's first responsibility is to
a. assess the client's injury
b. notify the physician
c. write up an incident report
d. report the incident to the nurse manager

16. When caring for a restrained client, the nurse at least would plan to assess the placement of the restraint and the condition of the restrained area at which interval?
a. ½ hour
b. 1 hour
c. 2 hours
d. 8 hours

17. When applying a restraint, which information must the nurse document? (Select all that apply.)
a. Type of restraint
b. Time applied
c. Condition of area to which restraint is applied
d. Family understanding of the restraint
e. Client response to the restraint

18. When assessing a client with upper extremity restraints, the nurse notes the right hand is pale and cold and the client is complaining that it pains. Which is the appropriate initial action for the nurse to take?
a. Loosen the restraint

(continued)

b. Remove the restraint

c. Notify the MD

d. Document findings

19. Which direction represents a task that an RN may legally delegate to an unlicensed assistant?
 a. "Decide if a less restrictive restraint will be effective for Ms. __."
 b. "Apply mitten restraints to Ms. __."
 c. "See if Ms. __ needs a restraint."
 d. "Check if Ms. __'s wrist restraint is affecting circulation to her hand."

20. Which interventions can the nurse use to help eliminate the need for restraints? (Select all that apply.)
 a. Orient at regular intervals to surroundings
 b. Have a clock in plain view
 c. Provide adequate sensory stimulation
 d. Void on a regular schedule
 e. Ambulate on a regular schedule

21. How often would the nurse manager expect assessment data related to the need for a restraint to be recorded in the client's record?
 a. Every shift
 b. Every 24 hours
 c. Every 48 hours
 d. Every 72 hours

22. One reason a nursing history is taken is to determine a client's level of wellness. Which of the following aspects might the nurse include in the history to determine if there are any underlying conditions that might threaten a client's safety? (Select all that apply.)
 a. Gait
 b. Development status
 c. Medications
 d. Vision

23. When caring for a client with an abscessed buttock infected with MRSA, which protective equipment would be used when removing the packing from the wound? (Select all that apply.)
 a. Respiratory protective device
 b. Mask
 c. Gloves
 d. Gown

24. Which new admission should the nurse plan to place in a private room with negative-pressure airflow?
 a. Client with rubella
 b. Client with strep throat
 c. Client with measles
 d. Client with TB of the bone

25. When caring for a client on droplet precautions, which protective equipment would the nurse use? (Select all that apply.)
 a. Respiratory protective device
 b. Mask
 c. Gloves
 d. Gown

ANSWERS & RATIONALES

TRUE & FALSE ANSWERS

Mark each of the following statements True or False. Correct all False statements in the space provided.

1. A tool used in risk management to report an accident or unusual happening is called an incident report. *True*
2. Risk management is a system of identifying potential hazards and eliminating them before harm occurs. *True*
3. Only the nursing department is involved in risk-management programs. *False*

 Risk management involves all departments within the agency including top management and the board of directors.

4. The abbreviation The Joint Commission stands for the "Joint Commission on Accreditation of Healthcare Organizations. *True*

5. A sentinel event is defined as an unexpected occurrence involving death or serious physical or psychological injury or risk of injury. *True*

6. The purpose of hand washing is to remove all microorganisms from the hands. *False*

   Hand washing reduces and controls the number of microorganisms.

7. Standard precautions are classified as tier one precautions and require the person to be in a private room. *False*

   Standard precautions do not require a person to be in a private room.

8. A client diagnosed with active tuberculosis would be placed on airborne precautions in conjunction with standard precautions. *True*

9. Contaminated hands are a prime cause of cross infection. *True*

10. The procedure used to eliminate all microorganisms, including pathogens and spores, is called surgical asepsis. *True*

11. One principle of surgical asepsis states that "edges of a sterile field or container are considered to be contaminated." *True*

12. A sterile field is an area free from microorganisms that is able to receive sterile and nonsterile items. *False*

    A sterile field will receive only sterile items; nonsterile items placed on a sterile field will contaminate the field.

13. Most medical errors are considered to be preventable. *True*

14. The nurse uses critical thinking in the assessment of actual and potential environmental risks to client safety. *True*

15. When assessing actual and potential environmental risks it is helpful for the nurse to get a sense of the client's daily routines at home. *True*

16. According to the National Fire Prevention Association, home fires are a major cause of death and injury. *True*

17. The risk of motor vehicle accidents is highest among teen drivers than any other age group. *True*

18. The Joint Commission for Accreditation of Healthcare Organization sets standards to address the nurse's responsibility for maintaining client safety. *False*

    The American Nurses Association (ANA) standards of nursing practice set the standards for nursing practice.

19. One of the first questions the nurse would ask when doing a "fall assessment" on a client would be "Does the client have a history of falling?" *True*

20. There are two types of disasters: man-made and natural. *True*

21. An earthquake is classified as a man-made disaster. *False*

    An earthquake is a natural disaster.

(continued)

22. "Agent-specific" approach to disaster planning focuses on preparing for disasters that are most likely to occur in a community. *True*

23. Communication is a major priority in disaster planning. *True*

24. The purpose of an Emergency Response Plan is to have an organizational structure and procedures in place to respond to major emergencies. *True*

25. Triage is the process for prioritizing which patients are to be treated first. *True*

26. Disaster triage is when decisions are based on identifying and treating the sickest individuals first. *False*

    Disaster triage is when decisions are based on doing the greatest good for the greatest number.

27. The first priority in a disaster is human safety. *True*

28. A hazardous material is a material capable of causing a harmful physical or health effect. *True*

29. Hazardous materials are removed from their original containers and placed in agency-specific containers for storage. *False*

    Hazardous substances need to be stored in their original containers.

30. The Center for Disease Control (CDC) has classified hazardous agents as Category A, B, or C. Category A is the most dangerous agent. *True*

31. The standard of "reasonable care" is used when emergency care is given in a health care setting. *False*

    "Reasonable care" standard is used in emergency situations that occur outside a health care institution.

APPLICATION ANSWERS

1. Which of the following events would be considered a "natural disaster?" (Select all that apply.)
   a. Flood
   b. Meteorological phenomena
   c. Fire
   d. Nuclear event

Rationale

Correct answers: a and b.

a. A flood is a natural disaster as it is the result of an ecological disruption.
b. A meteorological phenomena is also a natural disaster.

Incorrect answers: c and d.

c. A fire is an emergency situation caused by human beings.
d. A nuclear event is a man-made disaster.

2. When does a communicable, infectious disease outbreak management become disaster management?
   a. Once public health officials determine that the outbreak exceeds the capability and resources available to handle it
   b. At the beginning of the outbreak as communicable diseases are a serious threat to the population
   c. The disaster plan would need to be implemented only if the outbreak was a Category A biological agent
   d. When it is determined that the outbreak is an internal disaster

Rationale

Correct answer: a.

a. Disaster management would be put into place after public health officials recognize a communicable disease outbreak is occurring, determine the source, mode of transmission, and risk factors, and implement control measures and the outbreak exceeds their capacity and resources.

Incorrect answers: b, c, and d.

b. Public health officials would investigate and assess the situation first.

c. Any communicable disease outbreak could warrant the implementation of a disaster management plan.

d. Internal disease is a way that health care facilities often classify a disaster.

3. In handling a chemical, you accidentally spilled a small amount of the contents on your hand. What would be the best course of action for you to take?
   a. Immediately wash the affected hand and remove any clothing that the chemical might have come in contact with
   b. Call the Poison Control Center to determine what medication needs to be applied to the area to counteract the chemical
   c. Wrap your hand in a towel to protect it from exposure to the air
   d. Do nothing

Rationale

Correct answer: a.

a. Physical removal of the chemical is the highest priority because there is a direct relationship between contact time and effect for most chemical agents.

Incorrect answers: b, c, and d.

b. This might be done but is not necessarily the first course of action.

c. The most effective method is to dilute the chemical or reduce the amount of chemical on the skin.

d. Physical removal of the chemical is the highest priority, doing nothing is not the best course of action.

4. While making rounds, the nurse finds that a client's IV of Ringer Lactate was running at 75 ml/hr. The kardex stated that the IV ordered was D5W. The nurse's notes in the chart stated that the IV had been changed 2 hours ago and the drip rate had been set. The first thing the nurse would do is
   a. change the IV solution
   b. inform the person who hung the incorrect IV about the occurrence
   c. make out an incident report
   d. report the incident to the nurse in charge

Rationale

Correct answer: a.

a. The nurse's first action would be to change the IV solution to the solution that had been ordered.

Incorrect answers: b, c, and d.

b. Correcting the situation needs the nurse to be focused on improving delivery of care and not on placing the blame.

c. Making out an incident report would be one of the things the nurse would do later to record the incident.

d. The nurse would report the incident to the nurse in charge but it would not be the first thing that would done.

5. A planned program of loss prevention and liability control is called
   a. risk management
   b. critical pathways
   c. peer review
   d. quality assurance

Rationale

Correct answer: a.

a. Risk management is a planned program with the purpose of identifying risks, analyzing and prioritizing risks, and developing a plan to manage risks.

Incorrect answers: b, c, and d.

b. Critical pathways are guidelines that provide direction for optimum client care.

c. Peer review involves the evaluation of a person of equal status by a peer.

d. Quality assurance is an evaluation process with the purpose of assuring excellence in the health care provided to clients.

6. A client is admitted to the nursing unit with a diagnosis of mycoplasma pneumonia. The admitting physician did not order the client to be placed on any form of precautions. Which isolation precautions would be best for the client to be on?
   a. Transmission-based precautions
   b. Universal precautions
   c. Sterile precautions
   d. Standard precautions

Rationale

Correct answer: a.

a. Transmission-based precautions are used in addition to standard precautions when the person may have an "airborne", "droplet", or "contact" infection.

(continued)

Incorrect answers: b, c, and d.

b. Universal precautions interfere with the spread of bloodborne pathogens and are used in conjunction with other types of precautions.

c. Sterile asepsis eliminates all microorganisms from an area rendering it sterile.

d. Standard precautions are used in the care of all hospitalized clients regardless of the diagnosis.

7. Mr. Smith is one of the 10 clients on your team. You are making out the team assignment and must decide whom to assign Mr. Smith. The CNA is new to the unit and you have not worked with her that much; RN1 has been caring for two postoperative clients; RN2 will be attending a continuing education program for about 1 hour during the shift. Select the most appropriate staff member to take care of Mr. Smith:

a. RN2

b. CNA

c. RN1

d. Request a float nurse

Rationale

Correct answer: a.

a. Even though RN2 will be off the nursing unit for 1 hour, the individual would be the most appropriate staff member to care for Mr. Smith.

Incorrect answers: b, c, and d.

b. The CNA is new to the unit and you do not know the individual's ability to care for clients with infections and on precautions.

c. Assigning two postoperative clients and a client with an infection could spread the infection.

d. There is no need to request a float nurse as there are appropriate caregivers on the nursing unit to care for Mr. Smith and the other clients.

8. Which of the following activities would be an example of implementing medical asepsis? (Select all that apply.)

a. Mopping the floor

b. Hand washing

c. Covering hair with a cap

d. Wearing sterile gloves

Rationale

Correct answers: a and b.

a. Cleaning the environment to prevent the spread of microorganisms is a form of medical asepsis.

b. A basic technique in preventing and reducing the spread of infections is hand washing.

Incorrect answers: c and d.

c. and d are examples of surgical asepsis; they are activities a nurse would do to protect and maintain the sterile field.

9. Disinfection and sterilization processes are two methods of eliminating microorganisms. Place a "D" in front of the methods that are examples of disinfection and an "S' in front of methods that are examples of sterilization.

a. __D__alcohol

b. __S__moist heat

c. __S__ethylene oxide gas

d. __D__boiling water

Rationale

Correct answers: Disinfection—a and d.

a. Alcohol eliminates many microorganisms but not all; it is a chemical disinfectant.

d. Boiling water is not a method of sterilization as bacterial spores and some viruses resist boiling.

Correct answers: Sterilization—b and c.

b. Moist heat is steam under pressure (autoclave) and reaches temperatures above boiling point to kill pathogens and spores.

c. Ethylene oxide gas destroys spores and microorganisms by altering cell's metabolic processes.

10. A nurse would use surgical asepsis at the client's bedside in the following situations. (Select all that apply.)

a. Inserting an IV

b. Applying a sterile dressing

c. Inserting a urinary catheter

d. Suctioning the oropharynx and trachea

Rationale

Correct answers: a, b, c, and d.

a. c, d. The cavities are considered sterile; sterile technique is required to not introduce microorganisms into the client's body.

b. The application of a sterile dressing requires a sterile field to not introduce microorganisms.

11. A nurse fills out an incident report in situations when someone could have been or did get hurt. The incident report needs to maintain the same qualities as all other types of documentation. Important guidelines the nurse needs to follow are (select all that apply):

a. Document an objective description of the incident

b. Document accurate information about the incident

c. Document the incident in a timely manner

d. Document the information in an organized manner

Rationale

Correct answers: a, b, c, and d.

a. Objective information is from direct observation by the nurse and measurable; vague terms are discouraged as they suggest opinions instead of facts.

b. The use of measurable terms provides a fuller and more accurate picture of what occurred.

c. Recording the incident when it is still fresh in the nurse's mind will increase accuracy and decrease duplication.

d. Information is expected to be presented in a logical order to facilitate better communications.

12. A "sentinel event" is defined as
    a. an unexpected occurrence involving death or serious physical or psychological injury or risk of injury.
    b. an emergency treatment that is provided to a client without his/her consent.
    c. a situation where a client's behavior requires the use of restraints.
    d. a system of identifying potential hazards and eliminating them before harm occurs.

Rationale

Correct answer: a.

a. The Joint Commission on Accreditation of Healthcare Organizations states that such events are called "sentinel" because they need immediate investigation and response.

Incorrect answers: b, c, and d.

b. It is describing an emergency situation, such as performing cardiopulmonary resuscitation, on a client.

c. When a physical or mechanical device is needed to limit the freedom of movement of a client.

d. A system for identifying potential sources of risks is called risk management.

13. A safe environment is an environment that includes which of the following factors? (Select all that apply.)
    a. Basic needs are met
    b. Physical hazards are reduced
    c. Sanitation is maintained
    d. Nursing standards of care are implemented

Rationale

Correct answers: a, b, and c.

a. Physiological needs influence a person's safety, for example, sufficient oxygen.

b. Physical hazards place a person at risk for accidental injury or death, for example, motor vehicle accident.

c. Adequate disposal of human waste through a proper sewage system is vital to maintaining a safe environment.

Incorrect answer: d.

d. Nursing standards of care are legal guidelines defined in the Nurse Practice Acts.

14. Falls are one of the leading environmental hazards reported in hospitals. One of the most common occurrences that precipitates a client fall is
    a. getting out of bed to go to the bathroom
    b. leaving the side rails down
    c. experiencing stress, anxiety, and fatigue
    d. slipping on a wet floor

Rationale

Correct answer: a.

a. It is natural behavior to use the bathroom for elimination purposes.

Incorrect answers: b, c, and d.

b, c, d. Each of the three occurrences may contribute to client falls but are not the most common reason for falls.

15. If a client falls, the nurse's first responsibility is to
    a. assess the client's injury
    b. notify the physician
    c. write up an incident report
    d. report the incident to the nurse manager

Rationale

Correct answer: a.

a. The nurse's first responsibility is to the client.

Incorrect answers: b, c, and d.

b, c, and d. The nurse may perform each of the other activities, however, not as his/her first responsibility.

16. When caring for a restrained client, the nurse at least would plan to assess the placement of the restraint and the condition of the restrained area at which interval?
    a. ½ hour
    b. 1 hour
    c. 2 hours
    d. 8 hours

Rationale

Correct answer: b.

b. Proper placement of restraints as well as skin condition, color, temperature, and sensation of restraint area must be checked at least once every hour.

Incorrect answers: a, c, and d.

a. Half-hour intervals provide closer monitoring but the standard is 1 hour.

(continued)

c, d. These intervals are too long and make the risk of injury too great.

17. When applying a restraint, which information must the nurse document? (Select all that apply.)
    a. Type of restraint
    b. Time applied
    c. Condition of area to which restraint is applied
    d. Family understanding of the restraint
    e. Client response to the restraint

Rationale

Correct answers: a, b, c, d, and e.
All factors listed are required to be documented. Also required is the method used in applying the restraint and the times of assessments and the findings.

18. When assessing a client with upper extremity restraints, the nurse notes the right hand is pale and cold and the client is complaining that it pains. Which is the appropriate initial action for the nurse to take?
    a. Loosen the restraint
    b. Remove the restraint
    c. Notify the MD
    d. Document findings

Rationale

Correct answer: b.
b. The restraint is removed to prevent further tissue damage.

Incorrect answers: a, c, and d.
a. The potential for tissue damage still exists if the restraint is merely loosened.
c and d. These activities are done but neither is the initial response.

19. Which direction represents a task that an RN may legally delegate to an unlicensed assistant?
    a. "Decide if a less restrictive restraint will be effective for Ms. __."
    b. "Apply mitten restraints to Ms. __."
    c. "See if Ms. __ needs a restraint."
    d. "Check if Ms. __'s wrist restraint is affecting circulation to her hand."

Rationale

Correct answer: b.
b. Nurses may delegate application of restraints.

Incorrect answers: a, c, and d.
a, c, d. The nurse cannot delegate selection of type of restraint, determination of need for restraint, or assessment for complications. The nurse also cannot delegate assessment of a restraint's effect.

20. Which interventions can the nurse use to help eliminate the need for restraints? (Select all that apply.)
    a. Orient at regular intervals to surroundings
    b. Have a clock in plain view
    c. Provide adequate sensory stimulation
    d. Void on a regular schedule
    e. Ambulate on a regular schedule

Rationale

Correct answers: a, b, c, d, and e.
a, b, and c. These help keep the client oriented and thereby decrease the need for restraints.
d and e. These help prevent discomfort which can contribute to restlessness and undesirable activity.

21. How often would the nurse manager expect assessment data related to the need for a restraint to be recorded in the client's record?
    a. Every shift
    b. Every 24 hours
    c. Every 48 hours
    d. Every 72 hours

Rationale

Correct answer: b.
b. The need for a restraint must be reassessed and documented every 24 hours.

Incorrect answers: a, c, and d.
a. It is more often than required
c and d. These are not often enough according to regulations.

22. One reason a nursing history is taken is to determine a client's level of wellness. Which of the following aspects might the nurse include in the history to determine if there are any underlying conditions that might threaten a client's safety? (Select all that apply.)
    a. Gait
    b. Development status
    c. Medications
    d. Vision

Rationale

Correct answers: a, b, c, and d.
a. The nurse would observe the client's mobility and body alignment and assess if the client needed assistance with ambulation.
b. The client's development status may create threats to client safety.
c. Is the client on any medications that might lead to confusion, disorientation, or other types of risks?

d. Visual acuity, particularly in the elderly, as decreased vision may lead to client injury.

23. When caring for a client with an abscessed buttock infected with MRSA, which protective equipment would be used when removing the packing from the wound? (Select all that apply.)
   a. Respiratory protective device
   b. Mask
   c. Gloves
   d. Gown

Rationale

Correct answers: c and d.

c and d. A wound infection requires contact precautions and these require use of gown and gloves.

Incorrect answers: a and b.

a and b. Respiratory protective devices are used for airborne precautions. Masks may be used for airborne precautions and always for droplet.

24. Which new admission should the nurse plan to place in a private room with negative-pressure airflow?
   a. Client with rubella
   b. Client with strep throat
   c. Client with measles
   d. Client with TB of the bone

Rationale

Correct answer: c.

c. Negative-pressure airflow is used for airborne precautions. Measles is spread by airborne transmission and therefore negative-pressure airflow protection is required.

Incorrect answers: a, b, and d.

a, b, and d. None of these diseases are spread by airborne transmission therefore negative-pressure airflow is not needed. Rubella and strep throat are spread by droplets.

25. When caring for a client on droplet precautions, which protective equipment would the nurse use? (Select all that apply.)
   a. Respiratory protective device
   b. Mask
   c. Gloves
   d. Gown

Rationale

Correct answer: b.

b. Protection from droplet transmission requires use of a mask.

Incorrect answers: a, c, and d.

a, c, and d. Gloves and gown are required for contact transmission. Mask or respiratory protective device is needed to protect against airborne transmission.

CHAPTER 6

Test Plan Category:

Health Promotion and Maintenance—Part 1

Sub-category: **None**

Topics: **Ant/Intra/Postpartum and Newborn Care**

ANTEPARTUM PERIOD

TERMINOLOGY RELATED TO PREGNANCY

Gravida: The number of pregnancies a woman has had. It includes the present pregnancy (if she is pregnant now). It does not consider the length or the outcome of the pregnancy.

Primigravida: A woman who is pregnant for the first time or has been pregnant only once.

Multigravida: A woman who has had more than one pregnancy or who is pregnant now and has been pregnant before.

Para: The number of pregnancies a woman has had which ended after 20 weeks. No consideration is given to the outcome of the pregnancy, means of termination of the pregnancy, or number of children involved in the pregnancy. A current, undelivered pregnancy after 20 weeks does not add to the number of paras until after the pregnancy has ended. To prevent confusion, the number of paras may not be changed in the chart during the hospitalization for delivery. The number of paras cannot exceed the number of pregnancies.

Stillborn: A baby born dead after the age of viability (20 weeks gestation).

Nulliparas: A woman who may or may not have been pregnant before, but never delivered a term infant.

Multiparas: A woman who has delivered more than one baby after the age of viability (20 weeks gestation).

Abortion: Termination of a pregnancy prior to viability of the fetus. Abortions may be subdivided into elective and spontaneous types.

Elective: The purposeful termination of a pregnancy. Laws often govern when and how an elective abortion can be performed.

Spontaneous: The unplanned termination of a pregnancy. In lay terms, it is called a miscarriage.

TPAL: This acronym provides information about the obstetrical history of a woman. T refers to term births, P is for preterm births, A is for abortions, and L is for living children.

Chadwick's Sign: Bluish discoloration of the cervix due to increased vascularity in these tissues. Its value in determining pregnancy is moderate and thus it is a probable sign of pregnancy.

Goodell's Sign: Softening of the cervix, also due to increased vascularity. It is a probable sign of pregnancy.

Hegar's Sign: A softening of the isthmus or neck of the cervix. It is another probable sign of pregnancy.

Braxton Hicks: Also called false labor contractions, these contractions can be felt by the pregnant woman beginning around the twenty-eighth week. Braxton Hicks contractions are generally described as irregular and painless contractions.

Decidua: The pregnant endometrium of the uterus. The decidua may also be described in relation to the fetus. The decidua basalis lies directly under the fetus and is a component of the placenta. The decidua capsularis covers the developing fetus. The decidua vera is the part of the endometrium not in contact with the fetus.

Leopold's Maneuvers: A system of palpating the maternal abdomen at term that will assist in determining the fetal presentation and position.

PREGNANCY

- Conception occurs with the union of the sperm and ova.
- Both the sperm and the ovum will bring to the union a nucleus with 23 chromosomes, 22 somatic (body) chromosomes and a sex chromosome, either an X or Y from the sperm and an X from the ovum.
- When the sperm fertilizes the ovum, the sex of the baby is determined and the resulting zygote contains 46 chromosomes with the characteristics of both the mother and the father.
- The normal gestation lasts 40 weeks.
- The diagnosis of pregnancy is based on the signs of pregnancy. The signs of pregnancy are categorized as probable, presumptive, and positive based on their significance in the diagnosis.

SIGNS OF PREGNANCY

The three categories of the signs of pregnancy are

- presumptive
- probable
- positive

Presumptive Signs of Pregnancy

Presumptive signs of pregnancy are weak signs that can be caused by other conditions. Because these signs are subjective, they may easily be misinterpreted (see Table 6–1).

Table 6–1 Presumptive Signs of Pregnancy

Sign	Relationship to Pregnancy	Other Possible Interpretations
Amenorrhea	Menses usually ceases after conception but absence can be caused by other conditions including stress.	Women with low body fat such as athletes often have amenorrhea. In addition, stress, menopause, and endocrine disorders can contribute to the absence of menses.
Nausea and vomiting	During early pregnancy, nausea and vomiting is associated with the elevated hormone levels seen in pregnancy.	Emotional distress and viral or bacterial GI infections are a few of the causes of nausea and vomiting.
Urinary frequency	Due to the elevated hormones and pressure of the enlarged uterus and uterine contents on the bladder, urinary frequency is seen in early pregnancy and again in the last trimester.	Urinary tract infections, diabetes, and increased fluid intake can all lead to urinary frequency.
Quickening	Quickening refers to fetal movement and is usually felt by the pregnant woman between 16 and 20 wks of pregnancy. The early movements are often described as "butterfly wings."	Normal peristalsis and abdominal gas from gas-producing foods can be perceived as quickening. Women who want to be pregnant can imagine the feelings of quickening.
Fatigue	This subjective sign is a frequent complaint of the woman in the first trimester.	Stress, illness, and overwork can bring on this symptom.
Weight gain	Weight gain in early pregnancy is usually minimal.	Weight gain is associated with water retention secondary to hormonal changes.
Breast changes	The changes which are noted in the breast are tingling and fullness.	Monthly hormonal changes are often noted in the premenstrual period.

Probable Signs of Pregnancy

Probable signs of pregnancy are objective and can be noted by a trained health care professional. Probable signs are more frequently associated with pregnancy (see Table 6–2).

Positive Signs of Pregnancy

Positive signs of pregnancy cannot be misinterpreted by the client or the examiner. These signs are the definitive symptoms of pregnancy (see Table 6–3).

PREGNANCY TESTS

Human chorionic gonadotropin (HCG) is a hormone produced by the placenta and present in the maternal bloodstream and eventually excreted by the kidneys. This hormone is responsible for the maintenance of the pregnancy in the early period and is the basis for the pregnancy tests commonly used (see Table 6–4). False negatives can occur if the test is performed too early in the menstrual cycle. If urine samples are used for testing, the first morning voided is best as the hormone concentration will be highest.

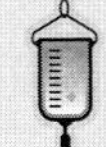

Clinical Alert

False negative results occur fairly frequently. If the results of the home pregnancy test are negative, the test should be repeated in a week if menstruation has not begun.

Table 6–2 Probable Signs of Pregnancy

Sign	Relationship to Pregnancy	Other Possible Interpretations
Abdominal enlargement	A feeling of abdominal fullness and tightening of clothes can be noted soon after the first period is missed.	Weight gain and tumors of the abdomen or uterus can also cause this symptom.
Changes in pelvic organs		
• Goodell's sign	• Due to increased vascularity, the examiner will notice a softening of the cervix.	• Any condition that increases the vascularity of the cervix including hormonal changes can cause this symptom.
• Hegar's sign	• Another symptom related to the increased vascularity of the isthmus (or neck) of the cervix is that the examiner will be able to compress the cervix to a minimum.	• Like Goodell's sign, this symptom may be associated with conditions such as infections.
• Chadwick's sign	• Due to the increased vascularity of the cervix, vagina, and vulva, the mucous membranes will assume a bluish coloration.	• Any condition increasing the blood flow to these tissues can give rise to this symptom.
Ballottement	Because the fetus floats in amniotic fluid, when the cervix is tapped, the fetus will float away from the cervix and then back toward the cervix producing a rebound tap felt by the examiner.	This symptom may also be associated with uterine polyps or tumors.
Braxton Hicks contractions	Most frequently felt by the pregnant woman during the third trimester, these painless, irregular contractions of the uterus are often termed false labor.	Some tumors may cause similar perceptions.
Uterine soufflé	This is the sound of blood flowing through the maternal side of the placenta; the rate will be the same as the maternal pulse.	Uterine tumors with increased uterine blood flow can also cause this symptom.
Pigmentation changes		
• Chloasma	• This refers to a flushing of the face of pregnant women.	• Oral contraceptives can lead to this symptom.
• Darkening of the areola of the nipples	• Darkening is more common in the dark-haired female and the primigravidas.	• Hormonal imbalances can cause this symptom.
• Linea nigra	• Beginning at the pubis, a dark line forms on the skin and progresses up the midline of the abdomen to the top of the fundus.	
Pregnancy tests	Various tests are available which detect the presence of human chorionic gonadotropin (HCG), a hormone produced by the placenta.	Hydatidiform mole and choriocarcinoma also respond to the tests.

Table 6–3 Positive Signs of Pregnancy

Sign	Relationship to Pregnancy	Other Possible Interpretations
Auscultation of fetal heart tones (FHTs)	FHTs can be heard as early as 10 wks with a Doppler ultrasound transducer and by 18–20 wks with a fetoscope. The FHTs must be differentiated from the maternal heart rate. FHTs usually run above 100 while maternal heart rates are slower.	None
Fetal movements felt by a trained examiner	The trained examiner is able to differentiate the fetal movements from abdominal gas.	None
Confirmed presence of a fetus	The presence of the fetus can be determined by ultrasound as early as 4 wks gestation.	None

ESTIMATION OF GESTATION

As soon as pregnancy is determined, the woman's first concern is to determine when the baby is due. The due date is called the Estimated Date of Confinement or EDC. There are several means of determining the EDC including Nagele's rule, fundal height, and the use of a gestational wheel.

Nagele's Rule

- It is the most common tool used to determine EDC.
- After determining the first day of the last menstrual period, the examiner would count back 3 months and add 7 days. For example, if the first day of the last menstrual period was September 1, the examiner would subtract 3 months $(9 - 3 = 6)$ and add 7 days. The sixth month is June, so the due date would be June 8.
- Inaccurate determinations occur when the date of the last menstrual period cannot be recalled. These are frequently associated with delays in seeking medical attention.

Table 6–4 Pregnancy Tests Commonly Used

Test	Tests	Diagnostic Period
Radioimmunoassay	Blood or urine	1 wk after fertilization
Enzyme-Linked Immunosorbent Assay (ELISA)	Blood or urine	10 d after fertilization or 5 d before first missed period
Home pregnancy tests	Urine	Varies

- EDC may be incorrectly defined when the woman missed a cycle before conceiving or had vaginal bleeding after conception. Some women will have a "light period" after conceiving while others have been known to continue to have cycles well into the pregnancy.

Fundal Height Measurement

- In fundal height measurement, the examiner measures the distance from the symphysis pubis to the top of the fundus.
- Measured in centimeters, the fundal height measurement corresponds well with the fetal age in the second and third trimester.
- Women carrying more than one fetus will appear to be further along in their pregnancy with this EDC determination.
- In situations with intrauterine growth retardation in the fetus or oligohydramnios (less than normal amounts of amniotic fluid), the pregnancy may be incorrectly dated as well.

The Gestation Wheel

- It is an easy to use tool to assist the practitioner in determining EDC.
- Since the system utilizes the first day of the last menstrual period, this method has the same difficulties as Nagele's rule.

PHYSIOLOGIC CHANGES IN PREGNANCY

A normal pregnancy lasts for approximately 40 weeks or 10 lunar months. The pregnancy can be divided into three distinct periods or trimesters. The changes in the woman's body can be related primarily to the hormones associated with pregnancy and the growth of the fetus (Table 6–5).

Table 6–5 The Sources and Functions of the Hormones Related to Pregnancy

Hormone	Source	Function
Follicle stimulating hormone (FSH)	Anterior pituitary	Stimulates ovarian activity and the production of the graafian follicle
Luteinizing hormone (LH)	Anterior pituitary	Stimulates the graafian follicle to release the ovum and convert to a corpus luteum
Prolactin	Anterior pituitary	Stimulates lactation after delivery
Oxytocin	Posterior pituitary	Stimulates uterine contractibility in labor Stimulates the "let-down" reflex or release of milk in the postpartum period
Estrogen	Corpus luteum/placenta	Promotes the thickening of the uterus Prepares the breasts for breast-feeding
Progesterone	Corpus luteum/placenta	Maintains the endometrium Suppresses uterine activity Prepares the breasts for breast-feeding Relaxes joints of pelvis allowing a slightly enlarged diameter of the birth canal and contributing to the characteristic waddling gait of the pregnant woman
HCG	Trophoblast/placenta	Maintains the corpus luteum to continue producing estrogen and progesterone preventing menstruation Once the placenta is producing HCG, the placenta will produce the hormones necessary to maintain the pregnancy
Human placental lactogen	Trophoblast	Antagonizes insulin maintaining a higher level of glucose in the maternal circulation to meet the needs of the growing fetus
Relaxin	Corpus luteum	Relaxes the uterus, inhibits uterine contractions
Prostaglandins	Various body tissues	Unknown

The hormones associated with pregnancy are estrogen, progesterone, and HCG. Both estrogen and progesterone are produced initially by the corpus luteum on the ovaries. The placenta will eventually take over control of the production of these hormones. While the trophoblast initially produces HCG, this hormone will also eventually be produced by the placenta.

Changes in the Reproductive Organs

Uterus

- In the nonpregnant state, the uterus is a small pear-shaped organ that weighs about 2 oz.
- At term, the pregnant uterus weighs about 2 lbs. Most of the growth is related to an enlargement of the uterine cells.
- The uterus is primarily a muscular organ and even in its stretched shape at the end of pregnancy, is very strong. The muscle fibers of the uterus are arranged in all directions, unlike the muscle fibers of the muscles of the arms or legs. The concentration of muscle fibers is particularly thick in the fundal area (top of uterus) giving the appearance of a hood and adding to the strength of the fundus.
- The accumulation of blood in the uterus adds to its enlargement. With the accumulation of blood, the uterus becomes a thick carpet in which the embryo can bury itself.
- The placenta development begins around 3 weeks after conception and is formed from fetal and maternal structures. It develops at the site where the embryo is attached to the wall of the uterus. It serves two functions: (1) provides nutrient exchange between the fetus and mother and (2) produces hormones that are essential for the maintenance of the pregnancy.
- Braxton Hicks contractions occur irregularly throughout pregnancy but become more noticeable late in pregnancy. At term, these contractions may be confused with labor contractions but differ from labor contractions in that the cervix does not dilate and the contractions usually cease with walking.

- In the nonpregnant state, the uterus lies completely in the pelvis. With the enlargement of the uterus and growth of the fetus, the uterus rises above the pelvis. The fundal height is related to the gestational age of the fetus as illustrated in the following box:

12 wks	Fundus rises out of the pelvis. It can be felt above the symphysis pubis
20 wks	Fundus reaches the umbilicus
36 wks	Fundus reaches the xiphoid process. Breathing is difficult
38–40 wks	Fundus drops down as the uterus settles back into the pelvis in preparation for labor. This is termed "lightening." The woman can now breathe easier, but has pressure on the bladder causing frequent urination

Cervix

- The cervix also is influenced to enlarge and thicken.
- The glandular tissue of the cervix becomes more active and produces thick mucus, which forms the mucous plug. This plug prevents the ascent of organisms into the uterus. Early in labor, this plug will be lost and will be described as "bloody show."
- With the increased vascularity, the cervix softens and takes on the distinctive blue discoloration. The diagnosis of pregnancy is often made as a result of observing these changes in the cervix. These changes in vascularity are described as Goodell's, Hegar's, and Chadwick's signs, which are used as pregnancy indicators.

Vagina

- Like the uterus and cervix, the vagina hypertrophies and displays increased vascularization.
- The cells of the vagina are active, producing the vaginal discharge (leucorrhea) that is common in pregnancy.
- The secretions of the vagina become more acidic providing protection from bacterial infections.

Ovaries

- In the nonpregnant state, the ovaries generally release one ovum per month. As the time of release approaches, the site on the ovary containing the ripening ovum is called a graafian follicle. Once the follicle ruptures and releases the ovum, the graafian follicle becomes the corpus luteum. If the ovum is not fertilized, the corpus luteum begins to shrink in about one week and eventually becomes a small scar on the ovary.
- If the ovum is fertilized, the cells that surround the fertilized ovum will begin to produce hormones that cause the corpus luteum to enlarge slightly and remain active in the production of hormones to maintain the pregnancy.
- Once the placenta is well established, it will become the main source of the hormones of pregnancy. The corpus luteum will then degenerate and serve no further function in pregnancy.
- Other than the activity of this corpus luteum, the ovaries remain quiet during the pregnancy and do not continue the cyclic maturation of ova.

Breasts

- The breasts increase in size and the glands will hypertrophy during the pregnancy in preparation for nourishing the newborn.
- Increased pigmentation can be noted in the areola and the Montgomery's follicles on the areola become prominent.
- Stretch marks, called striae, are visible on the breasts.
- By the second trimester, colostrum can be expressed from the breasts. This colostrum will be the first feedings for the breast-fed baby and is rich in antibodies.

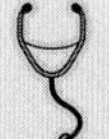

Assessment Alert

Tingling in the nipples and breast fullness are often the first subjective indicators of a pregnancy.

Respiratory System

- Oxygen requirements increase during pregnancy as the woman's body must provide for both the woman and the fetus.
- As the uterus increases in size, the uterus rises out of the pelvis and puts increasing pressure on the diaphragm.
- In response to the higher levels of estrogen and the pressure on the diaphragm, the ribs flare and the circumference of the chest increases.
- While the respiratory rate is only slightly increased during pregnancy, the tidal volume increases significantly.
- The respiratory center in the brain becomes more sensitive to carbon dioxide levels. Although respiratory function has improved slightly from the nonpregnant state, the woman may report feeling slightly short of breath during late pregnancy.

Cardiovascular System

- The pulse rate increases slightly during pregnancy. The blood pressure decreases during the first trimester and then returns to the prepregnant levels in the third trimester.
- The basal metabolic rate of the pregnant woman increases significantly in pregnancy. The workload of the heart

reaches its maximum around the thirty-second week of pregnancy. If the heart does not have the capacity to compensate, cardiac decompensation may occur. The pregnant cardiac client often delivers as she approaches the thirty-second week of pregnancy.

- Vena cava syndrome occurs when the pregnant woman near term lies in the supine position. The weight of the uterus compresses the inferior vena cava restricting blood returning to the heart. The woman will feel dizzy, be pale and clammy, and be hypotensive. This can be prevented by having the woman lie on her side rather than in the supine position. The left side-lying position is favored as it promotes blood return via the inferior vena cava.
- Both the number of blood cells and blood volume increase during pregnancy. The increase in volume exceeds the increase in the number of RBCs, changing the ratio of solids to liquids in the hemoglobin and hematocrit laboratory values. This change in ratio is the cause of the pseudoanemia seen in early pregnancy.
- The white blood cell count increases in number as the body protects itself from foreign invasion. The WBC count peaks during labor and early postpartum and then returns to the prepregnant level.
- Fibrin and clotting factor levels increase in pregnancy as another means of the body's self-protection. This change makes the woman more prone towards the development of venous thrombosis.

Gastrointestinal System

- Women often complain of nausea during early pregnancy. This nausea and its sometimes associated vomiting are termed "morning sickness" although the nausea may be felt anytime during the day. This morning sickness is thought to be caused by the levels of HCG. Morning sickness that leads to weight loss or when it continues into the second trimester is abnormal and should be evaluated.
- Changes in the mouth associated with pregnancy may include ptyalism (excessive salivation) and gingivitis due to an increase in the vascularity of the oral mucus membranes.
- Progesterone slows the motility of the GI tract in the second and third trimesters delaying gastric emptying. This along with the uterine displacement of the stomach and intestines may cause heartburn (pyrosis).
- Progesterone also slows peristalsis and promotes water absorption from the colon leading to constipation.
- Constipation and the weight of the pregnancy can cause hemorrhoids.

Urinary System

- Urinary frequency is a common problem in both the first and third trimester caused by the weight of the uterus. During the second trimester, the uterus rises out of the pelvis and relieves the pressure seen in the first trimester until the time the uterus returns to the pelvis in preparation for labor. This return to the pelvis is termed "lightening."
- Progesterone and its relaxation potential along with the weight of the uterus may lead to dilation of the ureters making the woman susceptible to urinary tract infections.
- The kidneys as a whole function at a higher capacity with higher glomerular filtration rates.

Musculoskeletal System

- Progesterone contributes to the relaxation of the pelvic joints. The pelvis, normally the stabilizing agent of the body, can no longer maintain the support system and the woman develops a waddling gait. This loosening of the joints provides for a slight increase in the diameter of the birth canal.
- The center of gravity of the body shifts due to the increased uterine weight. The body responds to this shift by increasing the curve of the lumbar spine and causing lordosis. These changes lead to a characteristic walk often termed "the pride of pregnancy." This change also leads to backache in the third trimester.

Integumentary System

- Pigment changes are the most noticeable changes occurring in the integumentary system. The pigment changes include chloasma, a facial rash, noticed primarily on the cheeks and forehead. This rash tends to be more prominent in a dark-skinned woman. Linea nigra is a dark line that develops on the midline of the abdomen and lengthens as the uterus grows.
- Striae or stretch marks occur as the connective tissue is damaged due to tissue stretching. During pregnancy, the striae may appear red but turn to silver after the completion of the pregnancy. Striae are most common on the abdomen, buttocks, thighs, and breasts.
- Hair growth is stimulated during pregnancy and the hair may appear more lustrous. After termination of the pregnancy, the hair follicle will assume a period of rest and the woman may notice some shedding of hair. By 6–12 months after the pregnancy, the hair will return to the prepregnancy appearance.

Endocrine System

- Influenced by the higher levels of estrogen during pregnancy and the increased needs of the pregnant body for nutrition, the endocrine glands increase their activities slightly and then return to their normal level of functioning in the immediate postpartum period.

Changes in Metabolism

- In general, the basal metabolic rate of the pregnant body increases over the nonpregnant state. This increase in metabolism is both a support of the growing fetus and a response to the increased metabolic needs of the fetus. Estrogen and progesterone both promote the retention of water allowing for a greater volume of blood. As the fetus grows, the demand for protein and carbohydrates increases. Weight gain during pregnancy is in response to the increase in fluid volume and growth of new tissues including the placenta and fetus. Typical weight gain is about 4 lbs in the first trimester and 15 lbs in the second and third trimester. Total weight gain averages about 30–35 lbs. Allowable weight gain varies according to the prepregnancy weight of the woman, but even the overweight woman is encouraged to gain an average of 25 lbs to ensure the fetus receives what it needs for growth. At the time of delivery, this 30–35 lbs weight gain can be divided up to the following:

—fetus ~8 lbs

—placenta ~2 lbs

—amniotic fluid ~2 lbs

—increase in body water (including blood volume) ~8 lbs

—increase in uterus and breasts ~5 lbs

—body stores ~5 lbs

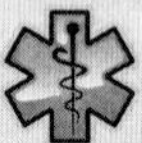

Nursing Intervention Alert

Monitoring weight gain and teaching the woman about the need for adequate nutrition for the fetus is a primary concern for the nurse in the obstetrical office.

Psychological Changes Associated with Pregnancy

Both the expectant mother and expectant father will have developmental tasks associated with the psychological maturation that comes with a pregnancy (see Table 6–6). Although each individual is different in how they handle the changes brought about by a pregnancy and birth of an infant, in general these changes can be divided into the three trimesters of pregnancy.

The Role of Other Family Members in an Expectant Family

Siblings

- Children's understanding and emotions related to the pregnancy vary according to the age and emotional maturity of the child. Young children will not understand the concept of pregnancy and may be surprised by the arrival of the new baby. Adolescents, on the other hand, may be fully aware of the concept of pregnancy and even feel embarrassment that their parents have so publicly shown that sexual relations are occurring.
- The acceptance of the new arrival will be affected by the age of the siblings as well as their present position in the family. Older children, especially in large families, may dread the addition as a new source of responsibilities. The youngest child may feel that their position in the family has been taken by the new baby. An only child may feel the loss of the parents' attention.
- Preparation of the siblings is important and dependent upon the ages of the children. Young children need to be prepared close to the event while older children can be told of the pregnancy earlier. Whenever possible, include the siblings in the planning. A young child may help fold and put away the new baby's clothes while an older child might enjoy listening to the baby's heartbeat. The older child should never be displaced by the new baby. If, for instance, the older child is still sleeping in a crib, the child should not be moved from the crib for the baby. Instead, the older child is moved from the crib well in advance of the birth and given a bed for "big boys" or "big girls."

Grandparents

- Pregnancy usually results in a closer, more supportive relationship between the expectant couple and their parents regardless of past issues.
- Difficulties for grandparents can relate to determining to what extent the expectant couple want them involved, conflicts with their own life and work demands, and ambivalence over aging as they assume this new role.

Culture

- The cultural values and beliefs of the mother and father as well as the extended family will affect every aspect of childbearing and childrearing.
- How the woman feels about her pregnancy will be influenced not only by her life situation but also by the values placed on pregnancy by her culture.
- Culture can influence the acceptance of the child into the family. For instance, in some cultures, boys are more valued and thus the birth of a girl may be seen as a negative life situation.
- Cultural practices may influence the well-being of the pregnant woman and her fetus. The practice of pica, eating of nonfood substances, may lead to nutritional deficiencies.
- Labor and delivery may be influenced by the cultural acceptance of medication.
- Childrearing beliefs such as an emotionally upsetting event "spoiling" the milk of a breast-feeding mother may lead to a sudden weaning of the infant.
- The nurse's role in working with clients of diverse cultural backgrounds and beliefs is to be open and acceptive of differences.

Table 6–6 Maternal and Paternal Tasks During Pregnancy

Trimester	Maternal Developmental Tasks	Paternal Developmental Tasks
First	• Accepting the fact of pregnancy is the primary concept in the first trimester. At this time, the mother is more aware of the fact that she is pregnant than that she is going to have a baby. The expectant woman becomes more aware of others around her who are pregnant. • Ambivalence is a key emotion even in the woman who has had difficulty achieving a pregnancy. Although she may be delighted to be pregnant, doubts may intrude. The woman may think she is not ready or the timing of the pregnancy was not right. • Along with ambivalence, the expectant woman may demonstrate mood swings that can be related at least in part to the hormonal changes occurring in the body. • Body image changes are perceived by the pregnant woman but may not be noticeable to an onlooker. Depending on her acceptance of pregnancy, the woman may look forward to "looking pregnant" or be embarrassed and try to hide or deny the changes.	• The expectant father will have difficulty accepting the fact of pregnancy. From his point of view, nothing has changed. The pregnancy is not obvious to onlookers and he is unable to perceive the influence of hormones that convinces the expectant mother that things are changing. • Some expectant fathers may develop some of the pregnancy symptoms that their partners are displaying including nausea, weight gain, backache, and fatigue. This condition is called couvades and is associated with expectant fathers who are more involved in the pregnancy and who assume a more active paternal role.
Second	• By the second trimester, the pregnant woman should have accepted the fact that she is pregnant. Now she has to accept the reality of the fetus. With fetal movements, the woman recognizes that her body now houses two people. The woman and her family may develop a pet name for the fetus. These names add to the reality that a new person exists. • As the pregnancy grows, the woman may become more introverted, wanting to spend time alone with her fetus. Now the pregnant woman notices new babies everywhere she goes as her focus turns from pregnancy to baby. • The pregnant woman is noticeably pregnant to the onlookers. The woman may now be acceptive of her pregnancy and delighted that others have noticed.	• Dependent on his outlook for the pregnancy, the father may be excited and looking forward to caring for his offspring or see the pregnancy as a negative event in his life. • Some men view the pregnancy of their spouses as a validation of their masculinity.
Third	• The pregnant woman has now accepted the fact of pregnancy and that the pregnancy will produce a new baby. The woman must now prepare herself for delivery and her role as a mother. • Nesting occurs, where the pregnant woman prepares the nursery and gathers baby supplies. • The woman may worry about how she will handle labor and delivery. She is eager to discuss these events with others and to learn what she needs to know to be successful. • As the physical discomforts of pregnancy increase, the woman begins to look forward to and wish for the end of the pregnancy. Women who deliver early may never reach this plateau and actually grieve for the loss of the pregnancy after delivery, even with a healthy child. • Body image again makes a change. The woman may feel that her body is huge and may feel a loss of sexual appeal. Physical discomforts of the third trimester may contribute to a negative body image.	• As the time of delivery approaches, the man may be concerned about how he will respond to labor and delivery. Some men choose not to be involved while other men want to be with their expectant spouses for every event. Although excited about the approaching labor and delivery, the man may worry about how he will handle himself. • The expectant father may also worry about the financial role that will be required of him. The medical costs as well as the costs of raising a child may be a source of worry to some men.
Postpartum	• The psychological changes occur during the postpartal period as well and can be described as "taking in, taking hold, and letting go." These changes will be discussed at a later point.	

- Nursing care that is planned to include this acceptance of cultural diversity will be more acceptable to the client and more successful in promoting the health and well-being of the childbearing and childrearing family.

ANTEPARTUM CARE

During the first prenatal visit, the pregnant woman's chief concerns will be the determination of her pregnancy and her due date. The nurse, on the other hand, has a multitude of data to collect and information to provide. During the first prenatal visit, nursing activities will include

- client history determination. Information gained in this interview will include, but not be limited to
  —personal data that may have an influence on the pregnancy. This will include age, marital status, ethnicity, and support system. The occupation of the woman will be a consideration for the safety of the woman and her fetus. Even the presence of a pet cat will be questioned as it may have a negative influence on the outcome of the pregnancy.
  —the attitude toward this pregnancy as well as expectations about delivery, child care, and infant nutrition.
  —previous and current medical history that may provide clues to issues that could arise during the pregnancy or delivery.
  —family medical history, which will suggest additional pregnancy-related issues.
  —previous obstetrical history beginning with the onset of menses and including contraceptive history, previous pregnancies and their outcomes as well as problems which arose during the pregnancy or delivery.
  —current history of this pregnancy, first day of last menses, use of medications including over-the-counter and street drugs and alcohol, drug allergies, and possible teratogenic exposures including X-rays and viral infections.
- mental preparation of the client for the events of this first prenatal visit including the pelvic examination and laboratory testing.
- physical assessments such as
  —checking for vital signs
  —head-to-toe assessment ending with pelvic examination
    - Encourage the woman to empty her bladder prior to examination
- pelvic examination, which includes checking for
  —signs and symptoms of pregnancy
  —fundal height
  —pelvic adequacy
    - Estimation of pelvic size in anticipation of delivery
- laboratory assessments such as
  —determining hemoglobin and hematocrit values or complete blood count
    - Pseudoanemia is a common finding as the client blood volume increase is greater than the increase in blood cells
  —ABO and Rh typing
  —urinalysis
    - Looking specifically for glycosuria and proteinuria
  —screening tests for
    - syphilis testing
    - gonorrhea culture
    - HIV
    - rubella titer
    - hepatitis B
    - sickle cell screen for selected clients
  —Pap smear

One of the major roles of the nurse in the obstetrical office or clinic will be "education." The nurse will provide information, on each prenatal visit, on topics including

- normal changes of pregnancy
  —best done on a monthly basis,
  —include physical changes for the woman, and
  —fetal growth and development.
- anticipatory guidance—during this and every prenatal visit, the nurse will be educating the woman about her body and her infant. There is a substantial amount of material to be shared with the pregnant woman and the nurse will need to present it in organized, small bits as the woman's pregnancy progresses. This will include
  —self-care
    - Hygiene: During pregnancy the glands of the body are more active. The pregnant woman will perspire more and have more vaginal secretions. The nurse will provide the client with the information that tub baths are allowed unless the membranes have ruptured. In late pregnancy, because of the changing body proportions, showers may be recommended as a safer activity. Soaking in hot tubs for prolonged periods of time is not recommended as studies have shown an increase in fetal anomalies associated with hot-tub use.
    - Clothing: All clothing should be loose and nonconstricting. The woman is encouraged to wear low-heeled, supporting shoes to reduce backache. A well-fitted support bra is recommended to promote the retention of breast shape.
    - Employment: Consider the activities involved in the job to determine the safety of working during pregnancy. Activities which might contribute to negative pregnancy outcomes include
      - prolonged standing which may lead to preterm delivery,
      - physical strain such as heavy lifting, and

- environmental factors which may be harmful to the fetus including inhalation of gases in an operating room.

- Travel: Consideration should be given to the length of time the pregnant woman will be unable to move around freely. In automobile travel, the pregnant woman should plan a short rest period from sitting every 2 hours. When traveling in a car, both the lap and shoulder belts should be worn with the lap belt positioned under the abdomen. If long trips are planned close to the due date, consideration should be given to the need for medical care at the destination.
- Exercise: The pregnant woman will want to continue her normal active lifestyle and should continue to participate in activities that maintain fitness and muscle tone.
  - As pregnancy advances, activities may need to be modified to promote the safety of the woman and her fetus. For instance, if the woman is a regular bicycle rider, as her central of gravity changes, the woman may need to consider other forms of exercise. Strenuous activities may need to be curtailed and activities that include an inherent risk may need to be avoided until after the pregnancy is complete.
  - Specific exercises may be added to the pregnant woman's regimen to assist with the discomforts of pregnancy and to prepare for delivery. The pelvic tilt exercise strengthens the back muscles and may reduce back strain. Kegal exercises will strengthen the perineal floor while sitting cross-legged will stretch the muscles of the inner thigh in preparation for delivery.
- Sexual relationships: Although there may be changes in the woman's sexual interest, sexual relations are considered safe during pregnancy. In late pregnancy, the enlarged uterus may require changes in position for intercourse.
  - Pregnant women are advised to avoid intercourse once the membranes have ruptured or if there is vaginal bleeding or a risk of preterm labor.

—nutritional guidance

- Pregnancy outcome is influenced by prepregnancy and pregnant nutrition.
- Maternal weight gain is important for adequate growth of the fetus.
  - Normal weight gain is around 30 lbs.
  - While once considered unnecessary for overweight women to gain during pregnancy, the current practice is for these women to gain up to 25 lbs.
  - When a woman is underweight prior to pregnancy, she needs to gain more than the recommended 30 lbs during pregnancy.
  - Women are concerned that gaining too much weight during pregnancy will lead to obesity. In a normal pregnancy, weight gain can be divided into the following:
    (1) fetus—7 lbs
    (2) placenta and amniotic fluid—4 lbs
    (3) increased blood volume—4 lbs
    (4) increase breast tissue—3 lbs
    (5) the remainder is maternal stores
  - Distribution of weight gain throughout the pregnancy:
    (1) first trimester: 2–5 lbs
    (2) second and third trimesters: 1 lb per week
  - The food pyramid remains the basic guide for food intake for pregnant women.
  - It is recommended that women increase their caloric intake by 300 kcal in the second and third trimester.
  - Supplements: While a good diet can provide all the elements needed for a successful pregnancy, many physicians place their pregnant women on supplements to ensure the adequacy of the diet. Supplements often include
    (1) multivitamins
    (2) folic acid
    (3) iron
    (4) calcium

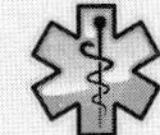

Nursing Intervention Alert

Remind the pregnant woman to take the iron supplement with juice as vitamin C will aid in absorption. Avoid taking iron with milk as it impairs absorption.

- Pica
  - Pica is the practice of eating nonfood substances such as laundry starch, dirt or clay, and ashes. It can also be taken to mean the ingestion of large quantities of nonnutritious dietary items such as ice. These practices may be supported by cultural beliefs and are often passed down through families. The purpose of eating the substance varies with the culture. For instance, some women eat laundry starch to "stiffen" the baby and make it stronger. In some cultures, ice is chewed to cut down on the food intake and keep the baby small to "make labor easier." In addition to affecting general nutrition, iron-deficiency anemia is a common problem among women who practice pica.

—warning signs: The pregnant woman is given a list of "warning signs" that require immediate notification of the physician (see Table 6–7).

Table 6–7 Warning Signs of Pregnancy

Symptom	Time of Occurrence	Possible Interpretations
Severe vomiting	Anytime, especially in the first and second trimesters	Hyperemesis gravidarum
Fever, chills	Anytime	Infection
Burning on urination	Anytime	Urinary tract infection
Abdominal cramping or pain	Anytime	Miscarriage, ectopic pregnancy, or abruptio placenta
Vaginal bleeding	Anytime	Miscarriage, ectopic pregnancy, abruptio placenta, or placenta previa
Sudden gush of fluid from the vagina, uterine contractions	Before 37 wks	Premature rupture of the membranes
Absence of fetal movement	Second and third trimesters	Fetal demise
Epigastric pain, muscular irritability, convulsions, headache, visual disturbances, or edema of face and hands	Second and third trimesters	Pregnancy-induced hypertension

—minor complaints of pregnancy and their relief: As the woman progresses through pregnancy, the nurse will provide instructions about the common complaints of pregnancy and will offer suggestions that will make the pregnant woman more comfortable (see Table 6–8).

SUBSEQUENT PRENATAL VISITS

After the first prenatal visit, pregnant women are generally seen once a month until the eighth month of pregnancy, when the women are seen twice a month. During the ninth month of pregnancy, women are generally seen once a week until delivery.

During these prenatal visits, the health care team will continue their assessment and education of the pregnant woman. During each visit, the woman will be assessed for

- weight gain
- vital signs
- uterine size
- FHTs (after the first trimester)
- edema and the presence of other complications
- glucose and protein in urine
- psychosocial adaptation

Periodically throughout the pregnancy, additional laboratory tests may be ordered to monitor for the development of a high-risk pregnancy. Table 6–9 lists the tests that will be ordered.

INTRAPARTUM PERIOD

SIGNS OF IMPENDING LABOR

Prior to the onset of labor, there will be changes occurring in the pregnant woman that can indicate the approach of labor. As the day of labor approaches, the fetus will most often settle in a head down (vertex) position. The pregnant woman may also notice a decrease in fetal activity, which can be at least partly due to the tightness of the uterus for the term fetus.

Lightening: Lightening is the settling of the presenting part into the pelvis. In the woman who is pregnant for the first time, this may occur two weeks prior to delivery. In the multipara client, lightening may occur closer to or with the onset of labor.

- As a result of the uterus moving down into the pelvis, the woman will note that breathing is easier as the top of the fundus is no longer at the level of the xiphoid process.

Table 6–8 Minor Complaints of Pregnancy and Nursing Interventions

Trimester	Complaint	Cause	Nursing Interventions
First	Nausea and vomiting (morning sickness) It can occur anytime during the day. It usually ends around the end of the first trimester.	Hormones—HCG	Consume small meals more often than thrice a day Eat dry crackers Do not mix liquids with solids Avoid fatty or highly seasoned foods Be aware that food/cooking odors may contribute to nausea
First	Breast tenderness	Estrogen and progesterone	Wear well-fitted bra
First and Third	Fatigue	Cause unknown Weight of pregnancy and nocturnal sleep deprivation may be contributing factors	Nap as needed
First and Third	Urinary frequency Nocturnal urination	Pressure of uterus on the bladder	Void as needed Decrease fluids as bedtime approaches
First	Ptyalism (excessive salivation)	Unknown	Suck hard candy Chew gum
Throughout	Leukorrhea	Hyperplasia of vagina and activity of cervical glands	Do not douche. Wear cotton-lined underpants to add to comfort
Second and third	Heartburn	Slowing of GI tract due to progesterone Pressure of growing uterus on stomach	Maintain good posture Do not lie down after meals Avoid spicy, fatty foods Eat small frequent meals Take antacids as recommended by physician
Second and third	Hemorrhoids and constipation	Pressure of uterus Slowing of peristalsis by progesterone	Use topical agents and sitz baths for hemorrhoids Increase fluid intake Add fiber to the diet Exercise Take stool softeners as recommended by physician
Second and third	Backache	Shift in center of gravity Lordosis Joint relaxation due to hormones	Maintain good posture Avoid high heels Select supportive shoes Do pelvic rock exercise Rest at frequent periods
Third	Leg cramps	Calcium/phosphorus imbalance	Take calcium supplements Dorsiflex foot when cramp occurs
Third	Postural hypotension/faintness Vena cava syndrome	Sudden changes in position Weight of uterus on ascending vena cava	Change positions slowly Prefer side-lying resting position Do not sleep on back
Third	Shortness of breath/dyspnea	Enlarging uterus	Maintain good posture Sleep in semi-Fowler's position

Table 6–9 Additional Tests Ordered During Pregnancy

Test	Source	Timing	Possible Findings
Alpha-fetoprotein (AFP)	Maternal blood or amniotic fluid	16–18 wks of pregnancy	AFP is a screening test for neural tube defects and Down's syndrome.
Glucose tolerance test (GTT)	Maternal blood	End of second trimester or when risk of gestational diabetes is recognized	A 1-hr or a 3-hr GTT may be done to determine the presence of gestational diabetes.
Indirect Coombs test	Maternal blood	28 wks gestation	In an Rh– mother, a positive indirect Coombs test could indicate the development of antibodies against the baby's blood.
Screening for group-B streptococcus	Vaginal and rectal swabs	35–37 wks gestation	Presence of group-B streptococcus in the vagina is associated with higher incidences of neonatal morbidity and mortality. A positive swab will result in prophylactic, intravenous antibiotic administration to the pregnant woman.
Percutaneous umbilical blood sampling	Intrauterine umbilical cord blood	Second and third trimesters	This test allows for prenatal diagnosis of inherited blood disorders, karyotyping of the fetus, and other fetal problems.
Chorionic villi sampling	Placental structure	8–10 wks	This sampling allows for evaluation of fetal chromosome makeup at an early date.
Amniocentesis	Amniotic fluid from the fetal sac through the maternal abdomen and uterus	After week 14 of pregnancy	Amniocentesis is used to identify genetic disorders.

- With lightening, there will be greater pressure on the bladder and urinary frequency will occur.
- Because of the presence of the gravid uterus in the pelvis, there will be venous stasis affecting the lower extremities.

Braxton Hicks Contractions: Although Braxton Hicks contractions have been occurring throughout the pregnancy, they become more noticeable and occur more frequently as labor approaches.

- Often referred to as "false labor," these contractions must be differentiated from "true labor" (see Table 6–10).
- Many women will be seen in the hospital for "false labor" and may feel embarrassed when sent home. It is not unusual to have the woman return hours later in true labor.

Bloody Show: This refers to the loss of the mucous plug.

- Pink tinged secretions are expelled with the softening of the cervix in preparation for labor.

Table 6–10 Differences between False Labor and True Labor

Sign	"False Labor"	"True Labor"
Contractions' regularity and frequency	Contractions are irregular and do not increase in frequency.	They are irregular in the beginning and then become more regular. The time between contractions shortens and contraction length increases while intensity heightens.
Location	They are felt in abdomen and groin. They may be uncomfortable and interfere with sleep.	They start in the back and extend to the abdomen.
Comfort measures	Walking usually lessens the discomfort.	Walking does not lessen the discomfort and may intensify the pain.
Differentiation	There is no change in cervix.	The cervix dilates and effaces.

- Onset of labor usually begins within 24 hours of the passage of the bloody show.
- The amount is relatively small and not to be confused with vaginal bleeding or with the blood-tinged discharge that may follow a vaginal examination.

Burst of Energy: Considered to be part of the "nesting" phenomena, the pregnant woman will experience a burst of energy days before going into labor.

- It is often seen as a time when the woman will complete the nursery preparations and prepare the household for her absence during delivery and postpartum.
- Pregnant women who experience a "burst of energy" should be cautioned not to overdo. The woman would be wise to conserve much of this energy to release during the labor process.

Rupture of the membranes: It is not uncommon for the membranes to rupture prior to the onset of labor contractions. This is termed Spontaneous Rupture of the Membranes (SROM).

- If the woman is at term, labor contractions will usually begin within 24 hours.
- The pregnant woman may confuse SROM with urinary incontinence. There are several tests to determine if the vaginal discharge contains amniotic fluid:
  —The vaginal secretions can be tested with nitrazine paper. Since amniotic fluid is alkaline while most body fluids including urine are acidic, the presence of a blue or green result indicates amniotic fluid is present in the discharge.
  —A second method is to place a drop of discharge on a slide and allow it to dry. When viewed under a microscope, a fern appearance indicates the presence of amniotic fluid.
- If the presenting part is not engaged, the gush of fluid may cause the umbilical cord to rush into the vagina. As the presenting part engages, the umbilical cord may be compressed between the pelvis and the presenting part, obstructing blood flow from the placenta to the fetus. The first nursing action following rupture of the membranes should be to listen to FHTs. Immediate notification of the physician is required if there is any change in the FHTs.
- If the woman is at term when the membranes rupture, it is the goal of the medical team to deliver the fetus within 24 hours of the rupture. Delay in delivery may lead to the development of an infection.

THE FOUR Ps OF INTRAPARTUM

The nurse in the obstetrical unit will need a clear understanding of factors that influence labor and delivery. These factors are often referred to as "the four Ps of intrapartum" which include the passenger, the passageway, the powers, and the psyche.

Passenger

Passenger refers to the fetus. Factors influencing the outcome of labor involving the passenger include the fetal lie, presentation, attitude, and position.

- Fetal lie—It compares the long axis of the fetus (the spinal column) to the long axis (spinal cord) of the mother.
  —Longitudinal lie: In this, the fetal spinal column is parallel to the maternal spinal column. The fetus in longitudinal lie may be either a cephalic or breech presentation.
  —Transverse lie: In this, the fetal spinal column is horizontal to the maternal spinal column. The fetus in transverse lie presents as a shoulder presentation. Vaginal delivery is impossible if this lie is maintained.
- Fetal presentation—It describes the part of the fetus that enters the maternal pelvis first. In a longitudinal lie, cephalic or breech presentation are the options. In a transverse lie, the fetal shoulder will enter the pelvis first.
  —Cephalic presentation describes an infant that presents itself head-first; it is the most common presentation.
  —Breech presentation describes an infant whose buttocks are the presenting part. Breech can further be divided into frank breech and complete breech:
- Frank breech describes an infant whose hips are flexed and the knees are extended, placing the infant's feet near the fetal head.
- Complete breech describes an infant whose hips and knees are flexed. In addition to the buttocks being noted on vaginal examination, the feet may also be felt. If during the delivery process, the fetus extends one or both feet, the feet will precede the buttocks and the delivery will be described as a footling breech or double footling breech.
  —Shoulder presentation is when the fetus is lying across the maternal abdomen. The infant cannot be delivered in this position.
- Fetal attitude—It compares the relationship of fetal parts to each other.
  —Flexed: Most infants present in the flexed attitude. If the fetus is in a cephalic presentation, the flexed attitude makes the occiput of the fetal skull the presenting part. This provides the smallest diameter possible for delivery. It is the most common attitude of the fetus.
  —Extension: In the cephalic presentation, but with an extended attitude, the forehead will be the presenting part. The diameter of the skull will be greater than the occiput and vaginal delivery will be more difficult.
  —Hyperextended: This fetus has tilted its head back. In the cephalic presentation, the face becomes the presenting part. This presents a wide diameter of the skull. Vaginal delivery is very difficult. The baby will usually have noticeable bruising of the face following this delivery.

- Fetal position—It refers to the relationship between the presenting part of the fetus and the maternal pelvis. The maternal pelvis is divided into four quadrants described as left anterior (LA), right anterior (RA), left posterior (LP), and right posterior (RP). In the flexed fetus presenting in the vertex lie, the occiput becomes the presenting part and is described as O. In the hyperextended attitude, the chin or M (for mentum) is the presenting part. If the fetus is in breech position, the sacrum (S) is the presenting part. For a transverse fetus, the scapula (SC) is described as the presenting part. The position will be described with three letters: mother's left or right, fetal presentation, then maternal anterior or posterior. Thus, a designation of ROA indicates a fetus in vertex position, flexed (to put the crown of the head down) longitudinal lie. The fetal crown faces the mother's right anterior.

Passageway

Made up of the birth canal and the maternal pelvis, the passageway can influence the delivery in either a positive or a negative manner. During early prenatal visits, the physician will have determined the type and adequacy of the maternal pelvis. In evaluating the pelvis, the true pelvis or area between the ischial spines will be the smallest internal diameter that the baby must pass through. There are four basic pelvis types:

- Gynecoid—the typical female pelvis provides the widest diameter in the true pelvis making delivery easier.
- Android—about one-fourth of all women have this form of pelvis. It is similar to the male pelvis with a narrow internal diameter making vaginal delivery difficult or impossible.
- Anthropoid—another one-fourth of all women will have this oval-shaped pelvis.
- Platypelloid—relatively rare, this pelvis is described as flat.

During the later part of pregnancy, the physician will estimate whether *this* fetus can be delivered vaginally through this pelvis. If in doubt, an X-ray can confirm the adequacy of the pelvis or the presence of cephalopelvic disproportionment.

The birth canal is composed of the cervix, vagina, and introitus. The cervix will dilate and efface during the first stage of labor. The normally thick cervix thins (effaces) and dilates (opens) to allow the fetus to pass. When the mother is 100% effaced and 10 cm dilated, the woman enters the second stage of labor. In primiparas, the cervix effaces and then dilates. In the multipara woman, the cervix effaces and dilates together, shortening the first stage of labor.

Powers

Power involves voluntary and involuntary powers that expel the fetus.

- Involuntary powers are responsible for the dilation and effacement of the cervix. The fundus contracts causing the cervix, normally about 3 cm long to be pulled up into the body of the uterus. As the cervix is pulled into the body of the uterus, the fetus is pushed down out of the uterus much like pushing your head through a turtleneck sweater. The contractions will be described in terms of frequency and duration, both of which increase as labor progresses.
- Voluntary powers, also called secondary powers, contribute to the delivery once the cervix is dilated or effaced. The conscious bearing down by the woman adds intraabdominal pressure to assist in expelling the fetus.

Psyche

The emotional state of the mother can affect the progress of labor. The woman who is able to relax with the contractions progresses faster than the woman who is fearful and resists the contractions, tightening nonlabor muscles. Many factors will affect the emotional state of the mother including the presence of a support person, childbirth preparation, and previous experiences. The nurse will work with the laboring woman to provide support and comfort measures. The environment should be controlled in terms of light, noise, and personnel. The nurse will need to provide information about the woman's labor progress to the laboring woman. During the latent period, the nurse can provide information on breathing that will assist the woman in managing her contractions better.

LABOR

Labor can be divided into four distinct stages.

First Stage of Labor

This stage begins with the onset of regular contractions and continues until the cervix is completely dilated and effaced. This is the longest stage of labor and can last for up to 20 hours in the primipara and still be considered normal. The first stage of labor is further broken down into three phases—latent, active, and transition (see Table 6–11).

Rupture of membranes

- On admission to the labor unit, the membranes may or may not be ruptured. The nurse can test for ruptured membranes by the following methods:
  - —test the vaginal discharge with nitrazine paper. If the paper turns blue or green, the membranes are ruptured.
  - —vaginal discharge can be spread on a slide and allowed to dry. When viewed under the microscope, a fern pattern will be observed.
- If not ruptured on admission, the membranes will rupture during labor. There is always the risk that the membrane rupture will cause the umbilical cord to precede the fetal presenting part and occlude the blood flow to the fetus. The first nursing activity following rupture of the membranes is always to take the FHTs.

Table 6–11 Phases of the First Stage of Labor

Phases of the First Stage of Labor and Corresponding Cervical Dilation	Contractions and Fetal Descent	Client's Behavior	Nursing Interventions	Pain Control
• Latent phase This phase extends from the onset of labor until the cervix is dilated to 3 cm.	• Contractions are irregular, mild in degree, widely spaced, and lasting less than 45 sec. This is the longest phase of the first stage of labor. • The mucous plug is lost. • The fetal head may be floating.	The client is • excited and talkative • able to read and converse with others between contractions	• Encourage the client to stay home as long as possible • Suggest walking and diversional activities • Admit to the labor unit and complete the paperwork • Review breathing exercises • Encourage to void q 2 hrs • Change position frequently • Take vital signs including FHT as per hospital routine, usually q 30 min during latent and active phases. The temperature can be taken every 4 hrs. • Limit vaginal examinations to reduce the risk of contamination.	Encourage the client to • relax • effleurage • walk • follow breathing techniques
• Active phase In this phase, there is 4–7-cm cervix dilation.	• Contractions are regular. • Their frequency increases to every 3–5 min. • Duration of each contraction lasts 30–45 sec. • The discharge increases slightly and consists of pink or bloody mucus.	• Labor becomes more intense. The woman is concentrating on her contractions. • She has a serious demeanor. • She does not want to be left alone. • She rests between contractions.	• Continue monitoring P, R, BP, and FHT q 30 min. • Encourage to void q 2 hrs. • Encourage ambulation and position changes. • Clear liquids orally. • Assist with personal hygiene.	• Ask client to follow breathing techniques • Provide opioid analgesia • Provide epidural analgesia
• Transitional phase In this phase, there is 8 cm to complete cervix dilation	• Contractions are strong. • They occur 2–3 min apart, each lasting up to 90 sec. • Discharge increases and is bloody.	The client • is nauseated • is irritable • has limited ability to concentrate • is concerned that she will lose control • sleeps between contractions	• The multipara may be moved to the delivery room. The primipara will continue in the labor room until dilation is complete. • Vital signs are monitored every 15 min. • Continue to encourage voiding to prevent a full bladder from slowing progress. • Stay with the client. • Prepare for birth.	• Same as above

- If membranes are ruptured for a prolonged period, there is a risk of an ascending infection. It is desirable to deliver the baby within 24 hours of rupture. If the membranes have been ruptured longer, monitor the woman's temperature closely. If attempts to hasten labor and delivery are unsuccessful, the physician may choose to perform a cesarean section.
- If the membranes do not rupture spontaneously, the physician may choose to rupture the membranes artificially. This is termed an amniotomy. An amniotomy may also be performed to assist with the onset of labor or to speed its progress. The physician uses a small sterile device to reach into the vagina and break the membranes. The nurse will immediately take FHT before providing personal hygiene for the mother.
- When the membranes rupture, the fluid should be assessed for color and consistency. Normal amniotic fluid is straw-colored and may contain vernix caseosa. The normal volume is about 1000 ml at term. Excessive amniotic fluid, polyhydramnios, is associated with fetal abnormali-

ties including GI obstruction and anencephaly. Diminished amniotic fluid, oligohydramnios, is associated with renal anomalies in the fetus.

- If the amniotic fluid is greenish-brown in color, the fetus may have passed meconium in utero, a sign of fetal distress.

Fetal assessments during intrapartum

During labor, the FHTs can provide essential information about fetal well-being and the fetal response to labor. The FHTs can be monitored intermittently with a fetoscope or with a Doppler ultrasound transducer. If more detailed information about the fetus is important, a fetal heart monitor can be applied to allow for continuous electronic monitoring of the fetus and provide additional information about the maternal contractions.

- *External fetal monitoring*: Fetal monitoring can be performed externally using sensors or transducers. This method is noninvasive. These devices are secured to the mother's abdomen with belts and provide continuous tracings comparing the FHT to the maternal contraction. The sensor that monitors FHTs is placed directly only at the spot on the maternal abdomen where the FHTs are best heard. In the cephalic presentation, this is usually on the lower abdomen. This device may need to be reapplied during labor as the fetal position changes. The second sensor, measuring the contractions, is applied over the fundus.
- *Internal fetal monitoring*: For more accurate monitoring of the fetus and contractions, an internal fetal monitor may be placed. Prior to placing an internal monitor, the mother's membranes will need to be ruptured and the cervix dilated at least 2 cm. The internal monitor will consist of two devices. An intrauterine pressure catheter will be placed in the uterus to measure the internal uterine pressure of the maternal contractions. A fetal scalp electrode will be attached to the presenting part by means of a sharp wire that punctures the skin of the presenting part. This device is less affected by maternal movement than the external fetal monitoring device but because of its nature, promotes the introduction of bacteria.
  - —Monitoring information to be noted include the baseline fetal heart rate. This information is acquired between uterine contractions. Normal FHT baseline is between 110–160 bpm.
  - —Baseline variability can also be obtained through both external and internal monitoring. It is expected that there will be beat-to-beat variability as well as long-term variability during the course of labor. Loss of variability can be attributed to factors such as hypoxia, fetal anomalies, and narcotic administration.
  - —Recurrent patterns in the FHTs include accelerations and decelerations. Accelerations (abrupt, short-term increases in the FHTs) are due to fetal movement and are usually considered a positive sign of fetal response. Decelerations refer to the decreases in the FHTs and can be divided into three general classifications:
    - Early decelerations are considered a normal response to pressure on the fetal head during contractions. These decelerations appear as a slightly delayed reverse mirror of the contraction. The heart rate drops slightly shortly after the beginning of the contraction and returns to baseline as the contraction ends.
    - Late decelerations have a similar appearance as early decelerations except the fact that they are more delayed in their onset following the beginning of a contraction and return to baseline later, after the contraction ends. These decelerations are thought to be due to uteroplacental insufficiency and are a nonreassuring pattern.
    - Variable decelerations are tracings showing the slowing of the fetal heart with no relation to the contraction. These decelerations are thought to be due to umbilical cord compression and are another nonreassuring pattern.

Anesthesia and analgesia for labor and delivery

Pain is a personal, subjective experience. Pain is a normal component of childbirth. Pain during labor can be attributed to pressure, stretching and distension of the pelvic organs and the birth canal as well as tissue ischemia of the uterine muscle as a result of the contraction. Many factors affect a woman's perception of labor pain and her response to it including cultural beliefs, childbirth preparation, anxiety, fetal position, and support system.

- Nonpharmacologic methods of pain relief are often based on the Gate Control method of pain relief. This theory explains that the pain message is carried to the brain by small diameter nerve fibers. Larger diameter nerve fibers carry other messages to the brain. In Gate Control, the "gate" allowing passage through the small diameter fibers is closed by sending messages through the larger diameter nerve fibers. Tactile stimulation is carried over these larger fibers so massage, either self-massage or massage by others, can be effective in reducing the pain messages that the brain receives.
  - —Self-massage involves the technique called effleurage, a light, stroking touch done over the abdomen.
  - —Counter pressure is particularly effective for back labor, when the fetal presenting part is in the posterior position.
  - —Hydrotherapy also provides tactile stimulation. The laboring woman may find a shower or a warm bath relaxing.
  - —Mental stimulation including imagery, soft music, and breathing techniques can be effective, reduce breath holding, and promote relaxation.
- Pharmacologic pain relief can be administered by many routes. Both analgesia and anesthesia may be used to assist the mother through the birth process. The analgesic can be systemic, regional, or local. With analgesic administration, there is always a concern that the fetus will be adversely affected during labor or after birth. In addition, improperly

used analgesics can slow or stop the progress of labor, especially during the latent period. Regional analgesics may hamper the woman's ability to push during the second stage of labor. On the other hand, a mother who is relaxed and comfortable during labor may progress at a more rapid rate as she allows her muscles to contract without resistance.

—Systemic analgesia and anesthesia

- Parenteral analgesia includes intravenous administration of opiods including fentanyl (Sublimaze), butophanol (Stadol), and nalbuphine (Nubain). These drugs cross the placenta and should not be administered when delivery is imminent as it may cause respiratory depression in the newborn. The nurse should always have naloxone (Narcan) available in case opiod reversal is necessary. Promethazine (Phenergan) may be added as an adjunctive drug to the opiod serving as an antiemetic.
- General anesthesia is rarely used in obstetrics. It may be utilized when immediate cesarean delivery is required in emergency situations since it provides more immediate access to the uterus. Respiratory depression may develop in the mother and/or the fetus, and with some general anesthetics, uterine relaxation may predispose the woman to postpartum hemorrhage.

—Regional analgesia: It refers to temporary loss of sensation and usually involves nerve blocks. Typical drugs used for the blocks include lidocaine (Xylocaine), bupivacaine (Marcaine), and other "caines." The advantage of regional analgesia is that the drug will have little or no effect on the fetus.

- Epidural blocks involve the threading of a catheter into the epidural space at the L5–S1 level and an anesthetic agent being injected. In addition to difficulty in moving lower extremities and potential urinary retention, the client will feel little urge to push.
- Spinal block has local anesthetic agents injected into the cerebral spinal fluid. Spinal blocks are used primarily for cesarean sections.

—Local analgesia: It is used during the second stage of labor to reduce the pain of delivery on the perineum and may be used for the episiotomy. The fetus will be minimally affected by local analgesia.

- Pudendal nerve block is used to relieve pain from the vulva and perineum. It does not relieve discomfort from labor contractions.

Second Stage of Labor

The second stage of labor begins with complete dilation and effacement and ends with the delivery of the fetus.

- The contractions are intense coming every 2–3 minutes and lasting up to 90 seconds. It is important that a rest period between contractions occur so that oxygenated blood can be delivered to the fetus.
- The woman will have the urge to bear down, increasing intra-abdominal pressure to help expel the fetus. Some women experience the urge to push prior to complete dilation and effacement. Other women may mistakenly believe that early pushing will shorten labor. The laboring client should use breathing techniques to resist the urge to push prior to complete dilation and effacement. Failure to resist can lead to a bruised fetus and maternal cervix.
- An episiotomy may be performed to prevent tearing of the perineum and to shorten the second stage of labor. An episiotomy is a surgical incision into the vagina and perineum to widen the birth outlet.

The cardinal movements of delivery

During labor and delivery, the fetus must move through the birth canal. By changing positions during the course of labor and delivery, the fetus attempts to maneuver through the birth canal. These steps occur in order and are

- engagement, descent, and flexion. These three movements occur almost simultaneously. The head flexes presenting the occiput, the fetus descends into the true pelvis, and engagement occurs.
- internal rotation. As the fetal head moves through the maternal pelvis, this rotation aligns the smallest diameter of the presenting part with the largest diameter of the maternal pelvis.
- extension. Once the head is through the pelvis, the fetus will extend his neck, and the head is delivered.
- external rotation. The next largest diameter of the fetus, the shoulder, is now in the pelvis. The fetus will turn again to slide the front shoulder out from the pelvis. With the fetal head outside the maternal body, observers can see this rotation.
- expulsion. As soon as the shoulders have passed the pelvis, the rest of the body will quickly slide through. This movement will happen quickly as the diameter of the body is much less than that which has already passed through the maternal pelvis.

Nursing care during the second stage of labor

The nurse's role of monitoring and supporting the woman continues in the second stage of labor. Vital signs, FHTs, and contraction assessments are monitored every 5 minutes. The client is positioned to promote delivery. Special birthing beds are used in many hospitals that allow a variety of positions for delivery. Positions that utilize gravity are beneficial. If the client will be placed in lithotomy position for delivery, it is important that both legs are placed in and removed from the stirrups simultaneously.

- The nurse and the client's support person will be assisting the laboring woman with her pushing technique. The nurse will need to provide simple, explicit instructions repeatedly as the woman's concentration is hampered. Breathing techniques will assist with the effectiveness of pushing and promote oxygenation.

- It is important that the laboring woman be kept informed of her progress and encouraged in her efforts. The support person may also need encouragement at this time.
- With delivery of the head, the nurse or physician will suction the oral cavity of the fetus.
- With full delivery, the physician or the infant's father will cut the umbilical cord.
- Until the cord is cut, the infant must be held at the level of the placenta to prevent a shift in the blood dynamics. The infant may be placed on the mother's abdomen at this time.
- Stimulation of infant respiration is a priority. A second priority is to warm the baby. The infant is wet and the room may be slightly cool (for the mother's and health care workers' comfort). Immediately wrap the baby in a warm towel and briskly rub. This will assist in drying and stimulate respiration at the same time.
- Allow the mother and father to see and touch their infant.
- The infant is usually placed in an over-bed warmer in mother's sight to continue the warming and stimulation. At this time, the nurse or the pediatrician will do a quick assessment, checking vital signs and looking for signs of distress, birth injuries, and birth defects. If the infant's condition allows, the baby should be returned to the parents as soon as possible.

Third Stage of Labor

The third stage of labor is termed "the stage of the placenta." Beginning with the birth of the baby, it ends with the delivery of the placenta.

- Immediately after the birth of the baby, the uterus can be palpated just below the umbilicus as a round, firm mass.
- After a short rest, contractions begin again.
- The uterus changes to a discoid shape.
- Usually within 5 minutes of the delivery of the baby, the placenta will separate.
- Separation of the placenta can be recognized by the following symptoms:
  —The umbilical cord protruding from the vagina will lengthen.
  —There will be a sudden increase in vaginal bleeding.
- Traction should never be applied to the umbilical cord to hasten delivery as it may cause the uterus to invert, a condition termed uterine prolapse. This will constitute a medical emergency that may have fatal consequences for the mother.

The placenta can separate first from the center and then to the edges or from the edges to the center. The method of separation will determine the appearance of the placenta at delivery. If the separation began at the center, the placenta will present with the fetal side of the placenta first. The fetal membranes give the placenta a shiny appearance; hence, this delivery is termed "shiny" shultz. If the placental separation begins at the edge, the placenta tends to deliver with the maternal side of the placenta first. This side is red and beefy in appearance and is termed a "dirty" duncan delivery. The physician will inspect the delivered placenta to determine its completeness. Retention of placenta pieces will inhibit normal involution and lead to postpartal hemorrhage.

Once the placenta is delivered, the episiotomy and any perineal lacerations will be repaired. Oxytocins are usually administered intravenously or intramuscularly to promote uterine contraction and decrease uterine bleeding.

The nurse will remove the client from the stirrups (if used) and the client will be transferred to a recovery bed. The fourth stage of labor is about to begin.

Fourth Stage of Labor

The immediate postpartal period is often termed "the fourth stage of labor." The woman, her support person, and the baby (if conditions allow) will be placed in a recovery room. The room will provide a degree of privacy for the new family while allowing the nurse to monitor the condition of the mother and infant. Immediately on arrival into the recovery room, the mother's vital signs will be taken. Her fundus and lochia will be assessed. Pericare will be provided. The mother will be given a clean gown and will appreciate a warmed blanket as chills and shaking are common. The woman will need assurance that this is a normal occurrence.

The nurse will continue to assess vital signs, fundus location and consistency, and amount and characteristics of the lochia every 15 minutes for the first hour, then if findings are normal, changing to every 30 minutes the next hour, and then hourly for the remainder of the recovery period.

Between assessments, the room should be dimly lit to allow the infant to open his or her eyes. This will be a quiet time for the new family to begin bonding. The mother may initiate breast-feeding if desired. This is an excellent time for the initial attempt at breast-feeding as the infant is awake and alert. After a short period of time, the baby may be transferred to the nursery to allow for a more thorough assessment and initiation of nursery procedures. The mother may request food at this time or the parents may want to notify other family members by phone. Some new mothers may choose to sleep during this short recovery period.

CESAREAN DELIVERY

Cesarean section refers to the surgical delivery of the infant. It can be a planned or an unexpected event. There are many factors that may lead to a cesarean delivery including the following:

- maternal factors
  —cephalopelvic disproportionment: It is a condition where the fetal head cannot be delivered through the maternal pelvis due to size discrepancies.
  —active genital herpes: Vaginal delivery may spread the infection to the newborn.

—failed induction: This refers to the case when the attempt to induce labor is unsuccessful and delivery is necessary.

—previous cesarean sections: It is no longer an exclusive factor. Previous cesareans, which involved a classic incision, are still considered to require a repeat cesarean.

- fetal factors
  —multiple gestation
  —transverse fetal lie
  —fetal distress
  —breech presentations
  —fetal anomalies such as hydrocephalus
- placental factors
  —placenta previa
  —umbilical cord prolapse
  —premature separation of the placenta

Emergency or unexpected cesarean deliveries can be extremely stressful for the woman and her family. There is the concern for the well-being of the fetus. In addition, the woman may feel that she failed in her womanly role of fetal delivery. The woman and her family will need to understand the reason for the cesarean delivery. They will need to be kept informed on the status of the fetus and the mother. The mother will need a chance in the postpartal period to reconcile her planned delivery to the actual event. This is usually accomplished by describing her delivery experience many times over the postpartal period. The nurse should assure the client that she did a good job in delivering her baby. In nonemergency cesarean deliveries, the father or support person may be allowed to accompany the woman, which will contribute to a more pleasant delivery experience. Regional or general anesthetics may be selected dependent upon the necessity of rapid access to the fetus.

Following a cesarean delivery, the mother will go to the recovery room (OB or surgical) and will be monitored during the recovery period. Like all postpartal women, the woman will need to have her vital signs, fundus, and lochia monitored along with her surgical incision. The abdomen will be very tender, so assessing the fundus is done gently and from the side but must still be monitored. Infants born by cesarean delivery are at greater risk for respiratory distress in the recovery period, so they may be immediately transferred to the newborn or high-risk nursery.

POSTPARTUM PERIOD

INVOLUTION

With the delivery of the fetus and placenta, the body of the woman begins the process of involution, returning to the nonpregnant state. All systems of the body are included in the involution process although the changes in the reproductive system are the greatest.

Nursing Assessments

Vital signs often may indicate the onset of postpartal complications:

- temperature above 100.4°F after the first 24 hours may indicate infection
- elevated pulse and blood pressure are associated with hemorrhage
- elevated blood pressure may indicate pregnancy-induced hypertension
- clients may develop orthostatic hypotension on arising after delivery

BUBBLE-HEB is a mnemonic used to remember the appropriate assessment of the postpartal client, where

B = breast
U = uterus
B = bladder
B = bowel
L = lochia
E = episiotomy

H = Homan's Sign
E = emotional status
B = bonding

Nursing Interventions

Nursing interventions during the postpartum period are aimed at promoting the involution, providing comfort, and teaching the woman to care for herself and her infant.

Uterus

- Gentle fundal massage promotes contraction of the uterus. Overmassage can cause a boggy fundus.
- Oxytocins may be ordered to promote involution: oxytocin (Pitocin), methylergonovine maleate (Methergine), and ergonovine maleate (Ergotrate).
  —Methergine and ergonovine promote the contraction of the cervix as well as the fundus and are therefore never given during labor.

Bladder

- Promote emptying the bladder every 2 hours while awake

Table 6–12 Changes in the Various Structures/Systems in the Postpartum Period

Structure/ System	Postpartal Activity	Variations from Normal
Uterus	There is a contraction of the uterine muscle resulting in descending level of the fundus • Immediately after delivery of the placenta, the fundus will be located midway between the symphysis pubis and the umbilicus • By day 1 postpartum, the fundus will have risen back to the level of the umbilicus • The fundus will descend 1 fingerbreadth a day until it is no longer palpable behind the symphysis pubis The contractions of the uterus will be felt by the new mother and are called "afterbirth pain." These are felt more fully • in the multipara • following delivery of a large baby or multiple fetuses • in the breast-feeding mother	When the fundus is higher in the abdomen than expected, bleeding will increase. Nursing activities will be aimed at promoting uterine contraction • The woman should be encouraged to void as a full bladder will prevent contraction of the uterus • While supporting the uterine body, the nurse will massage the fundus. Overmassage of the fundus can lead to a boggy fundus • Breast-feeding the baby will also promote uterine contraction Retained placenta segments will prevent uterine contraction; the fundus will be described as "boggy" and bleeding will be heavier than expected
Lochia	The bloody discharge following delivery is termed lochia. Lochia consists of blood, shed decidua, white blood cells as well as other debris. The discharge follows a predictable pattern: • Lochia rubra—dark red, bloody discharge with a musty, earthy smell occurs on days 1–3 postpartum • Lochia serosa—pink or brownish discharge that occurs on days 4–10 • Lochia alba—whitish discharge that persists typically for a couple of weeks but may persist for up to 6 wks Lochia often pools in the uterus when the mother is in bed. The first few times out of bed, the mother may note a sudden "gush" of lochia when she gets up Menstruation usually resumes about the eighth week postpartum for the non—breast-feeding mother and 12 wks for the breast-feeding mother. This first cycle is usually anovulatory	• Reverting to an earlier stage of lochial discharge can be a negative finding usually indicating the mother needs to reduce her activity level • Lochia with a foul smell can indicate uterine infection
Cervix	By the end of the first week postpartum, the cervix will have closed so that only a fingertip can be admitted	Continuous oozing of bright red blood can indicate a cervical laceration
Vagina	The vagina reverts to the nonpregnant state by 2 wks For several weeks following delivery, the vagina will have decreased lubrication due to low estrogen levels. When intercourse resumes, the woman may want to use a water-soluble lubricant for comfort	
Perineum	Labia may be swollen Episiotomy remains intact	Hematoma may form in the labia during the postpartal period Episiotomy may separate or become infected Hemorrhoids may be present due to pushing during delivery
Breasts	Prior to the birth of the baby, the woman may be able to express a small amount of a colorless liquid. With delivery, the volume will increase slightly. Milk production is dependent on the release of prolactin from the pituitary gland • The first milk is colostrum, which is rich in antibodies • By day 3, engorgement will occur where the breasts fill with milk. Breast milk is thin and appears bluish in color • By day 5–6, the let-down reflex will release milk when it is time to nurse the infant and the engorgement will diminish	Cracks and fissures in the nipples are not uncommon in the breast-feeding mother, usually thought to be the result of an infant who latches incorrectly • The nipples can be protected by assisting the infant to latch on correctly • Colostrum can be expressed and spread on the nipple as a protectant

(continued on next page)

Table 6–12 *(continued from previous page)*

Structure/ System	Postpartal Activity	Variations from Normal
Breasts	Early and regular stimulation of the breasts by nursing the infant will promote milk production and let-down which will ease engorgement For the non–breast-feeding mother, care should be taken to avoid breast stimulation, which will increase milk production and breast discomfort. Instructions for the non-lactating mother would include: • Wear a tight, well-fitting bra; it will suppress milk production • Avoid stimulating the breast. Do not handle the nipples and do not express the milk that develops • Stand in the shower so that water does not stimulate the breasts • For discomfort, the non–breast-feeding mother may be given NSAIDS and ice packs. Medications which suppress lactation are not usually given	• The mother should wash her hands before handling the breasts and feeding the infant to reduce the risk of infection Mastitis—It is the infection of the breast tissue • Causative factors include crackled nipples and lowered maternal immune levels • Symptoms include a hard, reddened, engorged area of the breast, fever, and other systemic symptoms of infection • Treatment includes antibiotics and antipyretics. Heat may be used to help milk let-down and ice may be used for comfort In most cases, breast-feeding will be continued despite the presence of mastitis as keeping the breast empty helps to prevent the growth of microorganisms
Cardiovascular system	High blood volume is no longer needed so fluid is eliminated by diuresis • Blood pressure remains consistent with pregnancy • Heart rate is usually slow (50–70 bpm) as the workload of the body has decreased • Homan's sign (test for thrombophlebitis) should be negative • An elevated WBC count may be a normal finding due to labor preparations by the body	• For the client with cardiac disease, this period of diuresis places the client at risk for cardiac failure • PIH can occur up to 48 hrs after delivery • Tachycardia is associated with excessive blood loss • Because the platelet count was high as the body prepared for labor, the client may be at risk for thrombophlebitis
Abdomen	Immediately after delivery, the skin will appear loose and flabby. Striae (stretch marks), which were red streaks during pregnancy, will fade to silver	
Urinary bladder	Diuresis will occur as the blood volume decreases to the nonpregnant state • Urinary output in the first 24 hrs may exceed 2000 ml	• Decreased bladder sensation and bladder tone makes the woman susceptible to a UTI during the postpartal period
Metabolism	The client will be hungry and thirsty after birth • The breast-feeding woman will need to increase her diet by 500 kcal/d and should have a fluid intake of at least 2000 ml/d	
Bowel function	• Normal bowel function returns by 2–3 wks postpartum • The client with an episiotomy may fear the bowel movement • Stool softeners may be ordered	• No suppositories are given if client had a third- or fourth-degree laceration

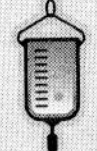

Clinical Alert

A full bladder will push the uterus up in the pelvis and interfere with contraction causing heavier lochia. Following labor and delivery, the woman may be less aware of a full bladder and needs to be reminded to void regularly.

Bowel

- Promote early ambulation
- Increase fluid and fiber in the diet

Comfort

- Episiotomy
  - —Apply ice pack to perineum (20 minutes on/10 minutes off) × 24 hours.
  - —Encourage sitz bath up to thrice a day beginning at 12 hours postpartum.
  - —Pericare
- After voiding or bowel elimination, spray the perineum with warm water.
- Apply clean peri-pad from front to back.
  - —Apply witch hazel or local anesthetics to the perineum.

—Teach the woman to contract her buttocks before sitting to reduce pressure on the perineum.

- After-birth pains and cesarean section incisional pain
  —Give ordered acetaminophen, NSAIDS, and opiods for pain control.
  —If mother is breast-feeding, encourage nursing the baby before taking opiods.

EMOTIONAL CHANGES—MATERNAL ADJUSTMENT

The typical emotional changes that postpartum client experiences can be divided into three sequential phases:

- taking in
  —occurs for the first 2 days postpartum
  —during this period, the mother is passive and preoccupied with her own needs
  —the woman needs to discuss the labor and delivery experience to assist in the integration of the planned experience with the reality of labor and delivery
  —nurses need to "mother" the mother so that she can move into the taking-hold phase
- taking hold
  —occurs in the second and third days postpartum
  —the mother is still concerned with her body functions
  —this is an excellent time for teaching about caring for herself and her infant
  —mood swings may be evident
- letting-go phase
  —beginning on about the fourth day of postpartum and proceeds through the postpartum period
  —the mother "lets go" of her old concept of herself to acquire the self-concept of being the mother of this infant
  —wants to be independent in caring for her infant

BONDING

- Bonding occurs most readily in the immediate postpartum period, but can also occur later.
- It is facilitated by close contact with the infant.
- It is facilitated by the infant opening his eyes and looking at the mother (dim the lights).
- Nursing assessments that indicate bonding is occurring include the following behaviors:
  —The mother begins exploring her infant with the fingertips, progress to the whole hand exploration, and finally enfolding the newborn in her arms.
  —She holds the infant face-to-face at a short distance from her face (*en face* position).
  —She speaks to the infant in a high-pitched soft tone.
- The father will also bond to the infant and should display interest in the infant.

POSTPARTUM BLUES

- This refers to a temporary mood depression that is fairly common in the early postpartum period.
- It is different from postpartum psychosis or postpartum depression, a serious emotional condition that occurs in some postpartum women.

CLIENT TEACHING

Prior to discharge from the maternity unit, the new mother will need information on how to take care of herself and her infant. Instructions should include:

- Maternal care
  —involution
  —breast care
  —resuming sexual relations
  —birth control
  —general health
- Newborn care
  —bathing and clothing
  —cord care
  —nutrition
    - breast-feeding
    - bottle feeding
  —immunizations and proper baby care
  —car safety

NEWBORN CARE

NEWBORN TRANSITION

The delivery of the newborn begins a period of transition for the infant. While in utero, the fetus has lived a parasitic lifestyle, totally dependent upon the maternal body for nutrients, oxygen, and even waste disposal. Suddenly with birth, the newborn must take over these functions. Health care workers monitor this transition beginning with the Apgar score.

Apgar Score

The newborn is assigned an Apgar score by the physician or the nurse at the delivery. Apgar scoring is performed at 1 minute and 5 minutes after birth. The score describes the success or difficulty with the transition. Five areas are scored and each area is scored as a 0, 1, or 2. The areas evaluated on the Apgar are

- A: activity (or muscle tone)
- P: pulse (or heart rate)
- G: grimace (reflex irritability)
- A: appearance (or skin color)
- R: respiratory effort

Since there are five areas evaluated and each area has a possible score of 0, 1, or 2, newborns can score anywhere from 0 to 10. The higher the score, the better the transition for the baby. Scores between 8 and 10 indicate a good extrauterine transition, while scores in the lower range indicate the newborn is struggling with the transition process and resuscitation efforts are needed.

Delivery Room Activities

As soon as the infant is delivered and the cord is clamped, he or she will be placed in an over-bed warmer. This device provides external heat while the infant is dried and evaluated. Two identification bands are placed on the infant with corresponding identification applied to the wrist of the mother and her significant other. In the over-bed warmer, an infant requiring resuscitation can receive the necessary treatment while avoiding the loss of body heat. An infant who has made a good transition can be monitored while the placenta is being delivered. This infant can then be wrapped in a warm blanket and given to the new mother for bonding. Some mothers choose to breast-feed the infant at this time. If the mother has received a minimum amount of analgesia, the infant will be awake, alert, and eager to feed. This period is termed the *first period of reactivity.*

Parent–Infant Bonding

Early parent–infant contact enhances the attachment process called bonding. Immediately after birth and the delivery of the placenta is a good time to promote bonding. The infant is awake and alert and the parents and infant can be provided time to become acquainted. Eye prophylaxis for the infant should be postponed until after this initial bonding period has occurred. The establishment of eye contact between parent and infant, a positive event promoting bonding, is enhanced by the *en face* position. The newborn's eyes are unaccustomed to bright lights and the infant will open his or her eyes more fully when the room is dimly lit. Private time should be provided to the new family. The new mother may choose to initiate breast-feeding, if she has not already, and the nurse will need to assist the new mother and baby in this activity. The new parent will initiate tactile contact with the fingertip touch but will progress to whole hand stroking followed by whole palm enclosing as the parent–baby relationship grows.

Eye Prophylaxis

Eye prophylaxis with an antimicrobial agent is required in all states in the United States to prevent the development of ophthalmia neonatorum. Ophthalmia neonatorum is an infection of the eye caused by the gonorrheal organism transmitted to the infant during the birth process. If untreated, ophthalmia neonatorum can result in blindness. Treatment consists of the instillation of silver nitrate, erythromycin, or other antimicrobials as prescribed by hospital protocols. This treatment may be delayed for up to 1 hour following birth to allow for parent–infant interaction.

Newborn Nursery Admission

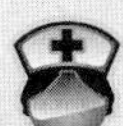

Practice Alert

Gloves are always worn when caring for a newborn until the first bath. This protects the health care worker from blood and body fluid exposure. The vernix, amniotic fluid, and bloody secretions are removed with the first bath.

On admission to the newborn nursery, all infants must have a complete physical assessment by the nurse. This assessment will continue to evaluate the child's transition as well as determine congenital problems and other conditions that can affect the infant's well-being. This assessment should be performed in a well-lit, distraction-free area. The baby will need to be observed without clothing so an external source of heat, such as an over-bed warmer, is necessary. The assessment should be organized and usually begins with the measurement of vital signs, height, and weight.

ASSESSMENT OF GESTATIONAL AGE

Ballard Score

The Ballard Score is an assessment tool that allows postnatal assessment of gestational age. This assessment is important to allow for monitoring for age-related problems. The Ballard Score should be performed within the first 24 hours after birth. It has two primary components: physical characteristics and neuromuscular maturation. The two areas together provide a maximum score of 50, which equates to a gestational age of 44 weeks+. The "New Ballard Score" has been updated to provide more accurate assessment of the very preterm infant.

PHYSICAL ASSESSMENT

General Appearance

Prior to the hands-on assessment, the nurse should do a general visual assessment noting, in particular, the respiratory effort. The infant who is struggling with respiration needs the assessment to be as invasion-free as possible to limit the stress on his body.

Table 6–13 Physical Assessment of a Newborn

Assessment Area	Normal Findings	Findings to Report
Skin • Color	• The skin is either all pink or the body is pink with blue extremities (acrocyanosis).	• Generalized or circumoral cyanosis, pallor, dusky red, or jaundiced at birth or shortly thereafter.
• Normal skin variations	• Vernix caseosa (white cheesy covering of the skin) in varying amounts will be observed at birth. This material has a protective quality. It will be removed during the initial bath or by being rubbed onto clothing and blankets. It is not necessary to remove it forcefully. • Mongolian spot: A dark bluish discoloration seen on the buttocks of dark-skinned individuals. This spot will fade by the age of 2 yrs. • Milia: Obstructed sebaceous glands seen on the face, most commonly on the nose. These white cysts should be left alone. • Lanugo: Fine, downy hair seen on the less mature newborn. • Erythema toxicum (newborn rash): White or yellow pustules with a red base. These may be widespread or limited. The rash comes and goes quickly appearing shortly after birth and continuing until about 5 d of life. • Mottling: Often associated with chilling, the skin color will appear patchy. • Petechiae: Small hemorrhages most commonly due to the pressures of labor and delivery. • Eccyhmoses: Bruises, usually from forceps. • Birthmarks: Birthmarks vary widely in appearance and location. • Telangiectatic nevi: More commonly known as "stork bites," they appear as flat, pink or red spots on the eyelids, between the eyes, under the nares, and at the nape of the eyes, under the nares, and at the nape of the neck. They generally fade by the age of 2 yrs.	• Skin lesions: May be caused by forceps or internal scalp monitors. These sites should be documented and watched for signs of infection.
Vital Signs • Temperature	• The initial method of assessing temperature may be with a rectal thermometer. In addition to providing a close approximation of core body temperature, this method assesses rectal patency. Normal rectal temperature is 97.7–99.7°F. • Axillary temperature ranges from 97.7–98.6°F.	• Subnormal temperatures can result from excessive heat loss during the delivery or nursery experience and may result in cold stress. Cold stress can lead to respiratory distress, jaundice, metabolic acidosis, and hypoglycemia. • Unlike an older infant, newborns most frequently display elevated temperatures due to an overheated environment, excessive clothing, or dehydration.
• Pulse	• Apical pulse rate is between 100 and 160. • Check peripheral pulses.	• Report bradycardia, tachycardia, irregularity, murmurs, and absent or peripheral pulses.
• Respiration	• Normal respiration is 30–60/min. The diaphragm is the major muscle of respiration. For a short period after birth, crackles and other sounds of moisture may be heard in the chest as the amniotic fluid present in the lungs is absorbed by the body.	• Report signs of respiratory distress, nasal flaring, grunting, gasping, and seesaw respirations. In addition, report apneic periods lasting longer than 15 sec, retractions, and bowel sounds heard in the chest.
Body Measurements • Length	• Measure from top of head to heel. Normal length is 19–21 in. (48–53 cm).	• Variations under the normal range could indicate intrauterine growth retardate (IUGR), gestational age discrepancies, and chromosomal abnormalities.
• Weight	• Normal weight is 2500–4000 g. The infant will lose approximately 10% of their body weight in the first 3 d of life and then start to gain. This weight loss is due to loss of maternal hormones, urination, and defecation.	• Variations include small for gestational age (SGA) and large for gestational age (LGA). Both conditions can indicate predelivery conditions that might affect the newborn's well-being.

(continued on next page)

Table 6–13 *(continued from previous page)*

Assessment Area	Normal Findings	Findings to Report
• Head	• The head circumference is measured at its greatest diameter. Average head circumference ranges from 33–36 cm and should be approximately 2 cm greater than the chest circumference. Chest circumference will exceed head circumference by the age of 5–7 mo. The head will represent a large percentage of the total length of the baby. The relatively large size of the head contributes to head injuries should the baby fall from an elevated position.	• Microcephaly—small head circumference. It is associated with mental retardation. • Hydrocephaly: The lay term is water on the brain. This condition is an accumulation of cerebral spinal fluid within the ventricles of the brain.
• Chest circumference	• Measured at the nipple line, the chest circumference measures approximately 31–34 cm.	• Excessively large chest circumference could indicate diaphragmatic hernia where the intestines have protruded through a hole in the diaphragm and have filled the chest cavity.
Head	The head will make up one-fourth of the total length of the newborn's body.	
• Shape	• Molding: The shape of the newborn's head will be affected by the delivery method. Babies born in vertex position will often have cone shaped heads due to the molding during labor. • Infants delivered in breech position and those delivered by cesarean section may have round heads.	• Premature infants are often described as "hammer heads" due to the predominance of the back skull. • Caput succedaneum is a generalized swelling of the head when the head is the presenting part. This is a normal variation and will disappear a few days after birth. • Celphalohematoma is bleeding into the periosteum of the bone. This often follows a difficult delivery and may not develop until a day after delivery. The celphalohematoma can be differentiated from caput by the fact that celphalohematoma never crosses a suture line. Although this will disappear, it may take months for it to fully resolve. Newborns with cephalohematomas are at risk for hyperbilirubinemia.
• Sutures	• Overlapping of the sutures is common due to molding. The frontal, coronal, sagittal, and lambdoidal sutures should be palpatable.	
• Fontanels	• With the baby lying quietly, the fontanel is palpated. • Anterior fontanel is located between the frontal, coronal, and sagittal suture. It is diamond-shaped and large. Parents term these fontanels as "soft spots" and fear they could damage the newborn's brain if they touch it. The anterior fontanel normally closes between 12 and 18 mo of life. • Posterior fontanel lies between the sagittal and lambdoidal sutures. It is small and triangular and may be difficult to locate due to molding. This fontanel normally closes at 2–3 mo of life.	• Bulging, tense fontanels can indicate hydrocephalus or increased intracranial pressure such as seen in intracranial hemorrhage. • Depressed fontanels are associated with dehydration.
Eyes • Color	• All newborns have blue or slate-blue eye color. As the newborn ages, the color will change to the permanent eye color of the child.	• Subconjunctival hemorrhage may be noted around the pupil and in the whites of the baby's eyes. This bleeding is caused by the pressure of delivery and will disappear in time.
• Appearance	• Epicanthic folds on the inner aspect of the eye are associated with selected ethnic groups.	• The presence of epicanthic folds in newborns not of ethnic decent is associated with chromosomal conditions such as Down's syndrome.
• Coordination	• Newborns do not coordinate eye movements well and often present with pseudostrabismus (or false cross eyes). This is not a concern during the newborn period and is not associated with strabismus later in life.	

(continued on next page)

Table 6–13 *(continued from previous page)*

Assessment Area	Normal Findings	Findings to Report
• Blink Reflex • Discharge • Pupils • Eyebrows	• Present • Normally there is no discharge from the eyes. • When a light is shined into the pupil, a round red or brownish red reflection can be seen. This is termed as the red reflex and is a visualization of the retina. • Two distinct eyebrows should be present.	• The eyes may appear swollen and have a slight discharge. This is attributed to the eye prophylaxis and is termed chemical conjunctivitis. • Absence of the red reflex could indicate congenital cataracts and should be reported to the physician. • The presence of a single connected midline eyebrow can indicate certain chromosomal abnormalities.
Ears • Placement • Appearance	• Draw an imaginary line from the inner canthus to the outer canthus of the eye and straight back toward the ear. The top of the auricle (helix) should be above this imaginary line. • Observe for the normal shape of the auricle. • The auricle should feel firm and return to its normal position when folded. This indicates a firm cartilage. • Check for the presence of an ear canal in both ears.	• Low-set ears are associated with renal disorders and mental retardation. • Ear tags (these may be removed during the nursery stay). Extra skin usually located in front of the ear. • Very soft cartilage in the auricle is associated with prematurity. • Bruises are not uncommon around the ear, especially in forceps delivery. Be sure to look for bruises or scratches behind the ear.
Nose	• The nose should be midline and free of discharge. • Infants are obligant nasal breathers. If anything occludes the nares, the baby will stop breathing. • The sneezing reflex is present and assists in clearing the airway. It does not indicate the newborn "is catching a cold."	• Snuffles (copious discharge) is associated with congenital syphilis. • Choanal atresia is a membrane or bony development that occludes the nares. It can be unilateral or bilateral. If bilateral, when the infant falls asleep, breathing will cease. Maintain the mouth in the open position until the atresia can be surgically corrected.
Mouth • Appearance • Reflexes • Tongue and gums • Palate	• It is pink in color. • It has a symmetrical movement. • Sucking and rooting reflexes are present at birth. • A short lingual frenulum gives the appearance of being "tongue tied." • Palate is intact. • Epstein's pearls are small white cysts located on the hard palate of newborns. These disappear a few weeks after birth.	• Transient circumoral cyanosis is not uncommon but may be associated with respiratory distress or hypothermia. • Asymmetrical movement of the mouth is associated with facial paralysis often due to the placement of the forceps. This can be a permanent or temporary damage. • The tongue may seem too large for the infant's mouth and protrude. This is associated with selected chromosomal abnormalities including Down's syndrome. • On occasion, a newborn is born with a tooth in the lower gum line. This is usually not the deciduous tooth, but a third tooth for that position. It is often removed. • Report cleft, unilateral, or bilateral, soft and hard palates.
Neck	• Neck is short.	• Webbed neck is associated with Turner's syndrome.
Chest • Appearance	• Chest is round in appearance.	

(continued on next page)

Table 6–13 *(continued from previous page)*

Assessment Area	Normal Findings	Findings to Report
• Nipples	• Prominent, swollen breasts may be present in both males and females due to maternal hormones. Nipples may excrete "witches' milk."	• Report supernumerary nipple(s) down chest.
• Expansion	• There is bilateral expansion. • Diaphragm is a major muscle of respiration.	• Retractions, nasal flaring, and "seesaw" respirations can be indicative of respiratory distress.
• Auscultation	• Breath sounds are clear; may be "wet" sounding immediately after birth. • Heart sounds consist of a regular rhythm.	• Bowel sounds heard over the chest could indicate diaphragmatic hernia. • Unilateral absence or diminished breath sounds could indicate failure of a lung to expand. • Tachycardia, bradycardia, and arrhythmias should be evaluated by a physician.
Abdomen • Appearance	• Abdomen is rounded and protruding.	• Distended abdomen could indicate bladder or bowel fullness—check voiding and BMs. • Scaphoid abdomen may be associated with diaphragmatic hernia. • Report bowel present on skin surface (open or covered by membrane), omphalocele, or gastroschisis. • Report red meaty mass located on abdomen and exstrophy of the bladder. Urine excreted onto skin can lead to excoriation.
• Auscultation	• Bowel sounds are present shortly after birth. Infant passes meconium stool within 24 hrs of birth.	
Back	• The back is intact. Spinal column is readily visible under the skin and should be straight.	• Report failure of the fetal notochord to close resulting in a bony defect (spina bifida) and a skin and nervous system defects ranging from mild (meningocele) to severe (myleomeningocele). • A dimple (pilonidal dimple) low on the sacrum may be observed in some babies. The dimple should be inspected to ensure there is no open connection to the nervous system. • Curvature of the spine (scoliosis) may be present at birth, usually secondary to a vertebral defect called hemivertebrae.
Genitalia • Female	• Are swollen in response to maternal hormones. • Urinary meatus is located behind clitoris with vagina opening behind meatus. • It may have a bloody discharge (pseudo menstruation) also due to maternal hormones. • Smegma is present between labia.	• Report ambiguous genitalia and enlarged clitoris. • Report abnormal placement of urinary meatus—hypospadias or epispadias.
• Male	• Penis: There is a urinary opening at tip of glans penis. Prepuce covers glans penis and is not fully retractable. Prepuce may be removed in circumcision procedure prior to discharge from the nursery. • Scrotum surface is covered with rugae. Two small movable testes can be palpated in scrotum.	• Report ambiguous genitalia • Report if the opening of urinary meatus is not on glans penis—hypospadias or epispadias. • One or both testes may be absent from scrotum. Testes may be observed in groin. The testes may descend after birth. • Scrotum is swollen and fluid filled—hydrocele. This usually regresses spontaneously.
• Urination	• Infant voids spontaneously within 24 hrs of birth. • Pink or rust colored stains in urine are result of uric acid crystals and are normal.	

(continued on next page)

Table 6–13 *(continued from previous page)*

Assessment Area	Normal Findings	Findings to Report
Anus	• Anus is intact. A rectal thermometer can be inserted with ease. • Infant should pass meconium stool within 24 hrs of birth.	• Report imperforate anus in which there is no connection between the anus and the rectum, varying from a membrane separation to a significant distance between the two. • Failure to pass meconium usually indicates GI obstruction disorders including Hirschsprung's disease (lack of sympathetic nervous system connection to the intestines).
Extremities	• Infant should move all extremities equally. • There are 5 fingers and 5 toes on each hand and foot. • Equal in number thigh skin folds and equal knee height is expected. No click is heard or felt when hips are abducted.	• Failure to move one or more extremities could indicate birth injuries such as a fractured clavicle. • Report supernumerary fingers or toes and webbed or fused fingers or toes. • Unequal skin folds or knee heights can indicate a unilateral dislocated hip. Presence of a hip click also indicates dislocated hips.
Reflexes	The expected reflexes are • moro • rooting • sucking/swallowing • tonic neck • grasp • Babinski	• Absence of any of the expected reflex should be evaluated. Immediately after birth, if the mother received narcotic analgesia, the baby may not respond fully.

TRANSITION

The period after birth is one of great transition for the infant. In the uterus, all the needs of the infant are met by the mother through the placenta. With birth, the infant will need to make changes in many systems in order to sustain life.

Cardiac and Respiratory Transition Changes

With the loss of the placenta, the infant will need to change both the function of the circulatory and respiratory systems.

Cardiac system

Three fetal structures of the circulatory system are no longer needed and if retained may even be detrimental. These structures are the foramen ovale, ductus arteriosus, and ductus venosis.

- *Foramen ovale* is an opening between the right and left atrium. This structure allows oxygenated blood entering the right atrium from the placenta to bypass the lungs and enter the body circulation by way of the left atrium. Because of the decrease in blood entering the right atrium from the inferior vena cava, the foramen ovale is structurally closed almost immediately after birth.
- *Ductus arteriosus* is a connection between the aorta and the pulmonary artery. Because the lungs are nonfunctioning, the lungs need very little blood prior to delivery. The ductus arteriosus allows the blood that entered the pulmonary artery from the right ventricle to bypass the lungs and enter the aorta. This structure closes functionally following birth as a result of the increased needs of the lungs. Structurally, the ductus may still be present for a period after birth and if respiratory distress occurs, may reopen. It is not uncommon in the preterm infant for a patent ductus arteriosus to be present.
- *Ductus venosis* is a shortcut through the liver for the oxygenated blood. With the loss of the placenta, this structure closes functionally with birth.

Respiratory system

- In utero, the fetus will "practice" breathing with prerespiratory movements. These occur irregularly and the fetus does not "practice" throughout pregnancy.
- With birth, respiratory movements must occur and continue.
- Some immature infants may demonstrate short apneic periods when they "forget" to breathe.
- In monitoring the respirations of a newborn, the monitor is often set to allow for "apneic periods" of 15 seconds before alarming as this is not an uncommon finding.
- In utero, the lungs will contain amniotic fluid. This is sterile fluid and causes no problems at delivery.
- With birth and the onset of respirations, the fluid is absorbed. Initially, the nurse may hear moist respirations on auscultation, but it should quickly clear up.

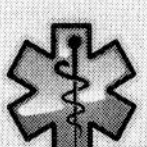

Nursing Intervention Alert

To reduce oxygen demand when the infant shows signs of respiratory distress, minimize the physical manipulation of the infant. Placing the infant in Trendelenburg position will cause gravity to put intestinal pressure on the diaphragm, the major muscle of respiration for the infant, increasing respiratory effort. A semi-Fowler's position with the head in "sniffing" position will best promote respirations.

- If the infant passes meconium in utero, the amniotic fluid in the lungs may contain meconium. This condition is called meconium aspiration and can create severe respiratory difficulties for the infant.

Hematologic System

- In utero, due to low oxygen tension, the fetus has a high hemoglobin and hematocrit.
- With delivery, the high levels of blood cells are no longer needed so the infant will begin breaking down the excessive numbers of cells.
- With the destruction of blood cells, bilirubin is released. As it is released from the RBC, the bilirubin is fat soluble and not easily eliminated from the body.
- The liver will convert this fat-soluble bilirubin (indirect or unconjugated bilirubin) to direct or conjugated bilirubin, a water-soluble bilirubin that will be excreted in the urine.
- If the liver is unable to convert this bilirubin efficiently due to liver stress or excessive breakdown secondary to bruising or injury, the unconjugated bilirubin will accumulate in the body (hyperbilirubinemia). The baby will appear jaundiced.
- When excessive unconjugated bilirubin builds up in the body, it will interfere with nutrition to the brain and can lead to brain damage, a condition called kernicterus.
- Infants who are premature or immature, those with birth trauma, maternal–fetal blood incompatibilities, and those who suffer cold stress are more likely to have higher levels of unconjugated bilirubin.

Elimination System

- It is normal for the fetus to void in utero and this liquid adds volume to the amniotic fluid. A fetus that passes meconium in utero is showing symptoms of distress.
- The infant should void and pass meconium within 24 hours of birth.
- Although the liver is functioning at birth, it is immature and takes several days to become fully active. Stressors on the infant, such as prematurity, cold stress, and bleeding and bruising problems will all affect the liver functioning.

TEMPERATURE MAINTENANCE

- At birth, the infant will be wet allowing loss of body heat. Drying quickly is extremely important to prevent cold stress.
- A mature infant will be better prepared to maintain body heat than a preterm infant.
- The nurse is responsible for ensuring conditions that maintain the normal body temperature of the infant. This includes frequent monitoring as well as activities designed to reduce the loss of body heat.
- Cold stress, a condition when the infant loses body heat, is extremely stressful on the body and will affect glucose metabolism and functioning of all body systems.

NEWBORN NUTRITION

Bottle Feeding

- The first feeding is usually glucose water or sterile water. This feeding substance is less irritating if the feeding should enter the lungs.
- Subsequent formula feedings should be every 3–4 hours.
- Nighttime feedings may be offered by the nursery personnel to allow the mother to rest.
- Commercially prepared formula offers the best nutrition to the bottle-fed baby as the companies producing formula have mimicked breast milk.
- The milk should be fed at room temperature and never heated in the microwave.

Breast-Feeding

- The first breast-feeding may occur in the delivery or recovery room.
- Unless the mother has received medication, the infant will be alert and eager to nurse.
- Colostrum is the first breast secretion. It is thin and watery and contains significant antibodies for the baby.
- Breast milk arrives at around the third day of life. It is bluish in appearance and is an ideal food for the human baby.
- Because it is easily digested, breast-fed babies often are hungry more frequently, eating at least every three hours.
- The infant will usually empty the breast within 5 minutes of sucking. Sucking is a pleasurable experience for the baby and the baby may continue to nurse when the breasts are empty.
- Throughout the breast-feeding experience, the baby will nurse more frequently with each growth spurt.

Parent Teaching

One of the main roles of the nurse in the maternity unit is client teaching. In addition to teaching the mother how to take care of herself, the nurse will provide instructions on infant care including bathing, warmth, holding, and immunizations.

- Nutrition: Infants should remain on formula or breast milk until 12 months of age for the best growth and development. Sterilization of the bottles are not usually required if sanitary conditions are present.
- The breast-feeding mother should be taught that the infant is probably getting adequate nutrition if it voids 6–8 times daily.

OBSTETRICAL COMPLICATIONS

ANTEPARTUM

Ectopic Pregnancy

- In ectopic pregnancy, the fertilized ovum implants in areas other than the endometrial lining of the uterus. The four types of ectopic pregnancy are
  —abdominal: The abdomen is usually unable to sustain the growing embryo.
  —tubal: The fallopian tube is the most common site of ectopic pregnancy. Tubal ectopic pregnancy places the client at risk for tubal rupture, which can be a life-threatening situation.
  —myometrial: It is also called placenta accreta. It is not usually recognized until delivery but will usually require a hysterectomy to stop hemorrhage.
  —cervical: Such low implantations are associated with placenta previa.
- Such pregnancy is not usually successful as areas outside of the uterus cannot sustain a full-term pregnancy.

Etiology: It usually occurs when tubal blockage prevents the fertilized ovum from passing through the fallopian tubes.

Precipitating factors: Pelvic inflammatory disease (PID), previous tubal surgery or tubal pregnancy, endometriosis, and congenital anomalies of the fallopian tubes.

S&S: Dependent upon location.

- Usual signs and symptoms of pregnancy are seen early in gestation
- There is a sharp one-sided pain
- There is adnexal (area over ovary and tube) tenderness
- Vaginal bleeding may or may not be present. (Bleeding may be occurring in the abdomen)
- With tubal rupture, abdomen becomes hard and rigid and signs of circulatory collapse occur. If it is not recognized and treated immediately, maternal death will occur

Dx: Transvaginal ultrasound is used to check for uterine pregnancy

Rx: Surgical removal of the products of conception is the most common treatment. An alternative medical treatment may be used if the tube has not ruptured. Methotrexate, a folic acid antagonist that inhibits DNA synthesis, may be administered IM to terminate the pregnancy in clients who desires future pregnancies

Nursing Process Elements

- Carefully assess all pregnant women to identify those with an ectopic pregnancy
- Provide emotional support for the woman undergoing either surgical or medical treatment for an ectopic pregnancy
- Provide emergency resuscitation including IV fluids and oxygen, and prepare for emergency surgery for the woman whose tube ruptures

Client teaching for self-care

- Methotrexate treatment will cause abdominal discomfort which must be differentiated from tubal rupture
- Teach client about pre- and postoperative self-care elements
- Refer client to a Fetal Demise Support Group

Hyperemesis Gravidarum

- Hyperemesis gravidarum refers to excessive vomiting during pregnancy.
- It can lead to electrolyte imbalances and dehydration.
- The resulting lack of nutrition may lead to fetal injury or death.
- Maternal death can also occur from the electrolyte imbalances and dehydration.

Etiology: It begins as morning sickness that progresses to severe vomiting. In addition to vomiting everything in the stomach, the woman may continue to retch even when the stomach is empty.

Precipitating factors: It is associated with higher levels of HCG including multiple pregnancies and molar pregnancies. It is seen more frequently in women with history of migraine headaches and motion sickness.

S&S:

- Dehydration with loss of skin turgor, diminished urine output, elevated hemoglobin, hematocrit, and BUN
  —can lead to hypovolemia, hypotension, and tachycardia
- Electrolyte imbalances including potassium loss which can cause cardiac arrhythmias
- Loss of hydrochloric acid which causes alkalosis
- Starvation which can cause protein and vitamin deficiencies

Dx: Based on above laboratory values and client history

Rx: Antiemetics and NPO are prescribed for 24–48 hours until retching has stopped and IV fluids until dehydration and electrolytes restored. Diet is returned slowly to full, but spicy and fatty foods are withheld. If hyperemesis is not controlled, the client may be placed on total parenteral nutrition (TPN)

Nursing Process Elements

- Monitor hydration status, skin turgor, urine output, and specific gravity of urine
- Monitor for signs of electrolyte imbalances
- Administer antiemetics and intravenous fluids as ordered
- If TPN is ordered, monitor for expected and untoward effects of treatment
- Provide emotional support
- Monitor weight

Client teaching for self-care

Instruct client to

- avoid fatty and spicy foods
- ingest liquids and solids separately

Hydatiform Mole

- Hydatiform mole is also called gestational trophoblastic disease or molar pregnancy.
- In molar pregnancy, conception occurs but in most cases, an embryo does not develop.
- The trophoblast proliferates and becomes filled with fluid-filled, grape-like clusters.
- Choriocarcinoma may develop from the trophoblastic tissue.

Etiology: In a complete mole, an empty ovum was fertilized making all chromosomal material coming from the father. In a partial mole, the embryo forms but dies prior to 9 weeks gestation. The embryo is found to have 69 chromosomes, the triploid number resulting from an ovum being fertilized by 2 sperms or by 1 sperm which had not undergone haploid division of chromosomes.

Precipitating factors: It occurs most often in the woman over 35 years of age, those with low protein intake, and those of Asian heritage.

S&S:

- Early pregnancy signs are present
- HCG levels are higher than expected
- Uterus grows more rapidly than expected
- Symptoms of pregnancy-induced hypertension (PIH) occurs in the second trimester
- Dark brown spotting occurs

Dx: Ultrasound diagnosis

Rx: Suction curettage is prescribed to remove the mole. HCG levels are monitored for 1 year after the termination of the pregnancy because of the risk of the development of choriocarcinoma

Nursing Process Elements

- Assess all first and second trimester women for signs of hydatiform mole
- Provide emotional support for the loss of the pregnancy
- Provide preoperative preparation for the curettage

Client teaching for self-care

- Instruct the client to use a reliable birth control method for 1 year after the curettage
- Provide instructions to avoid pregnancy so that the client can be monitored for the development of choriocarcinoma
- Refer the client to a Miscarriage Support Group

Abortion

- Abortion refers to the termination of pregnancy before the fetus is viable, usually before 20 weeks gestation.
- It may be elective (induced) or spontaneous.
- A spontaneous abortion in lay terms is called a miscarriage.
- The five types of spontaneous abortion are
  —threatened: There may be vaginal spotting and slight cramping but the cervix remains closed. It may stop spontaneously or progress to abortion.
  —imminent or inevitable: In this type, cervical dilation occurs and fetal loss is imminent.
  —complete: In complete abortion, entire products of conception are expelled.
  —incomplete: Although some of the products of conception are expelled, some remain in the uterus. A dilation and curettage are performed to empty the uterus.

—missed: In missed abortion, fetus dies in utero but is not expelled. Dilation and curettage are performed to remove the products of conception.

Etiology: Spontaneous abortions are natural events usually unrelated to the mother's activities.

Precipitating factors: Abortions are caused by fetal abnormalities due to a teratogenic agent or chromosomal abnormalities, implantation problems, hormonal insufficiencies, and uterine abnormalities.

S&S:

- Vaginal spotting
- Abdominal cramping

Dx: Differentiate the types of abortion, which determines treatment. Determine the viability of the fetus and the contents of the uterus with sonogram, HCG levels, and FHTs.

Rx:

- Threatened—avoid strenuous activities for 48 hours and intercourse for 2 weeks
- All other forms of abortion—dilation and curettage to remove the products of conception, if not fully expelled

Nursing Process Elements

- Preoperatively monitor blood pressure, pulse, and vaginal discharge frequently
- Retain all expelled tissue for examination
- Monitor FHTs if abortion is threatened
- Prepare for surgical procedure
- Obtain blood for type and cross match
- Provide emotional support

Client teaching for self-care

- Teach client that she was not responsible for miscarriage
- Refer client to Miscarriage Support Group

Incompetent Cervix

- Incompetent cervix refers to the premature dilation of the cervix.
- It usually occurs in the fourth or fifth month of gestation.
- It is a cause of repeated miscarriages.

Etiology: Cervix dilates due to the increasing pressure of uterine contents. It is not associated with uterine contractions.

Precipitating factors: The causal factors include cervical trauma, congenital anomalies of the cervix, and infection.

S&S:

- History of repeated miscarriages
- Painless second trimester cervical dilation
- Little to no vaginal bleeding
- Bulging membranes on vaginal examination

Dx: Serial ultrasounds demonstrate progressive effacement and dilation

Rx: Surgical suture insertion used to maintain closed cervix, performed early in pregnancy

- Shirodkar's operation (cerclage of the cervix)
- McDonald's procedure which uses sutures to reinforce the cervix
- Delivery may be by clipping the suture or cesarean delivery

Nursing Process Elements

- Carry out preoperative preparation
- Conduct postoperative monitoring of the woman, the uterus for contractions, and the fetus
- Provide emotional support

Preterm Labor

- Preterm labor is that which occurs after the twentieth week and prior to the thirty-seventh week of gestation.
- The risk for fetus is dependent upon gestational age; the earlier in gestation that labor occurs, the lesser will be the chances that the fetus will survive. Even if the infant survives, he or she is more likely to have resultant long-term sequelae including cerebral palsy, mental retardation, and visual problems.

Etiology: Unknown.

Precipitating factors: Numerous factors are associated with preterm labor including multiple gestations, incompetent cervix, abdominal trauma, urinary tract infections, low maternal weight, and substance abuse including cigarettes.

S&S:

- Persistent backache
- Vaginal spotting
- Feeling of pelvic pressure

Dx: Assessment of contractions by a trained practitioner, vaginal examination for cervical dilation and FHTs. Vaginal and urine cultures are often obtained to rule out infection

Rx: If the membranes have not ruptured, cervix is minimally dilated, and the fetus is not in distress, attempts will be made to halt labor. Bed rest is usually prescribed to reduce pressure on the cervix. Medications that may be administered include

- betamethasone (Celestone Soluspan)—given to mature fetal lungs. To be effective, the drug must be given 24 hours prior to delivery and
- tocolytics (medications to halt preterm labor)
  - —beta-adrenergic agonists such as ritodrine (Yutopar) and terbutaline sulfate (Brethine) and
  - —magnesium sulfate

Nursing Process Elements

- Obtain baseline hematocrit, serum glucose, sodium chloride, potassium, and pCO_2 levels
- Administer medications according to directions and physician's orders
- Monitor contractions, vaginal discharge, FHTs, and for negative effects of tocolytic drugs
- Administer betamethasone as ordered
- Provide emotional support

Client teaching for self-care

Once labor has been stopped, the woman will be discharged to be managed at home. Discharge teaching will include the following instructions:

- Take increased amounts of rest, varying from two to three extra rest periods a day to total bed rest; left-side lying is preferred
- Ensure proper medication administration, effects, and side effects. It is important to stress that medications must be taken on time
- Void every 2 hours to reduce pressure on the uterus
- Drink 8–12 glasses of water or juice per day. Avoid caffeine
- Avoid heavy lifting and strenuous activities
- Prohibit sexual activity
- Contact physician for cramping, increased pelvis pressure, low back pain, or unusual vaginal discharge. The clients are usually instructed to count contractions (even non-painful contractions) and report to physician if they are greater than five per hour

Pregnancy-Induced Hypertension (PIH)

- Pregnancy-induced hypertension is a condition of vessel spasm involving both large and small vessels.
- It was originally called toxemia of pregnancy.
- It usually occurs in the third trimester.
- This is a progressive disorder and is generally divided into two stages
  —preeclampsia: the period before seizures occur and
  —eclampsia: generalized seizure.
- HELLP Syndrome (hemolysis, elevated liver enzymes, and low platelet count) is associated with PIH and may cause
  —multiple organ failure and
  —high morbidity and mortality for client and fetus.
- With delivery, the condition resolves although seizures may occur for up to 48 hours after delivery.

Etiology: Unknown.

Precipitating factors: The client may be a primigravida, age under 20 or over 40, grand multipara (more than 5 pregnancies), or may have had multiple gestation.

S&S: Classic signs are hypertension, proteinuria, and edema.

- Hypertension
  —in preeclampsia, the readings are above 140/90
  —in eclampsia, the readings are 160/110
- Proteinuria
  —in preeclampsia, 1–2+
  —in eclampsia,—there is marked proteinuria, 3–4+
- Edema
  —in preeclampsia, weight gain is greater than 1 lb per week
  —in eclampsia, weight gain increases
- Oliguria
- Symptoms indicating the approach of eclampsia are

—epigastric pain
—visual or cerebral disturbances
—pulmonary and cardiac involvement
—hyperreflexia

Dx: Based on the presence of the classic three symptoms

Rx:

- Bed rest
- Diet high in protein, moderate sodium
- Antihypertensives
- Anticonvulsants

Nursing Process Elements

- Monitor blood pressure, pulse rate, and edema
- Monitor urine output, protein, and specific gravity
- Monitor daily weights
- Monitor FHTs and for signs of placental separation such as bleeding and uterine rigidity
- Assess lungs for pulmonary hypertension
- Monitor laboratory values including hematocrit, clotting factors, and liver enzymes
- Monitor for symptoms of approaching seizures such as severe headaches, hyperreflexia, and visual disturbances
- Be prepared if seizures should occur—have oxygen and suction available

Client teaching for self-care

- Mild preeclampsia may be managed at home. The client will be taught
  —bed rest, primarily on left side
  —to monitor weight, urine output, and urine protein
  —expected effects and untoward effects of medications
  —to monitor fetal movements and report decrease in movements

—to notify the physician immediately if signs of approaching symptoms or HELLP syndrome occur

Placenta Previa

- Placenta previa refers to the attachment of placenta in the lower uterine segment which
  —may occlude internal cervical os.
- During later weeks of pregnancy, as the uterus prepares for delivery and cervical dilation begins, placenta may be torn away from the endometrium. Painless bleeding occurs.
- There are three degrees of placenta previa:
  —complete: In this, the placenta covers the internal os. Successful delivery cannot occur by the vaginal route as placenta must separate before fetus can be delivered. Cesarean section delivery is required.
  —partial or marginal: In this, the placenta partially covers internal cervical os.
  —low lying: In this, the placenta is attached low in the uterus but not covering the cervical os.

Etiology: Unknown.

Precipitating factors: Previous history of placenta previa, multiparity, previous cesarean section(s), increasing maternal age, and cocaine use and smoking during pregnancy.

S&S:

- Painless vaginal bleeding occurring in the third trimester; bleeding is bright red

Dx: Ultrasound demonstrates location of placenta

Rx: Prior to term, bed rest with bathroom privileges, no vaginal examinations. Client usually has blood typed and cross-matched for transfusion. Delivery by cesarean section if complete placenta previa present. Low-lying and partial may attempt delivery under double set-up so that an emergency cesarean can be performed if fetal distress occurs

Nursing Process Elements

- Monitor pulse, blood pressure, and vaginal discharge
- Encourage bed rest with left side-lying position
- Monitor FHTs
- Provide emotional support

Client teaching for self-care

- Assist the family in planning bed rest at home to minimize activity
- Teach the client and family about the signs and symptoms that must be reported immediately

Abruptio Placenta

- Abruptio placenta refers to the premature separation of the normally implanted placenta.
- It is divided into three types:
  —marginal in which placenta separation occurs at the edge and blood escapes vaginally,
  —central in which placenta separates in the center with the margins attached and blood collects under the placenta so that there is no visible bleeding, and
  —complete in which there is total separation of the placenta with massive hemorrhage and loss of FHTs.
- There is an increased risk of developing disseminated intravascular coagulation (DIC), and diminished clotting factors, which increase the risk of hemorrhage.

Etiology: Unknown.

Precipitating factors: Hypertension and cocaine use during pregnancy, higher maternal age and parity, smoking, and abdominal trauma.

S&S:

- Sudden onset
- Dark bleeding or bleeding that may not be observed due to concealed bleed
- Severe abdominal pain
- Uterus is hard to touch
- FHTs may or may not be present
- Development of symptoms of shock and anemia dependent on the degree of separation

Dx: Based on symptoms. Usually an emergency situation

Rx: Dependent on the degree of separation and gestational age. Moderate to severe placental separation requires immediate cesarean section to salvage the fetus. Intravenous fluids are required to maintain blood volume. Client may require blood transfusions

Nursing Process Elements

- Start IV line and run fluid at ordered rate
- Draw blood for hemoglobin and hematocrit values, type, and crossmatch
- Monitor pulse, blood pressure, and FHTs (if present)
- Prepare client for immediate cesarean section
- Provide emotional support for client and family

Client teaching for self-care

Teach the client about

- signs and symptoms of placental separation
- risk factors, to promote a healthy pregnancy

Rh Incompatibility

- Rh incompatibility occurs when the pregnant woman is Rh− while fetus is Rh+.
- Rh+ blood has a protein not found in Rh− blood.

- Following exposure to Rh+ blood, the Rh− woman becomes sensitized and produces antibodies again the Rh+ protein.
- These antibodies can cross the placenta and attack the fetus.
- Maternal and fetal circulations are separate with minimal mixing of blood.
- Sensitization occurs when fetal blood enters the maternal circulation. This occurs primarily with delivery.
- Antibodies are produced after delivery and the woman is sensitized.
- With any subsequent pregnancy involving an Rh+ fetus, the small amount of blood that crosses the placenta will cause the pregnant woman to produce antibodies.
- These antibodies cross the placenta and attack the fetal blood.
- With the advent of Rh immune globulin (RhoGram or RhIgG), the incidence of fetal loss due to Rh incompatibility has decreased.

Etiology: The Rh− woman usually does not have problems with Rh incompatibility in the first pregnancy with an Rh+ fetus, but becomes sensitized in the following delivery and will have problems in all subsequent pregnancies with an Rh+ fetus.

Precipitating factors: The majority of the population has Rh+ blood. If a man with Rh+ blood fathers a child with a woman who is Rh–, the fetus could be Rh+.

S&S: Rh incompatibility problems are rarely seen now. If present, signs and symptoms would be

- antepartum
  —fetal hydrops: Fetus is severely anemic due to the destruction of the RBCs by the maternal antibodies. Severe edema and congestive heart failure will be present in the fetus. Fetal death is common
- after delivery
  —rapid onset of hyperbilirubinemia
  —continued anemia and congestive heart failure

Dx: Blood tests are done on the first prenatal visit to determine the mother's Rh

Rx: If mother is Rh–, screening for antibodies (Indirect Coomb's test) will be done at 28 weeks gestation. If the antibody titer is negative, the mother will receive Rh immune globulin. After delivery, if the father was Rh+ or paternal Rh status was unknown, the mother will receive additional Rh immune globulin. This occurs with every pregnancy that might include a Rh+ fetus. Rh immune globulin will also be given after abortions, ectopic pregnancies, chorionic villi sampling, and amniocentesis. Infant blood is screened for antibodies with the Direct Coomb's test

Nursing Process Elements

- Administer Rh immune globulin as ordered prenatally and within 72 hours of birth

Client teaching for self-care

- The mother needs to be taught about the condition and about the need for Rh immune globulin with every pregnancy of an Rh+ fetus or fetus of unknown Rh type

ABO Incompatibility

- The naturally occurring blood types are A, B, O, and AB. In considering blood types, consider the antigen in the blood (A or B) and the antibody (anti-A or anti-B) present.
  —Type A blood contains the A antigen and the anti-B antibody
  —Type B blood contains the B antigen and the anti-A antibody
  —Type AB blood contains the A and B antigens and no antibodies
  —Type O blood contains no antigens and both anti-A and anti-B antibodies
- ABO incompatibilities may occur in the first pregnancy or any subsequent pregnancies. It is not predictable as the mother who has one infant with an ABO incompatibility may not have problems with the next infant.
- It is usually a less severe problem than Rh incompatibility.

Etiology: Typically, it is caused when the mother is O and the baby either A or B. The maternal antibodies cross the placenta and attack the fetal blood.

S&S:

- Early development of jaundice in the infant

Dx: Direct Coomb's test on the infant blood

Rx: Phototherapy treatment

Nursing Process Elements

See hyperbilirubinemia

Client teaching for self-care

See hyperbilirubinemia

INTRAPARTUM

Dystocia

- Dystocia refers to difficult delivery.
- In dystocia, labor may be long and painful. Vaginal delivery may be impossible, requiring cesarean delivery.

Etiology: It may be caused due to the following factors:

- Fetal factors
  —difficult presentation: There is face or shoulder presentation or transverse lie.

—oversized fetus: The infant is of a diabetic mother or there is disparity in size of the mother and father.

- Maternal factors
  —small pelvis or other than gynecoid pelvis shape,
  —disparity in size of fetal head and maternal pelvis, cephalopelvic disproportionment (CPD),
  —full bladder,
  —low-lying placenta, and
  —emotional factors.

Precipitating factors: The client may be a very young primigravida or one with no prenatal care.

S&S:

- Failure to progress despite adequate time

Dx: Pelvimetry, ultrasound

Rx: May require a cesarean section

Nursing Process Elements

- Monitor labor progress
- Observe for nonreassuring pattern on fetal monitoring
- Provide emotional support
- Ensure physical and emotional preparation for surgery
- Provide postoperative care

Client teaching for self-care

- Potential CPD may be determined in early pregnancy. This pregnant woman can then be prepared emotionally and educationally for what to expect with a cesarean delivery
- The woman who experiences an emergency cesarean delivery will need an explanation of the cause, what happened, and emotional support

Prolapsed Cord

- In case of prolapsed cord, a loop of the umbilical cord precedes the presenting part into the birth canal and becomes compressed as the presenting part descends.
- It requires immediate intervention for a successful delivery.

Etiology: Prolapsed cord occurs most frequently when the membranes rupture prior to engagement of the presenting part.

Precipitating factors: Hydramnios (excessive amniotic fluid), multiple gestation, noncephalic presentation, small fetus, CPD, and placenta previa.

S&S:

- Fetal bradycardia
- Fetal monitoring demonstrates severe variable decelerations
- Umbilical cord is felt on vaginal examination

Dx: Based on fetal assessment and vaginal examination

Rx: Immediate cesarean delivery

Nursing Process Elements

- Keep all women in labor on bed rest until the presenting part has engaged (this reduces the chance that rupture of membranes will "wash" the cord ahead of the presenting part)
- Immediately upon rupture of the membranes, take the FHTs for one full minute
- If prolapsed cord is suspected
  —notify physician immediately
  —place the woman in Trendelenburg position
  —place a gloved hand in the vagina to elevate the presenting part off the cord
  —administer oxygen per mask to mother
  —if cord is protruding into room air, cover with a sterile saline moistened cloth to prevent drying
  —prepare the client for an emergency cesarean section
  —provide emotional support

Amniotic Fluid Emboli

- Amniotic fluid emboli is a nonpreventable cause of maternal mortality during delivery.
- It causes a sudden onset of respiratory distress and circulatory collapse.

Etiology: Amniotic fluid enters maternal circulation through a defect in the fetal membranes where it becomes an embolous when it reaches the lungs.

Precipitating factors: Associated with rapid delivery, oxytocin augmentation, abruptio placenta, and polyhydramnios.

S&S:

- Sudden onset of chest pain
- Cyanosis and dyspnea
- Tachycardia
- Hemorrhage
- Shock, coma, and death

Dx: Based upon symptoms

Rx: Immediate intervention is required to restore circulation. Cardiopulmonary resuscitation is started immediately, although it is not always successful. Prognosis is dependent upon the restoration of pulmonary circulation

Nursing Process Elements

- Carefully monitor all women in labor, especially those with precipitating factors
- Quick recognition and initiation of emergency interventions essential to the woman's survival
- Start intravenous fluids
- Provide oxygen

- Provide CPR as necessary
- Prepare for cesarean section if undelivered
- Prepare for blood transfusion and the insertion of a CVP line

Client teaching for self-care

- After successful resuscitation, the woman and her family will need to understand what has happened
- Emotional support should be provided for the woman and her family

POSTPARTUM

Postpartum Hemorrhage

- Postpartum hemorrhage can occur in the first 24 hours after delivery or up to 6 weeks after birth.
- There are numerous causes of hemorrhage including
  - —uterine atony,
  - —retained placenta,
  - —hematomas of the pelvic region,
  - —lacerations,
  - —subinvolution, and
  - —uterine inversion which is an unusual cause occurring at the time of delivery when the uterus prolapses through the cervix.

Etiology: It is caused by the failure of the uterus to contract to conserve maternal blood or loss of excessive blood during the postpartal period.

Precipitating factors: The factors responsible are overdistention of the uterus due to multiple gestation or polyhydramnios, rapid or prolonged labor, oxytocin augmentation, use of anesthesia, and grand multiparity. Uterine inversion is associated with traction on the umbilical cord prior to separation of the placenta at birth.

S&S:

- Excessive vaginal bleeding the amount of which varies dependent on the time of occurrence
- Decreasing blood pressure and increasing pulse
- Dropping hemoglobin and hematocrit
- Decreased urine output

Dx: Based on laboratory values and reports of vaginal discharge. Assessment of a boggy fundus could indicate subinvolution. Sonogram may demonstrate retained placental fragments

Rx: Dependent upon cause. Retained placenta will usually require dilation and curettage to manually remove the fragments. Oxytocins or Methylergonovine Maleate (Methergine) may be administered for subinvolution. Lacerations may require packing and/or suturing. Transfusions may be required if blood loss is extensive

Nursing Process Elements

- Assess vaginal discharge for color and amount. Question new mother about the frequency of pad changes and observe pads for the amount of blood
- Remind the new mother that after being in bed for a period of time and then arising, a gush of blood escaping the vagina is normal and due to pooling of blood in the uterus
- Assess fundus, provide bimanual massage—massage the fundus while supporting the cervix with the opposite hand
- Assess perineum for hematoma formation. Clients with developing hematomas will often complain of pain
- Have client void frequently as a full bladder will hamper uterine contractions
- Administer medications for uterine contraction as ordered
- Monitor vital signs
- Administer blood products as ordered

Client teaching for self-care

- Once the cause of the blood loss is determined and treated, the client may be discharged home. Prior to discharge, the nurse should teach the client about
  - —the reason for the blood loss
  - —foods that will promote blood formation
  - —medications, including iron administration
  - —the need for extra rest periods due to anemia

Postpartum Infection

- It is also called puerperal infection.
- It was once the major cause of maternal mortality.

Etiology: It is caused by introduction of an organism into the uterine or perineal tissues.

Precipitating factors: It is associated with prolonged rupture of the membranes (greater than 24 hours), postpartal hemorrhage, prolonged and difficult labor and delivery, internal fetal monitoring, frequent vaginal examinations, vacuum and forcep deliveries, and poor hygiene.

S&S:

- Temperature of 100.4°F or higher for 48 consecutive hours that do not include the first 24 hours after delivery, excluding the first 24 hours
- Pain
- Foul-smelling lochia

Dx: Based on signs and symptoms as well as laboratory findings

Rx: Appropriate antibiotic therapy

Nursing Process Elements

- Monitor vital signs
- Teach perineal care to promote cleanliness of area

- Administer antibiotics as ordered
- The client's infant may be isolated from other infants in the nursery
- The pediatrician should decide if the breast-feeding mother should nurse her infant as the antibiotics may be present in breast milk
- If breast-feeding is not recommended, the mother can pump her breasts and discard the milk. Once the antibiotic therapy has been completed, breast-feeding can be reinitiated

Client teaching for self-care

- Teach client good hygiene practices including frequent hand washing
- Discuss with the breast-feeding mother the issue of continuing nursing the infant while antibiotics are being administered. Assist client as necessary to maintain milk supply
- Instruct client to complete antibiotic therapy as ordered

Mastitis

- Mastitis is an infection of the breast tissue that occurs primarily in the lactating woman.
- It usually does not occur in the first week of lactation but may occur anytime during the remaining period of lactation.
- It is usually unilateral.

Etiology: The organism usually enters the breast tissue through cracks and fissures in the nipples. The source can be the infant's mouth or maternal hands.

Precipitating factors: One factor is that the infant latches incorrectly traumatizing the nipple. Other factors can include milk stasis, maternal fatigue, plastic-lined nursing pads which maintain moisture around the nipple, and incorrect infant-removal techniques.

S&S:

- Pain in the breasts
- Redness, heat, and swelling
- Fever
- Breast milk may diminish in quantity

Dx: Based on signs and symptoms, laboratory values, and breast-milk culture

Rx: Appropriate antibiotic therapy

Nursing Process Elements

- Observe the breast-feeding and assist the mother in positioning the infant correctly
- Encourage adequate rest and nutrition in the breast-feeding mother
- Encourage the mother to change infant positions while nursing to promote breast emptying
- Encourage the mother to wear a well-fitting, supportive bra
- Ice packs may promote comfort. Heat may be applied prior to nursing to promote let-down

Client teaching for self-care

- Teach the mother to wash her hands prior to handling the breasts
- Monitor the nipples for cracks and fissures
- Vitamin E ointment may be used on the nipples to maintain integrity. Colostrum and breast milk may also be applied to the nipple to promote integrity
- Teach the mother to allow the nipples to air dry after feeding
- Teach the mother about antibiotic administration including the need to complete the prescription. The pediatrician will determine the advisability of continued nursing while on the antibiotics

NEWBORN

Prematurity

- Prematurity refers to birth prior to 37 weeks gestation.
- The earlier in gestation that birth occurs, the less mature is the infant and the less likely to sustain extrauterine life.
- Prematurity affects all systems
    - —Respiratory: The infant has inadequate surfactant, a substance that helps maintain lung expansion. Lung development is inadequate for transfer of oxygen and waste products to and from the blood. Its brain is too immature to maintain continuous respirations. Bronchopulmonary dysplasia (BPD) is a long-term lung injury that results from high oxygen concentration and positive pressure respirator use to sustain life.
    - —Gastrointestinal: Suck and swallow reflexes of the infant are weak and ineffective. The immature digestive system is unable to digest and absorb nutrients. The basal metabolic rate is increased which means the nutrient requirement is higher per mass than more mature infant. The risk of NEC (necrotizing enterocolitis), a condition where the intestines may become ischemic and perforate secondary to diminished blood flow.
    - —Renal: The kidneys are unable to concentrate urine. Kidneys are too immature to modify pH predisposing the infant to metabolic acidosis.
    - —Integumentary: Its skin is thin and fragile and is easily damaged allowing bacteria to enter. There is inadequate fat for insulation making the infant prone to hypothermia.
    - —Cardiac: The ductus arteriosus, a fetal structure, may remain open after birth due to low oxygen tension. The PDA increases the blood volume entering the lungs leading to pulmonary congestion and eventually to congestive heart failure.

—Nervous: The tissues of the skull are fragile and easily damaged. Premature infants are prone to intracranial hemorrhage, which can lead to brain damage, seizures, and the development of hydrocephalus.

—Skeletal: Bones are not as fully mineralized as full term infants making them more susceptible to injury during the birth process.

Etiology: It is the birth of the infant prior to 37 weeks gestation.

Precipitating factors: The associated factors are multiple gestations, poor maternal nutrition, maternal smoking, or infection.

S&S: Numerous assessment findings are present in the preterm including:

- Skin appears thin and transparent. Blood vessels are easily visible.
- Lanugo may be noted in greater quantity than on a full term infant.
- Plantar creases are absent or only on the anterior portion of the foot. This must be assessed within 12 hours of birth for accuracy.
- Position tends to be primarily one of extension versus flexion in the full term infant.
- Areolar tissue increases with gestation age.
- Ear becomes more firm as gestational age increases due to presence of cartilage.
- Head may be described as "hammer head" due to the prominence of the back skull.

Dx: Ballard and Dubowitz gestation age assessment tools can determine the gestation age of the infant as maternal EDC may be incorrect, the baby may appear larger or smaller than expected based on "due date"

Rx: Careful attention should be paid to meeting all the needs of the infant. Total parenteral nutrition or gavage feedings will probably be necessary. Warmth must be maintained externally. Respirations will need support with oxygen, surfactant therapy, and possibly positive pressure respirators

Nursing Process Elements

- Ensure careful and frequent monitoring of all systems. Labs will be drawn frequently to monitor blood values, gases and electrolytes
- Place the infant in an external heat source such as an isolette or over-the-bed warmer where the body temperature can be maintained while allowing close observation of the neonate
- Pay careful attention to nutritional needs. Measure abdominal circumference to monitor for NEC
- Monitor vital signs and pO_2
- Provide oxygen, positive pressure respirators, and medications to maintain lung function and acid-base balance
- Carefully handle the infant due to friable skin
- Protect from infection
- Provide emotional support for infant and his family

Client teaching for self-care

- Prior to discharge, the parents will need to be able to handle all the infant's needs including feeding, respiratory support, and maintenance of temperature
- These infants may be discharged with special equipment including apnea monitors, tracheotomies and gastrostomy tubes and feedings. The parents will need to be comfortable handling all this equipment
- Teach client about infant CPR
- Teach about the need to protect the infant from infections
- Instruct about the signs and symptoms to report to the physician
- Provide knowledge about the need for RSV vaccine (respiratory syncytival virus) during winter months as premature infants are especially susceptible to the organism

Hyperbilirubinemia

- Due to low oxygen tension in fetal blood, the fetus has a high hemoglobin and hematocrit. This condition is known as hyperbilirubinemia.
- At birth, oxygen tension increases and the extra RBCs are no longer needed.
- The infant begins breaking down the excessive RBCs.
- As RBCs are broken down, indirect bilirubin is released.
- Indirect bilirubin (unconjugated) is fat soluble.
- The liver converts indirect bilirubin to direct bilirubin (conjugated), which is water soluble and can be excreted in the urine.
- In the normal newborn, the direct bilirubin reaches its peak at about three days of life and then starts to decrease. This is termed physiologic jaundice.
- In a child with hyperbilirubinemia, the indirect bilirubin level may start climbing within hours of birth or the level of indirect bilirubin is excessive interfering with brain function.
- Normal indirect (unconjugated) bilirubin levels are below 1.4 mg/dl.

Etiology: Following birth, the liver is unable to convert indirect bilirubin to direct bilirubin adequately. The indirect bilirubin builds up in the blood and collects in fat-rich tissues including the skin and the lining of the brain. When the indirect bilirubin level reaches toxic range, the brain will be affected. This bilirubin encephalopathy is called kernicterus. Any condition that stresses the liver will delay the conjugation and increase the risk of hyperbilirubinemia.

Precipitating factors: Causes of hyperbilirubinemia include Rh and ABO incompatibility, prematurity and immaturity, any injury which increases blood cell destruction such as bruising, petechiae, and hematomas, infant of a diabetic mother, cold stress, infection, and breast-feeding.

S&S:

- Yellow appearance to the skin—the skin discoloration begins on the face and spreads caudally. Sclera also appear yellow
- As kernicterus develops, additional symptoms may be seen, such as
  —poor feeding
  —high-pitched shrill cry
  —lethargy or irritability

Dx: Based on bilirubin levels

Rx: Phototherapy. Exchange transfusions are done only in the most extreme cases

Nursing Process Elements

- Provide phototherapy, which slowly converts the indirect bilirubin on the skin surface so that it can be excreted. It is important that the treatment be continuous. Removing the infant from the treatment for extended periods of time will slow the therapy
- Ensure that the child is nude except for genitalia covering
- Cover the eyes with occlusive pads
- Phototherapy converts on the exposed skin surface only; turn the infant frequently
- Use no lotions or oils on the infant's skin to prevent burning
- Provide extra water feedings
- Maintain body temperature within normal limits
- Provide diaper care frequently as the stools tend to be loose and irritating

Client teaching for self-care

- For the infant discharged prior to 3 days of life, the mother will need instructions on monitoring the skin color
  —Expose skin to the sunlight while maintaining body temperature. Care should be taken that the child does not receive a sunburn
  —Provide extra po water to aid in excretion

Infant of a Diabetic Mother

- Women with poorly controlled diabetes will have a fetus that developed in the presence of large amounts of glucose and will thus be large for gestational age (LGA).
- Women with a severe form of diabetes may have vascular deterioration, which leads to poor nutrition to the fetus. The fetus will be small for gestational age (SGA).
- Infants of diabetic mothers are usually immature in physiologic functions and will respond as an infant of a lesser gestational age.
- The placenta of an infant of a diabetic mother often begins to deteriorate prior to the ninth month of gestation causing preterm delivery and/or fetal death. Many physicians choose to deliver the infant prior to term to reduce this risk.
- Because of the size of the fetus, many infants of diabetic mothers are delivered by cesarean section.
- The fetus is accustomed to plentiful glucose in utero. At delivery, the glucose source is terminated abruptly. The infant pancreas may continue to produce insulin leading to hypoglycemia shortly after birth.
- Excessive glucose in utero has been shown to predispose the fetus to congenital defects.

Etiology: Glucose readily crosses the placenta. The fetal pancreas produces insulin and utilizes the glucose. Excessive glucose in the fetal cell is converted to glycogen and stored. Infants of diabetic mothers are often obese.

Precipitating factors: Any woman with a history of producing large babies (weighing over 9 lbs at birth) should be evaluated for diabetes.

S&S:

- LGA infant
- Development of hypoglycemia within hours of delivery
- Polycythemia
- Possible birth trauma due to size of the fetus
  —shoulder dystocia is common in vaginal deliveries
  —potential for fractured clavicle
- Symptoms of immaturity
  —difficulty maintaining body temperature
  —Hyperbilirubinemia
  —prone to respiratory distress syndrome

Dx: Based on Glucose Tolerance Test (GTT)

Rx: Close monitoring of diabetic condition throughout pregnancy, diet and insulin regulation of glucose, and close monitoring of fetus including stress and nonstress tests

Nursing Process Elements

- Assess gestational age using Dubowitz and Ballard on all infants
- Assess infants who are LGA or SGA for S&S of infant of diabetic mother
- Monitor blood glucose at birth and frequently. Provide early protein feedings
- Assist the IDM in maintaining body heat
- Observe for early onset of hyperbilirubinemia
- Assess for birth injuries and congenital defects

Client teaching for self-care

- Provide preventative teaching of pregnant diabetic to assist the mother in maintaining blood sugars as close to normal as possible

Cold Stress

- Loss of body heat is a major event for the newborn and can be life-threatening if not corrected.
- Nonshivering thermogenesis is the major source of heat production in the neonate and is based on brown-fat metabolism.
- Cold stress in the neonate will lead to other physiologic problems including hyperbilirubinemia, hypoglycemia, respiratory distress, and acidemia.

Etiology:

- The neonate loses body heat through evaporation, conduction, convection, and radiation
- The neonate attempts to maintain body heat through nonshivering thermogenesis

Precipitating factors: Premature and SGA infants have less brown-fat stores and thus are at greater risk for cold stress. LGA infants, although they have adequate fat stores, have immature neurologic functioning making them at greater risk for hypothermia.

S&S:

- Decreased skin temperature
- If cold stress has occurred, the neonate will have the following symptoms:
  —lethargy
  —poor feeding
  —hypoglycemia
  —pallor
  —apnea
  —hypotonia

Dx: Based on axillary or rectal temperatures

Rx: Restore body temperature. Intravenous fluids may be required to restore glucose levels

Nursing Process Elements

Prevention is preferable to treatment.

- Dry newborn immediately to reduce evaporative heat loss
- Use external heat source to maintain core body temperature after birth
- Maintain nursery temperature 1°C higher than neonate's temperature
- Locate bassinet away from outside windows
- Wrap snuggly in blankets
- Encourage mother to maintain covering

If cold stress has occurred

- Use external heat source to return skin temperature to desired range
- Monitor temperature more frequently than routine
- Monitor blood glucose
- Assess the neonate for respiratory distress
- Assist the infant in taking formula to restore blood sugar. The infant will be a poor feeder and lethargic

Client teaching for self-care

- Teach mother about the need to keep the infant warm without overheating
- Infants usually need one layer of clothing above adult's needs
- Head is a major source of heat loss and should be covered when out of doors in winter

WORKSHEET

SHORT ANSWER QUESTIONS

1. Discuss how para, gravida, and TPAL are determined on an obstetric client.
2. Discuss the process of determining due dates using Nagele's rule.
3. Describe the initial prenatal obstetrician visit and the frequency of the subsequent visit.
4. Describe the probable, presumptive, and positive signs of pregnancy and the interpretations of these signs.

(continued)

5. Describe the warning signs that pregnant women should immediately report to the physician and their implications.
6. Describe the factors that initiate the onset of labor.
7. Define the four stages of labor.
8. Describe the mother's emotions and attitude during the three phases of labor.
9. Identify the five areas evaluated on the Apgar score and the possible point value of each area.
10. List the three fetal structures of normal circulation during the gestation and what each structure does.

MATCHING QUESTIONS

Match the following:

1. ___ Lightening
2. ___ Quickening
3. ___ Crowning
4. ____ Engagement
5. ____ Station
6. ____ Attitude
7. ____ Lie
8. ____ Presentation
9. ____ Position
10. ____ Striae
11. ____ Engorgement
12. ____ Homan's sign
13. ____ BUBBLE-HEB
14. ____ Caput succedaneum
15. ____ Cephalohematoma

a. A mnemonic to guide the nurse's assessment of the postpartum woman
b. Explains the relationship between the fetal presenting part and the mother's pelvis
c. An assessment performed on the mother to determine the presence of thrombophlebitis
d. The presenting part is seen on the mother's perineum
e. Evaluates the relationship of the fetal presenting part to the ischial spines of the mother's pelvis
f. Compares the spinal cord of the fetus to the spinal cord of the mother
g. Fetal movement
h. Swelling of the scalp if the head was the presenting part
i. Determines which fetal part is entering the pelvis first for delivery
j. The filling of the breasts with milk
k. Stretch marks
l. Bleeding into the periosteum of the skull
m. The presenting part descends into the pelvis before the onset of labor
n. In a cephalic presentation, the largest diameter of the head is at the smallest diameter of the pelvis
o. The relationship of fetal parts to each other

APPLICATION QUESTIONS

1. A woman visits her obstetrician for a pregnancy test that is positive. In taking her history, she reports that she has been pregnant four times before. She has two children at home, one of which was born at 32 weeks gestation. She lost a set of twins at 14 weeks and another baby at 12 weeks. What is her para, gravida, and TPAL?
   a. G5, P4 (T1, P1, A2, L2)
   b. G5, P2 (T1, P1, A3, L2)
   c. G3, P2 (T1, P2, A2, L1)
   d. G3, P4 (T2, P3, A3, L2)

2. The obstetrician asks the nurse to determine the due date for a pregnant client on her first prenatal visit. The client reports that her last menstrual period began on February 5, 2007 and ended on February 10, 2007. What is her due date?
   a. November 5, 2007
   b. November 12, 2007
   c. November 10, 2007
   d. November 17, 2007

3. A pregnant woman at 14 weeks gestation calls the obstetrician's office to report that she has noted some vaginal discharge. The discharge is clear and without odor. The office nurse would instruct the client to
   a. wear a peri-pad to absorb the liquid, which is normal
   b. douche with water to see if that improves the drainage
   c. do nothing, as vaginal discharge in pregnancy is normal
   d. report to the physician's office immediately for assessment

4. While attending childbirth education class, a primigravida asks when she should go to the hospital. The nurse's best response would be:
   a. With the first contraction.
   b. One hour after the onset of labor.
   c. When she thinks her membranes have ruptured.
   d. As soon as she is sure she is in true labor.

5. A nurse is teaching a class of childbirth education to four women in late pregnancy. The women make the following statements. Which statement would most likely indicate that lightening has occurred?
   a. "I can feel my baby move."
   b. "It's hard to sleep at night—I have to lie on my side."
   c. "I feel like my lungs are being crowded by the baby."
   d. "I have to void frequently like I did in the first trimester."

6. A woman arrives at the labor unit in labor. She is talkative and smiling between contractions. Prior to completing the vaginal examination, the nurse would suspect the woman is in what phase/stage of labor?
   a. Latent phase
   b. Active phase
   c. Transition phase
   d. Second stage

7. Monitoring the client during labor is the nurse's responsibility. If the mother is not hooked up to a fetal monitor, the nurse would assess FHT at the following times: (Select all that apply.)
   a. on admission
   b. after each contraction
   c. immediately when the membranes rupture
   d. each time the mother's vital signs are taken
   e. as the mother enters each phase of labor

8. One minute after birth, the nurse performs an Apgar scoring on the newborn. The baby receives a score of 6. The mother asks what this score indicates. The nurse's response would be based on the knowledge that
   a. the higher the score, the more intelligent the baby will be
   b. low scores indicate a baby who has experienced birth trauma
   c. a score of 6 suggests an infant that needs immediate transfer to the high-risk nursery
   d. the score indicates how well or poorly an infant has transitioned from intrauterine to extrauterine life

9. A newborn is admitted to the newborn nursery. A new nurse will be caring for the infant. The charge nurse is explaining bloodborne precautions to the new nurse. The charge nurse would tell the new nurse to wear gloves for what activities? (Select all that apply.)
   a. Admission bath
   b. Daily bath
   c. Meconium diaper change
   d. Urine diaper change
   e. Any contact with the infant

(continued)

10. There has been a rush of difficult deliveries at your hospital and the hospital nursery currently has babies with the following abnormalities. Which infant should be monitored for increased intracranial pressure?
    a. Cephalohematoma
    b. Caput succedaneum
    c. Intracranial hemorrhage
    d. Cerebral petechiae

11. The nurse is assessing a client on the second day postpartum. The nurse would intervene if the fundus was located
    a. 2 fingerbreadth above the umbilicus
    b. 1 fingerbreadth below the umbilicus
    c. 2 fingerbreadths below the umbilicus
    d. 3 fingerbreadths below the umbilicus

12. A new mother is planning to bottle feed her infant. Instructions have been given to the mother to prevent milk production. The nurse observes all the following activities by the mother. Which activity indicates a lack of understanding?
    a. The mother is wearing a tight bra.
    b. The mother does not try to express the milk.
    c. The mother avoids handling or touching the nipples.
    d. The mother takes a long, hot shower with water hitting the breasts.

13. The new mother calls the obstetrician's office at 8 days postpartum to state that her lochia had returned to red in appearance although the volume has not increased. The nurse would recommend the mother to
    a. drink more milk
    b. rest more frequently
    c. avoid sexual activity
    d. increase her iron intake

14. A woman is at the obstetrician's office for her second prenatal visit. She has numerous complaints including all of the following. Which would require reporting to the physician?
    a. She has to void frequently.
    b. She is tired and wants to sleep all the time.
    c. She has a burning sensation when she urinates.
    d. Although she has not vomited, she feels nauseated most of the time.

15. At 20 weeks gestation, a pregnant woman is diagnosed with polyhydramnios. Which assessment finding contributed to this diagnosis?
    a. voids frequently
    b. blood pressure is 148/86
    c. quickening has not been noted
    d. the fundus is two fingerbreadths above the umbilicus

16. Following admission to the newborn nursery, a newborn's rectal temperature is found to be 98.0°F. His pulse is 146 and respirations are 36. Lung assessments include adventitious sounds. Immediate nursing interventions should be directed at
    a. warming the baby
    b. promoting bonding with the parents
    c. calming the infant to slow the heart rate
    d. percussion and postural drainage to clear the lungs

17. A pregnant woman at term is being admitted to the labor room in early labor. During the admission process, the woman's membranes suddenly rupture. Priority nursing activities at this time would include
    a. checking the fetal heart tones
    b. vaginal examination to determine dilation and effacement
    c. cleaning up the woman and making her comfortable
    d. completing the admission process so that all paperwork is completed before delivery

18. A fetus of a woman in labor is found to have a breech presentation, longitudinal lie, and a flexed attitude. In listening for fetal heart tones, the nurse would listen on the mother's abdomen
    a. below the umbilicus
    b. at the umbilicus
    c. above the umbilicus
    d. lateral to the umbilicus

19. A teenager is admitted at term to the labor unit in early labor. She has not attended any childbirth education classes. Her mother is present as her support person. The best time to discuss breathing techniques with this teenager is
    a. during the latent phase of labor
    b. as she approaches transition stage
    c. after delivery in anticipation of future pregnancies
    d. as she approaches each labor stage that requires a different breathing technique

20. A single mother has delivered an infant boy. Which behavior by the mother indicates that bonding is proceeding on schedule?
    a. The mother successfully breast-feeds the infant.
    b. The mother asks questions about the baby's condition.

c. The mother states: "I wanted a girl, but a boy will be OK too."

d. The mother progresses from touching the infant with her fingertips to whole hand touching.

21. The nurses in the delivery room reported a concern about the mother's reaction to her newborn. Mother and infant are moved to the recovery room. Which activity by the recovery room nurse will promote mother–infant bonding?
   a. Dimming the overhead lights.
   b. Allowing the father to stay with the family unit.
   c. Administering morphine to ensure that the woman is pain free.
   d. Limiting fundal assessments to allow the family unit time alone.

22. The nurse is discharging a breast-feeding mother and her infant from the hospital on the third day postdelivery. Discharge instructions relative to breast-feeding have been given by the nurse. Which statement by the mother indicates the correct information about breast-feeding?
   a. "Six to eight wet diapers indicate my baby is getting enough milk."
   b. "I need to limit my fluid intake so that I won't dilute my breast milk."
   c. "I can feed formula from a bottle during the nights until my milk comes in."
   d. "I should weigh the baby before and after feeding to determine if I have enough milk."

23. The nurse is checking the infants in the newborn nursery for hyperbilirubinemia. The nurse knows that the infants most likely to have hyperbilirubinemia are those who (Select all that apply.)
   a. are premature
   b. are full term
   c. have broken bones
   d. have chromosomal disorders
   e. have a large amount of bruising

24. A woman in late pregnancy is complaining of severe backaches. The nurse notes that the pregnant woman's posture displays lordosis. To reduce the backaches, the nurse would suggest
   a. wearing a girdle to support the back muscles
   b. wearing shoes with heels no higher than 1 inch
   c. performing the pelvic tilt several times during the day
   d. limiting the amount of walking that she does during the day

25. A teenager purchases a home pregnancy test. She later asks the nurse how these tests work. The nurse's response is that the pregnancy tests are based on which hormone?
   a. Oxytocin
   b. Estrogen
   c. Progesterone
   d. Human chorionic gonadotropin

ANSWERS & RATIONALES

SHORT ANSWER QUESTIONS

1. Discuss how para, gravida, and TPAL are determined on an obstetric client.

Answer

Para and gravida describe the pregnancies. Gravida stands for pregnancies and is a simple count of every pregnancy including the current one. Para refers to pregnancies terminated after the age of viability (usually considered 20 weeks). Para does not consider the survival of the fetus or the number of fetuses delivered. TPAL describes the infants. T is for term infants (born at 38+ weeks), P is for premature (above 20 weeks gestation up to 38 weeks gestation), A is for abortions, babies lost before 20 weeks gestation (includes therapeutic abortions and miscarriages), and L is a total of the living children.

(continued)

Think Smart/Test Smart

The terms gravida and para refer to pregnancies while TPAL describes the babies.

2. Discuss the process of determining due dates using Nagele's rule.

Answer
Beginning with the first day of the woman's last menstrual period, count back 3 months and add 7 days.

3. Describe the initial prenatal obstetrician visit and the frequency of the subsequent visit.

Answer
A pelvic examination determines presumptive and probable signs of pregnancy. The para, gravida, and TPAL status is determined as well as the due date. Urine will be checked for sugar and protein. Blood will be drawn for blood typing, rubella titer, and hemoglobin and hematocrit. Initial instructions will be given to the pregnant woman about activities to promote health and situations to avoid. The woman will return once a month until the ninth month when she will see the obstetrician every week.

4. Describe the probable, presumptive, and positive signs of pregnancy and the interpretations of these signs.

Answer
Presumptive signs of pregnancy are subjective signs and can be caused by many other conditions including the desire to be pregnant. Probable signs are objective signs and are more closely related to the probability of pregnancy. These signs can have alternative causes and may be misinterpreted as pregnancy. Positive signs of pregnancy refer to the acknowledgment of the presence of the fetus and will have no alternative causes.

5. Describe the warning signs that pregnant women should immediately report to the physician and their implications.

Answer
a. Vaginal discharge, which could indicate premature rupture of membranes.
b. Vaginal bleeding—although some women will continue to have a small amount of bleeding at the time of the normal menstrual period. The doctor will need to determine if the mother is experiencing placenta previa or abruptio placenta.
c. Abdominal pain—could indicate premature labor or abruptio placenta.
d. Temperature above 101°F—could indicate infection.
e. Vomiting, especially into the second trimester—could indicate hyperemesis.
f. Severe headache, dizziness, and spots before the eyes—could indicate pregnancy-induced hypertension.
g. Edema of the lower extremities—could indicate pregnancy-induced hypertension.
h. Epigastric pain—could indicate pregnancy-induced hypertension.
i. Burning on urination—could indicate UTI.
j. Absence of fetal movement—could indicate fetal demise.

6. Describe the factors that initiate the onset of labor.

Answer
Although the cause of labor onset is not fully understood, theories include the beginning of deterioration of the placenta that results in decreasing hormones, stretching of the uterus to its capacity, some factor from the mature fetus initiating labor, and the presence of prostaglandin.

7. Define the four stages of labor.

Answer
First stage is from the onset of labor to complete dilation of the cervix. It can be further broken down into three phases: latent (early labor), active (the period of primary work), and transition (as the dilation and effacement is completed). Second stage is from complete dilation of the cervix to delivery of the fetus. Third stage is the stage of the placenta, extending from the birth of the fetus to the delivery of the placenta. Fourth stage is the beginning of the postpartal period usually lasting from 1–4 hours.

8. Describe the mother's emotions and attitude during the three phases of labor.

Answer
Latent—Happy, excited, and talkative. Good time for teaching.
Active—Busy, concentrating on the contractions, woman is more dependent on others, only talks between contractions.
Transition—May develop nausea and vomiting. Client fears she is losing control. Often irritable and sleeps between contractions.

9. Identify the five areas evaluated on the Apgar score and the possible point value of each area.

Answer
Color, heart rate, reflex irritability, muscle tone, and respiratory effort. Each area may receive a score of 0, 1, or 2. Total scores can range from 0–10.

10. List the three fetal structures of normal circulation during the gestation and what each structure does.

Answer
Foramen ovale—a hole between the right and left atrium that allows the blood to bypass the lungs.
Ductus arteriosus—a connection between the pulmonary artery and the aorta that allows blood to bypass the lungs.
Ductus venosis—a connection from the umbilical vein that bypasses the liver delivering blood to the inferior vena cava.

MATCHING ANSWERS

Match the following:

1. m Lightening
2. g Quickening
3. d Crowning
4. n Engagement
5. e Station
6. o Attitude
7. f Lie
8. i Presentation
9. b Position
10. k Striae
11. j Engorgement
12. c Homan's Sign

a. A mnemonic to guide the nurse's assessment of the postpartum woman
b. Explains the relationship between the fetal presenting part and the mother's pelvis
c. An assessment performed on the mother to determine the presence of thrombophlebitis
d. The presenting part is seen on the mother's perineum
e. Evaluates the relationship of the fetal presenting part to the ischial spines of the mother's pelvis
f. Compares the spinal cord of the fetus to the spinal cord of the mother
g. Fetal movement
h. Swelling of the scalp if the head was the presenting part
i. Determines which fetal part is entering the pelvis first for delivery
j. The filling of the breasts with milk

(continued)

13. __a__ BUBBLE-HEB

14. __h__ Caput succedaneum

15. __l__ Cephalohematoma

k. Stretch marks

l. Bleeding into the periosteum of the skull

m. The presenting part descends into the pelvis before the onset of labor

n. In a cephalic presentation, the largest diameter of the head is at the smallest diameter of the pelvis

o. The relationship of fetal parts to each other

APPLICATION ANSWERS

1. A woman visits her obstetrician for a pregnancy test that is positive. In taking her history, she reports that she has been pregnant four times before. She has two children at home, one of which was born at 32 weeks gestation. She lost a set of twins at 14 weeks and another baby at 12 weeks. What is her para, gravida, and TPAL?
   a. G5, P4 (T1, P1, A2, L2)
   b. G5, P2 (T1, P1, A3, L2)
   c. G3, P2 (T1, P2, A2, L1)
   d. G3, P4 (T2, P3, A3, L2)

Rationale
Correct answer: b.
Para and gravida refer to pregnancies and pregnancies terminated after the age of viability. The woman is now pregnant and has been pregnant four times before—G5. She has delivered twice after the age of viability—P2. TPAL looks at babies. She had 1 term infant, 1 preterm infant, 3 abortions (one at 12 weeks and two at 14 weeks), and has 2 living children.

2. The obstetrician asks the nurse to determine the due date for a pregnant client on her first prenatal visit. The client reports that her last menstrual period began on February 5, 2007 and ended on February 10, 2007. What is her due date?
   a. November 5, 2007
   b. November 12, 2007
   c. November 10, 2007
   d. November 17, 2007

Rationale
Correct answer: c.
Count back 3 months from February and add 7 days.

3. A pregnant woman at 14 weeks gestation calls the obstetrician's office to report that she has noted some vaginal discharge. The discharge is clear and without odor. The office nurse would instruct the client to
   a. wear a peri-pad to absorb the liquid, which is normal
   b. douche with water to see if that improves the drainage
   c. do nothing, as vaginal discharge in pregnancy is normal
   d. report to the physician's office immediately for assessment

Rationale
Correct answer: d.
Vaginal discharge should be evaluated to ensure that the membranes have not ruptured. Only a physician can determine if discharge is normal or abnormal.

4. While attending childbirth education class, a primigravida asks when she should go to the hospital. The nurse's best response would be:
   a. With the first contraction.
   b. One hour after the onset of labor.
   c. When she thinks her membranes have ruptured.
   d. As soon as she is sure she is in true labor.

Rationale
Correct answer: d.
When the membranes rupture, labor should start. If it does not, ruptured membranes could increase the risk of infection. The woman would not go to the hospital with the first contraction. Women cannot always tell the difference between true and false labor. During first pregnancies, latent labor may last several hours and the woman would be more comfortable at home.

5. A nurse is teaching a childbirth education class to four women in late pregnancy. The women make the following statements. Which statement would most likely indicate that lightening has occurred?
   a. "I can feel my baby move."
   b. "It's hard to sleep at night—I have to lie on my side."
   c. "I feel like my lungs are being crowded by the baby."
   d. "I have to void frequently like I did in the first trimester."

Rationale

Correct answer: d.

When lightening occurs, the baby settles back into the pelvis putting pressure on the bladder. Response "a" refers to quickening. Women in late pregnancy have trouble sleeping. At about 36 weeks, the uterus reaches the level of the xiphoid process making breathing difficult.

6. A woman arrives at the labor unit in labor. She is talkative and smiling between contractions. Prior to completing the vaginal examination, the nurse would suspect the woman is in what phase/stage of labor?
   a. Latent phase
   b. Active phase
   c. Transition phase
   d. Second stage

Rationale

Correct answer: a.

In latent phase, the woman is excited to finally be in labor, is able to walk around comfortably and will read or talk to family members between contractions. During the active phase, the woman is serious, no longer laughing and talking but working. In transition phase, the woman may suddenly complain of nausea and will be irritable. The second stage of labor is the delivery phase.

7. Monitoring the client during labor is the nurse's responsibility. If the mother is not hooked up to a fetal monitor, the nurse would assess FHT at the following times: (Select all that apply)
   a. on admission
   b. after each contraction
   c. immediately when the membranes rupture
   d. each time the mother's vital signs are taken
   e. as the mother enters each phase of labor

Rationale

Correct answers: a, c, and d.

An initial assessment is a component of every admission. When the membranes rupture, it is critical to assess FHT as the cord may prolapse. Hospitals will have a routine periodic assessment of vital signs, which will include the FHT, typically every 30 minutes during active labor and every 15 minutes during transition. If FHT were taken after each contraction, the nurse would accomplish nothing else.

8. One minute after birth, the nurse performs an Apgar scoring on the newborn. The baby receives a score of 6. The mother asks what this score indicates. The nurse's response would be based on the knowledge that
   a. the higher the score, the more intelligent the baby will be
   b. low scores indicate a baby who has experienced birth trauma
   c. A score of 6 suggests an infant that needs immediate transfer to the high risk nursery
   d. the score indicates how well or poorly an infant has transitioned from intrauterine to extrauterine life

Rationale

Correct answer: d.

The Apgar score is an indication of how well the infant has transitioned, the higher the score, the better the transition. It does not predict outcome or future events.

9. A newborn is admitted to the newborn nursery. A new nurse will be caring for the infant. The charge nurse is explaining bloodborne precautions to the new nurse. The charge nurse would tell the new nurse to wear gloves for what activities? (Select all that apply.)
   a. Admission bath
   b. Daily bath
   c. Meconium diaper change
   d. Urine diaper change
   e. Any contact with the infant

Rationale

Correct answers: a, c, and d.

Gloves are always worn when the nurse may be exposed to blood or body fluids. Since at birth, the baby is covered with vernix and amniotic fluid and maternal blood, gloves should be worn then, but subsequent baths do not require gloving.

10. There has been a rush of difficult deliveries at your hospital and the hospital nursery currently has babies

(continued)

with the following abnormalities. Which infant should be monitored for increased intracranial pressure?

a. Cephalohematoma
b. Caput succedaneum
c. Intracranial hemorrhage
d. Facial petechiae

Rationale

Correct answer: c.

Caput succedaneum is swelling of the scalp but puts no pressure inside the skull. Both cephalhematoma and facial petechiae are bleeding on the outside of the skull. Only intracranial hemorrhage would increase intracranial pressure.

11. The nurse is assessing a client on the second day postpartum. The nurse would intervene if the fundus was located
    a. 2 fingerbreadth above the umbilicus
    b. 1 fingerbreadth below the umbilicus
    c. 2 fingerbreadths below the umbilicus
    d. 3 fingerbreadths below the umbilicus

Rationale

Correct answer: a.

The fundus should decrease 1 fingerbreadth per day. The woman who has the fundus 2–3 fingerbreadths below the umbilicus is progressing normally. One fingerbreadth is slightly above where we expect but the woman 2 fingerbreadths above the umbilicus is displaying subinvolution, might have a full bladder or uterine atony.

12. A new mother is planning to bottle feed her infant. Instructions have been given to the mother to prevent milk production. The nurse observes all the following activities by the mother. Which activity indicates a lack of understanding?
    a. The mother is wearing a tight bra.
    b. The mother does not try to express the milk.
    c. The mother avoids handling or touching the nipples.
    d. The mother takes a long hot shower with water hitting the breasts.

Rationale

Correct answer: d.

This activity will stimulate milk production. The other activities will not.

13. The new mother calls the obstetrician's office at 8 days postpartum to state that her lochia had returned to red in appearance although the volume has not increased. The nurse would recommend the mother to
    a. drink more milk
    b. rest more frequently
    c. avoid sexual activity
    d. increase her iron intake

Rationale

Correct answer: b.

The change from lochia serosa back to lochia rubra usually occurs when the mother is becoming more active and is overdoing herself.

14. A woman is at the obstetrician's office for her second prenatal visit. She has numerous complaints including all of the following. Which would require reporting to the physician?
    a. She has to void frequently.
    b. She is tired and wants to sleep all the time.
    c. She has a burning sensation when she urinates.
    d. Although she has not vomited, she feels nauseated most of the time.

Rationale

Correct answer: c.

All other findings are normal in early pregnancy. Burning on urination could indicate a urinary tract infection.

15. At 20 weeks gestation, a pregnant woman is diagnosed with polyhydramnios. Which assessment finding contributed to this diagnosis?
    a. voids frequently
    b. blood pressure is 148/86
    c. quickening has not been noted.
    d. the fundus is two fingerbreadths above the umbilicus.

Rationale

Correct answer: d.

Polyhydramnios is excessive amniotic fluid. The extra amniotic fluid will push the fundus higher than normal. At 20 weeks, the fundus should be at the umbilicus.

16. Following admission to the newborn nursery, a newborn's rectal temperature is found to be 98.0°F. His pulse is 146 and respirations are 36. Lung assessments include adventitious sounds. Immediate nursing interventions should be directed at
    a. warming the baby
    b. promoting bonding with the parents
    c. calming the infant to slow the heart rate
    d. percussion and postural drainage to clear the lungs

Rationale

Correct answer: a.

This baby's core body temperature is low. Cold stress will cause the baby to develop hypoglycemia. Bonding is important but warming the baby takes priority. Moisture in the lungs is common at admission to the nursery and the lungs will quickly absorb the moisture.

17. A pregnant woman at term is being admitted to the labor room in early labor. During the admission process, the woman's membranes suddenly rupture. Priority nursing activities at this time would include
    a. checking the fetal heart tones
    b. vaginal examination to determine dilation and effacement
    c. cleaning up the woman and making her comfortable
    d. completing the admission process so that all paperwork is completed before delivery

Rationale

Correct answer: a.

There is a danger that the umbilical cord could prolapse if the membranes rupture prior to full engagement so the priority action is to check fetal heart tones.

18. A fetus of a woman in labor is found to have a breech presentation, longitudinal lie and a flexed attitude. In listening for fetal heart tones, the nurse would listen on the mother's abdomen
    a. below the umbilicus
    b. at the umbilicus
    c. above the umbilicus
    d. lateral to the umbilicus

Rationale

Correct answer: c.

In a breech presentation, the fetal heart tones are heard above the umbilicus.

19. A teenager is admitted at term to the labor unit in early labor. She has not attended any childbirth education classes. Her mother is present as her support person. The best time to discuss breathing techniques with this teenager is
    a. during the latent phase of labor
    b. as she approaches transition stage
    c. after delivery in anticipation of future pregnancies
    d. as she approaches each labor stage that requires a different breathing technique

Rationale

Correct answer: a.

During the latent phase, the teenager is alert and able to learn. When labor is active, it is hard for a woman to concentrate.

20. A single mother has delivered an infant boy. Which behavior by the mother indicates that bonding is proceeding on schedule?
    a. The mother successfully breast-feeds the infant.
    b. The mother asks questions about the baby's condition.
    c. The mother states: "I wanted a girl, but a boy will be OK too."
    d. The mother progresses from touching the infant with her fingertips to whole hand touching.

Rationale

Correct answer: d.

A woman will explore the newborn first with fingertips, progress to whole hand and then to enclosing the infant in her arms. *En face* behaviors also indicate bonding is occurring.

21. The nurses in the delivery room reported a concern about the mother's reaction to her newborn. Mother and infant are moved to the recovery room. Which activity by the recovery room nurse will promote mother–infant bonding?
    a. Dimming the overhead lights.
    b. Allowing the father to stay with the family unit.
    c. Administering morphine to ensure that the woman is pain free.
    d. Limiting fundal assessments to allow the family unit time alone.

Rationale

Correct answer: a.

Dimming the lights will cause the infant to open his eyes. Studies have shown that the baby looking back at the mother promotes the mother's interest in her child.

22. The nurse is discharging a breast-feeding mother and her infant from the hospital on the third day postdelivery. Discharge instructions relative to breast-feeding have been given by the nurse. Which statement by the mother indicates the correct information about breast-feeding?
    a. "Six to eight wet diapers indicate my baby is getting enough milk."
    b. "I need to limit my fluid intake so that I won't dilute my breast milk."
    c. "I can feed formula from a bottle during the nights until my milk comes in."
    d. "I should weigh the baby before and after feeding to determine if I have enough milk."

Rationale

Correct answer: a.

Urine output is a good indicator of the supply of breast milk. A breast-feeding mother will need ample fluid

(continued)

intake to produce breast milk. Missing feedings will diminish the amount of breast milk. Home baby scales are usually not accurate enough to determine how much milk the baby is receiving.

23. The nurse is checking the infants in the newborn nursery for hyperbilirubinemia. The nurse knows that the infants most likely to have hyperbilirubinemia are those who (Select all that apply.)
    a. are premature
    b. are full term
    c. have broken bones
    d. have chromosomal disorders
    e. have a large amount of bruising

Rationale

Correct answers: a, c, and e.

Any condition that causes excessive bruising or affects the maturing of the liver will cause hyperbilirubinemia. In addition to those listed above, infants who are large for gestational age and those who suffer cold stress are more likely to have hyperbilirubinemia.

24. A woman in late pregnancy is complaining of severe backaches. The nurse notes that the pregnant woman's posture displays lordosis. To reduce the backaches, the nurse would suggest
    a. wearing a girdle to support the back muscles
    b. wearing shoes with heels no higher than 1 inch
    c. performing the pelvic tilt several times during the day
    d. limiting the amount of walking that she does during the day

Rationale

Correct answer: c.

Pelvic tilt exercises will strengthen the muscle supporting the pelvis necessary for posture. Wearing a girdle reduces the muscle support. Shoes should be flat. Walking is excellent exercise for the pregnant woman.

25. A teenager purchases a home pregnancy test. She later asks the nurse how these tests work. The nurse's response is that the pregnancy tests are based on which hormone?
    a. Oxytocin
    b. Estrogen
    c. Progesterone
    d. Human chorionic gonadotropin

Rationale

Correct answer: d.

HCG is the hormone produced by the chorionic villi and then the placenta. It is the basis for most pregnancy tests.

CHAPTER 7

Test Plan Category:

Health Promotion and Maintenance—Part 2

Sub-category: **None**

Topics: **Growth and Development**
Aging Process
Development Stages and Transitions
Expected Body Image Changes
Family Systems
Human Sexuality
Family Planning

GROWTH AND DEVELOPMENT

- Closely interrelated processes influenced by the inner forces of heredity and temperament and outer forces of family, peers, nutrition, life experiences, and environmental elements.
- In the child
  —There is a definite and predictable **sequence** of growth and development through which an individual normally proceeds (one crawls before he/she walk)
  —These patterns are universal, but individuals progress at their own **pace**
  —There are regular patterns in the **direction** of growth and development; cephalocaudal (head to toe) and proximodistal (center to periphery)
- In the aging adult
  —There is a decline of systems, both physical and sensory
  —There is a loss of fine motor skills

GROWTH

- Increase in body size—quantitative change
- Measurements are plotted on standardized growth charts and expressed as percentile of height, weight, head circumference, and body mass index (BMI) for age.

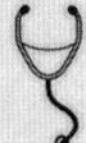

Assessment Alert

A child who is above the 95th or below the 5th percentile needs further evaluation.

DEVELOPMENT

- Increasing capacity to function at more advanced levels—qualitative change
- **Maturation:** the process of aging; increasing adaptability and competence in new situations allowing for relinquishing of existing behavior and the learning and integrating of new, more mature patterns of behavior
- **Critical or sensitive periods:** specific time period during which the environment has the greatest impact on the individual (i.e., if encouragement and stimulation to walk occurs at the critical period, walking will occur more easily than if at another time)

Think Smart/Test Smart

Prepare yourself to answer questions about growth and development from both a normal and an abnormal perspective growthe. Study the milestones of growth and development; this is the normal perspective. Next, stones change to the abnormal perspective by putting "is not" or "does not" in front of each of the normal developmental milestones.

Examples of questions from a normal perspective are "At what age would the nurse expect a child to ________" or "When assessing a 3-month old, which finding would the nurse expect?" Questions like these ask that you identify what constitutes normal development at a specific point in the lifespan. Examples of questions from an abnormal perspective are "When assessing a 3-month old, which finding indicates a need for further investigation?" and "Which behavior on the part of a 6-month old, suggests that a developmental delay or disability may exist?"

DEVELOPMENTAL STAGES

- Stages are approximate age ranges incorporating specific developmental changes and tasks
- The success or failure of achieving developmental tasks within a stage affects the ability to complete the stage and move on to the next stage
- Prenatal period: conception to birth
  —Rapid growth, development of body systems, and total dependency on maternal health
- Infancy period: Neonatal and infancy period from birth to 12 months
  —Initial adjustment to extrauterine life and subsequent rapid motor, social, and cognitive development, when mother and child develop a strong attachment influencing future adjustment and relationships
- Early childhood: Toddler and preschool period from 1 to 6 years
  —Begins with the child's first steps and a vocabulary of just a few words and extends until the child is physically and cognitively mature enough to start school. During these years, the child separates self from others, gains self-control, and develops social relationships outside of the home.
- Middle childhood: School-age period from 6 to 11 years
  —Child shifts away from family to the ever-increasing importance of peer relationships
  —Continual development and refinement of motor, language, and social skills
- Later childhood: 11–19 years preadolescent and adolescence
  —Rapid biological and psychosocial maturation accompanied by emotional turmoil and change
  —Begins at onset of puberty and extends until entry into the adult world
- Adulthood: Young adults from 20 to mid-to-late 30s, Middle adult from late 30s to mid-60s and older adult, 65 years and older
  —Young adulthood: crucial decisions made regarding career, marriage, and starting a family
  —Middle adulthood: life choices are reexamined and changes made if desired; time of giving back to the community and guiding the next generation
  —Older adulthood: time of adjustment to physical changes and losses and finding new ways to live and enjoy life

DEVELOPMENTAL TASKS

- Age related achievements, skills, or competencies normally occurring in a specific developmental stage
- The developmental tasks for each stage must be accomplished before progressing to the next stage
  —Physical tasks/motor development (e.g., learning to sit, crawl, walk)
  —Psychosocial tasks (e.g., learning trust, self-esteem)
  —Cognitive tasks (e.g., acquiring concepts of time and space, abstract thought)

DEVELOPMENTAL CRISIS

- Time when there is great difficulty in meeting the tasks of a specific developmental period

DEVELOPMENTAL AGE

- Achievement of specific developmental skills and tasks related to developmental stage

DEVELOPMENTAL THEORIES OF PERSONALITY, SOCIALIZATION, COGNITION, AND MORALS ARE:

- Freud's psychosexual theory of personality development
- Erikson's psychosocial theory of personality development
- Piaget's theory of cognitive development
- Kohlberg's theory of moral development

Freud's Psychosexual Theory of Personality Development

- Five stages each characterized by the inborn tendency of all individuals to reduce tension and seek pleasure (that which produces bodily pleasure is described as sexual)
- Each stage is associated with a particular conflict that must be resolved before the child can move successfully to the next stage
- Experiences during early stages determine an individual's adult adjustment patterns and personality traits
- Theory is grounded in the belief that two internal biologic forces, sexual and aggressive energies, drive psychological change in the child
- Motivation is to achieve pleasure and avoid pain created by these energies, which come into conflict with the reality of the world, thus facilitating maturational changes

Psychosocial Development (Erikson)

- Trust vs. mistrust (birth to 1 year)
- Infants whose needs for warmth, comfort, love, security, and food are met learn to trust. Infant's whose needs are significantly delayed or unmet, learn to mistrust
- Erikson reasons that the quality of parent–infant interactions determines development of trust or mistrust

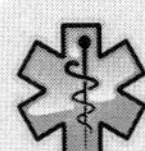

Nursing Intervention Alert

The nurse assesses the appropriateness and availability of experiences that will promote the development of trust.

Piaget's Theory of Cognitive Development

- Looks at age-related intellectual organization
- Defines cognitive acts as ways in which the mind organizes and adapts to the environment
- Four stages, each stage builds on accomplishments of the previous stage in a continuous, predictable, orderly process, however at an individualized rate

Kohlberg's Theory of Moral Development

- Focuses on the development of moral reasoning
- Attempts to explain how moral reasoning matures for an individual
- Children's moral development follows their cognitive development
- Moral development is a complicated process involving the acceptance of values and rules of society in a way that shapes behavior

DEVELOPMENTAL ASSESSMENT

- Essential component of the health assessment
- Developmental assessment tool: Denver Developmental Screening Test (DDST) revised, restandardized, and renamed the Denver II
- Denver II tool measures gross motor, fine motor, language, and personal- social development; does not measure intelligence
- Screening tests quickly and reliably identify infants and children whose developmental level falls below the expected norm and require further evaluation
- Means of recording present objective measurements for future reference

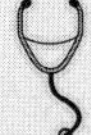

Assessment Alert

Caution: the tests are only as good as the examiner's expertise in administering them.

INFANCY PERIOD: BIRTH TO 12 OR 18 MONTHS

Newborn Infant or Neonate (birth to 1 month)

- **Apgar score:** Initial assessment of the newborn including heart rate, respiratory effort, muscle tone, reflex irritability and color at 1 and 5 minutes after birth. Each item is given a score of 0, 1, or 2. Total score of 0–3 is severe distress, 4–6 moderate distresses, and 7–10 good adjustment.

- **Weight:** Average birth weight = 2700–4000 grams (6–9 lbs).
  —10% of birth weight is lost in first few days of life, primarily through fluid losses and regained by the 2nd week;
- **Length:** Average birth length = 48–53 cm. (19–21 inches).
- **Head:** Average neonatal head circumference is 33–35 cm (13–14 inches) about 2–3 cm (1 inch) larger than chest circumference.
  —**Molding**, or overlapping of the soft skull bones, allows the fetal head to adjust to the diameter of maternal pelvis; the bones readjust within a few days producing a rounded appearance; molding may alter head circumference; head and chest circumference may be equal for first 1–2 days
  —**Fontanels**; Anterior diamond shape; Posterior fontanel triangular shape; (between the unfused bones of the skull); Fontanels should be flat, soft, and firm; may bulge when crying. The posterior fontanel closes at 2–3 months; anterior fontanel closes at 12–18 months

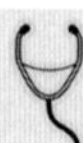

Assessment Alert

Bulging or depressed fontanels when infant is quiet indicates a potential problem and requires further evaluation.

—**Transitions to extrauterine life** include: physiologic onset of breathing, initiated by chemical and thermal stimuli; cough and sneeze to clear fluid present from intrauterine life; pressure changes in the heart and lungs; closure of fetal shunts; the foramen ovale; the ductus arteriosus; increased pulmonary blood flow
—**Heart rate**: 120–160 beats per minute and irregular for the neonate; count apical pulse for one full minute
—**Respiratory rate**: 30–60 breaths per minute and irregular; count for one full minute; neonates are abdominal breathers and obligate nose breathers

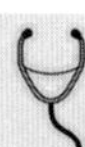

Assessment Alert

Signs of respiratory distress in newborn are: diminished breath sounds, periodic breathing with repeated apneic spells, wheezing, grunting, inspiratory stridor, persistent cyanosis.

- **Thermoregulation:** Newborns are subject to heat loss and stress from cold due to large body surface and thin subcutaneous fat; poor development of sweating and shivering mechanisms; poor temperature regulation. To compensate the infant has brown adipose tissue or *brown fat* which has a greater capacity for heat production than regular adipose tissue to help in heat regulation. Also, the flexed position decreases the amount of surface area exposed to the environment.
- **Elimination**
  —Meconium: infant's first stool should pass within the first 24–48 hours
  —Transitional stools usually appear by 3rd day after initiation of feeding
  —Milk stool appears by 4th day, by 2nd week elimination pattern associated with the frequency and amount of feeding. Breast fed-pasty, yellow, odor of sour milk; formula fed light brown, firmer consistency, stronger odor.
  —Urinary output 200–300 ml by the end of the 1st week
- **Neurological**
  —Assessment of reflexes is an essential component of the neurological assessment, along with assessment of posture, muscle tone, head control, and movement
- **Reflexes**
  —**Blink** reflex in response to light or touch; **corneal** reflex in response to touch; **pupillary** reflex in response to light or touch; reflexes persist for life
  —**Gag** in response to stimulation of posterior pharynx by food or tube; causes infant to gag; reflex persists for life
  —**Startle** in response to sudden loud noise; causes abduction of the arms with flexion of the elbow; disappears by 4 months
  —**Moro** in response to sudden loud noise; infant extends then flexes arms and fingers; decreases at 3–4 months, disappears at 6 months
  —**Sucking** in response to touching infant's lips; strong and coordinated; disappears at 3–4 months
  —**Rooting** in response to touching or stroking cheek along side of mouth; causes infant to turn head toward that side and begin to suck; disappears at 3–4 months
  —**Babinski** in response to stoking outer sole of foot upward from heel and across ball of the foot causes toes to hyperextend and hallux, big toe to dorsiflex; disappears after 1 year
- **Motor Development**
  —Movements are sporadic, symmetrical, and involve all extremities
  —Extremities flexes, knees flexed under abdomen
  —Turns head from side to side when prone; briefly lifts head off bed
  —Little head control
- **Sleep–wake pattern**
  —First hour of life quiet, alert, eyes wide opened with vigorous sucking

—Next 2–3 days sleeps most of the time, recovering from birth
—Sleep periods vary from 20 minutes to 6 hours, little day or night variation
—Wake newborn to feed q4hours (recommended by most practitioners)

- **Sensory**
  —Focus on objects 8–10 inches away and can perceive forms
  —Preference for human face apparent
  —Auditory systems function at birth
- **Cognitive Development**
  —Newborn learns to turn to the nipple
  —Learns that crying results in parents' response
- **Psychosocial Development**
  —Interactions during routine care between newborn and parent lay foundation for deep attachment

Nursing Process Elements

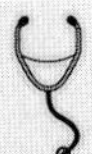

Assessment Alert

Deviations in growth and development require further evaluation, examples: absent reflex, hypotonia, hypertonia, limp posture, extension of extremities.

—Maintain open airway
—Stabilize and maintain body temperature
—Protect from infection
—Promote parent–infant attachment

- Early parent–infant interaction, close body contact, and breast-feeding encourages attachment.
- In the first hour of life, the newborn is quiet, alert, eyes wide-open and vigorously sucking, making this an opportune time to promote parent–child attachment.
- Bonding occurs when newborn and parent elicit reciprocal and complementary behavior.
- Attentiveness and physical contact are behaviors indicating successful parent–infant bonding.

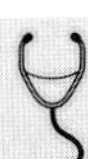

Assessment Alert

If newborn or mother experiences health complications after birth, attachment and bonding may be compromised.

Infant (1 month to 1 year)

- **Growth**
  —Infancy most rapid period of growth; especially during the first 6 months
  —Growth monitored by plotting on standardized growth chart
- **Weight**
  —Gains 5–7 oz. per week for first 6 months (150–210 g)
  —Birth weight doubles at 5–6 months
  —Weight gain slows during the second 6 months
  —Gains 3–5 oz (85–150 g) weekly for next 6 months
  —Birth weight triples by 1 year
- **Length**
  —Grows 2.5 cm (1 inch) per month for the first 6 months
  —Slows during the second 6 months
  —Grows 1.25 cm (½ inch) for second 6 months
  —Birth length increases by 50%, mainly in the trunk, by 1 year
- **Head Growth**
  —Posterior fontanel closes
  —Increases by 1.5 cm (1/2 inch) per month for the first 6 months and by 1.25 cm per month during the second 6 months
- **Chest Circumference**
  —Increases by 2–3 cm. for the first 6 months (1 inch less than head circumference)
  —Chest and head circumferences equal at 1 year
- **Vital Signs**
  —Heart rate 80–130
  —Respiratory rate 30–50 up till 6 months; 20–30 till 2 years
  —B/P 90/50 on average
- **Dentition**
  —Beginning signs of tooth eruption by 5–6 months
  —Chewing and biting 5–6 months
- **Sensory**
  —Rudimentary fixation on light or objects; ability to follow light to midline; and differentiates light and dark at birth
  —Hearing and touch are well developed at birth
  —Rudimentary color vision begins at 2 months and improves throughout the first year
  —Able to fixate on moving object 8–10 inches away, 45 degrees range at 1 month

Follows objects 180 degrees at 3 months
—Beginning hand eye coordination at 4 months
—Can fixate on very small objects at 7 months
—Begins to develop depth perception 7–9 months
—Able to discriminate simple geometric forms at 12 months

—Able to follow rapidly moving objects at 12 months

—Locates sound by turning head to side, looking in same direction at 3 months

- **Sleep**

—Most newborn infants sleep when not eating, being changed or bathed

—Most infants sleep 9–11 hours a night by 3–4 months

—Total daily sleep is approximately 15 hours

—Nighttime sleep hours and amount and length of naps vary among infants

Most infants take routine morning and afternoon naps by 12 months

- **Gross Motor Developmental Milestones**

—Lifts head 90 degrees when prone, sits with support at 3 months

—Good head control at 5 months

—Rolls completely over, good head control in sitting position, crawls on abdomen with arms at 6 months

—Attains sitting position independently, creeps on all four extremities, pulls self to standing position at 9 months

—Walks holding on to furniture cruising at 11 months

—Stands alone, takes one to two steps at 12 months

—Walks alone at 15 months

- **Fine Motor Developmental Milestones**

—Grasps and briefly holds objects and takes them to mouth at 3 months

—Uses palm grasp with fingers encircling object, transfers cube from hand to hand at 6 months

—Crude thumb-finger pincer grasp, bangs hand held cubes together at 9 months

—Places tiny object, such as raisin into container, makes marks with crayon at 12 months

—Builds tower of two cubes, scribbles with crayon at 15 months

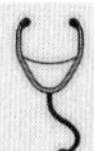

Assessment Alert

Head lag at 6 months requires further neurological evaluation.

An infant who does not pull up to a standing position by 11 or 12 months needs evaluation for dysplasia of the hip.

- **Cognitive Development (Piaget)**

—**Sensorimotor (birth to 2 years)**

—Learning takes place through the child's developing sensory and motor skills

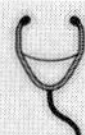

Assessment Alert

Infants need opportunities to develop and use their senses.

Visual, sensory, and tactile stimulation are as necessary as food for healthy development.

Nurses evaluate adequacy of these opportunities.

—The child progresses from reflexive activity to purposeful acts

—Initially the infant focuses on own body; discovers own body parts at 2–4 months; gradually shifts attention to objects in the environment

—Learning by simple repetitive behaviors: repeating pleasing actions; learning that sucking gives pleasure, leads to generalized sucking of fingers, rattle

—Prolonging interesting actions for reasons that result; grasping and holding becomes shaking, banging, and pulling. Shaking makes one noise, shaking more or less makes a different noise

—Imitates simple acts and noises

—Beginning understanding of object permanence, searches for dropped objects

- Can find partially hidden object at 6 months
- Briefly searches for dropped object; begins to understand object permanence 7–9 months
- Develops sense of object permanence at 10 months
- Searches for objects where seen last, even if not hidden at 12 months

- **Language Development**

—Vocalization is distinct from crying at 2 months

—Vocalizes to show pleasure; squeals at 3 months

—Laughs at 4 months

—Begins to imitate sounds at 6 months

—One syllable utterances *ma, da, mu, hi* at 6 months

—Chained syllables *baba, dada* at 7 months

—*Dada, mama* with meaning at 10 months

—Five word vocabulary at 12 months

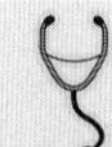

Assessment Alert

Language Developmental Milestone is: First words with meaning "dada," "mama" around 10 months.

- **Psychosocial Development (Erikson)**
  - —**Trust vs. Mistrust (birth to 1 year)**
  - —Infants whose needs for warmth, comfort, love, security, and food are met learn to trust. Infant's whose needs are significantly delayed or unmet, learn to mistrust
  - —Erikson reasons that the quality of parent–infant interactions determines development of trust or mistrust
- **Psychosocial Behaviors**
  - —Parents and infants develop a strong bond that grows into deep attachment as the parent cares for the newborn
  - —Stares at parents' face when parent talks to infant at 1 month
  - —Smiles socially at 2 months
  - —Recognizes familiar faces at 3 months
  - —Demands attention, enjoys social interaction with people at 4 months
  - —May show aggressiveness by occasional biting
  - —Plays peekaboo and pat-a-cake at 11 months
- **Fears**
  - —Begins to express fear; anticipates fear of mutilation, animal noises, the dark
  - —**Stranger anxiety** begins at around 6 months and intensifies in the following months, consistent stranger anxiety at 8 months
- **Psychosexual Development (Freud)**
  - —**Oral** stage (birth to 1 year)
  - —Actions center on oral activities. The infant sucks, tastes, bites, chews, swallows, and vocalizes for pleasure

Nursing Process Elements

- **Communication with Infant**
  - —Talking softly, singing, rocking, cuddling

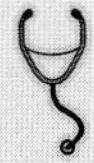

Assessment Alert

Assess the appropriateness and availability of experiences that will promote the development of trust.

- **Nursing Care of the Hospitalized Infant**
  - —Encourage parent to stay and provide care for infant; hospitalized infants experiencing repeated bodily intrusions, multiple caregivers, and separation from the parent are at risk for difficulty with establishing boundaries and building trust
  - —Diminish stranger anxiety by limiting the number of caregivers who have contact with the infant

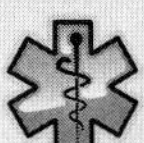

Nursing Intervention Alert

Parents of infants that are ill, have congenital defects, or who are hearing or visually impaired will need extra support and teaching on how to compensate and minimize developmental delay for those children. Nurses play an instrumental role in teaching, modeling interactions, and care for the compromised infant.

Preparing The Infant For Procedures

- Speak softly and handle gently, but firmly, have calm, unhurried approach
- Keep infant in view of parent; if possible have parent hold infant; upright position tolerated best; encourage parent to cuddle infant after procedure; if parent not available place familiar stuffed animal near infant
- **Diminish stranger anxiety**; have primary nurse perform or assist with procedure; limit number of strangers entering room during procedure
- **Sensorimotor** considerations; use sensory soothing measures; firm gentle handling and stroking; hugging and cuddling; soothing, calming, quiet voice
- Analgesics as needed
- Do not perform painful procedures in crib
- Expect older infants to resist; restrain safely if needed

Parent teaching

- **Caring for the infant:**
  - —Care of umbilicus and circumcision
  - —Support of thermoregulation in neonate
  - —Prevention of diaper rash, skin care
  - —Care of the teeth
    - Clean teeth with damp cloth
    - Frozen teething ring to reduce inflammation and manage pain
    - Tylenol may be given for teething pain disrupting sleep and feeding
    - Topical baby Ora Jel, benzocaine, may be used if instructions followed carefully
    - Prevent dental carries by avoiding having infant falling asleep with bottle, causing milk to linger, avoid apple juice bottles for older infants before sleep
    - Fluoride supplement at 6 months and up for breast or formula fed, if water supply not adequately fluorinated
    - Stress management/prevention of abuse/**shaken baby syndrome**

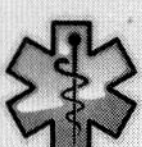

Nursing Intervention Alert

Alert parents to major causes of injury and death: aspiration of foreign objects, suffocation, falls, poisoning, burns, motor vehicular injuries, and teach prevention.

- **Safety:**
  - —Use federally approved infant car seat, teach proper installation facing rear, place in back seat, not in a seat with an air bag. Infants up to 9 kg (20 lb) and younger than 1 year should face rear
  - —Check bathing water temperature/formula temperature
  - —Ensure crib mattress fits snugly; no pillow or comforter in the crib
  - —Position supine or supported on side for sleep until infant can turn over because prone position may increase sudden infant death syndrome (SIDS). SIDS—sudden unexpected unexplained death of a seemingly healthy infant
  - —Only use pacifier with one-piece construction and loop handle
  - —Do not warm frozen breast milk in the microwave causing uneven warming and risk for burns; defrost in refrigerator, then run under warm water
  - —Never leave infant on raised, unguarded surface (may roll)
  - —Restrain in infant seat
  - —Remove bib before putting infant in crib
  - —Inspect toys for small removable parts
- **Older infant:**
  - —Keep phone number of poison control center posted near telephones or programmed in speed dial
  - —Be sure paint on furniture does not contain lead
  - —Teach danger of latex balloons
  - —Restrain in high chair
  - —Keep crib away from windows or other furniture
- **Child proofing the environment:**
  - —Install gates to block stairways
  - —Place safety plugs in electrical outlets
  - —Remove hanging electrical wires; remove tablecloths
  - —Use cabinet locks; use child protective caps
  - —Place cleaning solutions and medications out of reach
  - —Never leave child alone in bathtub
- **Infant nutrition:**
  - —Breast milk is a complete and healthful diet for the first 6 months; importance of breast-feeding mother being well nourished
  - —Support choice to use commercial iron fortified formula if breast-feeding not desirable to mother or not a feasible option; recommend mixing powdered formula with bottled water, if water supply has lead or other impurities
  - —No additional fluids needed during first 4–6 months, will fill infant up, not allowing for adequate nutritional calories
  - —Cows milk, imitation milks are **not acceptable**
  - —Breast milk or formula primary source of nutrition in second 6 months as well
  - —Gradual introduction of solid foods during second 6 months; starting with cereals, fruits, vegetables, and meats
  - —Finger foods: Teething crackers; zwieback can be given at 6 months, fresh fruit, at 8–9 months (not grapes); many table foods by 12 months
  - —Do not feed nuts, food with pits, hot dogs, or any foods that could block the airway or have risk of choking
  - —Honey not given in first year, a source of botulism
  - —Supplements include: vitamin D, iron by 4–6 months (fetal iron stores are depleted), vitamin B_{12} may be needed if mother's intake is inadequate
  - —Fluoride beginning at 6 months
- **Play, stimulation and toys (Birth to 6 months):**
  - —Importance of talking to infant at close range, singing to infant using soft tone, cuddling, caressing (enhance attachment), and rocking infant
  - —Place nude on soft surface and gently massage body and exercise extremities (swimming motion)
  - —Provide musical toys; rattles; soft cuddly stuffed toys; squeeze toys; toys with black and white designs and bright colors; hang musical mobiles within 8–10 inches from infant's face
  - —Place infant in front of unbreakable mirrors
  - —Use an infant seat; infant swing; cradle gym; and take for walks in stroller
  - —Allow infant to splash in tub
  - —Place on floor to encourage rolling over, crawling, and sitting, starting at 4 months and continue throughout infancy
  - —Encourage parent to teach language: Teach to repeat sounds infant makes, laugh when infant laughs, call by name, pick up infant, say "up"
- **Play, stimulation and toys (6–12 months):**
  - —Play hide and seek, peekaboo, hiding face in towel, pat-a-cake, bang a drum, give ball of yarn to pull apart, "catch running water," swimming in shallow baby pool or bathtub, play ball; rolling to child, take to place where can see animals, other children, people
  - —Put toys out of reach and encourage to get them

—Play with large toys with movable parts, noisemakers, stacking toys, blocks, pots, pans, push and pull toys, large puzzles with few pieces

—Read to infant: nursery rhymes, books with various textures, books with large bright pictures; encourage infant to turn pages

—Demonstrate building 2-block tower, stacking toys, placing objects into container

- **Discipline:**

—Consistently and promptly meeting infant's needs builds trust; does not "spoil" infant

—Setting limits is appropriate and will be required in establishing nighttime routine

—Corporal punishment is unacceptable

TODDLER (1–3 YEARS)

- Time of intense activity, exploration of the environment and discovery.
- Developmental tasks: acquisition of language and the ability to communicate verbally, learning socially acceptable behavior, coping with separation from parent, coping with delayed gratification, and controlling bodily functions
- Transition into toddlerhood begins when the child walks independently and extends until the toddler walks and runs with ease
- Development of motor skills allows the child to participate in dressing and feeding
- Sphincter control allows for toilet training

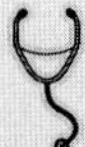

Assessment Alert

Parents report extreme frustration with setting limits and promoting independence at the same time. Be alert to risk for child abuse. Parenting classes are very helpful for support, valuable information, and socialization for the parent with other parents with similar challenges.

- **Physical Growth**

—**Growth** rate slows down during toddler years

—**Weight** average weight gain is 4–6 lbs. per year; (1.8–2.7 kg). The average weight of a 2-year old is 27 lbs (12.2 kg)

—**Height** average toddler grows 3 inches (7.5 cm) per year; average 2-year old is 34 inches (86.5 cm)

—**Head** circumference equals chest circumference for ages 1–2—Anterior fontanel closes at 18 months

—**Chest circumference** exceeds head circumference after age 2

- **Vital Signs**—cardiopulmonary system stabilizes

—Heart rate slows to approximately 110

—Respiratory rate slows to 25

—B/P average 90/50

- **Dentition**

—Primary dentition completed (20 deciduous teeth) by 2½ years

- **Sensory**

—Visual acuity: Binocular vision is fully developed; depth perception continues to develop

—Hearing, touch, taste, and smell become more refined and increasingly coordinated with each other

- **Elimination and Toilet Training**

—Gaining sphincter control

—Readiness for toilet training; stays dry for 2 hours; regular bowel movements; wants to have soiled diaper changed without delay; motor readiness

—Urinary output 500–1000 ml/day

- **Sleep**

—An average of 12 hours a day

—Most toddlers nap once a day until age 3 or 4

—Sleep problems related to fears of separation

—Bedtime rituals, and objects that represent security such as stuffed animals and special blanket are helpful

- **Gross Motor Development**

—Locomotion is the major gross motor development

—Walks independently by age 12–15 months, uses wide stance, protuberant abdomen, and hands out to the side for balance

—Walks up stairs, holding on to wall at first, both feet on the same step before continuing and when masters going up, is ready for the upright mode for going down the stairs by 2–2½ years

—Jumps with both feet at 2½ years

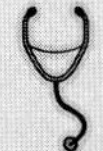

Assessment Alert

Walking independently is a developmental milestone.

- **Fine Motor Development**

—Can build towers by 2 years

—Draws lines at 2 years

—Ability to help with dressing/undressing at 18 months; can dress himself at 24 months

—Draws stick figures by 3 years

- **Safety**
  - —Many safety concerns in toddlerhood related to increasing motor development and the toddlers' exploration of the environment
- **Cognitive Development (Piaget)**
  - —Continued **sensorimotor stage** and beginning **preoperational thought**
  - —Actions become intentional and coordinated
  - —Tries new actions to see what happens and holds thought for later action
  - —**Object permanence**, retains image of person or object out of sight and senses self as separate from others, signals the transition to **preoperational thought (2–7 years)**, which is divided into **preconceptual** and **intuitive thought**
  - —Predominant characteristic of preoperational thought is **egocentrism**, which is the inability to recognize that others have a different point of view than their own; events and objects are understood in terms of their relationship to and the effect on the child
  - —Thinking is concrete and tangible, children can only reason with what they see or experience (perceptual thinking)
  - —**Preconceptual** (2–4 years) uses symbols, language, and play for representing ideas as well as recalling the past
  - —**Intuitive thought** (4–7 years) next section
  - —Transductive reasoning: Associates one event with a simultaneous event
- **Language**
  - —Language development continues; speech becomes understandable
  - —Gestures precede and then accompany language during toddlerhood
  - —Points to object and names, e.g., ball, body parts
  - —Comprehension much greater than number of words used
  - —One-word sentences at 1 year "up"
  - —Begins to use short 3-word sentences by 18–24 months "go bye bye"
  - —Uses pronouns "I", "you" at 24 months
  - —Uses first name by 24 months and first and last name by 30 months
  - —Simple sentences; beginning to use grammatical rules at 3 years
  - —Asks questions, "What's that? Who's that?" "Why"
  - —"That's mine," demonstrates desire for independence and control
  - —Favorite word is "no"
- **Moral Development (Kohlberg)**
  - —Preconventional stage
  - —Moral development is closely associated with cognitive abilities and is only beginning
  - —Does not understand concepts of right and wrong but learns to understand that some behaviors elicit positive feedback and other behaviors elicit negative feedback
- **Psychosocial Development (Erikson)**
  - —Autonomy vs. shame and doubt (1–3 years)
  - —Toddlers have an ever-increasing ability to control their bodies themselves, and the environment and need to express themselves and gain independence in areas where they are capable of assuming control. Empathetic guidance and support from parents allows for achievement of successful self-control without loss of self-esteem, thus avoiding shame and doubt
- **Psychosocial Behaviors**
  - —Increasing independence, ritualism, and negativism are hallmarks of toddlerhood
  - —Ritualism: provides comfort and a sense of reliability; has favorite toys, dolls or blanket, bedtime rituals
  - —Negativism: strongly expressed emotions "no"
  - —Temper tantrums; attention seeking behavior; teach to ignore
  - —Possessiveness; beginning awareness of ownership "mine"
  - —After stranger anxiety peeks start learning to tolerate separation from parent; transitional items such as special blanket during separation (nap)
  - —Sibling rivalry common when there is a new baby
  - —Differentiating self from others

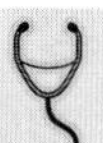

Assessment Alert

Behaviors and emotions of toddlerhood can be exasperating for parents:

Assess for the possibility of child abuse; signs of neglect, or mistreatment; provide parenting classes for teaching, reassurance, and support.

- **Discipline**
  - —Establish consistency in discipline
  - —Behavior is bad, not the child
  - —Ensure privacy, not shame inducing
  - —Time out, 1 minute per year of age
- **Fears**
  - —Loss of parents; separation anxiety
  - —Stranger anxiety
  - —Loud noises, e.g., vacuum cleaner
  - —Going to sleep
  - —Large animals

- **Play**
  - —Play is the work of the child
  - —Parallel play at 18 months, toddlers play alongside other toddlers
- **Psychosexual Development (Freud)**
  - —**Anal** stage (12 months to 3 years)
  - —Sphincter muscles develop and pleasure is centered on the anal region, the child gains pleasure from the elimination and retention of feces. The child is asked to withhold pleasure to meet parental expectations with toilet training.

Nursing Process Elements

- **Communicating with the Toddler**
  - —Use simple, short sentences
  - —Use concrete explanations
  - —Be sure nonverbal messages are consistent with spoken words and actions; do not smile while doing something painful; the child will think you enjoy hurting them
  - —Keep in mind the toddler understand words literally: "A little stick in the arm" they are imagining a twig from a tree in their arm
  - —Provide art supplies and encourage expression through drawing
  - —Play is a form of communication for the child; dolls are good for child to express family relationships
- **Nursing Care of the Hospitalized Toddler**
  - —Encourage parent to stay with child; rooming in
  - —Promote sense of autonomy by providing opportunities for choices; encouraging self-care as is able
  - —Involve the child in his care
  - —Maintain rituals and routine that child is accustomed to
  - —Provide the child with transitional objects (representation of the parent) from home, e.g., favorite doll, blanket
  - —Provide opportunities for play
  - —Prepare parents for regression to previous level of behavior, which is a primary defense mechanism used in response to stressful events
  - —Stages of separation anxiety in the toddler:

    Protest: prolonged crying for parent, rejects others, attempts to find parent,clings to parent when present

    Despair: disinterested in environment and play, decreased appetite, passive

    Detachment or denial: superficial adjustment, cheerful, shows interest, but remains detached
  - —Toddler has no concept of death; primary reaction is separation and loss

Preparing the Toddler for Procedures

- Encourage parent involvement as much as possible
- Communicate using gestures and behaviors; keep language simple; select words carefully, understands words literally (do not say "take B/P," say "check B/P")
- Prepare toddler almost immediately before procedure; keep teaching short 5–10 minutes
- Give toddlers information relevant to them only; how will this procedure affect them; what will they feel, see, hear, and taste (sensory aspects of procedure); the **egocentric** toddler is not interested in the experience of another
- Promote autonomy by providing opportunities for choices and encouraging the child to "help" as much as possible, holding bandages, tape etc.
- Allow toddler to touch and play with equipment that will come in contact with them; or use nurse's play kit
- Use play with dolls and puppets to demonstrate procedures; avoid favorite doll, child believes doll has feelings
- Use distraction; favorite toy; singing a song; blowing bubbles
- Keep frightening objects out of view; young children believe objects have life like qualities and can harm them (animism)
- Tell child it is ok to yell, cry or whatever to express discomfort verbally
- Expect treatments to be resisted and temper tantrums; use firm consistent approach; restrain safely if must
- Reward good behavior

Parent teaching

- **The toddler years:**
  - —Teach importance of attending parenting classes for information, support, and socialization
  - —Teach regarding common behaviors and thought processes in toddlerhood: desire to control, negativism, temper tantrums, ritualistic behavior, magical thinking
  - —Explain that unsuccessful attempts at control often result in negativism and temper tantrums; temper tantrums are attention seeking behavior
  - —Explain importance of ritualistic behavior and that it serves to master skills and decrease anxiety
  - —Explain how magical thinking (the child's belief that his own feelings and wishes affect events) leads to feelings of guilt; e.g., if child wishes that sibling would die and by chance sibling is hospitalized for illness, the toddler will feel intense guilt
  - —Teach to encourage independence but at the same time setting limits and giving guidance
  - —Teach on use of transitional objects, e.g., favorite blanket during separations

- **Care of teeth:**
  —Teach toddler to clean teeth with soft toothbrush and water (dislikes toothpaste), then floss
  —Do not use fluoridated toothpaste because it is dangerous if swallowed
  —Continue with fluoride supplementation, if water supply not adequate
  —Begin regular dental checkups
- **Nutrition:**
  —As growth periods slow, appetite diminishes and the toddler has periods of physiologic anorexia; small amounts of meat and vegetables are of greater nutritional value to the toddler than large servings of bread or potatoes
  —Do not overwhelm the toddler with large portions
  —Limit cow's milk to a maximum of 24 oz. a day; cow's milk is a poor source of iron and interferes with iron absorption, leading to iron deficiency anemia
  —Serve toddler using favorite dish, cup, and utensils (might refuse well-liked food if served in different dishes)
  —Serve toddler single foods instead of mixtures (such as stews); will often refuse two foods that are just touching each other
  —Serve a variety of nutritious foods, repeating them often so that they will be recognized by the toddler
- **Elimination and toilet training:**
  —Do not initiate toilet training during acutely stressful period, e.g., birth of a new baby, divorce
  —Reward desired outcomes

Nursing Intervention Alert

Guide and teach parents' signs of readiness for toilet training: motor readiness; stays dry for 2 hours; regular bowel movements, wants to have soiled diaper changed without delay.

Teach parents: need for patience and consistency; reward desired outcomes; avoid initiating toilet training during acutely stressful period, e.g., birth of new baby, divorce.

- **Safety: child proofing the environment, with increasing motor development:**
  —Place gates to block stairways
  —Place screens and bars on all open windows; safety locks on cabinets
  —Keep all toxic and dangerous items locked and out of child's reach: medications, cleaning products, knives, firearms, matches, plastic bags
  —Use of safety outlets
  —Remove all small objects with potential for aspiration; teach regarding danger in playing with and blowing up balloons
  —Move small kitchen appliances far back on the counter
  —Use tablecloth with caution because toddler will pull on it.
  —Teach parents dangers associated with outdoor play and prevention by not allowing child to play unsupervised; running after ball into traffic, playing in pile of leaves behind parked car; too close to the curb
  —Practice water safety, never leave child unattended even just for a moment, near pool, kiddy pool, bathtub, toilet
  —Use of federally approved car seat for size/weight (high incidence of deaths from MVA due to not using car seat or improper use)
- **Fears:**
  —Provide emotional support, simple explanations, and controlled desensitization
- **Play, stimulation and toys:**
  —Imitation is one of the most common forms of play
  —Toddlers change toys frequently due to their short attention span
  —Toddlers enjoy activities that provide mobility: riding toys, wagons, pull toys
  —Toddlers enjoy activities for fine motor development: finger painting, large piece puzzles, interlocking blocks

Parent teaching: moral development

- Teach parent that moral development is facilitated when parents use appropriate discipline measures:
  —Take advantage of every opportunity to praise appropriate behavior
  —Explain to the child simply why certain behaviors are unacceptable
  —Use distraction with the child to avoid inappropriate behavior

PRESCHOOL (3–5 YEARS)

- Refinement of all skills in preparation for formal education
- More effective communication and less negativity
- **Physical Growth**
  —Slower growth rate continues with continued refinement and coordination of fine and gross motor skills
  —Running, skipping, hopping, drawing
  —**Height** increases $2\frac{1}{2}$–3 inches a year (6.75–7.5 cm)
  —Birth length doubles at 4 years
  —**Weight** increases on average 5 lbs a year (2.3 kg)
- **Vital Signs**
  —Slight decrease in heart rate 70–110 and respiratory rate 20–30

- **Dentition**
  —20 deciduous teeth by age 3
- **Nutrition**
  —Nutritional requirements similar to toddler
  —Continues to reject mixed dishes
  —5-year old is aware of table manners, willing to try some new foods
- **Elimination**
  —For the most part independent with using toilet by end of preschool period, some children still have "accidents"
- **Sleep**
  —Sleeps 11–13 hours; may take afternoon nap till age 5
  —Extends bedtime rituals to delay sleep, 30 minutes or longer
  —Nighttime awakening and nightmares are not uncommon
  —Security object and night-light helpful
- **Gross Motor Development**
  —Coordination continues to improve; child is increasingly agile and graceful; good posture
  —Can learn to skate and swim
  —Rides tricycle; walks up stairs using alternate feet; stands on one foot for a few seconds by 3 years
  —Walks down stairs using alternate feet; hops on one foot by 4 years
  —Throws and catches a ball; skips using alternate feet; hops on alternate feet; jumps rope by 5 years
- **Fine Motor Development**
  —Preschooler developing self-care abilities: can use a toothbrush, lace shoes
  —Drawing increasing in sophistication; draws circles, may add facial features by 3 years
  —Laces shoes; copies a square; traces a diamond by 4 years
  —Hand dominance is established by 5 years
  —Ties shoelaces; handles scissors well; prints letters and numbers; manages fork and spoon by 5 years
- **Cognitive Development (Piaget)**
  —Preoperational period continues: Intuitive thought (ages 4–7)
  —Child exhibits intuitive thought process; aware that something is right but cannot say why
  —Thought process increasing in complexity, able to classify, increasing social interactions, and beginning awareness of cause and effect. Uses words appropriately but lacks real knowledge of their meaning
  —Beginning understanding of time at 3 years; greater understanding of time related to sequence of daily events at 4 years; using time oriented words with increasing understanding at 5 years
  —Uses own name and address by 5 years
  —Understands words literally; bad means bad person
  —The preschooler has **magical thinking**; thoughts are all powerful; if bad thought coincides with wished for event, e.g., wishes sibling were dead and sibling subsequently falls ill, the preschooler will experience extreme guilt
  —Begins to question and compare what parents think at 5 years
  —School readiness (attention span, easy separation from parent) around 5 years
- **Language Development**
  —3- and 4-word sentences at 3–4 years; using 4- and 5-word sentences by 4–5 years, termed telegraphic speech
  —The 3-year-old child asks many questions, talks constantly, uses pronouns correctly, plurals, and past tense of verbs, names objects and people they know, with a vocabulary of 900 words
  —The 4- and 5-year-old children use many more parts of speech, such as adjectives, prepositions, verbs; pattern of asking questions peaks and tells exaggerated stories
  —By the end of 5 years most children use all parts of speech correctly, have increased ability to describe things based on various properties, and have a vocabulary of over 2000 words
- **Moral Development (Kohlberg)**
  —Preconventional stage continues
  —Increasing ability to identify behaviors that elicit rewards or punishments and then labels these behaviors as right or wrong
  —Moral standards are those of others and does behaviors to receive rewards and avoid punishment
- **Psychosocial Development (Erikson)**
  —Initiative vs. guilt (3–6 years)
  —Curiosity and developing initiative leads to active exploration of the environment
  —Activities are attempted that might break the rules, impinge on the rights of others, or be beyond their capabilities, often resulting in unsuccessful outcomes and conflicts
  —Appropriate resolution of unsuccessful outcomes and conflict, will have a tremendous impact on whether the child feels good about himself/herself and moves forward, or is made to feel guilty by an overpunitive parent
  —Parents need to strike a balance between encouraging independence and setting limits. The child needs guidance on what he should and should not be doing
  —Successful completion of the earlier stages requires a loving family environment, allowing the child to engage in relationships beyond the family unit

- **Psychosocial Behaviors**
  - —Pervasive negativism and ritualism of toddlerhood diminishes gradually
  - —Egocentric in thought and behavior at 3 years; less egocentrism at 4 years; begins to tolerate other's perspective at 5 years
  - —Increased ability to separate comfortably from parents for short periods at 3 years, with increasing comfort for longer separations as getting closer to school age
  - —Less jealous of younger sibling at 3 years, (than toddler); sibling rivalry for older and younger siblings at 4 years
  - —Attempts to please parents and conform at 3 years; rebels if parents expect too much, "runs away from home" at 4 years; gets along better with parents at 5 years, seeks parents out for reassurance
- **Fears**
  - —Greatest number of imagined and real fears: dark, alone at bedtime, large dogs, ghosts, thunderstorms
  - —Body mutilation, pain, and people associated with painful experiences
- **Play**
  - —Play is the work of the child
  - —Associative play: children in a group, engaged in similar activities without rigid organization or rules
- **Psychosexual Development (Freud)**
  - —**Phallic** or **Oedipal** stage (3–6 years)
  - —Genitals are central; children recognize and are curious about the differences between the sexes. The boy becomes interested in the penis, and the girl becomes aware of the absence thereof. Exploration and imagination come into play and the child fantasizes about the parent as the first love.
  - —The developing superego (conscience) temporarily pushes these wishes aside as the resolution to this stage

Nursing Process Elements

- **Communicating with the Preschool Child**
  - —Very similar to toddler
  - —Use concrete explanations
  - —Be sure nonverbal messages are consistent with spoken words and actions; do not smile while doing something painful; the child will think you enjoy hurting them
  - —Keep in mind the preschooler understands words literally: "A little stick in the arm," he is imagining a twig from a tree in his arm
  - —Use nonthreatening words, say medicine under the skin, instead of shot
  - —Provide art supplies and encourage expression through drawing
  - —Plays with dolls and puppets to act out feelings
- **Nursing Care of the Hospitalized Preschool Child**
  - —Provide experiences and opportunities the child can master, to minimize regression (dependency), which is the child's primary defense mechanism in stressful situations. Success facilitates return to previously achieved more independent level of functioning
  - —Fears of bodily harm are now greater than fears of separation including: fear of the simplest intrusive procedure such as needles, fear of mutilation and castration, and pain
  - —Preschooler sees death as temporary and reversible, like going to sleep; may view death as punishment, fears the separation and abandonment
  - —Use adhesive bandages after giving injection or any opening to the skin; is afraid "insides will fall out"
  - —Encourage independence; provide opportunities for decision making; encourage self-care; praise and give rewards for accomplishments
  - —Protect from guilt; explain no one is to blame for illness
  - —Use puppets, dolls, nurse play kits, to demonstrate and act out and demonstrate procedures

Preparing the Preschool Child for Procedures

- Encourage parent to remain with child as much as possible
- Prepare preschool age shortly before procedure; 10–15 minute teaching sessions
- Encourage questions and praise suggestions
- Reassure preschooler that he or she is not responsible for illness and procedures are never a form of punishment; the child views illness as a punishment due to magical thinking
- Use puppets and dolls to demonstrate procedures; point out on drawing or doll where procedure is performed, emphasize that no other body part will be involved
- Play out experience (therapeutic play); play with equipment; use nurse kits
- Use noninvasive equipment when possible; tympanic temps and oral meds; allow child to wear underpants with gown; preschool child has fear of mutilation, castration, bodily injury; (stage of psychosexual conflict)
- Use adhesive bandages and Bandaids after injections, blood work, or any intrusive procedure with a break in the integrity of the skin. The preschooler believes an opening in the skin will allow the "insides of their body to leak out"
- Explain procedures using simple appropriate language for child's age; remember preschooler takes words literally; when you say "a little stick in the arm" the child is imagining a twig from a tree in their arm
- Use nonthreatening words; say I'm going to check your blood pressure instead of take your blood pressure; check how warm you are

- Provide opportunities for choices; opportunities to help out: hold gauze, remove bandage, tear tape, as the child strives for independence
- Allow child to maintain control as much as possible, own clothing, self-care, simple decision making
- Keep unfamiliar equipment out of view until it is needed because like in the toddler, the preschool child believes objects can perform without human direction and can jump up or bite at them on their own
- Tell child when procedure is completed, praise cooperation and give rewards

Parent/client teaching

- **The preschool years:**
  —Teach importance of attending parenting classes for information, support, and socialization
  —Teach regarding common behaviors and thought processes: child commonly has more fears in preschool than any other time. Fear of the dark, being left alone at bedtime, large dogs, other animals, ghosts, body mutilation and pain
  —Magical and animistic (inanimate objects taking on human attributes) thinking of toddlerhood continues and contributes to illogical fears
- **Care of the teeth:**
  —Teach child proper use of toothbrush and to brush twice a day
  —Supervise brushing and floss for child
  —Maintain routine dental care q6–12 m depending on presence or absence of caries
  —Obtain prompt evaluation by dentist in the event of trauma to teeth (common occurrence)
- **Elimination:**
  —Teach child proper hand washing and to flush
- **Safety:**
  —Preschoolers should be taught safety measures, as they can understand and will listen to precautions
  —Use belt positioned booster seat when child outgrows car seat (40–80 lbs); adult seat belts do not properly fit
  —Instruct on: pedestrian and street safety skills, proper use of playground equipment, fire safety, and pool and water safety
  —Preschooler is curious about fire, so matches, fire arms, must be keep out of reach
- **Socialization:**
  —Needs interactions with peers; benefits from social systems beyond parents, siblings, grandparents, and teachers
- **Discipline:**
  —Fair, but firm and consistent
  —Explain why behavior is inappropriate
  —Short time out to regain control and lessen intense feelings; 1 minute per year, 3-year-old child; 3 minutes time out
- **Fears:**
  —Play out fears with dolls
  —Night-light
  —Exposure to feared objects in controlled setting; desensitization
- **Play, stimulation and toys:**
  —Encourage activities and toys for physical development: jumping, running, climbing, tricycles, wagons, sand boxes
  —Choose activities for fine motor development: building blocks, puzzles, coloring, and painting
  —Most characteristic and enjoyable preschool activities and toys are for imitative, imaginative, and dramatic play; playing house, dress up, dolls, doll house, doing housekeeping chores, playing store, cars and trucks, doctor and nurse kits provide for hours of self-expression
  —Reassure parents that **imaginary playmates** are a normal healthy and useful part of the preschoolers play. It is okay to set a place at the table for the "friend" but do not allow the child to avoid responsibility by blaming something such as the mess in the room on the "friend"
  —Reading is an excellent activity that parent and child can do together (mutual activity)
  —Control time and content of TV or videos also teach parent that children enjoy and learn from educational programming and when watched together with parent becomes an interactive activity
  —Involve in household chores: picking up toys, clothing

SCHOOL-AGE (6–12 YEARS) ALSO KNOWN AS SCHOOL YEARS

- The transition from an informal playgroup or preschool to the structured formal education of the first grade marks the transition of the school years
- The school-aged child must learn to cope with new rules and expectations
- Continues to acquire new skills as well as continued refinement of skills in all areas of development
- **Physical Growth**
  —**Growth** from beginning of school-age years until preadolescence is gradual, steady pace, and slower than as compared with earlier years
  —**Weight** gain is from 4.5 to 6.5 lbs per year (2–3 kg)
  —**Height** increases an average of 2 inches per year (5 cm)

—Later middle years: diminishing fat and change in distribution pattern, slimmer appearance

—**Head circumference:** decrease in head circumference in relation to height; decrease in waist circumference in relation to height; and an increase in leg length in relation to height (indicators of physical maturity)

—**Body systems** becoming more mature: including the GI system, less stomach upsets, immune system, more competent in localizing an infection and producing an antibody–antigen response improves and strength increases substantially

—Independence in self-care is achieved

- **Dentition**

—Primary teeth lost and replaced by permanent teeth during school-age period

- **Sensory**

—Vision reaches maturity

- **Elimination**

—By age 6, most children have full bowel and bladder control

—Nocturnal enuresis (bed wetting) occurs in 15% of 6-year olds, 3% of 12-year olds

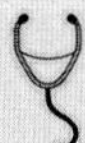

Assessment Alert

Problems with soiling should be referred to primary health provider.

- **Sleep**

—Typically require 9½ hours a night, (slowed growth rate) will require more sleep during adolescence

—Bedtime should be firmly established on school nights

—8–11-year-old children often resist going to bed; child may be unaware of fatigue, if they are allowed to stay up, they will be tired the next day

—Quiet activity before bedtime such as reading, listening to soft music facilitates sleep and establishes a positive bedtime pattern

- **Gross Motor Development**

—Increasingly active

—Steadier on their feet; more graceful; longer legs; lower center of gravity; improved posture; slimmer look; movement more fluid by 8–9 years

—Increasing strength and physical capabilities; however, muscles still functionally immature with risk of muscular damage due to overuse

—Bones continue to ossify (not mature yet) and yield to pressure

- **Fine Motor Development**

—Continual increasing dexterity

—Draws, prints, cuts, pastes, can sew by 6 years if needle is threaded

—Cursive writing 8–9 years

- **Cognitive Development (Piaget)**

—**Concrete operations** (7–11 years)

—Thought becoming increasingly logical and coherent

—Problem solving is systematic and concrete; based on tasks in the here and now (not in abstraction)

—Less egocentricity, seeing things from more than one perspective and enabling concentration on more than one aspect of a situation

—Masters concept of **conservation:** permanence of mass and volume, even if its shape or appearance changes; concept of reversibility, if $2 + 3 = 5$, $5 - 3 = 2$, $5–2 = 3$

—**Classification** becomes more complex, understanding that the same element can exist in more than one class at a time

- **Cognitive Skills**

—Concept of numbers by 6 years

—Knows right and left hand by 6 years

—Tells time by 6 years; develops understanding of more abstract time

—Understands places in relation to space—geography 8–9 years

- **Language Development**

—Realization that words have arbitrary rather than absolute meanings and that words can have more than one meaning

—Learns how to read; increasing ease during school-age years

- **Moral Development (Kohlberg)**

—Preconventional stage continues

—Instrumental relativist orientation: the child recognizes that there is more than one correct view; conforms to obtain rewards; becomes more flexible with time

- **Psychosocial Development (Erikson)**

—**Industry vs. inferiority (6–12 years)**

—The child needs to engage in tasks at which he can be successful and to acquire competence in his abilities. When success is recognized, he feels a sense of worth. If faced with failure, a sense of unworthiness ensues.

—A sense of accomplishment also involves the ability to cooperate with others to accomplish goals; peer approval is a strong motivating power; feelings of inferiority develop if he feels he cannot measure up to the expectations of others, resulting in withdrawal from school and peers

- **Psychosocial Behaviors**
  —Needs to engage in tasks that can be carried through to completion
  —More independence and increased ability to cooperate and share with others starting at 6 years
  —Rules and rituals have great importance
  —Conformity evidenced in mannerisms, clothing styles, and speech patterns
  —Considering others' points of view
  —Develops modesty at 8–9 years
  —Better behaved and easy to get along with at home at 8–9 years
  —Family increasingly important and meaningful at 10–12 years
- **Socialization**
  —Increasing importance and identification with peer groups; most important socializing agent; most important in gaining independence from parents
  —Prefers playing with groups of same sex 7–9 years; continues playing with groups of same sex, with increasing interest in the opposite sex 10–12 years
  —Talks about friends constantly; may have best friend 10–12 years,
- **Fears**
  —Most fears of earlier childhood resolving
  —May hide fears; does not want to be a "baby"
  —Fears include: intimidating teachers; not succeeding in school; something bad happening to parents
- **Play, Activities and Games**
  —Play competitive during school-age period
  —Play is a means to acquiring mastery over themselves, others, and the environment
  —May cheat to win
  —Activities that aid in growth and development include: team games, athletic activities, clubs, reading, music and art, complex board games and puzzles, sophisticated collections
- **Dishonest Behavior: cheating, lying, stealing**
  —**Lying:** may be exaggerated storytelling to impress others; difficulty differentiating between reality and fantasy; parents need to teach what is real and what is make believe
  —Might lie to escape punishment; older children may lie to meet expectations set by others; most children recognize that lying is wrong and outgrow it
  —**Cheating**: ages 5–6, cheat to win, do not want to lose a contest; do not understand that it is wrong; resolves as the child matures
  —**Stealing:** ages 5–8, limited understanding of property rights; when caught they "are sorry" and "they didn't mean to do it" but will do it again
  —Children do not take responsibility for these behaviors till the end of middle childhood. Have the child pay back the money or return the stolen object and teach the child respect for the property of others

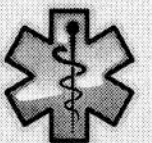

Nursing Intervention Alert

Teach parents the importance of modeling honest behavior and being conscious of setting a good example for children.

If stealing continues it can be an indication that something is seriously wrong, or lacking in the child's life, such as love and the child steals to fill the void; further help is needed.

- **Psychosexual Development (Freud)**
  —**Latency** period (6–12 years)
  —Time of tranquility between oedipal stage of early childhood and eroticism of adolescence. Children experience relationships with same sex peers following indifference of earlier years and preceding opposite sex fascination in adolescence
  —Sexual urges are submerged in the unconscious and energy is channeled into enthusiastic play and extensive learning

Nursing Process Elements

- **Communicating with the School-aged child**
  —School-aged children want explanations and reasons for everything; functional information; what something is used for, how is it used, why is it used
  —Give simple, concrete, accurate explanations
  —Encourage questions
  —Drawing for expression
  —Older school-aged children can use writing for expression
- **Caring for the Hospitalized School-aged child**
  —School-aged child believes outside forces are cause of illness
  —Monitor behavior and mood; primary defense mechanism in stressful situation is reaction formation (acts brave but is really frightened)
  —The nurse can help the child understand his illness and assume responsibility for his general health due to the child's increased sophistication in cognition and psychosocial development
  —Encourage child to talk about fears; common fears in school-aged children are fear of bodily injury, pain, illness, disability, and death

—Begins to see death as irreversible; may interpret it as destructive, scary, and/or violent

Preparing the School-aged Child for Procedures

- School-aged children want explanations for everything that will take place, how it will be done; where and why
- Give simple, concrete, accurate explanations and demonstrations; use diagrams and models
- Encourage questions and discussion before and after procedure; encourage verbalization of concerns (very concerned about threat or injury to their body)
- School-aged children are able to plan in advance for procedures; can tolerate longer teaching sessions, 20 minutes at a time or longer
- Encourage taking notes during teaching sessions
- Assign tasks the child can accomplish; encourage responsibility and participation collecting specimens, keeping records, handing practitioner equipment, removing bandages
- Provide opportunities for decision making, (e.g., preferred site, time of day to do procedure)
- Assist the child in taking control over the situation; teach relaxation techniques, suggest deep breathing

Client and parent teaching

- **The school age years:**
  —Teach parent importance of fostering a sense of industry in the child by encouraging and helping him or her to achieve success in school, sports, other activities
  —Teach parent importance of developing independence in the child, e.g., provide opportunities for child to make choices
  —Counsel parents about safety measures for latchkey children including: a list of emergency phone numbers, instruct child to tell callers that parent cannot come to the phone instead of saying they are not home, teach child basic first aid and safety

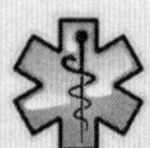

Nursing Intervention Alert

As children will be spending more and more of their time away from home, they will be confronted with many choices; food choices, activities, they may be offered cigarettes etc.

- Teach children about health, safety, nutrition, and exercise
- Teach older school-aged children about drugs, alcohol, cigarettes, STDs

- **Nutrition:**
  —Caloric needs are less than preschool years in relation to body size
  —What a healthy well balanced diet is; the food pyramid
  —Help child differentiate nutritious food from junk food
- **Gross motor development:**
  —Use backpack for books, distribute weight more evenly than tote bag
- **Safety:**
  —Proper use of seat belt while passenger in a vehicle
  —Safe pedestrian behavior
  —Use helmet for bicycle riding
  —How to swim; water safety; depth of water needed for diving
  —Potential burn hazards (matches, gasoline, firecrackers, cigarette lighters, bon fires, chemistry sets)
  —Procedures/proper behavior in the event of a fire
  —Hazards in regards to taking nonprescription drugs such as aspirin, antihistamines
  —Teach child about alcohol and drug abuse, cigarette smoking, and tobacco use. Teach child to say "no" if offered drugs or alcohol
- **Discipline:**
  —Set reasonable limits, keep rules reasonable
  —Provide explanations as to why behavior is inappropriate
  —Disciplinary technique should help control behavior
  —Withholding privileges is effective and fair
  —Include child in process of determining appropriate disciplinary measures
- **Play, activities and games:**
  —Importance of monitoring Internet use due to sexual predators, violence

PREADOLESCENT OR PREPUBERTAL 10–13 YEARS AND ADOLESCENCE 13 TO APPROXIMATELY 18

- Adolescence is the period of development during which the individual makes the transition from childhood to adulthood, with physiological and psychological maturation accompanied by turmoil and change
- **Physical Growth**
  —Reproduction becomes possible, referred to as puberty
  —Body mass increases to adult size
  —Fast period of growth
  —Girls mature earlier than boys
  —Girls: growth spurt begins between 9.5 and 14.5 years, height increase approximately 3 inches a year; slows at menarche; stops approximately at age 16, or 2–2.5 years after menarche

—Girls have fat deposited in thighs, hips, and breasts; pelvis broadens

—Boys: growth spurt starts between 10.5 and 16; height increases 4 inches a year; slows in late teens, between ages 18 and 20

—Boys become leaner with broader chest and have increased muscle mass

—Secondary sex characteristics

—Very conscious of changes in body

- **Vital Signs** approach adult norms

- **Sexual Development: Girls**

—Thelarche: appearance of breast buds, between 9 and 13.5

—Adrenarche: growth of pubic hair, 2–6 months afterward

—Menarche: initial menstruation, approximately 2 years after the first signs of puberty

- **Sexual Development: Boys**

—Testicular enlargement, between 9.5 and 14 years of age

—Growth of pubic hair

—Penile enlargement

—Axillary hair

—Facial hair

—Voice changes

- **Nutrition**

—Nutritional requirements peak during years of maximum growth; 10–12 in girls; 2 years later in boys

—Females have increased risk for eating disorders; ongoing nursing assessment needed

- **Sleep**

—During the time of growth spurts, increased activity, and overexertion the body requires more sleep

—The tendency to stay up late necessitates sleeping late whenever possible

- **Gross motor/Fine motor development**

—Gross motor at adult level: fine motor nearing adult level

- **Safety**

—Feelings of immortality contribute to taking risks

—Peer pressure significantly influences risk-taking behaviors; speeding to show off; doing drugs to be part of the gang; not cool to wear helmet

—Prone to motor vehicle accidents due to: reckless driving, speeding, driving under the influence of drugs or alcohol, failure to use seat belt; risk for diving and swimming accidents; bicycle and motorcycle accidents; sports injuries; misuse of firearms

- **Cognitive Development (Piaget)**

—Formal Operations (11 years to adulthood)

—Abstract thinking develops; uses abstract symbols, scientific reasoning, and formal logic; develops, constructs and tests hypotheses, and reflects on theoretical and philosophical matters

- **Language Development**

—Language development practically complete; vocabulary continually expanding

- **Moral Development (Kohlberg)**

—Transition to the **Conventional stage** between ages 10 and 13, in which the early adolescent seeks good relationships; wants approval of family; increased desire to please others; wants to be considered good by those persons whose opinions matter

—The middle adolescent has a society maintaining orientation: obedience to law and order in society; social order; respect for authority

—In the **Postconventional stage,** the later adolescent solves moral dilemmas by using an internalized set of moral principles that provide him with the resources to evaluate each situation

—There is social contract orientation: the concern with basic individual rights and following the laws of society; he recognizes the possibility of changing laws to improve society

—Universal ethical principle orientation: the last phase of the Postconventional stage and of the theory. Internal decisions of conscience define what is "right" based on abstract principles, like the Golden Rule, without clear rationale or universal principles. Kohlberg later termed this stage theoretical, as few people actually reasoned at this level

- **Psychosocial Development (Erikson)**

—Identity vs. Role Confusion (12–18 years)

—Adolescence is marked by many struggles and challenges. There are major decisions to be made, such as career choice and whether to marry. Identity development and separation from family are essential to successful resolution of this stage

- **Transition to Puberty**

—Young adolescents become very preoccupied with the rapid changes in their bodies and must make adjustments to handle them

—Boys must confront the sexual feelings and desires that accompany puberty

—Girls must deal with the appearance of secondary sex characteristics and menstruation

—Not every adolescent enters puberty at the same time, and there can be considerable inner conflict as each teenager worries about if he is normal

- **Socialization**

—Freedom from family domination is necessary to achieve full maturity

—Adolescents attempt to define their own identity, independent of their parents

—Social relationships serve as important functions in the maturation of identity

—Relationships with parents change from protection-dependency to mutual affection and equality

—Peer groups have a strong influence on teenagers' behavior and self-evaluation. Belonging to a group is of utmost importance

—Best friends provide support for each other and are an important stepping-stone toward development of intimate relationships in the future

—Increased interest in the opposite sex

—Sexual activity in older teens is high, reasons being to obtain pleasurable sensations, to satisfy curiosity and sexual drives, for affection, or to conform to peer pressure. By age 17, more than 50% of teenagers have had sexual intercourse

—Certain individuals become aware of same-sex attraction during the adolescent years, and the challenges that they face need to be addressed so that they can grow up mentally and physically healthy

—Leisure-time activities move from being family centered to peer centered, and teenagers learn to juggle their time to accommodate school, fun, and work

- **Discipline**

—Firm, reasonable limit setting appropriate

—Realistic rules regarding curfew, jobs, homework, and meals are needed

—Criticism or derogatory remarks should be minimized

—Positive behavior and accomplishments should be recognized

- **Fears/stressors**

—Homosexual feelings

—Not being normal or not developing normally

—Not belonging or not being accepted by group; being mocked by peers

- **Recreation**

—Sports, sports events and sports gear, computer and video games, musical events and disc/MP3 players, collectibles

- **Psychosexual Development (Freud)**

—**Genital** stage (Puberty through Adulthood)

—With maturation of reproductive system and sex hormones, earlier sexual urges reemerge

—Energies are invested into becoming emotionally independent, forming friendships, and finding adult sexual partner

Nursing Process Elements

- **Communicating with the Adolescent**

—Facilitate trust; talk to adolescent without parent

—Anticipate shifts in mood and identity

—Give undivided attention, listen, encourage open honest communication

—Try not to interrupt; be courteous, calm, and open-minded

—Try not to overreact

—Avoid disapproval, judging, criticizing, or giving advice; be nonjudgmental

—If taking a stand, make sure that the issue is important; remain open-minded and consider options, then make expectations clear.

—Ask adolescent to clarify meaning of expressions if not clearly understood due to teen culture

—Nonverbal means of communication can be expressed with spontaneous drawing, directed drawing, spontaneous play, directed play, (providing medical equipment or doll house for focused reasons) writing down thoughts and feelings, keeping a diary

- **Caring for the Hospitalized Adolescent**

—An adolescent's concerns during hospitalization include separation from peers, restricted independence, alterations in body image, and illness as punishment

—Potential reactions to hospitalization, therefore, include uncooperativeness, self-assertion, anger, and withdrawal. Defense mechanisms include denial and displacement (shifting focus from undesired objects or feelings to more acceptable ones)

—Adolescents may have numerous questions, psychosomatic complaints, and may question the adequacy of care

—Fear of mutilation and sexual changes should be addressed by providing counseling related to issues of puberty and health

—Older children and early adolescents view death as final and irreversible; may become interested in biological death and funerals

—A later adolescent begins to exhibit a mature understanding of death; may have difficulty coping with death of significant others

—Relate to an adolescent on his own level, respect his privacy, allow him to wear his own clothes and to decorate his room, and promote peer contact, by providing a telephone if possible, and allowing visits and calls

Preparing the Adolescent for Procedures

- Facilitate trust; talk to adolescent without parent
- Respect privacy and ensure confidentiality
- Have parent wait outside if adolescent prefers
- Encourage questions and verbalization of concerns
- Encourage participation

Client teaching

- Adolescence:
  - —Teach parent importance of positive reinforcement and limiting negativity and criticism
  - —Teach parent to be realistic when establishing family rules, e.g., curfew
  - —Teach parent that adolescents engage in risk-taking behaviors due to intense peer pressure and feelings of immortality
  - —Teach parent to encourage and empower child to stand up to peer pressure regarding risk-taking behaviors such as using drugs, cigarette smoking, and driving under the influence of alcohol
  - —Teach parent importance of talking to adolescent about techniques to prevent physical, emotional, and sexual abuse; talking to adolescent about safe sex, contraception, and STDs
- Nutrition:
  - —Adolescent caloric and protein requirements are higher now than at any other time in life; calcium and protein needed for skeletal and muscle growth
  - —Common deficiencies include iron, folate, and zinc (menstruation effects iron requirements)
  - —Dangers of poor eating habits, obesity, anorexia nervosa, and bulimia
- Safety and health promotion:
  - —Encourage discussions regarding standing up to peer pressure, drugs, alcohol, cigarette smoking, anger management and problem solving to avoid use of guns
  - —Prevention of physical, emotional, and sexual abuse
  - —Safe sex, contraception, STDs
  - —Encourage taking first aid course

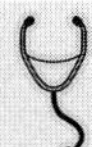

Assessment Alert

Be alert for risk factors for suicide: depression, substance abuse, history of a previous attempt (serious risk); any talk of suicide (must be taken seriously).

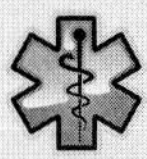

Nursing Intervention Alert

Adolescents who express suicidal thoughts with a specific plan need close observation and professional psychiatric evaluation. Prevent access to guns, razors, prescription, or over-the-counter drugs. Have adolescent sign a contract not to attempt suicide for agreed upon amount of time.

YOUNG ADULT (20 TO MID- TO LATE 30s)

- Challenges and rewards of young adulthood include: starting and raising a family, starting and advancing in a career, economic stability or instability, caring for aging parents
- **Physical Development**
  - —Completed by age 20, exception is the pregnant and lactating woman
  - —Natural process of maturation
  - —Lifestyle assessment: diet, exercise, cigarette smoking, alcohol consumption etc., to identify risks for chronic disease or accidents (routine component of physical examination)
- **Cognitive Development**
  - —Rational thinking steadily increases, educational, occupational, and life experiences dramatically increase conceptual and problem-solving skills
- **Moral Development (Kohlberg)**
  - —Postconventional stage, last stage identified, continues through adulthood
- **Psychosocial Development (Erikson)**
  - **—Intimacy vs. Isolation (young adult)**
  - —A strong sense of personal identity allows one to enjoy adult freedoms and responsibilities as well as love and care for another. When the individual is ready to share their life with another, this task is complete. Otherwise, isolation follows.
- **Other developmental tasks for the young adult**
  - —Unfinished tasks from previous stages should be revisited
  - —Separate from family of origin
  - —Decide whether to marry, begin a family, or remain single
  - —Identifying occupation that matches own qualities, abilities, and life goals
- **Sexual Development**
  - —Freud's last stage of psychosexual development, Genital, covers puberty through adulthood, with no special considerations for the maturing adult
  - —The young adult usually has the emotional maturity to complement the physical ability

MIDDLE ADULT (LATE 30s TO MID-60s)

- Transition into middle age occurs when changes in reproductive and physical abilities become apparent
- This may very well be a time of continuing transitions as individuals reexamine their life goals, life partner, and career

- Major life changes are often made to meet the person's needs, known as "midlife crisis"
- Have an abstract and realistic concept of death

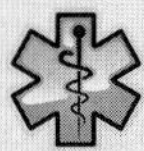

Nursing Intervention Alert

Nursing support, insightful counseling, and appropriate referrals promote resolution of midlife crisis with optimum outcome.

- **Physical Development**
  - —Beginning outward signs of aging such as: hair graying, balding in men (may begin earlier) wrinkles, thickening of the waist
  - —Decreasing visual acuity for many, Glaucoma not uncommon, some decreased hearing
  - —Menopause in women, Climacteric in men
  - —Lifestyle assessment: including diet, exercise, cigarette smoking, alcohol consumption etc. to identify risks for chronic disease or accidents; continues throughout adulthood
- **Cognitive Development**
  - —Rational thinking continues to increase
  - —Decline in cognition is rare
- **Psychosocial Development (Erikson)**
  - **—Generativity vs. Stagnation (middle adult)**
  - —The adult can now focus on raising the next generation, caring for others, and avoiding self-absorption and stagnation
- **Psychosocial Changes**
  - —Empty nest syndrome: Children moving away from home
  - —Reaching maturity: When an individual reaches physiological, psychological, cognitive maturation; feels comfortable with their abilities, accomplishments, and knowledge gained over the years; learns to accept and live with unsolvable problems, shortcomings, and own limitations; accepts constructive criticism, open to recommendations from others, yet not overly influenced or intimidated by others; and is accountable and accepts responsibility for his actions
- **Sexual**
  - —After departure of children from the home, many couples find increased marital and sexual satisfaction

OLDER ADULT (65 YEARS AND OLDER)

- **Physical Development**
  - —Changes in functioning and appearance
  - —Changes in strength and endurance
  - —Sensory changes
  - —Accepting self as an aging person
- **Cognitive Development**
  - —Active learning
  - —May be adjusting to actual declining memory or concern about possible declining memory in the future
- **Psychosocial Development (Erikson)**
  - **—Ego-Integrity vs. Despair (older adult)**
  - —Aging creates many losses with high risk of despair. Searching for meaning in life and meeting these challenges creates further opportunities for growth and integrity. Nurses can contribute to the valuing of older persons
- **Other Developmental Tasks of the Older Adult**
  - —Adjusting to many losses including: death of spouse, siblings, and friends
  - —Adjusting to loss of working role, loss of income
  - —Adjusting to loss of home, might need to move to less expensive, easier access, senior housing
  - —Adjusting to loss of caregiver role, if requires caregiving from children
  - —Adjusting to changing and redefined relationships with adult children
  - —Learning new ways in which to find quality of life
- **Adjusting to Retirement**
  - —A dramatic role change is coping with the loss of work outside the home
  - —Nursing evaluation and intervention is geared toward helping the individual pursue new interests and hobbies, get involved in volunteer activities, continue their education, and may be start a new business career that fits their new lifestyle
  - —Adjustment to living on a fixed income goes along with retirement

AGING PROCESS

- Number of older adults is increasing exponentially compared to any other age group, with the most dramatic increase in adults 85 years and older
- **Older adults** are divided into four groups:
  - —young-old, ages 64–74 years
  - —middle-old, ages 75–84 years

—old-old, ages 85–99

—centurions, age 100 and over

- Most body systems show progressive deteriorative changes to a greater or lesser degree with aging
- Extent and rate of change varies from individual to individual with lifestyle, stressors, and environmental conditions directly affecting the degree of change (decline) that is experienced
- These changes increase the older adults' vulnerability to multiple clinical conditions and disease

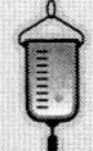

Clinical Alert

The response to stress and illness in the older adult is slowed, and less effective, and so a longer period is generally required for readjustment and return to baseline.

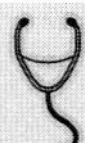

Assessment Alert

Classic signs and symptoms of diseases may be absent or atypical in the older adult.

Confusion, restlessness, and altered mental status are common symptoms and often the **only** symptoms with acute illness. For example, a UTI may present with confusion, loss of appetite, and fatigue, instead of the expected fever, dysuria, frequency, or urgency. An MI may present without chest pain.

- Normal aging changes are called **primary changes** and disease related changes are referred to as **secondary changes**

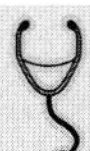

Assessment Alert

Distinguishing between primary (normative) aging changes and secondary (disease related) changes is integral to the nursing assessment of the older adult.

PRIMARY AGING CHANGES

- **Integumentary**

  Decreased elasticity; loss of subcutaneous fat; decreased sebaceous secretions ▶ wrinkles, sagging, dry thin fragile skin ▶ risk for skin breakdown

  Decreased vascular supply to nails ▶ thick brittle nails ▶ hard to cut

  Loss of melanin ▶ graying of hair

- **Musculoskeletal**

  Decreased muscle fibers; muscle mass; cartilage deterioration ▶ decreased strength and agility ▶ risk for impaired mobility

  Shrinkage of vertebral discs and narrowing of intervertebral space ▶ shortening of trunk

- **Respiratory**

  Reduced chest wall compliance; respiratory muscles atrophied ▶ reduced vital capacity; increased residual volume

  Decreased alveoli ▶ possible shortness of breath on exertion

  Decreased ciliary action ▶ reduced cough reflex ▶ risk for stasis of secretions ▶ increased susceptibility to infection

- **Cardiovascular**

  Endocardial thickening; thickened, more rigid heart valves ▶ decreased force of contraction ▶ risk for decreased cardiac output

  Decreased elasticity of arteries ▶ increased resistance to blood flow; mild increase in systolic B/P; cold extremities

- **Thermoregulation**

  Diminished subcutaneous tissue ▶ increased susceptibility to hypothermia

  Decreased efficiency of vasoconstriction ▶ diminished febrile responses to infections

  Decreased efficiency of sweating ▶ diminished acclimation to heat

- **Urinary**

  Decreased blood flow to the kidneys; decreased glomerular filtration rate; decreased number of functioning nephrons ▶ decreased renal function; increased serum creatinine and blood urea nitrogen; decreased creatinine clearance ▶ increased risk of infection; incontinence; and medication toxicity

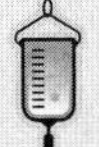

Clinical Alert

The decline in renal function results in inefficient excretion of active drug, allowing toxic drug levels to accumulate, placing the older adult at risk for **drug toxicity.**

Perineal muscle weakness in women > risk for urinary incontinence

Benign prostatic hypertrophy (BPH) > risk for urgency and frequency and risk for urinary incontinence

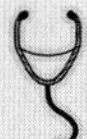

Assessment Alert

Urinary incontinence is a concern of many older adults. Rule out UTI, impaction, teach Kegel exercises.

- **Gastrointestinal**

  Decreased saliva, gastric acid, and digestive enzyme ▶ dry mouth; indigestion; risk for impaired absorption of nutrients and medications

  Decreased peristalsis ▶ delayed gastric emptying ▶ risk for constipation

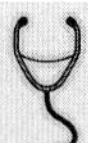

Assessment Alert

Gastrointestinal changes contribute to risk for malnutrition.

- **Neurological**

  Decreased neurons; dendrites; decreased size of brain ▶ delayed reaction ▶ may need more time needed for cognitive processes

  Decline in coordination of brain interactions ▶ causing a slowing of reaction time ▶ increased risk for accidents

  Decreased nerve endings ▶ decreased sensation ▶ risk for burns

  Pain, temperature, taste and touch are all dulled to some extent with aging

  Pain perception diminished ▶ risk for injury

  Taste buds atrophy and lose sensitivity ▶ nutritional risk

  Altered sleep stages and sleep patterns (increased difficulty falling asleep and staying asleep, and sleep may be less restful)

  seem to occur as part of normal aging

- **Vision**

  Reduced lens elasticity ▶ presbyopia

  Increased lens density ▶ difficulty seeing in dim light ▶ risk for injury

  Lens beginning to yellow ▶ colors perceived differently

- **Hearing**

  Nerve degeneration to inner ear ▶ high frequency tone loss; auditory reaction time increased ▶ risk for impaired communication

  Tympanic membrane ▶ atrophied, thickened ▶ many will experience some hearing loss ▶ risk for impaired communication

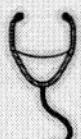

Assessment Alert

Impaired hearing might be more pronounced due to cerumen impaction. Inspect the inner ear and irrigate if warranted.

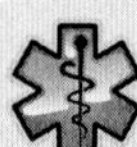

Nursing Intervention Alert

Sensory changes in vision and hearing lead to impaired communication and significantly increase the risk for isolation and loneliness.

- **Reproductive System**

  Hormone production diminished ▶ vaginal dryness ▶ dyspareunia ▶ increased risk of vaginal infection

  Decreased testosterone levels; decreased testicular volume; decreased sperm count ▶ possible change in libido

  —Impotence is a **secondary change** that may be related to medications, alcohol, diabetes, anxiety or other situations or conditions.

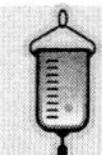

Clinical Alert

Many myths exist about sexuality and aging. If in good health, sexual desire and a satisfying sex life can extend well into the eighties and beyond.

- **Endocrine**

  —Primary change

  Decreased basal metabolic rate ▶ decreased temperature

FUNCTIONAL ASSESSMENT (SELF-CARE ABILITY)

Functional health and independence is described in terms of the ability to perform **Activities of Daily Living (ADLs) and Instrumental Activities of Daily Living (IADLs)**

- ADLs include bathing, dressing, toileting, and eating
- IADLs include more complex activities such as shopping, managing finances, housekeeping, cooking, managing medications, and the ability to use the telephone

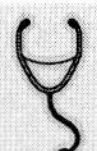

Assessment Alert

Change in functional status may be the only clinical indicator of acute illness, such as a subtle change in ambulation status.

BODY IMAGE

- Mental picture of one's own body
- Not necessarily consistent with a person's actual body structure or appearance
- Includes attitudes and emotions one has toward one's own body, perception of one's value and abilities, and the self in relation to others
- Gradually develops, evolves, and changes as a result of growth and development and the unique experiences from within the self, others, and realities of the world (cultural and societal values)
- Strongly influenced by perceptions of others' views, approval of others
- Actual or perceived change from the norm is cause for concern

BODY IMAGE DEVELOPMENT

Infancy

- Tasks in infancy contributing to body image:
  —Positive messages about body conveyed from caregiver to infant through meeting physical needs, pleasant and nurturing interactions, kissing and caressing which result in feelings of comfort, satisfaction, and internalization of positive messages about self
  —Interest in mirror image
  —Begins to differentiate between self and others

Toddler

- Tasks and practices contributing to body image:
  —Learns names of body parts and increasing usefulness of body parts
  —Looks in the mirror and makes verbal references about himself: "me big"
  —Recognition of gender differences by age 2, gender identity by age 3
  —Beginning comprehension of words used to describe physical appearance such as "big boy" or "pretty" influences view of his own body; positive body image is fostered by using positive language and avoiding labels such as "chubby thighs"
  —Increasing independence and separation from others
  —Learns control of body
  —Respect for the body contributes to positive body image; refer to body parts, especially those related to elimination and reproduction, by their correct names
- Awareness of body
  —Body integrity and boundaries are poorly understood and intrusive experiences are threatening
  —Toddler does not differentiate between nonviable body parts (such as feces) and essential body parts; reason toddler might be upset with flushing the toilet

Preschool

- Tasks and practices contributing to body image:
  —Significant advances in body image development
  —Increasing language comprehension, preschoolers learn that individuals have desirable and undesirable appearances "pretty" "ugly"
  —Reflect the opinions of others regarding their own appearance
  —Recognize differences in skin color and racial identity and are vulnerable to prejudices
  —Compare their size with their peers at age 5
- Awareness of body
  —Poorly defined body boundaries
  —Little knowledge of internal anatomy
  —Intrusive experiences are frightening, especially those that disrupt skin integrity; believes if the skin is "broken" the "insides can leak out," bandages "keep everything inside"
  —Sexual identity developing; sex role imitation, dressing up like mommy or daddy
  —Modesty and fear of mutilation often a concern

School-age

- Tasks and practices contributing to body image:
  —Body image strongly influenced not only by primary caregivers, but by increasing number of teachers and peers

- Awareness of body
  - —Relatively accurate and positive perception of the physical self; likes self less as gets older
  - —Acutely aware of own body and bodies of peers and adults
  - —Head very important to child's perceived image of self with the hair and eye color used to describe themselves
  - —Increasing awareness of deviations from the norm; physical impairments in hearing, vision or birthmarks assume great importance; if accompanied by unkind comments contribute to feelings of inferiority
  - —Important to teach school-aged child about bodily functions using correct information and terminology

Early Adolescence

- Secondary sex characteristics and rapid change in physical appearance heighten self-consciousness and concerns regarding body image
- Lost familiar body and feel uncomfortable with new body
- Either hide or advertise
- Continually comparing self with peers; most comfortable when just like peers
- Perceived or actual defects or deviations are threatening to the idealized image
- Time spent in front of the mirror to see what they look like to others
- Hormonal changes during adolescence influence body image
- Girls perceive increase in weight and changes in fat distribution as evidence of obesity and start fad dieting
- When there is a lag in physical maturation, girls feels out of place, left out;
- Boys feel weak and small compared with their more muscular peers, can no longer compete

Nursing Process Elements

- Compare adolescent's physical maturation with that of parents' and siblings' maturation, when extremes in growth are noted
- Start estrogen therapy before menarche to control height in extreme cases of tall stature if psychosocially indicated; begin growth hormone therapy in extreme cases of short stature if psychosocially indicated
- Listen to distressed adolescents, reassure them that they are normal, focus on positive aspects of personality and body
- Anticipate difficult behaviors or mood swings and support as needed
- Assess impact of physical changes and accompanying mood swings on family
- Teach client and family that hormonal changes are primary cause of changes in behaviors and will pass as body adjusts

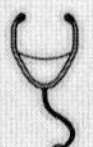

Assessment Alert

Early maturing boys and girls as well as late maturing boys have higher rates of risk taking behaviors than their peers.

Middle to Later Adolescence

- Rapid changes diminish, energies concentrated on making the body more attractive
- Needs the "perfect" body and the "right" clothes and hairstyle
- Practices facial expressions and postures and hair styles and agonizes over a pimple
- Later adolescents have a more secure body image
- Body image established during adolescence is retained throughout life

Young Adult

- Stable positive feelings about self
- **Pregnancy**
  - —Feel big, awkward, may feel unattractive
  - —Increase in breast size
  - —Begins to show during second trimester
  - —Feelings of well-being when baby moves, kicks, or heartbeat heard
  - —Desire for sexual activity may be influenced by body image

Middle Adult

- Accepts inevitable changes in appearance, such as graying of the hair, wrinkles, diminishing visual acuity
- Healthy lifestyle, i.e., physical exercise, balanced diet, and adequate sleep, contribute to a favorable body image

Older Adult

- How the older adult presents self impacts body image
- Changes in appearance threatening to body image: sagging skin, spotty skin pigmentation, loss of muscle tone, fat redistribution, shorter stature, hearing aid
- Changes in function threatening to body image: loss of sensation in a body part, incontinence, dependence on others for hygiene and grooming
- Increased difficulty in maintaining body image during illness

Nursing Process Elements

- Assess body image:
  —What aspects of your appearance do you like?
  —Are there any aspects of your appearance that you would like to change?
  —If yes, describe the changes you would like to make.
  —Long list of dislikes is problematic and requires intervention
- Encourage verbalization of feelings of client and family regarding changes in body
- Assist in fostering a sense of integrity and avoiding despair (Erikson)
- Assist with grooming and hygiene
- Assess impact on primary caregivers
- Suggest caregiver support groups

FAMILY SYSTEMS

CONCEPTS RELATED TO FAMILY FUNCTION

- Family is what the individual client says it is.
- Does not depend on legal or biological ties
- Types of families include nuclear, extended, single parent, blended, skip-generation, homosexual couples, cohabiting partners, multiadult, communal groups with children
- Families change and grow and can be described as going through developmental stages, each of which has tasks which need to be completed before the family can move successfully to the next stage, e.g., family with young children must successfully accept new members into the system; older family must accept shifting of generational roles
- Patterns of relationships in families determine roles and power within families: the resultant structure affects ability to cope and respond to stress
- Very rigid or very flexible structures can impede effective coping: very rigid by not allowing tasks to be assumed by others and very flexible because there are not clear and stable roles and so disintegration can occur in times of crisis
- Family function refers to the processes the family uses to achieve its goals, e.g., communication, goal setting, conflict resolution, use of resources including a social network, nurturing
- Psychological needs of family members must be met or dysfunctional family function results
- Clear, open communication supports effective family function including coping and conflict resolution
- Health promotion and disease prevention is determined strongly by family beliefs, values, and practices which in turn are significantly influenced by educational and economic level as well as cultural background

Nursing Process Elements

- When assessing a client within the context of family, the extent to which the family meets the individual's basic physical and psychological needs must be determined
- When the family is the client, family processes and relationships are the foci of assessment
- Assessment starts with finding out who constitutes the family, the client's attitude toward them, and the degree to which they can be involved
- Existing and potential internal and external resources and supports must be identified
- Collaboration with family members, which requires mutual respect and trust, is essential—all need to understand and agree on the plan of care
- Families need a sense of control; facilitate this by providing options not "musts" whenever possible and by asking for ideas or suggestions
- Help families identify their strengths and see how they will positively impact current coping
- Provide preparation and support for family caregiving: without this the risk of declining health in both the caregiver and receiver increases as does the risk of dysfunctional relationships and abuse
- Encourage caregivers and receivers to make decisions together; this gives the care receiver a sense of control, decreases risk of overprotective care, and promotes a positive feeling about caregiving

HUMAN SEXUALITY

- Feelings and attitudes about sex vary widely; sexual physiology has common features.
- **The Sexual Response Cycle** has four stages:

—**Excitement:** occurs with physical and psychological stimulation that causes parasympathetic nerve stimulation leading to arterial dilatation and venous constriction in the genital area. This increased blood supply leads to vasocongestion and increasing muscular tension. In women, the vasocongestion causes the clitoris to increase in size and lubricating fluid to be secreted. The vagina widens and increases in length. The nipples become erect. In men, penile erection occurs, the scrotum thickens, and the testes elevate. In both sexes, there is an increase in heart rate, respiratory rate, and blood pressure.

—**Plateau:** in women, the clitoris is drawn forward and retracts under the clitoral prepuce; the lower part of the vagina becomes extremely congested, and there is increased nipple elevation. In men, the vasocongestion leads to distension of the penis.

—**Orgasm:** as the shortest stage in the cycle, orgasm is usually experienced as intense pleasure affecting the whole body as the body suddenly discharges accumulated sexual tension. A vigorous contraction of muscles in the pelvic area expels blood and fluid from the area of congestion. In men, muscle contractions surrounding the seminal vessels and prostate project semen into the proximal urethra. The contractions are followed by propulsive ejaculatory contractions, occurring at the same time as the woman, which forces semen from the penis.

—**Resolution:** the period in which the external and internal genital organs return to an unaroused state. For men, a refractory period occurs during which further orgasm is impossible. Women do not go through this refractory period, so it is possible for woman to have additional orgasms immediately after the first. The resolution period usually takes 30 minutes for both men and women.

FAMILY PLANNING

Reproductive life planning, or family planning, includes all the decisions an individual or couple make about having children: whether and when to have children, how may children to have, and how they are spaced as well as counseling on contraception or on how to increase their fertility.

Contraception—natural and artificial methods used to prevent a pregnancy

Natural Family Planning—methods of conception regulation based on awareness of signs and symptoms of fertility during a menstrual cycle; do not involve introduction of chemicals or foreign material into the body

- **Abstinence** (celibacy)—only completely effective means of preventing pregnancy
- **Calendar (Rhythm) Method**—requires abstinence from coitus on the days of a menstrual cycle when the woman is most likely to conceive (3 or 4 days before until 3 or 4 days after ovulation); formulated after six menstrual cycles, the woman calculates her safe days by subtracting 18 from the shortest cycle documented representing her first fertile day; she subtracts 11 from her longest cycle which represents her last fertile day thereby giving her a window of fertility to initiate or prevent a pregnancy

Client teaching for self-care

—Keep a diary of six menstrual cycles in order to calculate "safe days"

—Avoid coitus or use a contraceptive such as vaginal foam during these days

—Calendar method has an ideal failure rate of 9%

- **Basal Body Temperature Method**—basal body temperature (BBT), which falls about 0.5 degrees just before the day of ovulation and at the time of ovulation rises a full degree, is monitored to determine when ovulation has occurred so that activity to produce a pregnancy can occur or she can refrain from having sex for 3 days to prevent pregnancy

Client teaching for self-care

—Take temperature each morning immediately after waking, before undertaking any activity, eating, or drinking

—Use a special BBT thermometer or a tympanic thermometer

—Record temperature each morning for at least 1 month

—Problems with this method arise because many factors can affect the BBT, e.g., temperature rise due to illness can be mistaken as the signal of ovulation; changes in daily schedule, such as starting an exercise program, can affect the BBT

—Women who work nights should take temperature after awakening from their longer sleep period, no matter what time of day

—Ideal failure rate is 9%

- **Cervical Mucus (Billings) Method**—this method used to predict ovulation is based on the properties of cervical mucous; before ovulation each month, the cervical mucous is thick and does not stretch when pulled; just before ovulation the mucous secretion increases and with ovulation, the mucous becomes copious, thin, watery, transparent, slippery, and stretches before the strand breaks; all the days the mucous is copious, or at least 3 days after the peak day, the woman is considered fertile

Client teaching for self-care

—Assess vaginal secretions daily or the change in cervical secretions can be missed

—Feel of vaginal secretions after intercourse is unreliable because seminal fluid has a watery, postovulatory consistency and can be confused with ovulatory mucus

—Ideal failure rate for this method is 3%

CHEMICAL BARRIERS

- **Oral Contraceptives (The Pill)**—composed of varying amounts of synthetic estrogen and/or progesterone; the estrogen acts to suppress follicle-stimulating hormone (FSH) and LH, thereby suppressing stimulation; progesterone acts to cause a decrease in the permeability of cervical mucus which limits sperm motility and access to ova
- **Mini-Pill**—contains progesterone only; does not allow the endometrium to develop fully, so implantation will not take place

Client teaching for self-care

—Must be prescribed by a physician, nurse practitioner, or nurse midwife after a physical examination and a Pap smear

—Contraindications to oral contraceptive use:

- breast-feeding and less than 6 weeks postpartum
- age 35 years or older and smoking 15 or more cigarettes a day
- multiple risk factors for arterial cardiovascular disease such as older age, cigarette smoking, diabetes, hypertension
- current or history of deep vein thrombosis or pulmonary embolism
- complicated valvular heart disease
- current or history of ischemic heart disease
- history of stroke
- major surgery that requires prolonged immobilization
- history of migraines with focal neurologic symptoms
- current breast cancer
- diabetes with neuropathy, retinopathy, vascular disease, or diabetes of more than 20 years duration
- severe cirrhosis
- liver tumors

—Major side effects are nausea, weight gain, headache, breast tenderness, breakthrough bleeding, monilial yeast infections, mild hypertension, depression

—Must take pills consistently and conscientiously; not a good method for those who are forgetful and/or noncompliant with regimens

—Women without risk factors may continue to use low-dose oral contraceptives until they reach menopause

—After stopping oral contraceptives, pregnancy may not be possible for 1 or 2 months, sometimes as long as 6–8 months, because the pituitary gland requires a recovery period before it begins gonadotropin stimulation again

—Ideal failure rate is under 1%

- **Implant Contraceptives (Norplant)**—low-dose progesterone-only device consisting of six soft Silastic capsules that are implanted under the skin of a woman's upper arm; the implant releases hormone over 5 years inhibiting ovulation

Client teaching for self-care

—Major advantage of this method of birth control is that it offers an effective and realistic alternative to oral contraceptives and their estrogen-related side effects

—Sexual enjoyment is not inhibited as may be the case with other contraceptive methods

—Implants can be used while breast-feeding without an effect on milk production

—Implants can be used safely in adolescents

—Return to fertility is rapid (1–3 months after removal)

—Failure rate is less than 1%

- **IM Injection (Depo-Provera)**—long-acting progestin inhibits ovulation for 3 months, reliable and convenient
  —Long-tern reliability without the estrogen-related side effects of oral contraceptives
  —No visible signs that a birth control method is being used
  —Can be used during breast-feeding because it contains no progesterone
  —Must return to the health care provider every 4–12 weeks for another injection
  —Return to fertility is often delayed by 6–12 months
  —Almost 100% effective
- **Intrauterine Device (Progestasert)**—a small plastic device, usually t-shaped, inserted into the uterine cavity; prevents conception by causing a local inflammatory reaction which is toxic to spermatozoa and blastocytes; the Progestasert releases progestin for 1 year and has to be replaced

Client teaching for self-care

—Advantages over other methods; only one insertion is necessary; only one expense; the device does not require daily attention; does not interfere with sexual enjoyment

—Appropriate for women who are at risk for complications associated with oral contraceptives or who wish to avoid some of the systemic hormonal side effects

—Can be used while breast-feeding

—Check after each menstrual flow that the IUD string is in place

—Must have yearly pelvic examination

—Failure rate can be as low as 0.1–1.5%

- **Vaginal Ring**—a silicone ring that surrounds the cervix and continually releases a combination of estrogen and progesterone; it is left in place for 3 weeks and then removed for 1 week to allow for menstruation

Client teaching for self-care

—Hormones released are absorbed directly by the mucous membrane of the vagina, thereby avoiding passing through the liver which is an advantage for those with liver disease

—Fertility returns immediately after removal of the ring

—Failure rate is 1%

- **Estrogen/Progesterone Patch**—transdermal patch that slowly and continuously releases a combination of estrogen and progesterone; applied once a week for 3 weeks; the 4th week is patch-free to allow for menstruation

Client teaching for self-care

—Efficiency of transdermal patches is the same as for oral contraceptives

—Can be concealed

—Mild breast discomfort and irritation at the application site may occur

—Remove and replace a loose patch immediately with a new one; if loose less than 24 hours, no backup contraception is required; if loose or missing for over 24 hours, a new patch is applied and a new 4-week cycle is started; a backup method of contraception should be used for the 1st week of the new cycle

- **Spermicides**—available over the counter as foams, gels, inserts (sponges), and on condoms

MECHANICAL BARRIERS

- **Diaphragm**—consists of a round, flexible spring (50–90 mm wide) covered with a domelike latex rubber cup; a spermicide is used to coat the concave side of the diaphragm before it is inserted deep into the vagina

Client teaching for self-care

—Do not use if allergic to latex

—Always empty bladder before insertion

—Increases risk of UTIs

—Inspect diaphragm for holes or tears by holding it up to a light source, or fill it with water and check for a leak

—Can be inserted up to 6 hours prior to intercourse

—Must be left in place for at least 6 hours after intercourse to be effective

—Wash the diaphragm with soap and water after use and dry thoroughly

—Place the diaphragm back into its storage case

—Have the diaphragm refitted for a weight loss or gain of 15 lbs. or after childbirth

—Failure rate is 20%

- **Cervical cap**—much smaller than the diaphragm, fits snugly over the cervix; used with a spermicide

Client teaching for self-care

—Do not use if allergic to latex

—Wait 30 minutes after insertion before engaging in sexual intercourse to be sure that a seal has formed between the rim and the cervix

—Leave in place for a minimum of 6 hours after sexual intercourse; can be left for up to 48 hours without additional spermicide being added

—Do not use during menses due to the potential for toxic shock syndrome; use an alternate method such as condoms during this time

—Inspect prior to insertion for cracks, holes, or tears

—Wash after use with soap and water, dry thoroughly, and store in its container

—Failure rate is 17%

- **Female condom**—cylinder of polyurethane enclosed at one end by a closed ring that covers the cervix and at the other end by an open ring that covers the perineum; expensive for frequent use and cumbersome

Client teaching for self-care

—Noisy during sex act

—For single use only

—Can be inserted up to 8 hours before intercourse

—Can be purchased over the counter

—Avoid wearing rings to prevent tears; long fingernails can also cause tears

—Protects against STIs

—Failure rate is 21%

- **Male condom**—latex rubber or synthetic sheath that is placed over the erect penis before coitus begins

Client teaching for self-care

—Do not use if either partner has a latex allergy

—Widely available at low cost

—Physiologically safe

—Decreases sensation for men

—Interferes with sexual spontaneity

—Protects against STIs

—Failure rate is 14%

EMERGENCY POSTCOITAL CONTRACEPTION

- **"Morning-After Pills"**—high-level estrogen pills that interfere with the production of progesterone, prohibiting implantation
  —Yuzpe regimen consists of the administration of two fixed-dose combination pills, taken within 72 hours of unprotected intercourse followed by two additional pills 12 hours later
  —"plan B" regimen is a progestin-only based where two pills containing high doses of levonorgestrel are taken (one pill immediately and one 12 hours later)

Client teaching for self-care

—Last chance to prevent a pregnancy: reduces risk of pregnancy for a single act of unprotected sex by almost 80%

—Sooner ECs (pills) are taken, the more effective they are

—Do not interrupt an established pregnancy

—Is a risk of ectopic pregnancy if ECs fail

—Side effects include nausea, vomiting, abdominal pain, fatigue, headache

- **Post-coital Intrauterine Device**—insertion of a copper-bearing IUD within 5 days of unprotected intercourse; the mechanism of action is unknown but is thought to interfere with fertilization

ABORTION is the interruption of pregnancy (induced or elective Ab) or expulsion of the product of conception (spontaneous Ab) before the fetus is viable; several types of abortion

- **Elective Termination of Pregnancy (Induced Abortion)**—procedure performed to deliberately end a pregnancy before fetal viability usually done in the case of an unwanted pregnancy; several methods employed (D&C, D&E, menstrual extraction, prostaglandin or saline induction, or administration of mifepristone and misoprostol)

SURGICAL METHODS OF FAMILY LIFE PLANNING (SEE CHAPTER 18 FOR NURSING CARE)

- **Tubal Ligation**—female sterilization; minor surgical procedure in which fallopian tubes are occluded by cautery, clamping, or blocking preventing passage of both sperm and ova; considered permanent
- **Vasectomy**—male sterilization; small incision is made on each side of the scrotum and vas deferens is cut and tied, cauterized, or plugged, blocking the passage of spermatozoa; considered permanent; failure rate of less than 1%

WORKSHEET

FILL IN THE BLANKS

Fill in the blank with the correct term.

Definitions related to Growth and Development

1. Control of the head proceeding to control over the torso and legs is known as ____________ development.
2. Development progressing from the center of the body to the extremities is called ____________ development.
3. Development progressing from mastery of simple operations to complex ones is called ____________ development.

(continued)

Fill in the blank with the appropriate number.

Milestones in Infancy

1. Good head control at _______ months
2. Attains sitting position independently at _______ months
3. Cruising at _______ months
4. Walks alone by _______ months
5. Grasp reflex fades and can actively hold rattle at _________ months
6. Crude pincer grasp at _______ months
7. First words with meaning _______ months
8. Builds 2-block tower at ________ months

Fill in the blank with the correct type of play.

1. Play alongside another, not with another is called ____________
2. Cooperative play is called ____________
3. Play is primarily _____ in infancy
4. Play is advancing to ___________ play in toddlerhood
5. Play is advancing to ___________ in the preschool child

TRUE & FALSE QUESTIONS

Concept of Death

1. The toddler has no concept of death.	___ T	___ F
2. The preschool child views death as temporary and reversible.	___ T	___ F
3. The younger school-aged child begins to see death as reversible.	___ T	___ F
4. The older school-aged child views death as final and irreversible.	___ T	___ F
5. The adolescent begins to exhibit mature understanding of death.	___ T	___ F

FILL IN THE BLANKS

Separation Anxiety

1. Separation anxiety is a major stress for the hospitalized child during which years?

   ____

2. Describe behavior exhibited for all 3 stages of separation anxiety:

   Protest: ____________________

   Despair: ____________________

   Detachment (denial): ____________________

3. Which of the 3 stages of separation anxiety is seen in prolonged separation?

   ____

Erikson's Theory of Psychosocial Development/Complete the list of developmental tasks and identify its stage

Developmental Task			Stage of Development
Autonomy	Vs.		
Trust	Vs.	Mistrust	Infancy
Industry	Vs.		
Identity	Vs.		
Initiative	Vs.		
Intimacy	Vs.		
Ego Integrity	Vs.		
Generativity	Vs.		

Freud's Psychosexual Theory of Personality Development/Fill in the blanks.

Conflict	Description	Developmental Stage
Oral		
		Toddler
Phallic or Oedipal		
	Time of tranquility	
Genital	Sexual emerges reemerge	

(continued)

Piaget's Theory of Cognitive Development/Fill in the blanks

Stage	Age	Characteristics/Description
1.	1–2 yrs	Learning takes place through developing sensory and motor skill
2.	2–4 yrs	**Preconceptual.** Object permanence is transition to preoperational thought. Egocentrism, concrete, tangible
	4–7 yrs	Aware something is right, cannot say why **Intuitive thought.** Simple classification
3.	7–11 yrs	Logical, systematic, concrete, based on tasks in the here and now, start seeing things from more than one perspective, *masters conservation, complex classification*
4.	11–adult	Abstract thinking, scientific reasoning, reflect on theoretical matters

APPLICATION QUESTIONS

1. Which of the following principles of growth and development is being addressed when the nurse teaches the parent that the infant will develop control of the head before control of the torso and legs?
   a. cephalocaudal
   b. proximodistal
   c. mass to specific
   d. simple to complex

2. Which is a sign of socialization that would be anticipated in a 6-month-old infant?
   a. social smile
   b. shows emotions such as jealousy
   c. begins to fear strangers
   d. smiles at mirror image

3. Which finding in an infant requires further evaluation?
   a. has a strong grasp at 1 month
   b. head lag at 6 months
   c. sits unsupported at 8 months
   d. pulls self to stand at 9 months

4. Which statement by a mother indicates the need for further teaching regarding infant nutrition?
   a. "I will feed the baby only commercially prepared infant formula for the first 6 months."
   b. "I will start skim milk and give an iron supplement at 6 months"
   c. "It is important for the mother to be well nourished when breast-feeding"
   d. "Solid foods are gradually introduced at around 5 or 6 months"

5. Which toy could appropriately be recommended for a 4-month-old infant?
   a. unbreakable mirror in a soft black and white frame
   b. large brightly colored balloon
   c. 5″ doll with removable clothing and shoes
   d. push-pull toy

6. When assessing a 5-month-old infant, which weight parameter indicates healthy growth?
   a. 10 lbs or more
   b. 15 lbs or more
   c. doubles birth weight
   d. triples birth weight

7. At which age do beginning signs of tooth eruption appear?
   a. 2–3 months
   b. 3–4 months
   c. 5–6 months
   d. 8–9 months

8. When discussing psychosocial development with a new parent group, the nurse presents Erikson's theory and identifies which task as the psychosocial task of infancy?
   a. trust versus mistrust
   b. oral versus anal
   c. sensation versus mobilization
   d. initiative versus guilt

9. Which is the best description of the function of the Denver II developmental assessment tool?
   a. measures fine and gross motor development and intelligence and is a means of recording measurements
   b. objectively measures cognitive development
   c. measures gross and fine motor, language and personal-social development and is a means of recording objective measurements
   d. measures psychosocial and cognitive development

10. When asked by a child's parent about Freud's theory of psychosexual development, which response by the nurse would be most accurate?
    a. Each stage of development is characterized by the inborn tendency of all individuals to reduce tension and seek pleasure and is associated with a particular conflict that must be resolved before moving on to the next stage
    b. Experiences during early childhood determine a child's pleasure-seeking behaviors but have little impact on later relationship and adjustment patterns
    c. Freud identified 8 stages of psychosocial conflicts and tasks that the individual strives to master from infancy through adulthood
    d. During the Latency stage of development patterns of pleasure, reward and guilt become established.

11. When assessing of an 11-month old, which the following developmental milestone achievements would the nurse expect to find as being the most recently achieved?
    a. Rolls completely over from back to abdomen
    b. Attains sitting position independently
    c. Walks holding on to furniture, cruising
    d. Develops crude thumb-finger pincer grasp

12. Which is the first stage of Piaget's theory of cognitive development?
    a. sensorimotor stage
    b. oral stage
    c. preoperational
    d development of trust

13. During the routine well check-up visit of an 18-month old, the mother asks the nurse the reason for her son's protruding abdomen. Which is a correct response for the nurse to give?
    a. Increased food intake at this age causes distention
    b. Underdeveloped abdominal muscles bulge
    c. Growth of the liver causes temporary protrusion
    d. It is uncommon in toddlers and requires further assessment

14. The nurse teaches the parent about readiness for toileting. Which event indicates that the time is not yet right for toilet training?
    a. Wakes up dry from a nap
    b. Stays dry for 2 hours
    c. Wants to have soiled diaper changed promptly
    d. Moves with family to new home with bathroom adjacent to bedroom

15. When discussing development with parents of a young child's play group, which would the nurse correctly identify as the psychosocial development task of the preschool child?
    a. Initiative versus guilt
    b. Autonomy versus shame and doubt
    c. Industry versus inferiority
    d. Identity versus role confusion

16. A preschooler is admitted to the hospital the day before scheduled surgery. Witch of the following actions will best help reduce the child's anxiety in this situation?
    a. have parent wait outside the room as child settles in
    b. begin preoperative teaching immediately; 30 minute session
    c. explain procedure in detail
    d. give the child dolls, puppets, and medical equipment to play out experience

17. According to Freud, which is the psychosexual stage of development of the preschooler?
    a. Phallic or oedipal stage
    b. Latency period
    c. Anal stage
    d. Genital stage

18. Which type of thought process is uncharacteristic of the 3-year-old child?
    a. Literal word interpretation
    b. Magical thinking
    c. Animistic thinking (inanimate objects take on human attributes)
    d. Intuitive thought

19. When assessing a preschooler, which description by the child of his or her parents would be considered typical?
    a. Persons who are in charge
    b. Persons who can do no wrong, practically perfect
    c. Old and rigid
    d. Necessary evil

(continued)

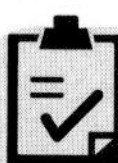

Think Smart/Test Smart

Note that the question asks for the uncharacteristic thought process. This means the one that would not be usual or expected in a 3-year old.

20. When exploring a 6-year old's concept of death, what would the nurse expect the child's perception to be?
    a. Death is punishment
    b. Death is a temporary state of sleep
    c. Death can be reversed
    d. Death probably lasts forever

21. Which behavior indicates that an adolescent is using formal thought?
    a. Uses abstract arguments for making a point
    b. Solves problems based on the here and now
    c. Uses language correctly without clear understanding of the meaning of words
    d. Is increasingly logical in thinking patterns

22. Which is the psychosocial task of the middle adult years?
    a. raising the next generation
    b. striving for identity
    c. sharing life with another
    d. searching for meaning in life

23. Which assessment finding related to the pulmonary function of an 89-year-old man who has come to the clinic for his annual checkup, would the nurse interpret as reflecting a normal age-related change?
    a. an increase in functional alveoli
    b. reduction of residual volume
    c. a decrease in vital capacity
    d. blood gases that show mild acidosis

24. Which is a normal sign of aging that may appear during assessment of the renal system of an 82-year old?
    a. concentrated urine
    b. microscopic hematuria
    c. occasional incontinence
    d. decreased glomerular filtration rate

25. An older gentleman who likes to eat tells the nurse that he has to use more salt than usual to make his food taste good. A possible explanation for this might be
    a. he has deceased sensitivity of his taste buds
    b. he needs more sodium to ensure good kidney function
    c. he is compensating for lost fluids
    d. he is confused due to his advancing age

ANSWERS & RATIONALES

ANSWERS FOR FILL IN THE BLANKS

Definitions related to Growth and Development

1. Control of the head proceeding to control over the torso and legs known is called <u>cephalocaudal</u> (head to tail) development.

2. Development progressing from the center of the body to the extremities is called <u>proximodistal</u> development.

3. Development progressing from mastery of simple operations to complex ones is called <u>mass-to-specific</u> development.

Milestones in Infancy

1. Good head control at 5–6 months
2. Attains sitting position independently at 9 months
3. Cruising at 11 months
4. Walks alone by 15 months
5. Grasp reflex fades and can actively hold rattle at 3 months
6. Crude pincer grasp at 9 months
7. First words with meaning 10 months
8 Builds 2-block tower at 12 months

Types of play

Although children engage in all types of play in each stage of development, the child adding new type of play to his repertoire

1. Play alongside another, not with another is called <u>parallel play</u>
2. Cooperative or interactive play is called <u>associative play</u>
3. Play is primarily <u>solitary</u> in infancy
4. Play is advancing to <u>parallel</u> play in toddlerhood
5. Play is advancing to <u>associative</u> in the preschool child

TRUE & FALSE ANSWERS

Concept of Death

1. The toddler has no concept of death. *True*
2. The preschool child views death as temporary and reversible. *True*
3. The younger school-aged child begins to see death as reversible. *False*
4. The older school-aged child views death as final and irreversible. *True*
5. The adolescent begins to exhibit mature understanding of death. *True*

ANSWERS FOR FILL IN THE BLANKS

Separation Anxiety

1. Separation anxiety is a major stress for the hospitalized child during which years?
   Middle infancy through preschool years

2. Describe behavior exhibited for all 3 stages of separation anxiety:
   Protest: cries for parent, inconsolable, attacks others, attempts to find parents, clings
   Despair: disinterested in the play or food, shows passivity, depression
   Detachment (denial): superficial adjustment, apparent interest, remains detached

3. Which of the 3 stages of separation anxiety is seen in prolonged separation?
   Detachment

Erikson's Theory of Psychosocial Development/Complete the list of developmental tasks and identify its stage

Developmental Task			Stage of Development
Autonomy	Vs.	Shame and doubt	Toddler
Trust	Vs.	Mistrust	Infancy
Industry	Vs.	Inferiority	School-age
Identity	Vs.	Role diffusion	Adolescence
Initiative	Vs.	Guilt	Preschool
Intimacy	Vs.	Isolation	Young adulthood
Ego Integrity	Vs.	Despair	Older adulthood
Generativity	Vs.	Stagnation	Middle adulthood

Freud's Psychosexual Theory of Personality Development/Fill in the blanks

Conflict	Description	Developmental Stage
Oral stage	Pleasure source centered on oral activities	Infancy
Anal stage	Interest centered on anal region; sphincter muscles develop	Toddler
Phallic or Oedipal	Genitals interesting and sensitive; recognize differences in the sexes; penis envy	Preschool
Latency period	Time of tranquility	School-age
Genital	Sexual emerges reemerge	Adolescence–adulthood

Piaget's Theory of Cognitive Development/Fill in the blanks

Stage	Age	Characteristics/Description
1. Sensorimotor	1–2 yrs	Learning takes place through developing sensory and motor skill
2. Preoperational	2–4 yrs	**Preconceptual.** Object permanence is transition to preoperational thought. Egocentrism, concrete, tangible
	4–7 yrs	Aware something is right, cannot say why **Intuitive thought.** Simple classification
3. Concrete operations	7–11 yrs	Logical, systematic, concrete, based on tasks in the here and now, start seeing things from more than one perspective, *masters conservation, complex classification*
4. Formal operations	11–adult	Abstract thinking, scientific reasoning, reflect on theoretical matters

APPLICATION ANSWERS

1. Which of the following principles of growth and development is being addressed when the nurse teaches the parent that the infant will develop control of the head before control of the torso and legs?
   a. cephalocaudal
   b. proximodistal
   c. mass to specific
   d. simple to complex

Rationale

Correct answer: a.

Incorrect answers: b, c, and d.

   b. proximodistal, midline to periphery.
   c. mass to specific (differentiation), simple operations precede complex ones.
   d. same as choice c.

2. Which is a sign of socialization that would be anticipated in a 6-month-old infant?
   a. social smile
   b. shows emotions such as jealousy
   c. begins to fear strangers
   d. smiles at mirror image

Rationale

Correct answer: c.

   c. stranger anxiety begins around 6 months

Incorrect answers: a, b, and d.

   a. social smile at 2 months.
   b. shows jealousy at 12 months.
   d. smiles at mirror image at 5 months.

3. Which finding in an infant requires further evaluation?
   a. has a strong grasp at 1 month
   b. head lag at 6 months
   c. sits unsupported at 8 months
   d. pulls self to stand at 9 months

Rationale

Correct answer: b.

   b. head lag at 6 months is an unfavorable developmental sign requiring further evaluation.
   a, c, and d are correct statements.

4. Which statement by a mother indicates the need for further teaching regarding infant nutrition?
   a. "I will feed the baby only commercially prepared infant formula for the first 6 months"
   b. "I will start skim milk and give an iron supplement at 6 months"
   c. "It is important for the mother to be well nourished when breast-feeding"
   d. "Solid foods are gradually introduced at around 5 or 6 months"

Rationale

Correct answer: b.

No cow's milk during first year, poor digestibility, lack of components needed for growth, no skim products either; infant needs fat for proper growth.

   a, c, and d are true statements.

(continued)

5. Which toy could appropriately be recommended for a 4-month-old infant?
   a. unbreakable mirror in a soft black and white frame
   b. large brightly colored balloon
   c. 5″ doll with removable clothing and shoes
   d. push-pull toy

Rationale

Correct answer: a.

Incorrect answers: b, c, and d.

   b. balloons are dangerous, they can be aspirated
   c. removable shoes of 5″ doll are too small, can choke
   d. pull-push toy for older infants when they can stand

6. When assessing a 5-month-old infant, which weight parameter indicates healthy growth?
   a. 10 lbs or more
   b. 15 lbs or more
   c. doubles birth weight
   d. triples birth weight

Rationale

Correct answer: c.

   c. doubles birth weight at 5–6 months.

Incorrect answers: a, b, and d.

   a. full-term infant should be over 10 lbs, but c is more accurate.
   b. if birth weight is 6 or 7 lbs, will be less than 15 lbs.
   d. triples birth weight at 1 year

7. At which age do beginning signs of tooth eruption appear?
   a. 2–3 months
   b. 3–4 months
   c. 5–6 months
   d. 8–9 months

Rationale

Correct answer: c.

   c. tooth eruption 5–6 months

Incorrect answers: a, b, and d.

8. When discussing psychosocial development with a new parent group, the nurse presents Erikson's theory and identifies which task as the psychosocial task of infancy?
   a. trust versus mistrust
   b. oral versus anal
   c. sensation versus mobilization
   d. initiative versus guilt

Rationale

Correct answer: a.

   a. trust versus mistrust is the psychosocial task in infancy.

Incorrect answers: b, c, and d.

   d. preschool
   b and c are terms from Freud and Piaget.

9. Which is the best description of the function of the Denver II developmental assessment tool?
   a. measures fine and gross motor development and intelligence and is a means of recording measurements
   b. objectively measures cognitive development
   c. measures gross and fine motor, language and personal-social development and is a means of recording objective measurements
   d. measures psychosocial and cognitive development

Rationale

Correct answer: c.

   c. denver II measures all items listed in c.

Incorrect answers: a, b, and d.

   a. intelligence is not measured.
   b. measures language.
   d. inaccurate.

10. When asked by a child's parent about Freud's theory of psychosexual development, which response by the nurse would be most accurate?
    a. Each stage of development is characterized by the inborn tendency of all individuals to reduce tension and seek pleasure and is associated with a particular conflict that must be resolved before moving on to the next stage
    b. Experiences during early childhood determine a child's pleasure-seeking behaviors but have little impact on later relationship and adjustment patterns
    c. Freud identified 8 stages of psychosocial conflicts and tasks that the individual strives to master from infancy through adulthood
    d. During the Latency stage of development patterns of pleasure, reward and guilt become established.

Rationale

Correct answer: a.

Incorrect answers: b, c, and d.

   b. Experiences during early childhood effect later adjustments and relationships.
   c. Erikson identified 8 stages of psychosocial conflicts from infancy through adulthood.
   d. During Latency (6–12 years), sexual urges are submerged into the unconscious and channeled into productive activities.

11. When assessing an 11-month old, which of the following developmental milestone achievements would the nurse expect to find as being the most recently achieved?
    a. Rolls completely over from back to abdomen
    b. Attains sitting position independently
    c. Walks holding on to furniture, cruising
    d. Develops crude thumb-finger pincer grasp

Rationale

Correct answer: c.

c. cruises at 11 months.

Incorrect answers: a, b, and d.

a. Rolls over back to abdomen at 6 months.

b. Attains sitting position independently at 8–9 months.

d. Develops crude thumb-finger pincer grasp at 9 months.

12. Which is the first stage of Piaget's theory of cognitive development?
    a. sensorimotor stage
    b. oral stage
    c. preoperational
    d. development of trust

Rationale

Correct answer: a.

Incorrect answers: b, c, and d.

b. oral stage is stage 1 of Freud's theory.

c. preoperational is the thought process for 1–2 years in Piaget's sensorimotor stage.

d. development of trust is Erikson's first stage of psychosocial development.

13. During the routine well check-up visit of an 18-month old, the mother asks the nurse the reason for her son's protruding abdomen. Which is a correct response for the nurse to give?
    a. Increased food intake at this age causes distention
    b. Underdeveloped abdominal muscles bulge
    c. Growth of the liver causes temporary protrusion
    d. It is uncommon in toddlers and requires further assessment

Rationale

Correct answer: b.

b. Undeveloped abdominal musculature gives the toddler the characteristic protruding abdomen.

Incorrect answers: a, c, and d.

a. During toddlerhood, food intake decreases.

c. Development of the liver does not cause the abdomen to protrude. d. Protruding abdomen is common in toddlers.

14. The nurse teaches the parent about readiness for toileting. Which event indicates that the time is not yet right for toilet training?
    a. Wakes up dry from a nap
    b. Stays dry for 2 hours
    c. Wants to have soiled diaper changed promptly
    d. Moves with family to new home with bathroom adjacent to bedroom

Rationale

Correct answer: d.

d. Moving is stressful and toilet training should not be initiated during stressful period.

Incorrect answers: a, b, and c.

a, b, and c are all signs of readiness for toilet training.

15. When discussing development with parents of a young child's play group, which would the nurse correctly identify as the psychosocial development task of the preschool child?
    a. Initiative versus guilt
    b. Autonomy versus shame and doubt
    c. Industry versus inferiority
    d. Identity versus role confusion

Rationale

Correct answer: a.

Incorrect answers: b, c, and d.

b. Is developmental task of toddlerhood.

c. Is task of school-aged child.

d. Is task of adolescence.

16. A preschooler is admitted to the hospital the day before scheduled surgery. Witch of the following actions will best help reduce the child's anxiety in this situation?
    a. have parent wait outside the room as child settles in
    b. begin preoperative teaching immediately; 30 minute session
    c. explain procedure in detail
    d. give the child dolls, puppets, and medical equipment to play out experience

Rationale

Correct answer: d.

Incorrect answers: a, b, and c.

a. parent should stay with the child.

b. Preoperative teaching is done shortly before the procedure; sessions should be no longer than 20 minutes.

c. no reason for detailed explanations, will only further frighten the child.

17. According to Freud, which is the psychosexual stage of development of the preschooler?
    a. Phallic or oedipal stage
    b. Latency period
    c. Anal stage
    d. Genital stage

(continued)

Rationale

Correct answer: a.

a. Phallic or oedipal stage, where genitals are central

Incorrect answers: b, c, and d.

b. Latency is school-age

c. Anal is toddlerhood

d. Genital is adolescent through adulthood

18. Which type of thought process is uncharacteristic of the 3-year-old child?
 a. Literal word interpretation
 b. Magical thinking
 c. Animistic thinking (inanimate objects take on human attributes)
 d. Intuitive thought

Rationale

Correct answer: d.

d. Intuitive thought (ages 4–7) is the 2nd phase of Piaget's preoperational period, increasing complexity in thought process and beginning ability to classify.

Incorrect answers: a, b, and c.

a, b, and c, are all characteristics of the 3-year-old child, and continue through preschool period.

19. When assessing a preschooler, which description by the child of his or her parents would be considered typical?
 a. Persons who are in charge
 b. Persons who can do no wrong, practically perfect
 c. Old and rigid
 d. Necessary evil

Rationale

Correct answer: b.

b. The preschooler sees parents as omnipotent, and enjoys and benefits from their guidance.

Incorrect answers: a, c, and d.

a. May be, but not adequate

c. Rigid, not a bad trait for the preschooler who likes order. Old is meaningless.

d. Maybe in adolescence

20. When exploring a 6-year old's concept of death, what would the nurse expect the child's perception to be?
 a. Death is punishment
 b. Death is a temporary state of sleep
 c. Death can be reversed
 d. Death probably lasts forever

Rationale

Correct answer: d.

d. The 6-year old begins to see death as irreversible.

Incorrect answers: a, b, and c.

a. Adolescent has mature understanding of death.

b and c. Preschool child sees death as reversible

21. Which behavior indicates that an adolescent is using formal thought?
 a. Uses abstract arguments for making a point
 b. Solves problems based on the here and now
 c. Uses language correctly without clear understanding of the meaning of words
 d. Is increasingly logical in thinking patterns

Rationale

Correct answer: a.

a. Adolescent using abstract thought.

Incorrect answers: b, c, and d.

b and d are stages of concrete operations, in school-aged child.

c. Preoperational stage using words appropriately, without clear understanding of their meaning

22. Which is the psychosocial task of the middle adult years?
 a. raising the next generation
 b. striving for identity
 c. sharing life with another
 d. searching for meaning in life

Rationale

Correct answer: a.

a. generativity versus stagnation.

Incorrect answers: b, c, and d

b. is seen in adolescence, identity versus role diffusion.

c. seen in young adulthood, intimacy versus isolation.

d. seen in the older adult, ego integrity versus despair.

23. Which assessment finding related to the pulmonary function of an 89-year-old man who has come to the clinic for his annual checkup, would the nurse interpret as reflecting a normal age-related change?
 a. an increase in functional alveoli
 b. reduction of residual volume
 c. a decrease in vital capacity
 d. blood gases that show mild acidosis

Rationale

Correct answer: c.

c. a decrease in vital capacity. Loss of elastic forces in the lung leads to an increase in residual volume and a decrease in vital capacity.

Incorrect answers: a, b, d.

None of the other options are age-related changes related to pulmonary function

24. Which is a normal sign of aging that may appear during assessment of the renal system of an 82-year old?
    a. concentrated urine
    b. microscopic hematuria
    c. occasional incontinence
    d. decreased glomerular filtration rate

Rationale

Correct answer: d.

Changes in the renal tubules cause a dramatic decrease in the glomerular filtration rate.

Incorrect answers: a, b, c.

None of the other options are normal age related changes.

25. An older gentleman who likes to eat tells the nurse that he has to use more salt than usual to make his food taste good. A possible explanation for this might be
    a. he has deceased sensitivity of his taste buds
    b. he needs more sodium to ensure good kidney function
    c. he is compensating for lost fluids.
    d. he is confused due to his advancing age

Rationale

Correct answer: a.

a. the taste buds begin to atrophy at age 40 and after age 60 there is an insensitivity to taste qualities. There are also studies that indicate that there are changes in the salt threshold in some elderly individuals.

Incorrect answers: b, c, d.

None of the other options would be correct or plausible explanations of the client's increased preference for salt.

CHAPTER 8

Test Plan Category:

Health Promotion and Maintenance—Part 3

Sub-category: **None**

Topics: **Health and Wellness**
Health Screening
Health Promotion Programs
Immunizations
Lifestyle Choices
High-Risk Behaviors
Principles of Teaching and Learning

HEALTH AND WELLNESS

HEALTH

- World Health Organization (WHO, 1948): "health is a state of complete physical, mental, and social well-being, not merely the absence of disease"; holistic definition
- ANA social policy statement (1980): "dynamic state of being in which the developmental and behavioral potential of an individual is realized to the fullest extent possible"; adds concept of moving toward optimal function
- Perception of what is health varies from individual to individual depending on his/her age, knowledge, expectations of self, and sociocultural background

WELLNESS

- Movement toward integration of human functioning; maximizing of potential; self-responsibility for health; increased self-awareness and satisfaction; wholeness of mind, body, and spirit.
- Seven aspects identified by Anspaugh, Hamrick, and Rosato are physical, social, emotional, intellectual, spiritual, occupational, and environmental.

Health Models

- Clinical Model—absence of S&S of disease indicates health; clients believing in this model are motivated toward healthy behaviors by a desire not to have a diagnosed disease
- Role Performance Model—health is the ability to perform normal societal roles, i.e., work; with this model, motivation for healthy behaviors is motivated by desire to be able to fulfill obligations at home, work, and in the community
- Adaptive Model—disease is a failure of the client's ability to adapt and treatment is aimed at restoring ability to adapt; the easier one can cope with changes in the internal

or external environment, the better is the state of health; motivated toward healthy behaviors by desire to alter self as situations change

- Eudaemonistic Model—health is the realization or actualization of potential; illness prevents this actualization; clients are motivated for health by joy and self-fulfillment.

Health Belief Models

- Health Belief Models identify factors that contribute to perceived state of health or risk of disease and hence there is probability of a client participating in an appropriate action plan for health.
- These are primarily concerned with clients' likelihood of engaging in health-protecting behaviors (preventative actions).

Factors Affecting Health

- Biologic factors—genetic makeup, age, sex, and developmental level
- Education
- Social network
- Health care—availability, accessibility, and cost
- Personal habits
- Economic status
- Family and cultural beliefs
- Physical environment—climate, noise, air, water supply, light, and exposure to toxic substances

HEALTH SCREENING

- The purpose of health screening is to identify risk factors or undiagnosed disease to allow for early intervention.
- Targeted screening—selected screening tests are based on person's age, gender, underlying health condition, or family history.
- Dangers of health screening are
  - —false positive results, which lead to more tests that may involve risk of complications, cost money, and cause anxiety;
  - —false negative results, which give false reassurance and may keep a person from seeing a physician.

SCREENING RECOMMENDATIONS FOR SPECIFIC AGE GROUPS

Neonate/infant

- Height/weight
- Growth and development (e.g., head circumference, Denver Developmental Screening Test)
- Urinalysis
- Hematocrit or hemoglobin
- Phenylketonuria (PKU) test (test for a genetically determined enzyme deficiency that causes mental retardation if not treated; testing mandated by state law shortly after birth)
- Blood lead level at 9–12 months
- Initial purified protein derivative (PPD) at 12 months

Toddler/preschooler

- Vision
- Hearing
- Growth and development (head circumference to age 2, DDST, speech and language)
- Height/weight
- Tuberculosis
- Blood pressure starting at 3 years
- Initial dental referral at 3 years
- Hematocrit or hemoglobin
- Cholesterol
- Lead
- Tuberculosis

School age children

- Vision
- Hearing
- Blood pressure
- Scoliosis
- Height/weight
- Tuberculosis (PPD)
- Dental
- Urinalysis
- Hematocrit or hemoglobin

Adolescents and young adults

- Sexually transmitted diseases

- Papanicolau smear
- Breast self-examination (Table 8-1)
- Testicular self-examination (Table 8-2)
- Blood pressure
- Vision
- Hearing
- Height/weight
- Dental
- Mental health (eating disorders, depression, schizophrenia)
- Tuberculosis (PPD)
- Urinalysis
- Hematocrit or hemoglobin

Early adult

- Physical examination: females without symptoms every 1–3 years; males without symptoms every 5 years
- Dental checkups: every 6 months
- Pap smear for cervical cancer
- Self-breast exam
- Clinical breast exam
- Baseline mammogram at 35 years
- Testicular self-exam

Middle adult

- Physical examination: annual for females; every 2–3 years for males
- Dental checkups: every 6 months
- Screening every 1–2 years for glaucoma starting at age 45 if family history of the disease
- Pap smear for cervical cancer
- Breast self-exam
- Screen for heart disease
- Colonoscopy
- Pelvic exam for uterine cancer
- Screen for prostate cancer
- Testicular self-exam
- HIV testing up to age 65

Over age 50

- Eye exam every 2–4 years, every 1–2 years over age 65
- Hearing test every 10 years
- Dental exam 1–2 times per year
- Blood pressure check at least every 2 years
- Cholesterol check every 5 years
- Diabetes screen every 3 years; every 1–3 years over age 65
- Annual skin exam (Table 8-3)
- Colorectal cancer screening: fecal occult blood test annually; sigmoidoscopy every 5 years; colonoscopy every 10 years
- Mammogram every 1–2 years
- Pelvic exam every 1–3 years (less often over 65 and if negative findings on previous screenings)
- Pap smear every 1–3 years
- Bone mineral density test at least once by age 65

Table 8–1 Client Teaching: Self Breast Examination

There are three parts to a self breast examination:

- Palpation of each breast while lying down so the breast tissue is spread more thinly over the chest wall.
- Inspection of the breast in a mirror with good lighting while standing with the arms in different positions
- Palpation of each axilla while sitting or standing with arms loosely at the side of the body.

Begin with palpation of the right breast

- Lying on the back, place the right arm up and behind your head.
- Use the pads of the middle three fingers of your left hand to palpate for nodules or changes in consistency.
- Move the finger pads in a circular motion feeling first with gentle then with increasing pressure so changes at all levels of the tissue can be felt.
- Progress in vertical lines going from your clavicle (collar bone) to the bottom of your ribs and from the middle of your side to your sternum (breastbone) in the middle of your chest being certain not to miss any areas.
- Remember a firm ridge felt at the bottom of each breast where it attaches to the chest wall is normal.

Repeat for the left breast.

Proceed to inspection of the breasts.

- Stand in front of a mirror and look for changes in the breast such as dimpling of the skin, prominent blood vessels, asymmetry, changes in size, pulling or deviation of the nipple inward or to one side, or nipple scaliness or discharge.
- Do this with hands on hips pressing down, arms loosely at sides, and with arms held up over the head.

Lastly. palpate each axilla.

Table 8–2 Client Teaching: Self Testicular Examination

- Perform once per month.
- Best done after a warm bath or shower because the scrotal skin is relaxed making it easier to feel the testes and find any lumps or changes in their size, shape or consistency.
- Examine the right and left testicle individually using both hands for each one.
- Place the index and middle finger of each hand on top of the testicle and the thumbs underneath; roll the testicle between the finger pads.
- Keep in mind that the epididymis may feel like a small bump on the upper or middle outer aspect of each testicle; this is normal.
- See your health care provider and report any unusual findings without delay.

HEALTH PROMOTION

- Health promotion is comprisesd of activities designed to develop human resources and behaviors that maintain or enhance well-being; enabling people to maximize physical, mental, and emotional potential through increased awareness, attitude change, and recognition of alternatives related to healthy lifestyle choices.
- The focus of health promotion is on changing personal behaviors and the environment.
- Current U.S. national health promotion and disease prevention objectives are identified in Healthy People 2010, Understanding and Improving Health, a publication of the Public Health Service of the US Department of Health and Human Services (See Table 8-4).

HEALTH PROTECTION

- Disease prevention or avoidance of health threats
- Interventions to prevent illness are as follows:
  —Primary prevention: these are the actions that focus on the prevention of health problems, e.g., health eduction programs.
  —Secondary prevention: these are the actions that focus on the early diagnosis and prompt treatment of health problems, e.g., control/treatment of early disease.
  —Tertiary prevention: these are the actions to minimize the effects of permanent, irreversible disease, or disability through interventions designed to prevent complications and deterioration.

Table 8–3 Client Teaching: Self Skin Examination

- Need a full length mirror, a hand held mirror, and a good light
- Systematically inspect **all** skin areas for new lesions, lesions that don't heal, and changes in existing lesions.
- Remember that signs of malignant change in moles are asymmetry, irregular border, altered color, surface or sensation, and size greater than a diameter of 6 mm.
  - Stand naked in front of the full length mirror and inspect the entire front of the body from head to toe.
  - Turn so your right side is facing the mirror, raise your right arm over your head, and inspect all skin on the right side of the body.
  - Repeat for the left side.
  - Standing with your back to the full length mirror, use the hand held mirror to inspect the skin on the back of the body including the back of the neck and behind the ears.
  - Sit down and examine the inner aspects of the legs, between the toes and the soles of the feet.
  - Inspect the skin between the fingers.
  - Use a comb to part the hair and inspect the scalp.
- See your health care provider without delay for any unusual findings.

PENDER'S HEALTH PROMOTION MODEL

This model analyzes the factors that influence person's behavior and lifestyle change as he/she seeks to improve well-being and maximize human potential. These factors can be classified into

- cognitive-perceptual factors—perceive importance of health;
- modifying factors—demographics, environment;
- factors that influence the likelihood of engaging in health promotion activities, i.e., internal and external cues to action such as mass media campaigns, reminders from doctors, newspaper and media ads.

HEALTH PROMOTION PROGRAMS

- Focus may be individual, family, or population (community)
- Types of health promotion/disease prevention activities
  —Information dissemination
    - Basic program to change attitudes, beliefs, and behaviors
    - Designed to raise level of awareness and knowledge to support client's ability to improve personal living conditions, make informed decisions about personal, family, and community health practices; and access health services appropriately
    - Uses health fairs, mass media, brochures, etc to inform clients about needed lifestyle changes and methods of enhancing quality of life
  —Health risk appraisal and wellness assessment: designed to provide motivation to change, i.e., reduce risk behaviors and adopt healthy behaviors

Table 8–4 Healthy People 2010

- National health objectives
- Overarching goals
  Increasing the quality and longevity of life
  —Eliminating disparities in health among different populations
- Enabling goals
  —Promote health behaviors
  —Protect health
  —Provide access to quality health care
  —Strengthen community prevention
- Defines public health priorities and 467 specific, measurable objectives aimed at improving health, which are grouped into 28 focus areas
  —Access to quality health services
  —Arthritis, osteoporosis, and chronic back conditions
  —Cancer
  —Chronic kidney disease
  —Diabetes
  —Disability and secondary conditions
  —Educational and community-based programs
  —Environmental health
  —Family planning
  —Food safety
  —Health communication
  —Heart disease and stroke
  —HIV
  —Immunization and infectious diseases
  —Injury and violence prevention
  —Maternal, infant, and child health
  —Medical product safety
  —Mental health and mental disorders
  —Nutrition and overweight
  —Occupational safety and health
  —Oral health
  —Physical activity and fitness
  —Public health infrastructure
  —Respiratory diseases
  —Sexually transmitted diseases
  —Substance abuse
  —Tobacco use
  —Vision and hearing
- Leading health indicators that reflect the major health issues that the nation needs to address
  —Physical activity
  —Overweight and obesity
  —Tobacco use
  —Substance abuse
  —Responsible sexual behavior
  —Mental health
  —Injury and violence
  —Environmental quality
  —Immunization
  —Access to health care

From Healthy People 2010; Understanding and Improving Health, 2nd ed., by US Department of Health and Human Services, 2000, Washington, DC; US Government Printing Office.

—Lifestyle and behavior change
  - Assist clients to take responsibility for health and make needed changes
  - Take extended periods of time

—Environmental control and safety programs such as those related to nuclear power plants, air and water pollution, and use of pesticides

—Environmental restructuring
  - focuses on physical, social, and economic environment;
  - aims to increase available options and support use of health-promoting behaviors;
  - supports other types of programs.

- Basic types of program by sponsorship/locale
  —Community programs such as screening or immunization programs offered by the health department; fire safety or CPR programs offered by the fire department or bicycle or auto safety programs offered by the police department
  —Programs offered by health care agencies such as those on testicular and self-breast examination by the American Cancer Society, or stop smoking, stress management offered by hospitals, or cardiac fitness offered by the American Heart Association
  —School-based programs such as those related to nutrition, dental hygiene, drug and alcohol abuse, sexual behavior, and child abuse
  —Work site programs such as accident prevention, hearing protection, fitness, and nutrition
  —Programs offered at senior citizen and retirement centers such as safe driving classes, vision screening, and blood pressure screening

Nursing Process Elements

- Assessment
  —In-depth assessment of client's health status is the foundation for health promotion
  —Health history and physical examination
  —Physical fitness assessment: muscle endurance, flexibility, body composition, and cardiorespiratory endurance
  —Lifestyle assessment: personal habits such as physical activity, use of safety precautions, eating habits, smoking, alcohol, and drug use
  —Health risk assessment
  —Spiritual assessment
  —Review of life stress, health beliefs, and social support systems
- Work with the client to develop a Health Promotion Plan using the steps identified by Pender
  —Identify most important health goals (These are broad goals such as reduce blood pressure to within recommended range)

Table 8–5 Stage Model of Health Behavior Change (Data from Prochaska et al., 1994.)

- Precontemplation—client does not see self as having problem; therefore needs no change; see others as having the problem and needing change
- Contemplation—client acknowledges problem and talks about change but is not ready to commit to action
- Preparation—person makes real plans to change; may have begun small changes
- Action-client implements strategies to change behavior; stage of greatest commitment of time and energy
- Maintenance—client integrates new behaviors into lifestyle warding off temptation to return to previous unhealthy behaviors and relapsing to the precontemplation or contemplation stage
- Termination—stage in which problem is no longer a temptation or threat; some behaviors may never be able to be terminated; they always require maintenance

—Identify behavioral or health outcomes related to each (These are specific indicators related to achievement of the goal, i.e., changes that are needed to achieve the goal such as lose weight; stop smoking; exercise regularly; decrease stress)

—Develop a plan for changes in behavior: options need to be examined and client assisted in selecting changes that are most acceptable based on personal values and preferences as well as expectations for success

—Reinforce benefits of change: having the client reiterate the benefits promotes ownership and commitment

—Consider interpersonal and environmental factors that both facilitate and inhibit the proposed changes: identify how facilitators can be used to reinforce the planned change and how barriers can be overcome

—Determine a time frame for instituting the planned behaviors; make sure it's realistic and schedule short-term goals, rewards, and reinforcement if possible

—Commit to behavior-change goals—often verbal but increasingly in the form of a written contract

- Use nursing strategies to promote implementation of a Health Promotion Plan

—Ensuring support to the client in regard to the behavior change; nurse may directly provide or facilitate receipt of support from others—social support network must be knowledgeable about client's needs and goals so nurse may meet with them at client's request

—Counseling to answer questions, review goals and activities; reinforce progress—in-person individual counseling; individual telephone counseling; group counseling, which also offers opportunity to learn from others

Table 8–6 Health Promotion for Specific Age Groups

Age Group	Health Concerns/Primary Prevention	Injury Prevention/High-Risk Behaviors
Infants	Low birth weight Congenital disorders Influenza SIDs Pneumonia	Accidents
Children	Nutrition Activity and exercise Sleep and rest Dangers of drugs and alcohol	Home safety, fire safety, firearm safety, safety of latchkey children Play safety: bicycles, skateboards and in-line skating, and water safety Lead poisoning Child abuse
Adolescents	Yearly health checkup Immunizations Unwanted pregnancy Health education	Unintentional injuries Homicide Substance abuse STIs Suicide
Early adulthood	Accidents, suicide, hypertension, substance abuse, STDs, domestic abuse, malignancies	Motor vehicle safety, sun protection, occupational safety, safe sex, smoking, stress, periodontal disease
Middle adulthood	Accidents, cancer, heart disease, obesity, alcoholism, mental health disorders	Motor vehicle safety, sun protection occupational safety, safe sex, smoking, stress, periodontal disease
Late adulthood	Accidents, arthritis, heart disease, pulmonary disease, pharmaceutical misuse, alcoholism, dementia, elder abuse, pneumonia, influenza, loss and depression	Risk of falls, inadequate caloric and/or roughage intake, inadequate exercise

—Teaching—must be based on client's need

—Facilitating modeling—helps the client identify a model that the client respects and can identify with in terms of factors such as age and background, to observe for ideas about behaviors and coping strategies; the client is not supposed to mimic the model

IMMUNIZATIONS

Immunizations provide protection from infectious disease by inducing a state of immunity.

TYPES OF IMMUNITY

- Active immunity: client makes antibodies that provide immunity.
- Passive immunity: client is given antibodies made by another human or animal to induce immunity.
- Naturally acquired active: body makes antibodies because of actual infection; immunity is lifelong.
- Naturally acquired passive: antibodies are produced by a mother and passed through the placenta and colostrum to the fetus/baby; immunity lasts 6–12 months.
- Artificially acquired active: vaccines or toxoids containing antigens are given to cause the person's body to produce antibodies; must be reinforced with periodic boosters.
- Artificially acquired passive: immune serum (serum-containing antibody) is injected in order to produce immunity; immunity is of short duration.

TYPES OF IMMUNIZATIONS

- Live Attenuated Vaccine
  —Pathogen is treated with heat or chemicals to reduce its virulence, but the organism is not killed.
  —Examples are MMR, varicella, rubella, and LAIV Influenza.
- Inactivated Vaccine
  —Bacterial endotoxins are treated with heat or formalin to yield a nontoxic, inactivated agent that is still antigenic.
  —Killed viral organisms or parts thereof are used in the vaccine to produce immunity.
  —Examples are IPV, DTaP, HBV, TIV influenza, and Hib.
- Immunoglobulins—blood and Immunity
  —Immunoglobulins provide passive immunity without stimulating an immune response.
  —Solutions that contain antibodies from large pools of human blood plasma are introduced into the body.
  —Immunoglobulins are used primarily for maintenance of immunity in immunodeficient people, and for passive immunity against hepatitis A and measles.
  —Specific Immunoglobulins contain high antibody titers of a specific antigen, e.g., Tetanus Ig, varicella-zoster Ig, and hepatitis B Ig.

Think Smart/Test Smart

As you study the information on immunizations, remember to keep clear in your mind that there are three sets of immunization guidelines: standard guidelines for children and adolescents, guidelines for children and adolescents that have not had immunizations in accord with the standard guidelines and therefore are behind, and guidelines for adults. Be sure to note "exceptions to the rule" such as live vaccines are contraindicated for immunosuppressed children except for MMR, which is given to children with HIV.

—Antibodies received by the fetus in utero through the placenta and by the newborn who is breastfed provide the infant with immunity for the first few weeks of life against most bacterial, viral, and fungal infections.

Recommended Vaccinations for Children and Adolescents

- Diphtheria, tetanus, pertussis (whooping cough) (DTaP)—five shot series from age 2 months to 6 years, and a booster shot at age 11–12 years
- Haemophilus influenza type B (Hib)—prevention against bacterial meningitis, pneumonia, and sepsis. Four shot series between ages 2 and 15 months
- Hepatitis B—three doses from birth to 18 months
- Measles, mumps, rubella (MMR)—two shots between ages 1 and 6
- Pneumococcal (PCA)—vaccination prevents fatal blood infections, pneumonia, and many ear infections. Four shots from 2—18 months
- Inactivated polio virus (IPV)—Four shots between 2 months and 6 years
- Varicella (Var)—One shot given between ages 1 and 6
- Hepatitis A (HepA)—two doses 6 months apart, at 1 year and at 18 months

See the following Recommended Childhood and Adolescent Immunization Schedule 2006 and the Recommended Immunization Schedule for Children and Adolescents Who Start Late or Who Are More Than 1 Month Behind 2006. For recommended adult immunizations, see Table 8-7.

DEPARTMENT OF HEALTH AND HUMAN SERVICES • CENTERS FOR DISEASE CONTROL AND PREVENTION

Recommended Childhood and Adolescent Immunization Schedule UNITED STATES • 2006

Vaccine ▼ Age ▶	Birth	1 month	2 months	4 months	6 months	12 months	15 months	18 months	24 months	4–6 years	11–12 years	13–14 years	15 years	16–18 years
Hepatitis B[1]	HepB	HepB		*HepB[1]*		HepB					HepB Series			
Diphtheria, Tetanus, Pertussis[2]			DTaP	DTaP	DTaP		DTaP			DTaP	Tdap		Tdap	
Haemophilus influenzae type b[3]			Hib	Hib	*Hib[3]*	Hib								
Inactivated Poliovirus			IPV	IPV		IPV				IPV				
Measles, Mumps, Rubella[4]						MMR				MMR			MMR	
Varicella[5]							Varicella				Varicella			
Meningococcal[6]							Vaccines within broken line are for selected populations		MPSV4		MCV4		MCV4 / MCV4	
Pneumococcal[7]			PCV	PCV	PCV	PCV			PCV		PPV			
Influenza[8]						Influenza (Yearly)					Influenza (Yearly)			
Hepatitis A[9]										HepA Series				

This schedule indicates the recommended ages for routine administration of currently licensed childhood vaccines, as of December 1, 2005, for children through age 18 years. Any dose not administered at the recommended age should be administered at any subsequent visit when indicated and feasible. ▇ Indicates age groups that warrant special effort to administer those vaccines not previously administered. Additional vaccines may be licensed and recommended during the year. Licensed combination vaccines may be used whenever any components of the combination are indicated and other components of the vaccine are not contraindicated and if approved by the Food and Drug Administration for that dose of the series. Providers should consult the respective ACIP statement for detailed recommendations. Clinically significant adverse events that follow immunization should be reported to the Vaccine Adverse Event Reporting System (VAERS). Guidance about how to obtain and complete a VAERS form is available at **www.vaers.hhs.gov** or by telephone, **800-822-7967**.

Range of recommended ages **Catch-up immunization** **11–12 year old assessment**

1. **Hepatitis B vaccine (HepB).** ***AT BIRTH:*** **All newborns** should receive monovalent HepB soon after birth and before hospital discharge. **Infants born to mothers who are HBsAg-positive** should receive HepB and 0.5 mL of hepatitis B immune globulin (HBIG) within 12 hours of birth. **Infants born to mothers whose HBsAg status is unknown** should receive HepB within 12 hours of birth. The mother should have blood drawn as soon as possible to determine her HBsAg status; if HBsAg-positive, the infant should receive HBIG as soon as possible (no later than age 1 week). **For infants born to HBsAg-negative mothers,** the birth dose can be delayed in rare circumstances but only if a physician's order to withhold the vaccine and a copy of the mother's original HBsAg-negative laboratory report are documented in the infant's medical record. ***FOLLOWING THE BIRTHDOSE:*** The HepB series should be completed with either monovalent HepB or a combination vaccine containing HepB. The second dose should be administered at age 1–2 months. The final dose should be administered at age ≥24 weeks. It is permissible to administer 4 doses of HepB (e.g., when combination vaccines are given after the birth dose); however, if monovalent HepB is used, a dose at age 4 months is not needed. **Infants born to HBsAg-positive mothers** should be tested for HBsAg and antibody to HBsAg after completion of the HepB series, at age 9–18 months (generally at the next well-child visit after completion of the vaccine series).
2. **Diphtheria and tetanus toxoids and acellular pertussis vaccine (DTaP).** The fourth dose of DTaP may be administered as early as age 12 months, provided 6 months have elapsed since the third dose and the child is unlikely to return at age 15–18 months. The final dose in the series should be given at age ≥4 years.
   Tetanus and diphtheria toxoids and acellular pertussis vaccine (Tdap – adolescent preparation) is recommended at age 11–12 years for those who have completed the recommended childhood DTP/DTaP vaccination series and have not received a Td booster dose. Adolescents 13–18 years who missed the 11–12-year Td/Tdap booster dose should also receive a single dose of Tdap if they have completed the recommended childhood DTP/DTaP vaccination series. Subsequent **tetanus and diphtheria toxoids (Td)** are recommended every 10 years.
3. ***Haemophilus influenzae*** **type b conjugate vaccine (Hib).** Three Hib conjugate vaccines are licensed for infant use. If PRP-OMP (PedvaxHIB® or ComVax® [Merck]) is administered at ages 2 and 4 months, a dose at age 6 months is not required. DTaP/Hib combination products should not be used for primary immunization in infants at ages 2, 4 or 6 months but can be used as boosters after any Hib vaccine. The final dose in the series should be administered at age ≥12 months.
4. **Measles, mumps, and rubella vaccine (MMR).** The second dose of MMR is recommended routinely at age 4–6 years but may be administered during any visit, provided at least 4 weeks have elapsed since the first dose and both doses are administered beginning at or after age 12 months. Those who have not previously received the second dose should complete the schedule by age 11–12 years.
5. **Varicella vaccine.** Varicella vaccine is recommended at any visit at or after age 12 months for susceptible children (i.e., those who lack a reliable history of chickenpox). Susceptible persons aged ≥13 years should receive 2 doses administered at least 4 weeks apart.
6. **Meningococcal vaccine (MCV4).** Meningococcal conjugate vaccine (MCV4) should be given to all children at the 11–12 year old visit as well as to unvaccinated adolescents at high school entry (15 years of age). Other adolescents who wish to decrease their risk for meningococcal disease may also be vaccinated. All college freshmen living in dormitories should also be vaccinated, preferably with MCV4, although **meningococcal polysaccharide vaccine (MPSV4)** is an acceptable alternative. Vaccination against invasive meningococcal disease is recommended for children and adolescents aged ≥2 years with terminal complement deficiencies or anatomic or functional asplenia and certain other high risk groups (see *MMWR* 2005;54 [RR-7]:1-21); use MPSV4 for children aged 2–10 years and MCV4 for older children, although MPSV4 is an acceptable alternative.
7. **Pneumococcal vaccine.** The heptavalent **pneumococcal conjugate vaccine (PCV)** is recommended for all children aged 2–23 months and for certain children aged 24–59 months. The final dose in the series should be given at age ≥12 months. **Pneumococcal polysaccharide vaccine (PPV)** is recommended in addition to PCV for certain high-risk groups. See *MMWR* 2000; 49(RR-9):1-35.
8. **Influenza vaccine.** Influenza vaccine is recommended annually for children aged ≥6 months with certain risk factors (including, but not limited to, asthma, cardiac disease, sickle cell disease, human immunodeficiency virus [HIV], diabetes, and conditions that can compromise respiratory function or handling of respiratory secretions or that can increase the risk for aspiration), healthcare workers, and other persons (including household members) in close contact with persons in groups at high risk (see *MMWR* 2005;54[RR-8]:1-55). In addition, healthy children aged 6–23 months and close contacts of healthy children aged 0–5 months are recommended to receive influenza vaccine because children in this age group are at substantially increased risk for influenza-related hospitalizations. For healthy persons aged 5–49 years, the intranasally administered, live, attenuated influenza vaccine (LAIV) is an acceptable alternative to the intramuscular trivalent inactivated influenza vaccine (TIV). See *MMWR* 2005;54(RR-8):1-55. Children receiving TIV should be administered a dosage appropriate for their age (0.25 mL if aged 6–35 months or 0.5 mL if aged ≥3 years). Children aged ≤8 years who are receiving influenza vaccine for the first time should receive 2 doses (separated by at least 4 weeks for TIV and at least 6 weeks for LAIV).
9. **Hepatitis A vaccine (HepA).** HepA is recommended for all children at 1 year of age (i.e., 12–23 months). The 2 doses in the series should be administered at least 6 months apart. States, counties, and communities with existing HepA vaccination programs for children 2–18 years of age are encouraged to maintain these programs. In these areas, new efforts focused on routine vaccination of 1-year-old children should enhance, not replace, ongoing programs directed at a broader population of children. HepA is also recommended for certain high risk groups (see *MMWR* 1999; 48[RR-12]1-37).

The Childhood and Adolescent Immunization Schedule is approved by:
Advisory Committee on Immunization Practices www.cdc.gov/nip/acip • American Academy of Pediatrics www.aap.org • American Academy of Family Physicians www.aafp.org

Recommended Immunization Schedule for Children and Adolescents Who Start Late or Who Are More Than 1 Month Behind

UNITED STATES • 2006

The tables below give catch-up schedules and minimum intervals between doses for children who have delayed immunizations. There is no need to restart a vaccine series regardless of the time that has elapsed between doses. Use the chart appropriate for the child's age.

CATCH-UP SCHEDULE FOR CHILDREN AGED 4 MONTHS THROUGH 6 YEARS

Vaccine	Minimum Age for Dose 1	Minimum Interval Between Doses			
		Dose 1 to Dose 2	Dose 2 to Dose 3	Dose 3 to Dose 4	Dose 4 to Dose 5
Diphtheria, Tetanus, Pertussis	6 wks	4 weeks	4 weeks	6 months	6 months[1]
Inactivated Poliovirus	6 wks	4 weeks	4 weeks	4 weeks[2]	
Hepatitis B[3]	Birth	4 weeks	8 weeks (and 16 weeks after first dose)		
Measles, Mumps, Rubella	12 mo	4 weeks[4]			
Varicella	12 mo				
Haemophilus influenzae type b[5]	6 wks	4 weeks if first dose given at age <12 months 8 weeks (as final dose) if first dose given at age 12-14 months No further doses needed if first dose given at age ≥15 months	4 weeks[6] if current age <12 months 8 weeks (as final dose)[6] if current age ≥12 months and second dose given at age <15 months No further doses needed if previous dose given at age ≥15 mo	8 weeks (as final dose) This dose only necessary for children aged 12 months–5 years who received 3 doses before age 12 months	
Pneumococcal[7]	6 wks	4 weeks if first dose given at age <12 months and current age <24 months 8 weeks (as final dose) if first dose given at age ≥12 months or current age 24–59 months No further doses needed for healthy children if first dose given at age ≥24 months	4 weeks if current age <12 months 8 weeks (as final dose) if current age ≥12 months No further doses needed for healthy children if previous dose given at age ≥24 months	8 weeks (as final dose) This dose only necessary for children aged 12 months–5 years who received 3 doses before age 12 months	CDC

CATCH-UP SCHEDULE FOR CHILDREN AGED 7 YEARS THROUGH 18 YEARS

Vaccine	Minimum Interval Between Doses		
	Dose 1 to Dose 2	Dose 2 to Dose 3	Dose 3 to Booster Dose
Tetanus, Diphtheria[8]	4 weeks	6 months	6 months if first dose given at age <12 months and current age <11 years; otherwise 5 years
Inactivated Poliovirus[9]	4 weeks	4 weeks	IPV[2,9]
Hepatitis B	4 weeks	8 weeks (and 16 weeks after first dose)	
Measles, Mumps, Rubella	4 weeks		
Varicella[10]	4 weeks		

1. **DTaP.** The fifth dose is not necessary if the fourth dose was administered after the fourth birthday.
2. **IPV.** For children who received an all-IPV or all-oral poliovirus (OPV) series, a fourth dose is not necessary if third dose was administered at age ≥4 years. If both OPV and IPV were administered as part of a series, a total of 4 doses should be given, regardless of the child's current age.
3. **HepB.** Administer the 3-dose series to all children and adolescents <19 years of age if they were not previously vaccinated.
4. **MMR.** The second dose of MMR is recommended routinely at age 4–6 years but may be administered earlier if desired.
5. **Hib.** Vaccine is not generally recommended for children aged ≥5 years.
6. **Hib.** If current age <12 months and the first 2 doses were PRP-OMP (PedvaxHIB® or ComVax® [Merck]), the third (and final) dose should be administered at age 12–15 months and at least 8 weeks after the second dose.
7. **PCV.** Vaccine is not generally recommended for children aged ≥5 years.
8. **Td.** Adolescent tetanus, diphtheria, and pertussis vaccine (Tdap) may be substituted for any dose in a primary catch-up series or as a booster if age appropriate for Tdap. A five-year interval from the last Td dose is encouraged when Tdap is used as a booster dose. See ACIP recommendations for further information.
9. **IPV.** Vaccine is not generally recommended for persons aged ≥18 years.
10. **Varicella.** Administer the 2-dose series to all susceptible adolescents aged ≥13 years.

Report adverse reactions to vaccines through the federal Vaccine Adverse Event Reporting System. For information on reporting reactions following immunization, please visit www.vaers.hhs.gov or call the 24-hour national toll-free information line 800-822-7967. Report suspected cases of vaccine-preventable diseases to your state or local health department.

For additional information about vaccines, including precautions and contraindications for immunization and vaccine shortages, please visit the National Immunization Program Website at www.cdc.gov/nip or contact 800-CDC-INFO (800-232-4636) (In English, En Español — 24/7)

Administration

- Be familiar with manufacturer's recommendation for proper storage and reconstitution of the vaccine.
- Check expiration dates.
- Excellent intramuscular injection technique must be used to avoid local reactions to the injection.
- When two or more vaccinations need to be given, the order of injections is arbitrary. They may be given sequentially or simultaneously by two people.
- Doses of live vaccines should be separated by a minimum of 30 days, but more than one live vaccine may be given on the same day.

Table 8–7 Adult Immunizations

Vaccine Name and Route	For Whom Vaccination Is Recommended	Schedule for Vaccine Administration (Any Vaccine Can Be Given with Another)	Contraindications and Precautions (Mild Illness Is Not a Contraindication)
Influenza	• Persons aged 50 yrs and older.		Contraindication Previous anaphylactic reaction to this vaccine, to any of its components, or to eggs.
Trivalent inactivated influenza vaccine (TIV) *Give IM*	• Persons with medical problems (e.g., heart disease, lung disease, diabetes, renal dysfunction, hemoglobinopathy, immunosuppression) and/or people living in chronic-care facilities. • Persons with any condition that compromises respiratory function or the handling of respiratory secretions or that can increase the risk of aspiration (e.g., cognitive dysfunction, spinal cord injury, seizure disorder, or other neuromuscular disorder). • Persons working or living with at-risk people. • Women who will be pregnant during the influenza season (December–March). • All health care workers and other persons who provide direct care to at-risk people. • Household contacts and out-of-home caregivers of children aged 0–59 mo. • Travelers at risk for complications of influenza who go to areas where influenza activity exists or who may be among people from areas of the world where there is current influenza activity (e.g., on organized tours). • Persons who provide essential community services. • Students or other persons in institutional settings (e.g., dormitory residents). • Anyone wishing to reduce the likelihood of becoming ill with influenza.	• Given every year in the fall or winter. • October and November are the ideal months to give TIV. • LAIV may be given as early as August. • Continue to give TIV and LAIV through the influenza season from December through March (including when influenza activity is present in the community) and at other times when the risk of influenza exists.	Precautions • Moderate or severe acute illness. • History of Guillain-Barré syndrome within 6 wks of previous TIV.
Influenza Live attenuated influenza vaccine (LAIV) *Give intranasally*	• Healthy, nonpregnant persons aged 49 yrs and younger who meet any of the conditions listed below: —Working or living with at-risk people as listed in the section above —Health care workers or other persons who provide direct care to at-risk people (except persons in close contact with severely immunosuppressed persons). —Household contacts and out-of-home caregivers of children ages 0–59 mo.		Contraindications • Previous anaphylactic reaction to this vaccine, to any of its components, or to eggs • Pregnancy, asthma, reactive airway disease, or other chronic disorder of the pulmonary or cardiovascular system; an underlying medical condition, including metabolic disease such as diabetes, renal dysfunction, and hemoglobinopathy; a known or suspected immune deficiency disease or receiving immunosuppressive therapy; history of Guillain-Barré syndrome.

(continued on next page)

Table 8–7 *(continued from previous page)*

Vaccine Name and Route	For Whom Vaccination Is Recommended	Schedule for Vaccine Administration (Any Vaccine Can Be Given with Another)	Contraindications and Precautions (Mild Illness Is Not a Contraindication)
	—Travelers who may be among people from areas of the world where there is current influenza activity (e.g., on organized tours). —Persons who provide essential community services. —Students or other persons in institutional settings (e.g., dormitory residents). —Anyone wishing to reduce the likelihood of becoming ill with influenza.		Precaution Moderate or severe acute illness.
Pneumococcal poly-saccharide vaccine (PPV) *Give IM or SC*	• Persons aged 65 yrs and older. • Persons who have chronic illness or other risk factors, including chronic cardiac or pulmonary disease, chronic liver disease, alcoholism, diabetes, CSF leak, as well as people living in special environments or social settings (including Alaska Natives and certain American Indian populations). Those at highest risk of fatal pneumococcal infection are persons with anatomic asplenia, functional asplenia, or sickle cell disease; immunocompromised persons including those with HIV infection, leukemia, lymphoma, Hodgkin's disease, multiple myeloma, generalized malignancy, chronic renal failure, or nephrotic syndrome; persons receiving immunosuppressive chemotherapy (including corticosteroids); those who received an organ or bone marrow transplant; and candidates for or recipients of cochlear implants.	• Routinely given as a one-time dose; administer if previous vaccination history is unknown. • One-time revaccination is recommended 5 yrs later for persons at highest risk of fatal pneumococcal infection or rapid antibody loss (e.g., renal disease) and for persons age 65 yrs and older if the 1st dose was given prior to age 65 and 5 yrs or more have elapsed since the prior dose.	Contraindication Previous anaphylactic reaction to this vaccine or to any of its components. Precaution Moderate or severe acute illness.
Hepatitis B (HepB) *Give IM* Brands may be used interchangeably.	• All adolescents; any adult wishing to obtain immunity. • High-risk persons, including household contacts and sex partners of HBsAg-positive persons; injecting drug users; heterosexuals with more than one sex partner in 6 months; men who have sex with men; persons with recently diagnosed STDs; patients receiving hemodialysis and patients with renal disease that may result in dialysis; recipients of certain blood products; health care workers and public safety workers who are exposed to blood; clients and staff of institutions for the developmentally disabled; inmates of long-term correctional facilities; and certain international travelers. • Persons with chronic liver disease.	• Three doses are needed on a 0, 1, 6 mo schedule. • Alternative timing options for vaccination include 0, 2, 4 mo and 0, 1, 4 mo. • There must be 4 wks between doses #1 and #2, and 8 wks between doses #2 and #3. Overall, there must be at least 16 wks between doses #1 and #3. • Schedule for those who have fallen behind: If the series is delayed between doses, DO NOT start the series over. Continue from where you left off.	Contraindication Previous anaphylactic reaction to this vaccine or to any of its components. Precaution Moderate or severe acute illness.

(continued on next page)

Table 8–7 *(continued from previous page)*

Vaccine Name and Route	For Whom Vaccination Is Recommended	Schedule for Vaccine Administration (Any Vaccine Can Be Given with Another)	Contraindications and Precautions (Mild Illness Is Not a Contraindication)
	Note: Provide serologic screening for immigrants from endemic areas. When HBsAg-positive persons are identified, offer appropriate disease management. In addition, screen their sex partners and household members, and give the first dose of vaccine at the same visit. If found susceptible, complete the vaccine series.		
Hepatitis A (HepA) *Give IM* Brands may be used interchangeably.	• Persons who travel or work anywhere except the United States, western Europe, New Zealand, Australia, Canada, and Japan. • Persons with chronic liver disease, including persons with hepatitis B and C; injecting and noninjecting drug users; men who have sex with men; people with clotting-factor disorders; persons who work with hepatitis A virus in experimental lab settings (not routine medical laboratories); and food handlers when health authorities or private employers determine vaccination to be cost effective. • Anyone wishing to obtain immunity to hepatitis A. Note: Prevaccination testing is likely to be cost-effective for persons older than age 40 yrs, as well as for younger persons in certain groups with a high prevalence of hepatitis A virus infection.	For Twinrix® (hepatitis A and B combination vaccine [GSK]), three doses are needed on a 0, 1, 6 mo schedule. Recipients must be of age 18 yrs or older. • Two doses are needed. • The minimum interval between doses #1 and #2 is 6 mo. • If dose #2 is delayed, do not repeat dose #1. Just give dose #2.	Contraindication Previous anaphylactic reaction to this vaccine or to any of its components. Precautions • Moderate or severe acute illness. • Safety during pregnancy has not been determined, so benefits must be weighed against potential risk.
Td, DTaP (Tetanus, diphtheria, pertussis) *Give IM*	• All adults who lack a history of a primary series consisting of at least three doses of tetanus- and diphtheria-containing vaccine. • A booster dose of tetanus- and diphtheria-containing toxoid may be needed for wound management as early as 5 yrs after receiving a previous dose, so consult ACIP recommendations.* • Using tetanus toxoid (TT) instead of Td or DTaP is not recommended. • In pregnancy, when indicated, give Td or DTaP in 2nd or 3rd trimester. If not administered during pregnancy, give DTaP in immediate postpartum period. ***For DTaP (tetanus- and diphtheria-toxoids with acellular pertussis vaccine) only:***	• For persons who are unvaccinated or behind, complete the primary series with Td (spaced at 0, 1–2 mo, 6–12 mo intervals). One dose of DTaP may be used for any dose if aged 19–64 yrs. • Give Td booster every 10 yrs after the primary series has been completed. For adults aged 19–64 yrs, a one-time dose of DTaP is recommended to replace the next Td. • Intervals of 2 yrs or less between Td and DTaP may be used if needed.	Contraindications • Previous anaphylactic reaction to this vaccine or to any of its components. • For DTaP only, history of encephalopathy within 7 days following DTP/DTaP. Precautions • Moderate or severe acute illness. • Guillain-Barré syndrome within 6 wks of receiving a previous dose of tetanus toxoid-containing vaccine. • Unstable neurologic condition. • Note: Use of Td or DTaP is not contraindicated in pregnancy. At the provider's discretion, either vaccine may be administered during the 2nd or 3rd trimester.

(continued on next page)

Table 8-7 *(continued from previous page)*

Vaccine Name and Route	For Whom Vaccination Is Recommended	Schedule for Vaccine Administration (Any Vaccine Can Be Given with Another)	Contraindications and Precautions (Mild Illness Is Not a Contraindication)
	• All adults younger than age 65 yrs who have not received DTaP. • Health care workers who work in hospitals or ambulatory care settings and have direct patient contact and who have not received DTaP. • Adults in contact with infants younger than age 12 month (e.g., parents, grandparents younger than age 65 yrs, child care providers, health care workers) who have not received a dose of DTaP.	Note: The two DTaP products are licensed for different age groups: Adacel (sanofi) for use in persons aged 11–64 yrs and Boostrix (GSK) for use in persons aged 10–18 yrs.	
Polio (IPV) *Give IM or SC*	Not routinely recommended for persons aged 18 yrs and older. Note: Adults living in the United States who never received or completed a primary series of polio vaccine need not be vaccinated unless they intend to travel to areas where exposure to wild-type virus is likely (i.e., India, Pakistan, Afghanistan, and certain countries in Africa). Previously vaccinated adults can receive one booster dose if traveling to polio endemic areas.	• Refer to ACIP recommendations* regarding unique situations, schedules, and dosing information.	Contraindication Previous anaphylactic or neurologic reaction to this vaccine or to any of its components. Precautions • Moderate or severe acute illness. • Pregnancy
Varicella (Var) (Chickenpox) *Give SC*	All adults without evidence of immunity. Immunity is defined as any one of the following: • a history of two doses of Var. • born in the United States before 1980. • history of varicella disease or herpes zoster based on health care provider diagnosis. • laboratory evidence of immunity or laboratory confirmation of disease.	• Two doses are needed. • Dose #2 is given 4–8 wks after dose #1. • If Var and either MMR, LAIV, and/or yellow fever vaccine are not given on the same day, space them at least 28 days apart. • If the second dose is delayed, do not repeat dose #1. Just give dose #2.	Contraindications • Previous anaphylactic reaction to this vaccine or to any of its components. • Pregnancy or possibility of pregnancy within 4 wks. • Persons immunocompromised because of malignancies and primary or acquired cellular immunodeficiency including HIV/AIDS. (see *MMWR* 1999, Vol. 48, No. RR-6.) Note: For those on high-dose immunosuppressive therapy, consult ACIP recommendations regarding delay time.* Precautions • If blood, plasma, and/or immunoglobulin (Ig or VZIG) were given in past 11mo, see ACIP statement *General Recommendations on Immunization** regarding time to wait before vaccinating. • Moderate or severe acute illness.
Meningococcal conjugate vaccine (MCV4) *Give IM*	• College freshmen living in dormitories. • Adolescents and adults with anatomic or functional asplenia or with terminal complement component deficiencies.	• One dose is needed. • If previous vaccine was MPSV4, revaccinate after 5yrs if risk continues.	Contraindication Previous anaphylactic or neurologic reaction to this vaccine or to any of its components, including diphtheria toxoid (for MCV4).

(continued on next page)

Table 8–7 *(continued from previous page)*

Vaccine Name and Route	For Whom Vaccination Is Recommended	Schedule for Vaccine Administration (Any Vaccine Can Be Given with Another)	Contraindications and Precautions (Mild Illness Is Not a Contraindication)
Polysaccharide vaccine (MPSV4) *Give SC*	• Persons who travel to or reside in countries in which meningococcal disease is hyperendemic or epidemic (e.g., the "meningitis belt" of sub-Saharan Africa). • Microbiologists who are routinely exposed to isolates of *N. meningitidis*.	• Revaccination after MCV4 is not recommended. • MCV4 is preferred over MPSV4 for persons age 55 yrs and younger, although MPSV4 is an acceptable alternative.	Precautions • Moderate or severe acute illness. • For MCV4 only, history of Guillain-Barré syndrome.
MMR (measles, mumps, rubella) *Give SC*	• Persons born in 1957 or later (especially those born outside the United States.) should receive at least one dose of MMR if there is no serologic proof of immunity or documentation of a dose given on or after the first birthday. • Persons in high-risk groups, such as health care workers, students entering college and other post–high school educational institutions, and international travelers, should receive a total of two doses. • Persons born before 1957 are usually considered immune, but proof of immunity (serology or vaccination) may be desirable for health care workers. • Women of childbearing age who do not have acceptable evidence of rubella immunity or vaccination.	• One or two doses are needed. • If dose #2 is recommended, give it no sooner than 4 wks after dose #1. • If MMR and either Var, LAIV, and/or yellow fever vaccine are not given on the same day, space them at least 28 d apart. • If a pregnant woman is found to be rubella susceptible, administer MMR postpartum.	Contraindications • Previous anaphylactic reaction to this vaccine or to any of its components. • Pregnancy or possibility of pregnancy within 4 wks. • Persons immunocompromised because of cancer, leukemia, lymphoma, immunosuppressive drug therapy, including high-dose steroids or radiation therapy. Note: HIV positivity is NOT a contraindication to MMR except for those who are severely immunocompromised. Precautions • If blood, plasma, and/or immunoglobulin were given in past 11 mo, see ACIP statement *General Recommendations on Immunization** regarding time to wait before vaccinating. • Moderate or severe acute illness. • History of thrombocytopenia or thrombocytopenic purpura. Note: If PPD (tuberculosis skin test) and MMR are both needed but not given on same day, delay PPD for 4–6 wks after MMR.
Human-papillomavirus (HPV) *Give IM*	All previously unvaccinated women through age 26 yrs.	• Three doses are needed. • Dose #2 is given 4–8 wks after dose #1, and dose #3 is given 6 mo after dose #1 (at least 12 wks after dose #2).	Contraindication Previous anaphylactic reaction to this vaccine or to any of its components. Precaution data on vaccination in pregnancy are limited; therefore, vaccination during pregnancy should be delayed until after completion of the pregnancy.
Zoster (shingles) (Zos) *Give SC*	A herpes zoster (shingles) vaccine was licensed in May 2006 for use in persons aged 60 yrs and older. ACIP recommendations for its use are pending. Refer to the package insert for details on its use.		

*For specific ACIP recommendations, refer to the official ACIP statements published in MMWR. To obtain copies of these statements, call the CDC-INFO Contact Center at (800) 232-4636; visit CDC's Web site at www.cdc.gov/nip/publications/ACIP-list.htm; or visit the Immunization Action Coalition (IAC) Web site at www.immunize.org/acip.

This table is revised periodically. Visit IAC's website at www.immunize.org/adultrules to make sure you have the most current version. IAC thanks William Atkinson, MD, MPH, from CDC's National Center for Immunization and Respiratory Diseases for his assistance. For more information, contact IAC at 1573 Selby Avenue, St. Paul, MN 55104, (651) 647-9009, or E-mail: admin@immunize.org.

Item #P2011 (9/06).

www.immunize.org/catg.d/p2011b.pdf.

Immunization Action Coalition 1573 Selby Avenue St. Paul MN 55104. E-mail: admin@immunize.org; Web: http://www.immunize.org/

- Procedures should be in place to deal with allergic/anaphylactic reactions to the vaccine.

Interventions

- To minimize local reactions:
  —use a needle with adequate length to inject the antigen deep in the muscle mass;
  —inject into the vastus lateralis or ventrogluteal muscle in infants; the deltoid muscle may be used in children over 18 months old or for infants receiving the HBV vaccine;
  —clear the needle after injecting the vaccine by using an air bubble.
- To minimize pain:
  —apply topical EMLA (eutectic mixture of local anesthetic) to the injection site and after injecting, cover the site with an occlusive dressing for 2.5 hours.
  —apply an EMLA patch, which requires no dressing.
  —Spray a vapocoolant (ethyl chloride or Fluori-Methane) directly on the skin or on a cotton ball, which is placed on the skin 15 seconds before injecting.
  —use a distraction, such as telling the child to "take a deep breath and blow and blow and blow until I tell you to stop."

Contraindications to Administering Vaccine

- All vaccines
  —Anaphylactic reaction or allergy to the vaccine or any of its components
  —Moderate or severe illness with or without a fever
  —Avoid giving live virus immunizations to children with an impaired immune system (except MMR for children with HIV), to children living with an immunosuppressed person, during pregnancy, and in women who may become pregnant within 3 months
  —Postpone giving live virus vaccines to children who have received passive immunity from blood transfusions or immunoglobulins, for 3–7 months
- DTaP
  —Severe adverse reactions from a previous DTaP immunization
  —Encephalopathy within 7 days of administration of previous dose of DTaP
  —Wait for at least 90 days after receiving immunoglobulins
  —Anaphylactic reaction or allergy to neomycin, streptomycin, or polymyxin B
- MMR
  —Pregnancy
  —Known altered immunocompetency (hematologic and solid tumors, congenital immunodeficiency, long-term immunosuppressive therapy) except HIV
  —Allergy to eggs and neomycin
- HBV
  —Anaphylactic reaction or allergy to common baker's yeast
- Var
  —Immunocompromised individuals (e.g., HIV, acute lymphocytic leukemia)
  —Pregnancy
- PCV
  —Allergy to vaccine components or anaphylactic response to previous dose
  —Acute, moderate, or severe illness with or without fever
- Influenza
  —Acute febrile illness
  —Egg hypersensitivity
- Hepatitis A (HAVRIX or VAQTA)
  —Sensitivity to alum or phenoxyethanol
- Haemophilus Influenza type B
  —No contraindications; quite safe

Precautions – Weigh Risks and Benefits Before Administering Vaccine

- DPaT –
  —Fever greater than 40.5°C (105°F) within 48 hours of vaccination with a prior dose of DTaP
  —Collapse or shock-like state within 48 hours of prior dose of DTaP
  —Seizures within 3 days of prior dose of DTaP
  —Persistent, inconsolable crying lasting 3 hours within 48 hours of prior dose of DTaP
  —Pregnancy
- IPV
  —Pregnancy
- MMR
  —Recent immunoglobulin administration.
  —MMR and immunoglobulin products should not be given simultaneously; if they must be given at the same time, give at different sites and revaccinate or test for seroconversion in 3 months.
  —If immunoglobulin is given first, MMR should not be given for 3–6 months, depending on the dose. If MMR is given first, immunoglobulin should not be given for 2 weeks.
  —Thrombocytopenia.

Side Effects/Allergic and Adverse Reactions

- DTaP
  —Usually occur within a few hours or days of administration, and are usually limited to local tenderness, erythema, and swelling at the injection site, low-grade fever; behavioral changes, and mild anorexia
  —Reactions are usually less severe when the deltoid site is used versus the vastus lateralis site

- —Severe adverse reactions include anaphylaxis, shock or collapse, fever greater than 102°F, and persistent crying
- IPV, Salk
  - —Site tenderness and irritability
- Hib
  - —Low-grade fever and mild local reactions at the injection site; usually resolve rapidly.
  - —Fever above 101.3°F may rarely occur.
- MMR
  - —Unfavorable reactions and vaccine related disorders can occur for 30–60 days
  - —Are usually mild; in older children and adults, reactions to rubella may be more troublesome. Include rash, itching, low-grade fever, and arthralgia
  - —Studies have found no association between MMR and autism

Client teaching for self-care

- Parents need to be informed about vaccine safety, and benefits and risks associated with their administration
- Lack of knowledge and unfounded fears may needlessly expose a child to the dangers of life-threatening diseases
- Each child should have an accurate immunization record, kept by both the parents and physician. Parents should be made aware of when vaccinations are due to be given
- Adolescents need to maintain their level of immunization by receiving booster shots when necessary

- Children at high risk should receive any of the following nonmandated vaccines, as necessary:
  - —Nonmandated vaccines
    - Meningococcal Polysaccharide Vaccine (MPSV4)—preferred for children of ages 2–10
    - Meningococcal Conjugate Vaccine (MCV4)—preferred for older children
      - For prevention of meningococcal disease, which can lead to high fever, deafness, and death
      - Recommended for children of 2 years and older with terminal complement deficiencies and anatomic or functional asplenia, incoming college students who will live in dormitories, and military recruits
      - Safety during pregnancy has not been established
    - Lyme Disease Vaccine
      - Recommended for those living in lyme endemic areas and for those infected with lyme disease, ages 15–70
      - Has been demonstrated to be safe for children 4–18 years old
    - Influenza Virus Vaccine
  - —Recommended for
    - children older than 6 months who have a chronic illness (cardiac or respiratory disorder, renal disease, diabetes mellitus), sickle cell disease, HIV, and children on long-term aspirin therapy;
    - adults who are elderly and frail;
    - health care professionals;
    - persons (family members, caregivers) who are in close contact with those at high risk.

LIFESTYLE CHOICES

- Healthy lifestyle is the choice of living behaviors, which maximize health and decrease risk of illness and death.
- Lifestyle choices are based on family experience with its ethnic, cultural, religious, and socioeconomic beliefs.
- Major risk factors related to illness and death are related to the Healthy People 2010 leading health indicators: age, heredity, diet, stress, exercise, smoking, alcohol use, environmental factors such as pollution, poverty, occupational hazards, unprotected sex, drunk driving, failure to wear seat belts in automobiles, helmets when riding motorcycles or bikes, helmets and knee and elbow protective gear when in-line skating.

GUIDELINES FOR HEALTHY LIVING

- *Eat a balanced diet* (see nutrition in Chapter 13 for further information including serving size and number)
  - —Select foods and number of daily servings of the five food groups based on the MYPyramid food guidance system produced by the US Department of Agriculture (MYPyramid.gov), which focuses on a balance between food eaten and energy expended in physical activity and recommends limited fat, sugar, and salt.
  - —Eat a variety of grains daily, at least half of which are whole grains, which provide complex carbohydrates. Approximately 60% of daily calories should be from carbohydrates and 80% of these from complex carbohydrates.
  - —Eat a variety of fruits and vegetables daily; they are rich in vitamins C and A, complex carbohydrates, and fiber. Daily diet should contain 20–30 g of fiber.
  - —Prepare, cook, serve, and store foods so they remain safe to eat.
  - —Select a diet that is low in saturated fat and cholesterol and moderate in total fat. Daily intake of cholesterol should be

less than 300 mg and fat intake 30% or less of total calories with not more than 10% from saturated fats.

—Select foods and beverages to moderate sugar intake.

—Choose and prepare foods with less salt. Limit daily intake to slightly less than one teaspoon per day.

—Use alcohol only in moderation: not more than two small glasses of wine, two cans of beer, or two drinks with not more than 1 ½ oz of alcohol per day each.

—Drink 5–8 glasses of water each day.

- *Maintain a healthy weight*

—Obesity is a chronic disease.

—Research has demonstrated relationships between obesity and coronary artery disease, hypertension, stroke, diabetes, arthritis, and selected cancers.

—Obesity and overweight is an increasing problem in the United States particularly in the Hispanic population.

—Ongoing balance between caloric intake and energy expended is the goal of weight control programs.

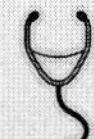

Assessment Alert

Best measure of weight is the BMI because it applies to men and women regardless of frame size or muscle mass.

BMI does not work for pregnant women, competitive athletes, or frail elderly.

—Loss of 1 lb of fat per week requires a 500-calorie deficit per day.

—Daily caloric requirement for men is about 2200 calories and for sedentary women and older adults about 1600 calories.

—Dieting with a marked reduction in daily calories results in an initial significant weight loss mainly due to water loss; more weight typically is then not lost for 7–10 days.

—Group support or a weight loss partner helps clients stick to the needed diet

—Diet teaching is most effective when the whole family or social group is involved especially if the client is not the cook.

—Drinking two or three glasses of water before each meal results in a feeling of fullness, which suppresses appetite.

- *Exercise regularly*

—Benefits of exercise

- Improves cardiovascular fitness
- Helps control weight
- Creates a sense of well-being
- Increases or maintains strength and endurance
- Increases or maintains flexibility
- Maintains bone mass
- Increases glucose tolerance; helps prevent Type II diabetes
- Increases proportion of HDLs
- Reduces concentration of triglycerides
- Reduces risk of coronary artery disease
- Helps prevent hypertension

—Types of exercise

- Aerobic: rhythmic, continuous use of large muscle groups, e.g., swimming, dancing, and walking
- Anaerobic: bursts of energy expended at intervals, e.g., weight lifting

—Muscular strength

- Ability to contract at or near maximum for a short period of time
- Best improved by activities that overload or gradually increase the resistance (load or weight) that muscles must move
- Three types of overload-based exercise are
    - isometric: muscles contract against an immovable object because resistance is so great; can be dangerous for people with hypertension; not generally used in strength training.
    - isotonic resistive: repetitively use muscles to move or lift specific fixed resistances or weights, e.g., weight lifting, resistance exercise machines; most common type of exercise done to build strength.
    - isokinetic: resistance moves only at a preset speed regardless of force applied so muscles are consistently overloaded throughout the range of motion; require expensive machines.

Strength training helps minimize the progression of osteoporosis and helps older adults maintain muscle mass and strength.

—Muscular endurance

- Ability to perform at submaximal levels for a long period of time
- Improved by activities requiring repeated muscular contractions of less than maximal degree, e.g., sweeping, raking, or pushing a lawn mower

—Flexibility

- Ability of joints to move with ease through their range of motion
- Maintained by stretching
- Static stretching: slow stretch held at the most extended point for 10–30 seconds
- Ballistic stretching: repetitive, bouncing, quick, and forceful stretches

—Guidelines for cardiorespiratory fitness exercise training (American Academy of Sports Medicine)

- Mode of activity: any continuous physical activity using large muscle groups; may be rhythmic and aerobic
- Frequency: three to five times per week

- Intensity: (amount of effort put into an activity) moderate
- Duration: 30–60 minutes
- Higher levels of frequency, intensity, and duration can be set for specific clients

Nursing Process Elements (exercise)

Determine client's current pattern of activity and exercise. Determine client's understanding ofthe need for exercise to maintain/attain optimum health

Client teaching for self-care

- Consult physician if over age 45 or with risk factors for cardiovascular disease before beginning an exercise program
- Warm up with stretching before aerobic exercise and allow for a cool-down period at the end to let the heart gradually return to normal rate; this helps prevent hypotension and syncope
- Wear proper clothing
- Use any equipment correctly
- Avoid exercising in extremes of temperature
- Suggestions to help clients adhere to an exercise program:
  —Select a simple, not a complex, exercise routine
  —Exercise with a friend or group
  —Have a scheduled time to exercise that fits with daily lifestyle
  —Start small and increase gradually
  —Incorporate music into exercise routine
- *Avoid smoking*
  —Tobacco smoking is the number one cause of preventable death in the United States (40,000 deaths per year)
  —Tobacco-related causes of death include lung cancer; COPD; bladder, renal, pancreatic, and female reproductive cancers; CAD, hypertension, PVD, and cerebrovascular disease
  —Second-hand smoke causes 3000 deaths per year from lung cancer and numerous fetal problems
  —Nicotine is an addiction. It causes release of epinephrine resulting in tachycardia, peripheral vasoconstriction, elevation of blood pressure, and a feeling of euphoria
  —Withdrawal effects include irritability, anger, anxiety, restlessness, hunger, decreased concentration, and cravings
  —Snuffing tobacco or smoking cigars or pipes is associated with cancer of the lip, tongue, mouth, larynx, and esophagus
  —Approaches to smoking cessation include 12-step support programs, psychotherapy, hypnosis, aversion therapy, acupuncture, and nicotine replacement by means of gums, patches, nasal sprays, or pills, which is designed to alleviate withdrawal symptoms.

Nursing Process Elements (smoking)

- Use the "four A" approach with clients who are smokers.
  —Ask about the client's smoking habit
  —Advise client to stop smoking
  —Assist client to develop a specific plan to stop smoking
  —Arrange follow-up and support

Client teaching for self-care

- During the first week of smoking cessation, stay away from places and activities where people smoke
- Try chewing regular gum, sucking hard candy, using imagery or engaging in deep breathing, or other relaxation routine to control cravings
- Do not smoke if using nicotine replacement therapy because of the risk of overdose: headache, abdominal pain, N&V, and in some cases severe hypotension and its sequelae
- Most at risk for deleterious effects of overdose are clients with heart problems
- *Act responsibly in regard to sexual activity to prevent STIs and unwanted pregnancies*
  —STIs are epidemic among young adults and teenagers
  —STIs tend to have more serious effects in women
  —STIs are associated in pregnant women with spontaneous abortion, prematurity, low birth weight, and congenital infection
  —Engage only in "safer" sex
- *Limit sun exposure*
  —UVA and UVB rays are both harmful to the skin; they cause premature aging with wrinkling and are directly related to the development of skin cancer.
  —Different skin types vary in sensitivity to the skin; sunscreens with an SPF of 15 are appropriate for all types.

Nursing Process Elements (sun exposure)

Assess client's skin type.
Assess client's lifestyle for degree of sun exposure.

Client teaching for self-care

- Use sunscreen with a sun protection factor of 15 every day applying it at least 30 minutes before sun exposure
- Wear a hat and long-sleeved clothing when out in sun to shield from rays
- Avoid being out in the sun between 10 a.m. and 3 p.m. when ultraviolet rays are most intense
- Reapply sunscreen (even water resistant) after swimming, strenuous exercise, or prolonged sunbathing
- Avoid tanning lamps and commercial tanning booths

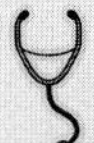

Assessment Alert

Photosensitivity rashes associated with medications have an abrupt onset and are bright red, symmetrical, and widespread. Medications that are associated with photosensitivity include certain tetracyclines, sulfas, antihypertensives, diuretics, oral hypoglycemics, psychotropic drugs, and NSAIDs.

- Avoid other risky behaviors: do not travel in an automobile without a seat belt; do not ride a motorcycle without proper training and a helmet; do not take infants and children in automobiles without proper car seats/seatbelts; do not in-line skate without a helmet and elbow and knee protectors; do not ride a bicycle without a helmet; do not abuse drugs or alcohol (see Chapter 12; do not remain in an environment with respiratory irritants without a protective mask or other device; do not remain in areas with loud sound without ear plugs; never dive in shallow water
- Research has linked dietary factors to the development of diseases such as heart disease, diabetes, and certain cancers

PRINCIPLES OF TEACHING/LEARNING

- Learning
  - —Acquisition of a new or changed behavior by an individual
- Factors influencing learning are
  - —motivation,
  - —readiness to learn,
  - —cognitive ability,
  - —sensory ability,
  - —environment,
  - —physical status,
  - —comfort level, and
  - —culture.
- Strategies to promote learning:
  - —Provide comfortable environment: free of distraction, private, nonjudgmental, and comfortable temperature
  - —Involve client and family in developing teaching plan
  - —Build on existing knowledge
  - —Use short-term goals
  - —Actively involve client
  - —Use multiple strategies
  - —Provide positive reinforcement
  - —Evaluate learning through return demonstration, observing subsequent behavior, written test, return explanation, and self-report
  - —Make client physically comfortable: pain free, empty bladder
- Areas of client teaching:
  - —About health problem
  - —About prescribed medications: name, dose, route, frequency, directions for taking (e.g., with water, food, on an empty stomach, do not take with foods, OTC, or prescribed medications), common side effects and how to manage them, adverse effects to be reported to health care provider, and expected effect
  - —About follow-up care: when and how reports of lab tests will be received, date and times of next visit, needed follow up lab tests intervals, how to make appointment
  - —Prevention and health promotion: screening guidelines, healthy lifestyle guidelines (each system—cigarette smoking, alcohol)
  - —Preoperative teaching
  - —Therapeutic interventions
  - —Community services/support groups applicable to condition

WORKSHEET

Mark each health-related activity as an example of primary, secondary, or tertiary prevention.

1. Screening for hearing deficits
2. Teaching about dangers of high-fat diets
3. Recreation program for children of working mothers
4. Use of neonatal intensive care units
5. Immunization of the elderly against pneumonia
6. Clinical breast examinations
7. Health fair exhibit about dangers of water pollution
8. Physical therapy for an accident victim
9. Colonoscopy to screen for bowel cancer
10. Removal of asbestos tile from buildings

Mark each factor listed below as a leading health indicator from Healthy People 2010 or not. Do this by writing Healthy People 2010 beside those that are and No by the side of those that are not.

1. Physical activity
2. Accident mortality
3. Overweight and obesity
4. Tobacco use
5. Cancer screening
6. Chronic disease morbidity
7. Substance abuse
8. Responsible sexual behavior
9. Mental health
10. Incidence of infectious disease
11. Injury and violence
12. Environmental quality

13. Deaths from heart disease
14. Immunization
15. Access to health care

Underline the types of health screening recommended for a school-aged child.

1. Lead
2. Vision
3. Hearing
4. HIV
5. Mental health
6. Blood pressure
7. Scoliosis
8. Height/weight
9. Bone density
10. Tuberculosis (PPD)
11. Dental
12. Urinalysis
13. Hematocrit or hemoglobin
14. Physical abuse
15. Blood sugar

FILL IN THE BLANKS

Fill in the blank spaces with the correct word or phrase to complete each statement.

1. What are the five stages of health behavior changes as described by Prochaska et al.?

   ____

   ____

   ____

(continued)

____

____

____

2. In-depth assessment of client's health status is the foundation for __________.

3. The purpose of __________ is to identify risk factors or undiagnosed disease to allow for early intervention.

4. The most basic type of health promotion program is one that disseminates information to __________.

5. In a healthy diet at least __________ of the daily intake of grains should be whole grains.

6. How many 8-oz glasses of water should an adult drink per day? __________.

7. BMI as a measure of weight cannot be used for clients who are __________, __________, or __________.

8. Most sedentary women and older adults need about __________ cal/d whereas men need about __________ cal/d.

9. Rhythmic, continuous exercise using large muscle groups is __________.

10. The two overarching goals of Healthy People 2010 are to __________ and to __________.

APPLICATION QUESTIONS

1. Why can infants born without an immune system survive for the first few months of their lives with no apparent problems?
   a. Limited antibodies are produced by bacteria in the infant's colon.
   b. The exposure to pathogens during this time is limited.
   c. Antibodies are passively received from the mother through the placenta and breast milk.
   d. The fetal thymus produced a limited number of antibodies during the eighth and ninth months of pregnancy.

2. The nurse explains to the mother of a child who has received a tetanus toxoid injection, that this vaccination confers which type of immunity?
   a. Lifelong active natural immunity
   b. Lifelong passive immunity
   c. Long lasting active immunity
   d. Temporary passive natural immunity

3. Why are live virus vaccines contraindicated for children receiving corticosteroid, antineoplastic, or irradiation therapy? These children
   a. Are be susceptible to infection because of their depressed immune response
   b. Have had the disease already or may have been immunized against it
   c. Are be unlikely to need this protection since they probably have a shortened lifespan
   d. Have an allergy to rabbit serum, which is used as is for these vaccines

4. The nurse is asked which immunizations a child, currently up-to-date on all primary immunizations, should receive before starting kindergarten. He is currently up to date on all the primary immunizations. Which boosters should the mother be told the child needs?
   a. IPV, Hep-B, and Td
   b. DTaP, Hep-B, and Td
   c. MMR, DTaP, and Hib
   d. DTaP, IPV, and MMR

5. The nurse is reviewing the immunization history of an 11-month-old baby boy. Which diseases should the nurse expect the child to already have been immunized against?
   a. Polio, pertussis, tetanus, and diphtheria
   b. Pertussis, tetanus, polio, and measles

c. Measles, mumps, rubella, and tuberculosis
d. Rubella, polio, measles, tuberculosis, and pertussis

6. Which is an example of primary prevention?
a. Testing neonates for sickle cell anemia
b. Admitting clients to an intensive care unit
c. Screening clients for osteoporosis
d. Speaking to community groups about radon exposure in the home

7. Which is an example of secondary prevention?
a. Physical therapy for a stroke client
b. Immunization of children against measles
c. Teaching about birth control
d. Screening for hypertension

8. Which is an example of tertiary prevention?
a. Occupational therapy for a client with spinal cord injury
b. PPD testing for tuberculosis
c. After school programs for at-risk youth
d. Vision checks

9. A client comes to the clinic complaining of a rash that suddenly appeared while she was sunbathing earlier in the day. Assessment shows that the rash is bright red, covers wide symmetrical areas of the body, and has no accompanying local or systemic symptoms. Which question would be most important for the nurse to ask?
a. Did you use a new brand of sunscreen?
b. Did you wash with perfumed soap before sunbathing?
c. What medications do you take?
d. Have you eaten any new foods in the last 24 hours?

10. The mother of an infant is questioning the nurse about the health care needed by her child. She expresses concern because of the number of people in her family with high blood pressure and asks when her baby's blood pressure will be checked. Which is the appropriate response for the nurse to give?
a. age 1
b. age 3
c. age 6
d. age 12

11. Which health model does a person subscribe to when his or her motivation to engage in healthy behaviors is the desire to avoid illness?
a. Clinical
b. Adaptive
c. Role Performance
d. Eudaemonistic

12. For which age groups would the nurse most appropriately plan to include a discussion of suicide as part of a health promotion program?
a. Children and teenagers
b. Teenagers and young adults
c. Young and middle adults
d. Middle and older adults

13. Which client could the nurse administer an MMR vaccine to?
a. A child with HIV
b. A woman who is trying to get pregnant.
c. A child whose father had a kidney transplant.
d. A 7-month pregnant woman

14. Which statement made by a client who is starting a smoking cessation program using a combination of nicotine replacement and hypnosis indicates the need for further teaching?
a. "I will try to use deep breathing and imagery to control cravings."
b. "I will suck hard candy when I get an urge for a cigarette."
c. "I will smoke just half a cigarette if I really feel out of control."
d. "I will stay away from places where people smoke during the next week."

15. Which direction regarding self-testicular examination is appropriate for a nurse to give a 20-year-old male client?
a. Do not examine your testicles for at least 12 hours after intercourse.
b. Examine both testicles simultaneously so one can be compared to the other.
c. Keep in mind there may normally be what feels like a small bump on the upper or middle outer side of the testis.
d. If one testicle appears larger than the other, see your physician immediately.

16. Which statement made by a client about self-breast examination indicates the need for health teaching?
a. "I palpate my breast carefully each month while standing in front of a mirror so I can see any changes in the contour or appearance of the skin."
b. "I use the finger pads of the three middle fingers of each hand to palpate my breasts."
c. "I use an up-and-down pattern of palpation on my breast and go all the way up until I reach my collar bone."

(continued)

d. "I press lightly, then with medium pressure, and then with firm pressure on each area of my breast as I examine it."

17. A client who has been told that her total cholesterol is too high and that a cholesterol-lowering drug is being prescribed for her says that different people normally have different cholesterol levels and that everyone doesn't need pills and she is not going to take the ordered medication. According to the Stage Model of health behavior change, which stage is she in?
   a. Precontemplation
   b. Contemplation
   c. Preparation
   d. Termination

18. How does the nurse begin to develop a Health Promotion Plan with a client?
   a. Involve a significant other
   b. Identify priority health goals
   c. Reinforce benefits of a change in health behaviors
   d. Obtain a commitment to a healthy lifestyle

19. Which are strategies that the nurse may employ to aid a client in implementing a Health Promotion Plan? Mark all that apply.
   a. ___Group counseling
   b. ___Telephone counseling
   c. ___Modeling
   d. ___Ensuring social support
   e. ___Teaching

20. Which statement best indicates that a client who needs to begin an exercise program to improve cardiorespiratory fitness is in the preparation stage of the Stage Model of health behavior change?
   a. "I never really liked exercise but maybe I could get to like it."
   b. "I think maybe I really do need to exercise; I get awfully short of breath going upstairs."
   c. "I asked my friend if she would be interested in going to an exercise class with me."
   d. "I asked my sister and she agrees exercise isn't always a good thing."

21. A mother states she will not allow her child to receive immunizations which contain live or attenuated organisms. Which immunizations could the child not receive?
   a. ___MMR
   b. ___HBV
   c. ___Varicella
   d. ___DTaP
   e. ___TIV influenza
   f. ___IPV

22. A client asks about receiving the hepatitis A vaccine because of upcoming travel to an underdeveloped country where the disease is endemic. The client particularly wants to know how many injections are needed and at what interval. Which is a correct response for the nurse to give?
   a. 2 injections @ 3 months apart
   b. 2 injections @ 6–18 months apart
   c. 3 injections @ 1 month apart
   d. 3 injections @ 3 months apart

23. What purpose does clearing the needle by injecting an air bubble after administration of an immunization serve?
   a. Decrease risk of an anaphylactic reaction
   b. Decrease pain during injection
   c. Minimize local reaction
   d. Ensure proper dose

24. Which information should be given to a 52-year-old client who is planning to start a cardiorespiratory exercise program?
   a. Consult your physician to obtain an exercise prescription
   b. Include only anaerobic activities
   c. Stretch at the completion of each exercise session
   d. Work up gradually to a maximum of 90 minutes five times per week.

ANSWERS & RATIONALES

Mark each health-related activity as an example of primary, secondary, or tertiary prevention.

1. Screening for hearing deficits *Secondary*

2. Teaching about dangers of high-fat diets *Primary*

3. Recreation program for children of working mothers *Primary*

4. Use of neonatal intensive care units *Tertiary*

5. Immunization of the elderly against pneumonia *Primary*

6. Clinical breast examinations *Secondary*

7. Health fair exhibit about dangers of water pollution *Primary*

8. Physical therapy for an accident victim *Tertiary*

9. Colonoscopy to screen for bowel cancer *Secondary*

10. Removal of asbestos tile from buildings *Primary*

Mark each factor listed below as a leading health indicator from Healthy People 2010 or not. Do this by writing Healthy People 2010 beside those that are and No by the side of those that are not.

1. Physical activity *Healthy People 2010*

2. Accident mortality

3. Overweight and obesity *Healthy People 2010*

4. Tobacco use *Healthy People 2010*

5. Cancer screening

6. Chronic disease morbidity

7. Substance abuse *Healthy People 2010*

8. Responsible sexual behavior *Healthy People 2010*

9. Mental health *Healthy People 2010*

10. Incidence of infectious disease

11. Injury and violence *Healthy People 2010*

12. Environmental quality *Healthy People 2010*

13. Deaths from heart disease

14. Immunization *Healthy People 2010*

15. Access to health care *Healthy People 2010*

Underline the types of health screening recommended for a school-aged child.

1. Lead

2. Vision

(continued)

3. Hearing
4. HIV
5. Mental health
6. Blood pressure
7. Scoliosis
8. Height/weight
9. Bone density
10. Tuberculosis (PPD)
11. Dental
12. Urinalysis
13. Hematocrit or hemoglobin
14. Physical abuse
15. Blood sugar

ANSWERS FOR FILL IN THE BLANKS

Fill in the blank spaces with the correct word or phrase to complete each statement.

1. What are the five stages of health behavior changes as described by Prochaska et al.?
   ___ Precontemplation ___
   ___ Contemplation ___
   ___ Preparation ___
   ___ Action ___
   ___ Maintenance ___
   ___ Termination ___

2. In-depth assessment of client's health status is the foundation for ___ health promotion ___.

3. The purpose of ___ health screening ___ is to identify risk factors or undiagnosed disease to allow for early intervention.

4. The most basic type of health promotion program is one that disseminates information to ___ raise level of awareness and knowledge ___.

5. In a healthy diet, at least ___ half ___ of the daily intake of grains should be whole grains.

6. How many 8-oz glasses of water should an adult drink per day? ___ 5–8 ___.

7. BMI as a measure of weight cannot be used for clients who are __________ pregnant __________, __________ competitive athletes __________, or __________ frail elderly __________.

8. Most sedentary women and older adults need about __________ 1600 __________ cal/d. whereas men need about __________ 2200 __________ cal/d.

9. Rhythmic, continuous exercise using large muscle groups is __________ aerobic __________ exercise.

10. The two overarching goals of Healthy People 2010 are to __________ increase the quality and longevity of life __________ and to __________ eliminate disparities in health among different populations __________.

APPLICATION ANSWERS

1. Why can infants born without an immune system survive for the first few months of their lives with no apparent problems?
   a. Limited antibodies are produced by bacteria in the infant's colon.
   b. The exposure to pathogens during this time is limited.
   c. Antibodies are passively received from the mother through the placenta and breast milk.
   d. The fetal thymus produced a limited number of antibodies during the eighth and ninth months of pregnancy.

Rationale

Correct answer: c.

Antibodies received by the fetus in utero through the placenta and by the breast-fed newborn via the mother's milk provide the infant with immunity against most bacterial, viral, and fungal infections for the first few weeks after birth. Thereafter, as the titer of maternal antibodies drops and the infant is not replacing them with his own antibodies, infection can and will occur

2. The nurse explains to the mother of a child who has received a tetanus toxoid injection that this vaccination confers which type of immunity?
   a. Lifelong active natural immunity
   b. Lifelong passive immunity
   c. Long lasting active immunity
   d. Temporary passive natural immunity

Rationale

Correct answer: c.

The tetanus toxoid vaccine has modified toxins that stimulate the body to produce antibodies against tetanus that last for up to 10 years, at which time a booster shot will be necessary. Only having the actual disease can provide lifelong natural immunity.

3. Why are live virus vaccines contraindicated for children receiving corticosteroid, antineoplastic, or irradiation therapy? These children
   a. Are be susceptible to infection because of their depressed immune response
   b. Have had the disease already or may have been immunized against it
   c. Are be unlikely to need this protection since they probably have a shortened life span
   d. Have an allergy to rabbit serum, which is used as is for these vaccines

Rationale

Correct answer: a.

Corticosteroids, antineoplastic drugs, and radiation all depress the immune system, either by slowing the immune response or by killing off fast dividing cells, including lymphatic tissue and bone marrow, where antibodies are produced, and the body might not be able to fend off an attack by live virus injected into the system. It is therefore contraindicated

4. The nurse is asked which immunizations a child, currently up-to-date on all primary immunizations, should receive before starting kindergarten. He is currently up-to-date on all the primary immunizations. Which boosters should the mother be told the child needs?
   a. IPV, Hep-B, and Td
   b. DTaP, Hep-B, and Td
   c. MMR, DTaP, and Hib
   d. DTaP, IPV, and MMR

Rationale

Correct answer: d.

Only DTaP, IVP, and MMR require booster shots for preschool children. HepB does not require a booster, and a Td booster is given at age 7–10, depending on when the vaccine was first given. Hib booster is given at age 12–15 months.

(continued)

5. The nurse is reviewing the immunization history of an 11-month-old baby boy. Which diseases should the nurse expect the child to already have been immunized against?
   a. Polio, pertussis, tetanus, and diphtheria
   b. Pertussis, tetanus, polio, and measles
   c. Measles, mumps, rubella, and tuberculosis
   d. Rubella, polio, measles, tuberculosis, and pertussis

Rationale

Correct answer: a.

DTaP and IVP are given at 2, 4, and 6 months. MMR is not administered till age 12 months.

6. Which is an example of primary prevention?
   a. Testing neonates for sickle cell anemia
   b. Admitting clients to an intensive care unit
   c. Screening clients for osteoporosis
   d. Speaking to community groups about radon exposure in the home

Rationale

Correct answer: d.

Primary prevention is speaking to community groups about radon exposure in the home. Testing for sickle cell anemia is an example of secondary prevention, using intensive care unit is an example of tertiary prevention, screening for osteoporosis is an example of secondary prevention.

7. Which is an example of secondary prevention?
   a. Physical therapy for a stroke client
   b. Immunization of children against measles
   c. Teaching about birth control
   d. Screening for hypertension

Rationale

Correct answer: d.

Screening for hypertension is an example of secondary prevention. Physical therapy for a client with a stroke is an example of tertiary prevention. Immunization against measles is an example of primary prevention. Teaching about birth control is also primary prevention.

8. Which is an example of tertiary prevention?
   a. Occupational therapy for a client with spinal cord injury
   b. PPD testing for tuberculosis
   c. After school programs for at-risk youth
   d. Vision checks

Rationale

Correct answer: a.

Occupational therapy for a client with a spinal cord injury is an example of tertiary prevention. PPD testing for tuberculosis is an example of secondary prevention. After school programs for at-risk youth is secondary and checking for visual problems is secondary prevention.

9. A client comes to the clinic complaining of a rash that suddenly appeared while she was sunbathing earlier in the day. Assessment shows that the rash is bright red, covers wide symmetrical areas of the body, and has no accompanying local or systemic symptoms. Which question would be most important for the nurse to ask?
   a. Did you use a new brand of sunscreen?
   b. Did you wash with perfumed soap before sunbathing?
   c. What medications do you take?
   d. Have you eaten any new foods in the last 24 hours?

Rationale

Correct answer: c.

Photosensitivity rashes associated with medications have an abrupt onset and are bright red, symmetrical, and widespread. Medications that are associated with photosensitivity include certain tetracyclines, sulfas, antihypertensives, diuretics, oral hypoglycemics, psychotropic drugs, and NSAIDs.

10. The mother of an infant is questioning the nurse about the health care needed by her child. She expresses concern because of the number of people in her family with high blood pressure and asks when her baby's blood pressure will be checked. Which is the appropriate response for the nurse to give?
   a. age 1
   b. age 3
   c. age 6
   d. age 12

Rationale

Correct answer: b.

The American Academy of Pediatrics recommends that blood pressure screening start at age 3 and be a part of every physical checkup thereafter.

11. Which health model does a person subscribe to when his or her motivation to engage in healthy behaviors is the desire to avoid illness?
   a. Clinical
   b. Adaptive
   c. Role performance
   d. Eudaemonistic

Rationale

Correct answer: a.

With the Clinical Model of health, motivation to engage in healthy behaviors is motivated by a desire to not have a diagnosed disease. In the Adaptive Model, motivation is based on a desire to alter self. In the Role Performance Model, motivation for healthy behavior derives from a desire to be able to fulfill responsibilities at work, in the home, and in the community. In the Eudaemonistic model, motivation for health comes from joy and self-fulfillment.

12. For which age groups would the nurse most appropriately plan to include a discussion of suicide as part of a health promotion program?
    a. Children and teenagers
    b. Teenagers and young adults
    c. Young and middle adults
    d. Middle and older adults

Rationale

Correct answer: b.

Suicide is a major risk among teenagers and young adults and needs to be addressed in health promotion programs. Primary areas of concern for children are fire safety, firearm safety and home safety; for middle adults, accidents are a major concern; and among older adults, the risk of falling is major.

13. Which client could the nurse administer an MMR vaccine to?
    a. A child with HIV
    b. A woman who is trying to get pregnant.
    c. A child whose father had a kidney transplant two months ago.
    d. A 7-month pregnant woman

Rationale

Correct answer: a.

The only live virus vaccine that is given to a child with HIV is the MMR. Live virus vaccines of which MMR is one are contraindicated for women who are pregnant or may become pregnant within 3 months, and for children living with an immunosuppressed person.

14. Which statement made by a client who is starting a smoking cessation program using a combination of nicotine replacement and hypnosis indicates the need for further teaching?
    a. "I will try to use deep breathing and imagery to control cravings."
    b. "I will suck hard candy when I get an urge for a cigarette."
    c. "I will smoke just half a cigarette if I really feel out of control."
    d. "I will stay away from places where people smoke during the next week."

Rationale

Correct answer: c.

Smoking while using nicotine replacement therapy is dangerous because of the possibility of nicotine overdose. It is most dangerous for those with cardiovascular problems and can lead to severe hypotension and prostration.

14. Which direction regarding self-testicular examination is appropriate for a nurse to give a 20-year-old male client?
    a. Do not examine your testicles for at least 12 hours after intercourse.
    b. Examine both testicles simultaneously so one can be compared to the other.
    c. Keep in mind there may normally be what feels like a small bump on the upper or middle outer side of the testis.
    d. If one testicle appears larger than the other, see your physician immediately.

Rationale

Correct answer: c.

The epididymis can feel like a small bump on the middle or upper, outer side of each testis. Intercourse is unrelated to testicular examination; testicles are best examined after a warm bath or shower when the scrotum is relaxed. Each testicle is examined separately using both hands. One testicle is normally larger than the other.

16. Which statement made by a client about self-breast examination indicates the need for health teaching?
    a. "I palpate my breast carefully each month while standing in front of a mirror so I can see any changes in the contour or appearance of the skin."
    b. "I use the finger pads of the three middle fingers of each hand to palpate my breasts."
    c. "I use an up-and-down pattern of palpation on my breast and go all the way up until I reach my collar bone."
    d. "I press lightly, then with medium pressure, and then with firm pressure on each area of my breast as I examine it."

Rationale

Correct answer: a.

The breast should be palpated while the client is lying down so that the breast tissue is spread over the chest wall making it as thin as possible and therefore making any abnormalities easier to feel. After palpating the breast lying down, the client stands in front of a mirror with the hands pressing down on the hips and observes for any changes in contour, size, dimpling, skin changes, or nipple changes.

17. A client who has been told that her total cholesterol is too high and that a cholesterol-lowering drug is being prescribed for her says that different people normally have different cholesterol levels and that everyone doesn't need pills and she is not going to take the

(continued)

ordered medication. According to the Stage Model of health behavior change, which stage is she in?

a. Precontemplation

b. Contemplation

c. Preparation

d. Termination

Rationale

Correct answer: a.

Precontemplation is the stage when persons deny they have a problem and therefore do not need to change. Contemplation is the stage in which the client admits to a problem and talks about it but is not ready to do anything about it yet. Preparation is the stage in which clients make real plans to change and may even have begun to make small changes. Termination is the stage at which the behavior is incorporated into the lifestyle and returning to prior unhealthy behaviors is no longer a temptation or threat.

18. How does the nurse begin to develop a Health Promotion Plan with a client?

a. Involve a significant other

b. Identify priority health goals

c. Reinforce benefits of a change in health behaviors

d. Obtain a commitment to a healthy lifestyle

Rationale

Correct answer: b.

Joint development of a Health Promotion Plan begins with identifying priority health goals. Involving a significant other can facilitate adherence to the plan but it is not the first step. Reinforcing the benefits of change is also important but it comes after needed changes are identified. The final step is obtaining commitment to the behavior-change goals – not to the broad concept of a healthy lifestyle.

19. Which are strategies that the nurse may employ to aid a client in implementing a Health Promotion Plan? Mark all that apply.

a. ___Group counseling

b. ___Telephone counseling

c. ___Modeling

d. ___Ensuring social support

e. ___Teaching

Rationale

Correct answers: a, b, c, d, and e.

All of these are strategies, which can facilitate adherence to a Health Promotion Plan.

20. Which statement best indicates that a client who needs to begin an exercise program to improve cardiorespiratory fitness is in the preparation stage of the Stage Model of health behavior change?

a. "I never really liked exercise but maybe I could get to like it."

b. "I think maybe I really do need to exercise; I get awfully short of breath going upstairs."

c. "I asked my friend if she would be interested in going to an exercise class with me."

d. "I asked my sister and she agrees exercise isn't always a good thing."

Rationale

Correct answer: c.

In the preparation stage, the client makes a real plan to change. Asking a friend if she would go with her is part of such a plan. Answers a and b are representative of the contemplation stage in which the client acknowledges a problem but is not yet willing to commit to change. Answer d is more representative of the precontemplation stage in which the client denies having a problem.

21. A mother states she will not allow her child to receive immunizations which contain live or attenuated organisms. Which immunizations could the child not receive?

a. __x___ MMR

b. ___HBV

c. __x___ Varicella

d. ___ DTaP

e. ___ TIV influenza

f. ___ IPV

Rationale

Correct answers: a and c.

Measles, mumps and rubella, and varicella contained live viruses which have been treated with heat or chemicals to decrease their virulence; they have not been killed. Hepatitis B virus vaccine, diphtheria, pertussis and tetanus, TIV influenza, and IPV contain inactivated or killed pathogens.

22. A client asks about receiving the hepatitis A vaccine because of upcoming travel to an underdeveloped country where the disease is endemic. The client particularly wants to know how many injections are needed and at what interval. Which is a correct response for the nurse to give?

a. 2 injections @ 3 months apart

b. 2 injections @ 6–18 months apart

c. 3 injections @ 1 month apart

d. 3 injections @ 3 months apart

Rationale

Correct answer: b.

Hepatitis A vaccine is given in two injections at 6–18 months apart.

23. What purpose does clearing the needle by injecting an air bubble after administration of an immunization serve?
    a. Decrease risk of an anaphylactic reaction
    b. Decrease pain during injection
    c. Minimize local reaction
    d. Ensure proper dose

Rationale

Correct answer: c.

Clearing the needle with an air bubble prevents leakage of vaccine back out through the needle tract and into surrounding tissue thereby minimizing local reaction. It does not decrease risk of anaphylaxis or decrease pain. It is not used to ensure proper dose.

24. Which information should be given to a 52-year-old client who is planning to start a cardiorespiratory exercise program?
    a. Consult your physician to obtain an exercise prescription
    b. Include only anaerobic activities
    c. Stretch at the completion of each exercise session
    d. Work up gradually to a maximum of 90 minutes five times per week

Rationale

Correct answer: a.

Clients over age 45 and those with risk factors for cardiac disease should consult a physician to determine the appropriate amount of exercise before beginning a program. Aerobic exercise involving continuous use of large muscle groups is effective in building cardiorespiratory reserve. Stretching should be done at the beginning of aerobic exercise and a cool down period at the end. Clients should start gradually but the recommended duration of exercise is 30–60 minutes three to five times per week.

CHAPTER 9

Test Plan Category:

Health Promotion and Maintenance—Part 4

Sub-category: None

Topic: Techniques of Physical Assessment

TECHNIQUES OF PHYSICAL ASSESSMENT

BIOLOGICAL SCIENCE FOUNDATION

- The basic sciences inform the techniques of physical assessment.
- Physical assessment techniques reveal information about underlying structures.

Etiology: Physical assessment is guided by symptoms reported by the client as well as the nurse's understanding of human anatomy, physiology, and pathophysiology. Physical assessment techniques provide important information to determine the etiology of client's complaints.

Precipitating factors: If present, may require examination of additional body systems.

The scientific principles of physical assessment techniques by system are

- skin:
  —structure
    - epidermis: keratin, melanocytes; appendages, hair, sebaceous glands, sweat glands, and nails
    - dermis: collagen and elastic tissue; location of epidermal appendages, nerves, sensory receptors, blood vessels, and lymphatics
    - subcutaneous tissue: adipose tissue for energy, insulation, and cushioning; mobility allows skin to slide over underlying structures

  —function
    - protection from penetration and invasion
    - temperature regulation
    - sensory perception
    - identification
    - communication
    - wound repair
    - absorption and excretions
    - production of vitamin D
- head:
  —structure
    - skull: cranium and facial bones

  - cranium: frontal, parietal, occipital, temporal connected by coronal, sagittal, and lambdoid sutures
  - face: 14 bones connected by sutures excluding the mandibular temporal joint
  - muscles: temporalis and masseter
  - lymph nodes: preauricular, postauricular, and occipital
  - children: anterior and posterior fontanels
- —function
  - protection of brain and sensory organs and expressions
- neck:
  - —structure
    - bones: cervical spine, hyoid, clavicle, and manubrium
    - muscles: sternocleidomastoid, trapezius, and the anterior and posterior triangles
    - arteries: internal, external, and common carotid
    - veins: internal and external jugular
    - lymph nodes: jugulodigastric, superficial cervical, posterior cervical, deep cervical, and supraclavicular
    - other: thyroid cartilage, cricoid cartilage, thyroid gland, and trachea
  - —function
    - head mobility and passage between head (brain) and body
- eyes:
  - —structure
    - visible: upper eyelid, palpebral fissure, lateral canthus, medial canthus, caruncle, pupil, iris, sclera, limbus, lower eyelid, and conjunctiva
    - muscles: medial rectus, superior oblique, superior rectus, lateral rectus, inferior rectus, and inferior oblique
    - lacrimal system: lacrimal gland, inferior and superior lacrimal puncta, lacrimal sac, and nasolacrimal duct
    - outer: sclera and cornea
    - middle: choroids, pupil, lens, and anterior chamber
    - inner: retina, macula, optic disk, and optic nerve
  - —function
    - central and peripheral vision
- ears:
  - —structure
    - external: helix, antihelix, tragus, antitragus, lobule, mastoid process, and external auditory canal
    - middle: tympanic membrane, malleus, incus, stapes, and eustachian tubes
    - inner: bony labyrinth, vestibule, semicircular canals, and cochlea
  - —function
    - hearing and equilibrium
- nose:
  - —structure
    - external: bridge, tip, nares, columella, vestibule, and ala.
    - nasal cavity: superior, middle, and inferior turbinates; septum; olfactory.
    - nerve: maxillary, frontal, and ethmoid and sphenoid sinuses.
  - —function
    - sense of smell and warm and filter external air flowing into lungs.
- mouth/throat:
  - —structure
    - hard and soft palates, tongue, pharynx, tonsil, frenulum, and teeth
    - glands: salivary, parotid, submandibular, sublingual, and submental.
  - —function
    - chew and begin digestion of food, enhance smell, swallowing, speech, and respiratory pathway.
- breasts:
  - —structure
    - located over pectoralis major and serratus anterior muscles, Tail of Spence extends into axilla.
    - central nipple consisting of erectile tissue and pigmented
    - nipples surrounded by darker areola with hair follicles and Montgomery tubercles; 12–25 glandular lobes contain alveoli that produce milk and transport it to the nipple. Men lack the milk-producing alveoli.
    - Cooper's ligaments provide support for each breast.
    - lymph nodes: pectoral, brachial, subscapular, midaxillary, internal mammary (women only), and superficial lymphatic.
  - —function
    - milk production and self-image
- respiratory:
  - —structure
    - upper airway: nasopharynx, oropharynx, laryngopharynx, and larynx
    - lower airway: trachea, bronchial tubes, bronchi, bronchioles, alveolar ducts, and alveoli.
    - right lung has upper, middle, and lower lobes; left lung with upper and lower only; both wrapped in visceral pleura.
    - parietal pleura lines thorax and sends pain signals with inflammation
    - pleural fluid between parietal and visceral pleurae allows for expansion and contraction.
    - bones: ribs, manubrium, sternum, and xiphoid process.

- muscles: diaphragm, external intercostal muscles, trapezius, sternocleidomastoid, and scalenes.
- blood vessels: pulmonary artery from right ventricle brings deoxygenated blood to alveolar capillaries where oxygen and carbon dioxide exchange occurs; oxygenated blood returns via pulmonary veins to left atrium.

—function

- acid—base balance, oxygenation

- cardiac:

—structure

- four chambers: right and left atria and right and left ventricle
- heart wall: myocardium, endocardium, epicardium; surrounded by pericardium with parietal and visceral layers, pericardial space and fluid
- blood vessels: inferior and superior vena cava and coronary sinus to right atrium; pulmonary artery to lungs; pulmonary vein from lungs to heart; aorta from heart to body
- valves: mitral, tricuspid (atrioventricular), aortic, pulmonic (semilunar)
- nerve conduction: sinoatrial node, atrioventricular node, bundle of His, Purkinje fibers

—function

- circulates blood cells, removes wastes, and provides oxygen and nutrients

- peripheral vascular:

—structure

- major blood vessels: arteries, arterioles, capillaries, venules, and veins
- pulses: temporal, carotid, brachial, radial, ulnar, femoral, popliteal, posterior tibial, and dorsalis pedis

—function

- circulates blood cells to periphery and temperature regulation

- gastrointestinal:

—structure

- hollow tube from mouth to anus; smooth muscle; pharynx, esophagus, stomach, small intestine, and large intestine
- organs aid in digestion: liver, pancreas, and gallbladder
- blood supply: through abdominal aorta to common iliac arteries; back to heart through gastric and splenic veins to portal vein to hepatic vein to inferior vena cava

—functions

- digests and absorbs nutrients, water, and electrolytes and eliminates wastes

- genitourinary:

—structure

- urinary tract: kidneys, nephrons, ureters, bladder, urethra, and antidiuretic hormone (ADH)
- functions: forms urine, maintains homeostasis, removes wastes, regulates acid—base, fluid, and electrolyte balance
- female genitalia
- external: vulva, mons pubis, labia majora, labia minora, clitoris, vestibule, vaginal introitus, urethral orifice, Skene's and Bartholin's glands, and perineum
- internal: vagina, uterus, ovaries, and fallopian tubes
- male genitalia: urethra, penis, scrotum, testicles, epididymis, vas deferens, seminal vesicles, prostate gland, and inguinal canal and ring

—functions

- intercourse, reproduction, and secondary sex characteristics

- musculoskeletal:

—structure

- muscles, tendons, ligaments, bones, cartilage, joints, bursae visceral, and skeletal and cardiac muscle types
- long, short, flat, irregular, and sesamoid bone types
- axial versus appendicular skeleton
- immovable and synovial joints

—functions

- shape, movement, protection of organs, support, RBC production, mineral salt storage, and cushioning

- neurological:

—structure

- central nervous system: brain and spinal cord
- brain: cerebrum, brain stem, cerebellum, meninges, and cerebrospinal fluid
- dermatomes
- peripheral nervous system: peripheral and cranial nerves
- autonomic nervous system: sympathetic and parasympathetic

—functions

- controls and regulates systems, interprets motor and sensory stimuli, maintains equilibrium, and provides enervation to visceral organs

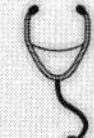

Assessment Alert

Although each body system is discussed separately, all body systems interact for proper functioning of the human body. Therefore, if there is a disorder in one system, more systems will eventually be affected. The acuity and chronic nature of the illness will determine how quickly the disorder is manifested in multiple systems.

Examples of assessment tools:

- Equipment such as stethoscope, otoscope, ophthalmoscope, sphygmomanometer, reflex hammer, and tuning fork
- Examiner's senses: smell, touch, vision, and hearing
- Special testing such as rebound tenderness or Apley's compression test

Examples of assessment questions:

Ask the client

- For more information about the complaint: onset, location, duration, severity, quality, associated symptoms, precipitating symptoms, and interventions that decrease the symptoms and situations in which the symptoms worsen.
- To localize the symptom by pointing to the location on his/her body.
- About all body systems. Often, a client does not understand the link between a symptom and a condition. In a complete review of systems, more information about associated symptoms or illnesses may be collected.
- About his/her perception of the problem. This may reveal an opportunity to reinforce a correct association between a symptom and an action or disease process or correct an erroneous association between a symptom and an action or disease process.
- To clarify information that is confusing or contradictory. For example, a client may have a cough and explain that this is due to foot pain. A further explanation is needed to determine the link, if it exists, between cough and foot pain.
- To correct any misperceptions in a summary of the complaint given by the nurse.

Rx: The etiology of a client complaint provides the basis for treatment. An accurate and thorough physical examination by the nurse helps to discern which treatments are most beneficial for each individual client.

Nursing care:

- The basic sciences inform the actions and interventions available for clients.
- Specific interventions for a specific client are guided by both the client's complaints and the objective physical findings.
- Assess all client complaints in intervals appropriate to the acuity of the problem.

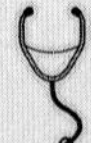

Assessment Alert

Beware of complaints that may be referred from one organ/tissue to a different location on the body. For example, knee pain may be due to a disorder in the hip and not the knee itself.

Client teaching for self-care

- Teaching about the underlying illness processes helps clients and families understand disease manifestations, progression, and treatment.
- Teaching should be geared toward the needs of the client and family. They should be encouraged to ask questions and repeat their understanding of the education provided by the nurse.
- Assessment of the client/family's education level, age, language, and readiness for learning are essential for effective client/family teaching about illness.
- Specific questions about prognosis, further treatment and expectations should be referred to the health care team responsible for the client's treatment goals. A discussion involving the broader health care team decreases the risk of miscommunication and seemingly contradictory information.

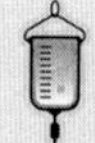

Clinical Alert

Avoid assessing the client according to what seems to be the most plausible explanation of his/her complaints. A focused, yet thorough examination will prevent loss of relevant assessment data and lead to effective and efficient interventions.

PSYCHOMOTOR SKILLS USED IN ASSESSMENT

The basic techniques of physical assessment are interviewing, inspection, palpation, percussion, and auscultation.

- Interviewing techniques
  —Use verbal and nonverbal clues to guide discussion
  —Ask open-ended questions to hear the client's story in detail
  —Use nonjudgmental comments
  —Repeat statements to ensure understanding and encourage clients to continue
  —Summarize information and have the client verify the summary
  —Clarify contradictory and vague points
  —Obtain assistance from other appropriate health care providers/resources when needed
- Observation
  —Use vision to compare contours for symmetry, movement, pulsations, and deformities

—Magnifying devices, such as an otoscope, allow for visualization of areas which otherwise would not be visible
—Includes observing behavior and whether it is consistent with the situation
—Begins from the first meeting with the client and continues until the nurse or client leaves the examination site.

- Palpation
  —Second skill used in assessment excluding examination of the abdomen.
  —Finger pads are sensitive to contour, texture, consistency, movement, and pulsations.
  —Point of maximal impulse is located using the palm of the hand.
  —Dorsal surface of the hand is sensitive to temperature.
  —Gentle touch is used to elicit tenderness and/or identify superficial lesions or structures.
  —Deep touch is used to identify lesions or tenderness deep within tissue.
  —Touch is also used to evaluate organs such as the liver, kidneys, and spleen.
- Percussion
  —Tapping on the finger of a hand placed over a person's skin.
  —Percussion "note" is used to determine if the area under the tapped finger is solid or air-filled.
  —Requires considerable practice to elicit an audible, clear percussion note, and to hear the difference in percussion notes.
    - Flat: over the thigh
    - Dull: over the liver
    - Resonant: over healthy lungs
    - Hyperresonance: over hyperinflated lungs
    - Tympanic: over the gastric air bubble or puffed-out cheek
- Auscultation
  —Use of a stethoscope to hear sounds within a structure
  —The last step in physical assessment, excluding the abdomen where it is the second step
  —Listen for
    - abnormal heart sounds such as murmurs;
    - abnormal vascular sounds such as a bruit;
    - bronchial, bronchovesicular, and vesicular breath sounds;
    - bowel sounds.
- Physical assessment begins with inspection, then palpation, percussion, and auscultation excluding examination of the abdomen.

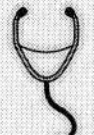

Assessment Alert

For the abdomen, inspection is followed by auscultation and percussion, then palpation. This sequence is necessary to prevent alteration of peristalsis and/or bowel sounds. To prevent muscle tensing that can interfere with palpation, ask client to take slow, deep breaths through the mouth. Have client void before percussing lower abdomen

Client teaching for self-care

- Explain the procedures or techniques used in physical assessment to the client.
- During the physical examination, step-by-step instructions prepare the client and result in increased cooperation.
- Determine which body systems may be tender for the client before starting the physical examination.
- Ensure privacy and comfort for the client.

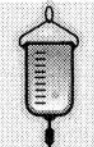

Clinical Alert

Always evaluate a tender area last. The exam may be altered or halted if the tender area is examined first.

Requirements for a Good Physical Examination

- Systematic approach
- Privacy but with good exposure of body parts
- Good lighting
- Proper equipment
- Comfortable room temperature
- Appropriate positioning of the client
- Bilateral comparison of body parts to identify variations
- Use of standard precautions

Choosing Appropriate Equipment and Technique

- The assessment techniques of interviewing, observation, palpation, percussion, and auscultation may need to be modified for the age and/or capabilities of the client.
- Equipment may also need to be modified such as the use of a larger BP cuff for larger clients or a smaller pediatric stethoscope for a child.

- The general, underlying physical assessment principles remain the same:
  - —observe the client from the moment he/she is visible;
  - —learn about the client's concerns and history through interviewing techniques;
  - —use palpation, percussion, and auscultation to gather further information about the physical condition of the client.

Variations in Physical Assessment Equipment and Techniques

- Infants
  - —Use smaller equipment such as a pediatric stethoscope.
  - —Infants generally will lie on an examining table during the exam.
  - —Restrain PRN firmly by immobilizing joint above and joint below area to be examined. To restrain head, extend arms above head and press toward midline.
  - —The otoscopic exam is the most traumatic and left until the end of the exam.
  - —Ears are pulled back and down to visualize the tympanic membrane.
  - —Use noises to distract the infant or to draw attention to a certain area. For example, if neck mobility is being examined, snapping fingers to one side of the head and then the other side will encourage the infant to turn the head side to side.
  - —Red reflex of the eyes is important to elicit, but further ophthalmologic examination may not be possible.
  - —Speak to the parents/guardians, but also speak directly to the infant. The infant may not be able to understand the words yet, but direct attention to the infant sets the stage for building rapport in the future.
  - —Ask the parent/guardian about pregnancy, labor, and delivery, feeding amounts and times, sleep, urinary and fecal excretion.
  - —The parent/guardian may help to stabilize a body part for injections.
  - —Ask the parent/guardian if they have any further questions or concerns.
- Toddlers
  - —Continue to use smaller equipment as for the infant.
  - —Ask the toddler and parent/guardian whether the toddler would like to sit on the parent's/guardian's lap or on the examining table. Depending on the exact age, the toddler may feel safer in a parent's/guardian's lap; if not in lap, keep caretaker in view.
  - —Ask the toddler and parent/guardian about day care, interests, food preferences, sleep, toileting, and safety practices.
  - —Perform parts of exam likely to cause crying last; otoscopic exam remains traumatic and is completed at the end.
  - —Ears are pulled back and down to visualize the tympanic membrane.
  - —Use noises, phrases, toys to distract or attract attention to a certain area.
  - —Red reflex of the eyes is important to elicit.
  - —Speak to the toddler and parent/guardian directly. Continue to build rapport with the toddler.
  - —Ask the toddler as well as the parent/guardian about any concerns or questions.
  - —Give clear, firm directions in age-appropriate language.
- Preschool children
  - —Continue to use smaller equipment
  - —Sits on the examining table
  - —May want to examine/explore equipment
  - —Ask about school or day care, food preferences, toileting, safety, sleep, friends, interests, and hobbies
  - —Repeat questions to the parent/guardian
  - —May examine the child systematically from head to toe
  - —Pull ear back and up to visualize the tympanic membrane
  - —Red reflex of the eyes is important, but further examination may be possible
  - —Ask the child as well as the parent/guardian about concerns or questions
- School-aged children
  - —Continue to use smaller equipment according to the size of the child
  - —Sits on the examining table
  - —Ask about school, friends, activities, food preferences, toileting, sleep, and safety
  - —Repeat questions to the parent/guardian
  - —Systematically examine the child from head to toe
  - —Pull ear back and up to visualize the tympanic membrane
  - —Perform full eye exam
  - —Ask the child as well as the parent/guardian about concerns or questions
- Adolescents
  - —Use adult-sized equipment unless the adolescent is small/petite for their age
  - —Sits on examining table
  - —Ask about school, friends, activities, nutrition, sleep, safety, sexual development, and goals
  - —Ask about the use of drugs and alcohol, risky behaviors
  - —Repeat questions to parent/guardian
  - —Question the adolescent alone at some point. Politely ask the parent/guardian to go to the waiting room
  - —Full examination, although genital exam is traumatic and left to the end
  - —Ask the adolescent as well as the parent/guardian about concerns or questions

- Older adult
  - —Adjust voice, if needed, and speak clearly so that the client hears and understands
  - —May not be able to get onto the examining table. If not, examination may be completed seated and standing.
  - —Adjust exam to possible body positions; help with positioning and change position slowly; may need rest periods.
  - —Elderly clients chill easily so draping is important.
  - —Ask client about support system, activities, nutritional intake, water intake, bowel pattern, voiding pattern, sensory deficits, safety, and future plans
  - —Ask client about concerns or questions
  - —Head to toe systematic examination
  - —Include supportive friends and family in interventions/care plans with client's permission
- Disabled clients
  - —Adjustments to equipment and techniques according to specific disability
  - —Often gentle approach and quiet manner will relax client
  - —Physical development will continue although outward appearance may resemble younger/older client
  - —Discuss condition and care plans with client and/or supportive caregivers

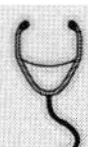

Assessment Alert

Adolescents may not admit to risky behaviors in front of parents/guardians. Interviewing adolescents alone is important. The information divulged between client and examiner is confidential unless deemed to be immediately harmful to the client or other person.

Examples of assessment questions:

Ask the client

- If he/she is comfortable?
- What other accommodations he/she might need?
- To listen to directions and explanations.
- Whether he/she can sit on the examining table?
- If he/she have any concerns or questions?

Nursing care:

- Nursing care differs according to age and/or disability.
- Nursing care is based on client's needs according to age and/or disability.
- Nursing care may require significant adaptation to meet the needs of a disabled client.

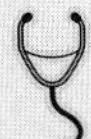

Assessment Alert

Be alert to S&S of physical and emotional abuse. It can occur at any age.

Client teaching for self-care

- The client's needs will be met through creative interventions.
- The client, his/her support system, and the nurse are all involved in meeting the client's health care needs.
- The client is entitled to a private interview with the nurse at any age.
- Information that threatens the safety of the client or those around him/her will be reported to the appropriate agencies.

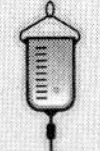

Clinical Alert

The nurse is ethically and legally compelled to act upon S&S that indicate a client's safety has been compromised. Reporting such S&S to appropriate community agencies is in the best interests of the client.

Includes subjective information (what the client said) and objective information (what the examiner observed).

- The health history is subjective information. It includes
  - —the chief complaint;
  - —history of the present illness;
  - —past history;
  - —family history;
  - —personal and social history; and
  - —review of systems.
- The physical exam is objective information. It includes a general observation, vital signs, and the following systems:
  - —skin;
  - —head, eyes, ears, nose, and throat;
  - —neck;
  - —thorax and lungs;
  - —breasts and lymph nodes;
  - —cardiovascular;
  - —abdomen;
  - —peripheral vascular;
  - —musculoskeletal; and
  - —neurological

Comprehensive Health History

- Chief complaint is the reason for the visit.
- History of the present illness
  - —It provides more information about the chief complaint.
  - —The client explains onset, character, location, duration, severity, alleviating factors, aggravating factors, and perception of the symptom.
- Past history
  - —Childhood and adult illnesses
  - —Immunizations
  - —Screening tests such as tuberculin test, mammogram, Pap smear, stools for occult blood, and lipid panel
  - —Medications and allergies
- Family history
  - —Age and health or cause of death
  - —Immediate relatives: parents, grandparents, siblings, children, and grandchildren
  - —Review family history of cardiac disease: hypertension, stroke, seizures, migraines, psychiatric illness, cancer, diabetes, thyroid disease, renal disease, substance abuse, and allergies
- Personal and social history
  - —Education level
  - —Occupation and financial situation
  - —Interests and hobbies
  - —Safety: both seatbelts, smoke detectors as well as feeling safe where they live, who they live with and where they work
  - —Household members, significant others, and children
  - —Diet and exercise: medications may be affected by diet. Iron, for example, is best absorbed with acidic substances like orange juice. Levothyroxine, a thyroid replacement hormone, is not absorbed well when taken with iron or calcium. Bananas have much potassium and a person with renal failure who is on a potassium-restricted diet should not eat potassium-rich foods like bananas.
  - —Religion and spirituality
  - —Sources of stress
- Review of systems: under each system, ask questions regarding
  - —general: usual weight, recent weight change, fatigue, weakness, and fever
  - —skin: rashes, lumps, sores, itching, dryness, color change, and changes in hair or nails
  - —head: trauma, headache, dizziness, and light-headedness
  - —eyes: vision changes, redness, spots, double vision, blurred vision, tearing, last eye exam, glaucoma, and pain
  - —ears: decreased hearing, trauma, discharge, pain, tinnitus, and vertigo
  - —nose: discharge, colds, stuffiness, allergies, itchiness, nose bleeds, and sinus infections
  - —throat: pharyngitis, teeth, gums, dentures, bleeding, sores, dryness, hoarseness, and last dental exam
  - —neck: lumps, swollen glands, goiter, stiffness, and pain
  - —breasts: pain, discharge, lumps, and self-examination practices
  - —respiratory: shortness of breath, wheezing, cough, sputum, hemoptysis, dyspnea, last chest X-ray, asthma, bronchitis, emphysema, pneumonia, tuberculosis, smoking, exposure to environmental chemicals, medications used to treat nasal congestion, cough, dyspnea, or other respiratory symptoms
  - —cardiovascular: palpitations, murmurs, chest pain or pressure, dyspnea, orthopnea, high BP, heart trouble, rheumatic fever, edema, and last EKG
  - —gastrointestinal: burping, cramping, diarrhea, constipation, last bowel movement, color and size of stools, hemorrhoids, pain, food intolerance, flatus, jaundice, gall-bladder problems, and hepatitis
  - —urinary: frequency of urination, dysuria, polyuria, nocturia, urgency, burning on urination, hematuria, infections, kidney stones, incontinence; for males, reduced force of stream, hesitancy, or dribbling
  - —genital:
    - male: hernias, discharge from penis, sores, testicular pain or pressure, sexually transmitted diseases, sexual habits, birth control methods, and exposure to HIV
    - female: age at menarche, last menstrual period, last gyn exam, pelvic pain or pressure, change in menstrual periods, spotting, premenstrual symptoms, discharge, itching sores, lumps, sexually transmitted diseases, exposure to HIV, birth control method, number of pregnancies, number and type of deliveries and abortions, complications during pregnancy, sexual habits, and exposure to diethylstilbestrol (DES) if born before 1971
  - —peripheral vascular: leg pain or cramps, varicose veins, and clots
  - —musculoskeletal: bone or joint pain, stiffness, arthritis, gout, backache, swelling, weakness, limited mobility, and trauma
  - —neurologic: fainting, blackouts, seizures, weakness, paralysis, numbness, tingling, and tremors

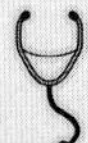

Assessment Alert

For all symptoms reported by the client, obtain information about time and type of onset; course; severity, precipitating and relieving factors; and associated S&S.

—hematologic: anemia, bruising, bleeding, and transfusions
—endocrine: thyroid problems, diabetes, heat or cold intolerance, sweating, thirst, hunger, and polyuria
—psychiatric: anxiety, nervousness, depression, tension, memory change, and tendency to suicide

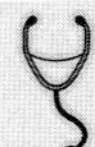

Assessment Alert

For clients who cannot report their history, interviewing family and significant others may provide pertinent information about the client's health history.

Complete Physical Examination

- General survey: observe general state of health, height, build, sexual development, weight, posture, motor activity, gait, dress, hygiene, grooming, odors, facial expressions, manner, affect, reactions, speech, awareness, and level of consciousness

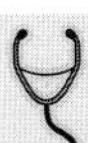

Assessment Alert

Hearing and/or vision loss can cause an inaccurate assessment of orientation; make sure client is using assistive devices. Response time to questions slows with age. Confusion is not a normal age change—if present, determine if rapid or gradual onset.

- Vital signs: measure temperature, pulse, respirations, BP, height, and weight
  —Oral temperature contraindicated if client is confused, disoriented, comatose, and unable to keep the mouth closed; has chills, history of seizures, recent oral surgery, oxygen by face mask or has smoked, chewed gum, or ingested hot or cold substances within the last 15 minutes.
  —Rectal temperature contraindicated if client cannot follow directions; stay still or has recent rectal surgery, hemorrhoids, or an inability to assume an appropriate position.
  —Apical pulse (midclavicular line at fifth intercostal space) taken in children less than 2 years and clients with an arrhythmia or on cardiac medication. Baseline pulse is obtained at least 10 minutes after activity.
  —Pulse is affected by factors that stimulate either the sympathetic nervous system (caffeine, stress, fever, pain, emotion) or the parasympathetic (vomiting, suctioning).
  —Baseline BP is taken at least 30 minutes after smoking, exercising, or ingesting caffeine. Other BPs allow 5-minutes rest; have arm at level of heart; no constriction of upper arm and do not take on side with mastectomy, IV, or hemodialysis access site.
  —Abnormal findings:
    - >10 mm difference in BP between right and left arm
    - >25 mm difference in systolic or >10 mm diastolic BP between sitting, lying, and standing positions
  —Fever occurs less often in geriatric clients but hypothermia occurs more often.

See Chapter 17 for normal BP, pulse, and respiratory rates for various age groups.

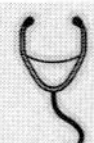

Assessment Alert

An unintentional weight loss of 5% or greater in a month, 7.5% or greater in 3 months, or 10% or more in 6 months in older person is a cause of serious concern.

- Skin
  —Assess color, lesions, edema, moisture, temperature, texture, and turgor
    - Color: assess general color as well as local or patchy variations (see Table 9–1.). In dark-skinned individuals, observe in areas of least pigmentation such as under the tongue, buccal membranes, or sclera.
    - Lesions: observe and describe the size (measure in metric), shape, distribution, pattern, color, margins of lesions (regular, irregular, clearly demarcated), raised or flat
    - Edema: palpate with finger pads; note location; determine if pitting or non—pitting; if pitting note 1+ (2-mm depression), 2+ (4 mm), 3+ (6 mm), and 4+ (8 mm)
    - Moisture: check for moistness or dryness using pads of fingers
    - Temperature: use back of hand to determine hot, warm, cool or cold
    - Texture: use pads of fingers to determine if smooth or rough
    - Turgor: pinch and lift a skin fold over the sternum or clavicle and note time until skin returns to original position. Normal is 5 seconds; tenting of more than 5 seconds in these areas is indicative of dehydration

Table 9–1 Assessment of Skin Color

Color Variation	Where to Observe	Clinical Notes	Interpretation
Pallor	Nail beds, lips, oral mucous membranes, palpebral Conjunctiva	Appears as dull ash or gray in black skin and dull yellow-brown in brown skin	Marked pallor occurs with syncope, shock, and anemia
Central cyanosis	Lips, buccal mucosa, tongue	Noticeable only when severe in dark skin	Anxiety, cold exposure, heart, lung, or blood disorder
Peripheral cyanosis Jaundice	Nail beds, skin of arms or legs Sclera, lips, hard palate, skin	Noticeable only when severe in dark skin Outer sclera of dark-skinned individuals may normally have a yellow tinge; jaundice involves whole sclera up to iris.	Liver disease, hemolysis of RBCs (yellow tinge to skin only, especially exposed areas occurs with uremia)
Erythema	All areas of skin and mucous membrane	Redness cannot be seen in dark skin; therefore, must palpate for heat as a sign of inflammation	Local inflammation, fever, blushing, alcohol intake, cold exposure
Bronze (brown)	Skin, palmar creases, nipples, genitalia		Addison's disease, pregnancy (face, nipples and genitalia only)

Think Smart/Test Smart

Remember the parameters of skin assessment by thinking of CLEM and the 3 Ts (color, lesions, edema, moisture, temperature, texture, and turgor).

- Head
  - —Observe for symmetry and evidence of trauma
  - —Hair distribution: male or female
  - —Amount: sparse, balding, or thick
  - —Texture: fine, coarse, brittle, or soft
  - —Palpate for tenderness and lesions
  - —Palpate the temporomandibular joint: in front of the ear where the temporal and mandibular bones articulate. Ask the client to open his/her mouth, move the jaw front, back and side to side. Palpate for crepitus, observe for pain or locking.
  - —Palpate the masseter and temporal muscles: palpate superiorly from the temporomandibular joint as you ask the client to clench his/her teeth. Palpate for tone, tenderness, and any lesions.
- Eyes
  - —Observe position, alignment, symmetry, extraocular movements, and visual fields
  - —Observe eye for tearing, discharge, presence of lesions, and condition of brows and lashes
  - —Palpate upper and lower lids and lacrimal glands and ducts for tenderness
  - —Inspect sclera and conjunctiva for color and vascular patterns and lesions
    - ▪ Separate lids with thumb and index finger and ask client to look up, down, and to the sides.
    - ▪ Use thumb to evert lower lid while client looks up to inspect palpebral conjunctiva
  - —Estimate distance vision and near visual acuity
    - ▪ Have the client read a clock or similar at a distance
    - ▪ Have client read a newspaper or similar at 14 inches from face
  - —Check clarity of cornea
    - ▪ Shine light from side into each eye; note smoothness and cloudiness
  - —Inspect pupil
    - ▪ Note size (in mm), shape, and symmetry
  - —Elicit red reflex
    - ▪ Ask the client to look over your shoulder/in the distance; shine a light into each pupil and look for a red reflection. Abnormal results occur with cataracts when either there is no red reflex or a white reflection rather than red.
  - —Test pupillary response to light
    - ▪ Ask client to look into distance; shine a bright light on one pupil bringing the light in from the side. Observe for constriction of the pupil into which the light is shone (direct response) and simultaneous constriction of other pupil (consensual response). Repeat on the other side.

—Test accommodation

- Hold a finger or pen 4–6 inches from client's nose. Ask client to look into distance and then look quickly at finger/pen. Observe for inward movement of both eyes and pupillary constriction.
- Normal findings are recorded as PERRLA (pupils equal, round, and reactive to light and accommodation).

—Test extraocular movements

- Directly in front of the client, ask her/him to follow your pen/finger with eyes only, not head.
- Draw a large letter "H" and observe each eye move in eight directions: up, down, lateral, medial, upper outer, upper inner, lower outer, and lower inner.

• Ears

—Inspect auricles and tragus for symmetry, color, and lesions

—Palpate the auricles and tragus for tenderness

—Inspect auditory canal; the canal should be smooth and pink without foreign bodies

—Inspect tympanic membrane, malleus, incus, stapes, umbo; using an otoscope, pull the ear up and back. The tympanic membrane appears pearly gray with a cone of light at 5 o'clock (left ear) or 7 o'clock (right ear). The cone of light is a triangular area with the base pointing toward the nose. The umbo may be seen as a central light area; the manubrium of the malleus runs superiorly from the umbo, the incus lies to one side of the manubrium, on the opposite side of the cone of light

—Perform the whisper test: cover one ear and whisper a two syllable word on the side not covered. The client should be able to tell you what was whispered. Repeat on the other side.

—If hearing is diminished, perform

- Weber: place a vibrating tuning fork (512 Hz) on top of the head. Ask the client if he/she can hear the sound and if it is louder in one ear over the other. Normal is equal in both the ears.
- Rinne: place a vibrating tuning fork (1024 Hz) behind the ear on the mastoid bone. Ask the client to tell you when he/she can no longer hear the sound. Move the tuning fork in front of the client's same ear and ask the client if he/she can hear the sound again. Since air conduction is longer than bone conduction, the client should hear the sound again when the tuning fork is placed in front of the ear.
- Abnormal results: conductive loss is indicated by lateralization of sound to the affected ear with the Weber and inability to hear the sound in the affected ear with the Rinne. Sensorineural loss is indicated by lateralization of sound to the healthy ear and inability to hear the sound in the ear on the Rinne.

• Nose

—Inspect and palpate external nose.

- Erythema and edema of nostril area may indicate allergy.

—Using a light source and a broad, short speculum, observe internal nasal mucosa, septum, and turbinates.

- Look for color of the mucous membrane, presence of drainage, and condition and position of the septum.
    - Erythema is seen with infection; paleness of the turbinates with allergy.
    - Watery drainage occurs with allergy; purulent with nasal or sinus infection
    - Perforations of the septum occur with chronic cocaine snorting
    - Deviated septum may be from trauma

—Palpate frontal and maxillary sinuses for tenderness; this may indicate sinusitis.

—Test bilateral nasal patency: ask the client to block one nostril and breathe in through the other nostril; repeat on the other side.

—Test sense of smell: ask the client to identify common scents such as cinnamon, vanilla, or coffee by blocking one nostril and breathing in with the other; repeat on the other side using a different scent.

• Mouth

—Inspect lips, oral mucosa, gums, and teeth

—Use a tongue blade and a good light to inspect all areas including under the tongue and under dental plates

—wearing gloves, grasp the tip of the tongue in a gauze pad and pull it left and right to inspect the sides

—note the condition of teeth

—palpate lips, oral mucosa, gums, teeth, and tongue for tenderness

—test tongue protrusion: ask the client to stick out his/her tongue, move side to side

—Observe for lateral deviation and fasciculations

• Throat

—Inspect hard and soft palates and pharynx.

—Inspect tonsils: grade 1 for tonsils less than one-quarter of the way between the anterior pillars and uvula, grade 2 for tonsils one-quarter to one-half the distance between the anterior pillars and uvula, grade 3 for tonsils one-half to three-quarters of the distance between the anterior pillars and uvula, grade 4 for touching tonsils.

—Test elevation of uvula: ask the client to open his/her mouth and say "ah." Observe elevation of the uvula. Deviation to either side is abnormal.

—Test gag reflex: use a tongue blade to gently touch the posterior one-third of the tongue to elicit the gag reflex.

- Neck
  - —Inspect for midline alignment of neck and trachea. Pleural effusion and pneumothorax causes trachea to shift to the unaffected side. Atelectasis causes shift to the affected side.
  - —Inspect for symmetry.
  - —Inspect for pulsations, especially on either side of the neck.
  - —Inspect for visible lymph nodes.
  - —Inspect for thyroid gland enlargement: thickening of the neck at the base.
  - —Palpate for tenderness and lymph nodes: preauricular, postauricular, occipital, tonsillar, submandibular, submental, posterior cervical, anterior cervical, deep cervical and supraclavicular. Have the client shrug his/her shoulders while palpating for supraclavicular nodes.
  - —Palpate for tracheal alignment.
  - —Palpate thyroid gland: deviate the trachea to one side and while the client swallows, palpate for the lobe of the thyroid gland on the side to which the trachea was moved. Repeat on the other side.
  - —Palpate carotid arteries for amplitude and rate of pulsations.
  - —Auscultate carotid arteries for bruits.
- Breasts
  - —Inspect female breasts with arms relaxed, elevated, and pressing against the hips.
  - —Palpate the breasts for lumps in a systematic pattern usually circular or linear. All lumps require further assessment.
  - —Palpate the anterior, deep, and posterior axillary nodes and epitrochlear nodes along the humerus.

Assessment Alert

Do not omit palpation of the Tail of Spence that extends from the breast into the axilla. The majority of cancerous breast lesions are found in this area

- Thorax and lungs: anterior and posterior
  - —Sit the client up to examine the chest.
  - —Be alert for difficulty breathing, shortness of breath, e.g., stopping to breathe in middle of sentences when speaking, hoarseness, and cough.
  - —Observe for abnormalities in rate or rhythm of breathing (e.g., tachypnea, bradypnea, shallow).
  - —Ask about use of inhalants, oxygen, and aerosols.
  - —Inspect the size and shape of the chest.
    - Anteroposterior diameter should be less than the transverse diameter (Normal ratio ranges from 1:2 to 5:7.).
    - Barrel chest: AP diameter equals the transverse; occurs with emphysema.
    - Pigeon chest: common deformity in which AP diameter is greater than the transverse.
  - —Inspect and palpate muscles and ribs .
    - Intercostal retraction may occur with asthma.
    - Intercostal bulging can occur with pneumothorax.
  - —Palpate the chest for tactile fremitus.
    - Ask the client to say 99 as you palpate three different levels of the chest for vibration due to the sound waves passing through open bronchi to the chest wall.
    - Tactile fremitus is decreased in atelectasis, emphysema, asthma, pleural effusion, and absent with pneumothorax; increased or normal with bronchitis, increased with bronchiectasis and over tumor mass.
  - —Palpate for equal respiratory excursion.
    - Place thumbs over the spinal processes of the 10th rib and lay hands, palm down and fingers spread, on the posterolateral chest; press palms inward so there is a thin layer of skin between the thumbs; ask client to take a deep breath; observe your thumbs for amount and symmetry of movement as the client inhales.
    - Asymmetrical expansion with movement on the affected side decreased with pneumonectomy, pneumothorax, pneumonia, pleural effusion, and atelectasis.
    - Bilateral symmetrically decreased expansion is seen in emphysema.
  - —Percuss the chest to determine the nature of the underlying tissue.
    - Dullness indicates solid or fluid-filled tissue; resonance over air-filled tissue; and tympany over tissue that is hyperinflated with air.
    - Atelectasis, lobar pneumonia, and pleural effusion cause a dull percussion note; dull over tumor mass.
    - Chronic asthma and pneumothorax cause hyperresonance.
  - —Determine diaphragmatic excursion.
    - Ask client to exhale and hold, then percuss from a point of resonance over the lung down toward the diaphragm until dullness is heard; mark this point.
    - Ask client to inhale and hold and repeat the above procedure.
    - Measure distance between two marks.
    - Normal is 3–6 cm.
    - Bilaterally decreased in emphysema.
    - Unilaterally (affected side) decreased with pleural effusion or pneumothorax.
    - Absent in atelectasis.

—Auscultate breath sounds.

- Use diaphragm of stethoscope to listen to 10 areas on the back; 8 on the anterior chest.
- Move stethoscope from side to side then down to allow comparison.
- When the stethoscope is placed at each location, ask the client to take a deep breath; observe for signs of hyperventilation and pause if needed.
- Three types of normal breath sounds are bronchial, bronchovesicular, and vesicular.
    - Tracheal: heard over the trachea; loud, high-pitched; expiration longer than inspiration.
    - Bronchovesicular: heard anteriorly on either side of the sternum and posteriorly between scapula; medium pitch; inspiration equals expiration.
    - Vesicular: heard over all normal lung tissue except in area of major bronchi; soft, gentle, low-pitch sound; inspiration is longer than expiration.
- Four types of abnormal or adventitious sounds:
    - Wheezes: high-pitched and continuous musical sounds
    - Gurgles: low-pitched and continuous musical sounds
    - Crackles: short, discrete, and crackling sounds
    - Friction rub: loud, dry, and creaking sound
    - If adventitious sounds are heard, note location, timing (if on inspiration or expiration), and if cleared by coughing, deep breathing, or change in position
    - Wheezes result from markedly narrowed bronchi; do not clear with coughing, may be inspiratory or expiratory; expiratory wheeze common in asthma
    - Gurgles result from fluid or mucus in large airways; may clear with coughing; more evident on expiration
    - Crackles result from sudden reinflation of groups of alveoli as in CHF and atelectasis; may or may not change with coughing; may be inspiratory or expiratory
    - Friction rub: inflammation of the pleura with resultant rubbing of the parietal against the visceral pleura; most marked on inspiration; does not clear with coughing

• Cardiovascular

—Inspect and palpate the precordium: look for heaves, thrills, and pulsations anterior to the heart.

—Locate the point of maximal impulse (PMI): palpate the fifth right intercostal space, midclavicular line. Someone with left ventricular hypertrophy will have a PMI displaced toward the axilla.

—Auscultate heart sounds in the following areas:

- Aortic: second right intercostal space, where the closure of the aortic valve is heard well (S2)
- Pulmonic: second left intercostal space, where the closure of the pulmonic valve is heard well (S2)
- Erb's point: third left intercostal space, midclavicular line, where anatomically S1 and S2 are heard well
- Tricuspid: fourth left intercostal space, sternal border, where closure of the tricuspid valve is heard well (S1)
- Mitral: fifth left intercostal space, midclavicular line, where closure of the mitral valve is heard well (S1)

—Note any abnormal heart sounds or murmurs.

- S3: during systole, blood moving from atria to ventricles, indicates moderate to severe congestive heart failure.
- S4: during diastole, atria contract as ventricles almost filled, indicates decreased compliance of ventricles.
- Murmurs are caused by regurgitation of incompetent valves or narrow openings caused by stenotic valves.
- Common diastolic murmurs: aortic regurgitation and mitral stenosis.
- Common systolic murmurs: aortic stenosis, mitral regurgitation, mitral valve prolapse.

—Measure jugular venous pressure in relation to the sternal angle.

- With the client's head elevated to approximately 45 degrees, find the jugular venous pulsations in the neck (venous pulsations change with breathing and movement, arterial do not).
- Using a straight edge, run a line from the sternal angle (junction of the manubrium and sternum) to the base the neck.
- Measure from the sternal angle to the highest level of pulsations. Normal is 3 cm. Higher pressures indicate increased venous pressure in the body. Low or absent values may indicate dehydration.

• Abdomen

—Inspect the abdomen for symmetry and lesions.

—Inspect for pulsations: the aorta is above the umbilicus and slightly to the left. Localize pulsations between fingers to measure the size of the abdominal aorta.

—Peristaltic waves: more easily seen in slender individuals in the lower half of the abdomen.

—Auscultate bowel sounds in all four quadrants: bowel sounds are "absent" when none are heard in 5 minutes, normal bowel sounds are 5–25 tinkles per minute; hyperactive bowel sounds in one quadrant, followed by hypoactive in the next quadrant may indicate an impending obstruction; later, bowel sounds decrease before the obstruction as well.

—Auscultate the aorta for bruits.

—Percuss the abdomen: in all four quadrants. The percussion sounds vary between tympany and dullness. Tympany is heard over the gastric air bubble and dullness is heard over organs.

—Determine location and size of liver.

- Percussion method: percuss downwards from the fourth right intercostal space midclavicular line until dullness is heard; this is the superior border of the liver. Percuss up from below the right costal margin midclavicular line until dullness is heard; this is the inferior border of the liver. Measure the distance between the borders. The normal size of the liver is 6–12 cm in the right midclavicular line.
- Scratch test: place the diaphragm of the stethoscope over where the client's liver should be. Begin scratching downwards from the fourth right intercostal space midclavicular line. The superior border of the liver has been reached when the auscultated sound becomes much louder. Scratch up from below the right costal margin midclavicular line; the inferior border of the liver has been reached when the auscultated sound becomes much louder. Measure the distance between the borders.

—Determine the location of the spleen: the spleen should be well hidden under the left costal margin. Percuss in the anterior axillary line, 10th intercostal space. Dullness indicates the inferior border of the spleen. Extension of dullness below the left costal margin indicates splenomegaly.

—Percuss for costovertebral angle (CVA) tenderness: the CVA is formed by the posterior edge of the ribs and the spinal column. Place a hand on this area and with the other hand in the form of a fist, strike the hand. Repeat on the other side. Positive CVA tenderness occurs when pain is elicited with percussion. This could be an indication of renal infections such as glomerulonephritis, pyelonephritis, etc.

—Lightly palpate the abdomen for superficial masses, tenderness: light palpation is up to 0.5 inches deep.

—Deeply palpate the abdomen: up to 2 inches deep.

—Palpate the liver: with the client recumbent, place your left hand posteriorly to lift the right rib cage. Ask the client to take a deep breath and position the edge of the right hand at the right costal margin. Ask the client to exhale and deeply palpate with the edge of the right hand under the costal margin while lifting the rib cage. The liver edge may be felt returning to its normal position as the client exhales. Perform palpation only after percussing the borders of the liver. Adjust hand position for hepatomegaly.

—Palpate the spleen: while standing at the recumbent client's right side, hook the left hand under the left rib cage. Using the edge of the right hand, ask the client to inhale deeply and begin to palpate deeply under the left costal margin. Ask the client to exhale. Palpate the spleen only after determining size and location by percussion. Do not palpate the spleen when it is enlarged as it is easily ruptured.

—Kidneys: attempt to capture the kidneys between both hands. Position one hand behind the client at the CVA. Place the other hand in the corresponding upper quadrant and attempt to capture a kidney between both hands. Repeat on the other side.

—Aorta: place fingers on the area of pulsation previously detected by inspection. Palpate for rhythm and amplitude.

—Palpate the inguinal nodes and femoral pulses: these are palpated in the groin along the crease formed by the thigh and hips. Normally, inguinal nodes are nonpalpable. Femoral pulses may be difficult to palpate. Check blood flow by assessing the lower extremities and checking capillary refill in the toes.

- Peripheral vascular

—Inspect the lower extremities for skin discoloration, varicose veins, edema; peripheral vascular disease is indicated by brown discoloration of the lower extremities, hair loss, achiness, edema, worsens with standing; peripheral arterial disease is indicated by cool extremities, hair loss, numbness, paresthesias, dry and scaly skin, and weak pulses.

—Palpate the popliteal, dorsalis pedis, and posterior tibialis pulses; popliteal pulse is found deep in the popliteal space behind the knee; dorsalis pedis is found on the top of the foot, proximal to the first digit, lightly palpated; posterior tibialis is found behind the medial malleolus grade pulses: 0 absent, 1+ weak/thready, 2+ normal, 3+ increased, 4+ bounding.

—Palpate for edema, tenderness grade edema: 0 absent, 1+ impression disappears <10 sec, 2+ impression lasts 10–15 seconds, 3+ up to 1 minute, 4+ 2–5 minutes.

- Musculoskeletal: including the spine

—For all muscles and joints

- Inspect for muscular symmetry, size, tone, and shape
- Compare bilateral muscles for strength, symmetry, equality, and resistance
- Grading muscle strength
  - 0 = no contraction
  - 1 = contraction, but no movement
  - 2 = contraction and movement, but not fully against gravity
  - 3 = full movement against gravity
  - 4 = partial movement against resistance
  - 5 = full movement against resistance
- Palpate joints for tenderness and alignment
- Test range of motion of joints

—Cervical spine

- Inspect head alignment and muscle and skin fold symmetry
- Palpate for tone, symmetry, tenderness, and spasm
  - Spasm may feel like hardened, tender areas in the neck

- Assess range of motion (ROM)
  - Flexion: touch chin to chest
  - Extension: look up to the ceiling
  - Lateral bending: touch each ear to shoulder
  - Rotation: turn the head to look over each shoulder
- Assess muscle strength: ROM with resistance
  - Trapezius: shrug shoulders and do not let the examiner push them down
  - Sternocleidomastoid: repeat lateral bending and rotation while the examiner applies a hand to resist the movement

—Thoracic and lumbar spine

- Inspect alignment, straightness, and curves
- Inspect for lordosis: hyperextension of lumbar spine
- Inspect for kyphosis: thoracic spine hump
- Inspect for scoliosis: standing look for curvature of the spine, flexed look for one side of the spine higher than the other
- Palpate the vertebral column and paravertebral muscles for tenderness
- Assess ROM
  - Flexion: bend forward as far as possible
  - Hyperextension: bend backward as far as possible
  - Lateral bending: bend side to side
  - Rotation: turn side to side
- Muscle strength of thoracic and lumbar spine is not routinely tested

—Shoulders

- Inspect size, shape, symmetry, and contour
- Inspect for nerve damage to scapula: ask the client to push against the wall while observing the scapula. There is nerve damage if the scapula "wings" or dislocates laterally.
- Palpate joint capsule and muscles
- Assess ROM
  - Flexion: brings arms forward
  - Hyperextension: bring arms back
  - Abduction: bring arm laterally away from the body
  - Adduction: bring arm across the body
  - Internal rotation: place both arms behind the back
  - External rotation: place both arms behind the head
- Assess muscle strength of shoulder girdle: repeat flexion, hyperextension, abduction, and adduction with pressure applied near the shoulder on each side.

—Elbows

- Inspect contour
- Inspect carrying angle: with the client standing, a line drawn from the shoulder and the relaxed position of the arm forms an angle of approximately 15 degrees
- Inspect for subcutaneous nodules
- Palpate for tenderness, swelling, and thickening
- Assess ROM
  - Flexion: bend the elbow and bring arm up to the body
  - Extension: extend the arm straight
  - Pronation: with arm extended, twist the hand down
  - Supination: with arm extended, twist the hand up
- Assess muscle strength: repeat flexion and extension with pressure applied near the elbow on each side

—Hands and wrists

- Inspect for contour, position, shape, number, and completeness of digits, and finger deviation
- Palpate joints for texture, swelling, tenderness, bogginess, nodules, and bony overgrowths
- Assess median nerve
  - Tinel sign: tap below the palm, over the middle of the wrist. If there is tingling or pain, there is median nerve irritation.
  - Phalen test: flex hands against each other for approximately a minute. If any tingling or pain develops in the wrist and fingers, there is median nerve irritation.
- Assess ROM
  - Flexion: move hands down from the wrist
  - Extension: move hands up to "stop traffic"
  - Opposition: touch the thumb to each finger on each hand
  - Abduction: fan the fingers out
  - Adduction: bring the fingers together
  - Rotation: move the wrists in a circular pattern
- Assess muscle strength
  - Grip: squeeze examiner's hands
  - Repeat flexion, extension, abduction, and adduction with resistance near the wrist on each side

—Hips

- Inspect for symmetry, size, and gluteal fold symmetry
- Palpate for stability and tenderness
- Assess ROM
  - Flexion: move leg forward at the hip
  - Extension: move leg back at the hip
  - Abduction: move leg laterally
  - Adduction: move leg across the body
  - Internal rotation: with the leg flexed at the hip and knee, move knee medially while moving the lower leg laterally
  - External rotation: with the leg flexed at the hip and knee, move knee laterally while moving the lower leg laterally

    - Assess muscle strength: repeat flexion, extension, abduction, and adduction with pressure applied above the knee
  - —Legs and knees
    - Inspect length, alignment, concavities, and contour
    - Palpate for swelling, tenderness, bogginess, and crepitus
    - Assess ROM
      - Flexion: bend the knee
      - Extension: straighten the leg
    - Assess muscle strength: repeat flexion and extension with pressure applied just below the knee
  - —Feet and ankles
    - Inspect contour and position
    - Inspect size and number of toes
    - Inspect alignment
    - Inspect ability to weight bear
    - Inspect arch of the foot
    - Palpate for heat, swelling, and tenderness
    - Assess ROM
      - Dorsiflexion: move foot and toes toward the head
      - Plantar flexion: move foot and toes away from the head (put your foot on the gas pedal)
      - Inversion: move foot medially
      - Eversion: move foot laterally
    - Assess muscle strength: repeat dorsiflexion and plantar flexion with pressure just below the ankle
- Nervous system
  - —Perform a mental status exam (See separate section below.)
  - —Test cranial nerve (CN) function, if not completed during the exam
    - Olfactory CN I: sensory nerve for smell. Test for odor identification (see nose)
    - Optic CN II: sensory and visual acuity. Test for visual acuity, visual fields, perform ophthalmologic exam (see eyes)
    - Oculomotor CN III, Trochlear CN IV, and Abducens CN VI: motor nerves for eye movement, pupil size, and eyelid opening. Assess for eyelid drooping, pupil size and equality, consensual response, accommodation, and extraocular eye movements (see eyes).
    - Trigeminal CN V: mixed motor and sensory for muscle tone and sensation. Inspect face for atrophy/tremors, palpate jaw for tone while client clenches teeth. Push down on chin and try to separate jaws. Test for pain by randomly touching the forehead, cheek, and chin with either a sharp or dull object or repeating on the other side. Test for sensation by lightly touching forehead, cheek, and chin with a cotton ball. Test corneal reflex by lightly touching cornea with cotton wisp while client looks straight ahead.
    - Facial CN VII: mixed motor and sensory for facial expressions and taste. Ask client to smile, frown, raise eyebrows, show upper and lower teeth, keep eyes closed against resistance, and puff out cheeks. Press puffed cheeks in and see if air escapes equally from both sides. Test tongue for salty and sweet sensations.
    - Acoustic CN VIII: sensory nerve for hearing and balance. Test hearing with whisper test, Weber and Rinne (see ears).
    - Glossopharyngeal CN IX: mixed sensory and motor nerve for taste and swallowing. Test tongue for sour and bitter sensations. Test gag reflex (see throat).
    - Vagus CN X: mixed sensory and motor nerve for swallowing and speech. Inspect palate and uvula for symmetry, inspect for swallowing difficulty, and evaluate guttural speech sounds (sounds made in the back of the throat such as g, k).
    - Spinal accessory CN XI: motor nerve for muscle strength of the trapezius and sternocleidomastoid. (see neck).
    - Hypoglossal CN XII: motor nerve for tongue strength. Inspect tongue for symmetry, tremors and atrophy, test tongue movement and strength. Evaluate lingual speech sounds (sounds made in the front of the mouth such as l, t, d, n)
  - —Coordination and fine motor skills
    - Test rapid alternating movements
      - Touch the thumb to each finger in rapid succession
      - Touch hands to thighs and flip back and forth rapidly
      - Evaluate: rhythm, flow, speed, and accuracy
    - Test balance
      - Observe gait.
      - Perform Romberg test: ask client to stand feet together and arms by the side of the body with eyes closed for 30–60 seconds. A problem with balance causes the person to step out or fall.
  - —Sensory function: ask the client to close his/her eyes and then test the following:
    - superficial touch: lightly touch several areas on upper and lower extremities with a cotton ball. The client states "yes" when touched.
    - superficial pain: using a broken tongue blade with the smooth side being "dull" and the broken side "sharp," randomly touch upper and lower extremities. The client states whether the sensation was sharp or dull.
    - vibration: place a vibrating tuning fork on a distal interphalangeal joint and then a distal metatarsal joint. Each time, ask the client to state whether

he/she feels anything and what it is. Repeat on the other side.

- joint position: as the examiner moves the client's finger up and down in a random pattern, the client identifies whether the finger is up or down. Repeat with a toe, then on the other side.
- stereognosis: place a familiar object in the client's palm (coin, paperclip, eraser, etc.). The client states what the object is. Repeat with a different object on the other side
- two point discrimination: using toothpicks, touch the client simultaneously and determine at what minimal distance on that body part does the client distinguish two objects. The most sensitive area is the tongue and the least sensitive are the upper arms and thighs.
- extinction phenomenon: simultaneously touch bilateral areas on the client's body, such as the upper arms. The client states if he/she was touched in one place or two.
- point location: lightly touch several areas on upper and lower extremities with a cotton ball. Each time, the client identifies where he/she was touched.

—Test reflexes

- Superficial
  - Plantar reflex: begin stroking the foot along the lateral edge then across the base of the metatarsals. In individuals over 2-years old, the toes should curl. A normal reaction in children less than 2-years old, the 1st digit dorsiflexes and the toes fan out.
- Deep tendon reflexes: tap a reflex hammer
  - Biceps: above the elbow joint anteriorly and observe for elbow flexion
  - Triceps: above the elbow joint posteriorly and observe for elbow extension
  - Brachioradial: above the wrist on the radial side and observe for forearm pronation/elbow flexion
  - Patellar: just below the patella and observe for lower leg extension
  - Achilles: above the heel posteriorly and observe for plantar flexion.

Complete History and Physical Examination

- Complete history and physical examination is performed when a new client is examined.
- It provides a database for future comparison.
- It documents changes over time with subsequent visits.

Focused History and Physical Examination

- Focused history and physical examination is performed when the client's visit is for a particular problem.
- It may occur before the complete history and physical is completed.
- It provides evidence to determine effectiveness of interventions.

Nursing care:

- Address the concerns of the client first.
- Obtain the complete history and physical examination information after the health care issue is addressed. The client may need to be seen at another time to collect this information.
- Compare condition to the client's documented baseline health history and physical examination information. Alert colleagues to deviations from baseline.

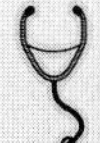

Assessment Alert

Allow the client to voice his/her concerns or questions at the beginning of the visit. The client's fears or misconceptions may be alleviated and result in a more efficient and effective examination.

Client teaching for self-care

- Explain procedures and tests to the client.
- Give clear guidance and directions.
- Describe normal findings to alleviate client's anxieties.
- Reschedule for a complete history and physical examination if the client has only time enough for a focused visit.

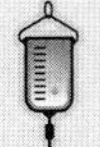

Clinical Alert

Clear and concise documentation of findings is necessary to provide a record of the client's baseline condition and function. Subsequent visits, when compared to the complete history and physical examination, may indicate steady decline or improvement.

MENTAL STATUS

- Mental status is defined as the expression of the person's cognition, mood, emotions, and personality.
- Seven parameters to assess are level of consciousness, appearance and behavior, speech and language, mood and affect, perception and thought content, insight and judgment, and cognition.
- Assessment continues throughout the entire history and physical examination.

Etiology: Many conditions such as infection, tumors, dementias, toxicities, drug or alcohol intoxication or withdrawal, metabolic imbalances, cerebrovascular accidents, myocardial infarctions, dehydration, and malnutrition may result in changes in mental status.

Precipitating factors: If mental status deviates from baseline, assess for acute illnesses or exacerbations of chronic conditions.

Assessment of mental status:

- Level of consciousness: graded from hypervigilant to alert to comatose.
- Appearance and behavior: note hygiene, grooming, dress, posture, and facial expressions.
- Speech and language: observe pronunciation, tone, volume, clarity, smoothness and rate of speech, comprehension, and the ability to follow verbal directions.
- Mood and affect: note body language and emotional responses to simple and more complex statements or questions.
- Perception and thought content: evaluate the logic and congruence of statements and their basis in reality.
- Insight and judgment: note understanding of situations, events, and the ability to draw conclusions.
- Cognition: evaluate short-term and long-term memory, praxis, visual-spatial skills, calculation, and abstraction.

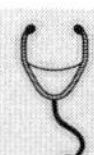

Assessment Alert

Delirium, clouded sensorium, in a client signifies a medical emergency. Immediately report delirium to the health care team responsible for the client.

Examples of assessment tools:

- Mini Mental State Examination (MMSE): brief, assesses multiple cognitive functions (orientation, memory, praxis, language, attention, calculation), widely used
- Confusion Assessment Method (CAM): tests for delirium
- Hopkins Competency Assessment Test: assesses ability to make decisions about health care
- Short Portable Mental Status Questionnaire (SPMSQ): assesses brain deficits

Examples of assessment questions:

Ask the client

- His/her name, where he/she is, and what time it is
- His/her date of birth, names and ages of children and grandchildren, and recent events.
- To add, subtract, divide, or multiply numbers. Begin with simple problems and advance to more complex with more steps.
- How two objects are similar or different (i.e., an apple and an orange are both fruit).
- To explain a proverb such as "he who hesitates is lost."
- What he/she would do if he/she saw flames coming from the neighbor's house?
- To draw a clock face with all the numbers and show 3 o'clock.
- To demonstrate how one brushes teeth, combs hair, or shaves.

Rx: The underlying cause for mental status change should be determined and treated. If the cause is not reversible, all efforts should be made to maintain function and assure safety.

Nursing care:

- Assess mental status whenever there is a change in the client's condition.
- Obtain baseline mental status when the client's condition is stable.
- Increase frequency of client evaluation when mental status is impaired.

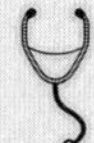

Assessment Alert

Beware of the client who has completed the MMSE enough times to have learned "the answers." Vary assessment questions and techniques in order to accurately assess mental status.

Client teaching for self-care

- Much teaching may be geared toward the family if the client is significantly impaired.
- The client will be assessed more frequently for maintenance of functions and safety until stable.
- A change in mental status indicates that further assessment and testing is required to determine a cause.
- If the underlying cause is reversible, all efforts will be focused on reversing the problem. If it is not reversible, all efforts will be focused on maintenance of function and client safety.

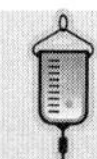

Clinical Alert

Age, culture, education, and language fluency will influence mental status testing. All questions should be individualized for the age, culture, educational level, and language of the client.

WORKSHEET

FILL IN THE BLANKS

Fill in the blank spaces with the correct word or phrase to complete each statement.

1. To assess the tympanic membrane in a 1-year-old child, you need to pull the pinna back and __________.
2. The last area to assess in a toddler is the __________.
3. During assessment of the eyes in a child less than 6-years old, you need to be able to see the __________ __________.
4. Preschoolers may already feel comfortable sitting on the __________ __________ rather than their parent's/guardian's lap during the physical examination.
5. The comfort and __________ of all clients should be ensured during the physical examination.
6. For an adolescent, the last area to be assessed is the __________ system.
7. Elderly clients may not be able to change __________ as easily as younger clients during the physical examination.
8. The skin produces vitamin __________.
9. The client's __________ of the problem is an important part of the health history.
10. The parasympathetic and sympathetic nerve pathways are part of the __________ nervous system.
11. The expression of a person's cognition, mood, emotions, and personality is called __________.
12. If the underlying cause of a mental status change is not reversible, the goal of care is to maintain __________.
13. The most sensitive part of the hand which is used for palpation is/are the __________.
14. The physical examination contains only __________ information.
15. The head is assessed for __________ and shape.

TRUE & FALSE QUESTIONS

Mark each of the following statements True or False. Correct all false statements in the space provided.

1. You should speak in a louder voice to all elderly clients. ___ T ___ F
2. When discussing an illness affecting one system, you would reinforce to the client that all body systems are interrelated. ___ T ___ F

(continued)

3. Elderly clients are never victims of abuse. ___ T ___ F
4. The Mini-Mental Status Examination is used to screen clients for cognitive dysfunction. ___ T ___ F
5. A reflex arc occurs when a sensory impulse travels to the spinal cord and a motor impulse is sent back out to the muscle. ___ T ___ F
6. The nurse may never divulge information gained during a client interview. ___ T ___ F
7. During the first year of life, the nervous system develops with increasing myelination. ___ T ___ F
8. Delirium is a medical emergency. ___ T ___ F
9. Baseline mental status is determined when the client is acutely ill. ___ T ___ F
10. At the end of the interview, a nurse should summarize what she heard from the client. ___ T ___ F
11. The ventral surface of the hand is most sensitive to temperature. ___ T ___ F
12. It is normal to hear tympany to percussion over the abdomen. ___ T ___ F
13. Subjective information is anything that the examiner observes. ___ T ___ F
14. The health history contains objective information. ___ T ___ F
15. The review of systems is necessary to prevent omission of important information. ___ T ___ F

MATCHING QUESTIONS

Match the following:

Organ	Function
1. Ear _____	a. Receives visual data
2. Eye _____	b. Circulates blood cells to body
3. Gall bladder _____	c. Maintains balance
4. Heart _____	d. Oxygen and carbon dioxide exchange
5. Large intestine _____	e. Wound repair
6. Liver _____	f. Produces bile
7. Lungs _____	g. Stores bile
8. Mouth _____	h. Absorbs water
9. Pancreas _____	i. Produces insulin
10. Skin _____	j. Begins digestion

MATCHING QUESTIONS

Match the following:

1. Abdomen _____	a. Trachea midline, thyroid nonpalpable
2. Extremities _____	b. Red mucosa, septum midline
3. Heart _____	c. Intact vibratory sense, deep tendon reflexes 2+
4. Lungs _____	d. No injection, uvula rises midline
5. Lymph nodes _____	e. No vascularities, warm, turgor intact
6. Neck _____	f. Full range of motion
7. Nervous system _____	g. Palpable in the occipital area, less than 1 cm, tender
8. Nose _____	h. Alternating tympany and dullness, liver 6 cm right midclavicular line
9. Skin _____	i. S_1S_2, no murmurs
10. Throat _____	j. Clear to auscultation

APPLICATION QUESTIONS

1. When assessing the abdomen, which sequence does the nurse follow?
   a. Palpation, percussion, auscultation, and inspection
   b. Inspection, palpation, percussion, and auscultation
   c. Percussion, inspection, auscultation, and palpation
   d. Inspection, auscultation, percussion, and palpation
2. Which action is correct for the nurse to take when examining the ear of an 18-month-old boy?
   a. Pulling the ear back and down
   b. Pulling the ear back and up
   c. Pulling the ear forward
   d. Looking into the ear without pulling it in any direction
3. When using an ophthalmoscope to assess a 3-year-old girl's eyes, for what does the nurse look?
   a. Optic disk
   b. Macula
   c. Red reflex
   d. Fovea centralis
4. At which age may a head to toe assessment first be done?
   a. Toddlers
   b. School-aged children
   c. Adolescents
   d. Adults
5. When assessing an adolescent, which structures would the nurse examine last?
   a. Head, eyes, ears, nose, and throat
   b. Neurological

(continued)

c. Musculoskeletal
d. Genitourinary

6. Adolescents should always be interviewed
   a. With and without their parents/guardians
   b. Only with their parents/guardians
   c. Only without their parents/guardians
   d. Once a year

7. Which type of abuse is the nurse most likely to discover when assessing the elderly?
   a. Physical abuse
   b. Emotional abuse
   c. Neglect
   d. Social

8. A child's interactions with his/her parent/guardian are important to observe because you learn about the child's:
   a. Relationship with the parent/guardian
   b. Level of functioning
   c. Neuromuscular functioning
   d. All of the above

9. During a skin assessment, a client asks a question about what the skin does. The nurse's response would be based on the knowledge that the functions of the skin include: (Mark all that apply.)
   a. ___Temperature regulation
   b. ___ Sensory perception
   c. ___Identification of the individual
   d. ___Protection

10. In order to localize a symptom, which direction should the nurse give a client?
    a. Point to where the symptom occurs.
    b. Come back when you are experiencing the symptom.
    c. Bring someone in with you who has witnessed you having the symptom.
    d. Tell me which body part is affected by the symptom.

11. When a client complains of right knee pain, which areas should the nurse examine?
    a. Only the right knee
    b. The right ankle, the right knee, and the right hip
    c. The left lower abdominal quadrant and the left knee
    d. The right leg and left arm

12. Which is the best approach to gathering information about diet as part of a client assessment?
    a. You don't eat much fatty food, do you?
    b. Tell me about your diet.
    c. Do you like potato chips?
    d. Do you eat three meals each day?

13. When percussing over organs, which percussion note would the nurse interpret as normal?
    a. Dull
    b. Flat
    c. Hyperresonant
    d. Resonant

14. Which test is an indicator of coordination?
    a. Rinne test
    b. Weber test
    c. Corneal reflex response
    d. Rapid alternating movement test

15. Which are components of a complete health history? Mark all that apply.
    a. ___ Chief complaint
    b. ___ History of the present illness
    c. ___ Past medical/surgical history
    d. ___ Family, personal, and social history
    e. ___ Review of systems
    f. ___ Physical exam

16. When shining a light in a client's eye, which reaction would the nurse interpret as normal? The pupils:
    a. Contract
    b. Dilate
    c. Move to the left
    d. Oscillate laterally

17. Which test is the nurse performing when a vibrating tuning fork is placed on top of a client's head and the client is asked if the sound is heard equally in both ears?
    a. Rinne test for bone and air conduction
    b. Romberg for balance
    c. Test for extinction
    d. Weber test for sound lateralization

18. When testing a client's ability to identify odors, the nurse is assessing the function of which cranial nerve?
    a. Facial
    b. Trigeminal
    c. Olfactory
    d. Spinal accessory

19. Which notation correctly indicates normal muscle strength?
    a. 0/5
    b. 5/5
    c. 5/10
    d. 10/10

20. During a presentation at a health fair, a client asks about the cause of presbyopia. On which information should the nurse's response be based? Presbyopia results when the
    a. lens becomes less flexible.
    b. iris does not open fully.
    c. retina is covered by a cataract.
    d. optic blood vessels are engorged.

21. A new mother asks how far her baby is able to see. Which is the correct response for the nurse to make?
    a. Across a 10 ft × 10 ft room
    b. Only distant objects
    c. Only within 2 in. of the eyes
    d. Objects to 1 ft away

22. Where would the nurse auscultate to best hear S1, the first heart sound?
    a. Apex of the heart
    b. Base of the heart
    c. Aortic area
    d. Third left intercostal space

23. A client with right heart failure asks what the right side of the heart does. The nurse's response is based on the fact that the right ventricle pumps deoxygenated blood through the
    a. pulmonary veins to the aorta
    b. aorta to the left atrium
    c. pulmonary arteries to the left ventricle
    d. pulmonary arteries to the lungs

24. When assessing the abdomen of a client who is complaining of diarrhea, which finding would the nurse expect?
    a. Absent bowel sounds
    b. Hypoactive bowel sounds
    c. Hyperactive bowel sounds
    d. Normal bowel sounds

25. While the nurse is trying to assess an infant's lungs, the infant is crying. Which conclusions should the nurse draw? Check all that apply.
    a. Airway is patent
    b. The infant may be distressed
    c. The infant is in need of emergency treatment
    d. Vocal cords are intact

ANSWERS & RATIONALES

ANSWERS FOR FILL IN THE BLANKS

Fill in the blank spaces with the correct word or phrase to complete each statement.

1. To assess the tympanic membrane in a 1-year-old child, you need to pull the pinna back and __ down ____.
2. The last area to assess in a toddler is the _____ ears _______.
3. During assessment of the eyes in a child less than 6-years-old, you need to be able to see the ___ red reflex ____.
4. Preschoolers may already feel comfortable sitting on the _____ exam table ______ rather than their parent's/guardian's lap during the physical examination.
5. The comfort and ____ privacy _____ of all clients should be ensured during the physical examination.
6. For an adolescent, the last area to be assessed is the ____ genitourinary _______ system.
7. Elderly clients may not be able to change ___ positions _____ as easily as younger clients during the physical examination.

(continued)

8. The skin produces vitamin ____ D _____.

9. The client's ____ perception _____ of the problem is an important part of the health history.

10. The parasympathetic and sympathetic nerve pathways are part of the ____ autonomic _____ nervous system.

11. The expression of a person's cognition, mood, emotions and personality is called ____ mental status _____.

12. If the underlying cause of a mental status change is not reversible, the goal of care is to maintain ___ function _____.

13. The most sensitive part of the hand which is used for palpation is/are the ____ finger pads _____.

14. The physical examination contains only _____ objective ______ information.

15. The head is assessed for ____ symmetry ______ and shape.

TRUE & FALSE ANSWERS

Mark each of the following statements True or False. Correct all false statements in the space provided.

1. You should speak in a louder voice to all elderly clients. *False*
   With aging the ability to hear high tones decreases (presbycusis). Therefore one should use lower tones when speaking to older clients; speaking more loudly tends to raise the tone of the voice and thus can make hearing more difficult.

2. When discussing an illness affecting one system, you would reinforce to the client that all body systems are interrelated. *True*

3. Elderly clients are never victims of abuse. *False*
   Persons of all ages are abused. Neglect is the most common type of abuse among the elderly.

4. The Mini-Mental Status Examination is used to screen clients for cognitive dysfunction. *True*

5. A reflex arc occurs when a sensory impulse travels to the spinal cord and a motor impulse is sent back out to the muscle. *True*

6. The nurse may never divulge information gained during a client interview. *False*
   Information can be divulged in accord with HIPAA guideline. Information can be shared with appropriate agencies when necessary to ensure the safety of the client and those around him or her.

7. During the first year of life, the nervous system develops with increasing myelination. *True*

8. Delirium is a medical emergency. *True*

9. Baseline mental status is determined when the client is acutely ill. *False*
   Beseline mental status is determined when the client is at his or her usual level of health and function.

10. At the end of the interview, a nurse should summarize what was heard from the client. *True*

11. The ventral surface of the hand is most sensitive to temperature. *False*
The dorsal surface of the hand (back of the hand) is most sensitive to temperature.

12. It is normal to hear tympany to percussion over the abdomen. *True*

13. Subjective information is anything that the examiner observes. *False*
Objective information is anything that the examiner observes.

14. The health history contains objective information. *False*
The health history contains subjective information.

15. The review of systems is necessary to prevent omission of important information. *True*

MATCHING ANSWERS

Match the following:

Organ	Function
1. Ear ___c___	a. Receives visual data
2. Eye ___a___	b. Circulates blood cells to body
3. Gall Bladder ___g___	c. Maintains balance
4. Heart ___b___	d. Oxygen and carbon dioxide exchange
5. Large intestine ___h___	e. Wound repair
6. Liver ___f___	f. Produces bile
7. Lungs ___d___	g. Stores bile
8. Mouth ___j___	h. Absorbs water
9. Pancreas ___i___	i. Produces insulin
10. Skin ___e___	j. Begins digestion

MATCHING ANSWERS

Match the following:

1. Abdomen ___h___	a. Trachea midline, thyroid non-palpable
2. Extremities ___f___	b. Red mucosa, septum midline

(continued)

3. Heart __I__	c. Intact vibratory sense, deep tendon reflexes 2+
4. Lungs __j__	d. No injection, uvula rises midline
5. Lymph nodes __h__	e. No vascularities, warm, turgor intact
6. Neck __a__	f. Full range of motion
7. Nervous system __c__	g. Palpable in the occipital area, less than 1 cm, tender
8. Nose __b__	h. Alternating tympany and dullness, liver 6 cm right midclavicular line
9. Skin __e__	i. S1S2, no murmurs
10. Throat __d__	j. Clear to auscultation

APPLICATION ANSWERS

1. When assessing the abdomen, which sequence does the nurse follow?
   a. Palpation, percussion, auscultation, and inspection
   b. Inspection, palpation, percussion, and auscultation
   c. Percussion, inspection, auscultation, and palpation
   d. Inspection, auscultation, percussion, and palpation

Rationale
Correct answer: d.
Palpation is last in order to prevent distortion of bowel sounds.

2. Which action is correct for the nurse to take when examining the ear of an 18-month-old boy?
   a. Pulling the ear back and down
   b. Pulling the ear back and up
   c. Pulling the ear forward
   d. Looking into the ear without pulling it in any direction

Rationale
Correct answer: a.
An infant's ear canal is positioned lower than older children and adults.

3. When using an ophthalmoscope to assess a 3-year-old girl's eyes, for what does the nurse look?
   a. Optic disk
   b. Macula
   c. Red reflex
   d. Fovea centralis

Rationale
Correct answer: c.
Often children will not remain stationary long enough to view further structures in the eye. Being able to view the red reflex rules out a congenital cataract.

4. At which age may a head to toe assessment first be done?
   a. Toddlers
   b. School-aged children
   c. Adolescents
   d. Adults

Rationale
Correct answer: b.
Some preschool-aged children may already be able to be examined head to toe as well.

5. When assessing an adolescent, which structures would the nurse examine last?
   a. Head, eyes, ears, nose, and throat
   b. Neurological
   c. Musculoskeletal
   d. Genitourinary

Rationale
Correct answer: d.
Developing adolescents find the genitourinary exam the most difficult.

6. Adolescents should always be interviewed
   a. with and without their parents/guardians.
   b. only with their parents/guardians.

c. only without their parents/guardians.
d. once a year.

Rationale

Correct answer: a.

Adolescents may not want to reveal risky behaviors in front of their parents/guardians.

7. Which type of abuse is the nurse most likely to discover when assessing the elderly?
   a. Physical abuse
   b. Emotional abuse
   c. Neglect
   d. Social

Rationale

Correct answer: c.

Neglect is the most common type of abuse against the elderly. Often, the elderly person does not want those close to them to help with physical functions or their caregivers may not be willing to perform incontinence and personal care.

8. A child's interactions with his/her parent/guardian are important to observe because you learn about the child's
   a. relationship with the parent/guardian.
   b. level of functioning.
   c. neuromuscular functioning.
   d. all of the above.

Rationale

Correct answer: d.

You learn about the child's relationship with the caregiver, what the child can or is allowed to do for him/herself and how the child manipulates the environment both physically and emotionally.

9. During a skin assessment, a client asks a question about what the skin does. The nurse's response would be based on the knowledge that the functions of the skin include (Mark all that apply.)
   a. ___temperature regulation
   b. ___sensory perception
   c. ___identification of the individual
   d. ___protection

Rationale

Correct answers: a, b, c, and d.

The skin regulates temperature through changes in its blood flow and through sweating. The skin provides sensory information through its nerve endings. Fingerprints allow for indentification of individuals. The skin and mucous membranes are the first line of defense against injury and invasion of microorganisms.

10. In order to localize a symptom, which direction should the nurse give a client?
    a. Point to where the symptom occurs
    b. Come back when you are experiencing the symptom
    c. Bring someone in with you who has witnessed you having the symptom
    d. Tell me which body part is affected by the symptom.

Rationale

Correct answer: a.

This gives the examiner an understanding of where the problem may be without the possibility of confusion due to terminology used by the client for various body parts. There are times when a client may need to return during the time a symptom is being experienced but this is not primarily to localize the symptom. There are also times such as in the case of loss of consciousness or a seizure when a witness can provide valuable information but again, this is not primarily directed at localizing the symptom.

11. When a client complains of right knee pain, which areas should the nurse examine?
    a. Only the right knee
    b. The right ankle, the right knee and the right hip
    c. The left lower abdominal quadrant and the left knee
    d. The right leg and left arm

Rationale

Correct answer: b.

Pain in the right knee may be referred from the right hip or right ankle.

12. Which is the best approach to gathering information about diet as part of a client assessment?
    a. You don't eat much fatty food, do you?
    b. Tell me about your diet.
    c. Do you like potato chips?
    d. Do you eat three meals each day?

Rationale

Correct answer: b.

This is an open-ended question which allows the client to describe the answer and say more than "yes" or "no."

13. When percussing over organs, which percussion note would the nurse interpret as normal?
    a. Dull
    b. Flat
    c. Hyperresonant
    d. Resonant

Rationale

Correct answer: a.

A flat percussion note is heard over bone, hyperresonant over over-inflated lungs and resonant over normal lung tissue.

14. Which test is an indicator of coordination?
    a. Rinne test
    b. Weber test
    c. Corneal reflex response
    d. Rapid alternating movement test

(continued)

Rationale
Correct answer: d.
Weber and Rinne are both hearing tests and corneal reflex response is an eye test.

15. Which are components of a complete health history? Mark all that apply.
    a. ___ Chief complaint
    b. ___ History of the present illness
    c. ___ Past medical/surgical history
    d. ___ Family, personal and social history
    e. ___ Review of systems
    f. ___ Physical exam

Rationale
Correct answers: a, b, c, d, e, and f.
The physical examination is not part of the health history.

16. When shining a light in a client's eye, which reaction would the nurse interpret as normal? The pupils:
    a. Contract
    b. Dilate
    c. Move to the left
    d. Oscillate laterally

Rationale
Correct answer: a.
Light causes the direct and consensual reactions of the pupil the light is shined on and the other pupil. The pupils should not dilate, move, or oscillate when light is shined on one or both.

17. Which test is the nurse performing when a vibrating tuning fork is placed on top of a client's head and the client is asked if sound is heard equally in both ears?
    a. Rinne test for bone and air conduction
    b. Romberg for balance
    c. Test for extinction
    d. Weber test for sound lateralization

Rationale
Correct answer: d.
For the Rinne test, the vibrating tuning fork is placed on the mastoid. No tuning forks are used in the Romberg test and in the test for extinction.

18. When testing a client's ability to identify odors, the nurse is assessing the function of which cranial nerve?
    a. Facial
    b. Trigeminal
    c. Olfactory
    d. Spinal accessory

Rationale
Correct answer: c.
The sensory function of the facial nerve relates to taste. The trigeminal nerve mediates light touch sensation. The spinal accessory nerve is a motor nerve tested by asking the client to turn the head against the resistance of the examiner's hand placed against the side of his or her chin and face and to shrug the shoulders against the resistance of the examiner's hands on them.

19. Which notation correctly indicates normal muscle strength?
    a. 0/5
    b. 5/5
    c. 5/10
    d. 10/10

Rationale
Correct answer: b.
Muscle strength is graded against gravity and resistance on a scale of 0–5 with 5 being normal and 0 being completely paralyzed. Grades of 4, 3, 2, or 1/5 indicate varying degrees of weakness.

20. During a presentation at a health fair, a client asks about the cause of presbyopia. On which information should the nurse's response be based?
    Presbyopia results when the
    a. lens becomes less flexible.
    b. iris does not open fully.
    c. retina is covered by a cataract.
    d. optic blood vessels are engorged.

Rationale
Correct answer: a.
The other answers are unrelated to the development of presbyopia, which is the decrease in ability to see near objects that occurs with age.

21. A new mother asks how far her baby is able to see. Which is the correct response for the nurse to make?
    a. Across a 10 ft × 10 ft room
    b. Only distant objects
    c. Only within 2 in. of the eyes
    d. Objects to 1 ft away

Rationale
Correct answer: d.
This is the distance between the mother's face and the infant in her arms.

22. Where would the nurse auscultate to best hear S1, the first heart sound?
    a. Apex of the heart
    b. Base of the heart
    c. Aortic area
    d. Third left intercostal space

Rationale

Correct answer: a.

The closing of the mitral and tricuspid valves forms the first heart sound. The apex of the heart is actually the bottom of the heart, where the left ventricle is found.

23. A client with right heart failure asks what the right side of the heart does. The nurse's response is based on the fact that the right ventricle pumps deoxygenated blood through the
    a. pulmonary veins to the aorta.
    b. aorta to the left atrium.
    c. pulmonary arteries to the left ventricle.
    d. pulmonary arteries to the lungs.

Rationale

Correct answer: d.

Blood flows from the right atrium through the tricuspid valve to the right ventricle through the pulmonic valve to the pulmonary arteries to the lungs, then back into the pulmonary veins to the left atrium, through the mitral valve to the left ventricle and through the aortic valve to the aorta and out to the body. The pulmonary arteries are the only arteries in the body that carry deoxygenated blood while the pulmonary veins are the only veins in the body that carry oxygenated blood.

24. When assessing the abdomen of a client who is complaining of diarrhea, which finding would the nurse expect?
    a. Absent bowel sounds
    b. Hypoactive bowel sounds
    c. Hyperactive bowel sounds
    d. Normal bowel sounds

Rationale

Correct answer: c.

Hypoactive bowel sounds may be a result of ileus or abdominal infection.

25. While the nurse is trying to assess an infant's lungs, the infant is crying. Which conclusions should the nurse draw? Check all that apply.
    a. Airway is patent
    b. The infant may be distressed
    c. The infant is in need of emergency treatment
    d. Vocal cords are intact

Rationale

Correct answers: a, b, and d.

If the infant can generate the sound of crying, vocal cords are intact and the airway is patent. The infant does not need emergency treatment for simply crying. The examination may be distressing to the infant.

CHAPTER 10

Test Plan Category:

Psychosocial Integrity—Part 1

Sub-category: **None**

Topics: **Mental Health Concepts**
Cultural Diversity
Coping Mechanisms
Religious and Spiritual Influences on Health
Situational Role Changes
Stress Management
Support Systems
Family Dynamics
Unexpected Body-Image Changes
Grief and Loss
End of Life

Psychosocial integrity is important for the promotion and support of the emotional, mental, and social well-being of the client, family, and significant others experiencing stressful events and acute or chronic illnesses.

CULTURAL DIVERSITY

- Culture is a shared system of beliefs, values, and behavioral expectations that influence daily living.
- Including the client's culture and ethnicity into the plan of care eliminates ethnocentrism—judging others by one's own standards of acting, believing, and thinking.
- Acculturation—also called cultural assimilation—occurs when a member of a cultural group adapts to the new dominant culture in order to survive.
- Cultural competence is a set of practice standards that ensures that clients of all cultures receive information about treatment in familiar ways, considering education, acculturation, and language.
- To maintain cultural competence, nurses must assess the client's health care practices including health-seeking behaviors, responsibility for health care, folklore practices, barriers to health care, and cultural responses to health and illness.
- Cultural competence standards in clinical practice include the use of interpreters, multilingual and multicultural staff that reflects the community, culturally sound psychological and diagnostic testing, recognition that cultural factors influence treatment compliance, availability of printed client education materials in the preferred language of the client, and documentation of how the client language needs were met.
- In addition to translation services, spiritual support and pastoral counseling should be made available to cross-cultural clients.
- A client's cultural influences on health care are many. The nurse must take these factors into consideration when planning nursing care.
  —Physiologic characteristics: Certain illnesses are associated with race and culture, such as sickle cell anemia in people of African or Mediterranean origin.
  —Psychological characteristics: A client may view some health care practices as irrelevant, whereas the nurse views the same practices as important. For example, the nurse may view a yearly mammogram in a Hispanic client with a past history of breast cancer as important, whereas the client views the procedure as interfering with God's ultimate plan.
  —Pain: Some cultures express pain openly and embrace measures to reduce pain, while other cultures remain stoic. The nurse must respect the client's cultural beliefs regarding pain. For example, Native Americans use relaxation such as meditation to help quell pain prior to using medications.
  —Mental health: Some cultures view mental illness as a stigma. For example, a traditional Chinese client may ignore symptoms of mental illness and thus not seek care due to the stigma associated with mental illness in the traditional Chinese culture.
  —Gender: In some cultures the male is the dominant figure, whereas the female is the dominant figure in other cultures. For example, in African-American families, the female typically makes the decisions for all family members.
  —Communication: Verbal and nonverbal communication techniques vary among cultures. For example, American culture emphasizes eye contact while speaking, whereas Arabs view this communication technique as impolite and aggressive. All written materials must be provided in the client's spoken language.
  —Personal space: Some cultures believe in maintaining physical distance while others prefer to be physically close to other humans. For example, Arabs prefer to sit and stand close to one another when talking, whereas Asians prefer distance between themselves and others.
  —Time: Being punctual for appointments is not important to all cultures. For example, some Asian cultures view being late as a sign of respect.
  —Food: Certain foods serve as dietary staples based on culture. Rice is a staple of the Chinese, and pasta is a staple of the Italians. The nurse should ask every client about food preferences and dietary practices.
  —Family support: Many cultures include family members in the health care decision-making process. For example, Chinese and Arab family members consult with the family's elders regarding health care advice.
  —Socioeconomic factors: Poverty impedes access to health care. Populations impacted by poverty include migrant farm workers, families living on welfare, and people living in isolated areas, such as the Appalachian Mountains.
- Many cultures rely on traditional healers to improve health outcomes. Healers may prescribe herbs, massage, heat and cold therapies, and acupuncture to alleviate pain and treat illness. Clients who use traditional healers may view health care providers as incompetent because they ask many questions and implement trial-and-error methods of healing.
- Cultural differences can affect responses to medications. For example, Asians require smaller doses of a drug because their bodies metabolize drugs at a slower rate. African-Americans may require larger doses of blood pressure medication.
  —Traditional herbal treatments may interfere with a prescribed medication's action.
  —Culture beliefs can affect compliance and response to a medication regimen. For example, an Asian client may prefer herbal tea over a sleeping medication to promote relaxation.

- A client's cultural practices can cause sensory deprivation, sensory overload, and sleep deprivation. The nurse asks the client what level of stimulation is acceptable to the client.
- Some cultures believe surgical intervention is the last option for treating illness. Clients of these cultures may be convinced that death will result due to surgery. This anxiety may increase the client's surgical risk.
  —For example, a client from a culture that believes bed rest is the best treatment for illness may refuse to participate in postoperative ambulation and exercises.
- Culture influences a client's reaction to grief and loss. In Western culture, families grieve privately and internalize their feelings of loss.
- During the nursing assessment, the nurse asks clients how they wish to be treated based on their cultural values and beliefs while remembering each client is an individual.
- The nurse's role in caring for culturally diverse clients is to understand the client's needs and to adapt care to meet those needs. The nurse must blend his or her own beliefs with those of the nursing profession and individual clients to deliver safe, considerate, and successful nursing care to all clients.
- Table 10–1 addresses cross-cultural perspectives of health.

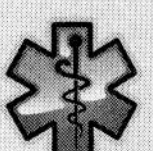

Nursing Intervention Alert

When delivering care to cross-cultural clients, the nurse must maintain the client's cultural mental health practices, facilitate effective verbal and nonverbal communication, and promote the client's understanding of treatment and the rationale behind the care received.

Table 10–1 Cross-Cultural Perspectives of Health

Culture	Family	Health Care Preferences	Health Care Concepts	Mental Illness	Communication Preferences	Health Promotion
African American	Matriarchal structure; many single-parent households headed by women	Traditional medicines; healers and voodoo priests; herbs	Health is freedom from pain and stress; a sense of well-being	Due to spiritual distress	Close personal space; present time over future	Protect against excessive cold Consume proper diet Maintain proper behavior Exercise in fresh air
Asian American	Hierarchical structure; loyal family members	Traditional medicines and healers; herbs	Balance of *yin* and *yang* to promote harmony	Stigma attached to mental illness; metabolic imbalance and organic problem	No physical contact; present time orientation	Maintain harmony with friends and family Consume a diet balanced with *yin* and *yang* foods
Hispanic	Nuclear structure; large extended family; strong church affiliation	Traditional medicines and healers; herbs; diagnostic techniques include exorcism	Ability to maintain role function; sense of well-being	Due to spells or bad spirits	Value physical presence and touch; present time orientation	Show aversion to health screenings and routine physicals because future is in God's hands
Native-American	Nuclear structure; large extended family	Traditional medicines and healers; herbs; diagnostic techniques include stargazing	Holistic approach to health: mind, body, spirit	Due to curse; holistic approach	Space important and has no boundaries; future over present time	Practise religious ceremonies and prayer Perform physical exercise and meditation
Arab	Patriarchal structure; men valued over women	Traditional medicines and healers	Turn to elders in the family for medical advice Health is freedom from pain	Due to physical or emotional trauma; attributed to supernatural beings	Formal manners; time orientation varies by religion	Value modern Western medical practices Care for personal hygiene Consume healthy diet

RELIGIOUS AND SPIRITUAL INFLUENCES ON HEALTH

- Every person has a spiritual dimension, which may be expressed formally or informally.
- Spirituality allows individuals to make sense of the cycle of life and death by offering hope and support.
- Spirituality is a search for the sacred.
- Religion is an expression of spirituality.
- Faith is the ability to draw on spiritual resources without requiring physical proof.
- Hope is responsible for a positive outlook even during the bleakest moments.
- Spiritual health occurs when the spiritual needs for meaning and purpose, love and belonging, and forgiveness are met.
- Spiritual assessment incorporates a holistic view of the client and addresses meaning and purpose in life, ability to recognize inner strengths, and self-concept.
- Many people seek support from their religious faith during times of illness.
- Religious beliefs can conflict with health care practices, as in the case of Muslims who view illness as fate instead of a condition in which action may be taken.
- Some people view illness as a punishment for sin, thus causing spiritual distress.
- In cases of spiritual distress, the nurse may explore with the client spiritual beliefs and practices, factors that challenge spiritual beliefs, and alternatives to reaffirm or modify beliefs.
- Nursing interventions to assist clients and their families meet their spiritual needs include offering support, facilitating the client's practice of religion, praying with a client and family, contacting a spiritual counselor, and resolving conflicts between treatment and spiritual beliefs.

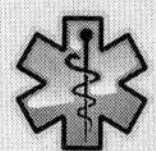

Nursing Intervention Alert

An objective explanation of alternative treatments and the predicted consequences of each may help the client determine acceptable treatment that does not conflict with religious beliefs.

STRESS MANAGEMENT

- Stress is a condition in which the human system responds to changes in its normal balanced state.
- A stressor is anything that is perceived as challenging, demanding, or threatening.
- A state of psychological stress results when resources are not available to reestablish balance.
- A person's age, developmental level, past experiences, support systems, and coping mechanisms influence adaptations to stress.
- Stress can cause illness and illness may precipitate stress.
- Prolonged stress can perpetuate ineffective coping and mental illness.
- Stress that affects the client also influences the family and significant others.
- Two main types of stress exist: developmental and situational.
- Developmental stress occurs as an individual progresses through the normal stages of growth and development.
- Situational stress is unpredictable and can occur at any time.
- The human body responds to stress by releasing epinephrine, norepinephrine, and other hormones that increase the metabolic rate and protect the immune system.
- Physiologic stressors include viruses, bacteria, fungi, drugs, alcohol, poison, heat/cold, radiation, trauma, electric shock, suppressed immune system, genetic disorders, acute and chronic illnesses, and the process of aging.
- Psychosocial stressors include trauma, accidents, lack of knowledge, fear, noise, uncertainty, and rapid changes in the world, which can include both real and perceived threats.
- See Table 10–2 for the physical and psychological responses to stress.
- Stress increases the client's chances of developing disease or illness.
- Clients who are under stress experience more depression, require more anesthesia and analgesia, and have lower immune functioning than those who experience minimal or no stress.

Table 10–2 Physical and Psychological Responses to Stress

Physical Responses	Psychological Responses
Dry mouth	Nightmares
Tachycardia	Irritability
Insomnia	Depression
Increased urinary frequency	Disturbed behavior
Muscle tension or pain	Anxiety
Headaches	Tearfulness
Loss of or excessive appetite	Inability to concentrate
Gastrointestinal distress	Increased use of nicotine, alcohol, and drugs
Fatigue	Impulsive behavior
Dizziness	Disturbed behavior
Change in menstrual cycle	Easily startled

- Clients who are able to cope with stress have better health outcomes. Coping mechanisms that help decrease stress are
  —exercise: Improves oxygenation, decreases heart rate, improves sleep, increases appetite, and produces a general sense of well-being.
  —music therapy: Relieves tension and promotes relaxation.
  —humor: Improves oxygenation, improves circulation, and reduces aggression.
  —pet therapy: Reduces depression.
  —art therapy: Invigorates the senses and reduces depression.
- See Table 10–3 for common stress management techniques.
- Inappropriate coping processes include alcohol and drug use, hostile behavior, denial, avoidance, and distancing.
- People who have hope, a strong sense of self, and effective support systems are better equipped to handle physical and psychosocial stressors.
- Stress is the wear and tear of life on an individual. Prolonged or unrelenting stress leads to anxiety.
- When a client encounters a stressful situation, three stages of reaction to stress occur: the alarm reaction stage, the resistance stage, and the exhaustion stage.
- In the alarm reaction stage, the stress stimulates the adrenal glands to produce adrenalin, which is needed for the "fight or flight" response.
- In the resistance stage, blood is shunted away from the digestive tract to areas needed for defense. Heart rate and respirations increase to circulate highly oxygenated blood to the muscles. If the client adapts to stress, the body relaxes and the systemic responses abate.
- In the exhaustion stage, the client fails to adapt to stress, depleting physical and emotional energy. As a result, the client develops anxiety, which may be classified as mild, moderate, severe, or panic.

Table 10–3 Common Stress-Management Techniques

Stress-Management Technique	Components
Relaxation	Rhythmic breathing, reduced muscle tension, altered state of consciousness
Meditation	Quiet surroundings, passive attitude, comfortable position, and a word or mental image on which to focus
Anticipatory guidance	Teaching to prepare the client for an unfamiliar or painful event; anticipatory socialization to prepare for a new role, such as parenthood
Guided imagery	Creation of a mental image, concentration on that image, decreased response to stimuli, such as painful stimuli
Biofeedback	Measurement device to measure mental control of the autonomic nervous system to control body responses, such as blood pressure, heart rate, and headaches
Progressive muscle relaxation	Tensing and releasing of muscles in sequence
Yoga	Combines rhythmic breathing and tensing and releasing of muscles

- Severe anxiety elicits cognitive, psychomotor, and physiologic responses, which include reduced perceptual fields, difficulty with problem-solving and completing tasks, feelings of dread, crying, headache, nausea and vomiting, tachycardia, chest pain, and ritualistic behaviors.
- Panic results in distorted perceptions, loss of rational thought, decreased ability to verbally communicate, delusions, hallucinations, suicidal thoughts, and dilated pupils. When a client is in a state of panic, the client's safety is a priority; immediate medical intervention is required.
- Without intervention, continued anxiety may cause both mental as well as physical illnesses.
- Stress precipitates adjustment disorders—feelings of depression or anxiety or combined depression and anxiety. Clients with an anxiety-adjustment disorder experience anxious feelings, nervousness, and worry.
- Anxiety-adjustment disorder can cause or worsen physical illness.
- Antidepressants, therapy, and support systems are beneficial in treating anxiety-adjustment disorder.

Client teaching for self-care

- Teach clients that spiritual components contribute to the holistic view of care
- Teach clients to recognize stressors and skills to manage the stressors
- Demonstrate relaxation techniques and their purpose in reducing stress
- Teach the client, family, and significant others to seek professional help if the client experiences panic

SUPPORT SYSTEMS

- Support systems lead people to believe they are loved, cared for, esteemed and valued, and belong to a network of communication and mutual obligation.
- Support systems provide emotional support that helps an individual identify and verbalize feelings, maintain a positive self-concept, and establish new relationships and social roles.
- Sources of support include families, significant others, friends, neighbors, religion, community organizations and resources, and support groups.
- Social networks assist with management of stress, thus improving health outcomes. Families and significant others provide love, a sense of sharing the burden, and information that helps the nurse in developing the plan of care.
- Friends and neighbors offer guidance, humor, and validation of feelings.
- Religion confirms values, beliefs, and spirituality.
- Community resources offer financial assistance, counseling, transportation, and education.
- Support groups provide an accepting environment, allowing exploration of problem-solving methods and implementation of new coping skills.
- Other support systems include encounter groups, assertiveness-training programs, and consciousness-raising groups.
- People who are loners, or lack support systems, are at high risk for ineffective coping with failure and illness.
- The nurse's role is to encourage client, family, and significant others' involvement in the health care decision-making process while promoting the independence of these individuals.
- The nurse uses therapeutic communication to evaluate client, family, and significant others' feelings about the diagnosis, illness, and treatment plan.

FAMILY DYNAMICS

- Family is defined as two or more people who are emotionally involved with each other and live together.
- Family is concerned with all aspects of a person's life, including meeting basic human needs to promote health.
- Researchers state that the role of the family is to help meet the basic human needs (health and survival) of its members while also meeting the needs of society.
- The nurse must respect all family structures and remember that there is no absolute "right" or "wrong" family structure. See Table 10–4 for the different types of family structures.
- Individuals with chronic mental illness who live at home with family drain financial, emotional, and personal resources, thus impacting the family's well-being.
- Stressors such as divorce, loss of employment, or death impact family functioning.
- The nurse assesses family dynamics by observing the communication and coping mechanisms utilized by the family.
- The nurse provides resources, such as group counseling, to assist in family functioning.

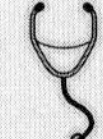

Assessment Alert

Ask all clients about their family structure to determine how the family will cope with the impact of the health condition. This information guides the nurse in creating each client's plan of care.

FAMILY FUNCTIONS

- Family functions are necessary for the growth of the individual and the family and for the maintenance of health.
- Physically, the family provides a safe, comfortable environment necessary for growth, development, and rest.
- The adults of the family use management skills to establish rules, make decisions about resources and finances, and plan for the future.

Table 10–4 Family Structures

Nuclear Family	Extended Family	Blended Family	Single-Parent Family	Other
Also called "traditional family"	Considered nontraditional	Also a "traditional family"	Considered nontraditional	Cohabitating family: Comprised of two unmarried adults living together
Comprised of two parents and their children; couples without children; or couples with grown children who no longer live at home	Comprised of aunts, uncles, cousins, and grandparents who live in close proximity to the nuclear family.	Comprised of parents who bring unrelated children from previous relationships together to form a new family	Comprised of one parent and his or her children	Binuclear family: Comprised of divorced parents who share joint custody of children
Parents may be heterosexual or homosexual; married or in a committed relationship	Extended family has their own nuclear family; the nuclear families within the extended family offer support to each other and share responsibilities	Parents may be heterosexual or homosexual; married or in a committed relationship	Parent may be separated, divorced, widowed, or never married	Dyadic nuclear family: Couple chooses not to have children
Comprised of biologic parents and children, adoptive parents and children, surrogate parents and children, or stepparents and children	Extended family may offer support to the nuclear family: child care, business partnerships, and sharing of household responsibilities	Comprised of parent and step-parent and biological and step-children	Majority are African-American and headed by women	Single adults: May not live with others, but are part of a family of origin
All members live in the same house until the children leave home as young adults	Some members of the extended family may live with the nuclear family; most commonly, a grandmother who lives with her children and grandchildren	All members live in the same house until the children leave home as young adults	Challenges include role shifts and financial concerns	Pets as family members: Many members of traditional and nontraditional families view pets as family members

- The reproductive function of the family is to raise children and set boundaries to distinguish the roles of adults and children within the family.
- Communication enhances the teaching of family beliefs, values, attitudes, and coping mechanisms.
- Providing emotional comfort and support helps family members endure stress and guides problem solving.
- Families teach their young the acceptable behaviors and cultural norms that enable them to interact with society.

FAMILY RISK FACTORS

- Family members can be placed at risk for health problems due to patterns of behavior, the environment in which the family lives, and genetic factors.
- Family members can be in several different developmental stages simultaneously, thus putting them at increased risk for altered health. See Table 10–5 for the risk factors that may alter family health.

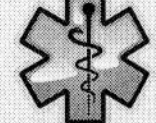

Nursing Intervention Alert

Nursing interventions for the family in health crisis include teaching using therapeutic communication skills, knowledge of family dynamics, referral to community financial and health care resources, and involvement of family members in the plan of care and implementation of care.

Table 10–5 Risk Factors for Altered Family Health

Biological Risks	Developmental Risks	Psychosocial Risks	Environmental Risks	Lifestyle Risks
Genetic predisposition to disease	Unmarried adolescent mothers	Inadequate income and resources, especially related to child care	Exposure to environmental toxins and pollutants including water and food pollution	Alterations in nutrition: more or less than body requirements
Birth defects	Older adults living alone or on a fixed income	Conflict among family members	Lack of knowledge to provide safe, clean living conditions	Chemical dependency: alcohol, drugs, and nicotine
Mental retardation	Families who have new babies	Lack of social support systems	Lack of resources to access healthcare	Inadequate hygiene: dental care

Client teaching for self-care

- Teach clients and their families how to access community resources to provide social support
- Teach clients and their families effective communication skills to strengthen family support
- Teach families the difference between coping mechanisms and defensive mechanisms to strengthen family communication and support
- Teach families stress management skills, relaxation techniques, and effective problem-solving skills to promote harmony
- Teach families to recognize risk factors and to access community resources in the presence of conflict or risk for altered psychosocial health
- Teach families techniques to implement roles and divide responsibilities among family members

COPING MECHANISMS

- Individuals use many methods to cope with their problems.
- The concept of coping is used interchangeably with the terms adaptation, defense, mastery, and adjustive reactions.
- Coping involves all of the behaviors individuals use, consciously or unconsciously, to deal with stress from threats to psychological integrity.
- When the stress involves the ego, coping reactions include complicated ego-defense mechanisms.
- Defense mechanisms are important for survival and are used in the process of coping (Table 10–6).
- Defense mechanisms are considered pathologic when they are used to deny, falsify, or distort perceptions of reality.
- Attack reactions attempt to overcome the stress-causing obstacle.
- Flight, withdrawal, or fear reactions include physical and psychological maneuvering to get rid of the threat.
- Compromise or substitution reactions occur when attack or flight options are not possible. These reactions involve accepting substitute goals or changing values.
- Tension-reducing reactions include aggression, regression, withdrawal, and repression.
- Individuals cope by crying, exercising, talking over their feelings, becoming angry or defensive, or withdrawing from a situation.
- These coping mechanisms are effective in maintaining emotional stability.

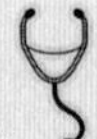

Assessment Alert

The following assessments are important to psychosocial health of the client, family, and significant others: support systems, available resources, psychological response to illness, and emotional reaction to illness.

- Past coping mechanisms may no longer be effective in adjusting to stressors later in life. See Table 10–7 for nursing actions to promote psychosocial health in older adults.

Table 10–6 Common Defense Mechanisms

Defense Mechanism	Definition	Example
Acting out	Use of action to deal with stress	A husband learns his wife is having an affair, and then goes to a bar where he engages in two fistfights.
Affiliation	Turning to others for support in times of conflict	A mother moves to the same city as her adult daughter after loss of a job.
Altruism	The gratifying self-serving of others to manage stress	Nurses serve others for unselfish reasons and gain gratification through giving.
Anticipation	Considering options and solutions in anticipation of future events	An athlete spends the hours before a race mentally rehearsing her race technique.
Compensation	Excelling in one area to counterbalance deficiencies in another area	A child with a heart condition that prohibits participation in sports excels in playing the violin.
Denial	Refusal to face an unpleasant reality as it exists	A client refuses to accept her diagnosis of multiple sclerosis.
Displacement	Placing feelings of hostility onto something or someone less threatening in the environment	After a man loses his job, he comes home and kicks the dog.
Fantasy	Substituting frustrated desires or relationships with daydreams and imagery	An unhappily married woman with four children imagines a life as a wildlife photographer.
Help-rejecting complaining	Repeated requests for help and advice from others that is then rejected; this behavior disguises covert feelings of hostility for others	A husband constantly complains of back pain to his wife, but refuses to take the wife's advice to receive medical treatment.
Humor	Emphasis on the amusing aspects of a situation	A client undergoing chemotherapy smiles and laughs when telling the nurse that she was so tired after the last treatment that she crawled into bed with her raincoat and rain boots still on.
Identification	Unconscious mimicking of an admired person	A high school girl dresses and speaks like her peer group's leader.
Intellectualization	Overuse of abstract thinking to minimize painful feelings	An alcoholic speaks of the illnesses associated with alcoholism to an Alcoholics Anonymous group, but never discusses his own fears associated with his alcoholism.
Introjection	Treating something that is outside the self as if it is inside the self	A child who fears monsters becomes a monster during play.
Isolation of affect	Separation of feelings from associated thoughts	A rape victim displays no emotion as she recounts the details of the rape to the police.
Omnipotence	Feeling or acting as if one have special powers or superiority over others	A scientist treats his team condescendingly.
Passive aggression	Indirect expression of aggression	A physically abused child repeatedly "forgets" his daily chores and begs forgiveness.
Projection	Attributing one's own unacceptable characteristics to another person or group	An egocentric teacher complains of her students' narcissism.
Rationalization	Using a socially acceptable explanation to justify unpleasant consequences	An obese client tells the nurse that he does not wish to be thin.
Reaction formation	Exaggerated adoption of opposite behaviors to those that are unpleasant	A couple that does not want its child before it is born becomes overly protective after the birth.

(continued on next page)

Table 10–6 *(continued from previous page)*

Defense Mechanism	Definition	Example
Regression	Returning to an earlier level of adaptation	An elderly client dresses like a child and insists on playing dolls.
Self-assertion	Direct expression of thoughts and feelings that are not manipulative or intimidating	A client informs the nurse that he appreciates the nurse's care.
Self-observation	Reflection of one's behavior, thoughts, and feelings, followed by appropriate behavior.	A client thinks about why she feels depressed, and then shares these feelings in group therapy.
Splitting	View of self and others as all good or all bad	A psychiatric client views the nurses in the facility as angels who are kind, while viewing the physicians as devils who wish to change the client's behavior and thinking.
Sublimation	Modification of a socially unacceptable impulse into an acceptable behavior	An aggressive young man becomes a star football player.
Suppression	Conscious inhibition of a thought or action	A victim of a near-fatal automobile accident does not think of the accident as he drives to work everyday.
Undoing	Attempt to dispel unacceptable behavior	An elderly client yells at the nurse, and then tells the nursing supervisor that the nurse is an outstanding employee.

Table 10–7 Psychosocial Health Promotion in Older Adults

Nursing Actions
Assess for abnormal responses to the aging process: anger, isolation, denial, and depression.
Be aware of major stressors: illness, hospitalization, and changes in living arrangements.
Assess support systems including cultural beliefs, spiritual values, and rituals.
Encourage use of support systems: family, friends, community resources, and pets to increase stimulation.
Set mutual goals; encourage the client to participate in the decision-making process.
Encourage life review and reminiscence.
Encourage self-care.
Consider the client's background, capabilities, interests, values and beliefs, culture, and lifestyle when planning care.
Facilitate individual, group, and family therapy when appropriate. Incorporate therapy goals into the plan of care.

Client teaching for self-care

- Teach older adults to focus on accomplishments instead of decline, to promote self-esteem
- Teach the older client that antidepressants may take 4–6 weeks to be effective in decreasing symptoms of depression
- Teach cross-cultural clients the importance of their heritage in self-care behaviors
- Teach clients how to differentiate coping mechanisms from defense mechanisms
- Teach client that coping mechanisms such as crying, kicking a chair, and yelling are normative behaviors
- Teach client that hitting others, hurting oneself, and destroying property are ineffective coping mechanisms
- Teach client that controlling anger by counting to 10, inhaling deeply through the nose and exhaling through the mouth, and diverting attention to another task, such as exercise, are healthy coping mechanisms

SITUATIONAL ROLE CHANGES

- Individuals play many roles both at home and in society.
- Role performance is a measure of how successfully an individual performs in a designated role.
- Role performance is easily compromised by illness and injury.
- An alteration in an individual's role performance can result in a situational role change.

Table 10–8 Disturbances in Self-Concept

Self-Concept Disturbance	Causes	Nursing Interventions
Disturbed body image	Weight changes: extreme thinness or obesity Changes in body image: amputation, mastectomy, scars, burns, colostomy, disfigurement, loss of vision, alopecia, and paralysis Use of ancillary devices: braces, canes, casts, and wheelchairs Development of secondary sex characteristics: aggressive development, delayed development	Allow client to express feelings about body image. Explore with the client perceptions of altered body image. Support the client through stages of grief, loss, and mourning. Implement play therapy with children to work through feelings of grief. Use open and accepting body language when interacting with clients. Encourage the client to participate in self-care activities. Intervene if the client's significant others negatively influence the client. Notice and voice positive physiologic characteristics.
Low self-esteem	Feelings of powerlessness, helplessness, and frustration Feelings of incompetence and inadequacy Feeling unloved or unapproved of by significant others Failure to live according to personal values or moral code Deficient knowledge: poor parenting skills, illiteracy	Allow the client to explore alternatives and make decisions. Listen to the client openly without instilling judgment. Teach the client to replace negative self-talk or thoughts with positive affirmations. Explore with the client alternative ways of viewing the same situation.
Ineffective role performance	Role conflict Role fatigue Rejection of role Multiple life stressors Physical and mental health changes Decline in motivation, commitment Decline in independence Loss of key roles: separation, retirement, or death of spouse or child	Allow client to express feelings about ineffective role performance. Facilitate grieving over valued roles that can no longer be performed. Explore new roles with the client. Facilitate options to alleviate stress and foster independence.
Disturbed personal identity	Unresolved crisis: divorce, loss of job, and abusive relationship Declining physical, mental, or sensory abilities Rejection by peers or group	Evaluate the client's coping strategy. Treat causes of disturbed personal identity: pain, substance abuse, and abusive living arrangement.

- Role changes may be due to death of a parent, spouse with chronic illness, or the aging process.
- Individuals whose roles are altered are at risk for disturbances in self-concept.
- Disturbances in self-concept may include the following diagnostic labels: *disturbed body image*, *chronic low self-esteem or situational low self-esteem*, *ineffective role performance*, and *disturbed personal identity*. See Table 10–8 for examples of disturbances in self-concept and related nursing interventions.
- The nurse's role is to assess client, family, and significant others' role changes, whether temporary or permanent.
- The nurse provides support to the client and/or family in coping with a new diagnosis, ongoing stressors, or role change.
- The nurse evaluates whether the client, family, and significant others have successfully adapted to situation role changes.

UNEXPECTED BODY-IMAGE CHANGES

- Body image is the subjective view an individual has about his or her physical appearance including body shape, size, weight, and proportions.
- Body-image disturbances are expected with any alteration in bodily appearance, structure, or function.
- See Table 10–8 for the causes and nursing interventions associated with body-image changes.

GRIEF AND LOSS

- Grief is the painful psychologic and physiologic response to any real or perceived loss.
- Grief accompanies any significant loss: death of a loved one and loss of self-esteem, identity, dignity, or self-worth.
- The manifestations of grief are found in Table 10–9.
- Grief has three basic stages: avoidance, confrontation, and reestablishment.
- Reestablishment is the gradual decrease of symptoms and adjustment to a different life.
- Kubler-Ross identified the five stages of grief as
  —denial: shock and disbelief regarding the loss
  —anger: expression of hostility which may be directed toward God, friends, relatives, or health care providers
  —bargaining: making attempts to negotiate to prevent or remove the loss
  —depression: sense of sadness, emptiness over the loss
  —acceptance: coming to terms with the loss
- The types of grief are anticipatory, acute, and complicated (Table 10–10).
- Factors influencing the grieving process include
  —culture and religion: Bereavement rituals have roots in the cultural and spiritual background of the person experiencing the grief and influences
    - the manner of public expression of the grief whether it is loud and expressive or quiet and hidden
    - the acceptable length of bereavement
    - outward display such as wearing black garments
    - funeral and burial rites and rituals

  —significance of the loss or death
  —cause of the loss or death
  —gender: In general, women are more overt with their expressions of grief and are more accepting of support
  —age and development: Ability to perceive permanence of death and the process in dealing with it differ according to age.
    - Infancy to 5 years—death is temporary and reversible
    - 5–9 years—develops sense of finality of death, believes own death can be avoided and may believe loss is related to own thoughts and actions
    - 9–12 years—death is inevitable, begins to understand own mortality
    - 12–18 years—may seem to reach "adult" perception of death but is emotionally unable to accept it
    - 18–45 years—attitude toward loss or death influenced by the religious and cultural beliefs
    - 45–65 years—accepts own mortality, experiences more deaths of close family members and peers
    - 65+ years—death may have multiple meanings ranging from freedom from pain to being with already deceased loved ones

Table 10–9 Manifestations of Grief

Physical Manifestations	Cognitive Manifestations	Behavioral Manifestations	Affective Manifestations
Weakness, anorexia, shortness of breath, dry mouth, gastrointestinal disturbances	Preoccupation with the deceased: conversations with the deceased	Inability to perform basic activities of daily living	Feelings of sadness, guilt, anger, loneliness, and helplessness
Fatigue, exhaustion, insomnia	Difficulty concentrating, focusing	Dragging through activities of daily living	Feelings of shock, disbelief, and denial
Decreased immune response	Disorientation to time and place	Old behavior patterns lose meaning	Impulse to use alcohol or drugs
Increased vulnerability to physical illness: myocardial infarction, hypertension, rheumatoid arthritis, malnutrition	Hallucinations: hearing voices, seeing the deceased	Despair, hopelessness	Loss of self-esteem; identity and role confusion
Increased vulnerability to mental illness: depression, alcohol abuse, drug abuse	Long periods of time spent reminiscing	Restless, disorganized behavior	Feelings of ambivalence about living

Table 10–10 Types of Grief

Anticipatory Grief	Acute Grief	Complicated Grief
Grief associated with impending death or loss	Painful experience associated with loss	Beyond the point of "normal" grief: major depressive disorder; posttraumatic stress disorder (PTSD)
Associated with depression or family withdrawal from the client	No clear ending	Associated with unresolved issues in the relationship with the person who died
Allows the client and family time to adapt to anticipated loss	May recur with holidays, birthdays, or other milestones	May be felt by those who experience an abortion or miscarriage

- Assessment of the grief process includes the grief experience of the mourner, factors that promote or inhibit working through the grief process, including cultural and religious norms, the mourner's ability to implement cognitive, behavioral, and emotional coping strategies.

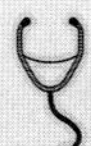

Assessment Alert

Loss and grief are personal: Each person proceeds through the grieving process differently and varying amounts of time are required.

- The plan of care for the person experiencing acute grief includes mobilizing personal and community resources, providing information about the grief process, and supporting the individual in grief work—means by which a person moves through the state of grieving, also known as bereavement.
- Table 10–11 discusses the nursing interventions associated with bereavement.

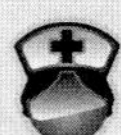

Practice Alert

Grief does not progress in an orderly manner through stages, but rather moves fluidly back and forth among the stages.

Think Smart/Test Smart

- Loss occurs when a valued person, object, or situation is changed or removed.
- Grief is the emotional reaction to loss. Bereavement is the state of grieving.
- Mourning is the period of acceptance of loss.
- Anticipatory grieving occurs when a person facing an impending loss begins to deal with the possibility of the loss or death.
- Dysfunctional grieving is related to the extended unsuccessful attempt to work through the process.

Table 10–11 Nursing Interventions for Bereavement

Allow adaptive denial	Denial is beneficial for a period of time
Remind of importance of meeting own needs and assist when necessary	Offer food, encourage rest, advocate for a sleeping aid
Ensure safety and prevent violence	Assess for thoughts of suicide or plans to harm others
Explore previous coping strategies	Identify strategies that have been successful in the past and encourage their use
Encourage open expression of feelings	Validate positive and negative feelings associated with loss
Promote interactions with others	Encourage increased social support including referrals to community bereavement resources
Teach information associated with grief	Provide information about the physical, cognitive, behavioral, and affective responses to grief
Explore spiritual issues	Facilitate spiritual support by including the spiritual or religious leader of choice in the plan of care

END-OF-LIFE CARE

- Death is defined as an irreversible cessation of circulatory and respiratory functions or of all functions of the entire brain, including the brain stem.
- Dying and death are unique to each individual.
- Physicians are usually responsible for deciding what, when, and how a client should be told about terminal illness.
- Palliative care is an approach to care for the seriously ill, which involves symptom management and psychosocial and spiritual support for diseases not responsive to treatment.
- Hospice is end-of-life care delivered in the client's home or a medical facility.
- Assisted suicide provides another person the means to end his or her own life.
- Terminal weaning is the gradual withdrawal of mechanical ventilation from a client with a terminal illness or irreversible condition with a poor prognosis.
- Palliative sedation differs from euthanasia in that its purpose is to relieve symptoms, not hasten death.
- The Dying Person's Bill of Rights ensures client safety, dignity, and care during the death process.
- Refer to Table 10–12 for the physiologic and psychosocial symptoms associated with dying.
- See Table 10–13 for the ethical and legal dimensions of end-of-life care.
- An organ donation consent card allows clients to donate functional organs, such as heart, corneas, liver, lungs, and kidneys.
- Assessment focuses on the client's and family's knowledge, perceptions, coping strategies, and resources.
- Table 10–14 discusses nursing interventions appropriate for dying clients and their families.

Table 10–12 Physiologic and Psychosocial Symptoms of Dying

Physiologic Symptoms	Psychosocial Symptoms
Inability to swallow	Denial and isolation
Decreased gastrointestinal and urinary tract activity	Anger
Bowel and bladder incontinence	Bargaining
Loss of motion, sensation, reflexes	Depression
Elevated temperature coupled with cold, clammy skin	Acceptance
Cyanosis	
Lowered blood pressure	
Irregular respirations; Cheyne–Stokes respirations	

Table 10–13 Ethical and Legal Dimensions

Advance Directives	Living will: provides specific instructions about the kind of health care that should be provided or foregone in particular situations. Durable power of attorney for health care: appoints an agent the client trusts to make decisions in the event of incapacity.
Do-Not-Resuscitate (DNR)/No-Code orders	No attempts are to be made to resuscitate a client who stops breathing or whose heart stops beating.
Comfort-Measures-Only order	The goal of treatment is comfortable, dignified death without implementation of life-sustaining measures.
Do-Not-Hospitalize order	Utilized by clients living in long-term care and assisted living facilities who do not wish to be hospitalized for aggressive treatments.

Table 10–14 Nursing Interventions at End of Life

Communicate openly with the client and family regarding the dying process.	Provide necessary information for the client and family to engage in the decision-making process regarding end-of-life care.
Be cognizant of death-related beliefs and practices of clients of other cultures.	Facilitate spiritual care at the client's and family's request.
Manage client pain and dyspnea with pharmacological and nonpharmacological interventions.	Provide nutrition and hydration as indicated or when appropriate.
Provide a safe environment for clients who are weak, confused, or delirious.	Provide pharmacological and nonpharmacological interventions for the management of depression.
Identify situational role changes and provide support.	Provide after-death care and bereavement support to the family.

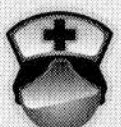

Practice Alert

It is not unusual for clients to die when the family has stepped away from the bed side for a brief moment.

Client teaching for self-care

Teach

- the client about signs of disturbed self-concept and tools to improve self-concept, such as replacing negative thoughts with positive thoughts
- the client to recognize and verbalize negative thoughts and behaviors associated with body-image disturbances
- clients to decrease environmental stressors, such as turning off the television or radio during periods of sensory overload
- clients to change environments or engage in activity, if appropriate during periods of sensory deprivation
- clients the purpose of grief work and its benefit during bereavement
- the dying client and family members the signs and symptoms of impending death, if appropriate
- client's family that hearing is usually the last sense to diminish during the dying process. Encourage family to talk to the dying client
- the client's family about bereavement resources and support available in the community

WORKSHEET

MATCHING QUESTIONS

Match the following (note that terms and/or descriptions may be used once, more than once, or not at all):

1. _____ Stress
2. _____ Introjection
3. _____ Self-assertion
4. _____ Displacement
5. _____ Ethnocentrism
6. _____ Acculturation
7. _____ Cultural competence
8. _____ Denial
9. _____ Regression
10. _____ Rationalization
11. _____ Repression
12. _____ Reminiscence

a. A technique for measuring mental control of body responses, such as blood pressure and heart rate

b. Treating something that is outside the self as if it is inside the self

c. Direct expression of thoughts and feelings that are not manipulative or intimidating

d. Occurs when a member of a cultural group adapts to the new dominant culture in order to survive

e. A search for the sacred; allows individuals to make sense of the cycle of life and death

f. Placing feelings of hostility onto something or someone less threatening in the environment

g. Two or more people who are emotionally involved with each other; may live together

h. A "traditional family" comprised of parents who bring unrelated children from previous relationships together to form a new family

(continued)

13. _____ Spirituality
14. _____ Coping
15. _____ Faith
16. _____ Biofeedback
17. _____ Family
18. _____ Nuclear family
19. _____ Blended family
20. _____ Body image
21. _____ Sensory perception
22. _____ Self-esteem
23. _____ Grief
24. _____ Palliative care
25. _____ Advance directive

i. The subjective view an individual has about his or her body shape, size, proportions, and weight

j. The painful psychological and physiological response to loss

k. Symptom management and psychosocial or spiritual support for diseases not responsive to treatment

l. A condition which can cause changes in the body's normal balanced state resulting in illness

m. Judging others by one's own standards of acting, believing, and thinking

n. Specific instructions about the kind of health care that should be provided or withheld in particular situations

o. The act of returning to a previous level of development

p. The process of keeping unacceptable ideas or impulses out of consciousness

q. Type of group therapy used to treat depression in older adults

r. The perception of one's competency, adequacy, or worth

s. The act of using socially acceptable or logical explanations to justify unpleasant thoughts or actions

t. A set of practice standards instituted by county health and mental agencies to ensure that all clients receive information with regard to education, background, and language

u. A "traditional family" comprised of two parents and their children

v. The refusal to face an unpleasant reality

w. Using conscious or unconscious behaviors to deal with stress

x. The ability to draw on spiritual resources without requiring physical proof

y. Provides another person with the means to end his or her own life

z. The conscious process of selecting, organizing, and interpreting data from the senses into useful information

FILL IN THE BLANKS

Fill in the blank space with the correct word or phrase to complete each statement.

1. Antidepressant drugs must be taken for ________ to ________ weeks before symptoms are relieved.
2. ________ is the unconscious mimicking of an admired person.
3. ________ is the attempt to dispel undesirable behavior.

4. When delivering care to cross-cultural clients, the nurse may require the use of an interpreter to ensure effective ________.

5. ________ is the expression of spirituality.

6. The two main types of stress are ________ and ________.

7. Teaching the client to prepare for an unfamiliar or painful event is called ________________.

8. Aunts, uncles, and grandparents who live in close proximity to the nuclear family are called an ________________.

9. A family that is comprised of divorced parents who share joint custody of children is called a ________ family.

10. Amputation, mastectomy, scars, burns, or other disfigurements may affect one's ________.

11. One who has feelings of inadequacy, incompetence, powerlessness, and frustration may be suffering from low ________.

12. Grief associated with impending death or loss is called ________________.

13. ________ is the irreversible cessation of circulatory, respiratory, and brain functions.

14. A ________________ for health care is an agent entrusted by the client to make decisions in the event of incapacity.

15. An order written by a physician which states that no attempts are to be made to resuscitate a client who stops breathing or whose heart stops beating is called a ________________ order.

TRUE & FALSE QUESTIONS

Mark each of the following statements True or False. Correct all false statements in the space provided.

1. Having conversations with the dead person can be a part of normal grieving. ____ T ____ F
2. Praying with the client is an acceptable nursing intervention to meet the client's spiritual needs. ____ T ____ F
3. Suppression is the unconscious inhibition of a thought or action. ____ T ____ F
4. Withdrawal from the dying client is a normal manifestation of anticipatory grieving. ____ T ____ F
5. Culture is a shared system of beliefs, values, and behavioral expectations that influence daily living. ____ T ____ F
6. The purpose of cultural competence is to ensure that all clients receive care. ____ T ____ F
7. Defense mechanisms are important for survival and are used in coping. ____ T ____ F
8. Developmental stress is unpredictable and can occur at any time. ____ T ____ F
9. Grief does not progress in an orderly manner through stages. ____ T ____ F
10. A couple who chooses not to have children is a binuclear family. ____ T ____ F

APPLICATION QUESTIONS

1. Maintaining the psychosocial health of the client is an important aspect of caring for the elderly. Which nursing actions should be taken to promote the psychosocial health of the elderly client? (Select all that apply.)
   a. Assess for abnormal responses to the aging process such as anger, isolation, or depression
   b. Encourage the use of support systems such as friends and family
   c. Encourage self-care
   d. Facilitate individual, group, or family therapy when appropriate

2. During a seminar on coping skills, the nurse is asked about the beneficial effects of humor. Which is a documented beneficial effect of humor around which the nurse should frame his or her reply?
   a. Lessened depression
   b. Increased relaxation
   c. Reduced aggression
   d. Improved sleep

3. What is the priority nursing concern when a client is in a state of panic?
   a. Maintenance of client safety
   b. Identification of the precipitating factor
   c. Preventing escalation of symptoms
   d. Provision of privacy

4. A widow of 10 days says to the nurse from hospice who has called to invite her to a grieving support group meeting "I feel like I am losing my mind. I see my husband in the house, in the yard, sometimes even at the store. I even find myself talking to him about things that happen." Which is the best response for the nurse to make?
   a. "If these things are still going on in 3 months then you may need to worry about losing your mind but you don't need to worry now."
   b. "That is a concern. Tell me more about what is going on with you."
   c. "I understand you find these events very disturbing but they are normal parts of the grieving process.
   d. "You need to relax; things will improve with time."

5. A client admitted for an exploratory laparotomy states he has never been so anxious—that he feels out of control. Which symptoms or physical findings might accompany this anxiety? (Select all that apply.)
   a. Headache
   b. Nausea and vomiting
   c. Tachycardia
   d. Chest pain

6. When asked why she does not take the prescribed antihypertensive medication, a client states she does not take medication to lower her blood pressure because she cannot swallow pills and they probably would not work anyway because her body was just meant to have a higher blood pressure than other people. This is an example of the use of which defense mechanism?
   a. Sublimation
   b. Rationalization
   c. Reaction formation
   d. Intellectualization

7. To provide culturally competent care, the nurse must assess the client's health care practices. Which factors should be included in the nurse's assessment? (Select all that apply.)
   a. Health-seeking behaviors
   b. Responsibility for health care
   c. Folklore practices
   d. Barriers to health care

8. When preparing a health-promotion presentation on stress and anxiety, which information could the nurse consider including because it is true? (Select all that apply.)
   a. Stress causes anxiety
   b. Prolonged anxiety may cause illness
   c. Severe anxiety may cause psychosis
   d. Severe anxiety may cause suicidal thoughts

9. Coping involves all of the conscious and unconscious behaviors used by individuals to deal with stress. Coping mechanisms are effective in maintaining emotional stability. Which coping mechanism is an ineffective mechanism?
   a. Hitting others
   b. Crying
   c. Yelling
   d. Kicking a chair

10. A nurse is caring for a client who is undergoing a major life crisis. Which self-care concepts should the nurse teach the client to enhance the client's ability to cope with the stress? (Select all that apply.)
    a. Teach the client that exercise can be a healthy coping mechanism
    b. Teach the client that hitting others, hurting oneself, and destroying property can be effective coping mechanisms

c. Teach the client to control anger by counting to 10 and breathing deeply
d. Teach the client to divert his or her attention to another task

11. Holistic nursing care involves addressing clients' physical, mental, emotional, and spiritual needs. Which nursing intervention assists clients and their families in meeting their spiritual needs?
a. Ensuring the confidentiality of the client
b. Notifying the physician of the family's presence
c. Resolving conflicts between treatment and beliefs
d. Resolving conflicts between family members

12. A preoperative nurse is preparing a client for surgery. While preparing the client, the nurse informs the client of what can be expected after surgery and how the client's pain will be controlled. Which stress-management technique is being utilized by the nurse?
a. Relaxation
b. Guided imagery
c. Progressive muscle relaxation
d. Anticipatory guidance

13. A labor and delivery nurse is caring for a client who is in the second stage of labor. The nurse instructs the client to create and concentrate on a mental image to help her to manage the pain of labor. Which stress-management technique is being taught to the client?
a. Relaxation
b. Guided imagery
c. Progressive muscle relaxation
d. Anticipatory guidance

14. A labor and delivery nurse is caring for a client who is in the final stage of labor. The nurse assists the client in focusing on the rhythm of her breathing and reducing muscle tension during her contractions. Which stress-management technique is being utilized by the nurse?
a. Relaxation
b. Guided imagery
c. Progressive muscle relaxation
d. Anticipatory guidance

15. A nurse is planning for the discharge of an elderly client from a hospital. Which statement made by the client would indicate to the nurse that the client lacks a support system at home?
a. "My sister and her husband are taking me home today."
b. "My church members have been sending cards and letters while I have been in the hospital."
c. "I am not sure how I am going to get to the grocery store after I get home."
d. "My neighbor is retired. We visit and have our meals together every day."

16. A family is defined as two or more people who are emotionally involved with each other and live together. A nuclear family is also called a "traditional family." Which families are considered nuclear families? (Select all that apply.)
a. Two biological parents and their children
b. Two parents and their adopted children
c. Two parents with grown children who no longer live at home
d. Two homosexual parents in a committed relationship and their adopted children

17. A psychiatric nurse is caring for a client who is involved in an emotionally abusive relationship. The nurse knows that the client may be at risk for which disturbances in self-concept? (Select all that apply.)
a. Disturbed body image
b. Low self-esteem
c. Ineffective role performance
d. Disturbed personal identity

18. Body image is the subjective view an individual has about his or her physical appearance including body shape, size, weight, and proportions. Which condition would put a client at risk for disturbed body image?
a. Urinary tract infection
b. Hyperlipidemia
c. Rheumatoid arthritis
d. High blood pressure

19. A hospice nurse is caring for the family of a client who has died 30 minutes ago. Which type of grief is the family experiencing in response to their loss?
a. Anticipatory grief
b. Acute grief
c. Complicated grief
d. Palliative grief

20. Loss occurs when a valued person, object, or situation is changed or removed. Grief is the painful psychological and physiological response to loss. Which phrase best describes the concept of mourning?
a. The emotional reaction to loss
b. The state of grieving
c. The period of acceptance of loss
d. The period of depression following a loss

(continued)

21. A client has just been admitted to a long-term care facility following the loss of a spouse. A nurse assesses the client and determines that the client is in a state of bereavement. Which nursing interventions for bereavement should be included in the client's plan of care? (Select all that apply.)
    a. Ensure safety and prevent violence
    b. Promote interactions with others
    c. Teach the client about the stages of grief
    d. Facilitate spiritual support by including the client's spiritual or religious leader

22. Death is defined as the irreversible cessation of circulatory, respiratory, and brain functions. Which are physiologic symptoms of impending death? (Select all that apply.)
    a. Bowel and bladder incontinence
    b. Anger
    c. Decreased blood pressure
    d. Cheyne–Stokes respirations

23. Death is defined as the irreversible cessation of circulatory, respiratory, and brain functions. Which are psychosocial symptoms of impending death? (Select all that apply.)
    a. Cyanosis
    b. Denial
    c. Bargaining
    d. Acceptance

24. A living will provides specific instructions about the kind of health care that an individual desires in particular situations. Some individuals desire that no attempt be made to resuscitate them if they stop breathing or if their heart stops beating. Which statement is true regarding a Do-Not-Resuscitate Order (DNR)?
    a. A DNR states that an individual does not wish to be hospitalized for aggressive treatments
    b. A DNR states that the goal of treatment is a comfortable, dignified death without implementation of life-sustaining measures
    c. A DNR appoints an agent the client trusts to make decisions in the event of incapacity
    d. A DNR must be written by a physician

25. A nurse in an intensive care unit is caring for a client who is dying. Which nursing interventions should be utilized in caring for the dying client and the client's family? (Select all that apply.)
    a. Encourage the family to talk to the dying client as hearing is usually the last sense to diminish during the dying process
    b. Communicate openly with the client and family regarding the dying process
    c. Provide a quiet, private environment for the client and family
    d. Provide after-death care and bereavement support to the family

ANSWERS & RATIONALES

MATCHING ANSWERS

Match the following (note that terms and/or descriptions may be used once, more than once, or not at all.)

1. __l__ Stress
2. __b__ Introjection
3. __c__ Self-assertion
4. __f__ Displacement
5. __m__ Ethnocentrism
6. __d__ Acculturation

a. A technique for measuring mental control of body responses, such as blood pressure and heart rate

b. Treating something that is outside the self as if it is inside the self

c. Direct expression of thoughts and feelings that are not manipulative or intimidating

d. Occurs when a member of a cultural group adapts to the new dominant culture in order to survive

e. A search for the sacred; allows individuals to make sense of the cycle of life and death

7. __t__ Cultural competence
8. __v__ Denial
9. __o__ Regression
10. __s__ Rationalization
11. __p__ Repression
12. __q__ Reminiscence
13. __e__ Spirituality
14. __w__ Coping
15. __x__ Faith
16. __a__ Biofeedback
17. __g__ Family
18. __u__ Nuclear family
19. __h__ Blended family
20. __i__ Body image
21. __z__ Sensory perception
22. __r__ Self-esteem
23. __j__ Grief
24. __k__ Palliative care
25. __n__ Advance directive

f. Placing feelings of hostility onto something or someone less threatening in the environment

g. Two or more people who are emotionally involved with each other; may live together

h. A "traditional family" comprised of parents who bring unrelated children from previous relationships together to form a new family

i. The subjective view an individual has about his or her body shape, size, proportions, and weight

j. The painful psychological and physiological response to loss

k. Symptom management and psychosocial or spiritual support for diseases not responsive to treatment

l. A condition which can cause changes in the body's normal balanced state resulting in illness

m. Judging others by one's own standards of acting, believing, and thinking

n. Specific instructions about the kind of health care that should be provided or withheld in particular situations

o. The act of returning to a previous level of development

p. The process of keeping unacceptable ideas or impulses out of consciousness

q. Type of group therapy used to treat depression in older adults

r. The perception of one's competency, adequacy, or worth

s. The act of using socially acceptable or logical explanations to justify unpleasant thoughts or actions

t. A set of practice standards instituted by county health and mental agencies to ensure that all clients receive information with regard to education, background, and language

u. A "traditional family" comprised of two parents and their children

v. The refusal to face an unpleasant reality

w. Using conscious or unconscious behaviors to deal with stress

x. The ability to draw on spiritual resources without requiring physical proof

y. Provides another person with the means to end his or her own life

z. The conscious process of selecting, organizing, and interpreting data from the senses into useful information

ANSWERS FOR FILL IN THE BLANKS

Fill in the blank space with the correct word or phrase to complete each statement.

1. Antidepressant drugs must be taken for 4 to 6 weeks before symptoms are relieved.
2. Identification is the unconscious mimicking of an admired person.
3. Undoing is the attempt to dispel undesirable behavior.
4. When delivering care to cross-cultural clients, the nurse may require the use of an interpreter to ensure effective communication.
5. Religion is the expression of spirituality.
6. The two main types of stress are developmental stress and situational stress.
7. Teaching the client to prepare for an unfamiliar or painful event is called anticipatory guidance.
8. Aunts, uncles, and grandparents who live in close proximity to the nuclear family are called an extended family.
9. A family that is comprised of divorced parents who share joint custody of children is called a binuclear family.
10. Amputation, mastectomy, scars, burns, or other disfigurements may affect one's body image.
11. One who has feelings of inadequacy, incompetence, powerlessness, and frustration may be suffering from low self-esteem.
12. Grief associated with impending death or loss is called anticipatory grief.
13. Death is the irreversible cessation of circulatory, respiratory, and brain functions.
14. A durable power of attorney for health care is an agent entrusted by the client to make decisions in the event of incapacity.
15. An order written by a physician which states that no attempts are to be made to resuscitate a client who stops breathing or whose heart stops beating is called a Do-Not-Resuscitate (DNR) order.

TRUE OR FALSE ANSWERS

Mark each of the following statements True or False. Correct all false statements in the space provided.

1. Having conversations with the dead person can be a part of normal grieving. *True*
2. Praying with the client is an acceptable nursing intervention to meet the client's spiritual needs. *True*
3. Suppression is the unconscious inhibition of a thought or action. *False*
   Suppression is the conscious inhibition of a thought or action.
4. Withdrawal from the dying client is a normal manifestation of anticipatory grieving. *True*

5. Culture is a shared system of beliefs, values, and behavioral expectations that influence daily living. *True*

6. The purpose of cultural competence is to ensure that all clients receive care. *False*
The purpose of cultural competence is to ensure that all clients receive information about treatment in familiar ways.

7. Defense mechanisms are important for survival and are used in coping. *True*

8. Developmental stress is unpredictable and can occur at any time. *False*
Developmental stress is somewhat predictable and occurs through the normal stages of growth and development. Situational stress is unpredictable and can occur at any time.

9. Grief does not progress in an orderly manner through stages. *True*

10. A couple who chooses not to have children is a binuclear family. *False*
A couple who chooses not to have children is a dyadic nuclear family.

APPLICATION ANSWERS

1. Maintaining the psychosocial health of the client is an important aspect of caring for the elderly. Which nursing actions should be taken to promote the psychosocial health of the elderly client? (Select all that apply.)
   a. Assess for abnormal responses to the aging process such as anger, isolation, or depression
   b. Encourage the use of support systems such as friends and family
   c. Encourage self-care
   d. Facilitate individual, group, or family therapy when appropriate

Rationale
Correct answers: a, b, c, and d.
All are appropriate nursing actions for promoting the psychosocial health of the elderly client.

2. During a seminar on coping skills, the nurse is asked about the beneficial effects of humor. Which is a documented beneficial effect of humor around which the nurse should frame his or her reply?
   a. Lessened depression
   b. Increased relaxation
   c. Reduced aggression
   d. Improved sleep

Rationale
Correct answer: c.
Humor has been shown to reduce aggression. Pet therapy and art therapy reduce depression. Music therapy promotes relaxation. Exercise improves sleep.

3. What is the priority nursing concern when a client is in a state of panic?
   a. Maintenance of client safety
   b. Identification of the precipitating factor
   c. Preventing escalation of symptoms
   d. Provision of privacy

Rationale
Correct answer: a.
Client safety is the priority. Identification of the precipitating factor may be important in understanding the event and in the prevention of recurrence. Preventing escalation of symptoms and provision of privacy are both important goals but do not take priority over client safety.

4. A widow of 10 days says to the nurse from hospice who has called to invite her to a grieving support group meeting "I feel like I am losing my mind. I see my husband in the house, in the yard, sometimes even at the store. I even find myself talking to him about things that happen." Which is the best response for the nurse to make?
   a. "If these things are still going on in 3 months then you may need to worry about losing your mind but you don't need to worry now."
   b. "That is a concern. Tell me more about what is going on with you."
   c. "I understand you find these events very disturbing but they are normal parts of the grieving process.
   d. "You need to relax; things will improve with time."

(continued)

Rationale

Correct answer: c.

Conversations with a deceased loved one and "seeing" the person in familiar places are normal manifestations of grief. By saying "I understand you find these events very disturbing", the nurse is acknowledging and accepting the client's distress as worthy of concern. Response "a" minimizes the client's concern and is trite in its manner. Response "b" although therapeutic in wording, is incorrect because the events are normal and not a cause for concern. Response "d" gives advice and utilizes a cliché.

5. A client admitted for an exploratory laparotomy states he has never been so anxious—that he feels out of control. Which symptoms or physical findings might accompany this anxiety? (Select all that apply.)
   a. ___Headache
   b. ___Nausea and vomiting
   c. ___Tachycardia
   d. ___Chest pain

Rationale

Correct answers: a, b, c, and d.

Headache, nausea and vomiting, tachycardia, and chest pain can all be manifestations of severe anxiety. Cognitive and psychomotor symptoms of severe anxiety include reduced perceptual fields, difficulty with problem solving and completing tasks, feelings of dread, crying, and ritualistic behaviors. Caution must be taken not to interpret physiological signs and symptoms as indicators of anxiety when, in fact, there is a pathophysiological cause.

6. When asked why she does not take the prescribed antihypertensive medication, a client states she does not take medication to lower her blood pressure because she cannot swallow pills and they probably would not work anyway because her body was just meant to have a higher blood pressure than other people. This is an example of the use of which defense mechanism?
   a. Sublimation
   b. Rationalization
   c. Reaction formation
   d. Intellectualization

Rationale

Correct answer: b.

Rationalization is the use of a socially acceptable explanation to justify unpleasant consequences. Sublimation is modification of a socially unacceptable impulse into an acceptable behavior Reaction formation is the exaggerated adoption of opposite behaviors to those that are unpleasant. Intellectualization is the overuse of abstract thinking to minimize painful feelings.

7. To provide culturally competent care, the nurse must assess the client's health care practices. Which factors should be included in the nurse's assessment? (Select all that apply.)
   a. Health-seeking behaviors
   b. Responsibility for health care
   c. Folklore practices
   d. Barriers to health care

Rationale

Correct answers: a, b, c, and d.

To provide culturally competent care, the nurse should assess the client's health care practices, which include health-seeking behaviors, responsibility for health care, folklore practices, barriers to health care, and cultural responses to health and illness.

8. When preparing a health-promotion presentation on stress and anxiety, which information could the nurse consider including because it is true? (Select all that apply.)
   a. Stress causes anxiety
   b. Prolonged anxiety may cause illness
   c. Severe anxiety may cause psychosis
   d. Severe anxiety may cause suicidal thoughts

Rationale

Correct answers: a, b, c, and d.

Stress causes anxiety, which, over time, may cause mental and/or physical illness. Severe anxiety can cause anxiety disorders and psychosis. Clients with severe anxiety may become suicidal.

9. Coping involves all of the conscious and unconscious behaviors used by individuals to deal with stress. Coping mechanisms are effective in maintaining emotional stability. Which coping mechanism is an ineffective mechanism?
   a. Hitting others
   b. Crying
   c. Yelling
   d. Kicking a chair

Rationale

Correct answer: a.

Hitting others, hurting oneself, and destroying property are ineffective coping mechanisms. Crying, yelling, and kicking a chair are normative behaviors.

10. A nurse is caring for a client who is undergoing a major life crisis. Which self-care concepts should the nurse teach the client to enhance the client's ability to cope with the stress? (Select all that apply.)
    a. Teach the client that exercise can be a healthy coping mechanism

b. Teach the client that hitting others, hurting oneself, and destroying property can be effective coping mechanisms
c. Teach the client to control anger by counting to 10 and breathing deeply
d. Teach the client to divert his or her attention to another task

Rationale

Correct answers: a, c, and d.
Exercise, anger management, and diversion are healthy coping mechanisms, which may enhance the client's ability to cope with stress.

11. Holistic nursing care involves addressing clients' physical, mental, emotional, and spiritual needs. Which nursing intervention assists clients and their families in meeting their spiritual needs?
a. Ensuring the confidentiality of the client
b. Notifying the physician of the family's presence
c. Resolving conflicts between treatment and beliefs
d. Resolving conflicts between family members

Rationale

Correct answer: c.
Nursing interventions to assist clients and their families to meet their spiritual needs include offering support, facilitating the client's practice of religion, praying with a client and family, contacting a spiritual counselor, and resolving conflicts between treatment and spiritual beliefs.

12. A preoperative nurse is preparing a client for surgery. While preparing the client, the nurse informs the client of what can be expected after surgery and how the client's pain will be controlled. Which stress-management technique is being utilized by the nurse?
a. Relaxation
b. Guided imagery
c. Progressive muscle relaxation
d. Anticipatory guidance

Rationale

Correct answer: d.
Anticipatory guidance involves preparing the client for an unfamiliar or painful event, such as surgery. By informing the client of what to expect, the nurse reduces the client's stress regarding the event.

13. A labor and delivery nurse is caring for a client who is in the second stage of labor. The nurse instructs the client to create and concentrate on a mental image to help her to manage the pain of labor. Which stress-management technique is being taught to the client?
a. Relaxation
b. Guided imagery
c. Progressive muscle relaxation
d. Anticipatory guidance

Rationale

Correct answer: b.
The nurse is teaching the client to use guided imagery to help the client manage the pain of labor.

14. A labor and delivery nurse is caring for a client who is in the final stage of labor. The nurse assists the client in focusing on the rhythm of her breathing and reducing muscle tension during her contractions. Which stress-management technique is being utilized by the nurse?
a. Relaxation
b. Guided imagery
c. Progressive muscle relaxation
d. Anticipatory guidance

Rationale

Correct answer: a.
The nurse is utilizing relaxation to help the client cope with the pain of labor. Relaxation technique utilizes rhythmic breathing, reduced muscle tension, and altered states of consciousness to help clients cope with stressors.

15. A nurse is planning for the discharge of an elderly client from a hospital. Which statement made by the client would indicate to the nurse that the client lacks a support system at home?
a. "My sister and her husband are taking me home today."
b. "My church members have been sending cards and letters while I have been in the hospital."
c. "I am not sure how I am going to get to the grocery store after I get home."
d. "My neighbor is retired. We visit and have our meals together every day."

Rationale

Correct answer: c.
When the client expresses concern about getting to the grocery store after returning home from the hospital, the nurse should be aware that the client may not have a support system at home to help.

16. A family is defined as two or more people who are emotionally involved with each other and live together. A nuclear family is also called a "traditional family." Which families are considered nuclear families? (Select all that apply.)
a. Two biological parents and their children
b. Two parents and their adopted children

(continued)

c. Two parents with grown children who no longer live at home

d. Two homosexual parents in a committed relationship and their adopted children

Rationale

Correct answers: a, b, c, and d.
All of these families are considered nuclear families.

17. A psychiatric nurse is caring for a client who is involved in an emotionally abusive relationship. The nurse knows that the client may be at risk for which disturbances in self-concept? (Select all that apply.)
   a. Disturbed body image
   b. Low self-esteem
   c. Ineffective role performance
   d. Disturbed personal identity

Rationale

Correct answers: b and d.
Victims of emotional abuse are at risk for developing low self-esteem and disturbed personal identity.

18. Body image is the subjective view an individual has about his or her physical appearance including body shape, size, weight, and proportions. Which condition would put a client at risk for disturbed body image?
   a. Urinary tract infection
   b. Hyperlipidemia
   c. Rheumatoid arthritis
   d. High blood pressure

Rationale

Correct answer: c.
Rheumatoid arthritis is a painful, inflammatory, autoimmune condition that results in the enlargement and/or gross disproportion of the joints. Clients who have rheumatoid arthritis are at risk for disturbances in body image.

19. A hospice nurse is caring for the family of a client who has died 30 minutes ago. Which type of grief is the family experiencing in response to their loss?
   a. Anticipatory grief
   b. Acute grief
   c. Complicated grief
   d. Palliative grief

Rationale

Correct answer: b.
The family is most likely experiencing acute grief; a painful experience associated with loss that has no clear ending.

20. Loss occurs when a valued person, object, or situation is changed or removed. Grief is the painful psychological and physiological response to loss. Which phrase best describes the concept of mourning?
   a. The emotional reaction to loss
   b. The state of grieving
   c. The period of acceptance of loss
   d. The period of depression following a loss

Rationale

Correct answer: c.
Mourning is the period of acceptance of loss.

21. A client has just been admitted to a long-term care facility following the loss of a spouse. A nurse assesses the client and determines that the client is in a state of bereavement. Which nursing interventions for bereavement should be included in the client's plan of care? (Select all that apply.)
   a. Ensure safety and prevent violence
   b. Promote interactions with others
   c. Teach the client about the stages of grief
   d. Facilitate spiritual support by including the client's spiritual or religious leader

Rationale

Correct answers: a, b, c, and d.
All of the nursing interventions should be included in the client's plan of care.

22. Death is defined as the irreversible cessation of circulatory, respiratory and brain functions. Which are physiologic symptoms of impending death? (Select all that apply.)
   a. Bowel and bladder incontinence
   b. Anger
   c. Decreased blood pressure
   d. Cheyne–Stokes respirations

Rationale

Correct answers: a, c, and d.
Bowel and bladder incontinence, decreased blood pressure, and Cheyne–Stokes respirations are all physiologic symptoms of impending death. Anger is a psychosocial sign of impending death.

23. Death is defined as the irreversible cessation of circulatory, respiratory, and brain functions. Which are psychosocial symptoms of impending death? (Select all that apply.)
   a. Cyanosis
   b. Denial
   c. Bargaining
   d. Acceptance

Rationale

Correct answers: b, c, and d.
Denial, bargaining, and acceptance are all psychosocial symptoms of impending death. Cyanosis is a physiologic symptom of dying.

24. A living will provides specific instructions about the kind of health care that an individual desires in particular situations. Some individuals desire that no attempt be made to resuscitate them if they stop breathing or if their heart stops beating. Which statement is true regarding a Do-Not-Resuscitate Order (DNR)?
   a. A DNR states that an individual does not wish to be hospitalized for aggressive treatments
   b. A DNR states that the goal of treatment is a comfortable, dignified death without implementation of life-sustaining measures
   c. A DNR appoints an agent the client trusts to make decisions in the event of incapacity
   d. A DNR must be written by a physician

Rationale

Correct answer: d.

A Do-not-Resuscitate order must be written by a physician. A Do-Not-Hospitalize order states that an individual does not wish to be hospitalized for aggressive treatments. A Comfort-Measures-Only order states that the goal of treatment is a comfortable, dignified death without implementation of life-sustaining procedures. A durable power of attorney appoints an agent the client trusts to make decisions in the event of incapacity.

25. A nurse in an intensive care unit is caring for a client who is dying. Which nursing interventions should be utilized in caring for the dying client and the client's family? (Select all that apply.)
   a. Encourage the family to talk to the dying client as hearing is usually the last sense to diminish during the dying process
   b. Communicate openly with the client and family regarding the dying process
   c. Provide a quiet, private environment for the client and family
   d. Provide after-death care and bereavement support to the family

Rationale

Correct answers: a, b, c, and d.

All of the nursing interventions are appropriate when caring for a dying client and his or her family.

CHAPTER 11

Test Plan Category:

Psychosocial Integrity—Part 2

Sub-category: **None**

Topics: **Therapeutic Communication**
Therapeutic Environment
Behavioral Interventions
Crisis Intervention

The nurse plays an important role in promoting and maintaining the psychosocial integrity of the client, family, and significant others. The nurse's success depends largely on the use of therapeutic communication, establishment of a therapeutic relationship, promotion of a therapeutic environment, implementation of behavioral interventions, and appropriate management of crises.

THERAPEUTIC COMMUNICATION

- Therapeutic communication is the foundation of an effective nurse–client relationship; it helps reduce stress, encourage insight, and support problem solving.
- Therapeutic communication involves both verbal and nonverbal communication.
- The nurse's use of therapeutic communication with clients and other nurses is essential for effective use of the nursing process. See Table 11–1 for the communication factors that influence the steps of the nursing process.
- The nurse builds a rapport with clients to further the nurse–client relationship. Good rapport facilitates open communication. See Table 11–2 for factors that promote trust in the nurse–client relationship.
- The nurse promotes trust by respecting the client's personal values, beliefs, and culture.
- The nurse maintains the client's culture by providing a language interpreter and including other members of the health care team who share the client's culture to assist in providing care.
- The nurse develops and maintains therapeutic relationships with the client, family, and significant others by allowing ample time for communication. He/she

Table 11–1 Communication Factors of the Nursing Process

Nursing Process Step	Communication Factors
Assessment	• Verbal and nonverbal communication is gathered. • Data enhances the client history and physical examination. • Data is passed on to appropriate team members through oral and written communication.
Nursing diagnosis	• Nurse communicates nursing diagnoses to other nursing professionals through written and spoken words.
Planning	• Communication among the client, nurse, and other health care team members occurs. • Oral and written communication is used to meet objectives and goals of the plan of care.
Implementation	• Verbal and nonverbal communication is used to teach, counsel, and support clients and their families. • The client communicates his/her ability or inability to meet targeted objectives. • Implementation of the plan of care is documented in the client's record.
Evaluation	• Client verbal and nonverbal cues verify whether client goals and objectives are achieved. • Communication guides revision of the plan of care.

communicates and delivers care in an unhurried and calm fashion.

- The nurse uses active listening, silence, touch, and humor to facilitate communication with the client, family, and significant others.
- Open-ended questions by the nurse encourage free verbalization from the client. This provides the nurse with specific, additional information that forms a basis for the plan of care.
- Therapeutic communication techniques provide support to the client, family, and significant others. See Table 11–3 for therapeutic communication techniques.
- Barriers to therapeutic communication negatively impact the nurse–client relationship. See Table 11–4 for barriers to therapeutic communication.
- Impaired verbal communication (NANDA nursing diagnosis) can affect every aspect of the client's life.
  —Impaired verbal communication is the state in which an individual experiences a decreased or absent ability to use or understand human language.
  —Communication in the older adult may be affected by
    - aphasia: the inability to recall words, understand what others are saying, or produce speech,
    - dysarthria: the inability to produce clear speech sounds,
    - voice problems: due to malfunction or removal of the larynx (voice box),
    - hearing impairment: presbycusis (hearing loss due to aging process); may hear speech, but is unable to understand distinct words or sounds,
    - other problems: memory loss, disorientation, loss of thought organization.
- Clients with special needs require specific communication techniques.
  —Visually impaired: Speak in a normal tone of voice; explain the reason for touching the client before doing so; keep the call light within easy reach; clean eyeglasses and confirm contacts are in place.
  —Hearing impaired: Face the client while speaking; demonstrate or pantomime ideas as appropriate; write ideas or use sign language; clean hearing aids and confirm proper placement.
  —Cognitively impaired: Maintain eye contact; keep communication simple and concrete; avoid open-ended questions; be client and allow time for the client's responses.
  —Unconscious client: The client can most likely hear even though there is no apparent response; assume the client can hear you; talk in a normal tone of voice; speak with the client before touching.
  —Client with a physical barrier (laryngectomy or endotracheal tube): Select a simple means of communication, such as eye blinks or hand squeezes; ensure that family and significant others are able to utilize the selected communication technique; allow time for the client's responses; ensure the client has an effective means of signaling for assistance (call bell or alarm).
  —Non-English speaking clients: Use an interpreter; speak in a normal tone of voice; speak in simple sentences; demonstrate or pantomime ideas; use accepting nonverbal communication cues.

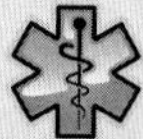

Nursing Intervention Alert

Clients suspected of a speech, language, or hearing deficit should be referred to a speech—language pathologist or audiologist.

Client teaching for self-care

The nurse teaches

- the client, family, and significant others the benefit of communicating in a therapeutic manner.

Table 11–2 Trust Builders in the Nurse–Client Relationship

Trust Builder	Rationale	Nursing Action
Specific objectives	Achieve a meaningful encounter with the client	• Perform a head-to-toe physical assessment • Discuss the client's feelings about a new diagnosis
Comfortable environment	Client and nurse comfort promotes interaction	• Provide proper lighting, a moderate temperature, and a relaxed, unhurried atmosphere
Privacy	Ensures a sense of security	• Draw curtains around the client's bed • Stand close to the head of the bed while speaking to the client in order to prevent conversations from being overheard by others
Confidentiality	Promotes a sense of security	• Inform the client who on the health care team will have access to the client's medical record.
Client-centered focus	Facilitates trust and decreases anxiety	• While inserting a Foley catheter, calm the client's anxiety with therapeutic communication instead of telling the client to quit distracting the nurse with conversation.
Nursing observations	Validates information	• Observe the client's hand shaking nervously as the client denies feelings of anxiety.
Conversation pacing	Decreases anxiety; assures complete information is gathered	• Allow an elderly client plenty of time to answer questions related to the health history
Personal space	Decreases anxiety	• Use touch while speaking to a visually impaired client
Pleasantness	Places the client at ease	• Smile • Look the client in the eye when speaking • Offer warm greetings
Respect	Facilitates open communication	• Offer open, frank communication without prejudice • Respect the client's culture, values, and beliefs by providing for a language interpreter as appropriate
Empathy	Facilitates achievement of goals	• Ask a dissatisfied client what the nurse may do to help • Validate the client's feelings of frustration and anger
Honesty	Decreases anxiety and facilitates achievement of goals	• Offer all available resources to the client • Assist the client in making informed health care decisions
Caring	Promotes feelings of acceptance	• Touch the client in a gentle manner • Address the client by name
Competence	Promotes trust and respect	• Communicate in an organized, professional manner

- the client, family, and significant others to recognize communication patterns and barriers to therapeutic communication.
- the client, family, and significant others techniques to build rapport with the goal of promoting health.
- the non-English speaking client, family, and significant others the importance of using a translator to ensure effective communication with the health care team.
- the family and significant others of elderly adults effective modes of communication.
- the family and significant others of clients with special needs effective modes of communication as well as revision of the modes based on evaluation.

Table 11–3 Therapeutic Communication Techniques

Technique	Purpose	Example
Broad openings	Encourages client to select topics for discussion; indicate acceptance by the nurse and value of the client's initiative.	"Is there something bothering you today?" "May I answer any questions or address any concerns you may have?"
Clarification	Asks the client to explain what he/she means to enhance the nurse's understanding; helps clarify the client's feelings, ideas, and perceptions; provides explicit correlation between the client's words and actions.	"Help me to understand. What do you mean when you say you've had enough of this?" "Are you saying that you are discouraged by the care you are receiving?"
Focusing	Questions or statements that help the client expand an idea; guides goal-directed communication.	"What other feelings are you experiencing besides the ones you just described?" "Let's go back to the part where you mentioned being sad. Can you tell me more about that?"
Humor	Comic enjoyment of the imperfect; brings repressed material to consciousness, tempers aggression, and reveals new options to promote insight.	The nurse follows the client's lead regarding humor. The nurse should never make jokes at a client's expense, but may want to validate the client's attempt at humor by smiling or laughing.
Informing	Provides information about the client's well-being and self-care during client education and teaching.	"If this is a good time for you, I'd like to go over the proper technique for insulin injections." "You look better today. The antibiotics given to you last night must be taking effect."
Listening	Active process of receiving information and examining client reactions to the messages received; nonverbally communicates the nurse's interest in the client.	The nurse remains quiet while the client is speaking. The nurse may occasionally interject phrases such as "Uh-huh," "I'm listening," and "Hmm" to indicate active listening.
Reflection	Direct back to the client his/her content, feelings, ideas, or questions; validates the nurse's understanding of what the client is saying; signifies empathy, interest, and respect for the client.	"I understand what you're saying. You're saying that living alone can be lonely at times." "I can understand why you would be upset by your family's reaction."
Restating	Repeats back to the client the main thought or idea expressed; demonstrates that the nurse is listening and validates the client's words.	"Let me make sure I have this right. You're saying that you no longer wish to undergo chemotherapy because it makes you so sick." "I heard you say that you are ready to be discharged. Let me convey your wish to the physician."
Sharing perceptions	Asks the client to verify the nurse's understanding of what the client is thinking or feeling; clarifies confusing communication; conveys the nurse's understanding to the client.	"It seems that you may be experiencing some feelings of anger. Is this correct?" "I sense that you are happy about your prognosis. Am I right?"
Silence	Therapeutic use of nonverbal communication; allows the client time to think, slows the pace of the conversation, and encourages the client to initiate communication while conveying the nurse's acceptance, support, and understanding.	The nurse looks at the client during periods of silence to nonverbally express interest and support.
Suggesting	Enhances problem-solving by offering the client alternative ideas; increases the client's options or choices.	"Have you ever considered walking with a cane for support?" "It may be helpful to leave the hallway light on at bedtime. This way, you won't have to stumble around in the dark when you have to use the bathroom in the middle of the night."
Theme identification	Identifies issues or themes experienced by the client repeatedly during the course of the client–nurse relationship; promotes the client's exploration and understanding of important problems.	"I've noticed that you become agitated every time your family comes to visit. Would you like to talk about this?"

Table 11–4 Barriers to Therapeutic Communication

Communication Barrier	Effect
Focusing on the diagnosis instead of the client	Increases client anxiety by not focusing on the whole client
Using slang terminology	Referring to the client as "honey" or "sweetie" instead of Mr., Mrs., or Dr. demeans the client
Using defensive language	Prohibits open and trusting communication; makes the nurse appear incompetent
Using clichés	Conveys lack of interest
Using closed questions	Asking questions that only require a yes or no answer prohibits discussion
Using questions containing the words why and how	Intimidates the client
Using probing questions	Causes client resentment and unwillingness to communicate further
Using leading questions	Produces answers that please the nurse while discouraging and intimidating the client
Giving advice	Prohibits client decision making and increases client dependence on the nurse
Casting judgment	Imposes the nurse's standards on the client
Changing the subject	Causes client frustration
Giving false assurance	Conveys lack of interest
Gossiping and spreading rumors	Undermines the nurse–client relationship; blocks effective team building

Other types of nontherapeutic communication involve verbal attack, rushing, minimizing, and taking sides.

THERAPEUTIC RELATIONSHIP

- This relationship is a nurse–client interaction that focuses on the client needs and is goal specific.
- Establishment of a therapeutic relationship is the basis of all nursing care of the clients with mental illness.
- There are three phases of therapeutic relationship:
  —Introduction
    - Establishes each person's role in the relationship.
    - May include making a contract with the client regarding goals and behavior.
    - Plan of care is developed with the client.

  —Working
    - Implementation of the care plan through the process of therapeutic alliance.

  —Termination
    - Review of the client's progress and development of plans for the immediate future.

THERAPEUTIC ENVIRONMENT

- The goal of the therapeutic environment, or therapeutic milieu, is to promote health and healing.
- The psychiatric unit serves as a social system in its own right. This social system incorporates.
  —a large work group that accepts the task of healing.
  —the activities of communal living, as clients must interact with each other daily with the task of promoting a community of healing.
- The principles of milieu therapy are that clients are active, not passive, participants in their lives; clients own their

behavior and environment; and clients are independent and self-sufficient.

- A therapeutic environment
  —promotes a fundamental respect of individuals, clients, and staff alike.
  —uses opportunities for communication between the client and staff for maximum therapeutic benefit.
  —encourages clients to act at a level equal to their ability and to enhance self-esteem.
  —promotes socialization.
  —provides opportunities for clients to be a part of the unit's management.
- The nurse's role is to support the five goals of a therapeutic environment as listed above, clarify boundaries for all clients, and assist clients in task completion to improve health.
- The nurse acts as a resource person, counselor, surrogate, and technical expert for the client.
- The nurse facilitates the basic concepts of a relationship: boundary development and maintenance, safety development, and trust development.
- Community meetings in the therapeutic environment serve to orient clients to the environment and define boundaries. In these meetings, the nurse defines the structure of the work the clients are to promote.
- Several factors are necessary for successful community meetings:
  —The leader defines the purpose of the meeting.
  —The leader provides structure and boundaries for the tasks.
  —The leader defines the tasks and explains how the clients can utilize the nurse in this role.
  —The leader focuses on the tasks.
  —The leader models acceptance.
- Safety and trust are important factors in the therapeutic environment.
  —Safety is developed by knowing what one's responsibilities are in a given situation.
  —Trust develops through actions that are consistent with an individual's or group's stated intent.
  —Clients need to know what is expected of them in order to feel safe.
  —Safety is promoted by clarifying client tasks.
  —Trust is the promotion of consistency between words and actions.
  —The nurse acts in a consistent manner to achieve objectives and promote trust.
  —The nurse ensures that his/her every interaction is a therapeutic one in order to promote safety and trust.
- Room assignments are based on the fragility of the client, the length of stay, client communication between roommates, the client's overall behavior, and the client's level of personal distress.

  For example, an anxious, verbal client would not be assigned to the same room as a nonverbal, catatonic client.
- In group therapy, the client defines himself/herself through human interaction and task accomplishment.
- Family therapy promotes health and functionality of the whole family system.
- Client recovery can be influenced by stressors. See Chapter 10 for information related to stress management.
- Family dynamics may also impact client recovery. See Chapter 10 for additional information on family dynamics.
  —Family rules are used to define behaviors and communication styles of family members. These impact how the family views and relates to institutions outside of the family. Ultimately, these influence the client.
  —Role confusion within a family or society at large impedes a client's recovery. For example, the eldest son assumes the patriarchal role of the family after the father's death.
  —Task confusion may result due to the birth of a child in the family resulting in neglect of other family members.
  —Mixed or double messages, such as when verbal and nonverbal messages conflict, can arrest a client's progression towards mental health.

Think Smart/Test Smart

Be aware that the terms therapeutic environment, therapeutic milieu, and milieu therapy are often used interchangeably.

BEHAVIORAL INTERVENTIONS

- The nurse assesses the client's appearance, mood, and psychomotor behavior. Examples of warning signs include disheveled appearance, inappropriate dress (shorts and t-shirt in winter), angry or withdrawn mood, and lack of physical coordination or difficulty speaking.

- The nurse assesses the mental health client for inappropriate or abnormal behavior. These behaviors may range from irrational anger to excessive happiness.
- The nurse assists the mental health client in achieving and maintaining self-control of behavior. Behavioral management techniques are effective in controlling behavior.
  —A contract may be used to hold a client accountable for his/her actions. The contract serves as a constant reminder of client tasks and goals.
  —Cognitive restructuring gives the client a greater degree of control over negative thinking by correcting these distortions or correcting thinking errors that precipitate the distortions, which result in inappropriate behavior.
  —Reframing is used to reinterpret irrational beliefs in a more realistic light.
  —Keeping a diary of significant events and associated feelings, thoughts, and behavior records the client's reaction to stressors.
  —Implementing relaxation and distraction techniques can decrease anxiety.
  —Trying alternative ways of behaving and reacting builds the client's sense of control and self-esteem.
  —Using positive reinforcement and positive language to praise the client when improvements are made.
  —Setting and enforcing limits and boundaries give clients a sense of security and what is expected of them.
- Anxiety is experienced by clients as they face new challenges or threatening situations.
- Anxiety impedes the client's healing. See Table 11–5 for nursing interventions to relieve client anxiety.

Table 11–5 Interventions to Relieve Client Anxiety

Discuss the importance of the client's safety and measures taken to ensure safety.
Explore and teach coping strategies such as visualization, imagery, breathing, and progressive relaxation.
Use distraction to relax and calm the client.
Listen actively to the client and encourage open discussion of feelings.
Use therapeutic communication techniques, and focus on positive remarks.
Use appropriate touch with client permission to demonstrate support.

- Clients who are disoriented are gently reminded of who they are, where they are, and what is expected of them. Conspicuous placement of clocks, watches, and calendars orient the client to time.
- Membership in group therapy promotes expression and exchange of ideas.
- The nurse leader of group therapy identifies behavior patterns of the members, promotes balance of the behavior patterns, and promotes self-esteem and socialization.
- The nurse continually evaluates the client, family, and significant others' ability to adhere to the treatment plan. Revisions to the plan are based on the nurse's evaluation.

CRISIS INTERVENTION

- A crisis is a situation that cannot be resolved by usual coping mechanisms.
- Psychosocial crises may be precipitated by acute or chronic illnesses, natural disasters, acts of violence, or emotional stress.
- During a crisis, the client, family, and significant others cannot function normally and require interventions to regain equilibrium.
- Symptoms of an impending crisis may include mood changes, impaired cognition, poor judgment and reasoning capabilities, and poor hygiene.
- Crisis intervention improves coping abilities. See Table 11–6 for the problem-solving techniques used during a crisis.
- The reason for the crisis may not always be clear to the client or the nurse. The nurse refers the client, family, and significant others to community resources, such as counseling and psychological evaluation to assist in understanding why the crisis occurred.
- Clients who experience psychosocial crisis are at risk for suicide. See Table 11–7 for the risk factors associated with suicide.
- Several factors protect clients from the risk of suicide such as
  —effective clinical care for mental, physical, and substance abuse disorders;
  —easy access to a variety of clinical interventions and support for help seeking;
  —family and community support;

Table 11–6 Crisis Problem-Solving Techniques

Technique	Factors
Identify the problem	Clients may have difficulty identifying the causative factor and may require assistance with this technique.
List alternatives	A solution to a problem is easier to ascertain when the many options are considered.
Choose from among alternatives	Each option is considered to help reach the best solution to the problem. The chosen alternative is based on the client's values and priorities.
Implement a plan	The chosen alternative is put into action. The nurse supports and encourages the client to execute the plan.
Evaluate the outcome	The effectiveness of the plan is evaluated to help guide future problem-solving efforts.

Table 11–7 Risk Factors for Suicide

Age: Younger than 20 years or older than 45 years, especially older than 65 years
Gender: Women make more attempts; men are more successful
Dysfunctional family: Experience with multiple losses while possessing limited coping skills
Family history of suicide
Family history of child maltreatment
History of mental disorders, particularly severe depression
Severe, intractable pain
Chronic, debilitating medical illnesses
Substance abuse
Severe anxiety
Overwhelming problems
Altered body image
Altered self-esteem
Detailed suicide plan
Previous suicide attempt(s)
Impulsive or aggressive tendencies
Barriers to accessing mental health treatment
Feelings of hopelessness and isolation
Loss: relational, social, work, or financial
Unwillingness to seek help due to stigma
Cultural and religious beliefs: belief that suicide is a noble resolution of a personal dilemma

—support from ongoing medical and mental health care relationships;

—skills in problem solving, conflict resolution, and nonviolent handling of disputes; and

—cultural and religious beliefs that discourage suicide and support self-preservation instincts.

- Suicidal clients often mistakenly believe they are doing their family and significant others a favor by committing suicide. This irrational belief drives suicidal behavior. Family members and significant others often blame themselves for the client's suicidal behavior.
- The symptoms of suicide include
  —depression;
  —expression of feelings of guilt;
  —tension or anxiety;
  —nervousness;
  —impulsiveness;
  —sudden change in behavior, especially calmness after a period of anxiety;
  —giving away belongings;
  —attempts to "get one's affairs in order";
  —direct or indirect threats to commit suicide;
  —direct attempts to commit suicide.
- Suicide attempts should always be taken seriously; dismissing them as attention-seeking behavior can have devastating consequences.
- Suicide precautions are ordered for clients who have either harmed themselves, verbalized intent to do so, or indicated, in an overt or covert manner, a wish to do so.
- Implementing suicide precautions includes placing the client in a private room close to the nurses' station.
- Remove all medications and other items considered unsafe, including glass or sharp items, nail polish remover or other alcohol-containing solutions, matches

or lighter, and any aerosol spray cans (i.e., hairspray). Similar items belonging to the client's roommate must also be removed, if placing the client in a private room is not an option.

- Once the crisis is managed, the client, family, and significant others should be aided in accessing recovery resources, such as social supports.

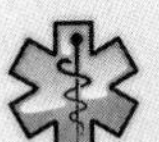

Nursing Intervention Alert

In crisis situations, nurses should facilitate referrals to a psychiatrist, psychiatric nurse specialist, hospital emergency department, or crisis center.

WORKSHEET

MATCHING QUESTIONS

Match the following:

Column A—Terms	Column B—Descriptions
1. _____ Aphasia	a. Asking the client to explain what he/she means to enhance the nurse's understanding of what the client is saying
2. _____ Dysarthria	b. A process that promotes the health and functionality of the family system
3. _____ Presbycusis	c. A behavioral management technique used to reinterpret irrational beliefs to more accurately reflect reality
4. _____ Conversation Pacing	d. The inability to recall words, understand what others are saying, or produce speech
5. _____ Clarification	e. A written agreement that holds a client accountable for his/her actions
6. _____ Reflection	f. Knowing what one's responsibilities are in a given situation
7. _____ Group Therapy	g. Manifestation of thoughts and feelings through gestures
8. _____ Family Therapy	h. Directing the client's feelings and ideas back to the client to validate the nurse's understanding of what the client is saying
9. _____ Contract	i. Sensitivity to what the client is experiencing
10. _____ Cognitive Restructuring	j. Use of all the senses to pick up verbal and nonverbal messages
11. _____ Reframing	k. Technique for reducing miscommunication and misunderstanding
12. _____ Anxiety	l. Promoted by consistency between words and actions
13. _____ Clarification	m. The inability to produce clear speech sounds
14. _____ Active Listening	n. A behavior management technique used to give the client greater control over negative thinking by correcting mental distortions
15. _____ Body Language	
16. _____ Trust	

(continued)

17. _____ Empathy

18. _____ Personal Space

19. _____ Crisis

20. _____ Safety

o. Allowing the elderly client plenty of time to answer health-related questions

p. Hearing loss due to the aging process

q. A situation that cannot be resolved by usual coping mechanisms

r. A manifestation of stress experienced by clients as they face new challenges or threatening situations

s. A process that promotes expression and the exchange of ideas; where the client defines himself/herself through human interaction and task accomplishment

t. Distance needed between self and other in order to feel comfortable

FILL IN THE BLANKS

Fill in the blank space with the correct word or phrase to complete each statement.

1. Clients suspected of having a speech or language deficit should be referred to a ________.
2. By informing the client of who will have access to the client's medical record, the nurse is ensuring ________.
3. The process of receiving information and examining the client's reactions to the messages received is a therapeutic communication technique known as ________.
4. ________ is the therapeutic use of nonverbal communication that allows the client time to think and slows the pace of the conversation.
5. A ________ provides socialization, promotes a fundamental respect for individuals, and provides opportunities for communication between the client and staff.
6. Cognitive restructuring, contracting, and reframing are ________techniques that are effective in controlling behavior.
7. During a ________, the client, family, and significant others cannot function normally and require interventions to regain equilibrium.
8. The symptoms of ________ include: depression, anxiety, impulsiveness, giving away belongings, and attempts to "get one's affairs in order."
9. Community meetings in the therapeutic environment serve to orient clients to the environment and ________.
10. ________develops through actions that are consistent with an individual's or group's stated intent.

TRUE & FALSE QUESTIONS

Mark each of the following statements True or False. Correct all false statements in the space provided.

1. Impaired verbal communication is the state in which an individual experiences a decreased or absent ability to use or understand human language. ___ T ___ F
2. Using touch while speaking to a visually-impaired client increases anxiety. ___ T ___ F
3. Giving advice, changing the subject, and using clichés are examples of barriers to therapeutic communication. ___ T ___ F
4. Family rules are used to define the behaviors and communication styles of family members. ___ T ___ F
5. Giving false reassurance conveys a lack of interest. ___ T ___ F
6. Asking why or how can be intimidating to the client. ___ T ___ F
7. Silence is nontherapeutic. ___ T ___ F
8. Using broad openings to conversation encourages client to select topic and indicates acceptance and value of the client's initiative. ___ T ___ F
9. Honesty promotes feelings of acceptance. ___ T ___ F
10. Maintaining a client's personal space helps decrease anxiety. ___ T ___ F

MATCHING QUESTIONS

Match the following:

Column A—Therapeutic Communication Techniques	Column B
1. _____ Validating	a. Encourages client to talk
2. _____ Restating	b. Rephrases and reviews key statements
3. _____ Focusing	c. Summarizes message in listener's own words
4. _____ Information Offering	d. Asks for explanation of vague response
5. _____ Sharing Impressions	e. Describes client's feelings as perceived by nurse and asks for corrective feedback
6. _____ Suggestive Collaboration	f. Redirects attention to a specific area
7. _____ Open-ended Questioning	g. Allows client to explore pros and cons of a proposed approach
8. _____ Reflecting	

(continued)

9. _____ Identifying Themes

10. _____ Clarifying

h. Explains purpose or components of an activity or procedure

i. Promotes identification and exploration of important problems

j. Directing back to the client his/her content, feelings, ideas or questions

APPLICATION QUESTIONS

1. A nurse is caring for a Hispanic client who speaks very little English. Which interventions by the nurse assist in meeting the client's therapeutic communication needs? Select all that apply.
   a. Providing a language interpreter
   b. Including Hispanic members of the health care team
   c. Providing client education materials written in Spanish
   d. Speaking in a normal tone of voice

2. A nurse in a long-term care facility is caring for an elderly client. The elderly client is experiencing bilateral hearing loss due to the aging process. Which is the correct term for the client's hearing loss?
   a. Aphasia
   b. Dysarthria
   c. Presbycusis
   d. Myopia

3. Clients with special needs require specific communication techniques. Which specific communication techniques should a nurse utilize when caring for a client who is cognitively impaired? Select all that apply.
   a. Maintain eye contact
   b. Keep communication simple and concrete
   c. Use open-ended questions
   d. Demonstrate or pantomime ideas

4. A nurse is caring for a client who has difficulty speaking. To which health care provider should the client be referred?
   a. Audiologist
   b. Physical therapist
   c. Surgeon
   d. Speech–language pathologist

5. Trust-building is an important nursing activity when establishing a nurse–client relationship. When a nurse draws the curtains around a client's bed, which trust builders are the nurse utilizing? Select all that apply.
   a. Providing a comfortable environment
   b. Ensuring client confidentiality
   c. Enhancing client privacy
   d. Providing a personal space

6. A nurse is recording the health history of a newly admitted client. The nurse asks the client to explain what he or she means when the client is providing health information. Which therapeutic communication technique is being utilized by the nurse?
   a. Informing
   b. Restating
   c. Clarification
   d. Reflection

7. A nurse is recording the health history of a newly admitted client. Which statement made by the nurse indicates that the nurse is using the therapeutic communication technique known as reflection?
   a. "I can understand why you are upset that you have been admitted to the hospital."
   b. "I'm listening."
   c. "You are only allowed to have one visitor at a time while in the hospital."
   d. "Have you ever considered a weight-loss program to help get your diabetes under control?"

8. Which actions by the nurse are barriers to therapeutic nurse–client communication? Select all that apply.
   a. Focusing on the diagnosis instead of the client
   b. Using slang terminology
   c. Using open-ended questions
   d. Giving advice

9. The goal of the therapeutic environment is to promote health and healing. Which statements are true regarding clients in a therapeutic environment? Select all that apply.
   a. Clients are active participants in their own lives
   b. Clients take ownership of their behavior and environment
   c. Clients are independent and self-sufficient
   d. Clients are responsible for safety and trust development

10. Room assignments on a psychiatric unit are based on which factors?
    a. The client's gender
    b. The client's fragility
    c. The client's race
    d. The client's length of stay

11. The nurse assists the mental health client in achieving and maintaining self-control of behavior. A commonly-used behavioral management technique is the use of contracts made with the client. Which statements are accurate regarding client contracts? Select all that apply.
    a. A contract gives a client greater control over negative thinking
    b. A contract may be used to hold a client accountable for his/her actions
    c. A contract serves as a constant reminder of client tasks and goals
    d. A contract promotes self-expression and the exchange of ideas

12. Clients who experience psychosocial crisis are at risk for suicide. Which are additional risk factors for suicide? Select all that apply.
    a. Younger than 20 years of age
    b. Older than 45 years of age
    c. Severe, intractable pain
    d. Substance abuse

13. During a crisis, the client and family cannot function normally and require interventions to regain equilibrium. In crisis situations, the nurse should facilitate referrals to which health care professionals? Select all that apply.
    a. A psychiatrist
    b. A psychiatric nurse specialist
    c. A hospital emergency department
    d. A crisis center

14. When caring for a client following a mastectomy, the nurse is positioning the affected arm. Which question is the most appropriate to ask?
    a. Does it hurt?
    b. Doesn't that feel good?
    c. That doesn't feel bad, does it?
    d. How does that feel?

15. During a dressing change, the client states, "My wife was really upset last night when she came to visit." The nurse says, "Your wound really looks good this morning." Of which block to therapeutic communication is this an example?
    a. Minimizing
    b. Rushing
    c. Giving false reassurance
    d. Changing the subject

15. A 90-year-old long-term care resident tells the nurse she has gotten three or four mosquito bites and they are swollen and very itchy. The nurse replies, "That's nothing; they'll be gone in a few days." What type of communication technique did the nurse use?
    a. Nontherapeutic minimizing
    b. Nontherapeutic use of cliché
    c. Therapeutic informing
    d. Therapeutic clarification

16. Which is an example of validation of a client's communication?
    a. "Would you tell me more about your feeling of light headedness?"
    b. "You said that the pain goes from your shoulder down your right arm?"
    c. "How would you describe your appetite?"
    d. "Putting it all together, you are feeling better today."

17. Which nursing approach would likely be most effective in decreasing anxiety in an elderly, visually impaired client during a health history?
    a. Pace the questions to allow plenty of time for answers
    b. Allow for increased personal space
    c. Reassure the client about the confidentiality of the information
    d. Ensure a private, comfortable environment

18. What does touching the client gently when performing a procedure or treatment communicate?
    a. Competence
    b. Client-centered focus
    c. Caring
    d. Pleasantness

(continued)

19. As a therapeutic technique, what purpose does humor serve?
   a. Helps put the nurse at ease with the client
   b. Lightens up a client who is too serious
   c. Tempers aggression
   d. Creates a sense of vitality

20. Which type of room accommodation would the nurse recommend for a suicidal client?
   a. Multibed room with active, alert clients
   b. Double room with a quiet, inactive client
   c. Private room near the nurse's station
   d. Private room at a quiet place on the unit

21. When caring for a client on suicide precautions, which items should the nurse remove from the room? Mark all that apply.
   a. Hand mirror
   b. Nail file
   c. Aerosol deodorant
   d. Alcohol based mouth wash
   e. Nail polish remover
   f. Matches

22. Clients with histories of which of the following factors are at increased risk for committing suicide? Mark all that apply.
   a. Substance abuse
   b. Impulsiveness
   c. Intractable, severe pain
   d. Family history of child abuse
   e. Altered body image

23. A client says to the nurse who is changing his ileostomy bag, "I think I should just die. I am a burden to everyone." Which is a therapeutic response?
   a. "There is no reason to feel that way, you are a good client."
   b. "I find it difficult to believe that you feel that way."
   c. "You shouldn't feel that way; your family loves you."
   d. "You feel like you are a burden?"

24. While discussing suicide as part of a health day program sponsored by a community group, the nurse is asked about signs that an individual is contemplating suicide. Which information could accurately be included in the nurse's response?
   a. The only signs of contemplated suicide are suicide notes, threats of suicide, and actual suicide attempts
   b. Giving away belongings, getting affairs in order such as paying off debts and preparing tax materials in advance, and sudden calm, directed behavior are often the signs of a decision to commit suicide
   c. Increase in use of alcohol, sudden interest in gambling or other "adult entertainment," or activities uncharacteristic of the person typically occur before a suicide
   d. There are no identifiable indications of potential suicide; persons can exhibit usual behavior and without warning kill themselves

ANSWERS & RATIONALES

MATCHING ANSWERS

Column A—Terms	Column B—Descriptions
1. __d__ Aphasia	a. Asking the client to explain what he/she means to enhance the nurse's understanding of what the client is saying
2. __m__ Dysarthria	b. A process that promotes the health and functionality of the family system
3. __p__ Presbycusis	c. A behavioral management technique used to reinterpret irrational beliefs to more accurately reflect reality
4. __o__ Conversation Pacing	d. The inability to recall words, understand what others are saying, or produce speech
5. __a__ Clarification	

6. h Reflection
7. s Group Therapy
8. b Family Therapy
9. e Contract
10. n Cognitive Restructuring
11. c Reframing
12. r Anxiety
13. k Clarification
14. j Active Listening
15. g Body Language
16. l Trust
17. i Empathy
18. t Personal Space
19. q Crisis
20. f Safety

e. A written agreement that holds a client accountable for his/her actions

f. Knowing what one's responsibilities are in a given situation

g. Manifestation of thoughts and feelings through gestures

h. Directing the client's feelings and ideas back to the client to validate the nurse's understanding of what the client is saying

i. Sensitivity to what the client is experiencing

j. Use of all the senses to pick up verbal and nonverbal messages

k. Technique for reducing miscommunication and misunderstanding

l. Promoted by consistency between words and actions

m. The inability to produce clear speech sounds

n. A behavior management technique used to give the client greater control over negative thinking by correcting mental distortions

o. Allowing the elderly client plenty of time to answer health-related questions

p. Hearing loss due to the aging process

q. A situation that cannot be resolved by usual coping mechanisms

r. A manifestation of stress experienced by clients as they face new challenges or threatening situations

s. A process that promotes expression and the exchange of ideas; where the client defines himself/herself through human interaction and task accomplishment

t. Distance needed between self and other in order to feel comfortable

ANSWERS FOR FILL IN THE BLANKS

1. Clients suspected of having a speech or language deficit should be referred to a speech—language pathologist.

2. By informing the client of who will have access to the client's medical record, the nurse is ensuring confidentiality.

3. The process of receiving information and examining the client's reactions to the messages received is a therapeutic communication technique known as active listening.

4. Silence is the therapeutic use of nonverbal communication that allows the client time to think and slows the pace of the conversation.

5. A therapeutic environment provides socialization, promotes a fundamental respect for individuals, and provides opportunities for communication between the client and staff.

(continued)

6. Cognitive restructuring, contracting, and reframing are <u>behavioral management</u> techniques that are effective in controlling behavior.

7. During a <u>crisis</u>, the client, family, and significant others cannot function normally and require interventions to regain equilibrium.

8. The symptoms of <u>suicide</u> include: depression, anxiety, impulsiveness, giving away belongings, and attempts to "get one's affairs in order."

9. Community meetings in the therapeutic environment serve to orient clients to the environment and <u>define boundaries</u>.

10. <u>Trust</u> develops through actions that are consistent with an individual's or group's stated intent.

TRUE OR FALSE ANSWERS

1. Impaired verbal communication is the state in which an individual experiences a decreased or absent ability to use or understand human language. *True*

2. Using touch while speaking to a visually-impaired client increases anxiety *False*
   Using touch while speaking to a visually-impaired client decreases anxiety.

3. Giving advice, changing the subject, and using clichés are examples of barriers to therapeutic communication. *True*

4. Family rules are used to define the behaviors and communication styles of family members. *True*

5. Giving false reassurance conveys a lack of interest. *True*

6. Asking why or how can be intimidating to the client. *True*

7. Silence is nontherapeutic. *False*
   Silence can be used therapeutically to allow client time to think and can encourage the client to initiate communication while conveying acceptance, support and understanding.

8. Using broad openings to conversation encourages client to select topic and indicates acceptance and value of the client's initiative. *True*

9. Honesty promotes feelings of acceptance. *False*
   Honesty decreases anxiety and facilitates goal achievement; caring promotes feelings of acceptance.

10. Maintaining a client's personal space decreases anxiety. *True*

MATCHING ANSWERS

Column A—Therapeutic Communication Techniques	Column B
1. __b__ Validating	a. Encourages client to talk
2. __c__ Restating	b. Rephrases and reviews key statements

3. __f__ Focusing
4. __h__ Information Offering
5. __e__ Sharing Impressions
6. __g__ Suggestive Collaboration
7. __a__ Open-ended Questioning
8. __j__ Reflecting
9. __i__ Identifying Themes
10. __d__ Clarifying

c. Summarizes message in listener's own words

d. Asks for explanation of vague response

e. Describes client's feelings as perceived by nurse and asks for corrective feedback

f. Redirects attention to a specific area

g. Allows client to explore pros and cons of a proposed approach

h. Explains purpose or components of an activity or procedure

i. Promotes identification and exploration of important problems

j. Directing back to the client his/her content, feelings, ideas or questions

APPLICATION ANSWERS

1. A nurse is caring for a Hispanic client who speaks very little English. Which interventions by the nurse assist in meeting the client's therapeutic communication needs? Select all that apply.
   a. Providing a language interpreter
   b. Including Hispanic members of the health care team
   c. Providing client education materials written in Spanish
   d. Speaking in a normal tone of voice

Rationale
Correct answers: a, b, c, and d.
The nurse assists in meeting the Hispanic client's therapeutic communication needs by providing a language interpreter, including Hispanic members of the health care team, providing client education materials written in Spanish, and by speaking in a normal tone of voice. It is an inappropriate tendency of some health care professionals to speak loudly to clients from other cultures.

2. A nurse in a long-term care facility is caring for an elderly client. The elderly client is experiencing bilateral hearing loss due to the aging process. Which is the correct term for the client's hearing loss?
   a. Aphasia
   b. Dysarthria
   c. Presbycusis
   d. Myopia

Rationale
Correct answer: c.
Presbycusis is hearing loss due to the aging process.

3. Clients with special needs require specific communication techniques. Which specific communication techniques should a nurse utilize when caring for a client who is cognitively impaired? Select all that apply.
   a. Maintain eye contact
   b. Keep communication simple and concrete
   c. Use open-ended questions
   d. Demonstrate or pantomime ideas

Rationale
Correct answers: a and b.
The nurse should maintain eye contact, keep communication simple and concrete, avoid open-ended questions, and be client when communicating with a client who is cognitively impaired. Demonstration or pantomiming ideas are not effective techniques for communicating with those who are cognitively impaired.

4. A nurse is caring for a client who has difficulty speaking. To which health care provider should the client be referred?
   a. Audiologist
   b. Physical therapist

(continued)

c. Surgeon
d. Speech–language pathologist

Rationale
Correct answer: d.
The client who is having difficulty speaking should be referred to a speech–language pathologist.

5. Trust-building is an important nursing activity when establishing a nurse–client relationship. When a nurse draws the curtains around a client's bed, which trust builders are the nurse utilizing? Select all that apply.
   a. Providing a comfortable environment
   b. Ensuring client confidentiality
   c. Enhancing client privacy
   d. Providing a personal space

Rationale
Correct answers: a, b, c, and d.
By performing the simple act of drawing the curtains around a client's bed, the nurse is providing a more comfortable environment, ensuring client confidentiality, enhancing client privacy, and providing a personal space; all of which aid the client in establishing a sense of trust with the nurse.

6. A nurse is recording the health history of a newly admitted client. The nurse asks the client to explain what he or she means when the client is providing health information. Which therapeutic communication technique is being utilized by the nurse?
   a. Informing
   b. Restating
   c. Clarification
   d. Reflection

Rationale
Correct answer: c.
Clarification is the therapeutic communication technique being utilized to ensure that the nurse has a clear understanding of what the client is saying.

7. A nurse is recording the health history of a newly admitted client. Which statement made by the nurse indicates that the nurse is using the therapeutic communication technique known as reflection?
   a. "I can understand why you are upset that you have been admitted to the hospital."
   b. "I'm listening."
   c. "You are only allowed to have one visitor at a time while in the hospital."
   d. "Have you ever considered a weight-loss program to help get your diabetes under control?"

Rationale
Correct answer: a.
The nurse is using reflection to direct the feelings that have been expressed back to the client; signifies empathy, interest, and respect for the client.

8. Which actions by the nurse are barriers to therapeutic nurse—client communication? Select all that apply.
   a. Focusing on the diagnosis instead of the client
   b. Using slang terminology
   c. Using open-ended questions
   d. Giving advice

Rationale
Correct answers: a, b, and d.
Barriers to therapeutic communication include: focusing on the diagnosis instead of the client; using slang terminology; and giving advice. Using open-ended questions is a therapeutic communication technique.

9. The goal of the therapeutic environment is to promote health and healing. Which statements are true regarding clients in a therapeutic environment? Select all that apply.
   a. Clients are active participants in their own lives
   b. Clients take ownership of their behavior and environment
   c. Clients are independent and self-sufficient
   d. Clients are responsible for safety and trust development

Rationale
Correct answers: a, b, and c.
Clients in a therapeutic environment are active participants in their lives, take ownership of their behavior and environment, and function independently and self-sufficiently. The nurse is responsible for facilitating safety development and trust development within the therapeutic environment.

10. Room assignments on a psychiatric unit are based on which factors?
    a. The client's gender
    b. The client's fragility
    c. The client's race
    d. The client's length of stay

Rationale
Correct answers: a, b, and d.
Room assignments on a psychiatric unit are based upon numerous factors which include: gender, fragility, length of stay, age, overall behavior, and level of personal distress.

11. The nurse assists the mental health client in achieving and maintaining self-control of behavior. A commonly-used behavioral management technique is the use of contracts made with the client. Which statements are accurate regarding client contracts? Select all that apply.
    a. A contract gives a client greater control over negative thinking
    b. A contract may be used to hold a client accountable for his/her actions
    c. A contract serves as a constant reminder of client tasks and goals
    d. A contract promotes self-expression and the exchange of ideas

Rationale

Correct answers: b and c.

A contract may be used to hold a client accountable for his/her own actions and serves as a constant reminder of client tasks and goals. Cognitive restructuring gives a client greater control over negative thinking by correcting the distortions. Group therapy promotes self-expression and the exchange of ideas.

12. Clients who experience psychosocial crisis are at risk for suicide. Which are additional risk factors for suicide? Select all that apply.
    a. Younger than 20 years of age
    b. Older than 45 years of age
    c. Severe, intractable pain
    d. Substance abuse

Rationale

Correct answers: a, b, c, and d.

Risk factors for suicide include: age younger than 20 years, age older than 45 years (especially over 65 years), severe intractable pain, and substance abuse.

13. During a crisis, the client and family cannot function normally and require interventions to regain equilibrium. In crisis situations, the nurse should facilitate referrals to which health care professionals? Select all that apply.
    a. A psychiatrist
    b. A psychiatric nurse specialist
    c. A hospital emergency department
    d. A crisis center

Rationale

Correct answers: a, b, c, and d.

In crisis situations, it is appropriate for the nurse to facilitate referrals to psychiatrists, psychiatric nurse specialists, hospital emergency departments, and crisis centers.

14. When caring for a client following a mastectomy, the nurse is positioning the affected arm. Which question is the most appropriate to ask?
    a. Does it hurt?
    b. Doesn't that feel good?
    c. That doesn't feel bad, does it?
    d. How does that feel?

Rationale

Correct answer: d.

"How does that feel?" is an open-ended question which encourages the client to respond as he/she desires. "Does it hurt?" requires only a yes or no response and hence has a limiting effect. "Doesn't that feel good?" and "That doesn't feel bad, does it?" are leading questions which predispose the client to the answer the nurse wants.

15. During a dressing change, the client states, "My wife was really upset last night when she came to visit." The nurse says, "Your wound really looks good this morning." Of which block to therapeutic communication is this an example?
    a. Minimizing
    b. Rushing
    c. Giving false reassurance
    d. Changing the subject

Rationale

Correct answer: d.

The nurse changed the subject rather than following up the client's statement with a therapeutic technique to encourage further identification and discussion of the problem.

16. A 90-year-old long-term care resident tells the nurse she has gotten three or four mosquito bites and they are swollen and very itchy. The nurse replies, "That's nothing; they'll be gone in a few days." What type of communication technique did the nurse use?
    a. Nontherapeutic minimizing
    b. Nontherapeutic use of cliché
    c. Therapeutic informing
    d. Therapeutic clarification

Rationale

Correct answer: a.

Saying that is nothing communicates unimportant and not deserving of attention. No cliché was used. No real information was provided about the client's health status or self-care. Clarification refers to asking a client to explain an unclear communication and is not relevant.

(continued)

17. Which is an example of validation of a client's communication?
    a. "Would you tell me more about your feeling of light headedness?"
    b. "You said that the pain goes from your shoulder down your right arm?"
    c. "How would you describe your appetite?"
    d. "Putting it all together, you are feeling better today."

Rationale

Correct answer: b.

Validating is rephrasing and reviewing key statements made by the client and allowing the client to confirm that the nurse accurately understood what was said. A is a question that focuses the client on a particular area. C is an open-ended question which encourages the client to share information. D is an example of summarizing.

18. Which nursing approach would likely be most effective in decreasing anxiety in an elderly, visually impaired client during a health history?
    a. Pace the questions to allow plenty of time for answers
    b. Allow for increased personal space
    c. Reassure the client about the confidentiality of the information
    d. Ensure a private, comfortable environment

Rationale

Correct answer: a.

Pacing conversation to allow plenty of time for the elderly client to answer questions without feeling rushed decreases anxiety. Allowing for the personal space desired by the client decreases anxiety but increasing or decreasing the preferred space can increase anxiety and sense of discomfort. Reassuring the client about confidentiality and providing privacy promotes a sense of security.

19. What does touching the client gently when performing a procedure or treatment communicate?
    a. Competence
    b. Client-centered focus
    c. Caring
    d. Pleasantness

Rationale

Correct answer: c.

Caring is communicated by gentle touch and addressing the client by name. Competence is communicated by an organized, professional manner. Client centered focus is evident when the nurse attends to the client's verbal and nonverbal behavior and responds to it rather than talking about personal concerns or conversing with another health care worker about other than the client. Pleasantness is communicated through smiling and warm greetings.

20. As a therapeutic technique, what purpose does humor serve?
    a. Helps put the nurse at ease with the client
    b. Lightens up a client who is too serious
    c. Tempers aggression
    d. Creates a sense of vitality

Rationale

Correct answer: c.

Humor can be used as a therapeutic technique to temper aggression, reveal new options and insights, and bring repressed material to consciousness.

21. Which type of room accommodation would the nurse recommend for a suicidal client?
    a. Multibed room with active, alert clients
    b. Double room with a quiet, inactive client
    c. Private room near the nurse's station
    d. Private room at a quiet place on the unit

Rationale

Correct answer: c.

A private room provides a controlled environment and being near the nurse's station allows for easy observation. A private room is a component of suicide precautions.

22. When caring for a client on suicide precautions, which items should the nurse remove from the room? Mark all that apply.
    a. Hand mirror
    b. Nail file
    c. Aerosol deodorant
    d. Alcohol based mouth wash
    e. Nail polish remover
    f. Matches

Rationale

Correct answer: all of the above.

Anything, glass, sharp objects, flammable liquids, or items in any way able to inflict injury must be removed from the room. This includes alcohol-based solutions and aerosol cans. If the client is not is in a private room, these types of items belonging to the other person in the room must also be removed.

23. Clients with histories of which of the following factors are at increased risk for committing suicide? Mark all that apply.
    a. Substance abuse
    b. Impulsiveness
    c. Intractable, severe pain
    d. Family history of child abuse
    e. Altered body image

Rationale

Correct answer: all of the above.

Substance abuse, impulsiveness, intractable, severe pain, family history of child abuse and altered body image are all risk factors for suicide.

24. A client says to the nurse who is changing his ileostomy bag, "I think I should just die. I am a burden to everyone." Which is a therapeutic response?
    a. "There is no reason to feel that way, you are a good client."
    b. "I find it difficult to believe that you feel that way."
    c. "You shouldn't feel that way; your family loves you."
    d. "You feel like you are a burden?"

Rationale

Correct answer: d.

This is a form of reflecting back the client's feelings. It allows for validation and shows interest and respect. It also invites additional communication on the part of the client. Responses a, b, and c are all nontherapeutic responses that are judgmental and trivialize the client's feeling. The "good client" is a cliché.

25. While discussing suicide as part of a health day program sponsored by a community group, the nurse is asked about signs that an individual is contemplating suicide. Which information could accurately be included in the nurse's response?
    a. The only signs of contemplated suicide are suicide notes, threats of suicide, and actual suicide attempts
    b. Giving away belongings, getting affairs in order such as paying off debts and preparing tax materials in advance, and sudden calm, directed behavior are often the signs of a decision to commit suicide
    c. Increase in use of alcohol, sudden interest in gambling or other "adult entertainment," or activities uncharacteristic of the person typically occur before a suicide
    d. There are no identifiable indications of potential suicide; persons can exhibit usual behavior and without warning kill themselves

Rationale

Correct answer: b.

Giving away belongings, getting affairs in order such as paying off debts and preparing tax materials in advance, and sudden calm, directed behavior are often the signs of a decision to commit suicide. Other signs are depression, expression of guilt feelings, tension, anxiety, nervousness, impulsiveness, and actual suicide attempts.

CHAPTER 12

Test Plan Category:

Psychosocial Integrity—Part 3

Sub-category: **None**

Topics: **Abuse/Neglect**
Chemical Dependency
Sensory/Perceptual Alterations
Psychopathology

MENTAL-HEALTH CONCEPTS

- Mental health is typically immeasurable by scientific standards.
- Influencing factors for mental health or disorder include inherited factors, biochemical influences, hormonal influences, family, culture, values and beliefs, cognitive abilities, spirituality, and worldview and perceptions.
- Protective defenses are the ways in which clients manage the negative aspects of life.
- A few defense mechanisms are repression, denial, rationalization, affiliation, and passive aggression.
- The nurse assesses factors that influence the client's perceptual, mental, emotional, and behavioral responses to internal and external stressors and crises.
- The nurse offers care to the mental-health client that is client-focused, goal-directed, and objective.
- The key to prevention and management of mental illness is stress reduction and adherence to an established treatment plan.
- Stress reduction and management decrease the occurrence of relapse in illness.

LEGAL OR ETHICAL PRINCIPLES IN MENTAL-HEALTH CARE

- Rights of the mentally ill client
  —Right to treatment
  —Right to refuse treatment
  —Right to informed consent
  —Right to privacy
  —Right to confidentiality
- Involuntary admission
  —Wishes of client regarding hospitalization must be respected unless client is a threat to self or others
  —Each state has laws that govern civil commitment process

—A person can usually be detained in a mental-health facility for 48–72 hours until a hearing can be conducted to determine if he or she should be committed

- Least restrictive environment
  —Restraints and seclusion may only be used to prevent client self-harm or harm to others
  —They are used only when all other physical and psychological means have failed
  —They are never used as a punishment
  —Criteria for the use of physical restraints include
    - examination by physician to determine need
    - physician's written order
    - application of restraints is for a specified duration only

SENSORY AND PERCEPTUAL ALTERATIONS

- Sensory perception is the conscious process of selecting, organizing, and interpreting data from the senses into useful information.
- Severe sensory alteration may be due to sensory overload, sensory deprivation, sleep deprivation, and cultural care deprivation. See Table 12–1 for the factors associated with sensory deprivation.
- Sensory overload, sleep deprivation, and cultural care deprivation may cause confusion and anxiety.
- Perception is influenced by sights, sounds, tastes, smells, body position, coordination, and equilibrium as well as past experiences, knowledge, and attitudes.
- Gross perceptual alterations result in hallucinations. A hallucination is a subjective disorder of perception in which an impression from one of the five senses is present in the absence of external stimuli.
- Delirium—a state of mental confusion and excitement characterized by disorientation for time and place—usually accompanies hallucinations.
- Clients experiencing sensory and perceptual alterations have difficulty establishing independent living arrangements.
- Limited communication and coping skills are common among individuals experiencing sensory and perceptual alterations. Stressors can greatly impact these individuals' ability to cope.

PSYCHOPATHOLOGY

- The nurse assesses the mental-health client for level of awareness, level of consciousness, behavior, appearance, memory, abstract reasoning, and language.
- Abnormal assessment findings include poor hygiene, inappropriate dress, disorientation, absent memory recall, and incoherent or illogical thought processes, which may be evidence of psychopathology.
- Several factors are associated with mental illness. See Table 12–2 for the factors associated with mental illness.

Table 12–1 Factors Associated with Sensory Deprivation

Perceptual	Hallucinations, delirium
Cognitive	Thought disorganization, decreased attention/concentration, slowness of thought, difficulty with problem solving and task performance
Emotional	Rapid mood changes, anxiety, panic, depression, nervousness, and jitteriness

- Many clients, their families, and significant others may have difficulty accepting the diagnosis of an acute or chronic mental illness.
  —Reactions may include disbelief, anxiety, confusion, and denial.
  —The nurse responds by offering support and information, dispelling myths and blame, and facilitating community resources and social supports.
- When caring for clients with mental illness, the nurse incorporates the client's beliefs, culture, spirituality, and religion into the plan of care.
- The nurse continually evaluates the ability of the client, family, and significant others to adhere to the treatment plan. Revisions to the plan are based on the nurse's evaluation.

ANXIETY DISORDERS

- Anxiety is a universal feeling; everyone experiences it at some time to some degree.
- Anxiety disorders are the most commonly seen psychiatric disorder.

Table 12–2 Factors Associated with Mental Illness

Desire to hurt self or others
Disorganized or disturbed thoughts
Extreme feelings of helplessness or hopelessness
Extreme negative thoughts
History of traumatic experience
Inability to accept reality or satisfy basic needs
Inability to derive pleasure from living
Ineffective coping mechanisms or stress management
Illness resulting from severe, unrelenting stress
Lack of support system
Personality traits associated with dysfunctional behavior

- These are classified as mild, moderate, or severe depending on the signs and symptoms.
- They can occur at any age and are more prevalent in women than men.

Etiology:

- Exact cause is unknown, often a combination of factors are involved.
- Several theories exist for the etiology of anxiety disorders.
- *Biological factors*
  - —Genetic predispostition is partially related to some anxiety disorders.
  - —Anxiety can result from improper functioning of the body systems responsible for the normal stress response.
  - —Some neurotransmitters have been associated with anxiety.
  - —Changes in the brain may be the origin of some anxiey disorders.
- *Psychological factors*
  - —The number and severity of stressors may overwhelm unconscious defense mechanisms and become dysfunctional.
  - —There is a correlation between parents' fears and those of children lending to the theory that fearful reactions are learned.

S&S:

- Varies according to the specific disorder

Dx:

- There are no diagnostic tests that definitively confirm anxiety disorders. Diagnosis is based upon manifestations of the disease with data obtained from a mental-status examination, psychiatric history, and careful clinical observation
- A thorough physical and psychiatric evaluation is needed to rule out other possible causes of the symptoms such as a brain tumor or thyroid disorder

GENERALIZED ANXIETY DISORDER

- Generalized anxiety disorder refers to anxiety that is persistent, overwhelming, uncontrollable, and out of proportion to the stimulus.
- It tends to be a chronic condition.
- It can vary from mild to severe.

Etiology:

- Exact cause is unknown.
- It is believed to have a genetic predisposition.

S&S: The client shows

- excessive physiological arousal including
  - —restlessness and inability to relax
  - —episodes of trembling and shaking
  - —shortness of breath
  - —tachycardia or palpitations
  - —sleep disturbances
  - —GI disturbances
  - —muscle tension
  - —headache
  - —cold, clammy hands
  - —dry mouth
- distorted thought processes and coping
  - —inability to concentrate
  - —excessive worry
  - —unrealistic assessment of problems
  - —procrastination
  - —poor problem solving

Rx:

- Often a combination of
  - —psychotherapy
  - —behavioral therapy
  - —relaxation therapy
  - —supportive counseling
  - —pharmacological therapy
    - Antianxiety agents
      - usually given for several weeks
      - should not take more than 6 weeks in order to reduce potential for abuse
    - Selective serotonin reuptake inhibitors (SSRIs)

- Tricyclic antidepressants
- Buspirone (Buspar)—drug of choice for clients with a history of substance abuse
  - differs from other antianxiety drugs in that it requires several weeks for the onset of therapeutic effect

Nursing Process Elements

- Attend to physical needs such as nutrition and rest
- Stay with the client while acutely anxious
- Encourage client to discuss feelings and thoughts that stimulate anxious reactions

Client teaching for self-care

- Provide nutritional teaching such as avoiding caffeine and alcohol
- Teach appropriate ways of managing anxiety
- Teach about medication administration and monitoring

PANIC DISORDER

- Panic disorder is the most severe form of anxiety.
- It is characterized by recurrent panic attacks with feelings of impending doom.

Etiology:

- Exact cause is unknown.
- It seems to have a family predisposition.

S&S: The client

- may have symptoms of an MI including chest pain, diaphoresis, and shortness of breath
- is unable to focus thoughts or to concentrate
- has a rapid speech
- has an exaggerated startle reaction
- is unable to remain still—fidgets and paces

Rx:

- A combination of therapies and client teaching
- Cognitive therapy
  —teaches the client to replace negative thoughts with realistic, positive thoughts
  —identifies triggers for the panic attacks
  —helps the client to understand that the panic attack is separate and independent of the trigger
- Behavioral therapy involving desensitization
- Relaxation techniques
- Pharmacologic therapy may include a combination of
  —antianxiety drugs especially benzodiazepines
  —antidepressants
  —beta blockers to control cardiac symptoms

Nursing Process Elements

- Stay with client while anxiety is acute
- Avoid using touch to calm client
- Provide a safe, calm, and nonstimulating environment
- Maintain a calm approach with attention to both verbal and nonverbal behavior
- Encourage client to express feelings
- Allow to move and pace as needed
- Administer and monitor effects of medication

Client teaching for self-care

Teach client about
- recognition of triggers
- alternative coping mechanisms
- medication administration and monitoring

OBSESSIVE-COMPULSIVE DISORDER

- Obsessions are persistent intrusive thoughts and ideas.
- Compulsion is the repeated performance of rituals or behaviors designed to prevent some event, divert unwanted thoughts, and decrease anxiety.

Etiology:

- Unknown.

S&S: The client

- has repetitive thoughts that increase stress
- has compulsive behaviors such as hand washing, counting, turning door lock a set number of times each time, etc.

The degree to which these thoughts and behaviors interfere with a person's ability to function determines if and when intervention is needed.

Rx:

- Primarily behavioral therapy
  —exposes client to the situation or object that triggers the obsessive thoughts and then encourages them to refrain from the compulsive behavior used to decrease anxiety
  —is very effective in most cases
- Relaxation techniques
- Social support such as support groups

Nursing Process Elements

- Identify situations that provoke the behaviors
- Allow the client to carry out the behavior until anxiety is decreased (unless behavior puts safety at risk)
- Set reasonable demands and limits on the client's behaviors and make their purpose clear
- Encourage the client to verbalize feelings and concerns

- Make a written contract to assist the client to gradually decrease the frequency of compulsive behaviors

PHOBIC DISORDERS

- A phobia is an irrational fear that persists although the person may recognize it as unreasonable.
- It can lead to panic level anxiety.
- There are many types of phobias including agoraphobia (fear of open spaces), social phobia (fear of situations in which one may be embarrassed), and xenophobia (fear of strangers).

Etiology:
- Unknown.

S&S: The client shows
- fear and avoidance of the object or situation which causes anxiety
- physical reactions such as trembling, GI distress, tachycardia including those associated with panic attacks

Rx:
- Desensitization therapy to gradually expose client to the feared object or situation while coaching on relaxation techniques
- Guided imagery is used to allow client to rehearse ways to relax while confronting the feared object or situation
- Modeling behavior has the client observe someone demonstrate appropriate behavior when confronting the feared object or situation
- Negative-thought stopping teaches the client to recognize negative thoughts, then use a distracting stimulus (such as snapping a rubber band worn on the wrist) and substitute an appropriate thought
- Pharmacologic therapy may be used with other therapies including
  —antianxiety drugs
  —antidepressants
  —beta blockers to reduce cardiac symptoms

Nursing Process Elements
- Do not trivialize client's fears
- Teach and assist with relaxation, guided imagery, and thought-stopping techniques
- Explore with client other ways to relieve stress
- Teach appropriate medication use

MOOD DISORDERS

- Mood disorder refers to the existence of persistent feelings that cause a wide span of both emotional and behavioral problems that hinder the client's psychosocial functioning.
- Depending on the type of disorder, the client experiences either intense high (manic) or low (depressed) mood states.
- Major depressive disorder and bipolar disorder are the primary mood disorders. Related disorders include diagnoses such as dysthymic disorder, cyclothymic disorder, postpartum depression, seasonal affective disorder (SAD), and schizoaffective disorder.

Etiology: There are basically three categories of theories:
- Genetic—Mood disorders occur more frequently in first-degree relatives than in the general population.
- Biological —Deficiencies or abnormalities in hormones or in the brain's neurotransmitters correlate with different mood disorders.
- Psychological—This category includes many theories that in essence fault the client or the family with the mood disorder. There is little use for these theories today.

S&S:
- Major depressive disorder: Two or more weeks of sad mood, lack of interest in life activities and at least four other symptoms such as
  —anhedonia or lack of enjoyment
  —feelings of guilt, helplessness, or hopelessness
  —decreased ability to concentrate and make decisions
  —sleep disturbances
  —appetite loss or overeating with related weight changes
  —lethargy
  —low self-esteem
  —thoughts of death and suicide
- Bipolar disorder: The client experiences extreme highs (mania) alternating with extreme lows (depression) with periods of normal mood interspersed between the highs and lows. Severe episodes of mania or depression can sometimes involve psychotic symptoms (hallucinations and delusions). Characteristics of mania include
  —elation and euphoria
  —agitation and irritability
  —hyperactivity and sleeplessness
  —poor judgment and high-risk behaviors
  —exaggerated sexuality
  —rapid thought and pressured speech

Dx:
- There are no diagnostic tests that definitively confirm mood disorders. Diagnosis is based upon manifestations of the disease with data obtained from a mental-status examination, psychiatric history, and careful clinical observation
- A thorough physical and psychiatric evaluation is needed to rule out other possible causes of the symptoms such as a brain tumor or thyroid disorder

Rx: The primary treatment of mood disorders is drug therapy to control the main symptoms. For persistent depression resistant to medication therapy, electroconvulsive therapy (ECT) may be helpful. In addition, other treatments such as psychotherapy, vocational counseling, and structured milieu therapy are needed to assist the client with social adjustment

- Drug therapy for major depression generally works by modifying the activity of relevant neurotransmitters. Selection of the appropriate antidepressant is often based on factors such as previous effectiveness of medication on client or family members and possible adverse effects. Many antidepressants have other uses including treatment of anxiety disorders, ADHD, and chronic pain.
  —SSRIs are often the first-line treatment for clients with depression
    - Examples are citalopram (Celexa), escitalopram (Lexapro), fluoxetine (Prozac), paroxetine (Paxil), and sertraline (Zoloft)
    - Effects can usually be seen after 1–3 weeks
    - Cause fewer side effects than other antidepressant medications
    - Common side effects include nausea, insomnia, nervousness, dry mouth, and sexual dysfunction

  —Atypical antidepressants are usually used when the client has an inadequate response to or intolerable side effects from SSRIs
    - Example of these antidepressants are venlafaxine (Effexor), bupropion (Wellbutrin), and nefazodone (Serzone)
    - Side effects vary with each individual medication but commonly include headache, dizziness, drowsiness, nausea, and vomiting

  —Tricyclic antidepressants (TCA) are one of the oldest classes of antidepressants.
    - Examples are amitriptyline (Elavil) and imipramine (Tofranil)
    - Effectiveness does not begin for 4–6 weeks and full therapeutic effects may not be reached for 6–8 weeks
    - Common side effects include dizziness, drowsiness, dry mouth, orthostatic hypotension, blurred vision, urinary retention, constipation, nausea, and headache
    - TCAs are the least expensive of the antidepressants

  —Monoamine oxidase inhibitiors (MAOI) are used infrequently because interaction with many common foods and medication causes hypertensive crisis
    - Examples are phenelzine (Nardil) and tranylcypromine (Parnate)
    - Maximum effectiveness takes 6 weeks
    - Side effects include dry mouth, blurred vision, constipation, urinary retention, sedation, weight gain, orthostatic hypotension, and nausea
- Electroconvulsive therapy

Nursing Process Elements

- Hypoactive clients
  —Eliminate need for decision making when possible; when a decision is needed, do not rush the client
  —Accept slowness; do not chastise
  —Encourage easily accomplished activities that do not require prolonged time or concentration
  —Monitor for constipation
- Hyperactive clients
  —Speak softly and slowly
  —Limit environmental stimuli
  —Be kind, firm, and matter of fact; do not argue, get angry, or engage in entertaining behaviors
  —Avoid long discussions and explanations
  —Engage in noncompetitive activities that utilize energy
  —Do not be demanding; it can result in a power play

PERSONALITY DISORDERS

- These are a group of disorders characterized by a pattern of behavior and thinking that noticeably differs from the cultural norm.
- These disorders result in problems with living rather than in clinical symptoms.
- Clients frequently see their behavior or thinking as the norm and do not see it as a painful or uncomfortable experience.

Etiology:

- Unknown although many believe it to be a combination of many factors including biological, social, developmental, and psychological.

S&S:

- Varies according to specific disorder

Dx:

- There are no diagnostic tests that definitively confirm personality disorders. Diagnosis is based upon manifestations of the disease with data obtained from a mental-status examination, psychiatric history, and careful clinical observation.
- A thorough physical and psychiatric evaluation is needed to rule out other possible causes of the symptoms such as a brain tumor or thyroid disorder.

ANTISOCIAL PERSONALITY DISORDER

- The antisocial personality disorder is characterized by selfishness, poor sexual adjustment, failure to accept social

norms, inability to maintain lasting relationships, irritability, and aggressiveness.
- Such a disorder predisposes the person to criminal behavior.

S&S: The client
- shows disregard for others feelings, rights, and society's values.
- has an impulsive and reckless behavior with a disregard for own and others' safety.
- shows a dishonest and deceitful behavior.
- is irritable and aggressive, may display passive-aggressive behavior.
- shows inability to maintain responsible functioning at work, school, or in family role.
- has a lack of shame, guilt, or empathy.
- displays manipulative behavior, seeking power and control.
- can be very charming on a superficial level.

Rx:
- Psychotherapy is treatment of choice
  —Goal is to help the client see connections between feelings and behaviors
- Supporting therapies include
  —group therapy
  —family therapy
  —support groups
  —pharmacologic therapy used to treat some of the symptoms the client may experience such as mood swings

Nursing Process Elements
- Set limits on client's behavior, may use a behavioral contract
- Hold client accountable for own behavior
- Reinforce positive behavior
- Avoid arguing with the client
- Anticipate and recognize manipulative behaviors
- Teach client social skills and what are socially accepted behaviors

BORDERLINE PERSONALITY DISORDER

Etiology:
- Unknown although 50% of those with this disorder have been victims of sexual abuse.

S&S: The client
- has instability in interpersonal relationships which are often intense and stormy, fears abandonment which is manifested in both clinging and distancing behaviors
- experiences extreme feelings of anger, depression and anxiety
- displays mood swings that are rapid and dramatic
- has self-image disturbance with feelings of unworthiness
- has lack of insight
- shows behavior that is often impulsive and unpredictable
- usually does not consider the consequences of own actions
- displays recurrent self-mutilating behavior or suicidal threats

Rx:
- Outpatient psychotherapy is treatment of choice supported by other treatments such as support groups

Nursing Process Elements
- Promote safety with a no-harm contract
- Help client to cope and control emotions with techniques such as journaling and identifying feelings
- Use and teach cognitive restructuring techniques
  —thought stopping
  —decatastrophizing
- Teach social and communication skills
- Set behavioral limits and personal boundaries
- Confront inappropriate behaviors
- Teach time structuring by making lists and written schedule of activities

Think Smart/Test Smart

Be aware that borderline personality disorder is sometimes referred to as emotional regulation disorder.

HISTRIONIC PERSONALITY DISORDER

S&S: The client
- is overly dramatic and displays intensely expressive behavior
- enjoys being the center of attention
- has a behavior that is lively, impulsive, and dramatic
- is overly concerned with appearance
- shows an overly flirtatious and seductive behavior
- is vain with much concern about appearance with possible exhibitionism
- has an intense affect
- does not tolerate being alone
- is egocentric, self-indulgent, and lacking in consideration of others

Rx:

- Individual psychotherapy with focus on solving client's problems rather than making permanent personality changes
- Pharmacologic therapy may be used to relieve some symptoms such as depression or anxiety

NARCISSISTIC PERSONALITY DISORDER

S&S: The client

- has an increased sense of self-importance
- has a constant need for attention and admiration
- lacks empathy and may use people to achieve own goals
- is self-absorbed and self-centered
- expects to be seen as superior
- is driven and goal oriented
- exaggerates talents, achievements, and self-importance
- expects special and favorable treatment

Rx:

- Most clients seek treatment when in a crisis and then terminate it when symptoms ease
- If willing to continue treatment, long-term psychotherapy is treatment of choice
- Group therapy is not effective because client often dominates group with need for attention and sense of superiority

Nursing Process Elements

- Always approach client in a matter-of-fact manner
- Avoid reinforcing inappropriate behavior and superior view of self
- Avoid defensiveness and arguing
- Focus on positive traits
- Teach appropriate social skills

PARANOID PERSONALITY DISORDER

S&S: The client

- is suspicious and distrusting of others' motives
- is unable to confide in others
- is unable to relax
- shows social detachment and aloofness
- displays hypersensitivity

Rx:

- Individual psychotherapy.
- Pharmacologic therapy on a limited basis to treat severe symptoms of anxiety, agitation, or depression.

Nursing Process Elements

- Establish an honest therapeutic relationship using a professional approach rather than a casual approach
- Listen to client's expression of feelings without becoming defensive or arguing
- Do not challenge the paranoid beliefs
- Identify behaviors that negatively impact relationships and how such behaviors affect others

SCHIZOID PERSONALITY DISORDER

S&S: The client

- shows social detachment and lack of close relationships
- shows emotional detachment
- has a lack of strong emotions with little outward sign of change in mood
- is unconcerned with others' feelings
- is indifferent to praise or criticism
- does not have close friends and is not at ease with people
- seldom feels pleasure

Rx:

- Short-term psychotherapy when individual seeks therapy
  —Usually will not seek therapy unless under extreme stress
- Group therapy
- Cognitive therapy
- Support groups
- Pharmacologic therapy as needed for overlapping disorders such as depression

DISSOCIATIVE DISORDERS

- Dissociative disorder refers to a disruption in functions of memory, consciousness, or identity.
- It is associated with exposure to an overwhelming traumatic event.
- In general, it is still a poorly understood phenomenon.
- It is classified as four types:
  —dissociative identity disorder
  —dissociative fugue
  —dissociative amnesia
  —depersonalization disorder

Etiology:

- Basically unknown but believed to be a defense mechanism used to cope with severe trauma.

S&S:

- Dissociative identity disorder
  —Presence of two or more distinct and unique personalities existing within the same person

—These personalities may not be aware of each other
—Each personality recurrently takes control of person's consciousness and behavior

- Dissociative fugue
  —Episodes of suddenly traveling away from home or work without any explanation and being unable to remember past or identity
  —May assume a new identity
- Dissociative amnesia
  —Inability to recall important personal information usually related to a traumatic or stressful event
  —Often does not recognize the inability to recall information
- Depersonalization disorder
  —Persistent or recurrent feeling of being detached from his or her mental processes or body
  —Feels as if watching self from a distance or living in a dream

Dx:

- There are no diagnostic tests that definitively confirm dissociative disorders. Diagnosis is based upon manifestations of the disease with data obtained from a mental-status examination, psychiatric history, and careful clinical observation

Rx:

- Individual psychotherapy
- Group therapy
- Cognitive behavioral therapy
- Pharmacologic therapy as needed for related symptoms such as depression or anxiety

Nursing Process Elements

- Establish trusting therapeutic relationship with client
- Encourage client to recognize use of defense mechanisms when faced with stressful situations
- Help client to develop effective coping skills
- Monitor for signs of possible self-harm or aggression toward others

SCHIZOPHRENIA

- Schizophrenia is a cluster of psychotic brain disorders that causes distorted and bizarre thoughts, perceptions, movements, emotions, and behavior.
- It is usually diagnosed in late adolescence or early adulthood.
- Subtypes of schizophrenia have similar features, but differ in their clinical presentations.
- Subtypes include paranoid, disorganized, undifferentiated, catatonic, and residual schizophrenia.
- It is often misunderstood by the public who may fear dangerous and uncontrollable behavior.

Etiology: Cause is uncertain, but several factors have been identified as having a high correlation with the development of schizophrenia. These include

- brain structure including imbalance in chemical neurotransmitters.
- genetic factors: studies show there is increased risk for the development of schizophrenia with a positive family history.
- psychological factors especially stress, with the presence of a genetic predisposition.
- environmental factors such as exposure to viruses in infancy or oxygen deprivation at birth.

S&S: Classified as positive, negative, and disorganized symptoms.

- Positive symptoms are those that are present but should be absent such as hallucinations. They indicate the person has lost touch with reality.
- Negative symptoms are those that reflect absence of normal characteristics such as apathy.
- Disorganized symptoms reflect abnormal thinking, inability to communicate, and strange behavior such as walking in circles or incoherent ramblings.

In general, the manifestations of schizophrenia are

- positive symptoms
  —hallucinations
  - false sensory perceptions that may involve any of the five senses
  - often manifests as voices the client hears

  —delusional ideation—a false belief with no basis in reality. Common types of delusions include
  - persecutory/paranoid—belief that "others" are following, tormenting, or planning to harm the client
  - grandiose—belief of being more important or of having powers others do not have
- negative symptoms
  —flat or blunted affect
  —poverty of speech
  —lack of self-care
  —social withdrawal
  —anhedonia: inability to experience pleasure or joy in life
- disorganized symptoms
  —abnormal speech patterns such as
  - word salad—jumbled words or phrases that are disconnected and make no sense to the listener ("See her dress, car, clouds, wall.")
  - clang associations—words that rhyme or sound alike ("Look at the cow, wow, how, pow.")

  - echolalia—imitation or repetition of what someone else says
- neologisms—inventing new words which are only meaningful to that person
- latency of response—longer than usual hesitation when responding to questions
- loose association and flight of ideas—rapid succession of incomplete ideas that are not connected
  —Bizarre behaviors, examples include inappropriate laughing, walking in circles, and repeated gestures

Dx:

- There are no diagnostic tests that definitively confirm schizophrenia. Diagnosis is based upon manifestations of the disease with data obtained from a mental-status examination, psychiatric history, and careful clinical observation.
- A thorough physical and psychiatric evaluation is needed to rule out other possible causes of the symptoms such as a brain tumor or thyroid disorder.

Rx: The primary treatment of schizophrenia is drug therapy to control the main symptoms. In addition, other treatments such as psychotherapy, vocational counseling, and structured milieu therapy are needed to assist the client with social adjustment.

- Drug Therapy—Use of antipsychotic drugs is a critical component in symptom reduction. Two categories of antipsychotics are available: conventional and atypical. In addition, anti-Parkinsonism medications are often used to prevent or manage extrapyramidal effects (EPS).
- Conventional or typical antipsychotic medications, for example, haloperidol (Haldol) and chlorpromazine (Thorazine)
  —effectively treat the positive symptoms but have no therapeutic effect on the negative symptoms.
  —are used less frequently mostly because they are only partially effective.

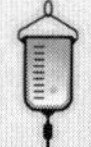

Clinical Alert

Typical antipsychotic medications haloperidol (Haldol) and fluphenazine (Prolixin) may be suggested for noncompliant clients because they are available in long-acting injection form.

- Atypical antipsychotic medications, for example, risperidone (Risperdal) and olanzapine (Zyprexa)
  —aid in relief of both positive and negative symptoms
  —are less likely to cause the side effects of EPS or tardive dyskinesia (TD)

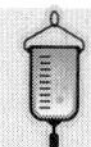

Clinical Alert

Clozapine (Clozaril) is an atypical antipsychotic medication that may cause agranulocytosis—a potentially fatal blood disorder marked by a very low WBC count. WBC counts must be performed every 2 weeks.

- Side effects of antipsychotic medications:
  —Sedation
  —Photosensitivity
  —Anticholinergic effects including orthostatic hypotension, tachycardia, dry mouth, constipation, blurred vision, and urinary retention (These side effects may lessen over time.)
  —EPS

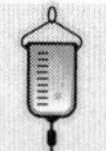

Clinical Alert

All EPS effects are reversible and can be treated with anticholinergic medications.

- Pseudoparkinsonism—includes shuffling gait, mask-like face, muscle stiffness, drooling, and difficulty in initiating movement
- Akathisia—characterized by restless movement, pacing, unable to remain still, report of inner restlessness
- Dystonia—characterized by spasms in particular muscle groups such as the neck muscles. May be accompanied by protrusion of the tongue and dysphagia. Laryngeal and pharyngeal spasms can compromise the client's airway causing a medical emergency
  —TD is a late-appearing side effect and includes manifestations such as involuntary and abnormal movements of the mouth, tongue, face, and jaw. It may progress to include the limbs

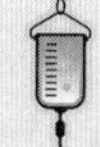

Clinical Alert

TD is an irreversible condition. Put these medications on hold and report findings to health care provider immediately.

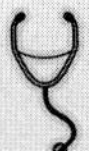

Assessment Alert

Administer the Abnormal and Involuntary Movement Scale (AIMS) to assess clients on antipsychotic medications.

—Neuroleptic malignant syndrome (NMS) is a potentially lethal side effect that requires emergency treatment. Manifestation include
- hyperthermia
- muscle rigidity
- tremors
- altered consciousness
- tachycardia
- hypertension
- incontinence

- Anti-Parkinsonism (anticholinergic) medications are often used to prevent or manage EPS of antipsychotic mediations. Examples include benztropine (Cogentin) and trihexyphenidyl (Artane).

Nursing Process Elements

- Assess for the manifestations of schizophrenia. Also assess for suicidal ideation and family/community support
- Promote safety. This includes observing for signs of increasing agitation.
  —Allow personal space
  —Monitor nutritional intake
  —Assist with ADLs as needed
  —Offer a quiet environment
  —Medicate as required
  —Avoid confrontations that may incite physical acting-out behavior that might necessitate restraint or seclusion

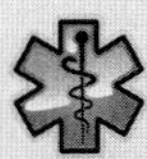

Nursing Intervention Alert

Use touch with caution. People with schizophrenia require a large personal space and often do not trust others. Touching could lead to an aggressive reaction.

- Establish a therapeutic relationship
  —Give clear explanations of rules and processes to follow
  —Use therapeutic communication
- Interventions for delusional thoughts
  —Initially, do not argue or try to convince the client that delusions are not real
  —Interact with the client in the here and now and on the basis of real things
  —Never convey that you believe the delusions
  —Later in the relationship and if the delusions are not fixed, nurse may interject doubt by presenting a factual account of the situation as he or she sees it
- Interventions for hallucinations
  —Provide protective supervision and appropriate space
  —Attempt to decrease the associated stimuli if possible
  —Avoid interacting as if the voices were real and let the client know you do not share the same reality. Say something like: "I know the voices are real to you, but I don't hear them."
  —Reassure client that you will not let anyone or anything hurt him or her while in the hospital
  —If client is frightened, do not ask for details of what is frightening; acknowledge you know he or she feels frightened; state that you cannot see or hear the frightening things; reaffirm belief that the client is safe
  —Attempt to determine if the voices are telling the client to do something harmful to self or others
  —If possible, engage in short periods of reality based conversation using simple concrete terms and as few words as possible because attention span is limited
  —Keep to simple, basic topics of conversation such as "What activities are planned for today?"
  —Do not share personal information or use terms such as "we", "us", or "let's." Must maintain separate identity from the client and not provide content for new imaginary figures or situations
  —Do not make promises that you may not be able to keep
  —Validate reality by orienting to time, place, and person, and who the staff are
  —Provide a structured, protective, and nonthreatening, environment with routine activities
  —Be alert for increasing anxiety and agitation then intervene as needed

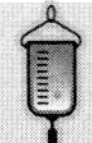

Clinical Alert

Remember, hallucinations are very real to the client and often cause them to be frightened and respond erratically.

- Promote socialization
  —If the client displays inappropriate behavior in public, attempt to redirect behavior or provide for privacy

—Remind and assist the client to attend to personal hygiene and appearance

—Identify family and community support

- Interventions for paranoia
  —Tell client what you are doing before you do it
  —Follow through on your word to promote trust
  —Do not argue or disagree; be matter of fact and accept what client says
  —Be aware of interpersonal discomfort and do not force closeness or social interaction
  —Limit number of staff members initially involved with client
  —Avoid competitive activities but encourage meaningful activities that can be easily done

Client teaching for self-care

Teach the client about

- how to manage illness and symptoms
- medication regimen
- importance of maintaining prescribed mediation regimen and regular follow-up with health care providers
- management of side-effects of medications
- never discontinuing medications abruptly
- avoiding alcohol and other drugs that are not prescribed
- need for self-care and proper nutrition
- social skills
- identifying stressful situations and ways to avoid or cope with them
- signs of relapse and what to do if they occur

Provide the client with names and contact information of community and supportive organizations and groups

Include teaching of all the above to the client's family and other support individuals

SOMATOFORM DISORDERS

- In somatoform disorders, anxiety is redirected into a somatic concern.
- The individual has excessive worry or complaints about physical illness without supporting physical findings.
- Physical signs and symptoms increase with psychosocial stress.
- Primary disorders include
  —somatization disorder
  —conversion disorder
  —hypochondriasis

Etiology:

- Exact cause is unknown.
- Thoughts about cause include theories related to
  —response to repression of emotions.
  —learned response: imitate behavior of a parent especially if secondary gains are reaped in response to the physical symptom.
    - Primary gain—direct external benefits that being sick provides such as relief of anxiety, conflict, or distress.
    - Secondary gain—internal or personal benefits received from others because one is sick such as attention form family and "special" treatment.

S&S:

- Somatization disorder
  —Multiple, usually vague physical complaints that suggest a physical disorder but have no physical basis
  —Most often complaints of GI, neurologic, cardiopulmonary, or reproductive problem
  —Often complaints involve multiple symptoms in more than one body system
  —History usually involves multiple examinations and work-ups by multiple physicians
- Conversion disorder
  —Physical symptoms such as blindness, paralysis, or inability to talk without a demonstrable physiologic basis
  —Tendency to not show concern about the symptom or limitation is a hallmark of the disorder. This is also called *la belle* indifference (French for "beautiful indifference")
  —Onset may occur at any age, but often begins in adolescence
- Hypochondriasis
  —Persistent belief that one has or is highly predisposed to get a serious disease
  —Usual focus is on one body system
  —Complaints do not fit a recognizable pattern of organic disease
  —Examination and reassurance by health provider does not relieve concerns

Dx:

- There are no diagnostic tests that definitively confirm a somatoform disorder. Diagnosis is based upon manifestations of the disease with the data obtained from a mental-status examination, psychiatric history, and careful clinical observation
- A thorough physical and psychiatric evaluation is needed to rule out other possible causes of the symptoms

Rx:

- Individual, group and family psychotherapy
- Relaxation techniques
- Pharmacological treatment as needed for related symptoms such as depression or anxiety

Nursing Process Elements

- Establish a supportive, therapeutic relationship
- Provide for physical needs when client is unable to do so, for example, if experiencing paralysis due to conversion disorder
- Encourage client to express feelings rather than repress or suppress them
- Assist client in finding ways to increase coping skills

MENTAL-HEALTH ILLNESS IN OLDER ADULTS

- Common mental-health illnesses in older populations include depression, delirium, and dementia. Table 12–3 discusses nursing strategies to manage mental-health illnesses in the older adult.
- Mental illness can be difficult for the elderly client to manage. Refer to Table 12–4 for nursing interventions to decrease stress and anxiety in the elderly client who is experiencing mental illness.

Table 12–3 Nursing Management of Mental-Health Illness in Older Adults

Illness	Factors	Symptoms	Treatment	Nursing Management
Depression	Most common mood disorder of old age; responsive to treatment; may be an early sign of chronic illness or the result of physical illness; often goes undiagnosed and untreated; alcohol abuse related to depression is significant in the elderly.	Feelings of sadness, fatigue, diminished memory and concentration; feelings of guilt or worthlessness; sleep and appetite disturbances; restlessness; and suicidal ideation	Selective-serotonin reuptake inhibitors: Paroxetine (Paxil) Tricyclic antidepressants: Nortriptyline (Aventyl), desipramine (Norpramin), doxepin (Sinequan) Arrange individual, group, or family therapy to explore feelings and utilize nonpharmacological treatment options when indicated.	Offer explanation of the illness and support for seeking treatment. Encourage expression of feelings and questions regarding treatment. Allow the client time to process any new information to decrease confusion. Encourage treatment for alcohol abuse and facilitate community resources.
Delirium	Begins with confusion and progresses to disorientation; is considered a medical emergency; secondary to physical illness, medications, alcohol toxicity, dehydration, fecal impaction, malnutrition, infection, head trauma, and sensory overload or deprivation; if left untreated, permanent brain damage can occur	Disorganized thinking, short attention span, hallucinations, delusions, fear, anxiety, and paranoia	Management varies depending on reason for the symptoms. Discontinue nonessential medications.	Provide a calm and quiet environment. Increase orientation by encouraging friends and family members to speak to and touch the client. Perform ongoing mental-status assessments to help evaluate treatment.
Dementia	Mostly affects elderly living in institutional settings; secondary to alcohol abuse, polypharmacy, and psychiatric disorders. Types of dementia include Alzheimer's disease, Parkinson's disease, AIDS-related dementia, Pick's disease.	Subtle in onset; forgetfulness, memory loss, depression, word-finding difficulty, absence of abstract thinking, impulsive behavior, difficulty maintaining activities of daily living, hostility, paranoia, suspicion, combativeness, agitation, night wandering	Medications: tacrine hydrochloride (Cognex), donepezil (Aricept), rivastigmine (Exelon)	Make certain eye glasses, hearing aids, etc., are in use to optimize ability to perceive environment. Determine how the client likes to be addressed and use consistently. Make face-to-face contact with the client. Keep the client in familiar environment. Assist with activities of daily living but do not let the client stop doing those things that he or she can.

(continued on next page)

Table 12–3 *(continued from previous page)*

Illness	Factors	Symptoms	Treatment	Nursing Management
				Remind client of what he or she can do, no matter how little. Explain physical procedures before carrying them out. Limit environmental stimuli to promote relaxation. Do not distress the client by asking a lot of questions or saying "Remember..." Prominently display clocks and calendars to orient to time. Provide a simple chart of daily activities. Encourage physical activity and communication. Use short, simple, and direct statements and talk about real, concrete, observable things. Promote independence in self-care activities. Reduce anxiety and agitation (see Table 12–4). To reduce confusion occurring at night (sun downing), leave a night light and radio on or have someone stay nearby.

Table 12–4 Nursing Interventions to Decrease Anxiety in Mentally Ill Older Adults

Provide an uncluttered, familiar, and noise-free environment
Remain calm and unhurried when delivering care to the client
For clients who become agitated, provide music, distraction, and stroking. Structure activities to provide distraction
Use clear, easy-to-understand language when communicating with the client
Promote independence in self-care activities. Organize daily activities into short, manageable tasks to give the client a sense of accomplishment
Balance activity and rest periods
Teach the client to listen to soft music or drink warm milk to induce sleep

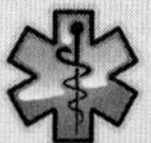

Nursing Intervention Alert

Anticholinergic, cardiac, and orthostatic side effects, as well as interactions with other medications require that antidepressants are prescribed and administered with care.

A summary of some common mental illnesses including their symptoms, treatments, and appropriate nursing interventions are given in Table 12–5.

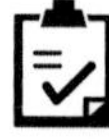

Client teaching for self-care

Summarizing the important points of client teaching, the nurse must teach

Table 12–5 Summary Comparison of Common Mental Illnesses

Mental Illness	Symptoms	Treatment	Nursing Intervention
Alzheimer's disease	• Forgetfulness or memory loss • Depression • Disorientation • Speech difficulties • Impulsive behavior • Difficulty performing activities of daily living • Personality changes • Agitation • Increase in physical activity • Sundowning	• Medications: cholinesterase inhibitors	• Maintain client safety • Reduce anxiety and agitation • Improve communication • Promote independence • Assist in socialization • Increase self-esteem • Manage sleep disturbance • Educate family and significant others
Borderline personality disorder	• Self-image rapidly changes • View self as evil or bad • Frequent changes in jobs, friendships, goals, values, and gender identity • Engage in impulsive, risky behavior • Inappropriate anger • Fear of being alone • Strong emotions that wax and wane frequently • Difficulty controlling emotions or impulses	• Psychotherapy • Medications: antidepressants, antipsychotics, and anxiolytics	• Encourage adherence to the treatment plan • Encourage regular attendance at therapy sessions • Explore client feelings of self-blame • Assist client in recognizing symptoms of compulsive behavior, such as substance abuse and facilitate community resources and support systems.
Bipolar disorder	• Manic episode: elevated mood (feeling extremely happy), irritability, anxiousness, rapid speech, decreased need for sleep, impulsive behavior, delusions, hallucinations, paranoia • Depressive episode: overwhelming feelings of emptiness or sadness, lack of energy, loss of interest in activities, impaired concentration, sleep disturbances, appetite disturbances, suicidal ideation	• Psychotherapy • Medications: antidepressants, anxiolytics, antimanics, anticonvulsants	• Maintain client safety • Assist client in recognizing symptoms of manic and depressive episodes • Explore client feelings of depression • Assist client in establishing behavioral boundaries • Facilitate community resources and support systems
Depression	• Feelings of sadness • Fatigue • Diminished memory and concentration • Feelings of guilt or worthlessness • Sleep disturbances • Appetite disturbances • Restlessness • Impaired attention span • Suicidal ideation	• Antidepressants • Psychotherapy • Electroconvulsive therapy	• Maintain client safety • Encourage client participation in decisions related to care • Encourage self-care • Consider the client's background, capabilities, interests, values and beliefs, culture, and lifestyle when planning care • Facilitate individual, group, and family therapy when appropriate. Incorporate therapy goals into the plan of care • Provide education to the client, family, and significant others
Schizophrenia	• Delusions • Hallucinations • Incoherent speech • Lack of emotions or inappropriate display of emotions • Paranoia • Social isolation • Poor hygiene • Lack of coordination	• Psychotherapy • Medications: antipsychotics	• Maintain client safety • Orient the client to surroundings and time • Encourage self-care • Assist in boundary compliance • Assist with communication • Encourage regular attendance at therapy sessions • Facilitate community resources and support systems

- the client, family, and significant others about the importance of functioning within the therapeutic environment and complying with boundaries
- the client about the importance of attending community meetings and therapy sessions
- the family to identify stressors and their impact on the client's recovery
- the client, family, and significant others about strategies to manage anxiety
- the family and significant others to gently orient the client to the surrounding environment and the present time
- the client about healthy ways to ease painful emotions, rather than to inflict self-injury
- the client, family, and significant others to recognize situations that trigger angry outbursts or impulsive behavior

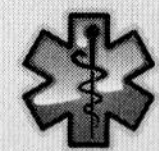

Nursing Intervention Alert

Smokers may need higher doses of antipsychotic medication because nicotine interferes with these medications.

CHEMICAL AND OTHER DEPENDENCIES

- Substance abuse results when the client is not able to cope with the burdens of life.
- Chemical dependency is significantly related to risk-taking behavior.
- Many clients deny or understate the degree to which they use alcohol and drugs. Refer Table 12–6 for commonly abused substances.
- The nurse may ask questions such as "What kind of alcohol do you enjoy drinking at a party?" to gather specifics about a client's behaviors.
- The nurse documents the specific type of substance ingested, inhaled, or injected (beer, crack cocaine, heroin, nicotine, caffeine, etc.) and the amount per day or week (12-12 oz beers a week for 3 years, 2 packs of cigarettes per day for 20 years).
- Alcohol abuse screening questionnaires such as CAGE, AUDIT, TWEAK, or SMAST can be used to elicit information about alcohol use.
- The nurse uses a nonjudgmental approach when questioning clients.
- The nurse understands that many clients who abuse substances take a variety of drugs simultaneously (alcohol, barbiturates, opioids, and tranquilizers).
- The nurse approaches substance abusers in a calm, consistent, and accepting manner because substance abuse impairs thought processes.
- The nurse assists the client, family, and significant others in identifying behaviors associated with chemical dependency and abuse.
- Clients who are aggressive or belligerent may require sedation.
- The nurse monitors appropriate clients for delirium tremens—the most severe form of alcohol withdrawal. Symptoms include anxiety, uncontrollable fear, tremor, irritability, agitation, hallucinations, and insomnia. This condition is life-threatening and requires immediate intervention.
- In the presence of delirium tremens or drug toxicity, the nurse maintains client safety, administers medications used in treatment, and promotes a quiet environment for recovery. The client's private room remains lighted to minimize the potential for hallucinations.
- The client is observed for suicidal behavior and is later referred to a rehabilitation center for treatment and counseling.
- The nurse helps the family members confront the situation, decrease their enabling behaviors, and motivate the client to obtain treatment.
- Some family members of substance abusers exhibit codependent behavior like exercising control over others, remaining involved and suffering with a client who has a drug problem, and struggling with the need to be needed. The nurse guides the family in breaking this unhealthy pattern.
- Social support services for the client, family, and significant others include Alcoholics Anonymous, Narcotics Anonymous, Al-Anon, Alateen, and church groups.
- The nurse works with the client, family, and significant others to prevent and prepare for relapse. Relapse is viewed and treated in the same way as chronic illness.
- Nonsubstance-related dependencies include gambling, sexual addiction, and pornography.

Table 12–6 Commonly Abused Substances

Substance	Effect of Substance	Effect of Withdrawal	Treatment	Nursing Interventionsn
Alcohol	Drunkenness, drowsiness, behavioral changes, poor judgment, coordination difficulty, slurred speech, aggression, inappropriate sexual behavior, nystagmus, memory problems, poor attention span, stupor, coma	Agitation, altered consciousness, aggressiveness, fear, anxiety, confusion, disorientation, delusions, hallucinations, insomnia, blackouts, acute psychosis, profuse sweating, tachycardia, hypertension, tachypnea, grand mal seizures, anorexia, nausea, abdominal cramps, vomiting, tremors	• Detoxification • Medication: benzodiazepines, anti-seizure medications • Psychotherapy • Behavior therapy • Twelve-step support groups • Halfway houses • Day or night hospitalization	• Maintain client safety • Monitor vital signs and neurologic status; notify physician of abnormal readings • Provide a quiet environment with a light on • Orient client to place, person, and time • Record I&O • Allow client to express fears and anxiety • Implement seizure precautions • Allow ambulation ad lib • Provide small, frequent, high-carbohydrate feedings • Provide support to the client, family, and significant others
Barbiturates Amobarbital (Amytal), pentobarbital (Nembutal), secobarbital (Seconal)	Sluggish coordination, emotional lability, aggressiveness, faulty judgment, nystagmus, diplopia, strabismus, decreased reflexes, ataxic gait, stupor, bradycardia, respiratory depression, decreased tendon reflexes	Anxiety, irritability, tachycardia, tachypnea, muscle pain, nausea, tremors, hallucinations, confusion, seizures, insomnia, vivid dreaming, coma, death	• Detoxification • Medications: slowly taper the abused barbiturate; sodium bicarbonate promotes excretion of barbiturates; use activated charcoal for overdose • Psychotherapy • Behavior therapy • Twelve-step support groups • Halfway houses • Day or night hospitalization	• Maintain client safety • Maintain airway • Monitor for alcohol abuse • Monitor vital signs and neurologic status; notify physician of abnormal readings • Provide a quiet environment with a light switched on • Orient client to place, person, and time • Control combative behavior • Allow client to express fears and anxiety • Implement seizure precautions
Benzodiazepines: Diazepam (Valium) Lorazepam (Ativan)	Sleepiness and deep sleep, slurred speech, poor coordination and falling, poor thought processes, weak comprehension, memory difficulty, poor judgment, mood swings, nystagmus, constricted pupils, tachypnea	Anxiety, panic attacks, rage, insomnia, nightmares, depression, dizziness, shaking, nausea, constipation, diarrhea, headache, muscle pain, sweating, tachycardia, paresthesia, seizures, death if combined with alcohol	• Detoxification • Medications: antagonist flumazenil (Romazicon); slowly taper the abused benzodiazepine • Psychotherapy • Behavior therapy • Twelve-step support groups • Halfway houses • Day or night hospitalization	• Maintain client safety • Monitor for alcohol abuse • Monitor vital signs and neurologic status; notify physician of abnormal readings • Monitor for dysrhythmias • Provide a quiet environment • Allow client to express fears and anxiety • Implement seizure precautions

(continued on next page)

Table 12–6 *(continued from previous page)*

Substance	Effect of Substance	Effect of Withdrawal	Treatment	Nursing Interventionsn
Cocaine Cocaine hydrochloride (sniffed), free-base cocaine (smoked), crack cocaine (small rocks that are smoked); cocaine may be injected intravenously	Euphoria, feelings of confidence, risk taking behavior, anorexia, inappropriate sexual behavior, tachycardia, tachypnea, hypertension, dilated pupils, nervousness, agitation, fever, inability to concentrate	Psychosis, hallucinations, delusions, depression, paranoia, ideas of persecution, hypervigilance, aggression, tremors, insomnia, fatigue, muscle pain, suicidal ideation, nausea, vomiting, general malaise	• Detoxification • Medications: antidepressants, antipsychotics • Charcoal to treat ingested cocaine • Psychotherapy • Behavior therapy • Twelve-step support groups • Halfway houses • Day or night hospitalization	• Ensure airway and ventilation • Maintain client safety • Monitor the client for alcohol and benzodiazepine use • Control seizures • Monitor cardiovascular status • Treat hyperthermia • Provide a quiet environment • Allow client to express fears and anxiety
Methamphetamines amphetamine (Benzedrine), dextroamphetamine (Dexedrine), MDMA (Ecstasy), methylphenidate (Ritalin)	Increased attention, decreased fatigue, increased activity, decreased appetite, euphoria, hyperthermia, tachycardia	Restlessness, insomnia, irritability, confusion, panic, paranoia, homicidal behavior, depression with suicidal ideation, hallucinations, nausea, vomiting, chills	• Detoxification • Medications: small doses of diazepam IV or haloperidol to combat CNS hyperactivity; treat seizures with benzodiazepines • Activated charcoal for overdose • Psychotherapy • Behavior therapy • Twelve-step support groups • Halfway houses • Day or night hospitalization	• Maintain client safety • Monitor for suicide attempts • Maintain airway • Maintain a calm, cool, quiet environment • Monitor vital signs and neurologic status; notify physician of abnormal readings • Allow client to express fears and anxiety
Nicotine Tobacco smoking, chewing, dipping	Mild euphoria, anorexia, feelings of relaxation, tachycardia, hypertension	Irritability, restlessness, difficulty in concentrating, insomnia, depression, increased appetite, weight gain	• Detoxification • Medications: nicotine gum, nicotine nasal sprays, nicotine patches • Psychotherapy • Behavior therapy • Support groups	• Maintain client safety • Monitor vital signs and neurologic status; notify physician of abnormal readings • Allow client to express fears and anxiety • Offer support to client, family, and significant others
Opioids Heroin, codeine, hydromorphone (Dilaudid), meperidine (Demerol), methadone, propoxyphene (Darvon), oxycodone (OxyContin), fentanyl (Sublimaze)	Temporary sense of well-being, poor coordination, drowsiness, light-headedness, impaired thought processes, confusion, memory difficulty	Gastrointestinal distress, anxiety, nausea, insomnia, muscle pain, fevers and chills, sweating, runny nose and eyes, tachypnea, coma, pinpoint pupils	• Detoxification • Medications: opiate antagonist naloxone (Narcan) IV in emergency situations; in morphine and heroin addicts, give methadone daily to stabilize the client; in other opioid addicts, slowly taper the abused opioid • Psychotherapy • Twelve-step support groups • Halfway houses • Day or night hospitalization	• Maintain client safety • Do not leave client unattended due to risk of lapsing into coma quickly • Maintain airway • Monitor for pulmonary edema • Monitor vital signs and neurologic status; notify physician of abnormal readings • Provide a quiet environment • Allow client to express fears and anxiety

- These addictions can cause stress, alcohol abuse, loss of income and assets, treatment nonadherence, malnutrition, safety risks related to associated alcohol usage and financial losses, and increased psychiatric problems such as depression.
- Pharmacological treatment strategies include mood stabilizers, serotonin reuptake inhibitors (SRIs), selective-serotonin reuptake inhibitors (SSRIs), and antipsychotics. Nonpharmacological treatment includes behavioral therapy to control obsessive compulsions.
- The nurse's role in management of the client who experiences dependency is to provide information and support to the client, family, and significant others, evaluate treatment measures and revise the plan of care as needed, and facilitate community resources and social support systems.

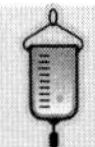

Clinical Alert

Alcohol withdrawal delirium is a life-threatening event that requires immediate intervention.

Client teaching for self-care

The nurse must teach

- the client, family, and significant others about the symptoms of chemical abuse and other dependencies
- family members and significant others about strategies to decrease codependent behavior
- the client, family, and significant others about how to access community resources and social supports
- the client, family, and significant others about the risk factors and signs of suicidal behavior, and to access help immediately if suicide is suspected

ABUSE AND VIOLENCE

ABUSE/NEGLECT

- Abuse and neglect can occur as physical, sexual, and psychological. Abuse and neglect occur at all ages and affect both genders from all socioeconomic, ethnic, and cultural groups.
- Few clients openly admit to abuse and neglect, especially elderly clients. The nurse should ask direct questions during the client's assessment. These questions should be asked in private, away from others. Refer to Table 12–7 for a list of questions to ask when assessing a client for abuse or neglect.
- All disabled and elderly clients should be assessed for possible abuse and neglect. Refer to Table 12–8 for the types of abuse and neglect directed at disabled and elderly clients.
- In caring for an elderly or disabled client who has experienced abuse or neglect, the nurse must enlist the interdisciplinary team to help the caregiver develop self-awareness, increased insight, and an understanding of the aging process and limitations of the disabled. The nurse also provides information to the client and caregiver regarding community resources and social supports.
- Domestic violence includes child abuse, elder abuse, and abuse of women and men.

Table 12–7 Abuse and Neglect Assessment Questions

Question
Sometimes women (or men or children) are forced into sexual activity. Has this ever happened to you? Has anyone ever suggested they wish to engage you in sexual activity even when you've resisted?
If the client is pregnant—Since you have been pregnant, have you been hit, slapped, kicked, or physically hurt in any other manner by someone?
Has anyone failed to help you when you needed help?
I noticed that you have a number of bruises. Can you tell me how they happened? Has anyone hurt you?
You seem anxious. Has anyone ever hurt you or threatened to do so? Are you ever afraid of anyone close to you, such as your partner, caretaker, or any other family member?
Sometimes clients tell me that they have been hurt by someone at home or work. Is this happening to you?
Has anyone ever prevented you from seeing your friends or family members?
Have you ever been pressured to sign papers you did not understand or did not wish to sign?

- Violence is rarely a one-time occurrence in a relationship; it usually continues and escalates in severity.
- Female survivors of sexual abuse have more health problems and undergo more surgeries than nonvictims.
- Victims of childhood sexual abuse experience more chronic depression, posttraumatic stress disorder, morbid obesity, marital instability, gastrointestinal problems, headaches, and greater reliance on health care services than nonvictims.
- Risk factors for abuse include high levels of stress or alcoholism in caregivers, evidence of violence, high emotions, and financial, emotional, or physical dependency.
- Client symptoms of abuse may include suicide attempts, drug and alcohol abuse, frequent emergency department visits, multiple injuries in various stages of healing, unexplained injuries, vague pelvic pain, insomnia, and depression.
- Client symptoms of neglect may include poor hygiene, unkempt appearance, hunger, dehydration, pain, inadequate clothing or shoes, unfilled medication prescriptions, missed appointments with healthcare providers, and lack of ancillary devices when warranted (cane, walker, eyeglasses, or hearing aid).
- When evidence indicates possible abuse or neglect, the nurse documents the events and provides drawings or photos of injuries. The nurse examines the entire surface of the client's body, assesses the client's interactions with significant others, and performs a mental-status examination.
- Sometimes, no obvious signs or symptoms of abuse or neglect are present.
- The nurse's primary concern is the safety of the client. The client is separated from the abuser, and the interdisciplinary team and community agencies work collaboratively to support the client.
- Alternative living arrangements may be necessary if the abuser or neglecter experiences mental illness.
- Caregivers who inflict abuse or neglect are relieved of their immediate duties by respite services. Support groups are helpful to these caregivers.
- The nurse evaluates the response of the client, family, and significant others to these interventions and updates the plan of care as necessary.

Table 12–8 Forms of Elder- and Disabled-Client Abuse

Physical violence
Personal neglect
Financial exploitation
Violation of rights
Denial of health care
Self-inflicted abuse

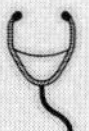

Assessment Alert

During the health history, the nurse explores the client's past coping patterns, perceptions of current stresses, and the client's expectations of family, friends, and caregivers in providing financial, emotional, and physical support.

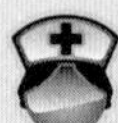

Practice Alert

The role of the nurse is not to prove the neglect or abuse, but to report it to an official agency.

Spouse or Partner Abuse

- Spouse or partner abuse may be emotional, physical, economic, sexual, or a combination which is very common.
- The most frequent abuse is that of a male on a female.
- Victims are more likely to abuse alcohol or drugs and to commit suicide.
- Attacks escalate in severity and frequency over time.
- Such abuse usually follows a cycle or pattern:
  —escalating tension
  —abuse
  —remorse, also called honeymoon period, in which the abuser
    - apologizes, promises it will never happen again
    - professes love for partner
    - often engages in romantic behaviors
    - tension-building phase begins again
  - The most dangerous period is when the victim leaves the abuser.

Nursing Process Elements

- Identify possible victims—SAFE questions
  —Stress/safety: Do you feel safe?
  —Afraid/abused: Are you ever afraid in your relationship?
  —Friends/family: Are they aware you have been hurt?
  —Emergency plan: Do you have a safe place to go and the resources you may need?
- Refer to appropriate resources
  —Police or legal aid
  —Local shelters
  —Support groups

Elder Abuse

- Elder abuse includes both abuse and neglect such as physical harm, sexual or verbal intimidation, emotional or physical neglect, and/or economic exploitation.

- The risk factors include declining strength and mobility, functional decline and dependence on others, being cared for by a family caregiver, and cognitive decline.
- Elders are often reluctant to reveal abuse out of fear of abandonment or retaliation.
- Perpetrators are usually family members.

S&S:

- Unexplained bruising, burns, or injuries
- Dehydration and malnutrition
- Oversedation
- Bruises, wounds, and pressure ulcers
- Unmet physical and medical needs
- Fearfulness
- Conflicting stories from client and caregiver
- Reports of restraints or being locked in a room

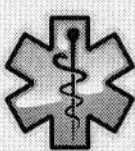

Nursing Intervention Alert

- Nursing intervention includes
  —assessing for signs of abuse or neglect
  —treating existing injuries
  —reporting abuse to appropriate authorities, for example, hotline or Adult Protective Services
- Refer to community agencies offering services to older adults and their families
  —Respite for caregivers
  —Support groups for caregivers

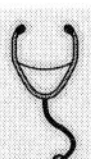

Assessment Alert

Demands of caring for a family member can exceed the caregiver's capacity for adjustment and result in anxiety, depression, and physical illness. Therefore, assessment for caregiver distress, provision of support and validation, teaching about the role of Support groups and Respite Care, and referral to appropriate community agencies for help are critical parts of the nursing role.

Sexual Abuse

- Sexual abuse ranges from sexual harassment to molestation and rape.
- Immediate consequences of rape include
  —physical injury
  —pregnancy and sexually transmitted diseases
  —rape-trauma syndrome
    - high level of anxiety
    - difficulty making decisions
    - flashbacks, violent dreams, and preoccupation with future danger
    - problems with intimate relationships
- In the long-term, the victim may experience posttraumatic stress disorder (PTSD), in which she
  —uses denial, repression, and suppression to cope with anxious feelings
  —shows symptoms including flashbacks, intrusive memories of the event, hopelessness, depression, nightmares, and outbursts of anger and rage

Nursing Process Elements

- Assess for sexualized behaviors in children
  —-"seductive" behavior used to gain affection
  —unusual curiosity regarding genitalia
  —decreased personal boundaries
  —extreme reaction to bathing
  —extraordinary fear of the opposite sex
  —unwillingness to participate in age-appropriate physical or social activity
- In the emergency department, gather evidence with permission of the victim following policies of facility and law enforcement
- Give as much control as possible to the victim during the assessment and evidence-gathering process
- Treat physical injuries
- Advise about potential for pregnancy and STDs
- Listen to the client discuss feelings about the assault
- Provide information about community services

Child Abuse

Signs of physical abuse

- Unexplained bruises or welts
  —Involve several different areas such as face, lips, and mouth or torso, back, buttocks, and thighs and show various stages of healing
  —Clustered in regular patterns often reflecting the shape of what was used to inflict injury, for example, belt, buckle, etc.
  —Often regularly appear after weekends, absences, or vacations
- Unexplained burns
  —Cigarette or cigar end shaped burns often on soles, palms, back, or buttocks
  —Immersion burns on hands and feet, appear like gloves or socks, round or donut shaped on buttocks
  —Shaped like an iron
  —Rope burns on arms, legs, neck, or torso

- Unexplained fractures particularly multiple and/or in various stages of healing
- Unexplained lacerations or abrasions especially to mouth, eyes, and external genitalia
- Reports of being injured by parents
- Expresses fear of going home
- Appears frightened of parents
- Exhibits either extreme aggressiveness or withdrawal
- Becomes apprehensive when other children cry
- Acts wary of contact with adults

Signs of physical neglect

- Always hungry
- Inappropriate dress
- Poor hygiene
- Consistent lack of supervision often for long periods of time and even when engaged in dangerous activities
- Uncared for medical or physical problems
- Abandonment
- Begging or stealing food
- Early arrival and late departure from school
- Fatigue
- Listlessness
- Alcohol or drug abuse
- Delinquency
- Reports lack of a caretaker

Risk factors for becoming an abusive parent

- Abused as a child
- Under significant stress
- Deficient in social and financial resources
- Uses inappropriate coping skills
- Lack of impulse control
- Anger and hostility
- Ambivalent toward parenthood
- Marital problems
- Mental illness
- Substance abuser
- Lack of knowledge regarding child development

Nursing Process Elements

- the client, family, and significant others about the signs of an impending crisis and effective problem-solving techniques to manage a crisis
- the client, family, and significant others about the signs of abuse and neglect, and to access help immediately if abuse or neglect are suspected
- caregivers about coping strategies to prevent abuse and neglect

Shaken Baby Syndrome

Shaken baby syndrome (SBS) is a form of physical abuse caused by rigorous shaking.

Risk factors

- Gender
- Financial stress
- Mental-health problems

S&S:

- Bulging fontanels
- Poor feeding
- Lethargy
- Seizures
- Retinal detachment
- Apnea

Nursing Process Elements

- Assure parents that age-appropriate play with infants will not cause injuries seen in SBS.

WORKSHEET

MATCHING QUESTIONS

Match the following (note that terms and/or descriptions may be used once, more than once, or not at all):

1. ___ Psychopathology a. Form of physical abuse

2. ___ Alzheimer's disease b. Screening tool for alcohol abuse

3. ___ Borderline personality disorder
4. ___ CAGE
5. ___ Bipolar disorder
6. ___ Depression
7. ___ Schizophrenia
8. ___ Suicide precautions
9. ___ Abuse
10. ___ Neglect
11. ___ Ecstasy
12. ___ Delirium tremens
13. ___ Shaken Baby Syndrome
14. ___ TWEAK
15. ___ Alateen
16. ___ Hallucinations
17. ___ Seasonal affective disorder
18. ___ Delirium
19. ___ Delusion
20. ___ Electroconvulsive therapy (ECT)

c. False belief with no basis in reality

d. Subjective disorder of perception

e. Social support service for teenagers

f. An effective treatment for some depressions, catatonia, mania, and schizophrenia

g. A mental illness characterized by manic episodes, irritability, and anxiety

h. State of mental excitement accompanied by disorientation to time and place

i. A common mental illness characterized by prolonged feeling of sadness, fatigue, diminished concentration, and feelings of guilt or worthlessness

j. A mental illness characterized by memory loss, disorientation, speech difficulties, or impulsive behaviors; treated with cholinesterase inhibitors

k. The most severe form of alcohol withdrawal; it is life-threatening and requires immediate intervention

l. A serious mental illness characterized by delusions, hallucinations, and paranoia

m. A mood disorder related to time of year

n. A behavior-management technique used to give the client greater control over negative thinking by correcting mental distortions

o. A commonly abused substance that produces increased attention, increased activity, decreased fatigue, decreased appetite, euphoria, and hyperthermia

p. A mental illness characterized by rapid changes in self-image, inappropriate anger, and difficulty controlling emotions or impulses; treated with antidepressants, antipsychotics, and anxiolytics

q. The act of withholding care from another individual; symptoms may include: poor hygiene, hunger, dehydration, or pain

r. Measures that are ordered for clients who have either harmed themselves, have verbalized the intent to do so, or have overtly indicated a wish to do so

s. Allowing the elderly client plenty of time to answer health-related questions

t. Hearing loss due to the aging process

(continued)

u. Screening tool for psychological abuse

v. Disorders of the psyche which may be characterized by disorientation, incoherent or illogical thought, or inappropriate dress

w. A manifestation of stress experienced by clients as they face new challenges or threatening situations

x. The most commonly abused substance in the United States

y. A process that promotes expression and the exchange of ideas where the client defines himself or herself through human interaction and task accomplishment

z. The act of harming another individual in a physical, sexual, and/or psychological way

FILL IN THE BLANKS

Fill in the blank spaces with the correct word or phrase to complete each statement.

1. ________ is a common mental illness affecting the elderly that is characterized by forgetfulness, memory loss, depression, disorientation, and impulsive behavior.
2. Bipolar disorder is characterized by an extreme elevation in mood called a ________.
3. ________ is sometimes referred to as an emotional regulation disorder.
4. Smokers may need higher doses of antipsychotic medications because ________ interferes with these medications.
5. ________ includes child abuse, elder abuse, and abuse of women and men.
6. Symptoms of ________ abuse include drowsiness, behavioral changes, slurred speech, and nystagmus.
7. ________ is given for an overdose of methamphetamines.
8. Desensitization therapy may be used in the treatment of ________ disorders.
9. Psychotherapy with the goal of helping the client see the relationship between feelings and behaviors is the treatment of choice for ________________.
10. Extrapyramidal effects of antipsychotic drugs can be treated with ________ medications.

TRUE & FALSE QUESTIONS

Mark each of the following statements True or False. Correct all false statements in the space provided.

1. Because they are available in long-acting injectable form, the antipsychotic drugs haloperidol (Haldol) and fluphenazine (Prolixin) may be used for noncompliant clients. ____ T ____ F
2. Persons with schizophrenia prefer a smaller personal space than usual. ____ T ____ F

3. Mood disorders are diagnosed based on clinical presentation because there are no definitive diagnostic tests. ___ T ___ F

4. Smokers may need lower doses of antipsychotic medications because of the interaction with nicotine. ___ T ___ F

5. Family reaction to a diagnosis of mental illness may include disbelief, anxiety, confusion, and denial. ___ T ___ F

6. Poor hygiene, inappropriate dress, disorientation, and absent memory recall may be evidence of psychopathology. ___ T ___ F

7. Strong emotions that wax and wane frequently and difficulty controlling these emotions are symptoms of Alzheimer's disease. ___ T ___ F

8. Schizophrenia is characterized by delusions, hallucinations, social isolation, and paranoia. ___ T ___ F

9. Abuse and neglect occur at all ages and affect both genders from all socioeconomic, ethnic, and cultural groups. ___ T ___ F

10. Common substance-related dependencies include alcohol, gambling, and pornography. ___ T ___ F

MATCHING QUESTIONS

Match the following (note that descriptions may be used once, more than once, or not at all):

1. ___ Diazepam (Valium)	a. Benzodiazepine antianxiety agent
2. ___ Escitalopram (Lexapro)	b. Monoamine oxidase inhibitor (MAOI) antidepressant
3. ___ Phenelzine (Nardil)	c. Benzodiazepine antagonist
4. ___ Sertraline (Zoloft)	d. Psychedelic
5. ___ Methylphenidate (Ritalin)	e. Selective serotonin reuptake inhibitor antidepressant
6. ___ Buspirone (Buspar)	f. Methamphetamine
7. ___ Tranylcypromine (Parnate)	g. Opiate antagonist
8. ___ Lorazepam (Ativan)	h. Antipsychotic
9. ___ Flumazenil (Romazicon)	i. Serotonin modulator antidepressant
10. ___ Naloxone (Narcan)	j. Tricyclic antidepressant
11. ___ Chlorpromazine HCl (Thorazine)	k. Alcohol deterrent
12. ___ Bupropion (Wellbutrin)	l. Antimania (mood stabilizing) agent
13. ___ Loxapine (Loxitane)	m. Anti-Parkinsonism agent

(continued)

14. ___ Amitriptyline HCl (Elavil)
15. ___ Disulfiram (Antabuse)
16. ___ Trazodone (Desyrel)
17. ___ Lithium carbonate (Eskalith)
18. ___ Benztropine (Cogentin)
19. ___ Nortriptyline HCl (Aventyl)
20. ___ Paroxetine (Paxil)
21. ___ Haloperidol (Haldol)
22. ___ Carbamazepine (Tegretol)
23. ___ Venlafaxine (Effexor)
24. ___ Fluphenazine (Prolixin)
25. ___ Valproic acid (Depokene)
26. ___ Fluoxetine (Prozac)
27. ___ Chlordiazepoxide (Librium)
28. ___ Risperidone (Risperdal)
29. ___ Alprazolam (Xanax)
30. ___ Clonazepam (Klonopin)
31. ___ Doxepin (Sinequan)
32. ___ Imipramine HCl (Tofranil)
33. ___ Clozapine (Clozaril)
34. ___ Olanzapine (Zyprexa)
35. ___ Citalopram (Celexa)

n. Anticonvulsant

o. Other antianxiety agent

p. Other antidepressant

APPLICATION QUESTIONS

1. Domestic violence is rarely a one-time occurrence in a relationship; it usually continues and escalates in severity. Which factors increase the risk of an individual becoming violent? (Select all that apply.)

   a. Alcoholism
   b. High stress levels
   c. Financial independency
   d. Physical dependency

2. Which symptoms are indicative of neglect? (Select all that apply.)
   a. Emergency department visits
   b. Missed appointments with health care providers
   c. Dehydration
   d. Unexplained injuries
3. A nurse in an Emergency Department (ED) is caring for a client who has been drinking alcohol everyday for the past 10 days. The client is drowsy, has slurred speech, and lacks coordination. As the client experiences alcohol withdrawal, which potential side effect concerns the nurse most?
   a. Anxiety
   b. Hypoglycemia
   c. Esophagitis
   d. Delirium tremens
4. Which nursing interventions are appropriate for a client experiencing alcohol withdrawal? (Select all that apply.)
   a. Provide a private, lighted environment for recovery
   b. Implement seizure precautions
   c. Orient the client to person, place, and time
   d. Provide small, frequent, high-carbohydrate feedings
5. A nurse in the Emergency Department is caring for a client who has been smoking crack cocaine. The client's pupils are dilated and the client is euphoric, tachycardic, and agitated. As the client experiences withdrawal from crack cocaine, which side effects should the nurse anticipate? (Select all that apply.)
   a. Psychosis
   b. Hallucinations
   c. Illusions
   d. Nausea and vomiting
6. Opioids are often prescribed by physicians for pain control and are commonly abused substances. Which medications are opioids? (Select all that apply.)
   a. Hydromorphone (Dilaudid)
   b. Meperidine (Demerol)
   c. MDMA (Ecstasy)
   d. Lorazepam (Ativan)
7. A nurse is discharging a client from a psychiatric unit who has been under suicide precautions. The nurse is providing discharge teaching to the client and the family. Which content would be appropriate for the nurse to teach? (Select all that apply.)
   a. Signs of an impending crisis
   b. Signs of suicidal behavior
   c. Signs of chemical abuse and dependency
   d. Signs of emotional abuse
8. Electroconvulsive therapy (ECT) is used as an effective treatment for which mental disorders? (Select all that apply.)
   a. Depression
   b. Severe catatonia
   c. Mania
   d. Schizophrenia
9. A nurse on a psychiatric unit is performing an initial assessment on the mental health of a client. Which assessment finding could be indicative of psychopathology? (Select all that apply.)
   a. Calm affect
   b. Disorientation
   c. Inappropriate dress
   d. Poor hygiene
10. A nurse in a long-term care facility is admitting an elderly client. The family informs the nurse that the client became forgetful a couple of years ago but now cannot remember family members' names and has become disoriented, impulsive, and easily agitated. Which common mental illness is most likely affecting the elderly client?
    a. Borderline personality disorder
    b. Bipolar disorder
    c. Schizophrenia
    d. Alzheimer's disease
11. A nurse in a psychiatric unit is caring for a client who engages in impulsive, risky behavior, has strong emotions that frequently wax and wane, and has difficulty controlling emotions and impulses. Which common mental illness is most likely affecting the client?
    a. Borderline personality disorder
    b. Bipolar disorder
    c. Schizophrenia
    d. Alzheimer's disease
12. A nurse in a psychiatric unit is caring for a client who is delusional, paranoid, and has been diagnosed with schizophrenia. Which type of medication is commonly used to treat schizophrenia?
    a. H2 inhibitors
    b. Cholinesterase inhibitors
    c. Antipsychotics
    d. Antiemetics

(continued)

13. A nurse is caring for an elderly client in a long-term care facility. The nurse knows that the client is most likely to experience which mental-health illness?
    a. Dementia
    b. Delirium
    c. Depression
    d. Dysgraphia

14. Antidepressant medications must be prescribed and administered with care, particularly when being given to elderly clients. Which adverse effects should the nurse anticipate when administering antidepressants to elderly clients? (Select all that apply.)
    a. Anticholinergic effects
    b. Cardiac effects
    c. Agitation
    d. Hostility

15. A nurse is caring for an elderly client who is experiencing dementia. Which assessment findings would the nurse expect? (Select all that apply.)
    a. Forgetfulness
    b. Memory loss
    c. Hostility
    d. Hallucinations

16. When speaking to a community group on the topic of dementia, which medications would be identified as currently being used in its treatment? (Select all that apply.)
    a. Nortriptyline (Aventyl)
    b. Donepezil (Aricept)
    c. Doxepin (Sinequan)
    d. Rivastigmine (Exelon)

17. Which statement made by a participant in a seminar on delirium indicates that additional clarification is needed?
    a. "If untreated, permanent brain damage can occur."
    b. "It is considered a medical emergency."
    c. "It mostly affects elderly living in institutional settings."
    d. "It may result in hallucinations."

18. For which client would the nurse expect the plan of care to include assessment using the Abnormal and Involuntary Movement Scale (AIMS)?
    a. Client with panic disorder
    b. Client with schizophrenia taking chlorpromazine (thorazine)
    c. Client with a mood disorder taking amitryptyline (Elavil)
    d. Client taking buproprion (Wellbutrin)
    e. Client taking paroxetine (Paxil)

19. Which assessment finding should the nurse interpret as indicative of agranulocytosis in a client taking clozapine (Clozaril)?
    a. Photosensitivity
    b. Tachycardia
    c. Low WBC
    d. Orthostatic hypotension

20. Which signs and symptoms are expected effects associated with withdrawal from oxycodone (OxyContin)? (Select all that apply.)
    a. Fevers and chills
    b. Runny nose and eyes
    c. Dilated pupils
    d. Paranoia
    e. Muscle pain
    f. Nausea
    g. Insomnia
    h. Tachypnea
    i. Hallucinations

21. When assessing a client for cocaine use, for which signs would the nurse observe? (Select all that apply.)
    a. Hypotension
    b. Tachycardia
    c. Tachypnea
    d. Dilated pupils
    e. Agitation
    f. Lack of concentration
    g. Slurred speech
    h. Poor coordination
    i. Hypervigilance
    j. Tremors

22. When caring for a client being withdrawn from barbiturate use, which nursing intervention is appropriate?
    a. Institute seizure precautions
    b. Keep the room dark and quiet
    c. Monitor for dysrhythmias
    d. Observe for suicide attempts

23. When discussing obsessive-compulsive disorder with the parents of a newly diagnosed child, the nurse bases the discussion of the compulsive behavior on the knowledge that the behavior serves to
    a. control unacceptable impulses
    b. dissipate excess energy

c. manipulate the environment
d. decrease anxiety

24. When reinforcing "negative thought stopping," which direction might the nurse give?
    a. When a negative thought occurs, immediately verbalize out loud an opposing positive thought.
    b. At least once per hour while awake, focus for 60 seconds on a positive thought.
    c. When a negative thought occurs, perform a distracting activity, and then think a positive thought.
    d. When you recognize a negative thought, repeat your positive mantra to yourself until the thought disappears.
25. When giving dietary instructions to a client for whom an MAO inhibitor has been prescribed, which foods would the nurse tell the client to avoid?
    a. Yellow vegetables, cereals and, chicken eggs
    b. Cheese, avocados, bananas, beer, and wine
    c. Beef, broccoli, cauliflower, and rice
    d. Mushrooms, salmon, celery, and grapefruit

ANSWERS & RATIONALES

MATCHING ANSWERS

Match the following (note that terms and/or descriptions may be used once, more than once, or not at all):

1. _v_ Psychopathology	a. Form of physical abuse
2. _j_ Alzheimer's disease	b. Screening tool for alcohol abuse
3. _p_ Borderline personality disorder	c. False belief with no basis in reality
4. _b_ CAGE	d. Subjective disorder of perception
5. _g_ Bipolar disorder	e. Social support service for teenagers
6. _i_ Depression	f. An effective treatment for some depressions, catatonia, mania, and schizophrenia
7. _l_ Schizophrenia	g. A mental illness characterized by manic episodes, irritability, and anxiety
8. _r_ Suicide precautions	h. State of mental excitement accompanied by disorientation to time and place
9. _z_ Abuse	i. A common mental illness characterized by prolonged feeling of sadness, fatigue, diminished concentration, and feelings of guilt or worthlessness
10. _q_ Neglect	j. A mental illness characterized by memory loss, disorientation, speech difficulties, or impulsive behaviors; treated with cholinesterase inhibitors
11. _o_ Ecstasy	
12. _k_ Delirium tremens	k. The most severe form of alcohol withdrawal; is life-threatening and requires immediate intervention
13. _a_ Shaken Baby Syndrome	

(continued)

14. b TWEAK

15. e Alateen

16. d Hallucinations

17. m Seasonal affective disorder

18. h Delirium

19. c Delusion

20. f Electroconvulsive therapy (ECT)

l. A serious mental illness characterized by delusions, hallucinations, and paranoia

m. A mood disorder related to time of year

n. A behavior-management technique used to give the client greater control over negative thinking by correcting mental distortions

o. A commonly abused substance that produces increased attention, increased activity, decreased fatigue, decreased appetite, euphoria, and hyperthermia

p. A mental illness characterized by rapid changes in self-image, inappropriate anger, and difficulty controlling emotions or impulses; treated with antidepressants, antipsychotics, and anxiolytics

q. The act of withholding care from another individual; symptoms may include: poor hygiene, hunger, dehydration, or pain

r. Measures that are ordered for clients who have either harmed themselves, have verbalized the intent to do so, or have overtly indicated a wish to do so

s. Allowing the elderly client plenty of time to answer health-related questions

t. Hearing loss due to the aging process

u. Screening tool for psychological abuse

v. Disorders of the psyche which may be characterized by disorientation, incoherent or illogical thought, or inappropriate dress

w. A manifestation of stress experienced by clients as they face new challenges or threatening situations

x. The most commonly abused substance in the United States

y. A process that promotes expression and the exchange of ideas where the client defines himself or herself through human interaction and task accomplishment

z. The act of harming another individual in a physical, sexual, and/or psychological way

ANSWERS FOR FILL IN THE BLANKS

Fill in the blank space with the correct word or phrase to complete each statement.

1. Alzheimer's disease is a common mental illness affecting the elderly that is characterized by forgetfulness, memory loss, depression, disorientation, and impulsive behavior.
2. Bipolar disorder is characterized by an extreme elevation in mood called a manic episode.
3. Borderline personality disorder is sometimes referred to as an emotional regulation disorder.
4. Smokers may need higher doses of antipsychotic medications because nicotine interferes with these medications.
5. Domestic violence includes child abuse, elder abuse, and abuse of women and men.
6. Symptoms of alcohol abuse include drowsiness, behavioral changes, slurred speech, and nystagmus.
7. Activated charcoal is given for an overdose of methamphetamines.
8. Desensitization therapy may be used in the treatment of phobic disorders.
9. Psychotherapy with the goal of helping the client see the relationship between feelings and behaviors is the treatment of choice for antisocial personality disorder.
10. Extrapyramidal effects of antipsychotic drugs can be treated with anticholinergic medications.

TRUE & FALSE ANSWERS

Mark each of the following statements True or False. Correct all false statements in the space provided.

1. Because they are available in long-acting injectable form, the antipsychotic drugs haloperidol (Haldol) and fluphenazine (Prolixin) may be used for noncompliant clients. *True*
2. Persons with schizophrenia prefer a smaller personal space than usual. *False*

Persons with schizophrenia prefer a larger personal space than usual; in fact, touch may precipitate aggression.

3. Mood disorders are diagnosed based on clinical presentation because there are no definitive diagnostic tests. *True*
4. Smokers may need lower doses of antipsychotic medications because of the interaction with nicotine. *False*

Smokers may need higher doses of antipsychotic medications because of the interaction with nicotine.

5. Family reaction to a diagnosis of mental illness may include disbelief, anxiety, confusion, and denial. *True*
6. Poor hygiene, inappropriate dress, disorientation, and absent memory recall may be evidence of psychopathology. *True*

(continued)

7. Strong emotions that wax and wane frequently and difficulty controlling these emotions are symptoms of Alzheimer's disease. *False*

Strong emotions that wax and wane frequently and difficulty controlling these emotions are symptoms of borderline personality disorder.

8. Schizophrenia is characterized by delusions, hallucinations, social isolation, and paranoia. *True*

9. Abuse and neglect occur at all ages and affect both genders from all socioeconomic, ethnic, and cultural groups. *True*

10. Common substance-related dependencies include alcohol, gambling, and pornography. *False*

Gambling and pornography are non–substance-related dependencies.

MATCHING ANSWERS

Match the following (note that descriptions may be used once, more than once, or not at all):

Column A	Column B
1. a Diazepam (Valium)	a. Benzodiazepine antianxiety agent
2. e Escitalopram (Lexapro)	b. Monoamine oxidase inhibitor (MAOI) antidepressant
3. b Phenelzine (Nardil)	c. Benzodiazepine antagonist
4. e Sertraline (Zoloft)	d. Psychedelic
5. f Methylphenidate (Ritalin)	e. Selective serotonin reuptake inhibitor antidepressant
6. o Buspirone (BuSpar)	f. Methamphetamine
7. b Tranylcypromine (Parnate)	g. Opiate antagonist
8. a Lorazepam (Ativan)	h. Antipsychotic
9. c Flumazenil (Romazicon)	i. Serotonin modulator antidepressant
10 g Naloxone (Narcan)	j. Tricyclic antidepressant
11. h Chlorpromazine HCl (Thorazine)	k. Alcohol deterrent
12. i Buproprion (Wellbutrin)	l. Antimania (mood stabilizing) agent
13. h Loxapine (Loxitane)	m. Anti-Parkinsonism agent
14. j Amitriptyline HCl (Elavil)	n. Anticonvulsant
15. k Disulfiram (Antabuse)	o. Other antianxiety agent
16. i Trazodone (Desyrel)	p. Other antidepressant

17. _l_ Lithium carbonate (Eskalith)

18. _m_ Benztropine (Cogentin)

19. _j_ Nortriptyline HCl (Aventyl)

20. _e_ Paroxetine (Paxil)

21. _h_ Haloperidol (Haldol)

22. _n_ Carbamazepine (Tegretol)

23. _p_ Venlafaxine (Effexor)

24. _h_ Fluphenazine (Prolixin)

25. _n_ Valproic acid (Depokene)

26. _e_ Fluoxetine (Prozac)

27. _a_ Chlordiazepoxide (Librium)

28. _h_ Risperidone (Risperdal)

29. _a_ Alprazolam (Xanax)

30. _a_ and _n_ Clonazepam (Klonopin)

31. _j_ Doxepin (Sinequan)

32. _j_ Imipramine HCl (Tofranil)

33. _h_ Clozapine (Clozaril)

34. _h_ Olanzapine (Zyprexa)

35. _p_ Citalopram (Celexa)

APPLICATION ANSWERS

1. Domestic violence is rarely a one-time occurrence in a relationship; it usually continues and escalates in severity. Which factors increase the risk of an individual becoming violent? (Select all that apply.)

   a. Alcoholism
   b. High stress levels
   c. Financial independency
   d. Physical dependency

Rationale

Correct answers: a, b, and d.

(continued)

Risk factors for abuse include: alcoholism; high stress levels; physical, emotional, and/or financial dependency; high emotions; and history of violence.

2. Which symptoms are indicative of neglect? (Select all that apply.)
   a. Emergency department visits
   b. Missed appointments with health care providers
   c. Dehydration
   d. Unexplained injuries

Rationale

Correct answers: b and c.

Symptoms of neglect may include missed appointments with health care providers, dehydration, hunger, poor hygiene, unkempt appearance, pain, unfilled medication prescriptions, and lack of adequate clothing, shoes, or ancillary devices.

3. A nurse in an Emergency Department (ED) is caring for a client who has been drinking alcohol everyday for the past 10 days. The client is drowsy, has slurred speech, and lacks coordination. As the client experiences alcohol withdrawal, which potential side effect concerns the nurse most?
   a. Anxiety
   b. Hypoglycemia
   c. Esophagitis
   d. Delirium tremens

Rationale

Correct answer: d.

The nurse monitors the client closely and is most concerned about delirium tremens—the most severe manifestation of alcohol withdrawal. Delirium tremens (DT) is characterized by anxiety, uncontrollable fear, tremor, irritability, agitation, hallucinations, and insomnia. This condition is life-threatening and requires immediate intervention.

4. Which nursing interventions are appropriate for a client experiencing alcohol withdrawal? (Select all that apply.)
   a. Provide a private, lighted environment for recovery
   b. Implement seizure precautions
   c. Orient the client to person, place, and time
   d. Provide small, frequent, high-carbohydrate feedings

Rationale

Correct answers: a, b, c, and d.

When caring for a client who is experiencing alcohol withdrawal, it is appropriate for the nurse to provide a private, lighted environment to reduce the potential for hallucinations, implement seizure precautions, orient the client to person, place, and time, provide small, frequent high-carbohydrate feedings, monitor vital signs and neurological status, record intake and output, and provide support to the client, family, and significant others.

5. A nurse in the Emergency Department is caring for a client who has been smoking crack cocaine. The client's pupils are dilated and the client is euphoric, tachycardic, and agitated. As the client experiences withdrawal from crack cocaine, which side effects should the nurse anticipate? (Select all that apply.)
   a. Psychosis
   b. Hallucinations
   c. Illusions
   d. Nausea and vomiting

Rationale

Correct answers: a, b, and d.

A client who is undergoing withdrawal from cocaine may experience side effects which include psychosis, hallucinations, delusions, depression, paranoia, ideas of persecution, hypervigilance, aggression, tremors, insomnia, fatigue, muscle pain, suicidal ideation, nausea, vomiting, hyperthermia and general malaise.

6. Opioids are often prescribed by physicians for pain control and are commonly-abused substances. Which medications are opioids? (Select all that apply.)
   a. Hydromorphone (Dilaudid)
   b. Meperidine (Demerol)
   c. MDMA (Ecstasy)
   d. Lorazepam (Ativan)

Rationale

Correct answers: a and b.

Hydromorphone (Dilaudid) and meperidine (Demerol) are opioids. MDMA (Ecstasy) is a form of methamphetamine. Lorazepam (Ativan) is a benzodiazepine.

7. A nurse is discharging a client from a psychiatric unit who has been under suicide precautions. The nurse is providing discharge teaching to the client and the family. Which content would be appropriate for the nurse to teach? (Select all that apply.)
   a. Signs of an impending crisis
   b. Signs of suicidal behavior
   c. Signs of chemical abuse and dependency
   d. Signs of emotional abuse

Rationale

Correct answers: a, b, and c.

It is appropriate for the nurse to teach the client and family about the signs of an impending crisis that could precipitate suicidal thoughts, the signs of suicidal behavior to help the family recognize risk for suicide, and signs of chemical abuse and dependency, which is commonly associated with suicidal behavior. There is nothing to suggest that the client has been emotionally abused or is an emotional abuser.

8. Electroconvulsive therapy (ECT) is used as an effective treatment for which mental disorders? (Select all that apply.)
   a. Depression
   b. Severe catatonia
   c. Mania
   d. Schizophrenia

Rationale
Correct answers: a, b, c, and d.
ECT may be used as an effective treatment for depression that does not respond to antidepressant pharmacotherapy, severe catatonia, mania, or schizophrenia.

9. A nurse on a psychiatric unit is performing an initial assessment on the mental health of a client. Which assessment finding could be indicative of psychopathology? (Select all that apply.)
   a. Calm affect
   b. Disorientation
   c. Inappropriate dress
   d. Poor hygiene

Rationale
Correct answers: b, c, and d.
Abnormal assessment findings that could be indicative of psychopathology include disorientation, inappropriate dress, poor hygiene, absent memory recall, and incoherent or illogical thought processes.

10. A nurse in a long-term care facility is admitting an elderly client. The family informs the nurse that the client became forgetful a couple of years ago but now cannot remember family members' names and has become disoriented, impulsive, and easily agitated. Which common mental illness is most likely affecting the elderly client?
    a. Borderline personality disorder
    b. Bipolar disorder
    c. Schizophrenia
    d. Alzheimer's disease

Rationale
Correct answer: d.
Alzheimer's disease is a common mental illness among the elderly and is characterized by memory loss, depression, disorientation, speech difficulties, impulsive behavior, personality changes, and agitation.

11. A nurse in a psychiatric unit is caring for a client who engages in impulsive, risky behavior, has strong emotions that frequently wax and wane, and has difficulty controlling emotions and impulses. Which common mental illness is most likely affecting the client?
    a. Borderline personality disorder
    b. Bipolar disorder
    c. Schizophrenia
    d. Alzheimer's disease

Rationale
Correct answer: a.
Borderline personality disorder is characterized by rapid changes in self-image, impulsive, risky behavior, inappropriate anger, fear of being alone, strong emotions that wax and wane, and difficulty controlling emotions and impulses.

12. A nurse in a psychiatric unit is caring for a client who is delusional, paranoid, and has been diagnosed with schizophrenia. Which type of medication is commonly used to treat schizophrenia?
    a. H2 inhibitors
    b. Cholinesterase inhibitors
    c. Antipsychotics
    d. Antiemetics

Rationale
Correct answer: c.
Antipsychotic medications are commonly used, usually in combination with other medications, to treat schizophrenia.

13. A nurse is caring for an elderly client in a long-term care facility. The nurse knows that the client is most likely to experience which mental-health illness?
    a. Dementia
    b. Delirium
    c. Depression
    d. Dysgraphia

Rationale
Correct answer: c.
Depression is the most common mental illness affecting clients in long-term care facilities.

14. Antidepressant medications must be prescribed and administered with care, particularly when being given to elderly clients. Which adverse effects should the nurse anticipate when administering antidepressants to elderly clients? (Select all that apply.)
    a. Anticholinergic effects
    b. Cardiac effects
    c. Agitation
    d. Hostility

(continued)

Rationale

Correct answers: a and b.

Antidepressants may cause anticholinergic, cardiac, and orthostatic side effects as well as interactions with other medications. Agitation and hostility are not side effects of antidepressant use.

15. A nurse is caring for an elderly client who is experiencing dementia. Which assessment findings would the nurse expect? (Select all that apply.)
    a. Forgetfulness
    b. Memory loss
    c. Hostility
    d. Hallucinations

Rationale

Correct answers: a, b, and c.

Forgetfulness, memory loss, and hostility are all signs of dementia in the elderly. Hallucinations are a sign of delirium—a medical emergency.

16. When speaking to a community group on the topic of dementia, which medications would be identified as currently being used in its treatment? (Select all that apply.)
    a. Nortriptyline (Aventyl)
    b. Donepezil (Aricept)
    c. Doxepin (Sinequan)
    d. Rivastigmine (Exelon)

Rationale

Correct answers: b and d.

Aricept and Exelon are commonly used in the treatment of dementia. Aventyl and Sinequan are tricyclic antidepressants.

17. Which statement made by a participant in a seminar on delirium indicates that additional clarification is needed?
    a. "If untreated, permanent brain damage can occur."
    b. "It is considered a medical emergency."
    c. "It mostly affects elderly living in institutional settings."
    d. "It may result in hallucinations."

Rationale

Correct answers: a, b, and d.

Delirium begins with confusion and progresses to disorientation over a brief time span. It is considered a medical emergency and, if untreated, may result in permanent brain damage. Hallucinations are a sign of delirium. Dementia mostly affects elderly living in institutional settings.

18. For which client would the nurse expect the plan of care to include assessment using the Abnormal and Involuntary Movement Scale (AIMS)?
    a. Client with panic disorder
    b. Client with schizophrenia taking chlorpromazine (Thorazine)
    c. Client with a mood disorder taking amitryptyline (Elavil)
    d. Client taking buproprion (Wellbutrin)
    e. Client taking paroxetine (Paxil)

Rationale

Correct answer: b.

Clients taking an antipsychotic medication should be assessed using the Abnormal and Involuntary Movement Scale (AIMS) because of the extrapyramidal side effects associated with these drugs. Thorazine is an antipsychotic and therefore the client taking it should be assessed with AIMS.

19. Which assessment finding should the nurse interpret as indicative of agranulocytosis in a client taking clozapine (Clozaril)?
    a. Photosensitivity
    b. Tachycardia
    c. Low WBC
    d. Orthostatic hypotension

Rationale

Correct answer: c.

Agranulocytosis is another name for neutropenia or a decrease in neutrophils

20. Which signs and symptoms are expected effects associated with withdrawal from oxycodone (OxyContin)? (Select all that apply.)
    a. Fevers and chills
    b. Runny nose and eyes
    c. Dilated pupils
    d. Paranoia
    e. Muscle pain
    f. Nausea
    g. Insomnia
    h. Tachypnea
    i. Hallucinations

Rationale

Correct answers: a, b, e, f, g, and h.

Fevers and chills, runny nose and eyes, muscle pain, nausea and other GI distress, insomnia, tachypnea, and coma can all occur with opiate withdrawal. In addition, pupils are pinpoint not dilated. Paranoia and hallucinations occur with withdrawal from methamphetamines.

21. When assessing a client for cocaine use, for which signs would the nurse observe? (Select all that apply.)

a. Hypotension
b. Tachycardia
c. Tachypnea
d. Dilated pupils
e. Agitation
f. Lack of concentration
g. Slurred speech
h. Poor coordination
i. Hypervigilance
j. Tremors

Rationale

Correct answers: b, c, d, e, and f.

Tachycardia, tachypnea, dilated pupils, agitation, and lack of ability to concentrate are all effects of cocaine use. Hypertension, not hypotension, is also an effect. Slurred speech and poor coordination are signs of benzodiazepine use. Hypervigilance and tremors are signs of cocaine withdrawal.

22. When caring for a client being withdrawn from barbiturate use, which nursing intervention is appropriate?
    a. Institute seizure precautions
    b. Keep the room dark and quiet
    c. Monitor for dysrhythmias
    d. Observe for suicide attempts

Rationale

Correct answer: a.

Seizures can occur with withdrawal from barbiturates and so seizure precautions must be implemented. The environment should be kept quiet but a light should be left on to aid orientation. Monitoring for dysrhythmias is an important nursing intervention for clients undergoing withdrawal from benzodiazepines or cocaine. Monitoring for suicide attempts is essential for clients withdrawing from methamphetamines.

23. When discussing obsessive-compulsive disorder with the parents of a newly diagnosed child, the nurse bases the discussion of the compulsive behavior on the knowledge that the behavior serves to
    a. control unacceptable impulses
    b. dissipate excess energy
    c. manipulate the environment
    d. decrease anxiety

Rationale

Correct answer: d.

Compulsive behaviors or rituals serve to prevent some event, divert unwanted thoughts, and decrease anxiety. Unless the behavior threatens safety, the client is allowed to carry it out until anxiety is decreased. Intervention is needed for compulsive behavior if it significantly impacts the person's ability to function.

24. When reinforcing "negative thought stopping," which direction might the nurse give?
    a. When a negative thought occurs, immediately verbalize out loud an opposing positive thought.
    b. At least once per hour while awake, focus for 60 seconds on a positive thought.
    c. When a negative thought occurs, perform a distracting activity, and then think a positive thought.
    d. When you recognize a negative thought, repeat your positive mantra to yourself until the thought disappears.

Rationale

Correct answer: c.

Negative thought stopping involves recognition of a negative thought followed by use of a distracting stimulus such as snapping an elastic band on the wrist, and then replacement with a positive thought.

25. When giving dietary instructions to a client for whom an MAO inhibitor has been prescribed, which foods would the nurse tell the client to avoid?
    e. Yellow vegetables, cereals and, chicken eggs
    f. Cheese, avocados, bananas, beer, and wine
    g. Beef, broccoli, cauliflower, and rice
    h. Mushrooms, salmon, celery, and grapefruit

Rationale

Correct answer: b.

Cheese, avocados, bananas, beer, and wine are rich in amines or amino acids, which can cause paradoxic hypertension when combined with an MAO inhibitor. Foods listed in other responses are not high in amines.

CHAPTER 13

Test Plan Category:

Physiological Integrity

Sub-category: Basic Care and Comfort

Topics: Complementary and Alternative Therapies
Assistive Devices
Elimination
Mobility/Immobility
Non-Pharmacological Comfort Interventions
Nutrition and Oral Hydration
Palliative/Comfort Care
Personal Hygiene
Rest and Sleep

COMPLEMENTARY AND ALTERNATIVE THERAPIES

- Complementary and alternative therapies (CATs) include methods of health promotion, health maintenance, disease prevention, and disease treatment that are not part of the standard North American approach to health care.
- These therapies mostly focus on the healing the person not curing the disease; stress the importance of mindfulness and attitude in healing; integrate culture and personal beliefs into the treatment regimen; and promote a general sense of well being and control in the client.
- Often CATs relieve symptoms but do not cure.

ACUPUNCTURE

- Acupuncture is based on belief that when Qi (energy) flow in the body is blocked, pain and dysfunction result in the affected organs.
- This therapy uses hair-sized needles to stimulate selected anatomic areas to restore energy flow to the linked internal organs.

- Research suggests it relieves pain through stimulation of high threshold sensory receptors, which in turn stimulate other CNS structures and result in the release of endorphins and increased cortisol levels.
- It is generally safe although infection and organ perforation can occur.
- It is contraindicated for those with clotting disorders, those who are pregnant, and those unable to cooperate such as children under 7 years of age and clients who are demented or under the influence of alcohol or narcotics.
- It is effectively used in relieving nausea related to anesthesia and chemotherapy, dental pain, headaches, menstrual cramps, osteoarthritis, low back pain, carpal tunnel syndrome, asthma, addiction, and also in stroke rehabilitation.

IMAGERY

- Imagery uses mental processes involving pictures and symbols to promote attitudinal, behavioral, and physiological reactions by opening communication among perception, emotion, and bodily changes.
- It can contribute to insight into concerns, support symptom management, and improve functional status.
- Clinical applications of this therapy include management of perioperative pain and anxiety, N&V related to chemotherapy, cancer pain, wound healing, asthma, stress, burnout, bulimia, and depression. It is also used to enhance immune function, improve client's outlook, and support the dying process.

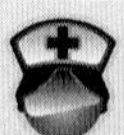

Practice Alert

Imagery alters brain-wave activity and can induce seizures in susceptible clients. Imagery alters blood glucose levels and so when used with diabetic clients, requires careful blood sugar monitoring—may be contraindicated for an unstable diabetic client. Imagery is contraindicated for use with clients with a history of psychosis.

MEDITATION

- Meditation refers to the deep contemplation associated with decreased heart and respiratory rates and decreased oxygen consumption.
- Twenty minutes of meditation per day decreases stress and renews energy.
- It is contraindicated for those fearing loss of control or with a history of psychosis.

YOGA

- Yoga is a mind–body therapy aimed at self-improvement through focused breathing, stretching, and meditation.
- In yoga, breath is seen as the link connecting mind, body, spirit, and emotion.
- It is effectively used against hypertension, menopausal symptoms, osteoporosis, and depression.

GROUP THERAPY

- Group therapy usually centers on a common theme: breast cancer survival, grieving, Alzheimer's caregiving, living with a laryngectomy, inflammatory bowel disease (IBD), or heart disease.
- This therapy offers mutual support, encouragement, and socialization.

BIOFEEDBACK

- Biofeedback involves the use of noninvasive electronic monitoring equipment to teach clients to regulate internal states such as blood pressure, heart rate, brain-wave patterns, or electrical muscular activity.
- It is effective in relieving hypertension, Raynaud's disease, migraine headache, and low back pain.

RELAXATION THERAPY

- Relaxation therapy is a basic stress-management technique.
- It involves either purposeful relaxation of specific muscles or use of breathing, words, or sounds to induce a general state of mental and muscular relaxation.
- It is easily used at the bedside.
- It is effective in managing chronic pain.

MASSAGE THERAPY

- Massage therapy manipulates skin, muscles, ligaments, tendons, and fascia through touch, stroking, friction, vibration, percussion, kneading, stretching, compression, and joint movement to promote healing/health.
- It reduces muscle tension, improves circulation, reduces blood pressure, decreases pain, improves mobility, relieves anxiety, and induces relaxation and a sense of well-being.
- It is commonly used in rehabilitation, postoperative, maternity, cancer, and hospice-care settings.

TOUCH THERAPIES

- Therapeutic touch involves manipulating the client's energy field without actually touching the body. The goal is to direct and balance the energy field surrounding the client, which is in interaction with the environment. Its uses include management of pain and anxiety, promotion of wound healing, and relaxation.

- Healing touch mobilizes the client's ability to heal by clearing, energizing, and balancing the client's energy field. It is widely used along with medical treatments.
- Reiki (universal life force energy) therapy involves energy drawn in through the top of the practitioner's head and directed out of the body by way of the practitioner's hands into the client through intentional touch over major body organs to promote healing.

HERBAL THERAPY

- Herbal products are natural but not necessarily safe.
- Herbal preparations vary depending on the part of the plant used, the time of harvest, and the quality of the soil and other growing conditions.
- Herbs frequently take a number of weeks to build up in the body and exert an effect because of their low potency.
- Herbal and dietary supplements are regulated as foods not drugs and hence lack quality standardization.
- Pharmacokinetic effects of herbs are not well understood so great caution is needed while using any herb or nutritional supplement especially during pregnancy or lactation or in combination with other medications (see Table 13–1 for commonly used herbs and related cautions).

Table 13–1 Commonly Used Herbs and Related Cautions

Herb	Action/Uses	Cautions
Black cohosh	Mild estrogen-like action; used for menstrual irregularities, menopausal symptoms, and stimulation of uterine contractions	Contraindicated in presence of estrogen dependent tumors
Butterbur	Migraine, chronic cough, asthma, and bladder spasms	May cause reaction in those allergic to ragweed or daisy
Chamomile	Various GI disturbances including constipation, diarrhea, dyspepsia, irritable bowel syndrome and diverticular disease	May cause reaction in those allergic to ragweed, asters, or chrysanthemums
Echinacea	Immune system enhancer; used to decrease duration and severity of viral and bacterial URIs; effectiveness decreases with prolonged use	Contraindicated by autoimmunedisease or immunosuppressive Rx Not appropriate for prevention of URIs Not to be used for more than 8 wks; recommended use: no more than 10 d
Elderberry	Topical use: decreases edema and inflammation Tea: Rx for colds and flu	
Feverfew	NSAID and antipyretic action; used for arthritis, fever, inflammation, prevention of migraines (no effect once headache has begun)	Caution with anticoagulants because it inhibits platelet activity Stop 2 wks before surgery
Garlic	Lowers cholesterol, increases HDLs and lowers BP (may take months of use); regulates blood glucose; decreases platelet adhesiveness; protects against vascular age changes; antibacterial	Caution with anticoagulants
Ginger	Motion sickness; digestive aid	Caution with anticoagulants as it can promote bleeding
Gingko	Antioxidant; improves circulation; decreases platelet aggregation; also used for intermittent claudication and dementia	Used with caution after trauma or surgery or in combination with anticoagulants
Ginseng	Increases resistance to stress, invigorates	Potentiates anticoagulants
Milkvetch	Immune system enhancer	Contraindicated by autoimmune disease
St. John's wort	Acts like monoamine oxidase (MAO) inhibitor to treat mild/moderate depression	Many drug interactions; contraindicated if MAO inhibitors are taken; can cause hypertension, headache, insomnia, cardiac dysrhythmias, nervousness, tremor, seizures, cerebrovascular accident (CVA) and myocardial infarction (MI).
Senna	Stimulates colon; used for constipation	Can potentiate cardiac glycosides
Saw palmetto	Anti-inflammatory/antiedema; used for benign prostatic hyperplasia (BPH)	None
Valerian root	Benzodiasapine-like effect on gamma aminobutyric acid receptors; used for restlessness and insomnia	Not recommended for chronic use

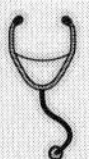

Assessment Alert

Ask all clients about the use of herbal products; consider an interaction with an herbal product whenever an adverse drug reaction occurs. Clients on anticoagulants are at particular risk for adverse reactions from concurrent herbal therapy especially from the use of quai, feverfew, garlic, ginseng, and gingko.

ASSISTIVE DEVICES

- Assistive devices are used to enhance a client's functional ability.
- They allow activities to be performed more independently.
- The available devices include those that aid eating, dressing, hygiene, mobility, writing, seeing, and performing household chores.
- No one device is suitable to all—clients need to be guided in trying different devices and models to find the one that works best for them.
- Excellent reviews, prepared by health care professionals, that compare different devices are available on the Internet and can serve as resources for clients. Table 13–2 discusses some assistive devices and their uses.

ELIMINATION

BOWEL ELIMINATION

Feces: Normally feces consists of 75% water and 25% solid; water is absorbed by the colon so the longer the waste products are in the colon the more solid stool will be; conversely the less time in the colon results in a more watery stool.

Age Variations in Stool

- Meconium: Black, tarry, odorless, sticky material found in the intestine of the full term fetus and passed by the newborn within 24 hours of birth.
- Transitional stool: Greenish-yellow, loose, mucus-containing stool passed after meconium for about a week.
- Normal infant stool: Yellow (bright yellow–gold and odorless in breast-fed infants; dark yellow–tan in cow's milk formula-fed infants), moist, and semisolid.
- Normal adult stool: Soft, formed, and brown.

Abnormal Stool

- Clay-colored or white: absence of the bile pigment due to obstruction, barium in the GI tract after a diagnostic test, or use of antacids.
- Black or tarry: bleeding from stomach or small intestine, ingestion of large amounts of red meat, dark green leafy vegetables, or licorice, ingestion of iron supplements or Pepto-Bismol.
- Red: colon or rectal bleeding.
- Gray–green: antibiotics

Defecation

- Defecation refers to the expulsion of feces from the rectum through the anus.
- Frequency of defecation varies from person to person: it ranges from several times per day to two or three times per week; infants often defecate after every feeding; frequency decreases with the introduction of solid food.
- Gastrocolic reflex is the increased peristalsis in the colon resulting in an urge to defecate when food enters the stomach; especially strong in the morning after breakfast.
- If urge to defecate is ignored, the urge usually does not recur for a few hours. If the urge is repeatedly ignored, rectum distends and accommodates so the urge to defecate is no longer felt and constipation can develop.
- Defecation is easiest in sitting position with thighs flexed.
- Ability to control defecation starts at about 18–24 months and daytime control is attained by 30 months.
- Normal defecation requires
  —a diet with adequate amounts of bulk to provide stool volume,
  —2000–3000 ml fluid daily to prevent excessive drying of intestinal contents as a result of reabsorption of water by colon,

Table 13–2 Examples of Assistive Devices and Their Uses

Functional Area	Examples of Assistive Devices
Eating	Silverware with widened or builtup handles to facilitate grasping Utensils with angled handles that can be used in either left or right hand to compensate for limited motion Utensils with straps that go over wrists to prevent dropping Raised rims for plates to facilitate getting food onto spoon or fork rather than being pushed off edge of plate Suction cups, rubber feet, or rubber mats for under dishes to prevent movement No-spill cups, double-handled cups, cups with spouts to compensate for poor coordination
Hygiene	Shower chair for those unable to stand and balance Tub or shower bars to aid getting in or out and maintain balance while bathing Hand-held shower attachment Soap on a rope to prevent dropping and need for bending Long-handled brushes to enable back and lower legs to be reached Battery-powered toothbrushes to decrease need for fine, coordinated movement
Toileting	Raised toilet seat to compensate for limited ability to bend at hips Raised toilet seat with arms to compensate for limited ability to bend at hips, difficulty with balance, and difficulty returning to a standing position
Dressing	Shoes and clothing with Velcro fasteners to allow one-handed closure and/or to compensate for lack of coordination Shoehorn with a long, tall handle to eliminate the need for bending Button hook for buttoning clothing to compensate for loss of motor function or coordination Dressing stick
Moving	Walkers with or without wheels, baskets, and seat mechanisms to provide support Straight canes for support and balance when walking or standing Quadripod canes for use in right or left hand for greater support and balance when walking or standing Curved canes with a lower hand grip for leverage in getting into and out of a sitting position Chairs with built-in hydraulic lifts to decrease need to bend and balance in order to sit and to decrease effort needed to stand Portable hydraulic lifts to aid sitting and rising to a standing position Crutches wheelchairs both motorized and hand driven
Seeing	Various nonglare, high-intensity floor and table lamps with goose necks for easy focus on work surface Magnifying devices with and without attached lights Transparent yellow sheets to be placed over print to reduce glare and make letters darker Templates with cutouts to guide writing such as in filling out checks
General functioning	Long-handled reachers with or without magnetic tip Telephones with large buttons Door handles that are elongated rather than knobs to allow easy grasping Appliances such as stoves with raised dial markings Cooking utensils with easy-grasp handles

—activity sufficient to stimulate peristalsis and maintain muscles needed to increase intra-abdominal pressure for defecation, and

—regular time for defecation and obedience to the urge to defecate.

- Factors which affect normal defecation:

—bland, low-residue diet has insufficient bulk to create volume of stool needed to stimulate the defecation reflex,

—irregular eating pattern,

—ingestion of foods that produce constipation (cheese, pasta, eggs, and lean meat), diarrhea (bran, prunes, chocolate, alcohol, and in some people, spicy foods and foods high in sugar), or flatus (cauliflower, cabbage, Brussels sprouts, beans, onion, bananas, and apples),

—inadequate fluid intake,

—inactivity, for example, lack of exercise, immobilization, and bed rest,

—ignoring the urge to defecate,

—emotions such as anxiety and anger often cause diarrhea while depression is associated with constipation,

—medications

- opioids, iron, some tranquilizers cause constipation

- stool softeners such as Colace (docusate sodium) facilitate defecation
- laxatives stimulate defecation; cathartics have a purgative effect
- types of laxatives are
  - bulk-forming: for example, methylcellulose (Citrucel), requires adequate fluid intake
  - stimulant: for example, bisacodyl (Dulcolax), cascara, castor oil; water is lost in stool due to rapid propulsion through intestine; may cause cramping; risk of fluid and electrolyte imbalance with prolonged use
  - lubricant: for example, mineral oil; risk of fat-soluble-vitamin (A, D, E, and K) deficiency with prolonged use
  - saline/osmotic: for example, milk of magnesia (MOM), magnesium citrate; draws water into intestine; risk of fluid and electrolyte imbalance especially in elderly and children with cardiac or renal problems, risk of impaired absorption of some fat-soluble vitamins
- Kaolin–pectin preparations (Kaopectate), diphenoxylate hydrochloride (Lomotil), and loperamide hydrochloride (Imodium) control diarrhea

Clinical Alert

Bismuth preparations used to treat "traveler's diarrhea" often contain aspirin and should not be given to children or adolescents with flu, chicken pox, or other viral infections because of the risk of Reye syndrome.

—General anesthesia blocks parasympathetic nervous stimulation of the colon causing decreased or absent peristalsis.

—Handling of gut during surgery causes ileus (cessation of peristalsis) for 24–48 hours.

—Spinal cord, head, or other injuries/diseases interfere with sensation, muscle control, or ability to respond to urge to defecate.

—Pain

Problems of Elimination:

- Constipation: Passage of dry, hard stool or no stool (see Chapter 17).
- Fecal impaction: Mass of hard stool in the rectum and above from prolonged stool retention and accumulation.
  - —S&S: Seepage of liquid stool and no passage of normal stool, nonproductive urge to defecate, rectal pain, anorexia, abdominal distention, and N&V.
  - —Dx: Palpation of hardened mass on digital examination of the rectum.
  - —Rx: Oil retention enema with cleansing enema in 2–4 hours followed by daily cleansing enemas, suppositories or stool softeners; if no results, manual extraction of feces.
- Diarrhea: Passage of abnormally liquid feces and/or abnormal frequency of defecation (see Chapter 17).

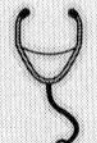

Assessment Alert

Diagnosis of constipation or diarrhea can only be made when there is deviation from the individual's normal pattern of elimination. What is constipation or diarrhea for one person may be normal for another

- Flatulence: Excessive flatus (gas) in the intestine.
- Bowel incontinence
  - —Loss of ability to voluntarily control passage of stool or flatus through the anal sphincter.
  - —Minor incontinence: inability to control passage of gas or minor soiling.
  - —Major incontinence: inability to control passage of normal feces.
  - —It may be due to impaired functioning of the sphincter or its nerve supply or inability to recognize the need to defecate.

Nursing Process Elements

- Assess stool for color, consistency, shape, amount, odor, and presence of abnormal material
- Determine frequency and pattern of elimination
- Assess toileting self-care ability
- For home care clients, assess access to and safety of toilet facilities, for example, lighting, does walker or wheel chair fit through doorway, need for raised toilet seat, etc.
- Provide privacy
- Schedule other care activities so as not to interfere with time for defecation
- Utilize best possible position and place for facilitation of defecation: toilet, bedside commode, bedpan with bed in high Fowler's position, bedpan with other position if no better option

- If laxatives are ordered in the form of suppositories, administer 30 minutes before usual defecation time or just after breakfast when the gastrocolic reflex is strongest

Client teaching for self-care

Teach the client about

- the importance of regular timing, diet and fluid needs, and exercise/mobility needs in maintaining normal defecation
- the foods and activities (gum chewing, drinking carbonated liquids, using a straw) that increase flatus; and foods that predispose to constipation or diarrhea
- the importance of avoiding overuse of OTC products for treatment of constipation or diarrhea

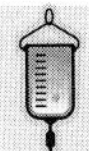

Clinical Alert

Laxatives should never be taken if nausea, cramps, colic, vomiting, or undiagnosed abdominal pain is present.

URINARY ELIMINATION

Voiding (Micturition)

- Voiding requires relaxation of abdominal and perineal muscles and the external urethral sphincter.
- The desire to empty bladder occurs in adult when 250–450 ml of urine accumulates in the bladder and in children when the accumulation is 50–200 ml.
- Patterns of urination are highly individualized.

Age Variations in Urine Production and Voiding

- The amount of urine produced varies with fluid intake and fluid loss through other routes as well as with the cardiovascular and renal status.
- Voluntary control is achieved between the age of 2 years and 5 years with daytime control acquired before nighttime control.
- Infants: 250–500 ml urine is produced per day with variation based on fluid intake; pale urine; specific gravity is 1.008 because immature kidneys cannot concentrate urine; voids up to 20 times per day.
- 12–24 months: kidneys mature and concentrate (specific gravity 1.010–1.025); urine is normal amber color.
- School age children: void 6–8 times per day
- Adults: void average of 5 times per day
- Older adults: capacity of bladder and ability to empty completely decreases with age resulting in frequency, nocturia, and increased risk of urinary tract infection (UTI).

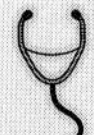

Assessment Alert

Normal adult kidneys produce urine at a rate of 60 ml/hr (1500 ml/d). Output less than 30 ml/hr must be reported as it may indicate low blood volume or renal disease.

Factors which affect normal voiding

- Lack of privacy can affect normal voiding.
- Upright sitting position is the most conducive to voiding.
- Sound of running water, or pouring water over the perineum can induce voiding.
- Increased fluid intake normally increases voiding; alcohol and caffeine inhibit antidiuretic hormone (ADH) secretion and result in increased urine production.
- Medications
  - —Diuretics move water out of the body by increasing production of urine
  - —Urinary retention can result from atropine, papaverine, phenothiazines, MAO inhibitors, Sudafed, hydralazine, methyldopate, levodopa, trihexyphenidyl, benztropine mesylate, propranolol, and hydrocodone
- Muscle tone of detrusor muscle is necessary for the bladder to fill and empty normally; loss of this muscle tone can result from prolonged use of indwelling catheters, which eliminate bladder filling and intermittent emptying.

Problems of Urinary Elimination

- Polyuria: Production of abnormally large amounts of urine; may result from excessive fluid intake, change in hormone levels postpartum, diabetes mellitus or insipidus, or chronic nephritis.
- Oliguria: Production of less than 500 ml of urine per day or less than 30 ml/hr.

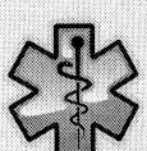

Nursing Intervention Alert

Oliguria can occur from lack of fluid intake or fluid loss by another route (diarrhea, diaphoresis, vomiting, burn injury, or drainage) but most often is a result of poor blood flow to the kidneys or impending renal failure. It should be reported promptly.

- Anuria: No production of urine by kidneys.
- Frequency: Voiding at frequent intervals; normal adult voids every 3.5–4 hours during the day and no more than once at night; occurs with UTIs, stress, pressure from pregnancy or an abdominal mass, increased volume of urine, and decreased bladder capacity.
- Nocturia: Voiding two or more times at night.
- Urgency: Feeling of immediate need to void even with little urine in bladder; occurs with irritation of the bladder and urethra; may be triggered by the sound of running water, an abrupt change in position or the feel of warm water on the skin.
- Dysuria: Painful or difficult voiding; usually accompanied by frequency and urgency creating the class triad of symptoms of UTI; dysuria at start of voiding suggests urethral inflammation while dysuria during or after voiding suggests bladder inflammation.
- Hesitancy: Difficulty initiating the stream; seen when urethra is partially blocked as with a urethral stricture or benign or malignant prostatic hypertrophy.
- Enuresis: Involuntary micturition in children beyond the time bladder control is normally achieved.
- Nocturnal enuresis: Involuntary release of urine during sleep; in adults it is generally due to a neurological problem.
- Urinary incontinence: Involuntary urination; risk factors include repeated UTIs, urinary tract surgery or trauma, sexual transmited infections (STIs), multiple vaginal births, musculoskeletal, neurological, or endocrine disorders, cognitive impairment, self-care deficit. The types of urinary incontinence are
  —total incontinence
    - constant, involuntary dribbling of urine
    - cause is neurological or related to trauma or anatomical abnormality
  —reflex incontinence
    - urine is retained in bladder and when pressure builds to a critical point, urine leaks out
    - causes include spinal cord injury and bladder neck obstruction
  —urge incontinence
    - urge to urinate is so strong that uncontrolled bladder emptying occurs
    - causes include spinal cord injury, bladder tumor, and bladder infection
  —stress incontinence
    - loss of small amounts of urine when intra-abdominal pressure is increased by activities such as laughing, coughing, sneezing, and physical straining
    - more common in women
    - causes include loss of tone in the pelvic muscles from obesity or aging, and childbirth injury
  —functional incontinence
    - inability to get to the bathroom to void as a result of physical or mental disability or environmental obstacles
- Urinary retention: Overdistention of bladder because of inability to expel urine; may have overflow voiding of 20–50 ml at frequent intervals; on palpation bladder is firm and distended and may be to one side of midline.

Nursing Process Elements

- Assess color, odor, and consistency of urine
- Measure urinary output; report output of less than 30 ml/hr in adults
- Assess color, texture, and turgor of skin as well as for edema when assessing urinary elimination status
- Facilitate voiding:
  —Position
    - standing for men, sitting upright for women is best. Sitting is better than lying down for men
  —Provide privacy
  —Have client press over suprapubic area to increase pressure on bladder
  —Run water; pour water over perineum, apply hot water bottle to lower abdomen
  —Administer ordered analgesics if pain is a problem
- Manage incontinence according to individualized need:
  —Teach Kegel exercises to women to strengthen pelvic floor muscles.
  —Institute timed voiding (habit training):
    - have client void at scheduled intervals; further enhance by prompting/encouraging to void as scheduled (prompted voiding)
  —Use a bladder-training program:
    - Set a voiding schedule based on the frequency of incontinence and have client void accordingly, for example, on waking in morning, then every 2 hours, on going to bed at night, and every 4 hours till morning
    - Have the client use slow, deep breathing to overcome the urge to go if sooner than the set schedule
    - Increase time between voiding gradually
    - Encourage fluid intake half an hour before scheduled voiding times
    - Restrict fluid intake in the evening
    - Avoid liquids such as citrus juices, caffeinated, and artificially sweetened drinks that irritate the bladder
- If any incontinence is reported, assess perineum for irritation from exposure to urine and initiate measures to maintain/restore skin integrity

Client teaching for self-care

Instruct client to

- maintain minimum daily fluid intake of 1500 ml
- decrease risk of UTI by
  —drinking 2000–3000 ml fluid per day to flush out the urinary tract
  —voiding every 2–4 hours and immediately after intercourse to wash bacteria away
  —avoiding tight-fitting, noncotton clothing that prevents air circulation to the perineal area
  —avoiding the use of irritating soaps or other products in the perineal area
  —females wiping front to back to prevent spread of intestinal bacteria to urethra and discarding tissue after each wipe
  —taking showers rather than baths
  —drinking two to three glasses of cranberry juice daily and ensuring adequate vitamin C in daily diet to increase acidity of urine

MOBILITY/IMMOBILITY

MOBILITY

Mobility is the ability to physically move about for work, pleasure, or exercise.

IMMOBILITY

- Immobility refers to the lack of movement or the inability to move without assistance.
- It affects the entire body both physically and psychosocially.
- Forced immobility, even for a short period of time affects multiple body systems. Immobility disrupts client's self-esteem (not being able to care for self); causes many emotional reactions, such as anger, apathy, regression, or frustration due to loss of control; causes change in perception of time or difficulty with problem solving due to a lack of stimuli.

Musculoskeletal System Effects

- Disuse osteoporosis: Loss of calcium (negative calcium balance) occurs when the body does not have the stress of weight bearing and can result in osteoporosis.
- Disuse atrophy: Muscles decrease in size (atrophy) when not used leading to a loss of both strength and muscle mass.
- Contractures: These occur as a result of the extremities not being used, such as with walking or self-grooming. The loss of movement to the muscles of the extremities leads to shortening of the muscle fibers, which is an irreversible condition except for surgical intervention.
- Stiff, painful joints: These result from shortening of tissue and a higher concentration of calcium at joints from being immobile.

Cardiovascular System Effects

- Decrease in cardiac reserve: Imbalance in the autonomic nerve system resulting from immobility leads to sympathetic activity without compensatory parasympathetic stimulation and causes an increase of heart rate with minimal exertion by the client.
- Increased use of the Valsalva maneuver: Clients typically hold their breath and strain against the closed glottis (Valsalva maneuver) when moving themselves in bed; this can cause cardiac arrhythmias in persons with a known cardiac history.
- Orthostatic hypotension: It occurs as a result of the loss of normal vasoconstriction in the lower extremities leading to pooling of blood in the lower extremities with a decrease in core blood pressure. Upon sitting or standing, the microcirculation fails to respond normally causing the client to feel dizzy as a result of a decrease in cerebral perfusion. A sudden increased heart rate is noted due to the body's response of protecting the brain from a sudden decrease in blood flow.
- Venous vasodilatation and stasis: Immobility results in the loss of the contraction and release of skeletal muscles in the lower extremities, which normally prevents pooling of blood in them.
- Dependent edema: Occurs as the serous component of blood is forced into the interstitial tissues.
- Thrombus formation: Shortened thromboplastin time and increased number of procoagulants lead to clot formation, which can result in an emboli, should the clot break loose.

Respiratory System

- Decrease in respiratory movement: Pressure of the body against a solid surface does not allow the lungs to expand fully due to the pressure of internal organs against the diaphragm. Immobility also decreases sighing with respirations secondary to muscle atrophy and lack of the exercise stimulus. Over time, these changes lead to a decreased vital capacity (maximum amount of air exhaled following a maximum amount of air inhaled) and shallow breathing.

- Pooling of respiratory secretions: Secretions from the lung are usually raised through coughing and changes in position, which are decreased with immobility. As a result, secretions pool in the respiratory tract.
- Hypostatic pneumonia: Pooled secretions impair gas exchange and provide an excellent medium for bacterial growth, which can result in hypostatic pneumonia.
- Atelectasis: It occurs when pooled secretions block a dependent area of the lung and the production of surfactant is decreased.

Metabolic System

- Decreased metabolic rate: Energy requirements of the body decrease with immobility.
- Negative nitrogen balance: Protein stores are depleted due to catabolism of muscle mass releasing more nitrogen than what is ingested.
- Anorexia: Decreased metabolic rate and catabolism lead to anorexia. Prolonged anorexia leads to severe negative nitrogen balance if protein intake is minimal.

Urinary System

- Urinary stasis: In a horizontal position, the client is forced to push against gravity resulting in incomplete emptying of the bladder and renal pelvis.
- Urinary retention: It results due to the loss of detrusor muscle tone with prolonged immobility.
- Urinary infection: It results from stasis of urine in the bladder and renal pelvis from both loss of gravity assistance for emptying and urinary retention; the client is at a higher risk for a urinary infection and the most common infection-causing organism is *Escherichia coli.*
- Urinary calculi: It is caused due to the loss of calcium from bone which results in alkaline urine containing large amounts of calcium, which crystallizes as calcium salts, becoming calculi in the renal pelvis.

Gastrointestinal System

- Constipation: Decreased peristalsis causes hardening of stool; muscle weakness and a horizontal position create difficulty in defecating.
- Increased use of the Valsalva maneuver to defecate causes increased intra-abdominal and intrathoracic pressure that impacts on the function of both the heart and circulatory system.

Integumentary System

- Decreased skin turgor and skin atrophy: Impaired hydration of the dermis occurs due to fluid shifts associated with immobility.
- Skin breakdown: Results from prolonged pressure, particularly over bony prominences, that decreases blood flow and delivery of oxygen and nutrients.

Nursing Process Elements

- Encourage or help to perform ROM
- Monitor for dehydration
- Monitor serum electrolytes (sodium, potassium, chlorine, and calcium)
- Assess for deep vein thrombosis (DVT)
- Apply compressive stockings (TEDS) or device (SCD)
- Encourage deep breathing and use of incentive spirometry
- Administer calcium and phosphorous supplements
- Monitor for infection
- Monitor bowel function
- Administer stool softener
- Encourage foods high in fiber
- Assess vulnerable body surfaces for changes in skin integrity
- Reposition at least every 2 hours
- Provide a pressure relief surface that is appropriate for client

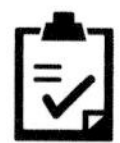

Client teaching for self-care

Teach client to

- reposition self at 15-minute increments when out of bed in chair
- replace fluids and maintain adequate protein and calcium intake in foods
- perform active ROM
- perform respiratory hygiene activities

NONPHARMACOLOGICAL COMFORT CARE/INTERVENTIONS

COMFORT

- Comfort refers to personal experiences of a client with physical, psychospiritual, social and environmental components, where
  —the physical component relates to bodily sensations,
  —the psychospiritual component relates to aspects of self or the meaning of life,
  —the social component relates to interpersonal relationships within and outside of the family, and
  —the environmental component relates to external conditions (e.g., noise, light, and climate) and events that impact the client.
- Absence of distress: This is the most basic degree of comfort.
- Positive feeling of ease: This is a higher degree of comfort.
- The promotion of comfort requires paying attention to all four components.

Nursing Process Elements

- Assess comfort level in all four areas.
- Identify sources of comfort and discomfort for the individual client
- Implement nursing actions designed to relieve discomfort and promote a positive sense of ease in each of the component areas of comfort
- Examples of comfort measures:
  — Physical
    - Apply lotion
    - Rub back
    - Offer fluids
    - Straighten sheets
    - Provide mouth, nail, and hair care
    - Elevate edematous parts
    - Maintain good body alignment to prevent pull on tissues and joints
      - Use pillow under arms of weak, paralyzed clients to prevent pull on shoulder joints
      - Use pillow to support upper leg for clients in side-lying position to prevent pull on hip
    - Apply heat and cold
      - Heat causes vasodilation, increased capillary permeability, increased cellular metabolism, and a quieting effect; cold causes vasoconstriction, decreased capillary permeability, decreased cellular metabolism, decreased inflammation, and a local anesthetic effect
      - Both heat and cold cause a rebound phenomenon: maximum vasodilation or vasoconstriction is followed by the reverse effect; therefore, intermittent application of heat and cold is needed to maintain the desired effect
      - Heat is used to support inflammation by increasing blood flow and softening exudates; increase joint range of motion and decrease joint stiffness; and reduce pain
      - Cold is used to relieve muscle spasm, decrease inflammation, decrease edema unrelated to inflammation, and decrease pain

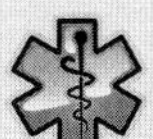

Nursing Intervention Alert

Do not use heat when active bleeding is present because vasodilation will increase bleeding; in the first 24 hours after trauma, because vasodilation and increased capillary permeability will increase edema and risk of bleeding; when edema unrelated to inflammation exists; or when skin is irritated and reddened.

Do not use cold on open wounds or when circulation is impaired because it can increase tissue injury; do not use on clients who exhibit an allergic type reaction on exposure to cold. Apply heat and cold with caution when the client has sensory impairment, cognitive impairment, altered circulation, or an open wound.

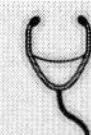

Assessment Alert

Assess skin area before applying heat or cold; reassess 15 minutes after application; stop application if an untoward response has occurred.

—Psychospiritual
- Be present
- Use soothing tones
- Be nonjudgmental and accepting
- Allow expression of feelings
- Exhibit empathy
- Use touch therapeutically
- Be efficient and coordinated in providing care
- Facilitate spiritual practices

—Social
- Promote communication with family/friends
- Suggest visiting
- Facilitate satisfying visits with family/friends by having client prepared for visit and avoiding interruptions

—Environmental
- Provide warm blanket
- Maintain quiet
- Open a window
- Adjust heat or air conditioning
- Maintain a tidy room

see Chapter 17 for management of pain, which is considered the fifth vital sign.

NUTRITION AND ORAL HYDRATION

ESSENTIAL NUTRIENTS

- Macronutrients: carbohydrates, proteins, lipids
- Micronutrients: vitamins, minerals
- Water

CARBOHYDRATES (CHO)

- Simple CHO (sugars)
  - —Monosaccharides or disaccharides
  - —Water-soluble
  - —Glucose is a monosaccharide, the simplest form of carbohydrate, and the energy source of cellular metabolism
  - —Sources: sugar, syrups, molasses, honey, fruit, and milk
  - —Energy yield: 4 kcal/g of CHO
- Complex CHO (starches and fiber)
  - —Insoluble, nonsweet CHO
  - —Polysaccharides
  - —Sources: bread, cereals, potato, rice, pasta, crackers, flour products, and legumes
  - —Fiber is a nondigestible, complex CHO, which provides roughage
- Functions of CHO
  - —Provides energy thereby sparing protein
  - —Essential for normal fat metabolism
  - —Promotes growth of normal flora in GI tract thereby supporting synthesis/absorption of vitamins K and B12
  - —Needed for the synthesis of nonessential amino acids
  - —Fiber supplies bulk to the diet stimulating peristalsis and maintaining bowel function
- CHO is stored as glycogen or converted to fat:
  - —glycogenesis
    - formation of glycogen from glucose
    - glycogen is stored primarily in liver and skeletal muscle
    - glycogen is converted back to glucose as needed for energy

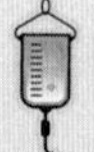

Clinical Alert

Processed CHOs have been extracted from the plants that produce them and concentrated, thereby removing other nutrients such as proteins, vitamins, and minerals leaving a high-calorie, relatively nutrient-poor foodstuff. Therefore, a healthy diet should contain natural as opposed to processed sources of CHO.

PROTEINS

- Proteins are composed of amino acids and contain nitrogen (amino acids are the simplest form of protein).
  - —Essential amino acids
    - There are nine different essential amino acids.
    - They cannot be made by body.
    - They must be taken in as part of diet.

—Nonessential amino acids
  - They can be made by the body.
  - Each does not have to be ingested as part of the diet.
- Complete proteins
  —These contain all nine essential amino acids.
  —Most animal proteins are complete: meat, fish, dairy products, and eggs.
  —Soy is the only complete vegetable protein.
- Partially complete proteins: These contain all essential amino acids but less than needed amount of one or more of them, Gelatin is a partially complete protein.
- Incomplete proteins
  —These do not contain one or more essential amino acids.
  —They are usually vegetable proteins.
  —Sources: dried beans and peas, peanut butter, seeds, fruits, vegetables, bread, cereal, rice, and pasta.
  —Client can utilize incomplete protein well by mixing with a small amount of complete protein, for example, cereal and milk, and pasta and cheese.
- Complementary proteins: incomplete proteins that when taken together make a complete protein, for example, corn and beans, peanut butter and wheat bread, and black beans and rice.
- Energy yield: 4 kcal/g.
- Functions of proteins
  —Maintenance of tissue and growth.
  —Regulation of body functions (enzymes are composed of protein).
- Protein metabolism
  —Anabolism: building of proteins from amino acids by cells.
  —Catabolism: breakdown of excess amino acids by liver for energy or conversion to fat.
  —Amino acids are not stored in body.
  —Nitrogen balance: state in which nitrogen intake equals output.
    - Negative nitrogen balance: output greater than intake.
    - Positive nitrogen balance: intake exceeds output.

LIPIDS

- Fats—name for lipids that are solid at room temperature.
- Oils—name for lipids that are liquid at room temperature.
- Fatty acids—building blocks (simplest form) of lipids.
  —Saturated fatty acids: all carbon atoms contain as many hydrogen atoms as possible
  —Unsaturated fatty acids:
    - monounsaturated
    - polyunsaturated
- Glycerides—glycerol molecule with up to three fatty acids attached (triglycerides refers to those that have three fatty acids attached).
  —Saturated triglycerides: glycerol with three saturated fatty acids.
    - Usually are in animal fats.
    - Usually solid at room temperature.
    - Example: butter, salt pork, etc.
  —Unsaturated triglycerides: glycerol with three unsaturated fatty acids.
    - Usually are in vegetable fats.
    - Usually liquid at room temperature.
    - Example: olive oil, corn oil, etc.
  —Energy yield: 9 kcal/g (concentrated energy source).

Function of Lipids

- Cellular transport
- Insulation
- Protection of vital organs
- Source of energy (9 kcal/gram)
- Vitamin absorption
- Transport of fat soluble vitamins

Cholesterol

- Cholesterol is a fat-like material.
- It is produced by the liver.
- It is found in animal products (egg yolk, milk, and organ meats).
- Use: formation of bile acids and steroid hormones; it is a component of cell membranes and other structures.

VITAMINS

- Small quantities of vitamins are required for metabolism.
- Vitamins cannot be made in the body.
- They must be taken in as part of diet.

Water-Soluble Vitamins

- Vitamin C (ascorbic acid) is needed for the formation of collagen in healing wounds and for absorption of iron; found in citrus fruits; deficiency results in impaired healing and scurvy.
- Vitamin B1 (thiamine) is essential for carbohydrate metabolism; found in enriched flour; deficiency causes beriberi.
- Vitamin B2 (riboflavin) is needed for the breakdown of fatty acids and amino acids for energy; found in milk and milk products; deficiency causes inflamed eyes, cracked lips, and a red, swollen tongue.
- Vitamin B5 (niacin) converts glucose to energy; found in enriched bread and wheat, and rice.

- Vitamin B6 (pyridoxine) is needed for the formation of RBCs and amino acids and for the metabolism of glucose; found in meats and whole grains.
- Vitamin B12 (cobalamin) is needed for protein metabolism and RBC formation; found only in meat, fish, cheese, and eggs; deficiency that occurs when the vitamin is not absorbed because of a lack of intrinsic factor in the stomach required for the absorption of vitamin B12 in the terminal ileum is called pernicious anemia.
- Folic acid (folacin) is essential to RBC development; it is found in organ meats and green, leafy vegetables. Its deficiency causes anemia.
- Pantothenic acid is a component of coenzyme A, which is necessary for metabolism of CHO, proteins, and fats and synthesis of cholesterol, steroid hormones, acetylcholine, and heme; found in foods such as liver, kidney, yeast, egg yolk, broccoli, and yogurt.
- Biotin is needed for synthesis of fatty acids, gluconeogenesis, energy production, and protein metabolism; found in brewer's yeast, egg yolk, organ meats, milk, soya, and barley.
- Water-soluble vitamins
  —cannot be stored in the body,
  —need to be ingested daily, and
  —can be lost from foods by boiling, sitting in water.

Fat-Soluble Vitamins

- Vitamin A (retinol) is necessary for good eyesight; found in yellow fruits and vegetables.
- Vitamin D (calciferol) is essential to bone health; it is manufactured in the body by the action of sunlight on substances in the skin and found in fortified milk and fish oils; deficiency causes rickets.
- Vitamin E (tocopherol) protects essential fatty acids and decreases destruction of RBCs; found in wheat germ.
- Vitamin K (menadione) is essential for the formation of prothrombin, and is therefore essential to clotting; manufactured by bacteria in the gut and found in green, leafy vegetables; deficiency results in bleeding problems.
- Fat-soluble vitamins
  —are stored in liver,
  —do not need to be ingested daily, and
  —excessive intake can result in hypervitaminosis for vitamins A and D.

MINERALS

- Major minerals (macrominerals): sodium (Na), chlorine (Cl), potassium (K), calcium (Ca), phosphorus (P), magnesium (Mg), and sulfur (S).
- Trace minerals (microminerals): iron (Fe), zinc (Zn), iodine (I), selenium (Se), copper (Cu), manganese (Mn), fluorine (Fl), chromium (Cr), and molybdenum (Mo).

DAILY ENERGY REQUIREMENT

Energy is needed

- for essential body functions,
- for additional physical activity, and
- to digest, absorb, transport, metabolize, and store nutrients.

IDEAL BODY WEIGHT

Weight recommended for optimal health is calculated using

- standardized weight tables and
- body mass index (BMI).

FACTORS AFFECTING NUTRITIONAL STATUS

- Age/development: nutritional needs increase during growth periods; decrease with old age and related risk of chronic disease (see Table 13–3 for detail).
- Gender: large muscle mass of men requires more calories and proteins; in women, menstruation requires additional iron, pregnancy and lactation require additional nutrients, calories, and fluids.
- Food preferences: both culturally determined and determined by the individual.
- Religious practices: fasting, avoidance of certain foods.
- Lifestyle factors: schedules, facilities for food preparation, level of exercise, and economic level.
- Physiological/health factors: problems such as difficulty in chewing (edentulous or poorly fitting dentures), swallowing (stroke), digesting (lactose intolerance), or absorbing nutrients (malabsorption syndromes).
- Therapeutic: effects or requirements of medications and treatments.
- Psychologic factors: under- or overeating in response to stress, depression; response to advertising

GUIDELINES FOR HEALTHY EATING

- Guiding principle: Eat a varied diet— heavy on fruits, vegetables, and grains, low in fat and cholesterol, moderate in everything else.
- Food-guide pyramid
  —It is the guide to daily food intake.
  —It identifies five food groups and recommends number of servings per day of each (see Table 13–4).
  —Variations of the standard pyramid are available for specific age groups and specific ethnic groups.

Table 13–3 Lifespan Nutritional Considerations

Birth to 1 Year	Period of greatest nutritional demand per unit body weight because it is period of most rapid growth Breast milk of formula; no cow's milk until 1 year; solid foods begun no earlier than 6 months because of risk of allergic reactions. Vitamin supplements and iron enriched foods are recommended; iron stores from birth deplete by 3–4 months.
PEDS Toddler	Can eat most adult foods and adjust to 3 meals per day Needs 1250 ml per 24 hours of fluid approximately Required calories decrease to 900--1800 kcal/d Table foods more nutritious than prepared toddler foods Toddlers may refuse certain foods or follow a certain ritual in eating
PEDS Preschooler	Snacks between meals for active children: cheese, fruits, raw vegetables, milk, and yogurt May rush through meals to play so need to monitor that nutritional needs are being met If in daycare or preschool, become informed about diet Needs 1500 ml per24 hours of fluid approximately
PEDS School-age child	Require 2400 kcal/d: 3 meals and 1--2 snacks Protein-rich food for breakfast essential to physical and mental demands of school 1750 ml per 24 hours of fluid To prevent obesity, monitor child's eating habits, provide balanced meals and lunches, healthy snacks, do not use food as reward, and promote regular exercise
PEDS Adolescent	Increased need for nutrients especially protein, calories, vitamins (groups B and D) and minerals (calcium and iron) particularly during growth spurt Typically have irregular eating patterns with frequent snacking or dieting Encourage healthy snacks; limit availability of junk food Be alert for developing problems such as anorexia nervosa, bulimia, and obesity
Young adult	Focus on dietary teaching to decrease risk of obesity, anemia, osteoporosis, and hypertension Number and size of nutrient servings for a healthy diet Females need 18-mg iron daily Need for calcium and vitamin D for bones
Middle age	Focus on adequate protein, calcium to prevent osteoporosis, and limit cholesterol to decrease risk of heart disease. 2000–3000 ml of fluid daily Caloric need decreased because of decreased metabolic rate and decreased activity so calories need to be limited to avoid obesity and decrease risk of diabetes, heart disease, and problems with mobility
Older adult	Nutritional needs are basically unchanged May need additional fiber Decreased smell, taste, saliva, and gastric acid, problems with chewing and swallowing may require dietary adjustments Economic, mobility, and psychological issues such as loneliness may result due to inadequate nutrition Encourage inclusion of high-nutrient foods in diet

VEGETARIAN DIETS

- Vegans—eat only plant foods, no meat, fish, eggs, and dairy products.
- Other variations allow dairy products (lacto-vegetarians); dairy products and eggs (lacto-ovo-vegetarians); eggs but no meat or dairy products (ovo-vegetarians); dairy products, eggs, and fish but not meat (pesco-vegetarians); only certain types of meat (partial vegetarians); and only fresh fruit, juice, nuts, honey, and olive oil (fruitarians—not an adequate diet).

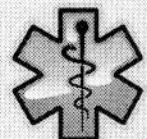

Nursing Intervention Alert

Vitamin B12 and iron are specific concerns for vegetarians. Brewer's yeast, B12-fortified foods, or B12 supplements should be included in diet. Foods rich in iron such as raisins, leafy green vegetables, whole grains, and iron-enriched foods should be ingested daily along with foods high in vitamin C, which promotes absorption of iron.

Table 13–4 Food Groups and Recommended Daily Servings

Age Group	Bread, Cereal Rice and Pasta	Vegetable Group	Fruit Group	Meat, Poultry, Fish, Beans,	Milk, Yogurt, Eggs, and Nuts	Fats, Oils, and Sweets and Cheese
Recommended servings	6–11	3–5	2–4	2–3		Use sparingly
PEDS Under 9 years					2–3	
PEDS Age 9–12 years					3 or more	
PEDS Teen					4 or more	
Adult					2 or more	
OB Pregnant					3 or more	
OB Lactating					4 or more	

NUTRITIONAL ASSESSMENT

Nutritional Screening

- Nutritional assessment is used to identify clients who are at risk of becoming malnourished. Once identified, more in-depth assessment is obtained.
- Screening tools for particular population groups such as the elderly, those with heart disease, and the pregnant have been developed.

Specific Methods of Obtaining Dietary Data

- 24-hour food recall—Client reports all food and beverage ingested in a typical 24-hour period.
- Food frequency record—Checklist of foods marked by the client as number of times eaten in a day, week, or month or marked as frequently eaten, seldom eaten, or never eaten. May include only foods suspected of being eaten in insufficient or excessive quantities.
- Food diary—Record of measured amounts of all food and fluids eaten in a specified time, usually 3–7 days.
- Diet history—Comprehensive analysis of type and amount of foods eaten and factors influencing their selection; obtained by a nutritionist or dietician.

Information reported on these tools can be analyzed against food pyramid recommendations to judge adequacy.

Physical Examination

- Obtain accurate height and weight measurements.
- Identify amount and direction of weight change: compare current body weight to usual body weight.
- Identify any weight change as intentional or unintentional.
- Observe for signs of malnutrition such as listless, tired appearance; dry, lackluster hair, pale, dry skin and nails; dull eyes with pale or reddened conjunctiva; swollen, smooth beefy-red or magenta tongue and swollen, spongy gums; swollen lips with cracks at the corners, slight musculature; irritability; and decreased reflexes.

Anthropometric Measurements

- Triceps skinfold measurement (TSF)
  —Determines fat stores.
  —Grasp skin on back of upper arm halfway between the elbow and the shoulder; place calipers 1 cm below fingers and record the size of the TSF to the nearest millimeter.
- Mid-arm circumference (MAC)
  —Measures fat, muscle, and skeleton.
  —Instruct client to let arm hang freely and bend elbow 90 degrees.
  —Measure circumference of upper arm at midpoint between elbow and shoulder.
  —Record in centimeters and to the nearest millimeter.

- Mid-arm muscle circumference (MAMC)
  —Using the above two measurements, determine MAMC by checking a table or using a formula.
- Compare to standard measurements.

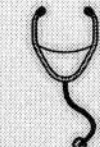

Assessment Alert

Changes in these measures occur slowly so they are used to monitor clients over months or years, not days or weeks. Measurements are affected by fluid status and normal age changes.

Laboratory Tests

- Serum proteins:used to estimate protein stores
  —Hemoglobin: low levels indicate iron-deficiency anemia; may or may not be dietary in cause.
  —Albumin: low albumin suggests long-term protein depletion as opposed to short-term depletion.
  —Transferrin: protein that transports iron from intestine through serum; decreases in response to protein lack more quickly than albumin.
  —Total iron-binding capacity: amount of iron in blood available to be bound; it provides an indirect measure of transferrin in the blood.
  —Prealbumin: responds most quickly of all the serum proteins to changes in nutrition; not routinely used because of expense.
- Urinary tests
  —Urinary urea nitrogen: compares nitrogen intake, calculated based on grams of protein intake, to nitrogen output calculated by the amount of urea (end product of amino acid metabolism) in the urine over 24 hours to provide a measure of protein catabolism and nitrogen balance.
  —Urinary creatinine: measures amount of creatinine (product of skeletal muscle metabolism; the more skeletal muscle, the more creatinine) excreted by kidney; reflects muscle mass, which decreases with malnutrition.
- Total lymphocyte count
  —Number of lymphocytes decrease as protein depletion occurs.

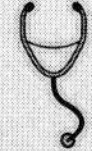

Assessment Alert

No one laboratory test is diagnostic of malnutrition—all findings can be due to a number of different causes.

TYPES OF DIETS

- Standard diet (house diet)
  —Balanced 2000 kcal diet based on the needs of a sedentary adult.
- Light diet
  —Plainly cooked.
  —No fat.
  —Limited fiber.
  —Used for persons not ready for full normal diet such as postoperative clients or those resuming eating full diet after an illness.
- Modified-consistency diets
  —Clear liquid diet
  - consists of clear liquids including broth and gelatin.
  - provides sugar; rests GI tract, relieves thirst, and prevents dehydration.
  - does not meet the need for protein, fat, vitamin, minerals, or calories.
  - is prescribed for short intervals only (24–36 hours).
  - is used postoperatively; as preparation for tests/surgery on GI tract; for GI infection/disease.

  —Full liquid diet
  - consists of foods liquid at body temperature including ice cream, yogurt, cream of wheat or rice cereal, pudding, and custard.
  - lacks in iron, protein, and calories; high in cholesterol.
  - is balanced with an oral supplement, such as Ensure, if required for more than a short time.

  —Soft diet
  - consists of foods that are easy to chew and swallow.
  - contains little fiber so is low-residue.

  —Pureed diet
  - is an adaptation of soft diet.
  - is prepared by adding liquid to foods and blending to create semi-solid consistency.
- Modified-nutrient diets
  —Low-sodium diet
  - Used in management of cardiovascular and kidney disease; portal hypertension.
  - Examples of food stuffs not allowed: Deli meats, bacon, ham; canned soups, bouillon, vegetables, and meats; table salt and salt based seasonings; olives; salted-snack foods; cheese and regular butter; gravies; frozen fish, pizza, and sausage products.

  —Potassium-rich diet
  - Used to replace potassium lost through the kidneys as a result of potassium-losing diuretics.
  - Foods rich in potassium include baked potato, cantaloupe, bananas, and oranges.

—Low-protein diet
- Used in management of hepatic encephalopathy and renal failure.
- Foodstuffs that are limited include meat, poultry, fish, cheese, eggs, and milk.

—High-protein diet
- Used whenever tissue needs to be built: after extensive burns, surgery, or malnutrition.
- All complete protein foods limited in low-protein diet are encouraged in a high-protein diet. Incomplete proteins are not useful in high-protein diets.

—Low-purine diet
- Used in the management of gout and certain types of kidney stones.
- Foods to be avoided include organ meats, sardines, anchovies, bouillon and other meat soups and gravies, and alcohol.

—Acid-ash diet
- Used in the prophylaxis and management of UTIs.
- Foods allowed include meat, fish, poultry, eggs, cereals, and cranberries, prunes, and plums; all other fruits are disallowed.

—Alkaline-ash diet
- Used to dissolve urinary stones composed of uric acid or cystine
- Foods allowed include fruits except cranberries, prunes, and plums, milk, vegetables, and carbonated vegetables.

—Modified kilocalorie diets

PARENTERAL AND ENTERAL NUTRITION

Parenteral Nutrition (Total Parenteral Nutrition, Intravenous Hyperalimentation)

- In parenteral nutrition, nutrient solutions are given directly into a high-flow central vein (e.g., through a central venous catheter into the superior vena cava) because they are hypertonic and need to be immediately diluted by the client's blood.
- This type of nutrition is used when GI tract is nonfunctioning.

Nursing Process Elements

- Assess for problems/risk for problems related to nutrition:
  —Signs of under- or overnutrition using anthropometric measures, laboratory data, physical characteristics, and dietary data
  —Anorexia
  —Dysphagia
  —Difficulty in chewing
  —Mobility problems that interfere with obtaining or preparing food or feeding self
- Stimulate appetite
  —Do not schedule unpleasant treatments for immediately before or after mealtime
  —Ensure clean, attractive environment free of odors or unpleasant sights
  —Make client comfortable for meals:
    - Encourage going to toilet
    - Instruct to wash hands
    - Provide mouth care
    - Provide a comfortable seat
    - Seat in a good position
    - Avoid constricting clothing or linens
    - Medicate for pain or other symptoms

  —Provide small portions of liked foods served neatly and attractively with clean utensils
  —Provide a stress-free social setting for meals when possible
- Assist with eating as needed:
  —Prepare food for eating: cut meat; butter bread; pour tea
  —Provide adaptive feeding aids to enable maximal independence (see section on "Assistive Devices")
  —Orient clients with impaired vision to type and location of foods and utensils. Describe location in terms of numbers on a clock face
  —If feeding client:
    - Create an unhurried environment
    - Make the client sit to feed if possible
    - Have client select order of foods fed
    - Provide manageable size bites
    - Allow sufficient time for swallowing
    - Offer fluids after every three or four bites of solid food
- Record intake, output, calorie count PRN, and document client's tolerance of the meal: difficulty in swallowing, nausea, and fatigue

Client teaching for self-care

Teach client about
- components of a healthy diet
- dietary/caloric requirements relative to the client's age, weight, and health status
- need for fluids
- food sources of specific nutrients

- giving special emphasis on complete and incomplete proteins and complementary food equations (for vegetarians)
  —grains + legumes = complete protein
  —legumes + nuts or seeds = complete protein
  —grains, legumes, nuts or seeds + dairy = complete protein
- how to read food labels
- proper food storage and preparation
- resources to aid in obtaining and preparing nutritious foods
- purpose of special diets as well as allowed and prohibited foods
- strategies to promote compliance with therapeutic diet
- alternatives to prohibited foods
- controlling desire to eat by using a "10-minute wait", drinking water, and taking a walk
- involving family members for support
- utilizing community resources and support groups

Enteral Nutrition

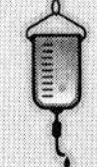

Clinical Alert

PEDS Orogastric tubes are used for infants because infants are obligatory nose breathers. Orogastric feedings are used for premature infants who have no gag reflexes, and therefore are at risk of aspiration if regular oral feedings are given.

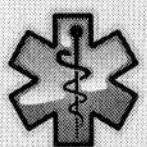

Nursing Intervention Alert

Bolus feedings can only be given into the stomach.

Enteral feedings are directly administered into the stomach or intestine by a nasogastric (through nose to stomach) tube, an orogastric (through mouth to stomach) tube, a nasoenteric (through nose into intestine) tube, a gastrostomy (through abdominal wall into stomach) tube, or a jejunostomy (through the abdominal wall into the jejunum) tube.

- Use nasogastric tubes (NG tubes) when
  —need for feedings is short-term,
  —gag and cough reflexes are intact, and
  —gastric emptying is normal.
- PEDS Use orogastric tube
  —for infants because infants cannot breathe through the mouth; they are obligatory nose breathers, and therefore the nostril can not be obstructed.
- Use a nasoenteric tube
  —for clients at risk for aspiration from the stomach such as restless, confused, or agitated clients; clients with an endotracheal tube or who have been recently extubated, and those with impaired cough or gag reflexes or decreased level of consciousness (LOC).
- Use a gastrostomy tube when
  —feedings will be needed for longer than 6–8 weeks.
- Use a jejunostomy tube when
  —feedings will be-long term and the risk of aspiration from the stomach is great.
- Types of gastrostomy/jejunostomy
  —Traditional
    - Tube is inserted surgically and sutured in place; in 10–14 days, when healing is complete, the tube can be removed and then reinserted for each feeding; when the tube is not in place a prosthetic cap is worn to cover the ostomy.
  —PEG or PEJ
    - Tube with rubber bumpers and an inflatable balloon to hold it in place is inserted through the abdominal wall with an endoscope; once healing has occurred, tube can be inserted without an endoscope.
- Schedule of feedings
  —Intermittent (300–500 ml several times daily)
  —Continuous (given over 24 hours via infusion pump to maintain a set rate)
  —Bolus feeding (type of intermittent feeding in which a syringe is used to rapidly administer the feeding)
  —Cyclic feedings (continuous feedings given over less than 24 hours, e.g., 12 or 16)
  —Only continuous feedings can be given into the intestine
- Formulas and feeding systems
  —The formulas are selected based on client needs: with a standard formula, there is 1 kcal/ml of solution with nutrients in specified proportions.
  —Feedings come in open and closed systems.
  —Open systems
    - Feedings are canned liquids or powders to be reconstituted.
    - Once opened, canned liquid formulas must be refrigerated and used within 24 hours.

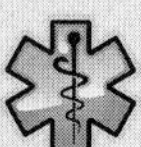

Nursing Intervention Alert

When formula must be reconstituted, sterile water is used to decrease the risk of contamination. The formula must be labeled with time, date, type of formula, and strength. Formula must be refrigerated and disposed of if more than 24-hours old.

—Closed systems consist of prefilled bags that are spiked with enteral tubing; these can be used within 24–36 hours.

—Feedings are given at room temperature unless otherwise prescribed.

Nursing Process Elements

- Assess bowel function by checking for bowel sounds before intermittent feedings and every 4–8 hours for continuous feedings
- Check order for type of feeding and rate
- Use enteral controller to regulate the amount of feeding the client is receiving
- Check expiration date of formula
- Label all equipment with name, date, rate, formula used, and the date when started
- Check tube placement by aspirating and checking pH of aspirate. Stomach secretions are usually green, tan, or off-white with a pH of 1–4 while intestinal secretions are yellow or brownish green stained with bile, with a pH up to 6

Think Smart–Test Smart

Recognize the fact that the appearance of secretions and measurement of pH cannot guarantee correct verification of tube placement. Secretions vary and sometimes secretions that are similar in appearance to GI secretions, can be aspirated from the respiratory tree. The pH can also vary and respiratory secretions can be as low as 6 and gastric secretions can be as high as 6 in clients with disorders of gastric acid secretion or who are taking medications to decrease it. The most reliable method of verifying tube placement is by X-ray visualization.

- Respiratory secretions are typically, though not always, 7 or higher
- If residual feeding of more than 100 ml for NG tube or more than 200 ml for gastrostomy tube is obtained on aspiration, hold feeding for 30 minutes to an hour and recheck. If it is still 100 ml/200 ml, contact physician.
- Place client in Fowler's position, or if contraindicated, in a right-sided position with head of bed elevated 30–45 degrees to prevent aspiration during feeding
- Flush tube with 30–50 ml of water before and after each feeding, to ensure patency
- Monitor for abdominal distention which can indicate intolerance of previous feedings; regurgitation and sense of fullness after feedings which can indicate need to decrease rate or amount of feeding; and for diarrhea or constipation which can develop due to the concentrated ingredients in the formula or the lack of bulk respectively
- Monitor for dumping syndrome if feedings are via a jejunostomy tube
- When administering medications, shut off feeding, give each separately and flush with water in between
- Do not mix medications with feeding formula
- Irrigate clogged tube with water or Viokase according to agency policy
- Document
  —date and time
  —amount of residual feeding
  —formula type, strength, and amount as well as any water instilled on the I&O sheet
  —client's tolerance of the procedure
  —any care of the stoma site
- Change disposable equipment every 24 hours
- If feeding is via an NG tube, check that the tube is securely taped, and not causing nasal irritation; if feeding is given through a gastrostomy or PEG tube, assess site for infection or skin breakdown
- Monitor for complications as aspiration, diarrhea, constipation, unplanned extubation, obstruction, or hyperglycemia
- When client requires long-term feeding at home, teach procedure to client or caregiver, arrange visits by home care RN

Before starting an enteral feeding, the client must be in a semi-Fowler's position for at least 30 minutes and the tube aspirated to check for residual feeding. If more than 100 ml of residual feeding is aspirated, the physician is notified. Following an *intermittent feeding*, the tube is flushed with 50 ml of water and the client remains in a sitting or right-side-lying position for 30–60 minutes.

When *continuous feedings* are administered, the tubing and container must be changed every 24 hours.

PALLIATIVE/COMFORT CARE

World Health Organization (WHO) definition of palliative/comfort care: "Approach which improves the quality of life of patients and their families facing life-threatening illness, through the prevention, assessment and treatment of pain and other physical, psychosocial, and spiritual problems."

- The focus is on the whole person, relieving distressing symptoms and improving quality of life.
- It utilizes an interdisciplinary team approach.
- It is provided along with other medical treatments.
- It incorporates complimentary and alternative approaches.
- It is not just end-of-life care; it starts at the time of diagnosis.
- It does not hasten or delay death.
- It provides a support system for remaining as active as possible until death.
- It offers support to family during client's illness and during grieving.

Refer to Chapter 16 for detailed discussion of relief of symptoms.

PERSONAL HYGIENE

- Factors that determine hygienic measures appropriate for a client include personal preferences (which may be culture-based), self-care ability, and skin condition
- Personal preferences of the client such as time and frequency of showering and/or bathing, type of oral care, usual hair and nail care, use of soaps, bath oils, lotions, powder, deodorant, etc., and products not used because of reactions such as dryness, itch, or rash

BATHING AND CARE OF THE SKIN

- Skin is the body's first line of defense so design and implement measures with the goal of maintaining an intact, healthy skin
- Skin sensitivity is greatest in infants, young children, older adults, and in under- and overweight persons
  - —Prevent/treat dry skin, which is easily damaged:
    - Limit bathing to once or twice per week
    - Limit or avoid use of soap; use cleansing cream
    - Avoid use of alcohol-based products
    - Apply lotions or creams
  - —Prevent injury to skin:
    - Protect from friction and shearing forces
    - Prevent scratching
    - Protect from excessive pressure

Nursing Process Elements

- Prevent irritation and infection:
  - —Wash from clean to dirty—for the perineum this means front to back
  - —When washing face, wash eyes first going from inner to outer canthus and using a different section of washcloth for each
  - —Rinse skin thoroughly to remove all soap residue
  - —Dry skin thoroughly but gently with special attention to skin fold areas such as under the breasts, groin, axilla, under the abdominal "apron" of overweight clients and between toes because bacteria grow best in warm, dark, and moist areas
- Check temperature of water carefully for clients who are confused or have poor circulation, as they may be unable to do so safely
- Do not leave children unattended in bathtub

Nursing Intervention Alert

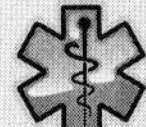

PEDS Neonates should be immediately dried and wrapped after bathing to prevent heat loss because heat is lost rapidly as a result of body surface area being large relative to body mass and because their temperature-regulating mechanisms are immature.

FOOT CARE

Proper foot care is critical for diabetic clients and others with poor circulation to the feet.

NAIL CARE

- Soak hands or feet if needed to soften nails before cutting or filing.
- Cut nails straight across at end of fingers or toes; then use file to round corners.
- File, do not cut, nails of diabetic clients and other clients with poor circulation.
- Do not trim nails low in corners because of the risk of ingrown nails.

ORAL CARE

Nursing Process Elements

- Assess for clients at risk for oral health problems:
  —Those unable to maintain oral hygiene: comatose, confused, and depressed
  —Those with dry oral mucous membranes: anxious, dehydrated, heavy smokers, alcohol users, mouth breathers, for example, those with a NG tube, oxygen, nasal packing, those with salivary-gland damage from radiation to the head or neck, and those taking medications such as tranquilizers (chlorpromazine, diazepam), anticholinergics, diuretics, and chemotherapeutic agents
  —Those with poorly cared for teeth or improperly fitting dentures

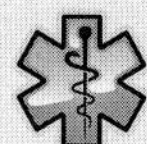

Nursing Intervention Alert

Hyperplasia of the gums is a side effect of phenytoin (Dilantin) so regular flossing and brushing with a soft brush is critical.

- Monitor for dryness of mucous membrane and for signs of glossitis and stomatitis
- Provide/assist/teach oral hygiene to clients PRN
- Assess the gag reflex before giving or delegating oral care
- Prevent aspiration when giving oral care to unconscious clients: turn head to side and lower head if possible; when using syringe to rinse, inject fluid into mouth gently to avoid forcing it into the throat; make sure all fluid is removed from mouth
- Avoid long-term use of lemon and glycerine swabs because of their drying effect and effect on tooth enamel
- Use only a water-soluble lubricant for lips or nares because aspiration of an oil-based lubricant can cause lipid pneumonia
- Use hydrogen peroxide in the mouth with caution as it can irritate mucosa and alter normal flora
- If delegating oral care, instruct regarding correct positioning, use of oral suction catheter if needed, and remind to report any changes in mucosa

REST AND SLEEP

- Rest: Cessation of work that provides for a period of relaxation in which the person is awake.
- Sleep: Physiologic state of full or partial unconsciousness during which the body suspends voluntary actions while the body rests and restores itself. The sleep cycle consists of two major stages:
  —Rapid eye movement (REM) sleep during which people dream.
  —Nonrapid eye movement (NREM): sleep which consists of 4 stages:
    - Stage 1: very light sleep characterized by drowsiness and relaxation, eyes roll from side to side, and heart rate and respirations decrease; lasts only moments and the client is easily woken.
    - Stage 2: light sleep with continued slowing of body functions; decline in temperature; eyes are still. Lasts 10–15 minutes and represents 40–45% of the total time the client is asleep.
    - Stage 3: further slowing of the heart and respiratory rates along with other body systems due to dominance of the parasympathetic system; client not easily aroused; skeletal muscles are relaxed; reflexes are diminished and snoring is common.
    - Stage 4: deep sleep (delta sleep) that lasts up to 30 minutes; heart and respiratory rates are 20–30% below normal waking hour rates; client is difficult to arouse, very relaxed with little movement and occasional dreaming. Body replenishes itself during stage 4.
    - REM sleep (paradoxical sleep): lasts 5–30 minutes and occurs about every 90 minutes. Brain is very active with its metabolism increased by nearly 20% and dreaming occurs. Client is difficult to arouse

but may wake spontaneously. Muscle tone is depressed, gastric secretions increased, and irregularities in both heart and respiratory rates may occur.

- A complete sleep cycle for adults lasts 1.5 hours and most experience 4–6 cycles during a 7–8 hour sleep.

SLEEP REQUIREMENTS

- PEDS Newborns: 16 hours of sleep per day typically divided into seven sleep periods.
- PEDS Infants can sleep up to 22 hr/d though 10–12 hours of sleep may be adequate.
- PEDS Toddlers sleep 10–12 hr/d and spend approximately 20–30% of sleep in REM. Preschool child sleeps 11–12 hr/d with REM sleep being 20–30% that of an adult.
- PEDS School-age children: 8–12 hour sleep with REM sleep decreasing to 20% of the cycle.
- PEDS Adolescents: 8–10 hours of sleep prevents unnecessary fatigue and susceptibility to infection. REM sleep continues to be 20%. Nocturnal emissions are experienced by adolescent boys.
- Young adults do well with 7–8 hours of sleep and by mid-adulthood can feel adequately replenished with as little as 6 hours of sleep with REM remaining at 20%.
- Many elderly clients require as little as 6 hours of sleep with the first REM period being longer at 20–25% of the sleep cycle. However, stage-4 sleep is decreased or absent resulting in a less restorative sleep. Older persons tend to wake more frequently during the night and have more difficulty falling back to sleep. Some older people experience confusion at night (sundown syndrome), which may be the result of a decrease in stimulation, change in sleep–wake cycle (circadian rhythm), or Alzheimer's disease.

Nursing Process Elements

- Determine client's sleep activity pattern
- Provide food or fluid that would facilitate sleep, such as milk or protein
- Provide a quiet, dark environment
- Limit activities that could interrupt sleep, such as taking vital signs
- Provide a back massage to promote comfort and rest
- Administer sleep or pain medication as appropriate
- Position an immobile client to facilitate muscle relaxation
- Support pressure-prone areas of the body
- Provide loose-fitting clothing

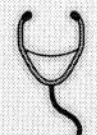

Assessment Alert

Factors affecting the client's ability to achieve adequate rest and sleep include pain, respiratory conditions that affect breathing pattern, gastric or duodenal ulcers (increased gastric secretions during sleep), endocrine disturbances (hyperthyroidism increases presleep time, hypothyroidism decreases stage-4 sleep, low estrogen levels), elevated body temperature, need to urinate, environment (too hot/cold, too much light, noise), fatigue, shift work, emotional stress, stimulants (caffeine, nicotine), alcohol, diet, and medications that disrupt sleep cycle (amphetamines, antidepressants, beta blockers, bronchodilators, decongestants, narcotics, and steroids).

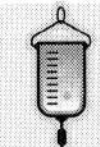

Clinical Alert

Milk and protein contain tryptophan, which is a precursor to serotonin and is thought to facilitate and maintain sleep.

Client teaching for self-care

Teach client

- that the five phases of sleep include REM (rapid eye movement, which is the time people dream) and NREM (nonrapid eye movement that includes two phases of deep sleep)
- to avoid or eliminate stressful situations prior to bedtime
- to void prior to going to bed
- to wear loose-fitting clothing
- to exercise regularly
- to avoid consuming alcohol, caffeine beverages, or a heavy meal at least 3 hours before bedtime
- to decrease fluid intake 2–3 hours prior to bedtime
- to maintain a regular bedtime and wakeup time always, including vacation and weekends
- when unable to sleep, to get up and do a nonstrenuous activity until sleepy

WORKSHEET

MATCHING QUESTIONS

Match the following (note that terms and/or descriptions may be used once, more than once, or not at all):

1. _____ A protein-sparing source of energy	a. Meditation
2. _____ A complex carbohydrate that promotes peristalsis	b. Vitamin C
3. _____ A fat which is filled with hydrogen atoms	c. Biofeedback
4. _____ An important component of cell membranes	d. Massage
5. _____ A fat-soluble vitamin	e. Saturated fat
6. _____ The form in which carbohydrates are stored in muscles and the liver	f. Glycogen
7. _____ Difficulty in swallowing	g. Black cohosh
8. _____ A comprehensive accounting of foods selected and eaten	h. Fiber
9. _____ A glycerol and three fatty acids	i. Atropine
10. _____ The transferring of universal life energy	j. Reiki therapy
11. _____ The improvement of blood flow secondary to muscle manipulation	k. Vitamin D
12. _____ A herb that exhibits mild estrogen-like action	l. Citrucel
13. _____ A complementary therapy that decreases respiratory rate and oxygen consumption	m. Diet history
14. _____ A herb that enhances immune functioning	n. Garlic
15. _____ A herb that decreases cholesterol and increases HDLs	o. Fecal impaction
16. _____ A complementary therapy that is contraindicated in the presence of clotting disorders	p. Hesitancy
17. _____ The decrease in muscle size associated with prolonged immobility	q. Tarry stools
18. _____ The self-regulation of physiologic processes	r. Dysphagia
19. _____ A common side effect of this medication is urinary retention	s. Acupuncture
20. _____ The presence of hard, dry stool in the rectum	t. *Echinacea*
21. _____ A bulk-forming laxative	u. Opioids
22. _____ Difficulty in starting a urinary stream	v. Carbohydrate

23. _____ A vitamin that acidifies urine	w. Triglyceride
24. _____ An indication of upper GI bleeding	x. Cholesterol
25. _____ A common side effect of this medication is constipation	y. Food intake
	z. Disuse atrophy

FILL IN THE BLANKS

Fill in the blanks with the correct word or phrase to complete each statement.

1. The client consumes a snack containing 15 g of carbohydrate, 5 g of protein, and 2 g of fat. The client has consumed ________ calories in this snack.
2. Three benefits of a clear liquid diet are: ________, ______________________, and ____________.
3. A curved cane with a lower handgrip is useful in helping the client perform which activity of daily living? ________________________.
4. A permanent shortening of muscle fibers, tendons, and ligaments is termed a _______________.
5. Four nonpharmacological comfort measures are
   a. ____
   b. ____
   c. ____
   d. ____
6. A written record of all foods consumed in a 3-day time period is called a ______________________.
7. The two nutritional deficiencies for which vegans are at greatest risk are ___________ and ___________.
8. During which stage of sleep is the brain most active? __________________.
9. Three assistive devices that the nurse could recommend to a client who has difficulty bending at the waist are
   a. ____
   b. ____
   c. ____
10. A client seeking to restore energy (Qi) flow to a specific body part would go to a practitioner of ______________________.
11. Four factors that the nurse would assess when determining a client's ability to achieve adequate rest and sleep are
   a. ____
   b. ____

(continued)

c. ______________________________

d. ______________________________

12. The nurse teaches the client that the minimum amount of fluid to consume daily is ______________ ml.

13. Laxatives are contraindicated in the presence of ____________.

14. List one nurse-initiated intervention that induces voiding. _____

15. An hourly urinary output of less than _______ ml must be reported to the physician immediately.

16. Vitamin ________ is manufactured by intestinal bacteria and is also found in green, leafy vegetables.

17. Vitamin ________ is essential for good eyesight.

18. Vitamin ________ protects essential fatty acids.

19. Clotting is impaired by a deficiency of vitamin ________.

20. Pernicious anemia results from a lack of vitamin ________.

21. The four factors that can contribute to disturbed sleep patterns are

a. ______________________________

b. ______________________________

c. ______________________________

d. ______________________________

TRUE & FALSE QUESTIONS

Mark each of the following statements True or False. Correct all false statements in the space provided.

1. Complete proteins are found only in animal-based food sources. ____ T ____ F
2. The total lymphocyte count decreases with protein depletion. ____ T ____ F
3. Nasogastric tubes are used for long-term enteral nutrition. ____ T ____ F
4. Older adults may require additional fiber in their diets. ____ T ____ F
5. Clients receiving palliative care must stop all medical treatments except pain control. ____ T ____ F
6. Lacto-ovo-vegetarians do not eat dairy or egg-containing foods. ____ T ____ F
7. Vitamin C promotes the absorption of carbohydrates. ____ T ____ F
8. Immobility is often accompanied by protein loss. ____ T ____ F
9. Atelectasis occurs when retained secretions become infected with bacteria. ____ T ____ F

10. Transitional stool is passed by newborns within 24 hours of birth. ___ T ___ F

11. Habit training for urinary incontinence requires placing the client on a planned voiding schedule. ___ T ___ F

12. A client can be easily aroused from stage-3 sleep. ___ T ___ F

13. Decreased stimulation is a cause of sundown syndrome. ___ T ___ F

14. Milk and protein if taken before bedtime will facilitate sleep. ___ T ___ F

15. The two age groups that require less than 8 hours of sleep are middle-aged adults and the elderly ___ T ___ F

APPLICATION QUESTIONS

1. Which statement made by a client following teaching about the importance of using only unsaturated fats when cooking indicates that information about which fats are unsaturated was understood?
   a. "I will use butter when cooking."
   b. "I will use olive oil when cooking."
   c. "I will use lard when cooking."
   d. "I will use palm oil when cooking."

2. When caring for a client taking phenytoin (Dilantin), the nurse assesses the client's mouth for which side effect of the drug?
   a. Gum hyperplasia
   b. Thrush
   c Dental caries
   d. Glossitis

3. When administering mouth care to an unconscious client, the nurse would place the client into which position?
   a. Dorsal recumbent
   b High-Fowler's
   c. Supine
   d. Side-lying

4. Which data should the nurse review to most accurately assess a client's protein stores?
   a. Urinary protein
   b. Triceps skinfold measurement
   c. Plasma albumin
   d. Height and weight

5. Which nursing order related to nutrition should be included in the plan of care for a client with limited vision?
   a. Assess for presence of the gag reflex
   b. Orient to type and location of foods and utensils
   c. Feed in the client's preferred order of eating
   d. Cut foods, then remove knife from tray

6. By which route does the nurse administer parenteral nutrition?
   a. Intravenous
   b. Nasogastric
   c. Intra-arterial
   d. Nasoenteric

7. The nurse performs range of motion exercises on an immobile client to avoid which complication associated with immobility?
   a. Urinary stasis
   b. Constipation
   c. Dependent edema
   d. Contractures

8. Which nursing intervention should receive priority when caring for an immobile client?
   a. Repositioning every 2 hours
   b. Assessing for dependent edema each shift
   c. Auscultating for bowel sounds daily
   d. Administering a calcium supplement twice a day

.(continued)

9. Which nursing intervention would best promote a client's psychospiritual comfort?
   a. Offering a back rub
   b. Maintaining a clean environment
   c. Encouraging expression of feeling
   d. Providing mouth and hair care

10. Use of a nasoenteric tube is the method of choice for the administration of enteral feedings when the client is at risk for which problem?
   a. Diarrhea
   b. Infection
   c. Aspiration
   d. Hyperkalemia

11. When teaching how to maintain healthy, intact skin, which direction would the nurse include?
   a. Bathe every day
   b. Apply lubricating lotions
   c. Briskly rub skin dry
   d. Use an alcohol-based skin splash weekly

12. A client states he is self-medicating with St. John's wort for mild depression. To assess for a common side effect of this OTC herb, which question should the nurse ask?
   a. "Have you experienced any abnormal bleeding?"
   b. "Have you had a rash or any other skin problem?"
   c. "How well do you sleep at night?"
   d. "Do you have any problems with constipation?"

13. Which direction should be included in the teaching plan for a client with orthostatic hypotension?
   a. Avoid use of the Valsalva maneuver
   b. Self-monitor blood pressure daily
   c. Limit use of table salt
   d. Change position slowly

14. Which conditions place a client at risk for oral health problems? (Select all that apply.)
   a. Coronary insufficiency
   b. Confusion
   c. Dehydration
   d. Obesity

15. Which suggestion would the nurse give to an older client who reports frequent waking at night with difficulty in falling back to sleep? (Select all that apply.)
   a. "Consume 5–10 oz of wine before bedtime."
   b. "Maintain a regular schedule of exercise."
   c. "Nap frequently during the day."
   d. "Get out of bed and read until sleepy."

16. The nurse would be cautious about including the alternative therapy of imagery in the plan of care for a client with which health problems? (Select all that apply.)
   a. Diabetes
   b. Asthma
   c. Psychosis
   d. Seizures

17. When caring for an unconscious client, the nurse implements nursing interventions directed at preventing which problems associated with immobility? (Select all that apply.)
   a. Pneumonia
   b. Osteoporosis
   c. Venous stasis
   d. Pressure ulcers

18. Which actions would the nurse take prior to initiating a NG tube feeding? (Select all that apply.)
   a. Check order for type and rate of feeding
   b. Wash hands
   c. Place client in the supine position
   d. Aspirate stomach contents and check pH

19. Which information regarding nutrition over the lifespan is correct? (Select all that apply.)
   a. Toddlers should be fed prepared toddler foods because they provide the best nutrition.
   b. The older adult's diminished taste and smell requires dietary adjustments.
   c. Menstruating females require additional daily iron.
   d. Middle-aged adults require additional calories to meet energy needs.

20. When delegating feeding of a client on a full liquid diet to a nonlicensed assistant, which items would the nurse include on the list of permitted foods? (Select all that apply.)
   a. Pudding
   b. Oatmeal cereal
   c. Yogurt
   d. Ice cream

21. Which of these nursing interventions would be most appropriate when monitoring an elderly client taking MOM (milk of magnesia) for the treatment of constipation?
   a. Assess serum electrolyte levels
   b. Administer supplemental B and C vitamins
   c. Instruct the client to limit physical activity
   d. Encourage the client to wear an incontinent pad

22. When obtaining a health history from a client with a history of liver disease, which new complaint would the nurse recognize as most pertinent?
    a. Pruritus
    b. Nausea
    c. Clay-colored stools
    d. Fatigue

23. When should the nurse plan to ambulate a client with constipation to the bathroom?
    a. As soon as the client wakes in the morning
    b. After the client has finished eating breakfast
    c. Immediately before eating dinner
    d. Prior to going to bed

24. A client's urinary output is 450 ml in 24 hours. Which term could the nurse use when documenting about the client's urinary elimination status?
    a. Anuria
    b. Oliguria
    c. Dysuria
    d. Nocturia

25. Which of the following statements, if made by a client, indicates correct understanding of self-care activities to decrease the likelihood of developing a urinary tract infection?
    a. "I will void every 6–8 hours."
    b. "I will take baths rather than showers."
    c. "I will perform pericare after each voiding."
    d. "I will void before and after sexual intercourse."

ANSWERS & RATIONALES

MATCHING ANSWERS

Match the following (note that terms and/or descriptions may be used once, more than once, or not at all):

1. v protein-sparing source of energy	a. Meditation
2. h A complex carbohydrate that promotes peristalsis	b. Vitamin C
3. e A fat which is filled with hydrogen atoms	c. Biofeedback
4. x An important component of cell membranes	d. Massage
5. k A fat-soluble vitamin	e. Saturated fat
6. f The form in which carbohydrates are stored in muscles and the liver	f. Glycogen
7. r Difficulty in swallowing	g. Black cohosh
8. m A comprehensive accounting of foods selected and eaten	h. Fiber
9. w A glycerol and three fatty acids	i. Atropine
10. j The transferring of universal life energy	j. Reiki therapy
11. d The improvement of blood flow secondary to muscle manipulation	k. Vitamin D
12. g A herb that exhibits mild estrogen-like action	l. Citrucel

(continued)

13. _a_	A complementary therapy that decreases respiratory rate and oxygen consumption	m. Diet history
14. _t_	A herb that enhances immune functioning	n. Garlic
15. _n_	A herb that decreases cholesterol and increases HDLs	o. Fecal impaction
16. _s_	A complementary therapy that is contraindicated in the presence of clotting disorders	p. Hesitancy
17. _z_	The decrease in muscle size associated with prolonged immobility	q. Tarry stools
18. _c_	The self-regulation of physiologic processes	r. Dysphagia
19. _i_	A common side effect of this medication is urinary retention	s. Acupuncture
20. _o_	The presence of hard, dry stool in the rectum	t. Echinacea
21. _l_	A bulk-forming laxative	u. Opioids
22. _p_	Difficulty in starting a urinary stream	v. Carbohydrate
23. _b_	A vitamin that acidifies urine	w. Triglyceride
24. _q_	An indication of upper GI bleeding	x. Cholesterol
25. _u_	A common side effect of this medication is constipation	y. Food intake
		z. Disuse atrophy

ANSWERS FOR FILL IN THE BLANKS

Fill in the blanks with the correct word or phrase to complete each statement.

1. The client consumes a snack containing 15 g of carbohydrate, 5 g of protein, and 2 g of fat. The client has consumed 98 calories in this snack.
2. Three benefits of a cleat liquid diet are relieves thirst, prevents dehydration, and rests the GI tract.
3. A curved cane with a lower handgrip is useful in helping the client perform which activity of daily living? Getting into and out of a sitting position.
4. A permanent shortening of muscle fibers, tendons and ligaments is termed a contracture.
5. Four nonpharmacological comfort measures are
   a. back rub
   b. mouth care
   c. therapeutic touch
   d. maintenance of a comfortable environment
6. A written record of all foods consumed in a 3-day time period is called a food diary.

7. The two nutritional deficiencies for which vegans are at greatest risk are vitamin B12 and iron deficiency.

8. During which stage of sleep is the brain most active? REM sleep.

9. Three assistive devices that the nurse could recommend to a client who has difficulty bending at the waist are

   a. soap on a rope
   b. shoehorn with a long handle
   c. long-handled bathing brush

10. A client seeking to restore energy (Qi) flow to a specific body part would go to a practitioner of acupuncture.

11. Four factors that the nurse would assess when determining a client's ability to achieve adequate rest and sleep are

    a. pain
    b. condition of the environment
    c. stress level
    d. alcohol use

    (Additional answers could be body temperature, medication taken, diet, endocrine, and respiratory status.)

12. The nurse teaches the client that the minimum amount of fluid to consume daily is 1500 ml.

13. Laxatives are contraindicated in the presence of nausea, cramps, colic, vomiting, or undiagnosed abdominal pain.

14. List one nurse-initiated intervention that induces voiding. Running water, pouring water over the perineum, stroking the inner thigh, etc.

15. An hourly urinary output of less than 30 ml must be reported to the physician immediately.

16. Vitamin K is manufactured by intestinal bacteria and is also found in green, leafy vegetables.

17. Vitamin A is essential for good eyesight.

18. Vitamin E protects essential fatty acids.

19. Clotting is impaired by a deficiency of vitamin K.

20. Pernicious anemia results from a lack of vitamin B12.

21. The four factors that can contribute to disturbed sleep patterns are
    a. pain
    b. respiratory conditions that affect breathing patterns
    c. gastric or duodenal ulcers (increased gastric secretions during sleep)
    d. endocrine disturbances (hyperthyroidism, hypothyroidism, low estrogen levels)

Answers may also include elevated body temperature, need to urinate, environment (too hot/too cold, too much light, noise), fatigue, shift work, emotional stress, stimulants (caffeine, nicotine), alcohol, diet, and medications that disrupt sleep cycle (amphetamines, antidepressants, beta blockers, bronchodilators, decongestants, narcotics, and steroids).

TRUE & FALSE ANSWERS

Mark each of the following statements True or False. Correct all false statements in the space provided.

1. Complete proteins are found only in animal-based food sources. *False*
   Complete proteins are found in animal-based food sources and soy.

2. The total lymphocyte count decreases with protein depletion. *True*

3 Nasogastric tubes are used for long-term enteral nutrition. *False*
   Gastrostomy tubes are used for long-term enteral nutrition.

4. Older adults may require additional fiber in their diets. *True*

5. Clients receiving palliative care must stop all medical treatments except pain control. *False*
   All medical treatments are provided for clients receiving palliative care.

6. Lacto-ovo-vegetarians do not eat dairy or egg-containing foods. *False*
   Lacto-ovo-vegetarians do eat dairy products and eggs.

7. Vitamin C promotes the absorption of carbohydrates. *False*
   Vitamin C promotes the absorption of iron.

8. Immobility is often accompanied by protein loss. *True*

9. Atelectasis occurs when retained secretions become infected with bacteria. *False*
   Hypostatic pneumonia occurs when retained secretions become infected with bacteria.

10. Transitional stool is passed by newborns within 24 hours of birth. *False*
    Meconium is passed by newborns within 24 hours of birth

11. Habit training for urinary incontinence requires placing the client on a planned voiding schedule. *True*

12. A client can be easily aroused from stage-3 sleep. *False*
    A client can be easily woken in stage-1 of sleep.

13. Decreased stimulation is a cause of sundown syndrome. *True*

14. Milk and protein if taken before bedtime will facilitate sleep. *True*

15. The two age groups that require less than 8 hours of sleep are middle-aged adults and the elderly. *True*

APPLICATION ANSWERS

1. Which statement made by a client following teaching about the importance of using only unsaturated fats when cooking indicates that information about which fats are unsaturated was understood?
   a. "I will use butter when cooking."
   b. "I will use olive oil when cooking."
   c. "I will use lard when cooking."
   d. "I will use palm oil when cooking."

Rationale
Correct answer: b.
Olive oil is an unsaturated fat.
Butter, lard, and palm oil are all saturated fats.

2. When caring for a client taking phenytoin (Dilantin), the nurse assesses the client's mouth for which side effect of the drug?
   a. Gum hyperplasia
   b. Thrush
   c. Dental caries
   d. Glossitis

Rationale
Correct answer: a.
Gingival hyperplasia is a common side effect of the drug Dilantin.

3. When administering mouth care to an unconscious client, the nurse would place the client into which position?
   a. Dorsal recumbent
   b. High-Fowler's
   c. Supine
   d. Side-lying

Rationale
Correct answer: d.
Placing the client in the side-lying position greatly decreases the risk of aspiration when performing oral hygiene on a comatose client.

4. Which data should the nurse review to most accurately assess a client's protein stores?
   a. Urinary protein
   b. Triceps skinfold measurement
   c. Plasma albumin
   d. Height and weight

Rationale
Correct answer: c.
Albumin is manufactured by the liver from dietary proteins. In the absence of other diseases, clients with adequate protein intake should have normal serum albumin levels.

5. Which nursing order related to nutrition should be included in the plan of care for a client with limited vision?
   a. Assess for presence of the gag reflex
   b. Orient to type and location of foods and utensils
   c. Feed in the client's preferred order of eating
   d. Cut foods, then remove knife from tray

Rationale
Correct answer: b.
Orienting the client to the food placement on the tray encourages independence in feeding and increases self-esteem in the client with limited vision.

6. By which route does the nurse administer parenteral nutrition?
   a. Intravenous
   b. Nasogastric
   c. Intra-arterial
   d. Nasoenteric

Rationale
Correct answer: a.
Parenteral nutrition is the nutrition administered directly into a vein.

7. The nurse performs range of motion exercises on an immobile client to avoid which complication associated with immobility?
   a. Urinary stasis
   b. Constipation
   c. Dependent edema
   d. Contractures

Rationale
Correct answer: d.
During periods of immobility, the muscle fibers shorten and atrophy, pulling the extremity into a position of flexion and fixation. Exercising the extremity can prevent this from occurring.

8. Which nursing intervention should receive priority when caring for an immobile client?
   a Repositioning every 2 hours
   b. Assessing for dependent edema each shift
   c. Auscultating for bowel sounds daily
   d. Administering a calcium supplement twice a day

Rationale
Correct answer: a.
Immobile clients are at a high risk for pressure ulcer development. Should this occur, the client is at an increased risk for infection and septicemia. Prevention of impaired skin integrity is a high priority.

(continued)

9. Which nursing intervention would best promote a client's psychospiritual comfort?
   a. Offering a back rub
   b. Maintaining a clean environment
   c. Encouraging expression of feeling
   d. Providing mouth and hair care

Rationale

Correct answer: c.

Encouraging clients to identify and verbalize their feelings is therapeutic.

10. Use of a nasoenteric tube is the method of choice for the administration of enteral feedings when the client is at risk for which problem?
    a. Diarrhea
    b. Infection
    c. Aspiration
    d. Hyperkalemia

Rationale

Correct answer: c.

Nasoenteric tubes deliver nutrients directly into the intestines, and therefore greatly reduce the risk for aspiration.

11. When teaching how to maintain healthy, intact skin, which direction would the nurse include?
    a. Bathe every day
    b. Apply lubricating lotions
    c. Briskly rub skin dry
    d. Use an alcohol-based skin splash weekly

Rationale

Correct answer: b.

Applying moisturizers to the skin prevents fluid loss and drying of the skin. Hydrated, supple skin can resist damage from pressure and other potentially damaging conditions better than dry skin.

12. A client states he is self-medicating with St. John's wort for mild depression. To assess for a common side effect of this OTC herb, which question should the nurse ask?
    a. "Have you experienced any abnormal bleeding?"
    b. "Have you had a rash or any other skin problem?"
    c. "How well do you sleep at night"
    d. "Do you have any problems with constipation?"

Rationale

Correct answer: c.

Insomnia is a common side effect of St. John's wort.

13. Which direction should be included in the teaching plan for a client with orthostatic hypotension?
    a. Avoid use of the Valsalva maneuver
    b. Self-monitor blood pressure daily
    c. Limit use of table salt
    d. Change position slowly

Rationale

Correct answer: d.

Clients with orthostatic hypotension experience a drop in blood pressure when changing positions. Changing positions slowly allows time for the blood pressure to equalize and reduces the occurrence of syncope.

14. Which conditions place a client at risk for oral health problems? (Select all that apply.)
    a. Coronary insufficiency
    b. Confusion
    c. Dehydration
    d. Obesity

Rationale

Correct answers: b and c.

Clients with confusion may be unable to perform proper oral hygiene or may not be able to verbalize oral problems. Dehydrated clients have dry oral mucus membranes, which may no longer serve as an effective barrier and may lead to infection.

15. Which suggestion would the nurse give to an older client who reports frequent waking at night with difficulty in falling back to sleep? (Select all that apply.)
    a. "Consume 5–10 oz of wine before bedtime."
    b. "Maintain a regular schedule of exercise."
    c. "Nap frequently during the day."
    d. "Get out of bed and read until sleepy."

Rationale

Correct answers: b and d.

These actions have been shown to be effective. Alcohol at bedtime may induce a sense of sleepiness initially but can interfere with the sleep cycle. Napping during the day makes one less sleepy at night and more likely to either have difficulty falling asleep or staying asleep.

16. The nurse would be cautious about including the alternative therapy of imagery in the plan of care for a client with which health problems? (Select all that apply.)
    a. Diabetes
    b. Asthma
    c. Psychosis
    d. Seizures

Rationale

Correct answers: a, c, and d.

Imagery has been shown to alter blood glucose levels and brain-wave activity. Imagery is contraindicated in clients with psychosis.

17. When caring for an unconscious client, the nurse implements nursing interventions directed at pre-

venting which problems associated with immobility? (Select all that apply.)

a. Pneumonia

b. Osteoporosis

c. Venous stasis

d. Pressure ulcers

Rationale

Correct answers: a, b, c, and d.

Unconscious clients are at risk for developing pneumonia secondary to decreased respiratory movement and pooling of secretions, osteoporosis secondary to lack of weight bearing, venous stasis secondary to lack of skeletal muscle activity, and pressure ulcers secondary to a reduction in blood flow to tissues due to pressure.

18. Which actions would the nurse take prior to initiating a NG tube feeding? (Select all that apply.)

a. Check order for type and rate of feeding

b. Wash hands

c. Place client in the supine position

d. Aspirate stomach contents and check pH

Rationale

Correct answers: a, b, and d.

The nurse must always determine that the correct feeding is being given by checking the order. Hand washing is necessary prior to any client care. Aspiration of stomach contents and checking the pH of the aspirate is necessary to determine tube placement. The head of the bed should be elevated 30–45 degrees to prevent aspiration during the feeding.

19. Which information regarding nutrition over the lifespan is correct? (Select all that apply.)

a. Toddlers should be fed prepared toddler foods because they provide the best nutrition.

b. The older adult's diminished taste and smell requires dietary adjustments.

c. Menstruating females require additional daily iron.

d. Middle-aged adults require additional calories to meet energy needs.

Rationale

Correct answers: b and c.

Older adults have a diminished sense of taste and smell. Diseases and medications exacerbate the problem. Menstruating females lose iron in the menstrual flow, and therefore require dietary supplementation. Prepared toddler foods are not as nutritious as the fresh food prepared at home. Caloric requirement decreases with middle age and change in activity and metabolism.

20. When delegating feeding of a client on a full liquid diet to a nonlicensed assistant, which items would the nurse include on the list of permitted foods? (Select all that apply.)

a. Pudding

b. Oatmeal cereal

c. Yogurt

d. Ice cream

Rationale

Correct answers: a, c, and d.

Oatmeal cereal is the only food listed that is not permitted on a full liquid diet.

21. Which of these nursing interventions would be most appropriate when monitoring an elderly client taking MOM (milk of magnesia) for the treatment of constipation?

a. Assess serum electrolyte levels

b. Administer supplemental B and C vitamins

c. Instruct the client to limit physical activity

d. Encourage the client to wear an incontinent pad

Rationale

Correct answer: a.

MOM is an osmotic laxative and can result in an electrolyte imbalance, particularly hypermagnesemia. MOM does not cause loss of B and C vitamins. Physical activity supports bowel function so limiting activity would tend to encourage constipation. MOM is a relatively gentle laxative and does not typically cause one to lose bowel control.

22. When obtaining a health history from a client with a history of liver disease, which new complaint would the nurse recognize as most pertinent?

a. Pruritus

b. Nausea

c. Clay-colored stools

d. Fatigue

Rationale

Correct answer: c

Clay-colored stools would indicate an obstruction to the flow of bile, a serious complication of liver disease.

23. When should the nurse plan to ambulate a client with constipation to the bathroom?

a. As soon as the client wakes in the morning

b. After the client has finished eating breakfast

c. Immediately before eating dinner

d. Prior to going to bed

Rationale

Correct answer: b.

(continued)

The gastrocolic reflex is strongest when food enters the stomach and is especially strong after breakfast. A bowel movement at this time is most likely a result of the stimulation of this reflex. Upon awakening, before dinner and at bedtime do not take advantage of this reflex.

24. A client's urinary output is 450 ml in 24 hours. Which term could the nurse use when documenting about the client's urinary elimination status?
    a. Anuria
    b. Oliguria
    c. Dysuria
    d. Nocturia

Rationale

Correct answer: b.

Oliguria is defined as a urinary output less than 500 ml in 24 hours. Anuria is the absence of urinary output by the kidney. Dysuria is painful urination and nocturia is the need to get up more than one time at night to void.

25. Which of the following statements, if made by a client, indicates correct understanding of self-care activities to decrease the likelihood of developing a urinary tract infection?
    a. "I will void every 6–8 hours."
    b. "I will take baths rather than showers."
    c. "I will perform pericare after each voiding."
    d. "I will void before and after sexual intercourse."

Rationale

Correct answer: d.

Voiding after sexual intercourse flushes out bacteria introduced into the urethra and bladder during intercourse. A normal adult voids every 3.5–4 hours. Taking a bath as opposed to a shower has the potential for introducing bacteria to the area of the urinary meatus. Pericare is not necessary; simply wiping front to back to avoid spreading *E. coli* or other organisms over the urinary meatus is sufficient.

CHAPTER 14

Test Plan Category:

Physiological Integrity

Sub-category: Pharmacological and Parenteral Therapies—Part 1

Topics: Dosage Calculation
Medication Administration
Pharmacological Agents/Actions
Pharmacological Interactions
Expected Effects/Outcomes
Adverse Effects/Contraindications and Side Effects
Pharmacological Pain Management

DOSAGE CALCULATION

THE MEDICATION ORDER

- The nurse is legally responsible for ensuring that the correct client receives the right medication at the right dose, at the correct time and by the ordered route.
- Proper interpretation of the medication order is essential.

Abbreviations

- The nurse must follow the institution's policy regarding the use of abbreviations in the medical record.
- Medication errors may occur as a result of a misinterpretation of an abbreviation.

Metric System

- The major system of weights and measures used in medicine is the metric.
- Conversions between units in the system are accomplished by simply moving a decimal point.
- The three basic units of the metric system are
  —meter (length),
  —gram (weight), and
  —liter (volume).
- The same prefixes are used with all three measures listed above.

- The prefixes also change the value of each of the basic units by the same amount.
- Four main prefixes:
  —Kilo, which identifies a larger unit of measure than the basics.
  —Centi, which identifies a smaller unit than the basic.
  —Milli, which identifies a smaller unit than the basic.
  —Micro, which identifies a smaller unit than the basic.
- When administering medications, convert units of measure within the metric system, for example, g to mg, and mg to μg.
- Four metric weights commonly used in medicine (from highest to lowest value) are as follows:
  —k = kilogram
  —g = gram
  —mg = milligram
  —μg = microgram
- Two units of volume in the metric system are as follows:
  —l = liter
  —ml = milliliter
- Each of these units differs in value from the next by 1000.
  —1 kg = 1000 g
  —1 g = 1000 mg
  —1 mg = 1000 μg
  —1 l = 1000 ml (1000 cc)

Conversion Rules for Metric System

- Conversion between the units is a matter of moving the decimal point three places because each of the units differs from the next by 1000.
- If you are converting from a larger unit of measure to a smaller unit of measure, the quantity must get larger, so move the decimal three places to the right (Example: 0.5 g = 500 mg).
- In metric conversions from smaller units to larger units of measure, the quantity will get smaller. Move the decimal three places to the left (Example: 520 mg = 0.52 g).

Common conversions to remember

—1 μg = 0.001 mg
—1 mg = 0.001 g
—1000 mg = 1 g

- In order to prevent medication errors, fractional dosages should be transcribed with a zero in front of the decimal point and unnecessary zeros are to be eliminated from dosages.

Examples:

—125 μg = _____ mg (0.125)
—0.25 mg = _____ μg (250)
—100 mg = _____ g (0.1)

The Apothecary and Household Measures

- The apothecary and household are the oldest of the drug measurement systems
- If a drug label contains an apothecary dosage, it will usually also contain a metric dosage equivalent
- The apothecary system of weights is based upon the grain (gr), which is the smallest unit in the system
- Common medications that may be ordered or labeled in grains are nitroglycerin, atropine, codeine, morphine, and aspirin
- gr 1 = 60 mg
- gr 15 = 1000 mg

Apothecary measures

- There are three apothecary measures for volume:

Liquids:

—minim (m, min)
—dram (dr)
—ounce (oz)

1 ounce = 30 ml
1 dram = 4 ml
1 minim = 1 drop approximately or 0.06 ml (1/16 of a dram)
15 minim = 1 ml approximately

Household measures

- Common household measures which may be used in medication calculation are as follows:

—Tablespoon (T or tbs) 1 T = 15 ml
—Teaspoon (t or tsp) 1 tsp = 5 ml
—Drop (gtt) 60 gtt = 1 tsp

Conversions from Apothecary to Metric

- When a medication dose is ordered using apothecary or household measures, it should be converted to metric.
- Use the equivalent: gr 1 = 60 mg.

Example:

gr 1/3 = _____ mg

$$\frac{\text{gr } 1}{60 \text{ mg}} = \frac{\text{gr } 1/3}{x \text{ mg}}$$

$$x = \frac{60}{3}$$

$$x = 20$$

- Remember, if you have less than 60 mg, the grain amount will be expressed as a fraction instead of a decimal number.

Example:

15 mg = gr ____

$$\frac{\text{gr } 1}{60 \text{ mg}} = \frac{\text{gr } 1/3}{x \text{ mg}}$$

$$60x = 15$$

$$x = \frac{15}{60}$$

$$x = \text{gr } {}^{1}/_{4}$$

Conversion from Household to Metric

- Examples to remember:
  —1 T = _____ ml (Answer: 15)
  —1 oz = _____ ml (Answer: 30)
  —1 t = _____ ml (Answer: 5)

Dosage Calculation: Ratio and Proportion Method

- A ratio consists of two numbers, which have a significant relationship to each other.
- While a ratio is an expression of a significant relationship between two numbers, a proportion takes this one step further, and is used to show the relationship between two ratios.
- Example: The physician has ordered 10 mg of a medication. The nurse has a solution containing 8 mg/1 ml.

$\frac{8 \text{ mg}}{1 \text{ ml}} = \frac{10 \text{ mg}}{x \text{ ml}}$	Check sequence of measurement units.
$\frac{8}{1} = \frac{10}{x}$	Drop the measurement units
$8x = 10$	Cross-multiply, keeping x on the left of the equation.
$x = \frac{10}{8}$	Remove the number on the left side of your equation by dividing 10 by the number in front of x.
$x = \frac{5}{4}$	Reduce the numbers by their highest common denominator—2. Divide the final fraction.
$x = 1.25$ ml	The x in the original proportion was ml, so the answer is 1.25 ml.

The ordered dosage of 10 mg is contained in 1.25 ml.

- It should be routine to check your math twice in dosage calculations.
- It is also necessary to assess each answer to determine if it seems logical. If 1 ml contains 8 mg, you will need a *larger* volume than 1 ml to obtain 10 mg. The answer obtained, 1.25 ml is larger, and, therefore, it is logical.
- You can prove that the proportion is true and your calculation correct by substituting your answer for x in the original proportion.

Solve this dosage calculation problem:

The physician orders digoxin (Lanoxin) 0.125 mg p.o. daily. The medication available is digoxin (Lanoxin) 0.5 mg/2 ml. What is the quantity of medication that the nurse should administer?

Answer:

$$\frac{0.5 \text{ mg}}{2 \text{ ml}} = \frac{0.125 \text{ mg}}{x \text{ ml}}$$

$$0.5\,x = 0.25$$

$$x = 0.5 \text{ ml}$$

Dosage Calculation: Converting Different Units of Measure to One Unit of Measure

- Doctor's order: Give 0.15 g of medication. The dosage strength available is 200 mg/ml. You have to convert the different units of measure to one unit of measure.
- Convert the 0.15 g to mg by moving the decimal point three spaces to the right. 0.15 g = 150 mg. Then solve for x. The ratio and proportion method can be used to solve all problems of fractional dosages. (Answer: 0.75 ml)

Solve this dosage calculation problem:

Remember to change to one unit of measure prior to calculating dose.

- The physician orders ampicillin (Principen) 0.5 g p.o. q 6 hour. The medication available is ampicillin (Principen) 125 mg/5 ml.
- What is the quantity of medication that the nurse should administer?

Change 0.5 g to 500 mg and then solve for x. (Answer: 20 ml)

Dosage Calculation: Converting pounds to kilograms

- There are 2.2 lbs in 1 kg
- To convert from lb to kg divide by 2.2
- Since you are dividing, the answer in kg will be smaller than the lb you are converting
- Answers are expressed to the nearest 10th.

Solve this dosage calculation problem:

Convert the weight of a 150-lb adult to kg.

Answer: $150/2.2 = 68.18 \cong 68.2$ kg

Dosage Calculation Based on Body Weight

- Individual dosages may be calculated in terms of μg/kg, mg/kg, or mg/lb/d
- The total daily dosage may be administered in divided doses, for example every 6 hours (4 doses), every 8 hours (3 doses) or every 12 hours (2 doses).

Dosage Calculation: Recommended Daily Dosage Range

Two-step procedure

- Calculate the total daily dosage range
- Divide the total daily dosage by the number of doses per day to obtain the actual dose administered at one time.
- Dosage discrepancies are much more critical if the dosage range is low, for example 4–6 mg, as opposed to high, for example 250 mg.
- To check the safeness of a dose ordered by the physician, calculate the correct dosage and compare it with the dosage ordered.

Solve this dosage calculation problem:

The physician orders amoxicillin (Amoxil) for a 50-lb child. The child is to receive this medicine p.o. tid. The usual dose range is 20–40 mg/kg/d in divided doses.

a. 50 lb = ______ kg

b. What is the lower daily dosage? ______

c. What is the upper daily dosage? ______

d. What is the lower dose for one dose? ______

e. What is the upper dose for one dose? ______

f. The dosage range is ______ mg to ______ mg per dose q 8 hours.

g. If the order is to give 400 mg q 8 hour, is this a safe dose? Why?

Answer:

- First, determine how many kg the client weighs: 50 lb/2.2 kg = 22.7 kg.
- Second, use 20 mg as your lower daily dosage and multiply that by 22.7 kg = 454 mg/d.
- Third, use 40 mg as your upper daily limit and multiple that by 22.7 kg = 908 mg/d.
- Fourth, using the 454 mg/d, divide by 3 to obtain the lower limit for one dose = 151.3 mg per dose.
- Fifth, using the 908 mg/d, divide by 3 to obtain the upper limit for one dose = 302.6 mg per dose.
- Sixth, you have determined that 151.3–302.6 mg is the safe dose range for this client.
- Seventh, 400 mg/8 hours is *not* a safe dose range for this client.

Dosage Calculation: Temperature Conversion

- To convert Celsius to Fahrenheit: multiply by 1.8 and add 32. (Or multiply by 9/5 and add 32)
- To convert Fahrenheit to Celsius: subtract 32 and divide by 1.8 (Or subtract 32, and multiply by 5/9).

Solve these problems:

37 °C	=	_____ °F	(Answer: 98.6)
34 °C	=	_____ °F	(Answer: 93.2)
107.6 °F	=	_____ °C	(Answer: 42)
105.8 °F	=	_____ °C	(Answer: 41)

Steps to Decrease Interpretation Errors

- Always place a zero before a decimal expression less than one.
- Never place a decimal point and zero after a whole number, because the decimal may not be seen and result in a 10-fold overdose.
- Avoid using decimals whenever whole numbers can be used as alternatives. Example: 0.3 g should be expressed as 300 mg
- Whenever possible, use the metric system rather than grains, drams, or minims.

Dosage Calculation: IV Flow Rate

- Most institutions require the use of an infusion controller or pump to assist with the delivery of intravenous infusions.
- However, there will be many times when the nurse will be responsible for calculating ml/hr or ml/min to safely administer intravenous medications or fluids.
- The size of the fluid drop is determined by the specific intravenous set being used.
- Macrodrip sets will vary among manufacturers and will deliver between 10–20 gtt/ml.
- Microdrip sets deliver 60 gtt/ml.

Information Needed to Calculate Intravenous Flow Rate

- The volume of solution to be infused
- The length of time of the infusion: converted to minutes: i.e., 1 hour = 60 minutes
- The drop factor of the infusion set being used: i.e., 15 gtt/ml

Formula to Calculate Flow Rates

$$\text{gtts/min} = \frac{\text{Volume (ml)} \times \text{Drop factor (gtt/ml)}}{\text{Time (min)}}$$

Solve this rate calculation problem:

- The physician orders an IV to infuse at 150 ml/hr. Calculate the drops per minute rate for a set with a drop factor of 10 gtt/ml.
- Do not forget to convert the hour to minutes.

Answer:

$$\frac{150 \text{ ml} \times 10 \text{ gtt/ml}}{60 \text{ min}}$$

Answer = 25 gtt/min

Solve this rate calculation problem:

- The physician orders 1000 ml D5 ½ NS to infuse over 8 hours.
- The nurse has an infusion set that delivers 15 gtt/ml.
- How many milliliters should the nurse administer per hour?
- How many drops per minute should the nurse administer?

Answer:

1000 ml/8 hours = 125 ml/hour

$$\text{Flow rate} = \frac{125\ \text{ml} \times 15\ \text{gtts/ml}}{60\ \text{min}}$$

Answer = 31 gtt/min

PHARMACOTHERAPY

BASIC CONCEPTS

- Pharmacology: The study of the physical and chemical properties of drugs, their origin, history, sources, and the ways in which drugs affect living organisms.
- Pharmacodynamics: Study of drugs and their mechanisms of action on living organisms.
- Pharmacokinetics: Study of the absorption, distribution, metabolism, and excretion of drugs.
- Pharmacodynamics: Mechanism of drug action.
  - —Drugs form chemical bonds with specific receptors within the body. This is the most common way in which drugs exert their action. A lock and key concept demonstrates the drug and receptor relationship. The bound drug elicits or blocks physiologic responses. Drugs that bind to the receptor and create a physiologic response are agonists. Drugs that bind to a receptor but do not elicit a response are called antagonists.
  - —Drugs may interact with enzymes by inhibiting the action of a specific enzyme.
  - —Drugs alter cellular functions. For example, an antibiotic slows or completely stops the growth and/or reproduction of microbial organisms.
  - —Drugs alter the chemical composition of body fluid. For example, antacids are designed to alter the acidity of the stomach contents.

Sources of Drugs

- Drugs may be derived from natural sources such as animals and plants.
- Drugs may be semisynthetically or synthetically produced in the laboratory to form pure products.
- Biotechnology plays an important role in mass-producing hormones and vaccines.

Factors Affecting Responses to a Drug

- Age of client: Variations in drug absorption, distribution, metabolism, and elimination may occur among all clients, but in particular, the pediatric and the geriatric.
- Body weight: Body surface area is a useful measure to determine if a specific dose of a drug would be appropriate for a specific client.
- Basal metabolic rate: Clients with high BMR may absorb, distribute, metabolize, and eliminate drugs more rapidly than clients with normal metabolic rates. In addition, clients with lower metabolic rates may be at risk for toxicity due to a slower absorption, distribution, metabolism, and excretion of drugs from their body.
- Disease States: Underlying disease states may affect a client's response to a drug by modifying factors such as, absorption, distribution, biotransformation, and excretion.
- Tolerance: May account for the need to increase dosage to maintain therapeutic effect.

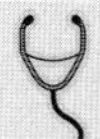

Assessment Alert

The very young and the very old clients are at a higher risk for drug toxicity.

Adverse drug effects

- Drugs may interact with other drugs, foods, and other substances.
- Over-the-counter drugs, herbal products, home remedies, and prescription drugs all may pose a threat.
- The nurse must be aware of all substances that a client may encounter and monitor the client for possible interactions.

—Side effects are undesirable effects resulting from the action of the drug. This is the most common type of adverse drug effects. Examples may include N&V, diarrhea, and rash. Side effects are generally predictable and manageable.

—Allergic reactions or hypersensitivity reactions are a response of the client's immunological system to the presence of that specific drug. Reactions may vary from mild (rash, hives, itching) to severe (difficulty breathing and shock).

—Drug toxicity may occur with any client. All drugs are capable of producing toxic effects. In monitoring the client, the nurse needs to be aware that sometimes drugs may accumulate faster than they are metabolized or eliminated. In addition, the very young and the older client are more susceptible to toxicity reactions.

—An idiosyncratic reaction is a genetically determined abnormal reaction to a normal dose of a drug. It can manifest as toxic, accelerated, or as an unusual response to a therapeutic dose.

—A teratogenic effect is one that will cause a structural defect in the unborn fetus whose mother took the drug. Drugs that cross the placenta may cause a teratogenic effect. The FDA requires that all prescription drugs absorbed systemically or known to be potentially harmful to the fetus be classified accordingly to five pregnancy categories (A, B, C, D, and X).

—Drug tolerance means that a client develops a resistance to the effects of the drug, thereby requiring an increased dose or increased frequency of administration.

Drug interactions

- A drug interaction occurs when the pharmacological effects of one drug are altered by another drug. This can cause an increase or a decrease in the actions of the drug.
- Synergistic interaction occurs if the administration of two or more drugs produces a pharmacological response that is greater than that which would be expected by the individual effects of either drug.
- Antagonistic interaction when the combination of two drugs results in effects that are less than if the two drugs had been given separately.
- Incompatibilities occur when two or more drugs or solutions are mixed together and an undesired chemical reaction occurs causing a precipitate, color change, or other physical deterioration to occur.

Measurement of drug concentrations in the body

- Peak drug level is the highest plasma concentration achieved by the administration of a drug at a specific time. Peak levels are drawn according to the type of drug and the route of administration. If the drug is an oral medication, it may be drawn within 1–3 hours after the drug was administered. If the drug was administered intravenously, the level may need to be drawn 10–30 minutes after administration.
- Trough drug level is the lowest plasma concentration of a drug. Trough levels are drawn immediately before the next dose of the drug is given.
- Minimum effective concentration—the minimum level required to elicit the desired effect.
- Minimum toxic concentration—minimum plasma level at which toxic effects of the drug are observed.
- Half-life is the time required by the body to metabolize half of the amount of the dose of the drug.

Controlled substances

- The manufacturing, prescribing, dispensing, and administration of controlled substances are regulated by the government as outlined in the Controlled Substance Act.
- The drugs identified as controlled substances are assigned to Schedules I–V according to their potential for abuse and dependence.

Controlled substances schedules

- Schedule I—High potential for abuse, no currently accepted medical use in the United States, and safety has not been established. Example: LSD.
- Schedule II—High potential for abuse, and may lead to severe psychological and physical dependence. Examples include oxycodone (OxyContin) and methylphenidate (Ritalin).
- Schedule III—Lower potential for abuse than Schedule I and Schedule II drugs, but abuse may cause moderate physical dependence or severe psychological dependence. Examples include hydrocodone/acetaminophen combination drugs (Vicodin), and hydrocodone/aspirin (Lortab).
- Schedule IV—Lower potential for physical or psychological dependence when compared with Schedule III drugs. Examples include alprazolam (Xanax) and diazepam (Valium).
- Schedule V—Lowest potential for physical and psychological dependence when compared with Schedule I–IV drugs. Examples include codeine/guaifenesin combination cough suppressants (Robitussin A-C) and diphenoxylate/atropine (Lomotil).

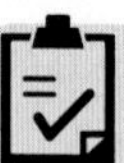

Think Smart/Test Smart

Remember, a peak is the pointed top of a mountain, thus a drug's peak is when the serum level is the highest. A trough is a depression; therefore the lowest serum level of a drug is the trough.

MEDICATION ADMINISTRATION

ASSESSMENT

Assessing the Client

- Medication history—The client should be asked for names of all medications he/she is taking (prescription, over-the-counter, herbals, home remedies, and alcohol). Ask client about adverse drug effects or allergies.
- Assess clients' understanding of their medications and the relationship of the medications to their illness.
- Conduct a physical assessment of the client. Obtain client's weight, height, BP, temperature, pulse rate, and respiratory rate. Assess general health, nutrition, and ability to perform activities of daily living.
- Assess growth and development issues related to the client's age. Explore emotional, cognitive, cultural, and socioeconomic concerns related to drug therapy
- Obtain information about social networks and resources to assist with self-care

Assessing the Drug

- Know the drug's classification, mechanism of action, indications, contraindications, safe dosages, adverse effects, S&S of toxicity, antidotes, and nursing implications
- Understand how to prepare the dose using correct administration techniques

Analyze the Information

- Obtain all relevant information regarding the client and the drug, evaluate the information, and make judgments and decisions to assist in formulating a nursing diagnosis.

NURSING DIAGNOSES

- Based upon the assessment and analysis of the data, the nurse will be able to make a conclusion regarding actual client needs and the risk for problems.

Planning

- Identify goals and outcome criteria.
- Goals should be client oriented, measurable, and realistic.
- Outcome criteria should be client oriented, apply to medications the client will receive, and assist in directing safe medication administration.
- Outcome criteria may address issues with drug preparation such as making sure all supplies are available, and providing for a clean and safe work area.

Implementation

- During the implementation phase, the nurse will put into effect the nursing care plan.
- The nurse needs to know the client information and the medication profile data in order to provide safe care.
- The nurse should always use the basic "Five Rights" of medication administration when implementing care for a client receiving medications.
- Remember to check the order, the label and the "Five Rights" at least three times before administration of the medication.

Evaluation

- After the nursing care plan has been implemented and the medication has been administered, the evaluation process continues as an ongoing part of the nursing process.
- The nurse is responsible for monitoring the client's responses to drug therapy at every part of the process.
- Identification of therapeutic responses, unexpected responses, adverse effects, and the need for continued client education are important nursing observations and judgments.

Five Rights of Medication Administration

Right drug

- After carefully checking the order and the drug label, select the correct medication
- Safe administration requires that the nurse be familiar with the drug's mechanism of action, indications, and contradictions for use, usual dosage, and side effects.

Right dose

- The nurse must check the dose and its safety in relation to the weight and age of the client.
- The nurse is responsible for correct dosage calculation and must be familiar with household measures, the apothecary system, and the metric system and be able to convert from one system to another.
- The nurse must have skills in using measuring devices, such as medicine cups, oral syringes, and parenteral syringes.

Right client

- Always compare the client's name and number on his/her identification band to the name and number on the medication administration record.
- Request that the client state his/her name.
- Remember to ask about allergies.
- If the client questions the appearance, dosage, or route, always recheck the order and medication before administering the dose.

Right time

- The nurse should always be aware of the institution's policy regarding routine medication times.
- The physician's order will specify the number of times a day the medication is to be given.
- The order may state the exact hours of administration or give general guidelines such as before or after meals.
- Take into consideration the drug's action, characteristics of the drug, possible interactions with other drugs or food, and the clients' daily schedule.
- At most institutions, the policy states that medication is administered within 30 minutes of the time it is ordered to be given.

Right route

- If the medication order did not specify the route, the nurse must clarify this with the physician. Remember, the route is part of a correctly written medication order.

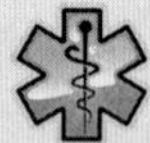

Nursing Intervention Alert

Always document the administration of medications immediately after you give them.

MEDICATION DOSAGE FORMS

- Tablet: A mixture of active and inactive ingredients pressed into a solid.
- Buccal tablet: A tablet that is placed in the mouth and held between the cheek and gum until dissolved and absorbed by the buccal mucosa.
- Sublingual (SL): Tablets are placed under the client's tongue until fully absorbed. Remind the client not to chew the tablet.

Sublingual and Buccal Routes:

—Medications are absorbed through the oral mucous membranes for rapid systemic effect.

—Instruct the client *not* to swallow these medications.

—Wear clean gloves if you place the medication in the client's mouth.

- Chewable tablets: These tablets are often used with children or adults who have difficulty swallowing. Remember that the drug may be absorbed faster than the oral tablet form that is designed to be swallowed.
- Enteric-coated tablets: Tablets are coated with a substance that prevents the tablet from dissolving in the stomach where gastric acid is present, but permits it to dissolve in the small intestine. Remind the client *not* to chew enteric-coated tablets.
- Timed or sustained-release tablets: Tablets are designed to release contents at specific timed intervals. Do not crush these tablets. Remind the client not to chew timed or sustained-release tablets.
- Capsules: The drug is enclosed in either a hard or soft soluble shell, usually made of gelatin. This gelatin shell dissolves in the stomach within 10–20 minutes.
- Lozenges: This solid dose form should always be dissolved slowly in the mouth. Often this form is ordered for the soothing effect it exerts on the oral mucus membranes.
- Oral solutions: A solution is a clear liquid preparation that contains one or more dissolved substances. The solution may have flavorings and color additives.
- Suspensions: Solutions that have solid drug particles mixed with, but not dissolved in, the fluid. Always shake suspensions thoroughly immediately prior to administration.

Nonoral Solutions

- Douche: Instillation of a medicated or nonmedicated solution into a body orifice.
- Injection: Instillation of a sterile solution administered intramuscular, intravenous, subcutaneous, intradermal, and epidural.
- Ophthalmic solution: Medicated or nonmedicated solution instilled onto the conjunctiva.
- Otic solution: Instillation of a medicated or nonmedicated solution into the ear.

Mouth Rinses

- After rinsing, some medications are expectorated but other medications may be swallowed
- Local anesthetic rinse agents area are indicated for painful mouth lesions
- "Swish and swallow": After rinsing mouth with medication, the client then swallows the medication
- Example of swish and swallow is an antifungal medication for a fungal infection of the mouth
- Always administer the mouth rinse and swish and swallow medications last

Topical Dosage Forms

- Ointments and creams: Most are used for the treatment of skin disorders.
- Transdermal therapeutic systems (Patches): A drug delivery system that allows for the drug to be absorbed through the skin and into the bloodstream.
- Implants: Medication filled pellets or capsules are surgically implanted under the skin.
- Lotions: Protect, soften, and provide relief from itching
- Liniments

—applied by rubbing

—provide relief from tight aching muscles

- Powders: applied for their soothing, drying action
- Aerosol foam: spreads drug over wide area

- Application of topical medication
  —Use clean gloves to apply medication to unbroken skin
  —Use sterile gloves to apply medication if the skin is open
  —Use cotton tipped applicators for small areas
  —Do not use tongue blades to apply medication
  —Use correct technique to apply medications from a tube
  —Use correct technique to apply medications from a jar
- Suppositories: This drug form is a semisolid substance and is usually inserted into the rectum, vagina, or urethra where it dissolves slowly to release the medication.

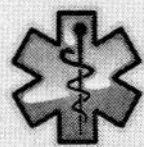

Nursing Intervention Alert

Always use a water-soluble lubricate on the suppository prior to insertion.

- Parenteral Products: Sterile solutions or suspensions packaged for use as an injection.
  —Ampules
  —Prefilled syringes
  —Vials

Administration of Medications to Client with Swallowing Difficulties

- Place client in high-Fowler's or a sitting position
- Provide sufficient fluid for swallowing
- Use special medicine and water glass which dispenses tablet and water at same time
- Use tablet divider to split the solid tablet into one or more pieces
- Use tablet crusher to reduce tablets to a powder and mix with juice, pudding, applesauce, etc.
- Empty powdered contents of regular capsules into a plastic medicine cup and mix with juice, pudding, or applesauce
- Obtain medications in liquid form
- Never divide or crush
  —Enteric-coated products
  —Sustained-action forms
  —Products that contain encapsulated beads or a wax matrix
  —Sublingual or buccal products
- Many sustained release (SR) preparations have time-release beads and can be sprinkled onto food, but the beads should never be chewed or bitten into.
- Some soft gelatin capsules can have a pinhole pricked in one end and the liquid squeezed out.

Parenteral Drug Administration: Advantages and Disadvantages

Definition

- Any route other than gastrointestinal
- Commonly used to indicate subcutaneous, intramuscular, intradermal, and intravenous routes

Advantages of parenteral routes

- Rapid, almost complete absorption of medication
- Gastric disturbances do not affect the medication
- Client does not have to be conscious to receive the medication

Disadvantages of parenteral routes

- Penetration of the skin increasing risk for infection
- Nerve damage
- Painful
- Potential for abscesses

Standard Precautions

- Wash hands before and after procedures, and between clients
- Wear gloves when performing any injection
- Carefully dispose of used gloves, needles, and syringes according to facility's policy.
- *Never* recap, remove, bend, or break needle after giving an injection.
- If accidentally exposed to body fluid by needle stick, always seek immediate treatment.
- Follow agency's procedures for care of clients with communicable diseases

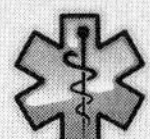

Nursing Intervention Alert

Proper hand washing is the single most important intervention in the prevention of the spread of organisms.

Calibration Scale of Syringes

- Tuberculin syringe: hundredths
- 3 cc syringe: tenths
- 5 cc, 6 cc, 10 cc, and 12 cc: two 10ths
- Syringes larger than 12 cc: full cc measures
- Minim scale
- First long calibration indicates zero
- Read calibrations from the top, or front ring, of the plungers suction tip

Needles for Injection: Gauge and Length

Intradermal

—26 or 27 gauge
—1/4–3/8 in. length
—Diagnostic purposes

Subcutaneous

—25–28 gauge
—1/2–5/8 in. length
—Frequently used for administration of insulin and heparin

Intramuscular

—21–23 gauge

—1–1 1/2 in. length

—Use the longer needles for medications that are irritating to tissues

—Use the larger diameter (smaller gauge) needle for viscous products

Intramuscular Injection

Sites

—Deltoid

—Dorsogluteal

—Ventrogluteal

—Vastus Lateralis

Considerations for site selection

- Muscle mass
- Adequate circulation
- Free of infection, breakdown, and scars
- Rotation of site
- Volume and type of medication

Subcutaneous Injection

Sites

—Middle lateral aspect of upper arm

—Abdomen: either side of umbilicus

—Upper posterior aspect of hips

—Middle and outer areas of thigh

Considerations for site selection

—Subcutaneous tissue mass

—Adequate circulation

—Free of infection, breakdown, and scars

—Rotation of site

—Type of medication

Intradermal Injection

Sites

—Inner aspect of forearm

—Upper chest

—Shoulder blades

Procedures for Administering Medications

Step-by-step procedures for the administration of oral rectal subcutaneous, intramuscular, intradermal, otic, and ophthalmic medications are given in Tables 14-1 through 14-12. Also included are procedures for medication administration via metered dose inhaler, and administration of nitroglycerine ointment, heparin, and various forms of insulin.

Table 14–1 Procedure for Administering an **Oral Medication**

• Check the medication order on the medication administration record (MAR) for completeness: ○ Client's name ○ Date ○ Name of medication ○ Dosage ○ Route ○ Frequency • Verify the medication listed on the MAR by comparing the MAR with the physician's order. • Check for any circumstances surrounding the administration of the medication to the client. For example, is the client NPO? • Check for a history of drug allergies. • Make sure you know the expected action, safe dosage range, special instructions for administration, and adverse effects associated with the medications ordered. • Assess the client's total drug profile for possible drug interactions. • Wash your hands. • Gather needed equipment: ○ Medicine cup (soufflé/plastic)		
Check 1. • Read the MAR: ○ Name of medication ○ Dosage of medication ○ Route by which medication is to be given ○ Date and time medication is to be given ○ Determine if medication has been given		
• Read the label on the medication container or unit dose package before removing it from the source. • Check expiration date.		
Check 2. • Pick up the medication container or unit dose package and compare the medication label with the MAR. ○ Name of medication ○ Dosage of medication • State the total amount of medication/volume of medication to be administered. • Remove the correct amount of medication.		
Check 3. • Compare the medication label with the MAR again. ○ Name of medication ○ Dosage of medication ○ Route by which medication is to be given ○ Date and time medication is to be given • Return medication to source. • Greet and identify the client. • Explain to the client what you are going to do. • Administer the medication. ○ Position the client in an upright position, if possible. ○ Give client a cup of water. ○ Stay with the client as he swallows the medication. • Document on the MAR. • Leave the client in a comfortable position. • Wash your hands.		

Table 14–2 Procedure for Administering Medication via **Subcutaneous Injection**

- Check the medication order on the MAR for completeness:
  - Client's name
  - Date
  - Name of medication
  - Dosage
  - Route
  - Frequency
- Verify the medication listed on the MAR by comparing the MAR with the physician's order.
- Check for any circumstances surrounding the administration of the medication to the client.
- Check for a history of drug allergies.
- Make sure you know the expected action, safe dosage range, special instructions for administration, and adverse effects associated with the medications ordered.
- Assess the client's total drug profile for possible drug interactions.
- Wash your hands.
- Gather needed equipment:
  - Alcohol prep pads
  - Tuberculin syringe
  - Needles: 25–28 gauge, 1/2–5/8 in. length

Check 1.

- Read the MAR.
  - Name of medication
  - Dosage of medication
  - Route by which medication is to be given
  - Date and time medication is to be given
- Determine if medication has been given.
- Read the label on the medication container or unit dose package before removing it from the source.
- Check expiration date.

Check 2.

- Pick up the medication container or unit dose package and compare the medication label with the MAR.
  - Name of medication
  - Dosage of medication
- State the total volume of medication to be administered.
- Draw up correct dosage of medication, maintaining asepsis:
  - Clean top of medication vial with alcohol prep pad and allow it to dry.
  - Discard alcohol prep pad.
  - Insert needle into vial through rubber stopper.
  - Inject air into vial.
  - Pick up vial with nondominant hand and withdraw correct volume of medication.
  - Expel any air bubbles.
  - Recheck volume of medication for accuracy.
  - Remove needle from vial.
  - Replace needle cap on sterile needle.

Check 3.

- Compare the medication label with the MAR again.
  - Name of medication
  - Dosage of medication
  - Route by which medication is to be given
  - Date and time medication is to be given
- Return medication to source.
- Greet and identify the client.
- Explain to the client what you are going to do.
- Close door and curtain.
- Provide adequate lighting.
- Put on gloves.
- Give the injection, maintaining asepsis:
  - Position the client for maximal comfort and locate the anatomical site for the injection.
  - Clean injection area with alcohol prep pad, using a circular motion, working from the site outward. Allow the site to dry.
  - Place alcohol prep pad between fingers of nondominant hand.
  - Remove the needle cap.
  - Using the thumb and index finger of your nondominant hand, pinch client's skin to elevate the subcutaneous tissue at selected site.
  - Insert needle in a dart-like-fashion at a 90-degree angle with your dominant hand, while maintaining pinched adipose tissue.
  - Using the *thumb* on your dominant hand, push *slowly* on the plunger to inject the medication.
  - Count 10 seconds before withdrawing needle.
  - Remove needle quickly and apply pressure to site with alcohol prep pad for 10 seconds.
  - Unless contraindicated, gently massage the injection site.
- Discard syringe and needle in "sharps" container.
- Remove and discard your gloves.
- Leave the client in a comfortable position.
- Wash your hands.
- Document on the MAR.

Table 14–3 Procedure for Administering **Heparin via Subcutaneous Injection**

- Check the medication order on the MAR for completeness:
  - Client's name
  - Date
  - Name of medication
  - Dosage
  - Route
  - Frequency
- Verify the medication listed on the MAR by comparing the MAR with the physician's order.
- Check for any circumstances surrounding the administration of the medication to the client. Assess the PTT results, if ordered.
- Check for a history of drug allergies.
- Make sure you know the expected action, safe dosage range, special instructions for administration, and adverse effects associated with the medications ordered.
- Assess the client's total drug profile for possible drug interactions.
- Wash your hands.
- Gather needed equipment:
  - Alcohol prep pads
  - Tuberculin syringe with needle.
  - Extra needle: 25–28 gauge, ½–5/8 in. length.

Check 1.
- Read the MAR.
  - Name of medication
  - Dosage of medication
  - Route by which medication is to be given
  - Date and time medication is to be given
- Determine if medication has been given.
- Read the label on the medication container or unit dose package before removing it from the source.
- Check expiration date.

Check 2.
- Pick up the medication container or unit dose package and compare the medication label with the MAR.
  - Name of medication
  - Dosage of medication
- State the total volume of medication to be administered.
- Draw up correct dosage of medication, maintaining asepsis:
  - Clean top of medication vial with alcohol prep pad and allow it to dry.
  - Discard alcohol prep pad.
  - Prepare syringe and needle.
  - Draw air into syringe equal to amount of medication to be given.
  - Insert needle into vial through rubber stopper.
  - Inject air into vial.
  - Pick up vial with nondominant hand and withdraw correct volume of medication.
  - Expel any air bubbles.
  - Recheck volume of medication for accuracy.
  - Remove needle from vial.
  - Replace needle cap on sterile needle.
  - Validate volume of medication in syringe with instructor.
  - Remove needle and discard in "sharps" container.
  - Apply new needle to syringe.
  - As a registered nurse, you will always validate strength and dose of heparin with another nurse.
- Create air lock with 0.2 ml of air, invert syringe, and tap air bubble to top of syringe.

Check 3.
- Compare the medication label with the MAR again.
  - Name of medication
  - Dosage of medication
  - Route by which medication is to be given
  - Date and time medication is to be given
- Return medication to source.
- Greet and identify the client.
- Explain to the client what you are going to do.
- Close door and curtain.
- Provide adequate lighting.
- Put on gloves.
- Give the injection, maintaining asepsis:
  - Position the client for maximal comfort and locate the anatomical site for the injection.
  - Cleanse, but do not rub injection site with alcohol prep pad. Allow the site to dry.
  - Place alcohol prep pad between fingers of nondominant hand.
  - Remove the needle cap.
  - Select an injection site on the abdomen outside a 2-inch radius around the umbilicus. Avoid scars, bruised areas, and previous injection sites. Using the thumb and index finger of your nondominant hand, pinch client's skin to elevate the subcutaneous tissue at selected site.
  - Insert needle in a dart-like-fashion at a 90-degree angle with your dominant hand, while maintaining pinched adipose tissue.
  - Do *not* aspirate.
  - Using the *thumb* on your dominant hand, push *slowly* on the plunger to inject the medication.
  - Count 10 seconds before withdrawing needle.
  - Remove needle quickly and apply pressure to site with alcohol prep pad for 10 seconds.
  - *Do not massage* or *rub* the site.
- Discard syringe and needle in "sharps" container.
- Remove and discard your gloves.
- Leave the client in a comfortable position.
- Wash your hands.
- Document on the MAR.

Table 14–4 Procedure for Administering **Insulin via Subcutaneous Injection**

- Check the medication order on the MAR for completeness:
  - Client's name
  - Date
  - Name of medication
  - Dosage
  - Route
  - Frequency
- Verify the medication listed on the MAR by comparing the MAR with the physician's order.
- Check for any circumstances surrounding the administration of the medication to the client. For example, is the client NPO? Verify blood glucose results.
- Check for a history of drug allergies.
- Make sure you know the expected action, safe dosage range, special instructions for administration, and adverse effects associated with the medications ordered.
- Assess the client's total drug profile for possible drug interactions.
- Wash your hands.
- Gather needed equipment:
  - Alcohol prep pads
  - Appropriate insulin syringe

Check 1.

- Read the MAR.
  - Name of medication
  - Dosage of medication
  - Route by which medication is to be given
  - Date and time medication is to be given
  - Determine if medication has been given
- Read the label on the medication container or unit dose package before removing it from the source.
- Check expiration date.

Check 2.

- Pick up the medication container or unit dose package and compare the medication label with the MAR.
  - Name of medication
  - Dosage of medication
- Determine the number of units of insulin to be administered.
- Draw up correct dosage of medication, maintaining asepsis:
  - Clean top of medication vial with alcohol prep pad and allow it to dry.
  - Discard alcohol prep pad.
  - Draw air into syringe equal to amount of medication to be given.
  - Insert needle into vial through rubber stopper.
  - Inject air into vial.
  - Pick up vial with nondominant hand and withdraw correct volume of medication.
  - Expel any air bubbles.
  - Recheck volume of medication for accuracy.
  - Remove needle from vial.
  - Replace needle cap on sterile needle.
  - Validate the type and dose of insulin with another nurse.

Check 3.

- Compare the medication label with the MAR again.
  - Name of medication
  - Dosage of medication
  - Route by which medication is to be given
  - Date and time medication is to be given
- Return medication to source.
- Greet and identify the client.
- Explain to the client what you are going to do.
- Close door and curtain.
- Provide adequate lighting.
- Put on gloves.
- Give the injection, maintaining asepsis:
  - Position the client for maximal comfort and locate the anatomical site for the injection.
  - Clean injection area with alcohol prep pad, using a circular motion, working from the site outward. Allow the site to dry.
  - Place alcohol prep pad between fingers of nondominant hand.
  - Remove the needle cap.
  - Using the thumb and index finger of your nondominant hand, pinch client's skin to elevate the subcutaneous tissue at selected site.
  - Insert needle in a dart-like-fashion at a 90-degree angle with your dominant hand, while maintaining pinched adipose tissue.
  - Using the *thumb* on your dominant hand, push *slowly* on the plunger to inject the medication
  - Count 10 seconds before withdrawing needle.
  - Remove needle quickly and apply gentle pressure to injection site with alcohol prep pad for 10 seconds.
  - Do not massage.
- Discard syringe and needle in "sharps" container.
- Remove and discard your gloves.
- Leave the client in a comfortable position.
- Wash your hands.
- Document on MAR and diabetic flow sheet.

Table 14–5 Procedure for **Mixing Two Types of Insulin:** Intermediate or Long-Acting Insulin with Regular Insulin

- Check the medication order on the MAR for completeness:
  - Client's name
  - Date
  - Name of medication
  - Dosage
  - Route
  - Frequency
- Verify the medication listed on the MAR by comparing the MAR with the physician's order.
- Check for any circumstances surrounding the administration of the medication to the client. Verify blood glucose results.
- Check for a history of drug allergies.
- Make sure you know the expected action, safe dosage range, special instructions for administration, and adverse effects associated with the medications ordered.
- Assess the client's total drug profile for possible drug interactions.
- Wash your hands.
- Gather needed equipment:
  - Alcohol prep pads
  - Appropriate insulin syringe

Check 1.
- Read the MAR.
  - Name of medication
  - Dosage of medication
  - Route by which medication is to be given
  - Date and time medication is to be given
  - Determine if medication has been given
- Read the label on the medication container or unit dose package before removing it from the source.
- Check expiration date.

Check 2.
- Pick up the medication container or unit dose package and compare the medication label with the MAR.
  - Name of medication
  - Dosage of medication
- State the number of units of each insulin dose to be administered and the total number of units to be administered.
- Invert and roll the bottle of intermediate or long-acting insulin between your hands, to mix the insulin. Do *not* shake the bottle.
- Clean the top of both insulin vials with alcohol prep pads and allow them to dry.
- Measure the same volume of air as you need of the intermediate or long-acting insulin and inject into the insulin vial. Withdraw the needle.
- Measure the same volume of air as you need of the regular insulin and inject into the insulin vial. Leave the needle in the vial, invert the bottle and withdraw the correct dosage, maintaining asepsis. (Rapid and short acting insulins are clear in color)
- Expel any air bubbles.
- Recheck volume of insulin for accuracy.
- Remove needle from vial.
- Validate volume of medication in syringe with another RN.
- Turn the bottle of intermediate or long-acting insulin upside down and reinsert the needle into this vial, maintaining asepsis.
- *Slowly* pull the plunger to withdraw the correct dosage of insulin. Remove the needle from the vial.
- Replace the needle cap on the sterile needle.
- Validate volume of medication in syringe with another RN.

Check 3.
- Compare the medication label with the MAR again.
  - Name of medication
  - Dosage of medication
  - Route by which medication is to be given
  - Date and time medication is to be given
- Return medication to source.

Table 14–6 Procedure for Administering Medication via **Intramuscular Injection**

- Check the medication order on the MAR for completeness:
  - Client's name
  - Date
  - Name of medication
  - Dosage
  - Route
  - Frequency
- Verify the medication listed on the MAR by comparing the MAR with the physician's order.
- Check for any circumstances surrounding the administration of the medication to the client.
- Check for a history of drug allergies.
- Make sure you know the expected action, safe dosage range, special instructions for administration, and adverse effects associated with the medications ordered.
- Assess the client's total drug profile for possible drug interactions.
- Wash your hands.
- Gather needed equipment:
  - Alcohol prep pads
  - Needles
  - Syringe

Check 1.

- Read the MAR.
  - Name of medication
  - Dosage of medication
  - Route by which medication is to be given
  - Date and time medication is to be given
  - Determine if medication has been given
- Read the label on the medication container or unit dose package before removing it from the source.
- Check expiration date.

Check 2.

- Pick up the medication container or unit dose package and compare the medication label with the MAR.
  - Name of medication
  - Dosage of medication
- State the total volume of medication to be administered.
- Draw up correct dosage of medication, maintaining asepsis:
  - Clean top of medication vial with alcohol prep pad and allow it to dry.
  - Discard alcohol prep pad.
  - Prepare syringe and needle.
  - Draw air into syringe equal to amount of medication to be given.
  - Insert needle into vial through rubber stopper.
  - Inject air into vial.
  - Pick up vial with nondominant hand and withdraw correct volume of medication.
  - Expel any air bubbles.
  - Recheck volume of medication for accuracy.
  - Remove needle from vial.
  - Replace needle cap on sterile needle.
  - Validate volume of medication in syringe with another RN.
- Create air lock with 0.2 ml of air, invert syringe, and tap air bubble to top of syringe.

Check 3.

- Compare the medication label with the MAR again.
  - Name of medication
  - Dosage of medication
  - Route by which medication is to be given
  - Date and time medication is to be given
- Return medication to source.
- Greet and identify the client.
- Explain to the client what you are going to do.
- Close door and curtain.
- Provide adequate lighting.
- Put on gloves.
- Give the injection, maintaining asepsis:
  - Position the client for maximal comfort and locate the anatomical site for the injection.
  - Clean injection area with alcohol prep pad, using a circular motion, working from the site outward. Allow the site to dry.
  - Place alcohol prep pad between fingers of the nondominant hand.
  - Remove the needle cap.
  - Using your nondominant hand spread the client's skin between your thumb and index finger, making it taut.
  - Insert needle in a dart-like-fashion at a 90-degree angle using your dominant hand.
  - Then, hold the barrel of the syringe steady with your nondominant hand while aspirating with your thumb and pointer finger of your dominant hand. If blood appears in the syringe, remove the needle, discard medication and begin the procedure over.
  - Using the *thumb* on your dominant hand, push *slowly* on the plunger to inject the medication.
  - Count 10 seconds before withdrawing needle.
  - Remove needle quickly and apply pressure to site with alcohol prep pad for 10 seconds.
  - Unless contraindicated, gently massage the injection site.
- Discard syringe and needle in "sharps" container.
- Remove and discard your gloves.
- Leave the client in a comfortable position.
- Wash your hands.
- Document on the MAR.

Table 14–7 Procedure for Performing an **Intradermal Injection**

- Check the medication order on the MAR for completeness:
  - Client's name
  - Date
  - Name of medication
  - Dosage
  - Route
  - Frequency
- Verify the medication listed on the MAR by comparing the MAR with the physician's order.
- Check for any circumstances surrounding the administration of the medication to the client.
- Check for a history of drug allergies.
- Make sure you know the expected action, safe dosage range, special instructions for administration, and adverse effects associated with the medications ordered.
- Assess the client's total drug profile for possible drug interactions.
- Wash your hands.
- Gather needed equipment:
  - Alcohol prep pads
  - Tuberculin syringe

Check 1.

- Read the MAR.
  - Name of medication
  - Dosage of medication
  - Route by which medication is to be given
  - Date and time medication is to be given
  - Determine if medication has been given
- Read the label on the medication container or unit dose package before removing it from the source.
- Check expiration date.

Check 2.

- Pick up the medication container or unit dose package and compare the medication label with the MAR.
  - Name of medication
  - Dosage of medication
- State the total volume of medication to be administered.
- Draw up correct dosage of medication, maintaining asepsis:
  - Clean top of medication vial with alcohol prep pad and allow it to dry.
  - Discard alcohol prep pad.
  - Prepare syringe and needle.
  - Draw air into syringe equal to amount of medication to be given.
  - Insert needle into vial through rubber stopper.
  - Inject air into vial.
  - Pick up vial with nondominant hand and withdraw correct volume of medication.
  - Expel any air bubbles.
  - Recheck volume of medication for accuracy.
  - Remove needle from vial.
  - Replace needle cap on sterile needle.

Check 3.

- Compare the medication label with the MAR again.
  - Name of medication
  - Dosage of medication
  - Route by which medication is to be given
  - Date and time medication is to be given
- Return medication to source.
- Greet and identify the client.
- Explain to the client what you are going to do.
- Close door and curtain.
- Provide adequate lighting.
- Put on gloves.
- Give the intradermal injection, maintaining asepsis:
  - Select a site on the inner surface of client's forearm, several finger-widths distal to his antecubital space.
  - Clean injection area with alcohol prep pad, using a circular motion, working from the site outward. Allow the site to dry. (Do *not* use iodine solution to cleanse the skin because it may interfere with interpreting the results of the skin test.
  - Holding the client's forearm in one hand, stretch the skin taut.
  - Hold the syringe at a 10–15 degree angle, with the bevel of the needle facing up.
  - Insert the needle just until the bevel is no longer visible.
  - *Slowly* inject the medication, and leave the needle in place for a few moments while watching for the development of a small blister (wheal).
  - When the wheal appears, withdraw the needle and apply *gentle* pressure. Do *not* massage.
  - When an intradermal injection is given for diagnostic purposes, a control wheal is made on the opposite arm.
- Discard syringe and needle in "sharps" container.
- Remove and discard your gloves.
- Leave the client in a comfortable position and advise not to rub or scratch the injection area.
- Wash your hands.
- Document on the MAR. Be sure to chart the correct location of the test and control sites.

Table 14–8 Procedure for Administering Medication via **Metered Dose Inhaler**

- Check the medication order on the MAR for completeness:
  - Client's name
  - Date
  - Name of medication
  - Dosage
  - Route
  - Frequency
- Verify the medication listed on the MAR by comparing the MAR with the physician's order.
- Check for any circumstances surrounding the administration of the medication to the client.
- Check for a history of drug allergies.
- Make sure you know the expected action, safe dosage range, special instructions for administration, and adverse effects associated with the medications ordered.
- Assess the client's total drug profile for possible drug interactions.
- Wash your hands.
- Gather needed equipment:
  - Correct metered dose inhaler
  - Spacer, if ordered

Check 1.
- Read the MAR.
  - Check name of medication.
  - Check dosage of medication.
  - Check route by which medication is to be given.
  - Check date and time medication is to be given.
  - Determine if medication has been given.
  - Read the label on the medication container or unit dose package before removing it from the source.
  - Check expiration date.

Check 2.
- Pick up the medication container or unit dose package and compare the medication label with the MAR.
  - Name of medication
  - Dosage of medication
- State the number of inhalations of medication ordered.

Check 3.
- Compare the medication label with the MAR again.
  - Name of medication
  - Dosage of medication
  - Route by which medication is to be given
  - Date and time medication is to be given
- Greet and identify the client.
- Explain to the client what you are going to do.
- Close door and curtain.
- Provide adequate lighting.
- Administer the medication.
  - Determine that client knows how to correctly use inhaler or provide the following instructions.
  - If the client has several different inhalers, administer the fast-acting bronchodilators first (Albuterol).
  - Shake the inhaler well immediately before each use.
  - Remove the cap from the mouthpiece.
  - Make sure the canister is fully inserted into the actuator.
  - If inhaler is brand new or has not been used for several days, spray three puffs into the air away from face and eyes.
  - Client should breathe out fully through his mouth, expelling as much air from lungs as possible.
  - Client should place mouthpiece fully into his mouth, holding the inhaler in its upright position.
  - Client should close his lips around the mouthpiece.
  - While breathing in deeply and slowly through his mouth, the client depresses the top of the metal canister with his index finger.
  - The client should hold his breath as long as possible.
  - Before exhaling, client should remove inhaler from his mouth.
  - Wait 2–5 minutes before second inhalation of medication. Shake inhaler again immediately before using and repeat previous steps for each inhalation ordered.
- Allow client to rinse mouth after using inhaler.
- Encourage client to use good oral hygiene.
- Observe client's oral mucosa and tongue for redness, white patches, and ulcerations.
- Assess client's respiratory rate, rhythm and ease of breathing.
- Rinse the inhaler thoroughly and frequently by:
  - Removing metal canister and cleanse the plastic case and cap by rinsing in warm running water once a day.
  - Dry the plastic case and cap and replace the canister.
- If a metered dose inhaler that contains a steroid medication is also ordered, wait approximately 15 minutes after the bronchodilator was administered before administering this inhaled medication. (This allows the airways to dilate and therefore more medication to be inhaled deeper).
- Leave the client in a comfortable position.
- Wash your hands.
- Document on the MAR.

Table 14–9 Procedure for Administering Medication to the Skin: **Nitroglycerin Ointment**

Procedure		
• Check the medication order on the MAR for completeness: ○ Client's name ○ Date ○ Name of medication ○ Dosage ○ Route ○ Frequency • Verify the medication listed on the MAR by comparing the MAR with the physician's order. • Check for any circumstances surrounding the administration of the medication to the client. Is the client hypotensive? • Check for a history of drug allergies. • Make sure you know the expected action, safe dosage range, special instructions for administration, and adverse effects associated with the medications ordered. • Assess the client's total drug profile for possible drug interactions. • Wash your hands. • Gather needed equipment: ○ Ruled nitroglycerin paper ○ Paper tape		
Check 1. • Read the MAR. ○ Check name of medication. ○ Check dosage of medication. ○ Check route by which medication is to be given. ○ Check date and time medication is to be given. ○ Determine if medication has been given. ○ Read the label on the medication container or unit dose package before removing it from the source. ○ Check expiration date.		
Check 2. • Pick up the medication container or unit dose package and compare the medication label with the MAR. ○ Name of medication ○ Dosage of medication • State the total amount of medication to be administered. • Put on gloves. • Using dose-determining applicator paper supplied with ointment, squeeze prescribed dose onto the applicator.		
Check 3. • Compare the medication label with the MAR again. ○ Name of medication ○ Dosage of medication ○ Route by which medication is to be given ○ Date and time medication is to be given • Return nitroglycerin tube to source. • Greet and identify the client. • Explain to the client what you are going to do. • Obtain client's BP and heart rate. • Remove ointment from previously used site before reapplication. Cleanse site with mild soap and water. • Rotate application sites to prevent dermal inflammation. • Place applicator paper with ointment side down onto desired site. Using the applicator, spread ointment in a thin, uniform layer. • Secure to client's skin with paper tape. • Remove gloves and wash hands. • After 5 minutes, check the client's BP. If there is a dramatic drop in BP or client complains of headache, notify the physician. • Document on the MAR. • Leave the client in a comfortable position.		

Table 14–10 Procedure for Administering **Otic Medication**

Procedure		
• Check the medication order on the MAR for completeness: ○ Client's name ○ Date ○ Name of medication ○ Dosage ○ Route ○ Frequency • Verify the medication listed on the MAR by comparing the MAR with the physician's order. • Check for any circumstances surrounding the administration of the medication to the client. • Check for a history of drug allergies. • Make sure you know the expected action, safe dosage range, special instructions for administration, and adverse effects associated with the medications ordered. • Assess the client's total drug profile for possible drug interactions. • Wash your hands. • Gather needed equipment: ○ Tissue, cotton balls, or gauze		
Check 1. • Read the MAR. ○ Check name of medication. ○ Check dosage of medication. ○ Check route by which medication is to be given. ○ Check date and time medication is to be given. ○ Determine if medication has been given. ○ Read the label on the medication container or unit dose package before removing it from the source. ○ Check expiration date.		
Check 2. • Pick up the medication container or unit dose package and compare the medication label with the MAR. ○ Name of medication ○ Dosage of medication • State whether medication is to be given in the right ear, left ear or both ears, and the number of drops ordered.		
Check 3. • Compare the medication label with the MAR again. ○ Name of medication ○ Dosage of medication ○ Route by which medication is to be given ○ Date and time medication is to be given • Greet and identify the client. • Explain to the client what you are going to do. • Close door and curtain. • Provide adequate lighting. • Administer the medication. ○ Put on gloves. ○ Warm the medication to body temperature by holding it in your hand for several minutes or placing the container into a small amount of warm water. ○ Ask the client to lie on one side, with the ear to be treated facing upward. ○ In an adult, pull the cartilaginous part of the pinna back and up. For children, pull pinna back and down ○ Without touching the dropper to the client's ear, place the drops into his/her ear canal. ○ Instruct the client to remain in this position for 5–10 minutes. ○ When the client sits upright, allow the remaining medication to flow out of the ear canal. Cleanse the external ear with dry cotton balls, tissue, or gauze. • Remove gloves and wash hands. • Document on the MAR. • Leave the client in a comfortable position. • Chart observations about the client's ear and his tolerance of the procedure.		

Table 14–11 Procedure for Administering **Ophthalmic Medication**

- Check the medication order on the MAR for completeness:
  - Client's name
  - Date
  - Name of medication
  - Dosage
  - Route
  - Frequency
- Verify the medication listed on the MAR by comparing the MAR with the physician's order.
- Check for any circumstances surrounding the administration of the medication to the client.
- Check for a history of drug allergies.
- Make sure you know the expected action, safe dosage range, special instructions for administration, and adverse effects associated with the medications ordered.
- Assess the client's total drug profile for possible drug interactions.
- Wash your hands.
- Gather needed equipment:
  - Tissues or gauze

Check 1.

- Read the MAR.
  - Check name of medication.
  - Check dosage of medication.
  - Check route by which medication is to be given.
  - Check date and time medication is to be given.
  - Determine if medication has been given.
  - Read the label on the medication container or unit dose package before removing it from the source.
  - Check expiration date.

Check 2.

- Pick up the medication container or unit dose package and compare the medication label with the MAR.
  - Name of medication
  - Dosage of medication
- Determine which eye is being treated. (Sometimes each eye is receiving a different treatment.)
- Remember that OS = left eye; OD = right eye; OU = both eyes.

Check 3.

- Compare the medication label with the MAR again.
  - Name of medication
  - Dosage of medication
  - Route by which medication is to be given
  - Date and time medication is to be given
- Greet and identify the client.
- Explain to the client what you are going to do.
- Close door and curtain.
- Provide adequate lighting.
- Administer the medication.
  - Put on powder free gloves.
  - Clean client's eyelids and lashes if necessary. Clean from inner canthus to outer canthus.
  - Ask the client to tilt his head slightly backward and to look up toward the ceiling.
  - Gently pull down his/her lower eyelid to form a pouch.
  - Squeeze the medication bottle to release the ordered number of drops into the middle of the exposed conjunctival sac. Do not touch the dropper tip to the eye.
  - Ask the client to close his eye gently and blink several times.
  - To prevent systemic effects of some medications, gently press on the inner angle of the eye against the client's nose.
  - Use tissue or gauze to wipe away excess medication.
- Instruct the client not to rub his eye.
- Remove gloves and wash hands.
- Document on the MAR.
- Leave the client in a comfortable position.
- Chart observations about the client's eye and his tolerance of the procedure.

Table 14–12 Procedure for Administration of a **Rectal Suppository**

• Check the medication order on the MAR for completeness: ○ Client's name ○ Date ○ Name of medication ○ Dosage ○ Route ○ Frequency • Verify the medication listed on the MAR by comparing the MAR with the physician's order. • Check for any circumstances surrounding the administration of the medication to the client. • Check for a history of drug allergies. • Make sure you know the expected action, safe dosage range, special instructions for administration, and adverse effects associated with the medications ordered. • Assess the client's total drug profile for possible drug interactions. • Wash your hands. • Gather needed equipment: ○ Water-soluble lubricant (KY Jelly) ○ Protective pad for bed, tissues ○ Bedpan		
Check 1. • Read the MAR. ○ Check name of medication. ○ Check dosage of medication. ○ Check route by which medication is to be given. ○ Check date and time medication is to be given. ○ Determine if medication has been given. ○ Read the label on the medication container or unit dose package before removing it from the source. ○ Check expiration date.		
Check 2. • Pick up the medication container or unit dose package and compare the medication label with the MAR. ○ Name of medication ○ Dosage of medication • Determine the amount of medication to be administered.		
Check 3. • Compare the medication label with the MAR again. ○ Name of medication ○ Dosage of medication ○ Route by which medication is to be given ○ Date and time medication is to be given • Greet and identify the client. • Explain to the client what you are going to do. • Close door and curtain. • Provide adequate lighting. • Administer the medication. ○ Put on gloves. ○ Ask client to turn onto his left side with his right leg flexed forward. ○ Open the package and lubricate the tip of the suppository with a small amount of water-soluble lubricant. ○ With your nondominant hand, separate the client's buttocks to expose the anus. ○ Ask the client to breathe in and out through his mouth while you are inserting the suppository. (This helps relax the sphincter muscles.) ○ Using a gloved, lubricated finger, insert the suppository into the client's rectum, tip first. ○ Advance the suppository past the anal sphincter. ○ Withdraw your finger and press the client's buttocks together for a few minutes. ○ Instruct the client not to push the suppository out. ○ Wipe excess lubricant from the client's anus. ○ Remove gloves and wash your hands. • Document on the MAR. • Leave the client in a comfortable position.		

PHARMACOLOGICAL AGENTS

Think Smart/Test Smart

As you review drugs and their classes, remember that the NCLEX-RN® is written in terms of nursing process. That means that you would not expect questions that ask: what is the action of Digoxin, what is a major side effect of digoxin, or what is a sign of digoxin toxicity. Phrased in terms of nursing process, these questions could be phrased as:

A client asks what digoxin will do for his heart. Which fact should serve as the basis for the nurse's response? (Way of asking for the therapeutic action of digoxin.) An alternate way of asking about the expected action of the drug is a question such as "When evaluating the effectiveness of digoxin for a client with congestive heart failure, which assessment data would the nurse gather?"

When teaching a client about her newly prescribed digoxin, which S&S would be correctly described as potential side effects of the medication?

Which symptoms should a client on digoxin be instructed to report immediately? (Way of asking what are signs of toxicity?)

Cardiac Glycosides

Example: digoxin (Lanoxin)

Drug Effects on Cardiac Action

- Positive inotropic: drugs that increase the force of contraction
- Negative inotropic: drugs that decrease the force of contraction
- Positive chronotropic: drugs that increase heart rate
- Negative chronotropic: drugs that decrease heart rate
- Positive dromotropic: drugs that increase the rate of electrical conduction through the myocardium
- Negative dromotropic: drugs that decrease the rate of electrical conduction through the myocardium

Mechanisms of Action

- Positive inotropic effect: increases the force of myocardial contraction
- Negative chronotropic effect: decreases the heart rate
- Negative dromotropic: decreases the rate of electrical conduction through the atrioventricular node

Common Uses

- Congestive heart failure
- Atrial fibrillation
- Atrial flutter
- Paroxysmal atrial tachycardia

Toxicity

- Gastrointestinal distress
  —Nausea
  —Vomiting
  —Anorexia
  —Diarrhea
  —Neurological effects
  —Restlessness and confusion
  —Headache
  —Weakness
  —Lethargy
  —Blurred vision, double vision, and decreased visual acuity
  —Colored vision and halo visual changes
- Cardiac effects
  Bradycardia (heart rate <60)
  Atrioventricular block
  Extrasystole (extra heart beats)

Monitoring Effects of Cardiac Glycoside

Nursing Process Elements

- Be familiar with client's baseline VS, electrolyte levels, and general health
- Assess the following before administering digoxin (Lanoxin)
  —Check serum digoxin, potassium, magnesium, and calcium levels
  —Take *apical* pulse for one full minute noting rate, rhythm, and quality.
  —Assess for toxicity
- Withhold digoxin (Lanoxin) and notify physician if:
  —Pulse rate <60
  —Significant change in pulse rate or rhythm
  —S&S of digoxin toxicity
  —Serum potassium level is less than 4 mEq/l
  —Serum digoxin level > 2 ng/ml (therapeutic range = 0.8–2 ng/ml)
- Monitor client's fluid intake and urinary output
- Monitor client's weight, signs of edema, lung, and heart sounds

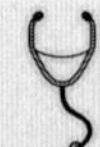

Assessment Alert

Take apical pulse for one minute prior to administering digoxin. Withhold digoxin and call physician if heart rate is less than 60 bpm.

Nursing Diagnoses

- Cardiac output: decreased
- Tissue perfusion: ineffective
- Knowledge deficit related to medications and disease

Client teaching for self-care

- Instruct how to count pulse
- Instruct to call physician if pulse < 60 or > 110
- Instruct to call physician if heart rhythm irregular
- Review S&S of toxicity and instruct to report them to physician
- Weigh each day and report > 2 lb gain per day
- Take digoxin (Lanoxin) as prescribed at same time each day

ANTIARRHYTHMICS

Mechanisms of Action

Varies depending on the antiarrhythmic class used

- Decreases the automaticity of cardiac tissue
- Alters the rate of conduction of electrical impulses
- Alters the refractory period

Common Uses

Suppression of arrhythmias

Common Adverse Effects

Differs among the different drugs

Monitoring Effects of Antiarrhythmics

Nursing Process Elements

- Assess heart rate and rhythm and BP prior to administration and throughout therapy
- Monitor ECG
- Monitor for adverse effects

Nursing Diagnoses

- Cardiac output is decreased
- Knowledge deficit related to medication and disease

Client teaching for self-care

- Instruct in how to obtain pulse rate, and to report changes in rate and rhythm to physician
- Instruct to take doses round the clock and what to do regarding missed doses and over-the-counter medications
- Advise regarding importance of follow-up appointments with health care provider

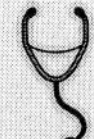

Assessment Alert

Take BP and heart rate prior to administering antiarrhythmic medications.

NITRATE VASODILATORS

Example: nitroglycerin (Nitrocot)

Mechanism of Action

- Relaxes smooth muscle
- Dilates venous and arterial blood vessels
- Reduces peripheral resistance
- Decreases venous return to the heart
- Reduces myocardial oxygen consumption
- Decreases BP
- Relieves and prevents angina (chest pain)

Common Uses

- Prophylaxis, treatment, and management of angina pectoris (chest pain)
- Congestive heart failure

Common Adverse Effects

- Hypotension
- Headache
- Dizziness
- Syncope

Forms of Nitrate Vasodilators

- Sublingual tablet
  —Place tablet under tongue to dissolve within 5 minutes
- Extended-release buccal tablet
  —Place tablet between lip and gum or between cheek and gum to dissolve over 3–5 hours
- Oral sustained-release tablet or capsule
- Translingual spray
  —Do not shake canister
  —Spray under tongue
  —Do not inhale spray
- Transdermal ointment
  —Use dose-determining applicator supplied with ointment
  —Nurse should wear gloves
- Transdermal Unit (patch)
  —Nurse should wear gloves
- Parenteral (IV)

Monitoring Effects of Nitroglycerin

Nursing Process Elements

- Be familiar with clients baseline VS
- Obtain BP, heart rate prior to administering medication
- Check BP and heart rate after administration (hypotension may occur)
- Assess chest pain using pain scale, and assess for associated symptoms: dyspnea, shortness of breath, jaw, arm, neck pain, nausea, and diaphoresis
- Assess for blurred vision, headache, and dry mouth
- Assess for topical reactions when using the ointment or transdermal unit

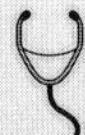

Assessment Alert

Take BP prior to and after administering nitroglycerin.

Nursing Diagnoses

- Pain: acute
- Tissue perfusion: ineffective
- Knowledge deficit related to medications and disease

Client teaching for self-care

- Instruct that sublingual tablets may be taken prophylactically 5–10 minutes prior to exercise or other stimulus known to trigger angina.
- Remind them to keep record of number of angina attacks, amount of medication taken, and precipitating factors.
- Instruct that contact with water (bathing, swimming) does not affect transdermal unit.
- Inform that the sublingual form can be taken while transdermal unit or ointment is in place.
- When chest pain occurs, take one nitroglycerine tablet as prescribed; if chest discomfort is not relieved in 3 minutes, call 911.
- Remind to report blurred vision, dry mouth, faintness, dizziness, flushing, or increase in frequency or severity of pain to physician.
- Explain to change positions slowly and avoid prolonged standing (postural hypotension)
- Inform that SL tablets should be kept in their original container and tablets need to be replaced every 6 months to assure potency.
- Advise to take medication as directed, avoid alcohol, and not to take over-the-counter medications without approval of physician.
- Encourage to keep follow-up appointments with health care provider.

ANTIHYPERTENSIVES

Diuretics

Mechanisms of Action

Thiazide diuretics

Example: hydrochlorothiazide (HCTZ)

—Inhibits sodium reabsorption in the distal tubule, thereby increasing excretion of water and sodium.

—Enhances excretion of magnesium, chloride, and potassium.

Loop diuretics

Example: furosemide (Lasix)

—Inhibits the reabsorption of sodium and chloride in the ascending loop of Henle

—Increases risk of hypokalemia (low potassium level)

—Reduces the ability of the kidneys to concentrate urine

—More potent than the thiazides in promoting sodium and fluid excretion

Potassium-sparing diuretics

Example: spironolactone (Aldactone)

—Promotes sodium and chloride excretion without concomitant loss of potassium

—Inhibits the action of the hormone aldosterone thereby causing diuresis

—Lowers BP by unknown mechanism

—Increases risk of hyperkalemia (increased potassium levels)

Common Uses

- Congestive heart failure
- Hypertension
- Renal failure
- Edema

Common Adverse Effects

- Hypokalemia (except potassium sparing diuretics)
- Hyponatremia
- Dehydration
- Postural hypotension
- Hyperglycemia

Monitoring Effects of Diuretics

Nursing Process Elements

- Be familiar with client's baseline VS
- Obtain BP and heart rate prior to administering medication
- Check BP and heart rate before and after administration
- Monitor for signs of hypokalemia
- Fatigue
- Muscle weakness and cramps
- Rapid irregular pulse
- Vomiting
- Shortness of breath
- Monitor fluid intake and urinary output
- In hospital, weigh client daily
- Monitor for
  —edema
  —abnormal lung sounds
  —extra heart sounds
- Assess for postural hypotension
- Monitor serum levels
  —Potassium
  —Sodium
  —Chloride
  —Glucose
  —Blood urea nitrogen (BUN)
- Assess for digoxin (Lanoxin) toxicity if dehydration or hypokalemia exists

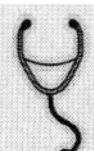

Assessment Alert

Take BP prior to and after administering diuretics. Always monitor electrolytes prior to administering diuretics.

Nursing Diagnoses

- Fluid volume: excess
- Knowledge deficit related to medications, disease, and nutrition

Client/family teaching

- Instruct regarding weighing at least once per week
- Remind to have BP monitored weekly
- Advise to follow dietary guidelines, especially regarding potassium and sodium
- Encourage to change positions slowly to avoid a decrease in BP (postural hypotension)
- Instruct to notify health care provider if experiencing muscle weakness or cramping, fatigue, or dizziness
- Advise to take medication as directed and to not take over-the-counter drugs unless approved by physician
- Encourage to keep follow-up appointments with health care provider

BETA-ADRENERGIC BLOCKING AGENTS

Example: propranolol (Inderal)

Think Smart/Test Smart

The generic names for the beta-blockers end in "lol," therefore, you will be able to identify the beta-blockers from a list of drugs.

Mechanisms of Action

- Reduction in heart rate
- Reduces force of cardiac contraction
- Slows electrical conduction
- Reduces myocardial irritability

Common Uses

- Management of cardiac arrhythmias
- Hypertension
- Tachyarrhythmias associated with digitalis toxicity
- Angina Pectoris

Common Adverse Effects

- Weakness: fatigue
- Impotence
- Concerns for use: Precautions
  —It may cause bronchoconstriction; therefore, its use may be contraindicated in clients with chronic pulmonary diseases
  —It may promote congestive heart failure therefore use cautiously in clients with risk for heart failure.

Monitoring Effects of Beta-Adrenergic Blocking Agents

Nursing Process Elements

- Assess heart rate and rhythm, BP prior to administration and throughout therapy

- Assess location, intensity, and duration of anginal pain and associated symptoms
- Monitor ECG
- Monitor for adverse effects

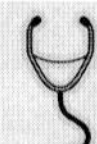

Assessment Alert

Always take BP and heart rate prior to administering beta-blockers.

Nursing Diagnoses

- Cardiac output, decreased
- Pain: acute
- Tissue perfusion: ineffective
- Knowledge deficit related to medication and disease

Client teaching for self-care

- Instruct in how to obtain pulse rate, and to report changes in rate and rhythm to physician
- Instruct to take doses round the clock and what to do regarding missed doses and over-the-counter medications
- Advise to report chest pain to health care provider immediately
- Advise regarding importance of follow-up appointments with health care provider

CALCIUM CHANNEL ANTAGONISTS

Example: nifedipine (Procardia)

Mechanisms of Action

- Relaxation of vascular smooth muscle and lowered BP
- Prevents or reverses spasms of coronary blood vessels
- Dilates coronary arteries and arterioles resulting in an antianginal effect
- Reduces myocardial oxygen consumption
- Slows electrical impulse conduction (supraventricular tachycardia)

Common Uses

- Prevention and treatment of angina pectoris
- Hypertension

Common Adverse Effects

- Hypotension
- Peripheral edema
- Dizziness
- Headache

Monitoring Effects of Calcium Channel Antagonists Agents

Nursing Process Elements

- Assess heart rate and rhythm, BP prior to administration and throughout therapy
- Assess location, intensity, and duration of anginal pain
- Monitor ECG
- Monitor for adverse effects

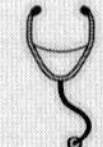

Assessment Alert

Always take the client's BP and heart rate before and after administering calcium channel antagonists.

Nursing Diagnoses

- Cardiac output, decreased
- Pain: acute
- Tissue perfusion: ineffective
- Knowledge deficit related to medication, disease

Client teaching for self-care

- Instruct in how to obtain pulse rate, and to report changes in rate and rhythm to physician
- Instruct to take doses around the clock and what to do regarding missed doses and over-the-counter medications
- Advise to report chest pain to health care provider immediately
- Advise regarding importance of follow-up appointments with health care provider

ANGIOTENSIN-CONVERTING ENZYME (ACE) INHIBITORS

Example: captopril (Capoten)

Think Smart/Test Smart

The generic names of the ACE inhibitors end in "pril," therefore, you will be able to identify them from a list.

Mechanism of Action

- Dilates peripheral arterioles
- Relaxes vascular smooth muscles
- Reduces peripheral resistance
- Interferes with conversion of angiotensin I to angiotensin II
- Dilates peripheral vessels thereby reducing BP

Common Uses

- Hypertension
- Congestive heart failure
- Arrhythmias (irregular heart rhythm)
- Angina Pectoris (chest pain)

Common Adverse Effects

- Hypotension
- Postural hypotension
- Dizziness, fainting, and headaches
- Drug-specific

Monitoring Effects of ACE Inhibitors

Nursing Process Elements

- Be familiar with client's baseline VS
- Obtain BP and pulse rate prior to administering medication
- Check BP and pulse rate after administration
- Monitor weight, edema, lung, heart sounds, and I&O
- Assess for postural hypotension
- Encourage client to rise slowly from lying to sitting position

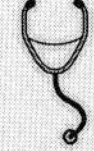

Assessment Alert

Always take the client's BP and heart rate prior to and after administering ACE inhibitors.

Nursing Diagnoses

- Tissue perfusion: ineffective
- Knowledge deficit related to medications and disease

Client teaching for self-care

- Instruct on monitoring BP weekly
- Remind to change positions slowly to prevent rapid decrease in BP
- Encourage to follow dietary restrictions: low sodium
- Instruct regarding reporting weight changes, edema, and dizziness to physician
- Emphasize importance of follow-up appointments with health care provider

ANTIMICROBIAL AGENTS

Classification of Antimicrobial Agents

- Bactericidal and bacteriostatic
  —Bactericidal agents have a killing action on the bacteria
  —Bacteriostatic agents inhibit the growth of bacteria permitting the host's immunological defenses to destroy the organism

Site of Action

- Agents that inhibit cell wall synthesis
- Agents that inhibit protein synthesis
- Agents that interfere with the permeability of the bacterial cell membrane
- Agents with antimetabolite action block or alter steps essential for the normal growth of the bacteria

Narrow or Broad Spectrum of Action

- Narrow spectrum
  —Effective against a limited number of organisms
  —Use when identity of organism and susceptibility of the antibiotic is known
  —Usually do not disrupt normal bacterial flora
- Broad spectrum
  —Act on a wide variety of organisms
  —Useful in treating infections when the identity and susceptibility to antimicrobial treatment of the infecting organism is unknown
  —However, they destroy the body's normal microbes and may permit superinfection and diarrhea

Adverse Effects

- Hypersensitivity reactions
  —Rash
  —Urticaria
  —Fever
  —Bronchospasm
  —Anaphylactic shock
- Organ toxicity
  —High doses and/or over long periods of time
  —Can involve liver, kidneys, central nervous system, etc
- Ototoxicity (detrimental effect on eighth nerve or organs of hearing)
- Hematological disorders
  —Anemia
  —Increased bleeding time

Major Classes

- Penicillins (beta-lactams)

Example: ampicillin (Polycillin)
  - —Bactericidal agents
  - —Inhibit the synthesis of the bacterial cell wall
  - —Narrow and broad-spectrum agents
- Cephalosporins
  - —Chemically and pharmacologically related to the penicillins
  - —Bactericidal or bacteriostatic effect
  - —Interferes with bacterial cell wall syntheses
  - —Four "generations" of cephalosporins
  - —Use caution when client has allergy to penicillins
- Tetracyclines:

Example: tetracycline (Tetracyn)
  - —Bacteriostatic
  - —Broad-spectrum agents
  - —Inhibits protein synthesis in the bacterial cell
  - —May interfere with normal calcification of temporary and permanent teeth and discolor developing teeth
  - —May interfere with bone growth
  - —Clients more susceptible to sunburn
- Macrolides:

Example: erythromycin (Ery-Tab)
  - —Bacteriostatic
  - —May be bactericidal in high concentrations
  - —Inhibits protein synthesis in the bacterial cell
- Aminoglycosides:

Example: gentamicin (Garamycin)
  - —Bactericidal or bacteriostatic
  - —Inhibits protein synthesis in the bacterial cell
  - —May produce nephrotoxicity and ototoxicity

Monitoring Effects of Antibiotics

- Take a careful medication history before administering antibiotics
- Know exactly why your client is receiving antibiotics
- If ordered, obtain specimen for culture and susceptibility *before* administering the antibiotic
- Know what a therapeutic response to antibiotic treatment would include for each specific client situation
- Administer oral doses of antibiotics on empty stomach or with food as specified
- Be aware of food–drug and drug–drug interactions, for example, penicillin can interfere with effectiveness of oral contraceptives.
- Monitor VS and S&S of infection
- Monitor WBC count, BUN, creatinine, and other laboratory values
- Observe for adverse effects
- Observe for S&S of superinfections

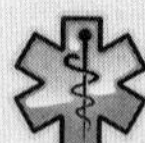

Nursing Intervention Alert

If cultures are ordered by the physician, always obtain the specimen prior to administering the first dose of antibiotic.

Nursing Diagnoses

- Infection: risk for
- Knowledge deficit related to medication or disease

Client teaching for self-care

- Advise to call health care provider if symptoms do not improve
- Remind to take all doses of the medication even if their symptoms are no longer present, and to follow instructions regarding taking medication with or without food
- Instruct to inform health care provider if diarrhea, vomiting occur, black, hairy growth develops on tongue, and vaginal irritation occurs
- Advise to keep all follow-up appointments with health care provider

ANTICOAGULANTS

Mechanism of Action

Parenteral anticoagulants

Example: heparin (Heparin Lock); enoxaparin (Lovenox)

- Exerts direct effect on blood coagulation (clotting) by enhancing the inhibitory actions of antithrombin III on several factors essential to normal blood clotting, thereby blocking the conversion of prothrombin to thrombin and fibrinogen to fibrin.
- Does not lyse existing thrombi but may prevent their extension
- Inhibits formation of new clots

Oral anticoagulant

Example: warfarin sodium (Coumadin)

- Indirectly interferes with blood clotting by depressing hepatic synthesis of vitamin K dependent coagulation factors: II, VII, IX, and X.

- Deters further extension of existing thrombi and prevents new clots from forming.
- Has no effect on platelets.
- Unlike heparin, action is cumulative and more prolonged.

Common Uses

Heparin and Lovenox

—Prophylaxis and treatment of venous thrombosis and pulmonary embolism (blood clot to leg or lung)

—Prevent thromboembolic complications arising from cardiac surgery and vascular surgery

—During acute stages of myocardial infarction (heart attack)

Coumadin

- Prophylaxis and treatment of deep venous thrombosis and pulmonary embolism (blood clot in leg or lung)
- Treatment of atrial fibrillation with embolization (irregular heart beat that may cause blood clots).
- An adjunct in treatment of coronary occlusion, cerebral transient ischemic attacks (heart attacks, near strokes)
- Prophylactic treatment for clients with prosthetic cardiac valves

Common Adverse Effects

- Bleeding
- Hematuria
- Tarry stools
- Excessive vaginal bleeding
- Abdominal, flank, or joint pain
- Headaches
- Changes in neurological status, restlessness
- Hematoma or bruising
- Vomiting blood
- Bleeding from the nose or gums
- Weak, rapid pulse rate
- Hypotension

Monitoring Effects of Heparin

Nursing Process Elements

- Before administration check coagulation tests, hemoglobin, hematocrit, and platelet counts.
- In general, the goal is to keep the activated partial thromboplastin time (aPTT) at 1.5–2.5 times its normal value of 35–45 seconds.
- Safely administer heparin via ordered route, i.e., subcutaneous injection, continuous intravenous infusion, or intermittent intravenous infusion.
- No intramuscular injections
- Observe for S&S of bleeding
- No aspirin containing products
- Use soft toothbrush and electric razor

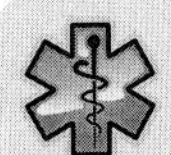

Nursing Intervention Alert

Always check the aPTT prior to administering heparin.

Monitoring Effects of Coumadin

- Before administration check coagulation tests, hemoglobin, hematocrit, and platelet counts
- In general, the goal is to maintain a prothrombin time (PT) of 1.5–2 times the control or reference value and maintain the international normalized ratio (INR) at a value of 2–3. The PT control value is generally 11–15 seconds
- The daily oral dose is based on the PT and INR results until maintenance dosage is established
- Observe for S&S of bleeding
- No intramuscular injections
- No aspirin containing products
- Medic alert identification
- Use soft toothbrush and electric razor

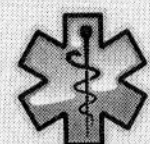

Nursing Intervention Alert

Always check the PT and INR prior to administering Coumadin.

Antidotes

- Heparin and Lovenox: Protamine sulfate
- Coumadin: Vitamin K (Aqua Mephyton)

Nursing Diagnoses

- Injury: risk for
- Tissue perfusion: ineffective
- Knowledge deficit related to medications, disease

Client teaching for self-care

- Instruct to use a soft toothbrush, electric razor, avoid contact sports
- Inform not to take medications containing aspirin or aspirin-like products without approval of physician

- Instruct about foods high in vitamin K (broccoli, collards, kale, spinach, cabbage, yogurt, milk, and green tea) and importance of not significantly increasing or decreasing daily intake of them
- Remind to report signs of bleeding to physician immediately: bleeding gums, bruising, blood in urine, feces, abdominal, joint or head pain, weak, rapid pulse, low BP, weakness, and restlessness
- Encourage to keep laboratory appointments to monitor coagulation factors and follow-up appointments with health care provider
- Request that a medical identification describing the anticoagulation medications be carried at all times

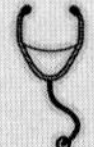

Assessment Alert

For clients receiving anticoagulation medications, always assess for S&S of bleeding.

ANTIDIABETIC AGENTS

Mechanisms of Action

Sulfonylureas

Example: glyburide: (DiaBeta)

- Directly stimulates functioning pancreatic beta cells to secrete insulin
- Increases sensitivity of peripheral insulin receptors resulting in increased insulin binding

Biguanide

Example: metformin (Glucophage, Glucophage XR)

- Increases glucose transport across cell membrane, with enhanced glucose utilization in skeletal muscles
- Increases the binding of insulin to its receptor and potentiating insulin action

Meglitinides

Example: repaglinide (Prandin)

- Stimulates release of insulin from the pancreatic islets

Thiazolidinediones

Example: rosiglitazone (Avandia)

- Improves target cell response to insulin
- Reduces cellular insulin resistance
- Decreases hepatic glucose output

Alpha-Glucosidase Inhibitors

Example: acarbose (Precose)

- Inhibits or delays the absorption of sugars from the intestinal tract

Mechanism of Action

Regular insulin

Example: (Humulin R)

- Enhances transmembrane passage of glucose across cell membranes
- Promotes conversion of glucose to glycogen

Common Uses

Oral hypoglycemic agent

- Noninsulin-dependent, type 2 diabetes mellitus

Insulin

- Insulin-dependent, type 1 diabetes mellitus

Common Adverse Effects

- Hypoglycemia

Rapid Acting Insulin

Example: insulin lispro (Humalog)

- Onset of action: within 15 minutes
- Peak action: 30–90 minutes
- Duration: 3–4 hours

Short-Acting Insulins

Example: Regular insulin (Humulin R)

- Onset of action: 30–60 minutes
- Peak action: 2–3 hours
- Duration: 3–6 hours

Intermediate-Acting Insulins

Example: NPH (Humulin N)

- Onset of action: 2–4 hours
- Peak Action: 6–10 hours
- Duration: 10–16 hours

Long-Acting Insulins

Example: Insulin glargine (Lantus), Insulin detemir (Levemir)

- Onset of action: 2 hours
- Peakless
- Duration: 24 hours

Fixed Combinations of N and R

Example: 1. 70/30 = 70% N and 30% R

- Onset of action: 30–60 minutes
- Peak action: Refer to N, R
- Duration: 10–16 hours

Fixed Combinations

Example: Humalog Mix 75/25 = 75% insulin lispro protamine and 25% insulin lispro

- Onset of action: within 15 minutes
- Peak action: 1–6.5 hours (average 2.5 hours)
- Duration: Refer to N and insulin lispro

Inhalation Agents

- Insulin human inhalation powder

Mechanism of Action: Incretin mimetics (Byetta)

- Enhances glucose-dependent insulin secretion
- Suppresses elevated glucagon secretion
- Slows gastric emptying

Monitoring Effects of Hypoglycemic Agents

Nursing Process Elements

- Be familiar with client's baseline blood glucose levels
- Monitor for S&S of hypoglycemia
  —Fatigue, restlessness
  —Cool, moist skin
  —Weakness and dizziness
  —Headache
  —Confusion, slurred speech
- Monitor for S&S of hyperglycemia
  —Flushed, dry skin
  —Increased urine output
  —Increased thirst
  —Increased appetite
  —Drowsiness
- Monitor blood glucose results as ordered

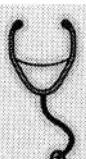

Assessment Alert

Assess the lower extremities and feet of clients with diabetes. Provide foot care and assure that client has shoes to wear while in the hospital.

Nursing Diagnoses

- Noncompliance
- Knowledge deficit related to medication, diet, and disease
- Nutrition: imbalanced

Client teaching for self-care

- Instruct in signs of hyperglycemia and hypoglycemia
- Instruct in actions to take for hyperglycemia and hypoglycemia
- Inform to carry a quick acting sugar product at all times
- Instruct in proper use of equipment for blood glucose testing
- Review the proper use of insulin syringes and pens, as well as proper technique for injection, storage and disposal of syringes
- Remind to rotate injection sites
- Review diet modifications, food item selections and substitutions, and alcohol restrictions
- Encourage to follow diet, medication, and exercise plan and to follow-up with regular appointments with health care provider

BRONCHODILATORS

Mechanisms of Action

Sympathomimetic agents

Example: albuterol (Proventil) and xanthine derivatives (theophylline [Uniphyl])

- Relax smooth muscle of bronchi and pulmonary vessels producing bronchodilation
- Increase vital capacity

Leukotriene receptor antagonists

Example: montelukast (Singulair)

- Decreases bronchial edema and inflammation
- Causes bronchodilation

Common Uses

- Prophylaxis and symptomatic relief of bronchial asthma
- Relieve bronchospasm associated with bronchitis and emphysema

Common Adverse Effects

- Tremor
- Tachycardia
- Nausea

Monitoring Effects of Bronchodilators

- Be familiar with client's baseline VS
- Monitor client's lung sounds, respiratory effort, and oxygen saturation percentages via pulse oximetry
- Monitor for cyanosis of lips, ear lobes, mucous membranes, and nailbeds

- Monitor theophylline plasma levels, if ordered. Therapeutic range is 10–20 μg/ml.
- Observe client for adverse effects
- Ensure that client uses metered dose inhaler correctly

Nursing Diagnoses

- Breathing pattern: ineffective
- Airway clearance: ineffective
- Knowledge deficit related to medications and disease

Client teaching for self-care

- Instruct in proper use of metered-dose inhaler and spacer. Remind to use the short-acting bronchodilator inhaler 5 minutes prior to the steroid dose inhaler
- Instruct in proper mouth care and cleansing of inhalers
- Inform to avoid smoke and all other respiratory irritants
- Remind to allow for rest periods before or between periods of activity
- Encourage to follow all medication and respiratory exercise regimes and keep appointments with health care provider

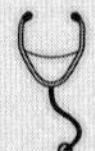

Assessment Alert

Inquire about the client's activities of daily living and modifications in their activities they have made as a result of frequent shortness of breath.

AGENTS AFFECTING GASTROINTESTINAL FUNCTION

Mechanisms of Action

Laxatives

Stimulant laxative:
Example: bisacodyl (Dulcolax)

- Increases motility of gastrointestinal tract by chemical irritation of the intestinal mucosa
- Increases the secretion of water into large and small intestines

Saline laxatives:
Example: magnesium hydroxide (milk of magnesia)

- Draws water through the intestinal wall by osmotic action increasing the fluidity of the stool and stimulates greater intestinal motility

Bulk-forming laxatives:
Example: psyllium hydrophilic (Metamucil)

- Absorbs fluid and the compound swells in the intestine, stimulating peristaltic action.

Lubricant laxatives:
Example: mineral oil

- Act as lubricant to facilitate passage of fecal mass through the intestines

Stool softeners:
Example: docusate sodium (Colace)

- Permits water and fat to penetrate and soften stool
- Detergent action lowers surface tension

Common Uses for Laxatives

- Prevent or treat constipation
- Prepare clients for a lower gastrointestinal X-ray series or surgery
- Reduce the strain of defecation in clients with cardiovascular disease or in postoperative clients
- Diagnose and treat parasitic infestations of the gastrointestinal tract
- Help remove unabsorbed poisons from the gastrointestinal tract

Guidelines for Laxatives

- Always assess the effectiveness of laxatives
- In selecting a laxative, consider the age and general condition of client
- In general, avoid use of stimulant laxatives in the elderly
- Follow bulk-forming laxatives with at least one glass of fluid to prevent gastrointestinal obstruction
- Never administer laxatives to clients experiencing abdominal pain, nausea, or vomiting until after consulting with physician
- Be aware of specific drug–drug and drug–food interactions
- Monitor frequent and prolonged laxative use

Mechanisms of Action

Histamine receptor antagonists

Example: famotidine (Pepcid)

- Inhibits the action of histamine at the histamine-sensitive H_2 receptor site of the parietal cells in the stomach
- Results in reduction in acid secretion

Proton pump inhibitors

Example: lansoprazole (Prevacid)

- Suppresses gastric acid secretion by inhibiting the gastric acid pump in the parietal cells of the stomach

Common Uses for Histamine Receptor Antagonists and Proton Pump Inhibitors

- Treatment of duodenal ulcer
- Treatment of gastric ulcer
- Gastroesophageal reflux disease
- Gastritis
- Erosive esophagitis

Adverse Effects of Histamine Receptor Antagonists and Proton Pump Inhibitors

- Diarrhea
- Headache

Monitoring Effects of Therapy

Nursing Process Elements

- Monitor symptoms of gastrointestinal distress:
  —Heartburn
  —Fullness in stomach and throat
  —Pain in abdomen or chest
- Monitor for signs of gastrointestinal bleeding:
  —Blood in stool
  —Vomiting dark-colored substance
  —Decrease in hemoglobin
- Be aware of drug–drug and drug–food interactions
- Monitor for adverse effects

Nursing Diagnoses

- Pain: acute
- Injury: risk for bleeding
- Knowledge deficit related to medication and disease

Client teaching for self-care

- Inform to avoid spicy foods, alcohol, aspirin, NSAIDs, and smoking
- Advise to continue taking medications even if symptoms are no longer present
- Instruct to call health care provider for any signs of bleeding: tarry stools, increase in abdominal or back pain

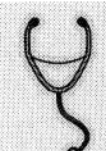

Assessment Alert

Obtain information about client's diet and modifications in food selection based on their frequent symptoms of heartburn or gastrointestinal distress.

PHARMACOLOGICAL PAIN MANAGEMENT

ANALGESIC, ANTIPYRETIC, AND ANTI-INFLAMMATORY AGENTS

Mechanisms of Action

Opioid analgesics

Example: morphine (Roxanol)

- Opioid and opioid-like agents bind onto opioid receptors found in the central nervous system and act to inhibit the transmission of pain impulses and alter pain perception
- Suppresses medullary cough centers
- Suppresses the motility of the gastrointestinal tract

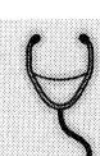

Assessment Alert

Always assess client's respiratory rate prior to and after administering morphine. Many institutional policies state that the nurse should not administer morphine to a client with a respiratory rate of less than 10 breaths per minute.

Salicylates

Example: aspirin (Ecotrin)

- Anti-inflammatory action: Inhibits prostaglandin synthesis (nonsteroidal anti-inflammatory drug (NSAID)
- Analgesic action: Acts peripherally to interfere with action of prostaglandins
- Antipyretic action: In addition to inhibiting prostaglandin synthesis, it lowers body temperature in fever by causing centrally mediated peripheral vasodilation and sweating
- Antiplatelet action: Aspirin (but not other salicylates) inhibits platelet aggregation, therefore, aspirin helps prevent strokes and myocardial infarction (heart attack)

Nonnarcotic analgesic and antipyretic

Example: acetaminophen (Tylenol)

- Produces analgesia by unknown mechanism, perhaps by action on peripheral nervous system
- Reduces fever by direct action on hypothalamus, peripheral vasodilation, and sweating

Nonsalicylates

Example: celecoxib (Celebrex)

- Newer NSAIDs inhibit prostaglandin synthesis by inhibiting COX-2
- Provides analgesic and anti-inflammatory effects
- Less adverse effects on the gastrointestinal system and less antiplatelet activity

Corticosteroids

Example: prednisone (Pred-Pak)

- Synthetic steroid used primarily for its glucocorticoid effects—anti-inflammatory agent
- Reduces the severity of inflammatory symptoms

Common Uses

Opioid analgesics

- Moderate to severe pain
- Cough suppressant
- Suppressing the motility of the gastrointestinal tract (diarrhea)

Salicylates

- Low to moderate pain
- Rheumatoid arthritis
- Osteoarthritis
- Reduction of fever
- Reduce incidence of stroke and myocardial infarction (heart attack)

Nonnarcotic analgesic and antipyretic

- Mild to moderate pain
- Reduction of fever
- Often a substitute for aspirin when aspirin is not tolerated

Nonsalicylates (NSAIDs)

- Osteoarthritis
- Mild to moderate pain
- Primary dysmenorrhea
- Reduction of fever

Corticosteroids

- Bronchial asthma
- Osteoarthritis
- Dermatitis
- Inflammatory conditions

Common Adverse Effects

Opioid analgesics

- N&V
- Constipation
- Pruritus (itching)
- Decrease in respiratory rate (Naloxone [Narcan] is opioid antagonist and reverses respiratory depression)

Salicylates

- Nausea
- Heartburn and stomach pain

Nonnarcotic analgesic and antipyretic

- Negligible with recommended dosage

Nonsalicylates (NSAIDs)

- Heartburn
- Nausea

Corticosteroids

- Insomnia
- Fluid retention
- Hyperglycemia
- Altered fat deposition causing "moon face"
- Weight gain
- Hypertension

Monitoring Effects of Therapy

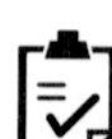

Nursing Process Elements

Opioid analgesics

- Be familiar with client's pain history
- Be familiar with client's baseline VS
- Monitor for respiratory depression, sedation, and orthostatic hypotension
- Assist client with ambulation activities
- Monitor for constipation and other adverse effects
- Evaluate level of pain relief

Salicylates

- Be familiar with client's pain history and baseline VS
- Do not administer aspirin to clients taking anticoagulants, those with gastric ulcers, pregnant women, or children with fever
- Observe for signs of bleeding (bleeding gums, bruising, bloody or dark stools, cloudy or bloody urine)
- If taking aspirin for prevention of stroke or heart attack, then observe for S&S of stroke or heart attack
- Evaluate for reduction of symptoms for which medication prescribed.

Nonnarcotic analgesics and antipyretics

- Be familiar with client's pain history and baseline VS
- Do not administer greater than 4 g of Tylenol in 24 hours to an adult because of risk of liver damage
- Evaluate for reduction of pain or fever after administration

Nonsalicylates (NSAIDs)

- Be familiar with client's pain history and baseline VS
- Monitor for S&S of gastrointestinal distress or bleeding
- Do not administer aspirin or acetaminophen concurrently with ibuprofen
- Evaluate for reduction of symptoms (relief of pain and stiffness, improved joint flexion)

Corticosteroids

- Be familiar with client's history and VS
- Be aware of exactly why the client is receiving a steroid medication
- Administer medication with food, and before 0900 if possible
- Monitor BP, fluid intake, urinary output, weight, and sleep pattern
- Monitor blood glucose, serum potassium levels as ordered
- Administer calcium supplements as ordered
- Observe for masked infection and delayed healing
- Inspect client's mouth for white patches, black furry tongue, painful membranes
- Assist client to plan a reasonable and safe range of activities
- Watch for changes in mood and behavior
- Do not abruptly discontinue medication
- Evaluate for reduction of symptoms for which medication was ordered

Nursing Diagnoses

- Pain: acute
- Body temperature: imbalance
- Knowledge deficit related to medications and disease

Client teaching for self-care

- Instruct that analgesics should be taken with food and may cause drowsiness.
- Inform that steroids may mask signs of infection, need to be taken with food, and calcium with vitamin D needs to be taken as long as steroids are prescribed.
- Instruct to take steroids exactly as directed by health care provider and to not abruptly stop taking medication.
- Advise to eat a diet high in protein, calcium, and potassium, but low in sodium while taking steroid medications.
- Instruct regarding assessing oral mucus membranes for redness and soreness while taking steroids.
- Remind parents not to administer aspirin to children with viral illnesses due to Reye's syndrome.
- Inform that aspirin and NSAIDs may cause an increase in bruising and bleeding and to report symptoms to health care provider. Must be discontinued 1 week before elective surgery.

ANTI-ALZHEIMER'S AGENTS

Cholinesterase Inhibitors

Example: donepezil (Aricept)

Mechanism of Action

- Enhances cholinergic function by increasing levels of acetylcholine

Common Uses

- Mild to moderate dementia associated with Alzheimer's disease

Common Adverse Effects

- Headache
- Diarrhea
- Nausea

Monitoring Effects of Therapy

- Assess memory, attention, language, and ability to follow directions or perform simple tasks.
- Assess for dizziness, headache, weight loss, diarrhea, nausea, and change in color of stools.

Nursing Diagnoses

- Injury: risk for
- Thought processes: disturbed
- Knowledge deficit related to medication and disease

Client teaching for self-care

- Advise to notify health care provider if symptoms worsen, if new symptoms appear or if adverse effects such as diarrhea, nausea, or headache occur
- Instruct in safe environment measures, and to be aware that dizziness may occur
- Encourage to keep follow-up appointments with health care provider

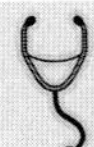

Assessment Alert

A home safety survey may need to be conducted in order to provide a safe, therapeutic environment.

ANTIANXIETY AGENTS

Example: alprazolam (Xanax)

Mechanisms of Action

Benzodiazepine group

- Slows nerve impulses by enhancing the activity of GABA

Common Uses

- Anxiety
- Panic attacks

Common Adverse Effects

- Dizziness
- Fatigue
- Drowsiness

Monitoring Effects of Antianxiety Agents

- Assess level of anxiety before and throughout therapy
- Monitor CBC, liver panel, BUN, and creatinine (Cr)
- Monitor for adverse effects: dizziness, drowsiness, and fatigue
- Assess coping mechanisms and resources available

Nursing Diagnoses

- Anxiety
- Injury: risk for
- Knowledge deficit related to medications and disease

Client teaching for self-care

- Instruct to not drive if drug causes drowsiness or dizziness
- Inform to avoid alcohol and other CNS depressants, and consult health care provider prior to changing medication regimen

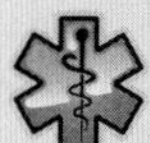

Nursing Intervention Alert

Always place call bell within client's reach, and keep bed in lowest position.

ANTICONVULSANTS

Example: phenytoin (Dilantin)

Mechanisms of Action

- Alters ion transport thereby limiting seizure propagation
- Improves AV conduction thus reducing incidents of arrhythmias

Common Uses

- Treatment and prevention of tonic-clonic seizures and complex partial seizures
- Treatment and prevention of arrhythmias

Common Adverse Effects

- Hypotension
- Nausea
- Rashes
- Diplopia
- Gingival hyperplasia
- Ataxia

Monitoring Effects of Anticonvulsants

- Assess type, duration, frequency, and characteristics of seizure activity
- Assess for adverse effects of medication: signs of gingival hyperplasia, rashes, fever, and vision changes
- Monitor serum phenytoin, CBC, platelet count, liver panel, calcium, and urinalysis
- Administer medications round the clock
- Implement seizure precautions

Nursing Diagnoses

- Injury: risk for
- Knowledge deficit related to medication and disease

Client teaching for self-care

- Instruct to follow the medication regime closely, and not consume alcohol
- Advise to carry medical identification at all times
- Instruct in proper oral hygiene practices and express need to have regular dental exams
- Advise that medication may cause drowsiness and should not drive until physician indicates that the seizures and the medication have provided a safe condition for such activities

ANTIDEPRESSANTS

There are two major classes: tricyclic antidepressants and selective serotonin reuptake inhibitors (SSRIs)

Examples: nortriptyline (Aventyl), paroxetine (Paxil)

Mechanisms of Action

Tricyclic antidepressants

- Potentiates the effect of norepinephrine and serotonin
- Possesses anticholinergic action

Selective serotonin reuptake inhibitors

- Inhibits uptake of serotonin in the CNS

Common Uses

- Treatment of depression

Common Adverse Effects

- Fatigue
- Drowsiness
- Blurred vision and dry eyes
- Dry mouth and constipation
- Hypotension

Monitoring Effects of Antidepressants

Nursing Process Elements

- Assess mental status, mood changes, and signs of suicide thoughts
- Monitor BP and heart rate
- Monitor serum drug levels, CBC, liver panel, and glucose

Nursing Diagnoses

- Injury: risk for
- Coping: ineffective
- Knowledge deficit related to medication and disease

Client teaching for self-care

- Inform family to observe for changes in mental status and notify physician
- Inform that medication should be taken as prescribed and not to abruptly discontinue medication, add any other CNS depressants or consume alcohol
- Instruct to inform physician if adverse effects occur
- Caution of teratogenic effect and notify physician immediately if pregnancy is planned or suspected
- Encourage to keep all follow-up appointments with health care providers

ANTIDIARRHEALS

Example: bismuth subsalicylate (Kaopectate)

Mechanisms of Action

- Increases intestinal absorption of fluids
- Decreases synthesis of prostaglandins in the intestines

Common Uses

- Diarrhea
- Indigestion: ulcer disease

Common Adverse Effects

- Constipation

Monitoring Effects of Antidiarrheals

Nursing Process Elements

- Assess frequency, amount, and consistency of stools
- Assess for nausea, abdominal pain, and indigestion
- Assess for electrolytes and fluid imbalance symptoms (dry mucous membranes, poor skin turgor, decrease urine output, fatigue, muscle weakness)
- Monitor serum electrolyte levels

Nursing Diagnoses

- Diarrhea
- Fluid volume deficit
- Knowledge deficit related to medication and disease

Client teaching for self-care

- Advise that medication may cause stools to change to a gray–black color while taking medication
- Instruct to contact health care provider if diarrhea continues or if experiencing muscle weakness, tremors, or dizziness

ANTIEMETIC AGENTS

Example: promethazine (Phenergan)

Mechanisms of Action

- Inhibits the chemoreceptor trigger zone in the medulla

Common Uses

- Treatment and prevention of N&V
- Allergic conditions
- Motion sickness
- Sedation

Common Adverse Effects

- Sedation
- Disorientation

Monitoring Effects of Antiemetic Agents

Nursing Process Elements

- Assess for N&V, and abdominal pain
- Assess for fluid volume deficit (dry mucous membranes, poor skin turgor, decreased urine output, and thirst)

- Monitor I&O
- Implement safety precautions to prevent falls

Nursing Diagnoses

- Fluid volume deficit
- Injury: risk for
- Knowledge deficit related to medication and disease

Client teaching for self-care

- Inform that medication may cause sedation and to take safety precautions to prevent accidents
- Instruct to take only sips of liquids and small meals to prevent nausea
- Advise to inform health care provider if condition continues

ANTIFUNGAL AGENTS

Example: fluconazole (Diflucan)

Mechanisms of Action

- Inhibits synthesis of fungal sterols
- Affects the permeability of the fungal cell membrane or protein synthesis within the cell

Common Uses

- Treatment of fungal infections
- Prevention of fungal infections

Common Adverse Effects

- abdominal discomfort

Monitoring Effects of Antifungal Agents

Nursing Process Elements

- Assess area of infection and document findings
- Obtain cultures, if ordered, prior to first dose
- Monitor CBC, liver function tests, BUN, and Cr

Nursing Diagnoses

- Infection: risk for
- Knowledge deficit related to medication and disease

Client teaching for self-care

- Instruct to take full course of medication even if symptoms are no longer present
- Advise to notify health care provider if symptoms do not improve, or if fever, pain, fatigue, or N&V occur

ANTIHISTAMINE AGENTS

Example: fexofenadine (Allegra)

Mechanisms of Action

- Blocks the effects of histamine at peripheral histamine-1 receptors

Common Uses

- Relief of allergic rhinitis
- Urticaria

Common Adverse Effects

- No common adverse effects

Monitoring Effects of Antihistamine Agents

Nursing Process Elements

- Assess allergy symptoms
- Maintain fluid intake of 2000 ml/d to provide hydration and decrease viscosity of secretions
- Provide an environment free of allergens

Nursing Diagnoses

- Airway clearance, ineffective
- Injury: risk for
- Knowledge deficit related to medication and disease

Client teaching for self-care

- Instruct in methods to reduce allergens in the environment
- Advise to take medication as directed and to call health care provider if symptoms do not improve

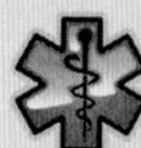

Nursing Intervention Alert

Apple, orange, and grapefruit juice will decrease the absorption of fexofenadine (Allegra).

ANTINEOPLASTIC AGENTS

Mechanisms of Action

Depends on specific agent used

- Interferes with folic acid metabolism resulting in inhibition of cell reproduction
- Competes with estrogen for binding sites

- Damages DNA before mitosis resulting in death of cells
- Inhibits DNA and RNA synthesis resulting in death of replicating cells

Common Uses

- Treatment of cancer
- Treatment of rheumatoid arthritis

Common Adverse Effects

- Nausea
- Alopecia
- Fatigue

Monitoring Effects of Antineoplastic Agents

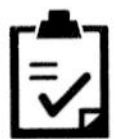

Nursing Process Elements

- Assess for symptoms of original tumor/disease
- Assess for signs of infection, bone marrow depression, stomatitis
- Monitor VS, I&O, weight, and fatigue
- Monitor CBC, platelet count, BUN, Cr, liver panel, and serum drug levels
- Encourage adequate oral intake and nutrition

Nursing Diagnoses

- Infection: risk for
- Nutrition: imbalanced, less than body requirements
- Knowledge deficit related to medication and disease

Client teaching for self-care

- Instruct to take medication as prescribed
- Advise to observe for signs of infection (fever, chills), cough, increased fatigue, increased pain, sore throat, gout, bleeding, red and sore oral mucous membranes, and difficulty breathing and to notify physician immediately
- Inform to avoid crowds and people with signs of illness
- Discuss options available in case hair loss occurs
- Encourage to schedule follow-up appointments with health care providers
- Advise to have laboratory tests done as prescribed
- Discuss community resources available

ANTIPARKINSON AGENTS

Mechanisms of Action

Anticholinergics

- Blocks cholinergic activity in the central nervous system and restores the balance of neurotransmitters

Dopamine agonists

- Converts levodopa to dopamine

Antiviral

- Increases the action of dopamine in the CNS

Catechol-O-methyltransferase Inhibitors

- Prevents the breakdown of levodopa

Common Uses

- Treatment of Parkinson's disease

Common Adverse Effects: Varies with specific drugs

- Blurred vision, dry eyes, and dry mouth
- Constipation
- Dizziness

Monitoring Effects of Anti-Parkinson Agents

Nursing Process Elements

- Assess for symptoms of Parkinson's disease (rigidity, tremors, movement difficulty, pill rolling, and shuffling gait)
- Monitor VS, assess for postural hypotension, assess oral mucus membranes
- Assess bowel and bladder function; maintain I&O record
- Assess for dizziness and implement safety precautions to prevent accidents

Nursing Diagnoses

- Mobility: impaired
- Injury: risk for
- Knowledge deficit related to medication, disease

Client teaching for self-care

- Encourage to take medication as prescribed
- Instruct to change position slowly so as to avoid a decrease in BP
- Advise to increase oral fluids, use gum, hard candy, or a saliva substitute to prevent dry mouth
- Encourage to keep appointments with health care providers

ANTIPLATELET AGENTS

Mechanisms of Action

- Glycoprotein IIb/IIIa inhibitors: eptifibatide (Integrilin)
- Platelet Aggregation Inhibitors: dipyridamole (Persantine)
- Platelet Adhesion Inhibitors: clopidogrel (Plavix)

Common Uses

- Prevention of myocardial infarction or stroke
- Treatment of acute coronary syndromes

Common Adverse Effects

- Dizziness
- Headache
- Bruising

Monitoring Effects of Antiplatelet Agents

Nursing Process Elements

- Assess VS
- Assess for signs of stroke or myocardial infarction
- Assess for signs of bleeding (venous and arterial access sites, hypotension, weak, rapid pulse, bruising)
- Monitor CBC, platelet count, coagulation studies, and Cr

Nursing Diagnoses

- Tissue perfusion: ineffective
- Injury: risk for
- Pain: acute
- Knowledge deficit related to medication and disease

Client teaching for self-care

- Instruct to take medication as prescribed and to avoid using over-the-counter medication containing aspirin or NSAIDs without prior approval from physician
- Advise to avoid using alcohol and tobacco products due to the vasoconstriction action
- Instruct to notify physician if signs of bleeding (bruising, headache, blood in urine, dark stools, headache, weakness)
- Encourage to keep appointments with health care providers

ANTIPSYCHOTICS

Example: risperidone (Risperdal)

Mechanisms of Action

- Alters dopamine and serotonin in the CNS

Common Uses

- Treatment of schizophrenia
- Acute manic episodes

Common Adverse Effects

- Dizziness, headache, sleep disturbances, and extrapyramidal reactions
- Visual changes, rhinitis, and rash
- Constipation, diarrhea, nausea, and dry mouth
- Dysmenorrhea

Monitoring Effects of Antipsychotic Agents

Nursing Process Elements

- Assess mental status, mood changes, and signs of suicidal thoughts
- Monitor for orthostatic hypotension, hypotension, hypertension, elevated temperature, respiratory distress, and ECG changes
- Monitor for extrapyramidal symptoms such as rigidity, muscle spasms, tremors, drooling, restlessness , and for facial twitching
- Monitor laboratory values: CBC, AST, and ALT

Nursing Diagnoses

- Injury: risk for
- Thought processes: disturbed
- Noncompliance
- Knowledge deficit related to medication and disease

Client teaching for self-care

- Instruct to take medication as directed and avoid alcohol and other CNS agents unless directed by physician
- Inform of adverse effects and importance of reporting them to the physician immediately
- Advise to change position slowly; avoid driving until approved by physician, and use sun protective products and clothing
- Instruct to use hard candy, gum, or mouth rinses to help prevent dry mouth
- Encourage to keep all follow-up appointments with health care providers

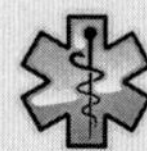

Nursing Intervention Alert

Advise client to use sunscreen and protective clothing to prevent photosensitivity reaction.

ANTIRETROVIRALS

Mechanisms of Action

- Protease Inhibitors: amprenavir (Agenerase)
  —Inhibits the action of HIV-I protease
- Nucleoside reverse transcriptase inhibitors: abacavir (Ziagen)
  —Converted to carbovir triphosphate which inhibits the activity of HIV-I reverse transcriptase
  —Nonnucleoside reverse transcriptase inhibitors: delavirdine (Rescriptor): Binds to reverse transcriptase and inhibits viral DNA synthesis

Common Uses

- Treatment of HIV infection in combination with other drugs

Common Adverse Effects

- Diarrhea and N&V
- Mood changes
- Rash

Monitoring Effects of Antiretroviral Agents

Nursing Process Elements

- Assess for changes in HIV symptoms or opportunistic infections
- Monitor for adverse effects
- Monitor laboratory values: viral load, CD4 cell count, glucose, CBC, and cholesterol levels
- Be aware of serious drug–drug interactions among the antiretroviral agents.

Nursing Diagnoses

- Infection: risk for
- Knowledge deficit related to medications and disease
- Noncompliance

Client teaching for self-care

- Instruct to take medication round the clock exactly as directed and to maintain dosing schedule
- Inform that these medications do not cure HIV or reduce the risk of spreading virus to others
- Instruct to use condom, do not share needles, and do not donate blood
- Inform not to use over-the-counter medication unless approved by physician
- Review adverse effects of all drugs and emphasize the importance of notifying physician if experiencing any of these
- Advise to keep all follow-up appointments with physician

Antirheumatic Agents

Example: etanercept (Enbrel)

Mechanisms of Action

- Binds to tumor necrosis factor (TNF) and blocks its interaction with cell surface TNF receptors

Common Uses

- Moderate to severe rheumatoid arthritis

Common Adverse Effects

- Respiratory tract infection
- Rhinitis, headache

Monitoring Effects of Antirheumatic Agents

Nursing Process Elements

- Assess joint swelling, redness, heat, pain, and range of motion
- Rotate injection sites and observe site for redness, heat, and swelling
- Assess S&S of upper respiratory infection, and chest pain

Nursing Diagnoses

- Pain: acute
- Mobility: impaired
- Knowledge deficit related to medication, disease

Client teaching for self-care

- Instruct regarding dilution of solution, proper injection technique, site rotation, and disposal of equipment
- Advise not to receive live vaccine immunizations while taking this medication
- Instruct to report signs of infection, dizziness, shortness of breath, chest pain, or other adverse effects to health care provider immediately
- Encourage to keep all follow-up appointments with health care providers

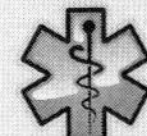

Nursing Intervention Alert

Latex allergy: Needle cover of diluent syringe contains latex.

ANTITUBERCULAR AGENTS

Example: rifampin (Rifadin)

Mechanisms of Action

- Suppresses RNA synthesis by preventing attachment of the enzyme to DNA and blocking RNA transcription in susceptible organisms

Common Uses

- Treatment of tuberculosis

Common Adverse Effects

- Red-orange discoloration of all body fluids
- Diarrhea, abdominal pain, N&V

Monitoring Effects of Antitubercular Agents

Nursing Process Elements

- Assess respiratory rate, pattern and effort, lung sounds, and amount and character of sputum
- Monitor CBC, liver and renal function studies, PPD test results, and sputum cultures
- Monitor for red–orange discoloration of body fluids

Nursing Diagnoses

- Infection: risk for
- Gas Exchange: impaired
- Airway clearance: ineffective
- Knowledge deficit related to medication and disease
- Noncompliance

Client teaching for self-care

- Inform to take medication as directed for the entire course of therapy even if symptoms have subsided and to avoid alcohol
- Instruct regarding red–orange discoloration of body fluids
- Advise of adverse effects and to report symptoms to physician
- Instruct to report fatigue, increase in cough, shortness of breath, fever, and chills to physician
- Encourage to keep follow-up appointments with physician

ANTIVIRAL AGENTS

Example: acyclovir (Zovirax)

Mechanisms of Action

- Inhibits viral DNA replication

Common Uses

- Treatment of herpes zoster (shingles)
- Treatment of herpes simplex virus types 1 and 2
- Treatment of genital herpes infections

Common Adverse Effects

- Headache and dizziness
- Nausea, vomiting, and diarrhea

Monitoring Effects of Antiviral Agents

Nursing Process Elements

- Assess skin lesions for redness, pain, edema, and exudates
- Monitor CBC, electrolytes, and liver function studies

Nursing Diagnoses

- Infection: risk for
- Skin integrity: impaired
- Pain: acute
- Knowledge deficit related to medication and disease

Client teaching for self-care

- Instruct to take medication as directed for the entire course of therapy.
- Advise that drug is not a cure, but will help manage symptoms.
- Explain methods to prevent spread of infection to others: Adequately cover lesions; wear loose fitting, cotton underwear for genital lesions and use a condom for sexual intercourse; wash hands after touching lesions; and apply ointment using a glove.
- Advise female clients to have annual pap smear due to increased risk of cervical cancer.
- Advise to avoid contact with children who have not had chicken pox, and avoid pregnant women.
- Encourage to keep all follow-up appointments with health care providers.

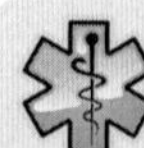

Nursing Intervention Alert

Monitor BUN and serum creatinine before and during treatment.

HORMONE AGENTS

Example: estrogens, conjugated (Premarin)

Mechanisms of Action

- Replacement of estrogen to promote normal development of female sex organs and secondary sex characteristics

Common Uses

- Hormone replacement therapy for moderate to severe vasomotor symptoms of menopause
- Prophylaxis of postmenopausal osteoporosis

Common Adverse Effects

- Edema, weight gain
- Hypertension, headache
- Breast tenderness, dysmenorrhea, or amenorrhea
- Nausea

Monitoring Effects of Estrogen Therapy

Nursing Process Elements

- Assess blood VS, edema, and weight gain
- Monitor I&O
- Monitor liver and lipid panels

Nursing Diagnoses

- Body image, disturbed
- Sexual dysfunction
- Knowledge deficit related to medication and disease

Client teaching for self-care

- Advise to take oral dose with food and follow the dosing schedule
- Instruct to report shortness of breath, vaginal bleeding, headache, pain, swelling in legs, weight gain, and visual changes to physician immediately
- Instruct to wear protective products during exposure to sunlight
- Review instructions for application of vaginal medication if prescribed: Emphasize to administer the medication at bedtime, remaining recumbent for at least 30 minutes after inserting drug
- Encourage to keep follow-up appointments with health care providers

CONTRACEPTIVE AGENTS

Example: norgestimate/ethinyl estradiol (Ortho Tri-Cyclen)

Mechanisms of Action

- Suppression of FSH and LH inhibits ovulation

Common Uses

- Prevention of pregnancy
- Regulation of menstrual cycle

Common Adverse Effects

- Weight changes

Monitoring Effects of Contractive Agents

Nursing Process Elements

- Assess BP, edema, and weight gain
- Assess for pain and swelling in extremities, headache, and abnormal vaginal bleeding
- Assess for high-risk sexual practices

Nursing Diagnoses

- Knowledge deficit related to medication
- Noncompliance

Client teaching for self-care

- Instruct to take medication as directed and keep oral medications in original container
- Advise to report pain in legs or chest, cough, and respiratory distress to physician immediately
- Advise to report edema, weight gain, mood changes, and fatigue to physician
- Inform to limit caffeine consumption and avoid tobacco products
- Remind client that this medication does not provide any protection against STD and to use appropriate barrier protection
- Encourage to keep follow-up appointments with health care provider

IMMUNOSUPPRESSANT AGENTS

Example: azathioprine (Imuran)

Mechanisms of Action

- Inhibits synthesis of DNA, RNA, and proteins

Common Uses

- Prevention of renal transplant rejection
- Treatment of rheumatoid arthritis

Common Adverse Effects

- Anemia, leukopenia, thrombocytopenia, and pancytopenia
- N&V and anorexia
- Chills and fever

Monitoring Effects of Immunosuppressant Agents

Nursing Process Elements

- Assess for signs of infection
- Assess joints for pain, heat, redness, edema, and limited mobility for clients with rheumatoid arthritis
- Monitor CBC, renal, and liver studies
- Protect client from visitors with risk for infecting client

Nursing Diagnoses

- Infection: risk for
- Knowledge deficit related to medication, disease

Client teaching for self-care

- Instruct to take medication as prescribed by physician. Emphasize importance of not stopping medication abruptly, and not taking over-the-counter medications without prior approval.
- Advise to report adverse effects to physician immediately: increase in fatigue, fever, chills, diarrhea, tarry stools, back or side pain, and cough.
- Advise to avoid crowds and contact with people who are sick.
- Encourage to keep follow-up appointments with health care provider

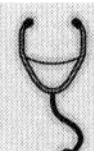

Assessment Alert

Report leukocyte counts of less than 3000 to physician and anticipate a dose reduction or drug to be temporarily discontinued.

Lipid Lowering Agents

Example: HMG-CoA Reductase Inhibitors: rosuvastin (Crestor)

Mechanisms of Action

- Reduces total cholesterol, LDL, and triglycerides and increases HDL

Common Uses

- Reduce lipids/cholesterol in order to decrease risk for myocardial infarction and stroke

Common Adverse Effects

- Indigestion, diarrhea, and constipation
- Rash

Monitoring Effects of Lipid-Lowering Agents

Nursing Process Elements

- Assess risk factors for stroke and myocardial infarction
- Obtain dietary history as well as food preferences
- Monitor serum cholesterol and triglyceride levels, and liver function tests
- Provide resources and suggestions for approved exercise activities

Nursing Diagnoses

- Knowledge deficit related to diet, medication, and disease risk factors
- Noncompliance

Client teaching for self-care

- Instruct in low cholesterol diet and appropriate exercise plan
- Advise to take medication as directed
- Advise to report adverse effects to physician: leg pain, muscle tenderness, weakness, fatigue, and fever
- Have regular eye examinations because of the risk of cataracts
- Encourage to keep follow-up appointments with health care provider

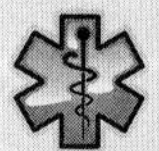

Nursing Intervention Alert

Grapefruit juice increases blood levels of most drugs in this class.

SEDATIVE/ HYPNOTIC AGENTS

Example: flurazepam (Dalmane)

Mechanisms of Action

- Depression of CNS, may be mediated by neurotransmitter GABA

Common Uses

- Management of insomnia

Common Adverse Effects

- Lethargy and daytime sedation
- Drowsiness

Monitoring Effects of Sedative/Hypnotic Agents

Nursing Process Elements

- Assess sleep history as well as daytime napping
- Assess for previous drug use for insomnia
- Monitor for postural hypotension
- Monitor daytime drowsiness and napping
- Implement safety precautions to prevent falls: bed in low position, call bell within reach, and supervised ambulation

Nursing Diagnoses

- Injury: risk for
- Sleep pattern: disturbed
- Knowledge deficit related to medication and safety
- Noncompliance

Client teaching for self-care

- Advise to take medication as directed
- Discuss relaxation techniques, cool, dark bedroom, quiet environment, avoiding caffeine, alcohol, and nicotine products
- Advise regarding safety measures: night light, phone, and glasses within reach
- Instruct to keep a sleep diary to help determine specific cause of insomnia
- Encourage to keep follow-up appointment with health care providers

SKELETAL MUSCLE RELAXANT AGENTS

Example: carisoprodol (Soma)

Mechanisms of Action

- Relaxation of skeletal muscles by depression of CNS

Common Uses

- Treatment of muscle spasm

Common Adverse Effects

- Dizziness and weakness
- Drowsiness

Monitoring Effects of Skeletal Muscle Relaxant Agents

Nursing Process Elements

- Assess muscle stiffness, tenderness, pain, and range of motion
- Assess for idiosyncratic reaction within first few minutes to one hour of dose: weakness, disorientation, blurred vision. Such reaction is temporary
- Implement safety measures to prevent falls

Nursing Diagnoses

- Mobility: impaired
- Injury: risk for
- Pain: acute
- Knowledge deficit related to medication and disease

Client teaching for self-care

- Advise to take medication as directed, and avoid driving until response to medication is established
- Instruct in safety measures to prevent falls: change positions slowly to prevent orthostatic hypotension
- Instruct to avoid alcohol and other CNS depressants
- Inform regarding adverse effects and to notify physician if symptoms occur
- Encourage to continue with other prescribed measures to prevent muscle spasms: heat or cold therapy, physical therapy, exercise, and relaxation techniques

THROMBOLYTIC AGENTS

Example: reteplase (Retavase)

Mechanisms of Action

- Activates plasminogen to degrade clot

Common Uses

- Acute coronary thrombosis

Common Adverse Effects

- Reperfusion arrhythmias

Monitoring Effects of Thrombolytic Agents

Nursing Process Elements

- Assess for bleeding at venous and arterial access catheters, check neurological status, abdominal and joint pain, hypotension, and weak and rapid pulse
- Assess for angina, nausea, pain radiating down arm or to jaw, and diaphoresis
- Monitor VS throughout therapy and maintain bed rest
- Monitor ECG continuously and assess for reperfusion arrhythmias
- Assess for hypersensitivity reaction (fever, dyspnea, wheezing, rash, and facial swelling)
- Monitor CBC, coagulation studies, cardiac enzymes, and liver panel.

Nursing Diagnoses

- Tissue perfusion: ineffective
- Pain: acute
- Injury: risk for
- Knowledge deficit related to medication and disease

Client teaching for self-care

- Inform of the goals of therapy and the monitoring routine
- Instruct to report any adverse effects immediately
- Explain the importance of maintaining complete bed rest during therapy

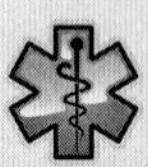

Nursing Intervention Alert

To prevent harm to the client, request that another RN check the physician's order, dosage calculations, and electronic infusion device settings.

IMMUNE GLOBULIN AGENTS

Example: RhoGAM

Mechanisms of Action

- Suppresses immune response of nonsensitized Rh negative clients who are exposed to Rh-positive blood

Common Uses

- Administered to a female client who is Rh negative after she gives birth to a child who is Rh-positive

Common Adverse Effects

- Anemia

Monitoring Effects of Immune Globulin Agents

Nursing Process Elements

- Assess VS throughout therapy
- Determine Rh factor of mother and baby
- Monitor for signs of intravascular hemolysis (chills, back pain, anemia)

Nursing Diagnoses

- Knowledge deficit related to medication

Client teaching for self-care

- Explain purpose and importance of medication: preventing hemolytic disease of the newborn

DRUG THERAPY FOR GERIATRIC CLIENTS

Anatomic and Physiological Factors

- Drug absorption
  - —Reduced gastric acidity may affect the way tablets dissolve
  - —Gastric emptying may be prolonged
  - —Rate of passage of drugs through the lower gastrointestinal tract may be slowed
  - —Elderly may use laxatives, which increase the passage of drugs, foods, and liquids through the intestines
  - —General reduction in blood flow to the intestines
  - —Topical absorption may be quicker because of thinner skin
- Drug Distribution
  - —Total body water is decreased in the older adult, which may increase the blood concentration of drugs and diminish the distribution of water-soluble drugs.
  - —Age-related loss of muscle tone due to atrophy, alters medications administered intramuscularly
  - — Total body fat content is increased in the older adult. Sedatives may be absorbed by the fatty tissue prolonging the effects of the drugs
  - —A decrease in protein-binding capability may be present in the older adult, therefore, drugs may accumulate rather than being excreted

- Drug metabolism
  —Blood flow to liver diminishes with age, which affects the rate of metabolism of drugs that are primarily metabolized by the liver
- Drug Excretion
  —Reduced blood flow to kidneys of older adults and the loss of nephrons reduces the ability of the elderly to excrete drugs and metabolites

Age Related Changes and Health Issues

- Sensory losses
- Vision loss
  —Difficulty reading instructions, directions, and labels
  —Difficulty distinguishing prescription bottles
- Hearing loss makes it difficult to hear directions and information given to them verbally
- Recent memory loss
  —Forget directions given by health care providers
  —Forget to stay on medication schedule
- Multiple medications due to chronic health problems
- More than one pharmacy filling the prescriptions
- Using over-the-counter medications and home remedies
- Failing to discard old medications
- Sharing medications with another person
- Economics
  —Not getting prescriptions filled
  —Ask physician for a sample of the drug
  —Ask pharmacist for a short-term supply

General Guidelines

- Obtain baseline measures
  —VS
  —Height
  —Weight
- Take a history of allergies and current use of prescription and nonprescription drugs
- Obtain information on
  —disabilities of client or others in the home,
  —home environment and safety,
  —social and family life, and
  —economic concerns.
- Make sure that clients responsible for self-medication are able to follow dosing schedule, open containers and obtain their prescriptions
- Follow the "Five Rights" of medication administration
- When giving oral medications, position client in an upright position
- Use liquid dosage forms if client has difficulty swallowing tablets or capsules
- Allow adequate time for client to take medication and fluids

Table 14–13 Class, Action, and Side effects of 75 Commonly Prescribed Medications*

Medication	Action	Side Effects
Accupril (quinapril)	ACE inhibitor used to treat hypertension and to decrease risk of CV disease	Rash, loss of taste, swelling of mouth, face, hands, feet, dizziness, fainting, chest pain, fast or irregular heartbeat, confusion nervousness, numbness and tingling in hands and feet, diarrhea, headache, tiredness, cough
Actonel (risedronate sodium)	Bisphosphonate used to treat postmenopausal osteoporosis	Stomach pain, bone or muscle pain, nausea, diarrhea, constipation, gas, leg cramps, bloated feeling, anxiety, depression, throat pain, heartburn, dysphagia, headache, weak muscles
Afeditab CR (nifedipine sustained-action—oral)	Calcium channel blocker used to treat hypertension, sometimes angina	Headache, dizziness, nausea, flushing, constipation, leg/muscle cramps, or sexual problems, edema of the ankles/feet, dyspnea, unusual weakness/tiredness, new or worsening chest pain, allergic reaction
Allopurinol	Xanthine oxidase inhibitor used to treat gout, high levels of uric acid in the body caused by certain cancer medications, and kidney stones	Rash, hives, itch, jaundice, drowsiness, diarrhea, N&V, stomach pain, headache

(continued on next page)

Table 14–13 *(continued from previous page)*

Medication	Action	Side Effects
Altace (ramipril)	ACE inhibitor used to treat hypertension and decrease cardiovascular risk	Rash, loss of taste, swelling of mouth, face, hands, feet, dizziness, fainting, chest pain, fast or irregular heartbeat, confusion nervousness, numbness and tingling in hands and feet, diarrhea, headache, tiredness, cough
Ambien (zolpidem)	Sedative/hypnotic used to treat insomnia	Daytime drowsiness, light-headedness, dizziness, clumsiness, headache, diarrhea, nausea, dry mouth, muscle aches or pain, tiredness, indigestion, joint pain, memory problems
Aricept (donepezil)	Cholinesterase inhibitor used to treat Alzheimer's disease	N&V, diarrhea, lack of coordination, rash, indigestion, headache, muscle aches, anorexia, stomach pain, chills, dizziness, drowsiness, dry or itching eyes, increased sweating, joint pain, runny nose, sore throat, lower extremity edema, insomnia, weight loss, facial flushing, unusual tiredness or weakness.
Avapro (irbesartan)	Angiotensin II receptor antagonist used to treat hypertension	Headache, dizziness, fever or sore throat (upper respiratory tract infection), diarrhea, back pain, cough, fatigue, stuffy nose
Cartia XT (diltiazem)	Calcium Channel Blocker used to treat hypertension, angina, and certain arrhythmias	Tiredness, brady or tachyarrhythmia, wheezing, cough, dyspnea, dizziness, numbness or tingling in hands or feet, swollen feet, ankles or legs, difficult urination, nausea, constipation
Celebrex (celecoxib capsules)	NSAID used to treat osteoarthritis, rheumatoid arthritis, and acute pain	Headache, indigestion, upper respiratory tract infection, diarrhea, sinus inflammation, stomach pain, nausea, gastric bleeding, kidney damage, liver damage, fluid retention
Cozaar (losartan)	Angiotensin II receptor antagonist used to treat hypertension	Headache, dizziness, fever or sore throat (upper respiratory tract infection), diarrhea, back pain, cough, fatigue, stuffy nose
Zestril (lisinopril)	ACE inhibitor used to treat hypertension and heart failure	Rash, loss of taste, swelling of mouth, face, hands, feet, dizziness, fainting, chest pain, fast or irregular heartbeat, confusion nervousness, numbness and tingling in hands and feet, diarrhea, headache, tiredness, cough
Tenormin (Atenolol)	Beta-adrenergic blocking agent used to treat angina, hypertension and to improve survival post MI	Bradycardia, drowsiness, fatigue, numbness and tingling of fingers or toes, dizziness, nausea, diarrhea, weakness, cold hands or feet, dry skin, eyes, mouth, hallucinations, nightmares, insomnia, headache, dyspnea, joint pain, confusion, reduced alertness, depression, impotence, abdominal pain, constipation, (life threatening: CHF, severe dyspnea, tachyarrhythmia, severe asthma)
Detrol (tolterodine)	Antispasmodic used to treat overactive bladder (OAB)	Change in vision, difficult, burning, or painful urination, frequency, bloody or cloudy urine, chest pain, dizziness, dry mouth, vomiting, abdominal pain, constipation, diarrhea, N&V, headache, flu-like symptoms, drowsiness, dry eyes, flatulence
Digoxin (Brand name: Lanoxin)	Cardiac glycoside used to treat heart failure, atrial fibrillation/flutter	Anorexia, diarrhea, extreme drowsiness, lethargy, disorientation, headache, fainting, vision changes

(continued on next page)

Table 14–13 *(continued from previous page)*

Medication	Action	Side Effects
Diovan (valsartan)	Angiotensin II receptor antagonist used to treat hypertension	Headache, dizziness, fever or sore throat (upper respiratory tract infection), diarrhea, back pain, cough, fatigue, stuffy nose
Diovan HCT (valsartan) (See Diovan)		
Doxazosin mesylate (Brand name: Cardura)	Alpha-adrenergic receptor blocker used for the control of hypertension and for benign prostatic hyperplasia	Headache, drowsiness, rash or pruritus, blurred vision, shortness of breath, dyspnea, chest pain, tachycardia, anorexia, constipation or diarrhea, abdominal pain, N&V, edema, joint or muscle aches, tiredness, orthostatic hypotension, headache, irritability, depression, dry mouth, stuffy nose, increased urination, drowsiness
Lisinopril (Brand names: Zestril, Prinivil) (See Zestril)		
Enalapril maleate (Brand names: Vasotec, Lexxel)	ACE inhibitor used to treat hypertension	Headache, dizziness, light-headedness, weakness, nausea, dry cough or blurred while adjusting to medication, fainting, decreased sexual ability, signs of infection (fever, chills, persistent sore throat), liver problems (jaundice, dark urine, stomach/abdominal pain, persistent fatigue, persistent nausea), allergic reaction
Evista (raloxifene)	Selective estrogen receptor modulator (SERM) used to treat and prevent osteoporosis	Thrombi, chest pain, bloody or cloudy urine, dysuria, frequency, infection, cold or flu-like symptoms, leg cramps, rash, edema of hands, ankles or feet, vaginal itching, joint or muscle pain, joint swelling, flatulence, upset stomach, vomiting, hot flashes, insomnia, white vaginal discharge, depression, unexplained weight gain, sweating, abdominal pain, diarrhea, anorexia, nausea, weakness, migraine, dyspnea, fever, congestion
Flomax (tamsulosin)	Alpha-1 antagonist with specificity to alpha-1A subtype receptors used in the management of BPH	Light-headedness, dizziness, headache, drowsiness, weakness, lethargy, nausea, palpitations
Fluoxetine HCL (Brand name: Prozac)	Selective serotonin reuptake inhibitor used to treat major depression, obsessive–compulsive disorder, panic disorder, posttraumatic stress disorder, bulimia nervosa	Allergic reaction: rash, pruritus, dyspnea, chest pain, drowsiness, nausea, cough or hoarseness, lower back or side pain, sores on lips or mouth, constipation or diarrhea, headache, anxiety, changed sexual desire or function, insomnia, dry mouth, unusual weakness or tiredness, vision changes, confusion, apathy, dyspnea, chills, black or tarry stools, fever, lymphadenopathy, arrhythmias, vomiting, skin rash, itching, abdominal pain, anorexia, yawning, tingling, skin burning or prickling, stuffy nose, changes in taste, tooth grinding, increased saliva, gas, heartburn, urinary changes, muscle or joint pain, menstrual changes, weight changes, loss of hair
Folic Acid (vitamin B 9)		Large amounts of yellow urine
Fosamax (alendronate)	A bisphosphonate (affects normal and abnormal bone resorption) used to treat and prevent osteoporosis	Abdominal pain, musculoskeletal pain, flatulence, acid regurgitation, esophageal ulcer, abdominal distention, gastritis, headache, fever

(continued on next page)

Table 14–13 *(continued from previous page)*

Medication	Action	Side Effects
Furosemide (Brand name Lasix)	Loop diuretic used to relieve peripheral edema from CHF, hepatic, and renal disease; relieve pulmonary edema; manage hypertension	Dizziness, mood change, fatigue, anorexia, diarrhea, arrhythmia, muscle cramps, hypotension, abdominal pain, weakness
Gemfibrozil (Brand name: Lopid)	Antihyperlipidemic drug used to treat hypertriglyceridemia and reduce risk of CAD	Indigestion, chest pain, sob, arrhythmia, N&V, diarrhea, stomach pain
Glucophage XR (metformin)	A nonsulfonylurea antidiabetic agent of the class biguanide, which improves the action of insulin	Stomach pain, diarrhea, vomiting, decreased appetite, gas, changes in taste, headache, weight loss, feeling of fullness, nausea
Glucotrol XL (glipizide)	Sulfonylurea, oral antidiabetic agent used in the management of type 2 diabetes	Dizziness, diarrhea, anorexia, stomach pain, heartburn, low blood sugar (hunger, anxiety, cold sweats, rapid pulse, shortness of breath)
Glyburide (Brand name: DiaBeta)	Sulfonylurea, oral antidiabetic agent, used in the management of type 2 diabetes	Dizziness, diarrhea, anorexia, stomach pain, heartburn, constipation, low blood sugar (hunger, anxiety, cold sweats, rapid pulse, shortness of breath)
Hydrochlorothiazide (Brand name: HydroDIURIL)	Thiazide diuretic used to treat hypertension and edema	Muscle cramps, blurred vision, severe abdominal pain, N&V, arrhythmia, weak pulse; dizziness, mood changes, headache, weakness, tiredness, weight changes, decreased sex drive, diarrhea, dry mouth, thirst
Hyzaar (losartan and hydrochlorazide)	Combination of losartan an angiotensin II receptor blocker and hydrochlorothiazide, a thiazide diuretic used to treat hypertension	(See losartan and hydrochlorothiazide for side effects)
Isosorbide dinitrate (Brand name: Isordil)	Nitrate used to prevent and treat angina pectoris	Headache, flushed face and neck, dry mouth, N&V, fainting, tachycardia, restlessness, blurred vision, dizziness
Klor-Con (potassium supplement)		Skin rash, swollen salivary glands, diarrhea, nausea, abdominal pain, bone and joint pain, numbness or tingling in hands or feet, vomiting, dizziness
Lescol (fluvastatin)	CoA reductase inhibitor used to reduce serum cholesterol and triglyceride levels	Aching muscles, fever, blurred vision, constipation, nausea, tiredness, weakness, dizziness, skin rash, headache, diarrhea, heartburn
Lescol XL (fluvastatin)	CoA reductase inhibitor used to reduce serum cholesterol and triglyceride levels	Aching muscles, fever, blurred vision, constipation, nausea, tiredness, weakness, dizziness, skin rash, headache, diarrhea, heartburn
Levothyroid (levothyroxine)		Tremor, headache, irritability, insomnia, appetite changes, diarrhea, leg cramps, menstrual irregularities, fever, heat sensitivity, unusual sweating, weight loss, nervousness, hives, rash, vomiting, chest pain, rapid and irregular heartbeat, SOB
Proventil (albuterol)	Bronchodilator used in the prevention and treatment of asthma symptoms	Nervousness, tremors, headache, insomnia, nausea

(continued on next page)

Table 14–13 *(continued from previous page)*

Medication	Action	Side Effects
Lisinopril-HCTZ	ACE inhibitor plus a thiazide diuretic used to treat hypertension, heart failure and edema	Rash, loss of taste, swelling of mouth, face, hands, feet, dizziness, fainting, chest pain, fast or irregular heartbeat, confusion nervousness, numbness and tingling in hands and feet, diarrhea, headache, tiredness, cough. Also muscle cramps, blurred vision, severe abdominal pain, N&V, arrhythmia, weak pulse; dizziness, mood changes, headache, weakness, tiredness, weight changes, decreased sex drive, diarrhea, dry mouth, thirst
Lotrel (benazepril and amlodipine)	ACE inhibitor and calcium channel blocker used to manage hypertension	Headache, dizziness, nausea, flushing, constipation, leg/muscle cramps, or sexual problems, edema of the ankles/feet, dyspnea, unusual weakness/tiredness, new or worsening chest pain, allergic reaction, rash, loss of taste, swelling of mouth, face, hands, feet, dizziness, fainting, chest pain, fast or irregular heartbeat, confusion, nervousness, numbness and tingling in hands and feet, diarrhea, cough
Lovastatin (Brand name: Mevacor)	Antihyperlipidemic CoA reductase inhibitor used to reduce serum cholesterol level	Aching muscles, fever, blurred vision, constipation, nausea, tiredness, weakness, dizziness, skin rash, headache, diarrhea, heartburn
Metoprolol (Brand names: Lopressor, Toprol XL)	Cardio-selective oral beta adrenergic blocking agent used to treat hypertension, angina, cardiac arrhythmias, myocardial infarction, migraine and pheochromocytoma among other problems	Tiredness, dizziness, diarrhea, depression, shortness of breath, bradycardia, itching, rash, other GI symptoms including vomiting
Miacalcin (calcitonin)	Calcium regulator drug used to treat PTH excess or high serum calcium levels	Allergic reaction/nasal inflammation, dryness, crusting, sores, irritation, itching, redness; swollen, runny, stuffy nose; small amount of nasal bleeding, discomfort tenderness, back and joint pain, headache, mild nose bleed, flushing, nausea, sinus infection
Nexium (esomeprazole)	Proton pump inhibitor used to treat GERD	Diarrhea, stomach pain, nausea, anorexia, headache, heartburn, muscle pain, skin rash, drowsiness
Norvasc (amlodipine)	Non-antiarrhythmic calcium channel blocker used to treat angina and essential hypertension	Constipation, dizziness, light-headedness, headache, nausea, hypotension, peripheral edema, bradycardia, AV block, pulmonary edema, shortness of breath, asthenia
Plavix (clopidogrel)	Platelet inhibitor used to prevent stroke, MI, or vascular death in clients with arteriosclerosis and in those who have had a stoke or MI. Also used for those undergoing CABG or PCI	Severe bleeding, chest pain, general body pain, red or purple spots on skin, diarrhea, stomach ache, back pain, dizziness, heartburn, muscle aches, symptoms of a cold, unusual bleeding or bruising, arrhythmia, shortness of breath, pedal edema, hematemesis, fainting, menometrorhaggia, headache, joint pain, mild weakness
Potassium chloride (Brand names: K-Dur, K-Lor, Slow-K)	Potassium supplement	Nausea, vomiting, diarrhea, rash, tingling in hands or feet, anxiety

(continued on next page)

Table 14–13 *(continued from previous page)*

Medication	Action	Side Effects
Pravachol (pravastatin)	Antihyperlipidemic used to lower serum cholesterol and triglyceride levels	Aching muscles, fever, blurred vision, constipation, nausea, tiredness, weakness, dizziness, skin rash, headache, diarrhea, heartburn
Premarin (conjugated estrogen)	Estrogen used to treat female hypogonadism, primary ovarian failure, menopausal symptoms, abnormal uterine bleeding associated with hormone imbalance and with no organic cause, vaginal dryness and dyspareunia. It is also used as palliative treatment for prostatic cancer, male breast cancer, and nonestrogen dependent female breast cancer	Profuse bleeding, painful or swollen breasts, pedal edema, rapid weight gain, anorexia, nausea, stomach cramps or bloating, breast lumps or discharge, changes in vaginal bleeding (more, less spotting, prolonged), migraine, dizziness, contact lens intolerance, vomiting, mild diarrhea, headache, change in sex drive, slow weight gain
Prevacid (lansoprazole)	Proton pump inhibitor used to treat active duodenal ulcer, erosive esophagitis, GERD, H pylori, hypersecretory disorders	Headache and diarrhea
Propoxy-N/APAP	Narcotic analgesic with acetaminophen used for mild to moderate pain	Irregular or slow heartbeat, dyspnea, wheezing, dizziness, drowsiness, tiredness, headache, lightheaded ness, N&V, stomach cramps, overexcitement, black tarry stools, bloody or cloudy urine, painful or frequent urination, fast, slow or pounding heartbeat; hallucinations; dyspnea, wheezing; back or side pain, tinnitus, rash, sore throat, facial edema, fever, oliguria; trembling; uncontrolled muscle movements, unusual bleeding or bruising, jaundice, feeling depressed, pale stools
Proscar (finasteride)	5-alpha reductase inhibitor used to shrink the prostate in symptomatic BPH and in much smaller doses is used to treat male pattern baldness	Decreased volume of ejaculation, back or stomach pain, headache
Ranitidine (Brand name: Zantac)	Histamine 2 receptor antagonist used in the management of peptic ulcer disease, GERD, and erosive esophagitis	Dizziness, headache, diarrhea, decreased sex drive, unusual milk flow in women, hair loss
Triamterene/HCTZ (Brand name: Diazide)	Potassium sparing diuretic and hydrochlorothiazide used	Nausea or mild vomiting, anorexia, stomach cramps, mild diarrhea- dizziness, muscle cramps, headache, skin sensitive to sun, dry mouth, decreased sex drive
Verapamil (Brand name: Calan)	Calcium channel blocker used to treat hypertension, angina, and certain arrhythmias	Tiredness, bradyarrhythmia or tachyarrhythmia, wheezing, cough, dyspnea, dizziness, numbness or tingling in hands or feet, swollen feet, ankles or legs, difficult urination, nausea, constipation
Viagra (sildenafil)	Oral erectile dysfunction agent taken an hour before sexual activity, a major contraindication of which is the concurrent use of nitrates	Headache, flushing, stomach upset, stuffy or runny nose, back pain, muscle aches, urination problems, blurred vision, changes in color perception, light sensitivity, rash, dizziness, prolonged erection, diarrhea

(continued on next page)

Table 14–13 *(continued from previous page)*

Medication	Action	Side Effects
Warfarin	Oral anticoagulant used after heparin therapy in the treatment of thrombosis and embolism; used prophylactically for clients at risk for thrombosis or embolism, e.g., those with venous stasis, atrial fibrillation or prosthetic heart valves	Bloating, flatulence, rash, hives, itch, blurred vision, sore throat, easy bruising, bleeding, hematuria, back pain, jaundice, fever, chills, fatigue, weakness, dysuria, oliguria, bleeding gums, menometrorhaggia
Xalatan (latanoprost)	Antiglaucoma prostaglandin	Eye itch, mild pain, redness, feeling of something in the eye, decreased vision, dryness or tearing, lid crusting, sensitivity to light, discharge, color or other vision changes, increased hair growth
Anagrelide (Brand name: Agrylin)	Antiplatelet agent used to reduce platelet counts in clients with essential thrombocytopenia	Headache, palpitations, diarrhea, asthenia, edema, nausea and abdominal pain
Azathioprine (Brand name: Imuran)	IV immunosuppressant antimetabolite to prevent rejection of renal transplants and to treat rheumatoid arthritis unresponsive to other therapy	Infection, GI distress, secondary malignancies
Azithromycin (Brand name: Zithromax)	Macrolide antibiotic used to treat lower respiratory tract infection, nongonococcal urethritis and cervicitis, skin infections, acute otitis media, pharyngitis, tonsillitis, helicobacter pylori infection	Nausea, vomiting, abdominal pain, diarrhea (GI effects less than with erythromycin), allergic reactions
Clindamycin (Brand name: Cleocin)	Very toxic lincosamide antibiotic active against a wide range of aerobic, gram-positive cocci and several anaerobic gram positive and gram-negative organisms	Nausea, vomiting, abdominal pain, maculopapular rash, erythema, pruritus, hypersensitivity reactions, thrombocytopenia, eosinophilia, neutropenia, which may be heralded by sore throat or fever
Atomoxetine (Brand name: Straterra)	Selective norepinephrine reuptake inhibitor used in the management of Attention deficit hyperactive disorder (ADHD)	Risk of suicide. In children: suppression of normal weight and height patterns, dyspepsia, nausea, vomiting, fatigue; in adults: constipation, dry mouth, nausea, anorexia, dizziness, insomnia, sexual dysfunction, urinary hesitation or retention, dysmenorrheal
Paxil (paroxetine)	SSRI used for depression, OCD, panic disorder, anxiety	Central nervous system: asthenia, dizziness, headache, insomnia, somnolence, tremor, nervousness, suicidal behavior, anxiety, paresthesia, confusion, agitation; cardiovascular: palpitations, vasodilation, orthostatic hypotension; EENT: sensation of lump or tightness in the throat; gastrointestinal: dry mouth, nausea, constipation, diarrhea, flatulence, vomiting, dyspepsia, dysgeusia, increased or decreased appetite, abdominal pain; musculoskeletal: myopia, myalgia, myasthenia; genitourinary: ejaculatory disturbance, sexual dysfunction, urinary frequency; skin: diaphoresis, rash and pruritus; and yawning

(continued on next page)

Table 14–13 *(continued from previous page)*

Medication	Action	Side Effects
Lexapro (escitalopram)	SSRI used in the management of major depressive disorder	Nausea, dry mouth, trouble sleeping, loss of appetite, weakness, tiredness, drowsiness, dizziness, increased sweating, or yawning, nervousness, unusual high energy/excitement, suicidal thoughts, tremor, decreased interest in sex, changes in sexual ability
Xanax (alprazolam)	Benzodiazepine used to control anxiety	Respiratory depression, drowsiness, hallucinations, confusion, agitation, rash, itching and sensitivity to sunlight
Cymbalta (duloxetine hydrochloride)	Selective serotonin and norepinephrine reuptake inhibitor used to treat major depressive disorders and neuropathic pain related to diabetic peripheral neuropathy	Nausea, which improves in a few weeks, dry mouth, constipation, decreased appetite, fatigue, sleepiness, increased sweating
Zoloft (sertraline)	Selective serotonin reuptake inhibitor used to treat depression	Nausea, anorexia, diarrhea, sweating, insomnia, nervousness, anxiety, drowsiness, fatigue, dizziness, headache, suicidal thoughts and behavior
Oxycodone hydrochloride (Brand names: OxyContin (timed release preparation), OxyIR (rapid release preparation), Roxicodone)	Oral opioid analgesic used for moderate to severe pain	Clouded sensorium, dizziness, euphoria, light-headedness, physical dependence, sedation, somnolence, bradycardia, hypotension, constipation, nausea, vomiting, urinary retention, respiratory depression, diaphoresis, pruritus
Effexor (venlafaxine)	Newer generation antidepressant chemically unrelated to all other available antidepressants	Asthenia, headaches, somnolence, dizziness, nervousness, insomnia, suicidal behavior, anxiety, tremor, abnormal dreams, paresthesias, agitation, hypertension, tachycardia, blurred vision, nausea, constipation, dry mouth, anorexia, vomiting, diarrhea, dyspepsia, flatulence, abnormal ejaculation, impotence, urinary frequency, urinary retention, diaphoresis, rash, weight loss, yawning, chills, infection
Terazosin (Brand name: Hytrin)	Alpha-adrenergic blocking agent used in the management of hypertension and benign prostatic hypertrophy (BPH)	Light-headedness, dizziness, headache, drowsiness, weakness, lethargy, nausea, palpitations, reflex tachycardia, orthostatic hypotension, nasal congestion, inhibition of ejaculation
Timolol (Brand name: Blocadren)	Nonselective beta-adrenergic blocking agent used to treat hypertension, angina, and arrhythmias. Also used post-myocardial infarction, to prevent migraine headaches; and as an ophthalmic preparation to treat glaucoma by lowering intraocular pressure (IOP)	Cognitive dysfunction, depression, hallucinations and psychosis with high doses; hypoglycemia in clients with Type I diabetes; diarrhea, weight gain and with abrupt withdrawal, risk of MI, ventricular arrhythmias, severe hypertension
Zyrtec (cetirizine)	Antihistamine used in the management of seasonal and perennial allergy and for hives	Drowsiness, fatigue, headache, nausea, abdominal pain
Gabapentin (Brand name: Neurontin)	Anticonvulsant used to control seizures and to relieve post herpetic neuralgia	Drowsiness, dizziness, unsteadiness, fatigue, vision changes, weight gain, nausea, dry mouth, constipation

(continued on next page)

Table 14–13 *(continued from previous page)*

Medication	Action	Side Effects
Amoxicillin (Brand names: Amoxil, Biomox)	Antibiotic in the penicillin group used to treat infections due to *H. influenzae, N. gonorrhoeae, E. coli*, pneumococci, streptococci, and certain strains of staphylococci	Nausea, vomiting, mild diarrhea, irritation of the mouth or throat

*Medications in this table are listed by either generic or brand name depending on how they are most often ordered based on lists prepared by Blue Cross and Blue Shield of Texas, AARP and the American Pharmaceutical Association.

If the listed name is generic, it is followed by one or more brand names identified as such in parentheses. If the listed name is a brand name, the generic name follows in parentheses and can be identified as such by its lower case first letter. Side effects are listed in general order of frequency.

WORKSHEET

Solve the following calculation problems:

1. gr 1/100 = _____ mg
2. 0.25 mg = gr _____
3. 100 mg = _____ g
4. 0.01 mg = _____ µg
5. 95°F = _____ °C
6. 40°C = _____ °F
7. 6 oz = _____ ml
8. ½ oz = _____ ml
9. 1 half-pint carton of milk = ___ ml
10. 1 dr = _____ ml
11. 1 T = ____ ml
12. A 2-liter bottle of 7 Up = ____ml
13. 1 T = _____ t
14. 1 l = _____ qt (approx.)
15. Order: promethazine (Phenergan) 20 mg p.o.
    Stock: 10 mg scored tablets
    Dose: __________

(continued)

16. Order: furosemide (Lasix) 0.04 g p.o. every day
    Stock: 20 mg scored tablets
    Dose: ____________

17. Order: levothyroxine (Levothroid) 100 μg p.o. qid
    Stock: scored tablets 200 μg
    Dose: ____________

18. The physician orders cefazolin (Ancef) 750 mg. The nurse has Ancef 330 mg/ml. How many ml should the nurse administer? Answer: ________

19. The physician orders digoxin (Lanoxin) 0.125 mg p.o. every day. The nurse has digoxin 0.25 mg per tablet. How many tablet(s) should the nurse administer? Answer: ______

Convert the kilograms to pounds or pounds to kilograms.

20. 150 lb ________

21. 130 lb ________

22. 114 lb ________

23. 99.2 kg ________

24. 71.8 kg ________

25. The physician orders 1000 ml D5¼ NS to be infused over 6 hours. The nurse will be using a 20 gtt/ml infusion set.
    a. At how many milliliters per hour will the nurse infuse the solution? Answer:______
    b. At how many drops per minute will the nurse set the flow rate? Answer:________

26. The physician orders morphine (MS Contin) gr ¼ p.o. q 6 hour p.r.n. The medication available is morphine 30 mg per scored tablet. How many tablets will the nurse administer? Answer:_______

27. The physician orders amoxicillin (Trimox) 7.5 ml q 8 hour. The amoxicillin on hand is 125 mg/5 ml.
    How many mg will the client receive per dose? Answer:______
    How many mg will the client receive per day? Answer: ______

28. The physician orders Amoxicillin (Amoxil) for a 70-lb child. The child is to receive this medicine p.o. 4 times per day. The usual dose range is 20 to 40 mg/kg/d in divided doses.
    a. 70 lb = _____ Kg
    b. What is the lower daily dosage? ______
    c. What is the upper daily dosage? ______
    d. What is the lower dose for one dose? ______
    e. What is the upper dose for one dose? ______
    f. The dosage range is ______ mg to ______ mg per dose q 8 hours.
    g. If the order is to give 450 mg q 6 hr, is this a safe dose? ______ Why? ________

29. The physician orders theophylline (Uniphyl) 20 mg/kg/24 hours to be administered p.o. every 6 hours. How many milligrams would you administer per dose to a client weighing 126 lb? Answer:_________

30. The physician orders cephapirin (Cefadyl) 400 mg IM every 6 hr. The 500-mg vial of powdered medication reads: "To prepare solution add 2 ml sterile water. Provides an approximate volume of 2.2 ml of a 225 mg/ml solution." How many milliliters will you administer for one dose? Answer:________

FILL IN THE BLANKS

Fill in the blank spaces with the correct word or phrase to complete each statement.

1. The physician orders digoxin (Lanoxin) 0.25 mg p.o. stat. You have digoxin 0.125 mg scored tablet. How many tablet(s) should you administer? Answer: ________
2. Prior to administering digoxin, the nurse checks the serum level. What is the therapeutic range for the digoxin serum level for a client receiving digoxin? Answer: ________________
3. Prior to administering digoxin, the nurse checks the serum potassium level. What is the normal range for the serum potassium level? Answer: ______________
4. The nurse has a vial of heparin (Calcilean) 10,000 unit/ml. The client is to receive 7000 units sc bid. How many ml(s) should the client receive per dose? Answer: ______________
5. What type of syringe will the nurse use to administer heparin subcutaneously? Answer: _______________
6. What is the normal range for a serum PTT level for a client who has NOT received an anticoagulant? Answer: ____________________
7. The client is to receive morphine sulfate 8 mg intramuscular for pain. The nurse has Morphine Sulfate 10 mg/ml. How many ml(s) will the nurse administer? Answer: ________
8. What size needle would the nurse use to administer this intramuscular injection for a client who is 5 ft 6 in. tall and weighs 125 lb?
   Gauge: ______________, length: ________________
9. The physician orders Lasix (furosemide) 30 mg p.o. every day. You have Lasix 20 mg scored tablets. How many tablet(s) will you give? Answer: ________
10. Name the primary laboratory test that you would closely monitor prior to administering Lasix. Answer: ______________
11. The client may receive nitroglycerin tablets (Nitrostat) gr 1/100 sublingual for chest pain. How many mg = gr 1/100? Answer: ________
12. Which one VS would you monitor closely before and after the administration of nitroglycerin? Answer: ___________________________
13. The nurse is to administer insulin lispro (Humalog) and NPH insulin (Humulin N) at 0730.
    (a) Which insulin should be drawn into the syringe first? Answer: ______________________
    (b) What is the onset of action of Humalog? Answer: ____________________
    (c) What is the onset of action of NPH insulin? Answer: __________________________
14. List the five rights of medication administration.
    a. ________________________
    b. ________________________
    c. ________________________
    d. ________________________
    e. ________________________
15. The client is to receive regular insulin (Humulin R) subcutaneous before each meal. The physician has written an order to administer the insulin using this formula: $\frac{BG-120}{40}$

    Your client's blood glucose is 368. How many units of insulin will you administer? Answer: __________

TRUE & FALSE QUESTIONS

Mark each of the following statements True or False. Correct all false statements in the space provided. ____ ____
T F

1. Pharmacokinetics is the study of the absorption, distribution, metabolism, and excretion of drugs. ____ T ____ F

2. The rate of drug absorption, distribution, metabolism, and elimination for each specific class of drug is basically the same for all clients. ____ T ____ F

3. The nurse should always take into consideration the drug's action, characteristics of the drug, possible interactions with other drugs or food, and the client's daily schedule prior to administering medications. ____ T ____ F

4. If the client questions the appearance, dosage, or route, the nurse should fully explain the process of checking the drug three times, assure the client that it is the correct medication, and request that the client speak to the physician if they are uncomfortable with the medication routines. ____ T ____ F

5. When administering medications to a client with difficulty swallowing, the nurse may reduce the risk of aspiration by placing the client in a high-Fowler's or a sitting position if condition allows, provide sufficient fluid for swallowing, divide or crush tablets which are not enteric coated or sustained release, or obtain medications in liquid form when available. ____ T ____ F

6. Always assess the client's respiratory rate prior to and after administering morphine. Many institutional policies state that the nurse should not administer morphine to a client a respiratory rate of less than 10 breaths per minute. ____ T ____ F

7. Aspirin—a member of the salicylate drug classification—possesses the actions of anti-inflammatory, analgesic, antipyretic, and antiplatelet, and, therefore, may be administered for many different reasons. ____ T ____ F

8. The drug donepezil (Aricept), a member of the cholinesterase inhibitor classification, acts by enhancing cholinergic function by decreasing the levels of acetylcholine.

9. When advising clients about the drug, fexofenadine (Allegra), the nurse should inform them to take it with 6–8 oz of orange juice daily. ____ T ____ F

10. When monitoring the effects of antineoplastic agents, the nurse should assess for signs of infection, monitor VS and WBC count, encourage adequate oral intake and nutrition, inform client to avoid crowds and people with signs of illness, and explore options with client for possible loss of hair. ____ T ____ F

____ T ____ F

11. When providing education to a client who is taking the antipsychotic medication, risperidone (Risperdal), the nurse should instruct the client to change positions slowly, drink alcohol in moderate amounts only, use sun protective products and clothing, and to use hard candy, gum, or mouth rinses to help prevent dry mouth. ____ T ____ F

FILL IN THE BLANKS

Fill in the blank spaces with the correct word or phrase to complete each statement.

1. List three instructions to include in client/family teaching for a client who is taking the antiretroviral medication, amprenavir (Agenerase).
   a. ____________________
   b. ____________________
   c. ____________________

2. List two possible nursing diagnoses for a client taking the antirheumatic agent, etanercept (Enbrel).
   a. ____________________
   b. ____________________

3. Describe three nursing interventions the nurse should include in a care plan for a client taking the antitubercular agent, rifampin (Rifadin).
   a. ____________________
   b. ____________________
   c. ____________________

MATCHING QUESTIONS

Match the following:

Drug Classification	Drug Action
1. _____ Immunosuppressant agents: azathioprine (Imuran)	a. Using its glucocorticoid effects, reduces inflammation
2. _____ Lipid lowering agents: rosuvastin (Crestor)	b. Activates plasminogen to degrade clot
3. _____ Sedative/hypnotic agents: flurazepam (Dalmane)	c. Inhibits DNA, RNA, and proteins
4. _____ Thrombolytic agents: reteplase (Retavase)	d. Potentiates the effects of norepinephrine and serotonin
5. _____ Immune globulin agents: RhoGAM	e. Reduces total cholesterol, LDL, and triglycerides and increases HDL
6. _____ Tricyclic antidepressants: nortriptyline (Aventyl)	f. Suppresses immune response of nonsensitized Rh negative clients who are exposed to Rh positive blood
7. _____ Corticosteroid: prednisone (Pred-Pak)	g. Increases the binding of insulin to its receptors and potentiates the action of insulin
8. _____ Antidiabetic agents: Biguanide (Glucophage)	h. Management of insomnia

MATCHING QUESTIONS

Match the following:

1. _____Carisoprodol (Soma)	a. Alzheimer's Disease
2. _____Fluconazole (Diflucan)	b. Prevention of stroke
3. _____Amprenavir (Agenerase)	c. N&V
4. _____Phenytoin (Dilantin)	d. Acute coronary thrombosis
5. _____Naloxone (Narcan)	e. Asthma
6. _____Promethazine (Phenergan)	f. Muscle spasm
7. _____Albuterol (Proventil)	g. Depression
8. _____Reteplase (Retavase)	h. Anxiety
9. _____Risperidone (Risperdal)	i. Seizure disorders
10. _____Donepezil (Aricept)	j. HIV
11. _____Nortriptyline (Aventyl)	k. Fungal infection
12. _____Alprazolam (Xanax)	l. Respiratory depression
13. _____Dipyridamole (Persantine)	m. Schizophrenia

APPLICATION QUESTIONS

1. A physician has prescribed enteric-coated tablets for the client. The nurse knows the following is true about enteric-coated tablets:
   a. The tablets should be administered with antacids.
   b. The tablets are designed to carry drugs that may irritate the stomach.
   c. The tablets are designed to dissolve in the stomach.
   d. The tablets should be crushed.
2. The nurse is providing care for a client with mild liver damage due to hepatitis. The nurse is aware that this client may need reduced dosages of medications because
   a. the client's kidneys cannot eliminate medications at the usual rate.
   b. the drugs may accumulate in the client's body and produce toxicity.
   c. the rate of absorption will increase allowing more of the drug to enter the bloodstream.
   d. liver damage may cause drugs to bind to plasma proteins.
3. Which of the following oral dosage forms should not be disrupted?
   a. Enteric-coated and sustained-action medications
   b. Sustained-action and intravenous medications

c. Products containing a wax matrix and subcutaneous medications

d. Enteric-coated tablets and all capsules

4. The physician has ordered nitroglycerin gr 1/200 for a client experiencing angina. How many milligrams of nitroglycerin (Nitrostat) are in one tablet of gr 1/200?
   a. 0.05 mg
   b. 0.005 mg
   c. 3 mg
   d. 0.3 mg

5. A client is to receive Synthroid (levothyroxine) 100 μg p.o. every day. The medication label states: Synthroid 0.05 mg per scored tablet. How many tablet(s) should the nurse administer?
   a. ½ tablet
   b. 1 tablet
   c. 2 tablets
   d. 3 tablets

6. The physician orders meperidine (Demerol) for a postoperative client weighing 145 lb. If the recommended dose for meperidine (Demerol) is 6 mg/kg/24 hours, how much should be administered as a single dose four times daily?
   a. 220 mg
   b. 98.8 mg
   c. 22.6 mg
   d. 65 mg

7. The physician orders Lasix (furosemide) 40 mg p.o. for a client who has fluid volume excess. The medication label states: Lasix 20 mg per scored tablet. How many tablet(s) should the nurse administer?
   a. ½ tablet
   b. 1 tablet
   c. 2 tablets
   d. 3 tablets

8. The physician orders gentamicin (Garamycin) for a child weighing 88 lb. If the dose range is 6–7.5 mg/kg/d, and the child is to receive the medication tid, what is the therapeutic range for a single dose for this child?
   a. 20–40 mg
   b. 50–70 mg
   c. 80–100 mg
   d. 110–130 mg

9. The physician ordered penicillin (Penicillin G) 250,000 units intravenously. The nurse has on hand penicillin 20,000,000 units in 20 ml. How many ml contains the ordered dose?
   a. 0.25 ml
   b. 4 ml
   c. 16 ml
   d. 25 ml

10. The physician ordered digoxin (Lanoxin) 0.125 mg p.o. every day. The nurse has digoxin 0.25 mg scored tablets. How many tablet(s) should the nurse administer?
    a. ½ tablet
    b. 1 tablet
    c. 1½ tablet
    d. 2 tablets

11. Which of the following classes of drugs would most likely predispose a client to digitalis toxicity?
    a. Salicylate analgesics
    b. Tetracycline antibiotics
    c. Diuretics
    d. Barbiturates

12. The nurse is providing care for a client who is receiving digoxin (Lanoxin). Which of the following symptoms should the nurse recognize as digoxin (Lanoxin) toxicity?
    a. Hyperkalemia
    b. Increased hunger
    c. Constipation
    d. Visual disturbances

13. A client comes to the clinic complaining of unexplained black and blues and bloody appearing urine. Which type of medication is it most important to find out if the client is taking?
    a. Antibiotic
    b. Antipruritic
    c. Antianemic
    d. Anticoagulant

14. A client was admitted to the hospital with pneumonia. The physician ordered "Zinacef, (a second generation cephalosporin) 2 g IV q 8 hour." While preparing to administer the first dose of Zinacef, the nurse notices that this client has a penicillin allergy. The best action by the nurse is to
    a. administer the Zinacef as ordered but watch the client carefully for any signs of an allergic reaction.
    b. ask the pharmacist if another antibiotic can be substituted for the Zinacef.
    c. administer the Zinacef as ordered.
    d. hold the Zinacef and notify the physician of the client's allergy to penicillin.

(continued)

15. The physician prescribes an antihypertensive medication for your client. As a nurse, you would instruct the client to
    a. limit fluid intake to 1200 ml daily.
    b. increase activities, but limit foods high in magnesium.
    c. take a laxative along with the antihypertensive mediation.
    d. change positions slowly, and sit up for a few minutes before rising from a lying position.

16. A client, who is 6-months pregnant, comes to the physician asking for a prescription for a tetracycline type medication to treat her acne. Your response should be
    a. "Tetracycline, if taken during pregnancy, may be deposited in the bones and teeth of the fetus."
    b. "The effect of tetracycline is decreased during pregnancy."
    c. "Tetracycline may cause renal failure if taken during pregnancy."
    d. "Taking tetracycline during pregnancy may cause your teeth to discolor."

17. You have just finished instructing your client on measures to help the body fight infections. Which of the following statements by your client would lead you to believe he needs additional instruction regarding the antibiotics?
    a. "I will make sure I get adequate rest."
    b. "I know I must continue to eat a balanced diet and drink lots of fluids."
    c. "I will take my medicine until I no longer have a fever."
    d. "I will wash my hands often."

18. The nurse should provide client education as an integral component of client care. Clients taking captopril (Capoten) should be informed that they may experience a common adverse effect of the angiotension-converting enzyme inhibitors (ACE inhibitors) such as
    a. Persistent cough
    b. Increased appetite
    c. Hypertension
    d. Sedation

19. A client was prescribed both heparin (Calcilean) and warfarin (Coumadin) by the physician. When preparing to administer both of these anticoagulants, what rationale would the nurse consider appropriate?
    a. It takes 12–24 hours before the action of oral anticoagulants is evident.
    b. Heparin (Calcilean) is more effective when used with warfarin sodium (Coumadin).
    c. By administering an oral anticoagulant with heparin (Calcilean), the client needs less frequent administration of heparin.
    d. The client is less likely to experience adverse effects

20. The nurse needs to administer two types of insulin to the client. Which of the following is the correct procedure for mixing two types of insulin in the same syringe?
    a. Withdraw the regular insulin prior to any other type of insulin.
    b. Withdraw the regular insulin after other types of insulin.
    c. Draw each of the insulin medications in a separate syringe then combine the two.
    d. Withdraw one half dose of the regular insulin prior to the other insulin, and then withdraw the remaining dose of the regular insulin.

21. A client was diagnosed with a thrombus in her left leg. The physician has ordered Coumadin (warfarin) 7.5 mg p.o. every day. The client's prothrombin time (PT) is 20 and the International Normalized Ratio (INR) is 2.4. The nurse has Coumadin (warfarin) 5 mg scored tablets. What should the nurse plan to do?
    a. Administer 1/2 tablet because the PT and the INR are in a safe range.
    b. Administer one tablet because the PT and the INR are in a safe range.
    c. Administer 11/2 tablets because the PT and the INR are in a safe range.
    d. Do not administer Coumadin because the PT and the INR are too high.

22. The physician orders digoxin (Lanoxin) 0.25 mg p.o. every day. The nurse has digoxin 0.125 mg scored tablets. The client's serum digoxin level is 1.4 and his potassium level is 4.2. What should the nurse plan to do?
    a. Administer ½ tablet.
    b. Administer 2 tablets
    c. Do not administer the digoxin because the client's digoxin level is too high.
    d. Do not administer the digoxin because the client's potassium is too low.

23. If the nurse is to administer both an inhalation bronchodilator and an inhalation corticosteroid, which of the following is true?
    a. The bronchodilator should be used first.

b. The corticosteroid should be used first.
c. The order of use does not matter.
d. It is a good idea to alternate which product is used first.

24. When the nurse is monitoring the effects of bronchodilators, which of the following should be included?
a. Monitor for cyanosis of lips, earlobes, nail beds and mucous membranes, and monitor theophylline levels.
b. Be familiar with client's VS, and monitor their bowel sounds and respiratory effort.
c. Observe client for cyanosis, rapid respiratory rate, and monitor magnesium levels.
d. Observe client for adverse effects and ensure that he uses metered-dose inhalers correctly every hour.

25. When administering medication using a metered-dose inhaler the nurse should
a. require the client to rinse mouth before using inhaler.
b. monitor client's respiratory rate and bowel sounds.
c. observe client's oral mucosa and tongue for redness and white patches
d. encourage client to use a hard bristle toothbrush.

26. The bulk-forming laxatives should always be taken with
a. 30 ml orange juice.
b. 45 ml milk.
c. 4 oz of any liquid.
d. 240–300 ml of water or juice.

27. When administering proton pump inhibitors to a client, the nurse understands that they act by
a. suppressing gastric acid secretion by inhibiting the gastric pump in the parietal cells of the stomach.
b. reducing gastric acid production by inhibiting the leukotriene activity in the stomach.
c. increasing gastric acid secretion by increasing the gastric pump output.
d. increasing gastric acid production by inhibiting the gastric pump in the stomach.

28. Client teaching regarding long-term corticosteroid therapy should include:
a. the need for periodic blood glucose assessment
b. the need to take the medication late in the day to avoid insomnia
c. the possibility of enhanced wound healing
d. the need for a diet low in iron

29. Clients receiving long-term corticosteroid therapy may require dietary modifications. Which of the following statements is true about special diets for long-term corticosteroid therapy?
a. A potassium-restricted diet may be needed due to sodium and water retention.
b. A low-protein, low-carbohydrate diet may be needed to correct negative nitrogen balance.
c. A potassium-restricted diet may be needed due to potassium retention.
d. Increased calcium is encouraged to help prevent osteoporosis.

30. Anatomic and physiological factors that affect drug absorption in the elderly include
a. Increased rate of passage of drugs through the lower gastrointestinal tract.
b. Decreased gastric emptying, thus increasing the time medications remain in stomach.
c. Increased gastric acidity affects the way tablets dissolve.
d. Thinner skin surface delays absorption of topical drugs.

31. Factors that may place elderly people at risk for medication related problems include
a. vision loss, hearing loss, and using the same pharmacy so accurate profiles may be kept.
b. memory loss, hearing loss, and using the same pharmacy so that prescriptions errors may be caught easily.
c. recent memory loss, vision loss, and taking multiple medications due to chronic health problems.
d. maintaining accurate profile at the pharmacy, asking physician for a sample of the prescription to assess the medications effects, and following the pharmacist's instructions.

32. A serious concern in health care is the development of increasing numbers of antibiotic-resistant strains of bacteria. To help prevent this problem, clients should be taught to
a. complete the entire prescription of antibiotics
b. share their antibiotic prescription with other family members with the same symptoms
c. stop taking their antibiotic medications when they begin to feel better
d. request a prescription for antibiotics from the physician when they have a viral infection

(continued)

33. The nurse monitors the client for adverse effects of medications. What is a major disadvantage of using broad-spectrum antibiotics to treat infections?
    a. They are only effective against a small number of microorganisms.
    b. They destroy normal flora, enabling superinfections to develop.
    c. They are not effective against viruses.
    d. They are more likely to cause an allergic reaction.

34. The nurse receives a medication order with no route specified. What is the best action by the nurse?
    a. Give the medication orally because that is the most common route.
    b. Ask the client how he usually takes the medication.
    c. Call the physician to clarify the order.
    d. Ask another nurse which route to use.

35. The physician orders nitroglycerin (Nitro Bid) 0.4 mg SL now. Which of the following options would indicate that the nurse correctly administered the medication?
    a. Tablet placed under the client's tongue and client instructed to allow medication to dissolve.
    b. Tablet given to the client with 8 oz of water after checking BP and heart rate.
    c. Tablet given to the client with 4 oz of juice to assist with masking bitter flavor.
    d. Tablet placed under client's tongue and client instructed to chew slowly to assist with absorption.

36. When administering intramuscular medication to a client who is 5 ft 6 in. tall and weighs 118 oz, which of the following needles should the nurse select?
    a. 27 gauge, 1 in.
    b. 23 gauge, 2 in.
    c. 25 gauge, 1½ in.
    d. 22 gauge, 1 in.

37. Which of the following rights do clients have in regard to medication? The right to
    a. know the names of the other clients on the hall.
    b. refuse medication and know the names of their medication.
    c. information concerning side effects of the medications they are taking at home only.
    d. know all of the medication that the nurse administers to all the clients.

38. What direction should the nurse give to a client in regard to the use of NSAIDs prior to scheduled surgery?
    a. Take as usual as long as recommended dose is not exceeded.
    b. Do not take after midnight the day of surgery.
    c. Gradually taper to zero during the week prior to surgery.
    a. Discontinue 7 days prior to elective surgery.

39. The nurse should instruct the client taking an antilipemic about the regular need for which type of examination?
    a. Colonoscopy
    b. Dental
    c. Ophthalmic
    d. Hearing

40. Which question should be asked of a young adult female for whom penicillin has been ordered?
    a. Do you drink milk?
    b. Are you allergic to shellfish?
    c. Do you take birth control pills?
    d. Have you ever had vaginitis?

ANSWERS & RATIONALES

Answers for the calculation problems:

1. gr 1/100 = 0.6 mg

2. 0.25 mg = gr 1/240

3. 100 mg = 0.1 g

4. 0.01 mg = 10 μg

5. 95 °F = 35°C

6. 40 °C = 104°F

7. 6 oz = 180 ml

8. ½ oz = 15 ml

9. 1 half-pint carton of milk = 240 ml

10. 1 dr = 4 ml

11. 1 T = 15 ml

12. A 2-liter bottle of 7 Up = 2000 ml

13. 1 T = 3 t

14. 1 L = 1 qt (approx.)

15. Order: promethazine (Phenergan) 20 mg p.o.
Stock: 10 mg scored tablets
Dose: 2

16. Order: furosemide (Lasix) 0.04 g p.o. every day
Stock: 20 mg scored tablets
Dose: 2

17. Order: levothyroxine (Levothroid) 100 μg p.o. qid
Stock: scored tablets 200 μg
Dose: ½

18. The physician orders cefazolin (Ancef) 750 mg. The nurse has Ancef 330 mg/ml. How many ml should the nurse administer? Answer: 2.3

19. The physician orders digoxin (Lanoxin) 0.125 mg p.o. every day. The nurse has digoxin 0.25 mg per tablet. How many tablet(s) should the nurse administer? Answer: ½

Convert the kilograms to pounds or pounds to kilograms.

20. 150 lb 68.2 kg

21. 130 lb 59.1 kg

22. 114 lb 51.8 kg

23. 99.2 kg 218.2 kg

24. 71.8 kg 158 kg

25. The physician orders 1000 ml D5 ¼ NS to be infused over 6 hours. The nurse will be using a 20 gtt/ml infusion set.
a. At how many milliliters per hour will the nurse infuse the solution? Answer: 167 ml/hr
b. At how many drops per minute will the nurse set the flow rate? Answer: 56 gtt/min

(continued)

26. The physician orders morphine (MS Contin) gr ¼ p.o. q 6 hour p.r.n. The medication available is morphine 30 mg per scored tablet. How many tablets will the nurse administer? Answer: ½

27. The physician orders amoxicillin (Trimox) 7.5 ml q 8 hour. The amoxicillin on hand is 125 mg/5 ml.
    a. How many mg will the client receive per dose? Answer: 187.5
    b. How many mg will the client receive per day? Answer: 562.5

28. The physician orders Amoxicillin (Amoxil) for a 70-lb child. The child is to receive this medicine p.o. 4 times per day. The usual dose range is 20–40 mg/kg/d in divided doses.
    a. 70 lb = 31.8 kg
    b. What is the lower daily dosage? 636 mg
    c. What is the upper daily dosage? 1272 mg
    d. What is the lower dose for one dose? 159 mg
    e. What is the upper dose for one dose? 318 mg
    f. The dosage range is 159 mg to 318 mg per dose q 8 hours.
    g. If the order is to give 450 mg q 6 hour, is this a safe dose? Answer: No. Why? Too high of a dose.

29. The physician orders theophylline (Uniphyl) 20 mg/kg/24 hours to be administered p.o. every 6 hours. How many milligrams would you administer per dose to a client weighing 126 lb? Answer: 126/ 2.2 = 57.3 kg ⇒ 57.3 ⇒ 20 = 1146 mg/day ⇒ 1146/ 4 = 286.5 mg.

30. The physician orders cephapirin (Cefadyl) 400 mg IM every 6 hours. The 500-mg vial of powdered medication reads: "To prepare solution add 2-ml sterile water. Provides an approximate volume of 2.2 ml of a 225-mg/ml solution." How many milliliters will you administer for one dose? Answer: 3.9

ANSWERS FOR FILL IN THE BLANKS

1. The physician orders digoxin (Lanoxin) 0.25 mg p.o. stat. You have digoxin 0.125 mg scored tablet. How many tablet(s) should you administer? Answer: Two tablets.

2. Prior to administering digoxin, the nurse checks the serum level. What is the therapeutic range for the digoxin serum level for a client receiving digoxin? Answer: 0.8–2.0 ng/ml.

3. Prior to administering digoxin, the nurse checks the serum potassium level. What is the normal range for the serum potassium level? Answer: 3.5–5.3 mEq/L.

4. The nurse has a vial of heparin (Calcilean) 10,000 unit/ml. The client is to receive 7000 units sc bid. How many ml(s) should the client receive per dose? Answer: 0.7 ml.

5. What type of syringe will the nurse use to administer heparin subcutaneously? Answer: Tuberculin.

6. What is the normal range for a serum PTT level for a client who has NOT received an anticoagulant? Answer: 25–45 seconds.

7. The client is to receive morphine sulfate 8 mg intramuscular for pain. The nurse has Morphine Sulfate 10 mg/ml. How many ml(s) will the nurse administer? Answer: 0.8 ml.

8. What size needle would the nurse use to administer this intramuscular injection for a client who is 5 ft. 6 in. tall and weighs 125 lb?
Answer: Gauge: 21–23 , length: 1 in.

9. The physician orders Lasix (furosemide) 30 mg p.o. every day. You have Lasix 20 mg scored tablets. How many tablet(s) will you give? Answer: 1½ tablets.

10. Name the primary laboratory test that you would closely monitor prior to administering Lasix.
Answer: Serum potassium level.

11. The client may receive nitroglycerin tablets (Nitrostat) gr 1/100 sublingual for chest pain. How many mg = gr 1/100?
Answer: 0.6 mg.

12. Which one VS would you monitor closely before and after the administration of nitroglycerin? Answer: Blood pressure.

13. The nurse is to administer insulin lispro (Humalog) and NPH insulin (Humulin N) at 0730.
(a) Which insulin should be drawn into the syringe first? Answer: lispro (Humalog).
(b) What is the onset of action of Humalog? Answer: Within 15 minutes.
(c) What is the onset of action of NPH insulin? Answer: Within 2–4 hours.

14. List the five rights of medication administration.
a. Client
b. Drug
c. Dose
d. Route
e. Time

15. The client is to receive regular insulin (Humulin R) subcutaneous before each meal. The physician has written an order to administer the insulin using this formula: $\frac{BG - 120}{40}$
Your client's blood glucose is 368. How many units of insulin will you administer? Answer: 6.2 (say 6) units.

TRUE & FALSE ANSWERS

1. Pharmacokinetics is the study of the absorption, distribution, metabolism, and excretion of drugs. *True*

2. The rate of drug absorption, distribution, metabolism, and elimination for each specific class of drug is basically the same for all clients. *False*
The rate of drug absorption, distribution, metabolism, and elimination may be affected by underlying disease states, age, body weight, or basal metabolic rate.

3. The nurse should always take into consideration the drug's action, characteristics of the drug, possible interactions with other drugs or food, and the client's daily schedule prior to administering medications. *True*

(continued)

4. If the client questions the appearance, dosage, or route, the nurse should fully explain the process of checking the drug three times, assure the client that it is the correct medication, and request that the client speak to the physician if they are uncomfortable with the medication routines. *False*

   The nurse should recheck the physician's orders, reevaluate the medication record, perform the "five rights" and "three checks" again, and obtain more information from client if needed prior to making a decision to administer the medication.

5. When administering medications to a client with difficulty swallowing, the nurse may reduce the risk of aspiration by placing the client in a high-Fowler's or a sitting position if condition allows, provide sufficient fluid for swallowing, divide or crush tablets which are not enteric coated or sustained release, or obtain medications in liquid form when available. *True*

6. Always assess the client's respiratory rate prior to and after administering morphine. Many institutional policies state that the nurse should not administer morphine to a client with a respiratory rate of less than 10 breaths per minute. *True*

7. Aspirin—a member of the salicylate drug classification—possesses the actions of anti-inflammatory, analgesic, antipyretic, and antiplatelet, and, therefore, may be administered for many different reasons. *True*

8. The drug donepezil (Aricept), a member of the Cholinesterase Inhibitor classification, acts by enhancing cholinergic function by decreasing the levels of acetylcholine. *False*

   Donepezil acts by increasing the levels of acetylcholine.

9. When advising clients about the drug, fexofenadine (Allegra), the nurse should inform them to take it with 6–8 oz of orange juice daily. *False*

   Apple, orange, and grapefruit juice will decrease the absorption of fexofenadine (Allegra).

10. When monitoring the effects of antineoplastic agents, the nurse should assess for signs of infection, monitor VS and WBC count, encourage adequate oral intake and nutrition, inform client to avoid crowds and people with signs of illness, and explore options with client for possible loss of hair. *True*

11. When providing education to a client who is taking the antipsychotic medication, risperidone (Risperdal), the nurse should instruct the client to, change positions slowly, drink alcohol in moderate amounts only, use sun protective products and clothing, and to use hard candy, gum, or mouth rinses to help prevent dry mouth. *False*

    Clients taking risperidone should avoid drinking alcohol.

ANSWERS FOR FILL IN THE BLANKS

1. List three instructions to include in client/family teaching for a client who is taking the antiretroviral medication, amprenavir (Agenerase).

   Answers may include: Instruct to take medication round the clock exactly as directed to maintain dosing schedule. Inform that these medications do not cure HIV or reduce the risk of spreading virus to others. Instruct to use condom, not to share needles, and not to donate blood. Inform not to use over-the-counter medication unless approved by physician. Review adverse effects such as diarrhea, N&V, mood changes, and rash. Advise to keep all follow-up appointments with health care providers.

2. List two possible nursing diagnoses for a client taking the antirheumatic agent, etanercept (Enbrel).
   Answers may include: Pain: acute, mobility: impaired, deficient knowledge related to medication and disease.

3. Describe three nursing interventions the nurse should include in a care plan for a client taking the antitubercular agent, rifampin (Rifadin).
   Answers may include: Assess respiratory rate, pattern and effort, lung sounds, and amount and character of sputum before and after administration of medication. Monitor CBC, liver and renal function studies, PPD test results, and sputum cultures. Assess for common adverse effects of the medication such as diarrhea, abdominal pain, nausea, vomiting, and red–orange discoloration of body fluids. Instruct client to report increase in fatigue, cough, shortness of breath, fever, and chills to health care provider.

MATCHING ANSWERS

Drug Classification	Drug Action
1. _c_ Immunosuppressant agents: azathioprine (Imuran)	a. Using its glucocorticoid effects, reduces inflammation
2. _e_ Lipid lowering agents: rosuvastin (Crestor)	b. Activates plasminogen to degrade clot
3. _h_ Sedative/hypnotic agents: flurazepam (Dalmane)	c. Inhibits DNA, RNA, and proteins
4. _b_ Thrombolytic agents: reteplase (Retavase)	d. Potentiates the effects of norepinephrine and serotonin
5. _f_ Immune globulin agents: RhoGAM	e. Reduces total cholesterol, LDL, and triglycerides and increases HDL
6. _d_ Tricyclic antidepressants: nortriptyline (Aventyl)	f. Suppresses immune response of nonsensitized Rh negative clients who are exposed to Rh positive blood
7. _a_ Corticosteroid: prednisone (Pred-Pak)	g. Increases the binding of insulin to its receptors and potentiates the action of insulin
8. _g_ Antidiabetic agents: Biguanide (Glucophage)	h. Management of insomnia

MATCHING ANSWERS

1. _f_ Carisoprodol (Soma)	a. Alzheimer's Disease
2. _k_ Fluconazole (Diflucan)	b. Prevention of stroke
3. _j_ Amprenavir (Agenerase)	c. N&V
4. _I_ Phenytoin (Dilantin)	d. Acute coronary thrombosis

(continued)

5. _l_ Naloxone (Narcan)	e. Asthma
6. _c_ Promethazine (Phenergan)	f. Muscle spasm
7. _e_ Albuterol (Proventil)	g. Depression
8. _d_ Reteplase (Retavase)	h. Anxiety
9. _m_ Risperidone (Risperdal)	i. Seizure disorders
10. _a_ Donepezil (Aricept)	j. HIV
11. _g_ Nortriptyline (Aventyl)	k. Fungal infection
12. _h_ Alprazolam (Xanax)	l. Respiratory depression
13. _b_ Dipyridamole (Persantine)	m. Schizophrenia

APPLICATION ANSWERS

1. A physician has prescribed enteric-coated tablets for the client. The nurse knows the following is true about enteric-coated tablets:
   a. The tablets should be administered with antacids.
   b. The tablets are designed to carry drugs that may irritate the stomach.
   c. The tablets are designed to dissolve in the stomach.
   d. The tablets should be crushed.

Rationale
Correct answer: b.
Answer (b) is correct; the coating prevents the tablet from dissolving in the stomach where gastric acid is present and allows these more irritating medications to be carried to the small intestines to dissolve. Answer (a) is incorrect because the antacids may change the pH of the stomach to a more neutral or alkaline environment and allow the tablet to dissolve in the stomach. Answers (c) and (d) are incorrect because the tablet is designed to dissolve in the small intestine, and should never be crushed.

2. The nurse is providing care for a client with mild liver damage due to hepatitis. The nurse is aware that this client may need reduced dosages of medications because
   a. the client's kidneys cannot eliminate medications at the usual rate.
   b. the drugs may accumulate in the client's body and produce toxicity.
   c. the rate of absorption will increase allowing more of the drug to enter the bloodstream.
   d. liver damage may cause drugs to bind to plasma proteins.

Rationale
Correct answer: b.
Answer (b) is correct because clients with liver damage may experience a decrease in the ability to metabolize drugs, thus the drugs accumulate in the body and may cause toxicity. Answer (a) does not relate to liver failure. Answer (c) is incorrect because absorption occurs prior to metabolism in the liver. Answer (d) is incorrect because the chemical properties of a drug are what determine how the drug is bound or distributed.

3. Which of the following oral dosage forms should not be disrupted?
   a. Enteric-coated and sustained-action medications
   b. Sustained-action and intravenous medications
   c. Products containing a wax matrix and subcutaneous medications
   d. Enteric-coated tablets and all capsules

Rationale
Correct answer: a.
Answer (a) is correct because enteric-coated and sustained action drugs should not be divided or crushed. Answers (b), (c), and (d) all have one option that may be disrupted, thus making them the incorrect choice.

(continued)

4. The physician has ordered nitroglycerin gr 1/200 for a client experiencing angina. How many milligrams of nitroglycerin (Nitrostat) are in one tablet of gr 1/200?
   a. 0.05 mg
   b. 0.005 mg
   c. 3 mg
   d. 0.3 mg

Rationale

Correct answer: d.

Answer (d) is correct:

$$\frac{\text{gr } 1/200}{x \text{ mg}} = \frac{\text{gr } 1}{60 \text{ m}}$$

$$1\,x = 60/200$$

$$x = 0.3 \text{ mg}$$

5. A client is to receive Synthroid (levothyroxine) 100 μg p.o. every day. The medication label states: Synthroid 0.05 mg per scored tablet. How many tablet(s) should the nurse administer?
   a. ½ tablet
   b. 1 tablet
   c. 2 tablets
   d. 3 tablets

Rationale

Correct answer: c.

Answer (c) is correct: Change the 100 μg to 0.1 mg, then set up your ratio.

0.1 mg/x tablet = 0.05 mg/1 tablet

0.05 x = 0.1

x = 2 tablets

6. The physician orders meperidine (Demerol) for a postoperative client weighing 145 lb. If the recommended dose for meperidine (Demerol) is 6 mg/kg/24 hours, how much should be administered as a single dose four times daily?
   a. 220 mg
   b. 98.8 mg
   c. 22.6 mg
   d. 65 mg

Rationale

Correct answer: b.

Answer (b) is correct. Determine the client's weight in kg: 145 lb/2.2 = 65.9 kg, then work the problem. 65.9 kg × 6 mg = 395.4 mg per 24 hours. Divide 395.4 by 4 doses per day = 98.8 mg per single dose.

7. The physician orders Lasix (furosemide) 40 mg p.o. for a client who has fluid volume excess. The medication label states: Lasix 20 mg per scored tablet. How many tablet(s) should the nurse administer?
   a. ½ tablet
   b. 1 tablet
   c. 2 tablets
   d. 3 tablets

Rationale

Correct answer: c.

Answer (c) is correct: 40 mg/x tablet = 20 mg/1 tablet

20 x = 40

x = 2 tablets

8. The physician orders gentamicin (Garamycin) for a child weighing 88 lb. If the dose range is 6–7.5 mg/kg/d, and the child is to receive the medication tid, what is the therapeutic range for a single dose for this child?
   a. 20–40 mg
   b. 50–70 mg
   c. 80–100 mg
   d. 110–130 mg

Rationale

Correct answer: c.

Answer (c) is correct: Determine the client's weight in kg: 88 lb/2.2 kg = 40 kg

To determine the range, take the dose range and multiply it by the client's weight: 6 mg × 40 kg = 240 mg/kg/d is the lower range. For the upper range: 7.5 mg × 40 kg = 300 mg/kg/d. To find a single dose, divide each of the doses by 3 because it was ordered tid. 240 mg/3 = 80 mg per dose. 300 mg/3 = 100 mg per dose. Therefore, the single dose range is 80–100 mg.

9. The physician ordered penicillin (Penicillin G) 250,000 units intravenously. The nurse has on hand penicillin 20,000,000 units in 20 ml. How many ml contains the ordered dose?
   a. 0.25 ml
   b. 4 ml
   c. 16 ml
   d. 25 ml

Rationale

Correct answer: a.

Answer (a) is correct:

250,000 units/x ml = 20,000,000/20 ml

20,000,000x = 5,000,000

x = 0.25 ml

10. The physician ordered digoxin (Lanoxin) 0.125 mg p.o. every day. The nurse has digoxin 0.25 mg scored tablets. How many tablet(s) should the nurse administer?
   a. ½ tablet
   b. 1 tablet
   c. 1½ tablet
   d. 2 tablets

(continued)

Rationale

Correct answer: a.

Answer (a) is correct: 0.125 mg/x tablet = 0.25 mg/1 tablet

$0.25x = 0.125$

$x = ½$ tablet

11. Which of the following classes of drugs would most likely predispose a client to digitalis toxicity?
    a. Salicylate analgesics
    b. Tetracycline antibiotics
    c. Diuretics
    d. Barbiturates

Rationale

Correct answer: c.

Answer (c) is correct because many diuretics increase the excretion of potassium from the body and a decreased level of potassium increases the risk of digoxin toxicity. Answers (a),(b), and (d) do not predispose a client to digoxin toxicity.

12. The nurse is providing care for a client who is receiving digoxin (Lanoxin). Which of the following symptoms should the nurse recognize as digoxin (Lanoxin) toxicity?
    a. Hyperkalemia
    b. Increased hunger
    c. Constipation
    d. Visual disturbances

Rationale

Correct answer: d.

Answer (d) is correct because it is a common symptom of digoxin toxicity. Other symptoms include fatigue, anorexia, blurred or double vision, nausea, confusion, and bradycardia. Answers (a), (b), and (c) are not symptoms of digoxin toxicity.

13. A client comes to the clinic complaining of unexplained black and blues and bloody appearing urine. Which type of medication is it most important to find out if the client is taking?
    a. Antibiotic
    b. Antipruritic
    c. Antianemic
    d. Anticoagulant

Rationale

Correct answer: d.

Answer (d) is correct because a side effect of anticoagulant therapy is abnormal bleeding, which can manifest in many ways two of which are as gross blood in the urine and easy bruising.

14. A client was admitted to the hospital with pneumonia. The physician ordered "Zinacef, (a second generation cephalosporin) 2 g IV q 8 hour." While preparing to administer the first dose of Zinacef, the nurse notices that this client has a penicillin allergy. The best action by the nurse is to
    a. administer the Zinacef as ordered but watch the client carefully for any signs of an allergic reaction
    b. ask the pharmacist if another antibiotic can be substituted for the Zinacef
    c. administer the Zinacef as ordered
    d. hold the Zinacef and notify the physician of the client's allergy to penicillin

Rationale

Correct answer: d.

Answer (d) is the best answer. Often, a client who has an allergy to Penicillin will experience an adverse effect to the cephalosporin class of antibiotics because they are chemically and pharmacologically similar. Therefore, for the safety of the client, the nurse should always call the physician. The answers of (a), (b), and (c) are not appropriate actions for the nurse to take with this client situation.

15. The physician prescribes an antihypertensive medication for your client. As a nurse, you would instruct the client to
    a. limit fluid intake to 1200 ml daily.
    b. increase activities, but limit foods high in magnesium.
    c. take a laxative along with the antihypertensive mediation.
    d. change positions slowly, and sit up for a few minutes before rising from a lying position.

Rationale

Correct answer: d.

Answer (d) is correct. Many of the antihypertensive medications cause orthostatic hypotension. Therefore, the nurse should instruct the client regarding sudden movements and about rising slowing to prevent a decrease in BP and prevent client injury. Answers (a), (b), and (c) are not appropriate instructions in regards to medications for hypertension.

16. A client, who is 6-months pregnant, comes to the physician asking for a prescription for a tetracycline type medication to treat her acne. Your response should be
    a. "Tetracycline, if taken during pregnancy, may be deposited in the bones and teeth of the fetus."
    b. "The effect of tetracycline is decreased during pregnancy."

c. "Tetracycline may cause renal failure if taken during pregnancy."
d. "Taking tetracycline during pregnancy may cause your teeth to discolor."

Rationale

Correct answer: a.

Answer (a) is correct because the tetracycline medications are contraindicated during pregnancy because the drugs may interfere with normal calcification of temporary and permanent teeth and discolor developing teeth of the fetus. The drug may also interfere with bone growth of the fetus. Answers (b) and (c) are incorrect. Answer (d) is incorrect because the medication affects the developing teeth of the fetus and children younger than 8 years of age, not the adult.

17. You have just finished instructing your client on measures to help the body fight infections. Which of the following statements by your client would lead you to believe he needs additional instruction regarding the antibiotics?
    a. "I will make sure I get adequate rest."
    b. "I know I must continue to eat a balanced diet and drink lots of fluids."
    c. "I will take my medicine until I no longer have a fever."
    d. "I will wash my hands often."

Rationale

Correct answer: c.

Answer (c) is correct. The question is asking how the nurse would know the client needs additional instruction or that the client does not understand. If the client thinks he should stop taking his antibiotics when he no longer has a fever, then he needs additional education. Answers (a), (b), and (d) are all good measures to help fight or prevent infection, therefore, these do not indicate he needs more instruction.

18. The nurse should provide client education as an integral component of client care. Clients taking captopril (Capoten) should be informed that they may experience a common adverse effect of the angiotension-converting enzyme inhibitors (ACE inhibitors) such as
    a. Persistent cough
    b. Increased appetite
    c. Hypertension
    d. Sedation

Rationale

Correct answer: a.

Answer (a) is correct. A persistent cough is a common adverse effect of ACE Inhibitors. Answers (b), (c), and (d) are not common adverse effects of ACE Inhibitors.

19. A client was prescribed both heparin (Calcilean) and warfarin (Coumadin) by the physician. When preparing to administer both of these anticoagulants, what rationale would the nurse consider appropriate?
    a. It takes 12–24 hours before the action of oral anticoagulants is evident.
    b. Heparin (Calcilean) is more effective when used with warfarin sodium (Coumadin).
    c. By administering an oral anticoagulant with heparin (Calcilean), the client needs less frequent administration of heparin.
    d. The client is less likely to experience adverse effects

Rationale

Correct answer: a.

Answer (a) is correct. In many situations the client is receiving heparin intravenously and the physician prescribes the addition of Coumadin for several days prior to discontinuing the heparin. For oral anticoagulants, their effect is usually not evident for 12–24 hours after therapy has begun. Therefore, the client is receiving the heparin while the effects of the Coumadin are beginning to become evident. After the laboratory work shows evidence that the oral anticoagulants are effective, then the physician will discontinue the heparin therapy. Answers (b),(c), and (d) are not correct.

20. The nurse needs to administer two types of insulin to the client. Which of the following is the correct procedure for mixing two types of insulin in the same syringe?
    a. Withdraw the regular insulin prior to any other type of insulin.
    b. Withdraw the regular insulin after other types of insulin.
    c. Draw each of the insulin medications in a separate syringe then combine the two.
    d. Withdraw one half dose of the regular insulin prior to the other insulin, and then withdraw the remaining dose of the regular insulin.

Rationale

Correct answer: a.

Answer (a) is correct. The nurse withdraws the regular (clear) insulin first so as to not contaminate the regular insulin vial with the other types of insulin. Answers (b) and (d) risk the chance to contaminate the regular insulin vial. Answer (c) indicates that the nurse is wasting time and supplies, as well as the insulin syringes do not have a detachable needle, thus, the nurse can not add solution from one syringe to another syringe.

21. A client was diagnosed with a thrombus in her left leg. The physician has ordered Coumadin (warfarin)

(continued)

7.5 mg p.o. every day. The client's prothrombin time (PT) is 20 and the international normalized ratio (INR) is 2.4. The nurse has Coumadin (warfarin) 5 mg scored tablets. What should the nurse plan to do?

a. Administer ½ tablet because the PT and the INR are in a safe range.
b. Administer one tablet because the PT and the INR are in a safe range.
c. Administer 1½ tablets because the PT and the INR are in a safe range.
d. Do not administer Coumadin because the PT and the INR are too high.

Rationale

Correct answer: c.

Answer (c) is correct. The PT and the INR values are in a normal range for a client who is receiving oral anticoagulant therapy. Therefore, you need to determine the dose the nurse will administer. 7.5 mg/x tablet = 5 mg/1 tablet

$5x = 7.5$

$x = 1½$ tablet

22. The physician orders digoxin (Lanoxin) 0.25 mg p.o. every day. The nurse has digoxin 0.125 mg scored tablets. The client's serum digoxin level is 1.4 and his potassium level is 4.2. What should the nurse plan to do?
    a. Administer ½ tablet.
    b. Administer 2 tablets
    c. Do not administer the digoxin because the client's digoxin level is too high.
    d. Do not administer the digoxin because the client's potassium is too low.

Rationale

Correct answer: b.

Answer (b) is correct. The serum digoxin level of 1.4 is within normal limits for a client taking digoxin (0.8–2.0). The potassium level of 4.2 is within normal limits (3.5–5.3). Therefore, you need to determine the dose the client will receive.

0.25 mg/x tablet = 0.125 mg/1 tablet

$0.125x = 0.25$

$x = 2$ tablets

23. If the nurse is to administer both an inhalation bronchodilator and an inhalation corticosteroid, which of the following is true?
    a. The bronchodilator should be used first.
    b. The corticosteroid should be used first.
    c. The order of use does not matter.
    d. It is a good idea to alternate which product is used first.

Rationale

Correct answer: a.

Answer (a) is correct. The nurse should administer the bronchodilator inhaler first so that the medication can dilate the bronchioles prior to the administration of the inhalation corticosteroid medication. It is best to wait 5–10 minutes after the administration of the bronchodilator inhaler before administering any other inhaled medications.

24. When the nurse is monitoring the effects of bronchodilators, which of the following should be included?
    a. Monitor for cyanosis of lips, earlobes, nail beds and mucous membranes, and monitor theophylline levels.
    b. Be familiar with client's VS, and monitor their bowel sounds and respiratory effort.
    c. Observe client for cyanosis, rapid respiratory rate, and monitor magnesium levels.
    d. Observe client for adverse effects and ensure that he uses metered-dose inhalers correctly every hour.

Rationale

Correct answer: a.

Answer (a) is correct. When the nurse is monitoring the effects of medications, the S&S of the disorder that these medications are treating are included in the assessment. With bronchodilators, the S&S of the disorder are respiratory system related. Theophylline is a medication that promotes bronchodilation, and the physician often orders serum theophylline levels to be drawn. Answers (b) and (c) have distracters such as bowel sounds and magnesium levels which are not associated with monitoring the effects of bronchodilators. Answer (d) is incorrect because the nurse would not administer the inhaler every hour as this would be an overdose.

25. When administering medication using a metered-dose inhaler the nurse should
    a. require the client to rinse mouth before using inhaler.
    b. monitor client's respiratory rate and bowel sounds.
    c. observe client's oral mucosa and tongue for redness and white patches
    d. encourage client to use a hard bristle toothbrush.

Rationale

Correct answer: c.

Answer (c) is correct. Some of the inhaled medications are steroids and may cause irritation or oral candidiasis. Answer (a) would not be the best answer, although there may be situations where the nurse may need the client to rinse their mouth before using the inhaler. Answer (b) is incorrect because the bowel sounds are not a component of this assessment. Answer (d) is incorrect because if there is a situation that may cause oral irritation, the client should be instructed to use a soft bristle toothbrush.

26. The bulk-forming laxatives should always be taken with
   a. 30 ml orange juice.
   b. 45 ml milk.
   c. 4 oz of any liquid.
   d. 240–300 ml of water or juice.

Rationale
Correct answer: d.
Answer (d) is correct. The nurse should administer a bulk-forming laxative with 240–300 ml of water or juice to prevent gastrointestinal obstruction. Answers (a), (b), and (c) are not enough volume.

27. When administering proton pump inhibitors to a client, the nurse understands that they act by
   a. suppressing gastric acid secretion by inhibiting the gastric pump in the parietal cells of the stomach.
   b. reducing gastric acid production by inhibiting the leukotriene activity in the stomach.
   c. increasing gastric acid secretion by increasing the gastric pump output.
   d. increasing gastric acid production by inhibiting the gastric pump in the stomach.

Rationale
Correct answer: a.
Answer (a) is the correct action of medications in the drug classification of proton pump inhibitors. Answer (b) is incorrect because leukotriene activity is not an action of these medications. Answers (c) and (d) are incorrect because gastric acid is decreased, not increased with this classification.

28. Client teaching regarding long-term corticosteroid therapy should include
   a. the need for periodic blood glucose assessment
   b. the need to take the medication late in the day to avoid insomnia
   c. the possibility of enhanced wound healing
   d. the need for a diet low in iron

Rationale
Correct answer: a.
Answer (a) is correct because an adverse effect of corticosteroid therapy is hyperglycemia. Answer (b) is incorrect because it is generally recommended that a client on long-term corticosteroid therapy take their medication early in the day to help prevent insomnia. Answer (c) is incorrect because one of the adverse effects is delayed wound healing and masking of infections. Answer (d) is incorrect because there are no recommendations to decrease iron intake.

29. Clients receiving long-term corticosteroid therapy may require dietary modifications. Which of the following statements is true about special diets for long-term corticosteroid therapy?
   a. A potassium-restricted diet may be needed due to sodium and water retention.
   b. A low-protein, low-carbohydrate diet may be needed to correct negative nitrogen balance.
   c. A potassium-restricted diet may be needed due to potassium retention.
   d. Increased calcium is encouraged to help prevent osteoporosis.

Rationale
Correct answer: d.
Answer (d) is correct. Clients on long-term corticosteroid therapy are at risk for osteoporosis due to an increased excretion of calcium. Therefore, calcium supplements are very important. Answers (a), (b), and (c) are incorrect as the client may need a high-carbohydrate, high-protein diet and foods high in potassium to maintain adequate nutrition.

30. Anatomic and physiological factors that affect drug absorption in the elderly include
   a. increased rate of passage of drugs through the lower gastrointestinal tract.
   b. decreased gastric emptying, thus increasing the time medications remain in stomach.
   c. increased gastric acidity affects the way tablets dissolve.
   d. thinner skin surface delays absorption of topical drugs.

Rationale
Correct answer: b.
Answer (b) is correct. In older adults gastric emptying is slowed and takes a longer time, therefore the medication remains in the stomach longer. Answers (a) and (c) are incorrect due to drugs taking longer to absorb in older adults, and gastric acid production is decreased in the older adult. Answer (d) is incorrect because thinner skin surfaces actually increase absorption of topical medications.

31. Factors that may place elderly people at risk for medication related problems include
   a. vision loss, hearing loss, and using the same pharmacy so accurate profiles may be kept.
   b. memory loss, hearing loss, and using the same pharmacy so that prescriptions errors may be caught easily.

(continued)

c. recent memory loss, vision loss, and taking multiple medications due to chronic health problems.
d. maintaining accurate profile at the pharmacy, asking physician for a sample of the prescription to assess the medications effects, and following the pharmacist's instructions.

Rationale

Correct answer: c.

Answer (c) is correct. These changes may occur in the older adult and many older clients are on eight or more medications per day. Answers (a) and (b) are incorrect, even though the cognitive and sensory changes are possible, using the same pharmacy for all the prescriptions helps prevent medication related problems. Answer (d) is incorrect because these are examples of methods that help prevent medication related problem.

32. A serious concern in health care is the development of increasing numbers of antibiotic-resistant strains of bacteria. To help prevent this problem, clients should be taught to
    a. complete the entire prescription of antibiotics
    b. share their antibiotic prescription with other family members with the same symptoms
    c. stop taking their antibiotic medications when they begin to feel better
    d. request a prescription for antibiotics from the physician when they have a viral infection

Rationale

Correct answer: a.

Answer (a) is correct. Nurses should instruct clients to complete the entire course of therapy of antibiotics. Answer (b) is incorrect. Clients should be instructed not to share any of their medications with another individual. Answer (c) is incorrect. Clients should be instructed to take the full course of therapy and not to stop taking their antibiotics when they feel better. Answer (d) is incorrect. Antibiotics are not the correct treatment for viral infections.

33. The nurse monitors the client for adverse effects of medications. What is a major disadvantage of using broad-spectrum antibiotics to treat infections?
    a. They are only effective against a small number of microorganisms.
    b. They destroy normal flora, enabling superinfections to develop.
    c. They are not effective against viruses.
    d. They are more likely to cause an allergic reaction.

Rationale

Correct answer: b.

Answer (b) is correct. Broad-spectrum antibiotics may destroy normal flora in the client's mouth and gastrointestinal tract, causing oral candidiasis and diarrhea. Answer (a) is incorrect. Broad-spectrum antibiotics are effective against a large number of organisms. Answer (c) is not the best answer to the question because antibiotics are not effective against viruses. Answer (d) is not accurate information.

34. The nurse receives a medication order with no route specified. What is the best action by the nurse?
    a. Give the medication orally because that is the most common route.
    b. Ask the client how he usually takes the medication.
    c. Call the physician to clarify the order.
    d. Ask another nurse which route to use.

Rationale

Correct answer: c.

Answer (c) is correct. The nurse should always call the physician to verify the route. Answers (a), (b), and (d) are incorrect and do not constitute safe nursing practice.

35. The physician orders nitroglycerin (Nitro Bid) 0.4 mg SL now. Which of the following options would indicate that the nurse correctly administered the medication?
    a. Tablet placed under the client's tongue and client instructed to allow medication to dissolve.
    b. Tablet given to the client with 8 oz of water after checking BP and heart rate.
    c. Tablet given to the client with 4 oz of juice to assist with masking bitter flavor.
    d. Tablet placed under client's tongue and client instructed to chew slowly to assist with absorption.

Rationale

Correct answer: a.

Answer (a) is correct. The order is for the tablet to be administered SL (sublingual). Answers (b), (c), and (d) indicate that the client is to swallow the medication.

36. When administering intramuscular medication to a client who is 5 ft 6 in. tall and weighs 118 lb, which of the following needles should the nurse select?
    a. 27 gauge, 1 in.
    b. 23 gauge, 2 in.
    c. 25 gauge, 1½ in.
    d. 22 gauge, 1 in.

Rationale

Correct answer: d.

Answer (d) is correct. The client is 5 ft 6 in. tall and only weighs 118 lb, which indicates that the client is probably slender without excess body fat. A 22-gauge needle is the normal size gauge for medications that are not viscous, and a 1-in. needle should be the correct length for the client's body built. Answer (a) is incorrect because the 27 gauge is too small for an intramuscular injection. Answer (b) is incorrect because the length of 2 in. is too long for this client's height and weight indicators. Answer (c) is incorrect because the gauge is too small for an intramuscular injection and the length is too long for this client's height and weight indicators.

37. Which of the following rights do clients have in regard to medication? The right to
    a. know the names of the other clients on the hall.
    b. refuse medication and know the names of their medication.
    c. information concerning side effects of the medications they are taking at home only.
    d. know all of the medication that the nurse administers to all the clients.

Rationale

Correct answer: b.

Answer (b) is correct. Clients have the right to know the names, doses, adverse effects, contraindications, indications, etc. of all their medications and they have the right to refuse medication. Answer (a) is incorrect because it violates client confidentiality in most institutions. Answer (c) is incorrect only because it indicates "at home only" in the answer. Answer (d) is incorrect because it violates the rights of other clients.

38. What direction should the nurse give to a client in regard to the use of NSAIDs prior to scheduled surgery?
    a. Take as usual as long as recommended dose is not exceeded.
    b. Do not take after midnight the day of surgery.
    c. Gradually taper to zero during the week prior to surgery.
    a. Discontinue 7 days prior to elective surgery.

Rationale

Correct answer: d.

Answer (d) is correct. NSAIDs should be discontinued 1 week prior to elective surgery because of their anticlotting effect.

39. The nurse should instruct the client taking an antilipemic about the regular need for which type of examination?
    a. Colonoscopy
    b. Dental
    c. Ophthalmic
    d. Hearing

Rationale

Correct answer: c.

Answer (c) is correct. An association has been found between the use of antilipemics and the development of cataracts so regular eye examinations are recommended. Antilipemics are not known to affect the large bowel, teeth, or hearing.

40. Which question should be asked of a young adult female for whom penicillin has been ordered?
    a. Do you drink milk?
    b. Are you allergic to shellfish?
    c. Do you take birth control pills?
    d. Have you ever had vaginitis?

Rationale

Correct answer: c.

Answer (c) is correct. Penicillin can inhibit the effectiveness of oral contraceptives so a backup form of birth control is needed when taking penicillin.

CHAPTER 15

Test Plan Category:

Physiological Integrity

Sub-category: Pharmacological and Parenteral Therapies—Part 2

Topics: Parenteral/Intravenous Therapy
Central Venous Access Devices
Blood and Blood Products
Total Parenteral Nutrition

INTRAVENOUS THERAPY

INDICATIONS FOR INTRAVENOUS THERAPY

- Administer intravenous medications
- Maintain fluid volume and electrolyte balance
- Replace fluid volume and electrolyte losses
- Provide nutritional support

ADVANTAGES OF INTRAVENOUS THERAPY

- Faster absorption and distribution of drugs and fluids
- Provision of access route for a client who is unconscious, NPO
- Provision of access route for delivery of medications and fluids in an emergency
- Administration of medications that are only available in intravenous parenteral form

DISADVANTAGES OF PARENTERAL THERAPY

- Potential for local and systemic complications
- Allergic reaction to a medication, fluid product
- Hypervolemia
- Painful for client

LOCAL COMPLICATIONS OF INTRAVENOUS THERAPY

- Phlebitis: inflammation of vein causing pain at site, redness, and heat along the length of vein
- Thrombosis: blood clot inside vein causing the infusion to slow or stop, swelling, tenderness, redness, and heat along the vein
- Infiltration: leaking of intravenous fluid or medication into the extravascular tissue causing edema and coolness at or above the insertion site

- Infection of site: caused by invasion of microorganisms and site may be warm, red, swollen, and painful
- Extravasation: caused by the leakage of a vesicant substance into the extravascular tissue. Edema and coolness are signs of extravasation at or above the insertion site

Think Smart/Test Smart

In the above list of local complications of intravenous therapy, signs and symptoms of the complications are presented with slightly different, but interchangeable wordings, any of which might be used as part of an NCLEX-RN test question. For example, it states that "infiltration causes edema and coolness at or above the insertion site." This could have been stated as "edema and coolness are signs of infiltration" or "edema and coolness occur at or above the site."

When testing knowledge of these facts, ways to ask questions include

When assessing an IV site for infiltration, for which signs would the nurse observe?

When assessing an IV site, the nurse notes the area above the site is swollen and cool. How should the nurse interpret this assessment data?

SYSTEMIC COMPLICATIONS OF INTRAVENOUS THERAPY

- Circulatory overload: Excess circulating fluid caused by fluids infusing at a faster rate than client can accommodate.
  —Assess for shortness of breath, increased respiratory and heart rate, elevated blood pressure, edema, and distended jugular veins.
- Allergic reaction: Client may be allergic to medication, intravenous solution, or intravenous catheter.
- Sepsis: Caused by microorganisms entering the circulatory system.
  —Assess for chills, fever, tachycardia, hypotension, change in level of consciousness, and leukocytosis.
- Catheter embolism caused by a piece of the catheter breaking off and entering the circulation.
  —Assess for pain along the vein, hypotension, weak, rapid pulse, a change in level of consciousness.

VASCULAR ACCESS DEVICES

SHORT PERIPHERAL CATHETER

- It is inserted into veins of the hand and forearm of adults: dorsal, and basilic, cephalic
- Three fourths of an inch to 1¼ inch in length, 14–26 gauge
- Rotation to different sites after 72 hours
- Use 18 gauge for blood administration

MIDLINE CATHETER

- It is inserted through the basilic vein at the antecubital area, with catheter tip located in the upper arm at the axilla level
- 6–8 inch in length, single, double, and triple lumens
- Rotation to different sites after 3–4 weeks
- It is used for clients who will receive intravenous medications over several weeks

PERIPHERALLY INSERTED CENTRAL VENOUS ACCESS DEVICE

- It is inserted through the basilic or cephalic veins with the catheter tip located in the superior vena cava
- 40–60 cm in length
- Chest X-ray is required prior to use
- Rotation to different sites may not be necessary for months/year
- It is used for clients who receive intravenous medications over a long period of time, and parenteral nutrition

NONTUNNELED CENTRAL VENOUS ACCESS DEVICE

- It is inserted through the jugular or subclavian veins, with the catheter tip located in the superior vena cava

- 15–20 cm in length, double or triple lumens
- Chest X-ray is required prior to use
- It is used for short term, acute situation, not for home care

TUNNELED CENTRAL VENOUS ACCESS DEVICE

- It is surgically inserted with the distal catheter tip located in the superior vena cava and the proximal end is tunneled subcutaneously to an exit site on the client's trunk
- It is used when intravenous therapy is long term and will be used frequently

IMPLANTED PORTS

- Implanted ports are surgically placed in the upper chest or upper arm area with the catheter inserted into the subclavian or internal jugular veins
- Nurse accesses the port using a noncoring needle, therefore, the client may experience discomfort with each access
- It is used when intravenous therapy needs will be long term

CLIENT PREPARATION FOR INTRAVENOUS THERAPY PROCEDURES

Client teaching for self-care

Preinsertion of Catheter

Provide information to the client about

- the physician's order for infusion therapy
- rationale for infusion therapy
- specific type of therapy ordered
- expected time frame therapy may be needed
- validate allergy information with client
- type of catheter, tubing, dressing, and rate controlling device required
- expected location of venipuncture and insertion of catheter
- postinsertion X-ray if a central venous catheter is inserted
- specific type of activity limitations
- signs or symptoms the client should report to the health care provider

Initiation of Intravenous Therapy Using a Peripheral Vascular Access Device

- Review physician's order for intravenous therapy.
- Review client's allergies.
- Review type of fluid and medication to be administered.
- Assess client for history of CVA, mastectomy, orthopedic injuries or surgery, lymphedema, or impaired circulation in area of expected venipuncture. Avoid these areas.
- Introduce yourself to client.
- Identify the correct client by checking the armband against the physician's order and use a second agency approved method of client identification.
- Conduct client education regarding the venipuncture and infusion therapy.
- Gather necessary equipment: vascular access device, tourniquet and dressing kit, intravenous solution and administration tubing if ordered, rate-controlling device if needed.
- Wash hands using approved agency procedure.
- Explain to client what you are doing throughout procedure.
- Provide privacy.
- Assess venipuncture locations and note areas of edema, previous venipunctures, veins that are sclerotic or phlebitic, or any areas of inflammation.
- Apply tourniquet 3–4 inches above the expected insertion site and tighten enough so that only venous, not arterial, blood flow is impeded. Release tourniquet within 4 minutes of application and wait at least 2 minutes before reapplying.
- Use other interventions to locate appropriate vein when needed. Place extremity below the level of the client's heart and apply warm compress, ask client to make a fist or open and close his hand several times.
- After locating an acceptable vein, release tourniquet, prepare supplies and equipment and prep insertion site for venipuncture. Remember to be aware of tape, latex, iodine, or shell fish allergies.
- Set up all the necessary supplies on the overbed table, cut tape to a desired length, open packages of alcohol, povidone-iodine or aqueous chlorhexidine gluconate, gauze, and transparent dressing.
- Apply gloves.
- Reapply the tourniquet to client's extremity.
- Remove the needle cover of over-the-needle catheter and inspect the catheter.
- Anchor the selected vein below the intended insertion site using your thumb and pull the skin taut.
- Hold the vascular access device by the needle hub flash chamber, with the bevel up and insert the needle into the skin at an angle of approximately 20 degrees.

- Observe the flash chamber for a blood return.
- Upon entering the vein and seeing the blood return, lower the device flush to the skin and advance the catheter tip further into the vein.
- Release the tourniquet.
- Remove the needle, and connect the vascular access device to the selected intravenous tubing.
- Secure the catheter and tubing to prevent dislodgement.
- Open the flow clamp to the intravenous solution or flush the catheter with saline solution to check for infiltration.
- Dress the insertion site per agency protocol.
- Discard the needle in the sharps container.
- Remove gloves, discard them properly, and wash hands.
- Label the insertion site with date, time, type and size of device, and your initials.
- Remind client of any activity restrictions, and to report signs and symptoms.
- Inquire if client has any questions or concerns.
- Document on client's medical record: insertion date and time of insertion, the extremity and vein used, type and size of device, the type and rate of solution administered, rate controlling device in use, as well as the client response.

Administration and Monitoring of Intravenous Therapy Using a Peripheral Vascular Access Device

- Review physician's order and select correct solution using the "5 Rights" of medication administration.
- Observe solution for clarity and note integrity of container; do not use if cloudy or otherwise not clear or if seals on container have been broken.
- Accurately calculate and set infusion rate.
- Use electronic infusion device as institution designates, especially important for infants and other clients at risk for fluid overload.
- Apply time-tape to fluid container to assist in monitoring flow rate accuracy.
- Assess flow rate every hour.
- Assess the catheter site for early signs of local reactions: infiltration, phlebitis, thrombosis, infection, and extravasation.
- Assess client for systemic reactions: allergic reactions, circulatory overload, sepsis, and catheter embolism
- Use aseptic techniques when performing venipuncture, applying or changing dressing, changing or accessing tubing, and accessing catheter
- Determine patency of catheter prior to injection of intravenous medications
- Document type of fluid and medication infusions, infusion rate, site assessment, I&O, and client's reaction.
- Document central venous access infusion rate/type/and I&O.

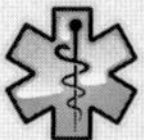

Nursing Intervention Alert

Always monitor intravenous flow rate and infusion site at least every hour.

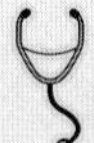

Assessment Alert

Monitor client for sign of infection at catheter insertion site: redness, swelling, heat, pain, and drainage.

Removal of a Peripherally Inserted Vascular Access Device

- Review physician's order to discontinue intravenous therapy
- Review client's allergies
- Introduce yourself to client
- Identify the correct client by checking the armband against the physician's order and use a second agency approved method of client identification
- Provide information to the client regarding removing the catheter
  - —The physician's order to discontinue infusion therapy
  - —Rationale for discontinuing the infusion therapy
  - —Procedure used to remove the dressing and catheter
  - —Expected discomfort associated with procedure
  - —Site care after catheter is removed: keep site clean and dry
  - —Signs or symptoms the client should report to the health care provider: redness, warmth, discomfort, and drainage
  - —Specific type of activity limitations
- Gather necessary supplies
- Wash hands using approved agency procedure
- Explain to client what you are doing throughout procedure
- Provide privacy
- Assess venipuncture location and note areas of edema, veins that are sclerotic or phlebitic, or any areas of inflammation
- Turn off rate controlling device, and clamp intravenous tubing
- Prepare dressing supplies
- Don gloves
- Remove tape, and loosen edges of transparent dressing carefully, using alcohol or adhesive remover if necessary
- Stabilize catheter while removing dressing completely
- Hold gauze over the insertion site while gently removing the catheter: do not pull on catheter if resistance is met
- Inspect catheter to ensure entire catheter has been removed
- Apply pressure to insertion site for 1 minute or until there is no bleeding

- Assess site and apply dressing per agency protocol
- Dispose of device in sharps container
- Remove gloves, discard them properly, and wash hands
- Inquire if client has any questions or concerns
- Document on client's medical record: date and time of removal, the extremity and vein used, type and size of device, condition of catheter upon removal, as well as the client response

Initiation of Intravenous Therapy Using a Centrally Inserted Vascular Access Device

- Review physician's order for intravenous therapy.
- Review client allergies.
- Review type of fluid and medication to be administered.
- Introduce yourself to client.
- Identify the correct client by checking the armband against the physician's order and use a second agency approved method of client identification.
- Conduct client education regarding the venipuncture and infusion therapy. Instruct client that physician may request that he/she perform a Valsalva maneuver at a point during the procedure. Instruct client that he/she will need to take a deep breath, hold it and bear down for 10 seconds when instructed to do so by the physician.
- Gather necessary equipment: central venous access device, insertion and dressing kit, sterile gown, masks, sterile gloves, intravenous solution and administration tubing if ordered, rate-controlling device. Wash hands using approved agency procedure.
- Explain to client what the physician and nurse are doing throughout procedure.
- Provide privacy.
- Apply mask, cap, goggles, gown, and gloves.
- Assist physician during procedure as needed.
- Monitor client's condition during and after catheter insertion.
- Apply dressing per agency protocol.
- Inquire if client has questions or concerns.
- Document the insertion date and time, type, size and length of catheter, the name of physician who inserted the catheter, and the client's response to the procedure.
- Follow physician orders regarding obtaining a preinfusion chest X-ray.
- Monitor client's condition and report results of chest X-ray to the physician.

Administration and Monitoring of Intravenous Therapy Using a Centrally Inserted Vascular Access Device

- Review physician's order and select correct solution using the "5 Rights" of medication administration.
- Explain therapy to client and family.
- Assess client's vital signs, I&O, weight.
- Observe expiration date and clarity of solution.
- Accurately calculate and set infusion rate.
- Administer using an electronic infusion device and monitor rate of infusion every hour. Maintain accurate rate of flow.
- Assess client for systemic reactions: allergic reactions, sepsis, and catheter embolism.
- Identify potential misconnections through risk assessment of all existing catheters.
- As part of the handoff communication, follow standardized "line reconciliation" process.
- Educate all clinical and nonclinical staff about the hazards of misconnecting tubing and devices.
- Maintain aseptic techniques when changing solution, accessing tubing, and dressing.
- Inspect catheter insertion site for redness, swelling, heat, drainage.
- Assess for signs of infection: elevated temperature and WBC, chills, redness at catheter site.
- Document fluid and medication infusions, I&O, and client's reaction.

Removal of a Centrally Inserted Nontunneled Vascular Access Device

- Obtain certification by your agency to perform procedure
- Review physician's order to discontinue the centrally inserted vascular access device intravenous therapy
- Review client allergies
- Introduce yourself to client
- Identify the correct client by checking the armband against the physician's order and use a second agency approved method of client identification
- Conduct client education regarding removing the catheter. Review the Valsalva maneuver with client
- Gather necessary supplies: dressing kit, mask, gloves, suture removal kit
- Wash hands using approved agency procedure
- Explain to client what you are doing throughout the procedure
- Provide privacy
- Assess venipuncture location and note areas of edema, redness, or warmth
- Turn off rate controlling device, and clamp intravenous tubing
- Prepare dressing supplies
- Position the bed in Trendelenburg or flat position, according to agency protocol and client condition
- Don gloves and mask
- Remove tape, and loosen edges of transparent dressing carefully, using alcohol or adhesive remover if necessary

- Stabilize catheter while removing dressing completely
- Cleanse the insertion site and surrounding area with alcohol and povidone-iodine (if client is not allergic)
- Carefully remove sutures
- Hold gauze over the insertion site and ask the client to perform the Valsalva maneuver while gently removing the catheter: do not pull on catheter if resistance is met
- Ask client to breathe normally
- Apply pressure to insertion site for 2 minutes or until there is no bleeding
- Apply dressing per agency protocol, making sure that air can not enter the site area
- Observe catheter for length, integrity, drainage
- Dispose of device in sharps container if catheter is intact and no signs of infection are present
- Remove gloves, discard them properly, and wash hands
- Inquire if client has any questions or concerns
- Document on client's medical record: date and time of removal, type and size of device, condition of catheter upon removal, as well as the client response

RATE-CONTROLLING DEVICES

General Principles for Properly Using a Rate-Controlling Device

- Monitor the client's infusion rate and insertion site carefully during intravenous therapy.
- Be aware that rate-controlling devices may malfunction, therefore, always monitor the client and assess the functioning of the device often.
- Know how to correctly operate the device.
- Understand that controllers use a sensor to count drops, and monitor the flow of the fluid, and they rely on gravity to create fluid flow.
- Be aware that pumps create fluid flow under pressure, and are more accurate than controllers.
- Always respond quickly to an alarm from a rate-controlling device. Never silence the alarm and do not follow up on why the alarm is occurring. Always troubleshoot the device and determine the specific problem quickly.

PARENTERAL FLUIDS

- Normal plasma osmolarity is approximately 290 mOsm/l
- Parenteral fluids with similar characteristics are isotonic
- Parenteral fluids with less than 250 mOsm/l are hypotonic
- Parenteral fluids with greater that 350 mOsm/l are hypertonic

Isotonic Solutions

- 0.9% saline (normal saline)
- 5% dextrose in water (D5W)
- Ringer's lactate
- 5% dextrose in 0.225% saline (D5¼ NS)

Hypotonic Solutions

- 0.45% Saline (½ NS)

Hypertonic Solutions

- 5% dextrose in 0.9% normal saline (D5NS)
- 5% dextrose in 0.45% normal saline (D5 ½ NS)
- 5% dextrose in Ringer's lactate (D5 RL)
- 10% dextrose in water (D10W)

PARENTERAL NUTRITION

TOTAL PARENTERAL NUTRITION

Solutions may contain

- Dextrose
- Amino acids
- Trace elements
- Vitamins and minerals
- Emulsified fats
- Heparin, insulin, and other medications specific for client

TYPES OF PARENTERAL NUTRITION

Peripherally Administered Parenteral Nutrition

- It is infused through a peripheral venous catheter
- Ten percent dextrose solution with vitamins, minerals, trace elements, and electrolytes added
- 10% or 20% lipid emulsions

Centrally Administered Parenteral Nutrition

- It is infused through a central venous access device
- Greater than 10% dextrose solution with vitamins, minerals, trace elements, electrolytes, and insulin added
- 10–20% lipid emulsions

INDICATIONS FOR TOTAL PARENTERAL NUTRITION (TPN THERAPY)

- Inadequate oral intake or need for NPO status for extended period of time
- Increased metabolic needs
- Bowel obstruction
- Inflammatory bowel disease and related intestinal disorders
- Radiation enteritis
- Preterm or newborn infants who require surgery
- Severe malnutrition disorders

MONITORING EFFECTS OF TOTAL PARENTERAL NUTRITION THERAPY: NURSING IMPLICATIONS

- Explain therapy to client and family.
- Assess nutritional status, daily weights, vital signs, and I&O.
- Assess for signs of infection: elevated temperature and WBC, chills, redness, edema, warmth, and drainage at catheter site.
- Monitor electrolyte levels/assess for signs of electrolyte imbalances.
- Assess oral mucosa and provide frequent mouth care.
- Compare solution contents with those listed in the physician's order.
- Check expiration date and clarity of TPN solution; do not use if expired or cloudy.
- Administer using an electronic infusion device and monitor rate of infusion every hour. Maintain accurate rate of flow. Do not try to "catch up" solution if infusion rate was slower than intended.
- Keep solution cold, warm to room temperature before administering.
- Discontinue use of any solution not infused within 24 hours.

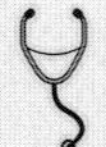

Assessment Alert

Monitor client's blood glucose levels every 6 hours, or as designated by the institutional policy.

- Administer insulin as ordered; may be needed because of the large amount of glucose in the TPN solution.
- Do not stop TPN suddenly due to high glucose content; if TPN administration is interrupted, give 5–10% dextrose to prevent hypoglycemia.
- Maintain aseptic technique when changing solution and tubing every 24 hours and dressing every 24 hours if using gauze or every 48–72 hours per agency policy.
- Position client flat when changing dressing and tubing.
- Tape connections securely.
- Assess for symptoms of hyperglycemia: weakness, headache, thirst, nausea, and fast respirations.
- Assess for complications: fluid overload, especially in the elderly, air embolism, osmotic diuresis or shifts of electrolytes caused by high glucose formulas.
- Monitor for pneumothorax, hemothorax or injury to brachial plexus due to insertion of central venous caterer.
- Encourage client activities.
- If needed, teach client/caregiver about administration of TPN, for example, hand washing, care of equipment, aseptic technique and provide a 24-hour phone number to call for any problems.

BLOOD AND BLOOD PRODUCTS

WHOLE BLOOD

- It is administered in incidents such as acute hemorrhage where a client has lost greater than 25% of their total blood volume
- Volume for transfusion is approximately 450–500 ml

PACKED RED BLOOD CELLS (PRBCs) AND FROZEN RED CELLS

- PRBCs and frozen RBCs are administered to clients with decreased hemoglobin (usually less than 7) from loss of blood related to trauma or surgery or to clients with conditions that affect red blood cell production who are symptomatic

- Volume of component for transfusion is 250–325 ml per bag
- These are infused within 2–4 hours

PLATELETS

- Platelets are administered to clients with bleeding due to thrombocytopenia or platelet dysfunction, platelet counts less than 20,000 (normal = 150,000–350,000)
- Volume of component for transfusion ranges from 200–300 ml per bag
- Platelets are infused over 15–30 minutes using the designated administration set

FRESH FROZEN PLASMA

- Fresh frozen plasma is administered to clients with clotting disorders who are actively bleeding or at high risk for bleeding
- Volume of component for transfusion is approximately 200 ml
- It is infused immediately after thawing over a 15–30 minute time frame

CRYOPRECIPITATE

- Cryoprecipitate is administered to clients with a decreased fibrinogen levels of less than 100 mg/dl
- Volume of component for transfusion is 10–20 ml per unit
- It is infused in a 15–30 minute time frame

COAGULATION FACTOR CONCENTRATES

Factor VIII

—Factor VIII is administered to clients with hemophilia A (congenital factor VIII deficiency) or von Willebrand's disease who are bleeding or preparing for an invasive procedure

Factor IX

—Factor IX is administered to clients with hemophilia B (Christmas disease), factor IX deficiency who are bleeding or preparing for an invasive procedure

Antithrombin III

—Antithrombin III is administered to clients with a congenital antithrombin III deficiency who have an acute risk of a venous thrombo-embolic event

IMMUNE SERUM GLOBULINS

- Nonspecific immune serum globulins are administered to prevent infection in clients with
  —poorly functioning immune systems: HIV infection
  —chronic lymphocytic leukemia
  —following bone marrow transplantation
- Specific immune serum globulins are administered to provide immunity prior to or following exposure to disease specific antigens
  —Hepatitis B immune globulin
  —Varicella-zoster immune globulin
  —Rh immune globulin
  —Cytomegalovirus immune globulin
  —Lymphocyte immune globulin

GRANULOCYTES (WHITE CELL)

- Granulocytes are administered to replace WBCs in clients with severe neutropenia and a life threatening infection.
- Volume of component for transfusion is approximately 400 ml of plasma
- These are infused within a 50–60-minute time frame.
- Severe reactions may occur. Monitor vital signs, level of consciousness, and respiratory status every 15 minutes throughout transfusion.

ALBUMIN

- Albumin is administered to clients as an expansion of plasma volume to correct fluid volume deficit
- Replacement of albumin is done for clients with renal or liver disease
- It mobilizes fluid from extravascular tissues back into the intravascular space

BLOOD TYPING AND CROSSMATCHING PRIOR TO TRANSFUSION OF BLOOD

General Principles

- Blood typing and crossmatching must be completed prior to a blood transfusion
- The physician will order the client's blood to be typed and crossmatched and a specimen will be drawn from the client and sent to the lab for testing and comparison with donor blood
- Typing is a process that determines the blood type (A, B, AB,O)

- Crossmatching is a process that correctly matches compatibilities between the blood types of the recipient and the donor
- Individuals with type O blood are considered "universal donors", but may only receive type O blood
- Clients with type A should only receive type A blood, but may receive type O in an emergency
- Clients with type B should only receive type B blood, but may receive type O in an emergency
- Clients with type AB blood are "universal recipients: and should only receive type AB blood but may, in an emergency, receive all four types of blood.
- Clients who have Rh-positive blood may receive a transfusion from an Rh-positive or Rh-negative donor
- Clients with Rh-negative blood should not receive Rh-positive blood
- Blood is also tested for the Rh determination, antibodies, HIV, hepatitis, and other viruses

TRANSFUSION REACTIONS

Allergic Transfusion Reaction

- Allergic transfusion reaction is caused by foreign plasma proteins
- Its signs and symptoms may include urticaria, itching, bronchospasm, and anaphylaxis.
- It occurs at anytime during infusion and up to 24 hours after transfusion
- Treatment may include stopping transfusion temporarily and administering antihistamines.

Hemolytic Transfusion Reaction

- Hemolytic transfusion reaction is caused by ABO or Rh incompatibility.
- Its signs and symptoms may include chest or back pain, fever, chills, shortness of breath, headache, change in level of consciousness, and hypotension.
- Treatment includes stopping infusion, send blood component and administration set to the lab, follow the institution's transfusion reaction protocol for follow-up lab samples, monitoring vital signs and observing client for shock.

Circulatory Overload

- Circulatory overload is caused by fluid volume excess and may be precipitated if blood product is infused too rapidly. Older adults are a high-risk population group for this problem.
- Its signs and symptoms include dyspnea, hypertension, tachycardia, distended jugular veins, and a change in level of consciousness.
- Treatment includes slowing or stopping infusion, administering diuretics, monitoring I&O.

Febrile Transfusion Reaction

- Febrile transfusion reaction is caused by recipient antibodies reacting with white cell antigens in the blood component
- Its signs and symptoms include fever, chills, nausea, vomiting, tachycardia, and hypotension
- Treatment may include stopping the infusion and managing the symptoms

Bacterial Transfusion Reaction

- Bacterial transfusion reaction is caused by bacteria introduced into the component at the time of collection or during processing or storage
- Its signs and symptoms include fever, chills, hypotension, and tachycardia
- Treatment includes immediately stopping the transfusion, following the protocol for transfusion reaction at the institution, blood cultures and broad spectrum antimicrobial agents may be prescribed

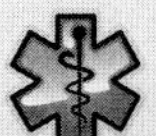

Nursing Intervention Alert

Always follow the institution's policy if a transfusion reaction occurs. There will be a step-by-step protocol to implement.

MONITORING EFFECTS OF BLOOD AND BLOOD PRODUCT ADMINISTRATION: NURSING IMPLICATIONS

Pretransfusion Care

- Assess vital signs, laboratory values.
- Review physician's order for blood products.
- Perform venipuncture and insert an 18-Ga catheter if peripheral line is required.
- Obtain blood products from blood bank.
- Follow institutional policy for verifying product with another RN, verify client's name and blood type, and compare product with transfusion record, client's chart and identification band. Check the expiration date on the component.

Transfusion Care

- Prime the appropriate blood product administration set. Use only 0.9% Normal saline if dilution or piggyback solution is required. Use standard precautions.
- Do not administer any medications using the blood administration tubing while blood is infusing.
- Assess vital signs before beginning the transfusion.
- Determine the infusion rate per hour and gtt/min. During the first 15 minutes, administer the blood component slowly.
- Remain with client during the first 15 minutes of the transfusion and obtain another set of vital signs.
- Place call bell within client's reach and instruct to call if experiencing pain at infusion site, back or chest pain, chills, fever, shortness of breath, or any other concern.
- Document blood component type and unit number, time infusion started, and vital signs.
- Monitor client every 30 minutes throughout transfusion for adverse reactions and obtain vital signs.

Posttransfusion Care

- Assess vital signs
- Assess for adverse reactions
- Discontinue the transfusion using standard precautions
- Document transfusion stop time, vital signs, and assessment finding related to adverse reactions
- Continue to monitor client for delayed adverse reactions

Client Controlled Analgesia (CCA)

Analgesic administered from a pump-controlled syringe attached to an IV line.

Patterns of administration

- Basal rate: small amount of drug administered continually without client action
- Client controlled dosing only: Medication administered only when the client pushes button
- Basal rate plus client dosing: small amount of analgesic administered continually with additional amount given when client pushes the button

Dose

- Total amount of analgesic that can be delivered to the client in a set period of time is determined by the health care provider.
- A "lockout" period prevents the client from getting too much medication too soon even if the button is repeatedly pushed.

Use

Control of acute pain postoperatively or posttrauma; control of chronic pain related to diseases such as cancer and sickle cell crisis.

Nursing Process Elements

- Explain PCA to clients.
- Caution others not to push button for client.
- Allay fears of becoming addicted. Explain that often less medication is taken because medication is given when needed without a wait and pain does not have a chance to become severe.
- Assess for sleepiness and bradypnea, which are signs of overmedication.
- Assess for restlessness and complaints of discomfort, which are signs of insufficient medication.
- Assess for medication side effects including nausea, pruritus, and difficulty urinating.
- Assist client as needed with activities such as changing clothes or getting out of bed.
- Instruct client to report:
  —Excessive sleepiness
  —Vomiting
  —Unmanageable pain
  —Pain, warmth, redness, edema or bleeding of the IV site.
  —Increased blood in the tube going to the pump.
  —No more medication in the pump.

EPIDURAL INFUSION

- Delivery of a local anesthetic and a narcotic analgesic via a computer-controlled pump directly into the epidural space at either a steady rate or in response to client-controlled dosing.
- Blocks impulse transmission in sensory nerves thereby blocking pain as well as heat, cold, and pressure without affecting movement.
- Client may experience transient mild weakness, tingling, or numbness in the tissues below the level of the block.

Use

- Postoperative pain management
- Chronic pain management

Advantages of Epidural Infusion

- Provides more consistent pain management
- Reduces amount of opioid requirement overall

- Decreases client sedation
- Increases client's ability to be active, cough, and deep breathe after surgery

Contraindication

Bleeding problems

Complications of Epidural Infusion

- Infection
- Bleeding at catheter site
- Leakage of cerebral spinal fluid
- Opioid related adverse effect such as respiratory depression, hypotension, urinary retention, constipation

Nursing Process Elements

- Review physician's order and select correct solution using the "5 Rights" of medication administration.
- Explain therapy to client and family.
- Assess client's pain level, vital signs, I&O: pain level should be checked on coughing or moving to judge effectiveness of block.
- Monitor client's respiratory rate and pattern frequently.
- Assess for signs of urinary retention and constipation.
- Assess motor power and sedation level.
- Observe expiration date and clarity of solution.
- Accurately calculate and set infusions rate.
- Administer using an electronic infusion device and monitor rate of infusion every hour. Maintain accurate rate of flow.
- Assess client for systemic reactions: allergic reactions, sepsis, and catheter embolism.
- Identify potential misconnections through risk assessment of all existing catheters.
- As part of the handoff communication, follow standardized "line reconciliation" process.
- Educate all clinical and nonclinical staff about the hazards of misconnecting tubing and devices.
- Maintain aseptic techniques when changing solution, accessing tubing, and dressing.
- Inspect catheter insertion site for redness, swelling, heat, and drainage.
- Assess for signs of infection: elevated temperature and WBC, chills, redness at catheter site.
- Document fluid and medication infusions, I&O, pain assessment, and client's reaction.
- Position/reposition as needed to prevent skin damage related to impaired sensation.
- Change position slowly in relation to gravity because of the risk of hypostatic hypotension.
- Have naloxone (Narcan), sodium chloride 0.9% diluent and injection equipment immediately available (Cox, 2001).

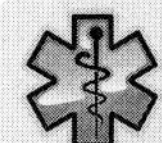

Nursing Intervention Alert

Nurses should follow the "line reconciliation" process by rechecking tubing and catheter connections, tracing all client tubes and catheters to their sources for correct route, and labeling all tubes and catheters at the point(s) of connection.

WORKSHEET

MATCHING QUESTIONS

Match the types of blood product with the specific client condition requiring an infusion of a blood product.

Blood Product	Condition
1. ______ Whole blood	a. Thrombocytopenia
2. ______ Packed red blood cells	b. Client lost > 25% of total blood volume
3. ______ Platelets	c. Fibrinogen levels < 100
4. ______ Cryoprecipitate	d. Hemoglobin < 7

MATCHING QUESTIONS

Match the types of parenteral fluids with the specific category of osmolarity.

Parenteral Fluid	Category of Osmolarity
5. ______ D5W	a. Hypertonic
6. ______ 0.45% Normal saline	b. Hypotonic
7. ______ D51/2 Normal saline	c. Isotonic
8. ______ Ringer's lactate	

MATCHING QUESTIONS

Match the types of intravenous catheters with the site of insertion.

Types of Catheters	Insertion Sites
9. ______ Midline catheter	a. Surgically inserted with the distal catheter tip located in the superior vena cava and the proximal end tunneled subcutaneously to an exit site on the client's trunk
10. ______ Peripherally inserted central venous catheter	b. Ports are surgically placed in the upper chest or upper arm area with the catheter inserted into the subclavian or internal jugular veins
11. ______ Nontunneled central venous access device	c. Inserted through the basilic vein at the antecubital area, with catheter tip located in the upper arm at the axilla level.
12. ______ Tunneled central venous access device	d. Inserted through the basilic or cephalic veins with the catheter tip located in the superior vena cava
13. ______ Implanted ports	e. Inserted through the jugular or subclavian veins, with the catheter tip located in the superior vena cava.

MATCHING QUESTIONS

Match the blood types with the blood transfusion products.

Client's Blood Type	Blood Product for Transfusion
14. ______ A	a. B
15. ______ B	b. Rh-negative donor

16. ______ AB
17. ______ O
18. ______ Rh-positive
19. ______ Rh-negative

c. O
d. A
e. Rh-positive donor
f. AB

MATCHING QUESTIONS

Signs & Symptoms

20. ______ dyspnea, cough
21. ______ chills, fever
22. ______ edema, restlessness
23. ______ nausea, vomiting
24. ______ urticaria
25. ______ bronchospasm

Type of Reaction

a. Circulatory overload
b. Pyrogenic (febrile)
c. Allergic

TRUE & FALSE QUESTIONS

Mark each statement True or False on the line provided. Correct each false statement in the space provided.

1. When inserting a peripheral IV access device, the tourniquet should be applied tightly enough to dilate the vein and suppress arterial blood flow. ___ T ___ F
2. When entering the skin and cannulating a vein with a vascular access device, the position of the needle is bevel up. ___ T ___ F
3. For a client who has an allergy to shell fish, the nurse should not use iodine to cleanse the skin prior to an intravenous catheter insertion. ___ T ___ F
4. When removing an intravenous catheter, the nurse should cover the venipuncture site with an alcohol swab and hold pressure on the site until the bleeding stops. ___ T ___ F
5. The nurse should monitor the client receiving intravenous fluid every hour or more frequently if needed. ___ T ___ F
6. Line reconciliation procedure is used when clients have an epidural infusion. ___ T ___ F

(continued)

7. Development of chest and back pain in a client receiving a blood transfusion are symptoms of circulatory overload. ___ T ___ F

8. If TPN administration must be interrupted, an infusion of normal saline should be immediately begun. ___ T ___ F

9. When priming a blood administration set, 0.9% normal saline should be used if dilution is required. ___ T ___ F

10. Clients with type A, B or AB blood may receive type O in an emergency. ___ T ___ F

FILL IN THE BLANKS

Fill in the blank space with the correct word or phrase to complete each statement.

1. The nurse is preparing to administer an intravenous medication, the best method to correctly identify the client is to ______________________.

2. The single most important method of preventing the spread of nosocomial infections is______________________.

3. Common indications for epidural infusions include__________ and __________.

4. Three advantages of epidural infusions include__________, __________, and __________.

5. Three complications of epidural infusions include __________, __________, and __________.

6. The nurse is documenting the care provided to a client who has an epidural infusion. What type of information would the nurse include in the documentation? __________

7. The physician ordered an intravenous infusion of 1000 ml of D5 1/2 NS to infuse over 8 hours. The drop factor for the administration set is 10 gtt/ml. Calculate the gtt/min. __________

8. The nurse is preparing to administer an intravenous infusion of 500 ml D5W with 20,000 units of heparin. The physician ordered the delivery of 1200 units of heparin per hour. How many milliliters per hour will the nurse administer in order to deliver 1200 units of heparin per hour to the client?

9. After insertion of a central venous access device, the physician will order a __________ prior to beginning infusion of fluid via the catheter.

10. The nurse should follow the "line reconciliation" process by performing the following checks and assessments:__________

11. For how long should the nurse remain with a client when a blood transfusion is started? __________

12. Client preparation for a peripherally inserted vascular access device includes assessing for conditions or situations which may lead to complications. Identify three areas of concern: __________

13. Describe the information the nurse should include in the documentation after removing a peripheral vascular access device. __________

14. How often should blood glucose levels be checked when a client is started on TPN? __________

15. A client receiving a blood transfusion has a shaking chill and complains of back pain. What should be the nurse's first action? __________

APPLICATION QUESTIONS

1. The nurse is preparing to insert a peripheral access device in a client's right lower arm. In order to dilate the veins of that extremity, the nurse asks the client to (Check all that apply)
   a. elevate his hand above his heart
   b. open and close his fist several times
   c. lower his arm below the level of his heart
   d. remain seated or lying in bed with warm compresses on area for 5–10 minutes
   e. allow the tourniquet to remain in place for 4 minutes while the nurse examines the arm
2. The client who is receiving an opioid analgesic via an epidural infusion becomes heavily sedated and has a respiratory rate of eight breaths per minute. The nurse anticipates the physician ordering which of the following medications?
   a. Abacavir (Ziagen)
   b. Bupivacaine (Marcaine)
   c. Naloxone (Narcan)
   d. Oxymorphone (Numorphan)
3. The nurse is preparing to administer morphine sulfate to the client for complaints of postoperative pain. The most important nursing assessment to perform prior to administering the medication would be to
   a. Assess respiratory rate and pattern
   b. Assess for urinary output and edema
   c. Assess capillary refill and skin color
   d. Assess pain level and cranial nerve # 1
4. The nurse is transcribing the physician orders and has difficulty reading one of the entries. The best action of the nurse is to
   a. clarify the order with another nurse
   b. call the physician who wrote the order and ask for clarification
   c. ask the pharmacist for clarification
   d. refer the matter to the Charge Nurse
5. The physician orders an infusion of 1000 ml of D5 ¼ NS to be infused at 50 ml/hr. The nurse begins the infusion at 0700. What time will the infusion be completed?
   a. 1100
   b. 1700
   c. 0100
   d. 0300
6. The physician ordered an antibiotic to be administered to the client and the pharmacy prepared the medication in a solution of 50 ml NS. The medication solution should be administered over a 20-minutes period of time. The rate controlling device the nurse

(continued)

will be using has to be programmed in ml/hr. At how many milliliters per hour will the nurse set the rate-controller device in order to administer the medication in 20 minutes?
a. 50 ml/hr
b. 100 ml/hr
c. 150 ml/hr
d. 200 ml/hr

7. The client is receiving an intravenous solution and may be experiencing a hypersensitivity reaction. Which of the following actions by the nurse is correct?
a. Stop the infusion, discontinue the IV, and observe the client carefully
b. Slow the infusion to 30 ml/hr, assess the client, and call the physician
c. Slow the infusion to 30 ml/hr, administer an antihistamine, and call the physician
d. Stop the infusion, keep the vein open with NS at 30 ml/hr, assess the client, and call the physician.

8. When monitoring clients who are receiving intravenous infusions, the nurse should include which of the following interventions in the plan of care? (Check all that apply)
a. Monitor all clients receiving intravenous solutions for circulatory overload: assess for rapid heart rate, dyspnea, cough, restlessness, and edema
b. Monitor all client receiving intravenous fluids for pyrogenic reactions: chills, fever, nausea, and vomiting
c. Throughout the infusion, monitor client for signs of infiltration and phlebitis
d. Monitor vital signs every 4 hours or more frequently, noting signs of orthostatic hypotension
e. Assess jugular vein distention, capillary refill, and heart and lung sounds
f. Monitor urinary output, daily weight, trends in weight loss or gain, edema, or signs of dehydration

9. When preparing a client for a blood transfusion, the nurse should consider for which of the following? (Check all that apply)
a. Blood typing and crossmatching must be completed prior to a blood transfusion
b. Clients with type A should only receive type A blood, but may receive type O in an emergency
c. Clients with type B should only receive type B blood, but may receive type A in an emergency
d. Clients with type AB blood are "universal recipients: and should only receive type AB blood but may, in an emergency, receive all four types of blood

10. The nurse is preparing to remove a central venous catheter and identifies which of the following interventions as appropriate care: (Check all that apply)
a. Position the bed in Trendelenburg or flat position, according to agency protocol and client condition
b. Review the Valsalva maneuver with client
c. Cleanse the insertion site and surrounding area with alcohol and povidone-iodine (if client is not allergic)
d. Carefully remove sutures
e. Document on client's medical record: date and time of removal, type and size of device, condition of catheter upon removal, as well as the client response

11. The physician orders fluconazole (Diflucan) 100 mg per mouth. The oral solution has 200 mg/5 ml. How many milliliters should the nurse administer?
a. 2.5 ml
b. 5 ml
c. 7.5 ml
d. 10 ml

12. Digoxin (Lanoxin) 0.125 mg by the intravenous route has been ordered for a client with atrial fibrillation. The client's potassium level is 3.1. The digoxin (Lanoxin) is available in a dose of 0.5 mg/2 ml. Which of the following actions by the nurse is appropriate?
a. Administer 0.5 ml and call the physician about the hyperkalemia
b. Administer 1 ml and call the physician about the hypokalemia
c. Administer 0.125 ml and call the physician about the hyperkalemia
d. Hold the digoxin and call the physician about the client's hypokalemia

13. Indications for Intravenous Therapy include: (Check all that apply)
a. Administer intravenous medications
b. Maintain fluid volume and electrolyte balance
c. Replace fluid volume and electrolyte losses
d. Provide nutritional support

14. Which of the following is correct about the administration of whole blood?
a. Administered in incidents such as acute hemorrhage where a client has lost greater than 25% of total blood volume

b. Volume of component for transfusion is 250–325 ml per bag
c. Administered to clients with bleeding due to thrombocytopenia or platelet dysfunction, platelet counts less than 20,000 (normal = 150,000–350,000)
d. Administered to clients with clotting disorders who are actively bleeding or at high risk for bleeding

15. Which of the following is correct with regards to the administration of cryoprecipitate?
 a. Administered to clients with a decreased fibrinogen level of less than 100 mg/dl
 b. Administered to clients with hemophilia A (congenital factor VIII deficiency) or von Willebrand's disease who are bleeding or preparing for an invasive procedure
 c. Administered to clients with hemophilia B (Christmas disease), factor IX deficiency who are bleeding or preparing for an invasive procedure
 d. Administered to clients with a congenital antithrombin III deficiency who have an acute risk of a venous thrombo-embolic event

16. A hemolytic transfusion reaction is caused by
 a. Fluid volume excess and may be precipitated if blood product is infused too rapidly.
 b. ABO or Rh incompatibility
 c. Recipient antibodies reacting with white cell antigens in the blood component
 d. Bacteria introduced into the component at the time of collection or during processing or storage

17. The nurse should monitor the client every hour or more frequently when the client is receiving an intravenous infusion. The complication of circulatory overload may cause the following symptoms:
 a. Less than 2 second capillary refill, headache, and hypertension
 b. Edema, decreased urinary output, increased respiratory rate, and hypotension
 c. Shortness of breath, increased respiratory and heart rate, hypertension, edema, and distended jugular veins
 d. Decreased level of consciousness, edema, hypotension, and dilated pupils

18. When providing care for a client with a tunneled central venous access device, the nurse is aware that the catheter is
 a. inserted through the jugular or subclavian veins, with the catheter tip located in the superior vena cava
 b. surgically inserted with the distal catheter tip located in the superior vena cava and the proximal end tunneled subcutaneously to an exit site on the client's trunk
 c. inserted through the basilic or cephalic veins with the catheter tip located in the superior vena cava
 d. inserted through the basilic vein at the antecubital area, with catheter tip located in the upper arm at the axilla level

19. Indications for TPN therapy include which of the following conditions? (Check all that apply)
 a. Inadequate oral intake or need for NPO status for extended period of time
 b. Increased metabolic needs
 c. Bowel obstruction
 d. Inflammatory bowel disease and related intestinal disorders
 e. 2-day episode of nausea, vomiting, and diarrhea
 f. Preterm or newborn infants who require surgery
 g. Severe malnutrition disorders

20. Peripherally administered parenteral nutrition may be
 a. infused through a peripheral venous catheter and contain 10% dextrose solution with vitamins, minerals, trace elements, and electrolytes added
 b. infused through a central venous access device and contain greater than 10% dextrose solution with vitamins, minerals, trace elements, electrolytes, and insulin added
 c. infused through a venous access device and contain greater than 20% dextrose solution with vitamins, trace elements, and insulin added
 d. infused through a 20-Ga angiocath in the basilic vein and contain 5% dextrose solution and potassium 20 mEq

21. The physician orders 1000 ml D5 ¼ NS with Potassium 40 mEq to be administered over 8 hours. The administration set has a drop factor of 15 gtt/ml. How many milliliters per hour and drops per minute should the nurse administer this infusion?
 a. 100 ml/hr, 25 gtt/min
 b. 100 ml/hr, 31 gtt/min
 c. 125 ml/hr, 38 gtt/min
 d. 125 ml/hr, 31 gtt/min

22. The physician orders ampicillin (Ampicin) 500 mg in 100 ml D5W to infuse over 30 minutes. The nurse sets the rate controller device to deliver the medication

(continued)

over 30 minutes. The rate controller device must be set at how many milliliters per hour?

a. 50 ml/hr
b. 100 ml/hr
c. 150 ml/hr
d. 200 ml/hr

23. When providing care for a client who is receiving peripherally administered parenteral nutrition, the nurse includes which of the following in the plan of care: (Check all that apply)

a. Assess the catheter insertion site for redness, swelling, heat, and drainage.
b. Assess nutritional status, daily weights, vital signs, and intake and output ratio
c. Administer 20% dextrose solution with vitamins, minerals, trace elements, and electrolytes added
d. Assess for signs of infection: elevated temperature and white blood cell count, chills, and redness at catheter site
e. Maintain accurate rate of flow and complete entire infusion on time increasing rate to "catch up" if necessary
f. Maintain aseptic techniques when changing solution and tubing every 24 hours

24. The physician has ordered a transfusion of packed red blood cells to your client. Which of the following actions should be included to provide safe care during the transfusion? (Check all that apply)

a. Use only 0.45% normal saline to prime the tubing or dilute the blood products
b. Assess vital signs before beginning the transfusion, 15 minutes after beginning the infusion, and every 30 minutes to 1 hour during transfusion.
c. Flush tubing with normal saline to administer intravenous medications throughout transfusion
d. Place call bell within client's reach, instruct client to call if experiencing shortness of breath, and request that the nurse aide remain with the client during the first 15 minutes of the transfusion
e. Monitor client every 30 minutes throughout transfusion for adverse reactions and assessment of vital signs

25. The client has had a peripheral intravenous device in the left hand for three days. The nurse's assessment for local complications of intravenous therapy includes which of the following? (Check all that apply)

a. Phlebitis
b. Thrombosis
c. Circulatory overload
d. Allergic reaction to medications
e. Infiltration
f. Infection at catheter site
g. Extravasation

ANSWERS & RATIONALES

MATCHING ANSWERS

Blood Product	Condition
1. _b_ Whole blood	a. Thrombocytopenia
2. _d_ Packed red blood cells	b. Client lost > 25% of total blood volume
3. _a_ Platelets	c. Fibrinogen levels < 100
4. _c_ Cryoprecipitate	d. Hemoglobin < 7

Parenteral Fluid	Category of Osmolarity
5. _c_ D5W	a. Hypertonic

6. b 0.45% normal saline
7. a D51/2 normal saline
8. a Ringer's lactate

b. Hypotonic

c. Isotonic

Types of Catheters

9. a Midline catheter
10. d Peripherally inserted central venous catheter
11. e Nontunneled central venous access device
12. a Tunneled central venous access device
13. b Implanted ports

Insertion Sites

a. Surgically inserted with the distal catheter tip located in the superior vena cava and the proximal end tunneled subcutaneously to an exit site on the client's trunk

b. Ports are surgically placed in the upper chest or upper arm area with the catheter inserted into the subclavian or internal jugular veins

c. Inserted through the basilic vein at the antecubital area, with catheter tip located in the upper arm at the axilla level.

d. Inserted through the basilic or cephalic veins with the catheter tip located in the superior vena cava

e. Inserted through the jugular or subclavian veins, with the catheter tip located in the superior vena cava.

Client's Blood Type

14. d, c A
15. a, c B
16. a, f, c, d AB
17. c O
18. b, e Rh-positive
19. b Rh-negative

Blood Product for Transfusion

a. B

b. Rh-negative donor

c. O

d. A

e. Rh-positive donor

f. AB

Signs & Symptoms

20. a dyspnea, cough
21. b chills, fever
22. a edema, restlessness
23. b nausea, vomiting
24. c urticaria
25. c bronchospasm

Type of Reaction

a. Circulatory overload

b. Pyrogenic (febrile)

c. Allergic

TRUE & FALSE ANSWERS

1. When inserting a peripheral IV access device, the tourniquet should be applied tightly enough to dilate the vein and suppress arterial blood flow. *True*

2. When entering the skin and cannulating a vein with a vascular access device, the position of the needle is beveled up. *True*

3. For a client who has an allergy to shell fish, the nurse should not use iodine to cleanse the skin prior to an intravenous catheter insertion. *True*

4. When removing an intravenous catheter, the nurse should cover the venipuncture site with an alcohol swab and hold pressure on the site until the bleeding stops. *False*

   When removing an intravenous catheter, the nurse should cover the venipuncture site with a gauze pad and hold pressure on the site until the bleeding stops.

5. The nurse should monitor the client receiving intravenous fluid every hour or more frequently if needed. *True*

6. Line reconciliation procedure is used when clients have an epidural infusion. *True*

7. Development of chest and back pain in a client receiving a blood transfusion are symptoms of circulatory overload. *False*

   Development of chest and back pain in a client receiving a blood transfusion are symptoms of a hemolytic reaction; signs and symptoms of circulatory overload include dyspnea, hypertension, tachycardia, distended jugular veins, and a change in level of consciousness.

8. If TPN administration must be interrupted, an infusion of normal saline should be immediately begun. *False*

   If TPN administration must be interrupted, an infusion of 5–10% dextrose is given to prevent hypoglycemia.

9. When priming a blood administration set, 0.9% normal saline should be used if dilution is required. *True*

10. Clients with type A, B, or AB blood may receive type O in an emergency. *True*

ANSWERS FOR FILL IN THE BLANKS

1. The nurse is preparing to administer an intravenous medication, the best method to correctly identify the client is to <u>compare the name and number on client's identification band with the name and number on his medical record</u>.

2. The single most important method of preventing the spread of nosocomial infections is <u>proper hand washing</u>.

3. Common indications for epidural infusions include <u>postoperative pain management</u> and <u>chronic pain management</u>.

4. Three advantages of epidural infusions include: <u>provides more consistent pain management</u>, <u>reduces amount of opioid requirement overall, decreases client sedation</u>, and <u>increases client's ability to be active, cough, and deep breathe after surgery</u>.

5. Three complications of epidural infusions include: <u>infection</u>, <u>bleeding at catheter site</u>, and <u>leakage of cerebral spinal fluid, opioid related adverse effect such as respiratory depression, hypotension, urinary retention, constipation.</u>

6. The nurse is documenting the care provided to a client who has an epidural infusion. What type of information would the nurse include in the documentation?
Document fluid and medication infusions, i& o, pain assessment, and client's reaction.

7. The physician ordered an intravenous infusion of 1000 ml of D5 1/2 NS to infuse over 8 hours. The drop factor for the administration set is 10 gtt/ml. Calculate the gtt/min. Answer: 21 gtt/min.

8. The nurse is preparing to administer an intravenous infusion of 500 ml D5W with 20,000 units of heparin. The physician ordered the delivery of 1200 units of heparin per hour. How many milliliters per hour will the nurse administer in order to deliver 1200 units of heparin per hour to the client? Answer: 30 ml/hr.

9. After insertion of a central venous access device, the physician will order a chest X-ray prior to beginning infusion of fluid via the catheter.

10. The nurse should follow the "line reconciliation" process by performing the following checks and assessments: rechecking tubing and catheter connections, tracing all client tubes and catheters to their sources for correct route, and labeling all tubes and catheters at the point(s) of connection.

11. For how long should the nurse remain with a client when a blood transfusion is started? Answer: 15 minutes.

12. Client preparation for a peripherally inserted vascular access device includes assessing for conditions or situations which may lead to complications. Identify three areas of concern: Assess client for history of cva, mastectomy, orthopedic injuries or surgery, lymphedema, or impaired circulation in area of expected venipuncture.

13. Describe the information the nurse should include in the documentation after removing a peripheral vascular access device: Document on client's medical record: date and time of removal, the extremity and vein used, type and size of device, condition of catheter upon removal, as well as the client response.

14. How often should blood glucose levels be checked when a client is started on TPN? Answer: Every 6 hours or as required by agency policy.

15. A client receiving a blood transfusion has a shaking chill and complains of back pain. What should be the nurse's first action? Answer: Discontinue the transfusion keeping the line open with normal saline.

APPLICATION ANSWERS

1. The nurse is preparing to insert a peripheral access device in a client's right lower arm. In order to dilate the veins of that extremity, the nurse asks the client to: (Check all that apply)
   a. elevate his hand above his heart
   b. open and close his fist several times
   c. lower his arm below the level of his heart
   d. remain seated or lying in bed with warm compresses on area for 5–10 minutes
   e. allow the tourniquet to remain in place for 4 minutes while the nurse examines the arm

Rationale
Correct answers: b, c, d, and e.
These answers are interventions used to dilate veins. Answer a is incorrect because raising the hand above the heart will not dilate the veins.

2. The client who is receiving an opioid analgesic via an epidural infusion becomes heavily sedated and has a respiratory rate of eight breaths per minute. The nurse anticipates the physician ordering which of the following medications?
   a. abacavir (Ziagen)

(continued)

b. bupivacaine (Marcaine)
c. naloxone (Narcan)
d. oxymorphone (Numorphan)

Rationale

Correct answer: c.

Answer c is correct because Narcan is an antidote for opioids and reverses CNS depression and respiratory depression related to opioid overdosage. a, b, and d are not opioid reversal agents.

3. The nurse is preparing to administer morphine sulfate to the client for complaints of postoperative pain. The most important nursing assessment to perform prior to administering the medication would be to
   a. assess respiratory rate and pattern
   b. assess for urinary output and edema
   c. assess capillary refill and skin color
   d. assess pain level and cranial nerve # 1

Rationale

Correct answer: a.

Answer a is correct because morphine sulfate is an opioid analgesic which depresses respiratory rate. Answers b, c, and d are not assessment findings which are directly related to the effects of morphine sulfate.

4. The nurse is transcribing the physician orders and has difficulty reading one of the entries. The best action of the nurse is to
   a. clarify the order with another nurse
   b. call the physician who wrote the order and ask for clarification
   c. ask the pharmacist for clarification
   d. refer the matter to the Charge Nurse

Rationale

Correct answer: b.

Answer b is correct. Always clarify the orders with the physician who wrote the orders. Answers a, c, and d are incorrect—these people did not write the order and thus are not the best people to clarify the order.

5. The physician orders an infusion of 1000 ml of D5 ¼ NS to be infused at 50 ml/hr. The nurse begins the infusion at 0700. What time will the infusion be completed?
   a. 1100
   b. 1700
   c. 0100
   d. 0300

Rationale

Correct answer: d.

Answer d is because 1000 ml of solution will take 20 hours to infuse at 50 ml/hour.

6. The physician ordered an antibiotic to be administered to the client and the pharmacy prepared the medication in a solution of 50 ml NS. The medication solution should be administered over a 20 minute period of time. The rate controlling device the nurse will be using has to be programmed in ml/hr. At how many milliliters per hour will the nurse set the rate-controller device in order to administer the medication in 20 minutes?
   a. 50 ml/hour
   b. 100 ml/hour
   c. 150 ml/hour
   d. 200 ml/hour

Rationale

Correct answer: c.

Answer c is correct. The solution will have to infuse at a rate of 150 ml/hour to instill 50 ml over the 20 minutes.

7. The client is receiving an intravenous solution and may be experiencing a hypersensitivity reaction. Which of the following actions by the nurse is correct?
   a. Stop the infusion, discontinue the IV, and observe the client carefully
   b. Slow the infusion to 30 ml/hr, assess the client, and call the physician
   c. Slow the infusion to 30 ml/hr, administer an antihistamine, and call the physician
   d. Stop the infusion, keep the vein open with NS at 30 ml/hr, assess the client, and call the physician.

Rationale

Correct answer: d.

Answer d is correct. The client may be experiencing a reaction to the solution, therefore, the nurse stops that solution, but maintains intravenous access with an infusion of NS. Assessing the client and calling the physician are standard procedures for safe care.

8. When monitoring clients who are receiving intravenous infusions, the nurse should include which of the following interventions in the plan of care? (Check all that apply)
   a. Monitor all clients receiving intravenous solutions for circulatory overload: assess for rapid heart rate, dyspnea, cough, restlessness, and edema
   b. Monitor all client receiving intravenous fluids for pyrogenic reactions: chills, fever, nausea, and vomiting
   c. Throughout the infusion, monitor client for signs of infiltration and phlebitis
   d. Monitor vital signs every 4 hours or more frequently, noting signs of orthostatic hypotension

e. Assess jugular vein distention, capillary refill, and heart and lung sounds
f. Monitor urinary output, daily weight, trends in weight loss or gain, edema, or signs of dehydration

Rationale

Correct answer: All answers are correct..

All answers are correct. All of these assessments are important when providing care for a client receiving intravenous therapy.

9. When preparing a client for a blood transfusion, the nurse should consider for which of the following? (Check all that apply)
   a. Blood typing and crossmatching must be completed prior to a blood transfusion
   b. Clients with type A should only receive type A blood, but may receive type O in an emergency
   c. Clients with type B should only receive type B blood, but may receive type A in an emergency
   d. Clients with type AB blood are "universal recipients: and should only receive type AB blood but may, in an emergency, receive all four types of blood

Rationale

Correct answers: a, b, and d.

Answers a, b, d are correct. Answer c is incorrect because clients with type B blood may only receive types B and O.

10. The nurse is preparing to remove a central venous catheter and identifies which of the following interventions as appropriate care: (Check all that apply)
   a. Position the bed in Trendelenburg or flat position, according to agency protocol and client condition
   b. Review the Valsalva maneuver with client
   c. Cleanse the insertion site and surrounding area with alcohol and povidone-iodine (if client is not allergic)
   d. Carefully remove sutures
   e. Document on client's medical record: date and time of removal, type and size of device, condition of catheter upon removal, as well as the client response

Rationale

Correct answer: All answers are correct..

11. The physician orders fluconazole (Diflucan) 100 mg per mouth. The oral solution has 200 mg/5 ml. How many milliliters should the nurse administer?
   a. 2.5 ml
   b. 5 ml
   c. 7.5 ml
   d. 10 ml

Rationale

Correct answer: a.

Answer a is correct. The ratio of 200 mg per 5 ml yields a dose of 100 mg per 2.5 ml

12. Digoxin (Lanoxin) 0.125 mg by the intravenous route has been ordered for a client with atrial fibrillation. The client's potassium level is 3.1. The digoxin (Lanoxin) is available in a dose of 0.5 mg/2 ml. Which of the following actions by the nurse is appropriate?
   a. Administer 0.5 ml and call the physician about the hyperkalemia
   b. Administer 1 ml and call the physician about the hypokalemia
   c. Administer 0.125 ml and call the physician about the hyperkalemia
   d. Hold the digoxin and call the physician about the client's hypokalemia

Rationale

Correct answer: d.

Answer d is correct. The potassium level is too low to administer digoxin. Hypokalemia places the client at a higher risk for digoxin toxicity.

13. Indications for Intravenous Therapy include: (Check all that apply)
   a. Administer intravenous medications
   b. Maintain fluid volume and electrolyte balance
   c. Replace fluid volume and electrolyte losses
   d. Provide nutritional support

Rationale

Correct answers: a, b, c, and d.

Answers a, b, c, and d are correct.

14. Which of the following is correct about the administration of whole blood?
   a. Administered in incidents such as acute hemorrhage where a client has lost greater than 25% of total blood volume
   b. Volume of component for transfusion is 250–325 ml per bag
   c. Administered to clients with bleeding due to thrombocytopenia or platelet dysfunction, platelet counts less than 20,000 (normal = 150,000–350,000)
   d. Administered to clients with clotting disorders who are actively bleeding or at high risk for bleeding

(continued)

Rationale

Correct answer: a.

Answer a is correct. Answer b is incorrect because the volume is not enough. Whole blood is usually about 450–500 ml. Answer c is incorrect because it is describing the purpose of platelet administration. Answer d is incorrect because it is describing when it is appropriate to administer fresh frozen plasma.

15. Which of the following is correct with regard to the administration of cryoprecipitate?
    a. Administered to clients with a decreased fibrinogen level of less than 100 mg/dl
    b. Administered to clients with hemophilia A (congenital factor VIII deficiency) or von Willebrand's disease who are bleeding or preparing for an invasive procedure
    c. Administered to clients with hemophilia B (Christmas disease), factor IX deficiency who are bleeding or preparing for an invasive procedure
    d. Administered to clients with a congenital antithrombin III deficiency who have an acute risk of a venous thrombo-embolic event

Rationale

Correct answer: a.

Answer a is correct. Answer b is incorrect because it describes the conditions for administering Factor VIII. Answer c is incorrect because it describes conditions to administer Factor IX, d is incorrect because it describes the conditions to administer Antithrombin III

16. A hemolytic transfusion reaction is caused by
    a. Fluid volume excess and may be precipitated if blood product is infused too rapidly.
    b. ABO or Rh incompatibility
    c. Recipient antibodies reacting with white cell antigens in the blood component
    d. Bacteria introduced into the component at the time of collection or during processing or storage

Rationale

Correct answer: b.

Answer b is correct. Answer a is the cause of circulatory overload. Answer c is the cause of febrile transfusion reaction. Answer d is the cause of bacterial transfusion reaction.

17. The nurse should monitor the client every hour or more frequently when the client is receiving an intravenous infusion. The complication of circulatory overload may cause the following symptoms:
    a. Less than 2 second capillary refill, headache, and hypertension
    b. Edema, decreased urinary output, increased respiratory rate, and hypotension
    c. Shortness of breath, increased respiratory and heart rate, hypertension, edema, and distended jugular veins
    d. Decreased level of consciousness, edema, hypotension, and dilated pupils

Rationale

Correct answer: c.

Answer c is correct. It describes the symptoms associated with circulatory overload.

18. When providing care for a client with a tunneled central venous access device, the nurse is aware that the catheter is
    a. inserted through the jugular or subclavian veins, with the catheter tip located in the superior vena cava
    b. surgically inserted with the distal catheter tip located in the superior vena cava and the proximal end tunneled subcutaneously to an exit site on the client's trunk
    c. inserted through the basilic or cephalic veins with the catheter tip located in the superior vena cava
    d. inserted through the basilic vein at the antecubital area, with catheter tip located in the upper arm at the axilla level

Rationale

Correct answer: b.

Answer b is correct. Answer a is location for a nontunneled central VAD. Answer c is the location for a peripherally inserted central VAD. Answer d is the location for a midline catheter.

19. Indications for TPN therapy include which of the following conditions? (Check all that apply)
    a. Inadequate oral intake or need for NPO status for extended period of time
    b. Increased metabolic needs
    c. Bowel obstruction
    d. Inflammatory bowel disease and related intestinal disorders
    e. 2 day episode of nausea, vomiting, and diarrhea
    f. Preterm or newborn infants who require surgery
    g. Severe malnutrition disorders

Rationale

Correct answers: a, b, c, d, f, and g.

Answers a, b, c, d, f, g are correct. Answer e usually does not necessitate TPN, only oral hydration or basic intravenous therapy replacement fluids.

20. Peripherally administered parenteral nutrition may be
    a. infused through a peripheral venous catheter, and contain 10% dextrose solution with vitamins, minerals, trace elements, and electrolytes added
    b. infused through a central venous access device, and contain greater than 10% dextrose solution with vitamins, minerals, trace elements, electrolytes, and insulin added
    c. infused through a venous access device and contain greater than 20% dextrose solution with vitamins, trace elements, and insulin added
    d. infused through a 20 Ga angiocath in the basilic vein and contain 5% dextrose solution and potassium 20 mEq

Rationale

Correct answer: a.

Answer a is the correct answer. Answer b is describing a centrally administered parenteral nutrition. Answer c contains too high of a concentration of dextrose. d is describing a solution which can be administered via a peripheral venous access device.

21. The physician orders 1000 ml D5 ¼ NS with Potassium 40 mEq to be administered over 8 hours. The administration set has a drop factor of 15 gtt/ml. How many milliliters per hour and drops per minute should the nurse administer this infusion?
    a. 100 ml/hr, 25 gtt/min
    b. 100 ml/hr, 31 gtt/min
    c. 125 ml/hr, 38 gtt/min
    d. 125 ml/hr, 31 gtt/min

Rationale

Correct answer: d.

Answer d is correct. 1000 ml/8 hr = 125 ml/hr. 125 ml/60 min X 15 = 31 gtt/min.

22. The physician orders ampicillin (Ampicin) 500 mg in 100 ml D5W to infuse over 30 minutes. The nurse sets the rate controller device to deliver the medication over 30 minutes. The rate controller device must be set at how many milliliters per hour?
    a. 50 ml/hr
    b. 100 ml/hr
    c. 150 Ml/hr
    d. 200 ml/hr

Rationale

Correct answer: d.

Answer d is correct answer. 100 ml: 30 minutes: X ml: 60 minutes

23. When providing care for a client who is receiving peripherally administered parenteral nutrition, the nurse includes which of the following in the plan of care: (Check all that apply)
    a. Assess the catheter insertion site for redness, swelling, heat, and drainage.
    b. Assess nutritional status, daily weights, vital signs, and intake and output ratio
    c. Administer 20% dextrose solution with vitamins, minerals, trace elements, and electrolytes added
    d. Assess for signs of infection: elevated temperature and white blood cell count, chills, and redness at catheter site
    e. Maintain accurate rate of flow and complete entire infusion on time increasing rate to "catch up" if necessary
    f. Maintain aseptic techniques when changing solution and tubing every 24 hours

Rationale

Correct answers: a, b, d, and f.

Answers a, b, d, and f are correct. All of these answers should be included in care planning for this client. Answer c is incorrect because the nurse should not administer greater than a 10% dextrose solution peripherally. Answer e is incorrect because the nurse should not increase the rate or "catch up" the solution as this may cause fluid overload or hyperglycemia.

24. The physician has ordered a transfusion of packed red blood cells to your client. Which of the following actions should be included to provide safe care during the transfusion? (Check all that apply)
    a. Use only 0.45% normal saline to prime the tubing or dilute the blood products
    b. Assess vital signs before beginning the transfusion, 15 minutes after beginning the infusion, and every 30 minutes to 1 hour during transfusion.
    c. Flush tubing with normal saline to administer intravenous medications throughout transfusion
    d. Place call bell within client's reach, instruct client to call if experiencing shortness of breath, and request that the nurse aide remain with the client during the first 15 minutes of the transfusion
    e. Monitor client every 30 minutes throughout transfusion for adverse reactions and assessment of vital signs

Rationale

Correct answers: b and e.

Answers b and e are correct. These are appropriate interventions to use when administering blood products.

(continued)

Answer a is incorrect because the nurse should only use 0.9% normal saline solution when administering blood products. Answer c is incorrect because the nurse should start an additional intravenous infusion is the client needs intravenous medications throughout the administration of blood products. Answer d is incorrect because the nurse should remain with the client during the first 15–30 minutes of the transfusion.

25. The client has had a peripheral intravenous device in the left hand for three days. The nurse's assessment for local complications of intravenous therapy includes which of the following? (Check all that apply)

    a. Phlebitis
    b. Thrombosis
    c. Circulatory overload
    d. Allergic reaction to medications
    e. Infiltration
    f. Infection at catheter site
    g. Extravasation

Rationale

Correct answers: a, b, e, f, and g.

Answers a, b, e, f, and g are correct. These answers are all local complications. Answers c and d are examples of systemic complications of intravenous therapy.

CHAPTER 16

Test Plan Category:

Physiological Integrity

Sub-category: Reduction of Risk Potential—Part 1

Topics: Diagnostic Tests
Laboratory Values
Therapeutic Procedures
Monitoring Conscious Sedation
Potential for Complications of Diagnostic Tests/Treatments/Procedures

DIAGNOSTIC TESTS

CARDIOVASCULAR SYSTEM

Electrocardiogram (ECG, EKG)

- Recording of the electrical activity of the heart
- Standard EKG is 12-lead EKG

Indications: To assess for dysrhythmias, myocardial ischemia, and myocardial infarction

Preparation: Shaving the skin may be required to allow adequate adhesion of the electrodes.

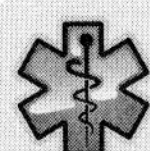

Nursing Intervention Alert

Remind the client not to speak or move during the recording to avoid the occurrence of artifact on the EKG strip.

Procedure: Monitoring electrodes are placed on the left arm, right, arm, and left leg; a grounding electrode is placed on the right leg, and six electrodes are positioned across the chest.

Echocardiogram

- A type of ultrasound, which focuses on cardiac structures.

Indications: To evaluate heart muscle and valves and to calculate ejection fraction of the heart

Preparation: No preparation is needed. Inform the client the test is not painful.

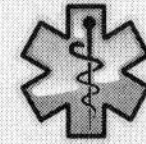

Nursing Intervention Alert

Remind client to remain still during the test to ensure clear imaging.

Procedure: A water-based gel is applied to the chest wall. The transducer is placed on the skin and moved to provide clear images of the cardiac structures. Recordings of images are made with the client supine and when turned on the left side (which brings the heart closer to the chest wall).

Cardiac Nuclear Scan (Myocardial Perfusion Scan)

- Involves the use of a radiopharmaceutical to perform diagnostic imaging examinations on the heart.
- In a thallium scan healthy cardiac tissue absorbs the thallium first, ischemic tissue absorbs it more slowly, and infarcted tissue does not absorb it at all. Similar testing can be done using other radioisotopes (Cardiolite, Myoview).
- It may be done in conjunction with an exercise stress test on a treadmill (exercise electrocardiography).
- For clients unable to exercise, the heart can be stimulated through the use of medications such as adenosine and dipyridamole, thus effectively simulating the effects of exercise on the heart.

Indications: To assess for ischemic heart disease, cardiac vessel patency, and cardiac wall functioning

Preparation: No solid food for 6 hours before the test. No nicotine on the day of the test.

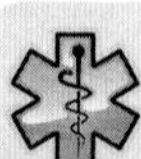

Nursing Intervention Alert

For exercise testing with adenosine: No caffeine for 12–24 hours prior to the test and no theophylline medications (such as Theo-Dur, aminophylline) for 24–48 hours before the test.

Procedure: A radioactive isotope is injected into a vein. Radioactive isotopes attach to red blood cells and pass through the heart in the circulating blood. The radioactive isotope can be traced through the heart using a special scanner. The images may be combined with an electrocardiogram. There are generally two phases to this test: exercise scan and resting scan. During the exercise portion of the test, the client will be injected with the isotope when 85–90% of maximum heart rate has been reached. The client will continue exercising for 1–2 minutes to distribute the isotope and is then immediately scanned. The client will be rescanned 3–4 hours after resting.

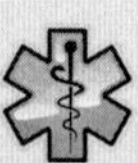

Nursing Intervention Alert

Bronchospasm may occur during exercise testing with adenosine or dipyridamole. This may be reversed with administration of aminophylline.

Nursing Process Elements

Special Considerations

- Have the client dress in comfortable clothes and wear walking shoes if an exercise stress test is going to be done.
- Educate the client concerning where the test will be performed and that he will have an IV, EKG monitor, and blood pressure cuff on during the testing.
- Obtain an accurate weight and baseline EKG.

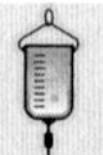

Clinical Alert

Nuclear medicine procedures are generally contraindicated for pregnant women and lactating mothers.

Cardiac Catheterization

- Involves the injection of a contrast medium through a catheter in the femoral or brachial artery
- Abnormalities of the coronary arteries or valves may be able to be treated during the cardiac catheterization
  - —*Percutaneous Transluminal Coronary Angioplasty (PTCA):* A balloon is inflated at the area of arterial narrowing
  - —*Stenting:* A metal mesh tube placed over the balloon will expand during angioplasty and lock into place to hold the artery open

Indications: To evaluate congenital disorders, coronary arteries, and function of heart muscle and valves

Preparation: The client is to fast for 8 hours prior to the procedure. A complete blood count and coagulation studies such as PT and PTT are obtained. Allergies to iodine, shellfish, or contrast medium dye must be reported. Any medications which might prolong bleeding must also be reported. Signed informed consent is obtained, and preprocedure sedation is administered as ordered.

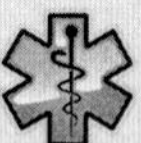

Nursing Intervention Alert

Inform the client that intense flushing may be experienced for 15–30 seconds during injection of the contrast medium.

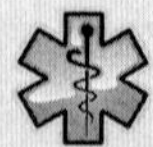

Nursing Intervention Alert

Clients who are taking metformin should discontinue the medication 2 days prior to the cardiac catheterization to avoid the possibility of lactic acidosis occurring. After the procedure, renal function should be assessed for adequacy prior to resuming the medication.

Procedure: An IV is started and EKG monitor applied. The puncture site is cleansed and anesthetized. The needle puncture is made; a guide wire is inserted through the needle; and the catheter is then inserted over the guide wire into the artery. Fluoroscopy is used to view the position of the catheter, and when in the correct position, contrast dye is injected. Images are taken as the dye moves through the vasculature and chambers of the heart. If abnormalities such as narrowing of a coronary artery are noted, treatment such as PTCA or stenting may be done.

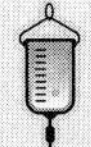

Clinical Alert

Generally contraindicated for those allergic to iodine, shellfish, or contrast medium dye, those with bleeding disorders, those with renal failure, and pregnant women.

Nursing Process Elements

Special Considerations

- Pressure must be maintained on the entry site and the affected extremity immobilized for 8–12 hours, unless a metal clip is used to seal the site. In this situation, ambulation is allowed in 1 hour.
- Vital signs, urinary output, and condition of the affected extremity (color, movement, temperature, sensation, and pulses) are monitored frequently per institutional protocol.

HEMATOLOGIC/IMMUNOLOGIC SYSTEM

Bone Marrow Biopsy

- Removal of a sample of bone marrow from the iliac crest or sternum

Indications: To investigate abnormal blood counts and to assess for the presence of systemic disease in the bone marrow

Preparation: No fasting is required prior to the test. The client is provided information about the procedure, noting discomfort occurs primarily when the puncture site is anesthetized and during removal of the marrow sample. Baseline coagulation laboratory studies are completed. A signed informed consent is obtained, and preprocedure sedation is administered as ordered.

Procedure: The client is assisted into a prone or lateral position. The puncture site is cleansed and anesthetized. A small incision is often made, and a large bore needle is inserted into the bone. Samples of liquid and other bone marrow are obtained. The needle is removed and pressure applied to the site for 10–15 minutes.

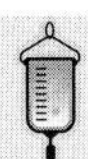

Clinical Alert

Generally contraindicated for clients with bleeding disorders, and for those unable to cooperate during the procedure.

Nursing Process Elements

Special Considerations

- Assess the client for signs of hemorrhage (change in vital signs, bleeding from puncture site, and pain)
- If possible, the client should remain on bedrest for 1 hour postprocedure.

RESPIRATORY SYSTEM

Pulse Oximetry

- A noninvasive study of arterial blood oxygen saturation using a probe or clip attached to a sensor site, most commonly the fingertips or ear lobe.
- Normal oxygen saturation is 95–100%

Indications: Often used to monitor the oxygen saturation of arterial blood during surgical procedure, diagnostic testing, and mechanical ventilation

Nursing Process Elements

- Assess for interfering factors such as excessive light, excessive pigmentation, nail polish, peripheral vascular disease, hypothermia, hypotension, and vasoconstriction.
- Place the transducer over the finger so that the light beams and sensors are opposite each other.
- Assess the site for skin irritation at least every 4 hours; check transducer site as needed.

ARTERIAL BLOOD GASES

Pulmonary Function Test

- Uses a spirometry device to measure pulmonary volumes and capacities
  - —*Tidal volume:* normal volume of air inspired/expired during normal respiration
  - —*Vital capacity:* maximum amount of air exhaled after a maximal inspiration

Indications: To evaluate ventilatory function, to determine cause of dyspnea, to assess effectiveness of medication, and to rule out obstructive or restrictive disease process

Nursing Process Elements

- Perform test before meals
- Explain the position: may be upright with a nose clip or in a plethysmograph or an airtight box (no need for nose clip). Reassure the client that although he/she may experience claustrophobia, he will be able to communicate with the technician
- Discuss with the client that he may receive bronchodilators

- Explain the importance of following directions so that the test can be done faster
- Instruct to the client to keep tight seal around the mouthpiece to ensure accurate result.

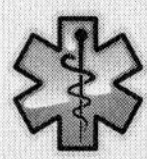

Nursing Intervention Alert

Instruct the client to use no bronchodilators and not to smoke for 6 hours prior to the test. If the client receives bronchodilators during the test then ask the client to take his/her normal dose after 4 hours.

Purified Protein Derivatives (PPD) Test

- Intradermal injection of purified protein derivatives to detect tuberculosis (TB) infection or to detect any previous sensitization of tubercle bacillus

Indications: To detect previous exposure to TB. If positive result, diagnosis of TB includes client history and presentation, chest X-ray, and sputum for AFB (acid-fast bacilli)

Nursing Process Elements

- Make sure to mark the area after administration of the test
- Document site of administration in the chart
- Result is read within 48–72 hours
- Measure induration (raised area) not erythema (redness)
  - —5 mm or above is considered positive if the client is immunocompromised.
  - —10 mm or above is considered positive for client who has other risk factors such as health care workers, people living in crowded areas, BCG vaccinated clients, teachers, and clients with lower economic status.
  - —15 mm or above is considered for clients with no known risk factors.

Sputum Culture

Indications: To identify and differentiate causative organism and to identify effective antibiotics

Nursing Process Elements

- Advise the client to cough deeply to produce specimen
- Avoid sending saliva
- Avoid mouthwashes before specimen is obtained.

Sputum Cytology

Indication: To identify abnormal cells

Nursing Process Elements

- Send the specimen in formalin or as ordered.

Chest X-ray

Indications: To evaluate gross lung presentation, and to aid in diagnosis of pneumonia, tuberculosis, and carcinoma

Nursing Process Elements

- Assess for pregnancy
- Protect radiation sensitive areas such as thyroid and reproductive organs

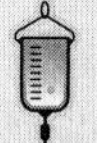

Clinical Alert

Assess for pregnancy. X-rays are generally contraindicated for clients who are pregnant.

Lung CT Scan

- Provides cross-sectional view of the lung segments by passing an X-ray beam from a computerized scanner through the lung at different angles and depth.

Indication: To assess abnormalities including masses or lesions

Preparation:

- Obtain an informed signed consent
- The client is to fast for 4 hours prior to the test
- Assess for allergy to contrast medium dye
- Explain to the client that the equipment may make him feel claustrophobic. He/she should not move during the procedure, relax, and breathe normally during the procedure.

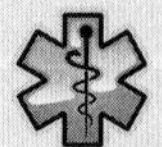

Nursing Intervention Alert

Clients who are taking metformin should discontinue the medication 2 days prior to the CT scan to avoid the possibility of lactic acidosis occurring. After the procedure, renal function should be assessed for adequacy prior to resuming the medication.

Bronchoscopy

- Involves direct visualization of larynx, trachea, and bronchi through the use of a fiberoptic bronchoscope

Indications: To view abnormalities seen on X-ray, to obtain specimens for examination, and for foreign body removal

Preparation:

- Obtain signed informed content
- The client is to fast for 12 hours prior to the procedure
- Dentures are removed.
- Preprocedure medication includes an anticholinergic to decrease bronchial secretions and a medication such as midazolam for sedation and relief of anxiety
- Explain that a local anesthetic will be sprayed in the throat

Nursing Process Elements

- Place client in supine or semi-Fowler position as ordered
- Observe for complications such as hemorrhage, subcutaneous emphysema and dyspnea, bronchospasm, pneumothorax, and laryngeal edema
- Discourage coughing, talking, and smoking for a few hours
- Administer oxygen as ordered
- Inform the client that sore throat and hoarseness of the voice may occur temporarily after the procedure

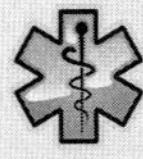

Nursing Intervention Alert

After the procedure, withhold fluids and food until the gag reflex returns.

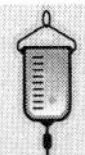

Clinical Alert

Generally contraindicated for clients with severe respiratory failure and clients who cannot tolerate interruption of high-flow oxygen.

GASTROINTESTINAL SYSTEM

Gastric Analysis

- Examination of stomach contents

Indications: Most often done to check for presence and amount of HCl (high in peptic ulcer disease, absent in pernicious anemia, should be decreased after vagotomy); can also document presence of occult blood, malignant cells, and parasites

Preparation: Light meal or fluids evening before then NPO after MN; no smoking in the morning of test because it stimulates HCl secretion

Procedure: Stomach contents aspirated via NG tube using a syringe and gentle suction; if production of HCl is being measured, this is the baseline amount. Subsequently, aspirations are repeated every 15–20 minutes for 1–2 hours usually after a stimulus such as a carbohydrate meal, 50 ml of caffeine or alcohol, or an injection of histamine is given.

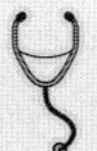

Assessment Alert

Check for history of allergies; may contraindicate use of histamine.

Whenever histamine is used, monitor pulse and blood pressure; expect client to experience a hot, flushing sensation.

Upper GI Series/Lower GI Series (Barium Enema)

- Fluoroscopic examination of the GI tract through the use of barium sulfate
  - —Upper GI: visualizes the esophagus, stomach, and small intestine
  - —Lower GI: visualizes the large intestine

Indications:

- *Upper GI:* To evaluate dysphagia, regurgitation, epigastric pain, and hematemesis
- *Lower GI:* To evaluate lower abdominal pain, changes in bowel habits, and blood in stools

Preparation:

- *Upper GI:* Fasting for 8 hours required prior to test.
- *Lower GI:* A liquid diet for 24 hours prior to test, use of stool softeners, laxatives, and enemas as ordered the evening before and morning of the test, and NPO for 8 hours prior to the test.

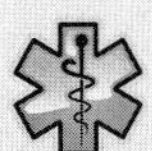

Nursing Intervention Alert

If both upper and lower GI series are to be done, the lower GI series should be done first so that barium from the upper GI series does not obscure lower GI images.

Procedure:

- *Upper GI:* The client drinks a milkshake-type solution containing barium sulfate. Movement of the barium is viewed fluoroscopically and spot films are taken throughout the passage of the barium from the pharynx through the small intestine.

- *Lower GI:* A preliminary film is taken with the client supine to check for adequacy of bowel prep. If adequate, the client is turned to the side and a rectal tube is inserted. Barium is allowed to flow slowly into the large intestine until it is full. Movement of the barium is viewed fluoroscopically and spot films are taken throughout the passage of the barium to the ileocecal valve.

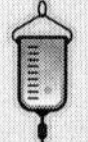

Clinical Alert

Generally contraindicated for intestinal obstruction, perforated GI tract (a water-soluble contrast medium [Gastrografin] would be needed), and pregnant women.

Nursing Process Elements

Special Considerations

- Encourage fluid intake to promote excretion of the barium.
- Reinforce to client the need to evacuate all of the barium. A cathartic may be ordered. Instruct the client to check all stools for barium and to notify the health care provider if the barium is not expelled within 2–3 days.

Oral Cholecystogram

- X-ray visualization of the gallbladder

Indications: To evaluate gallbladder function; to diagnose gallstones or other disease

Preparation: Ingest usual amount of dietary fat in days preceding test to empty bile from gallbladder. Fat free supper and Telepaque tablets containing contrast medium are taken the night before. Observe NPO after midnight. The fat free supper prevents contraction of gallbladder and allows dye to accumulate.

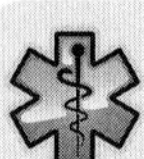

Nursing Intervention Alert

Give the Telepaque tablets 5 minutes apart with small amounts of water to minimize nausea. There are usually six or more tablets (dose is calculated according to body weight).

Procedure: X-ray is taken; if gallbladder with stones is seen, procedure is over. Otherwise a fatty meal is given to stimulate gallbladder contraction and more films are taken in 15–20 minutes.

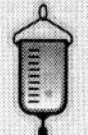

Clinical Alert

Complications include severe diarrhea and vomiting with dehydration; anaphylaxis if client is allergic to iodine in dye, liver and kidney damage if dye is not properly excreted.

Cholangiogram

- Visualization of bile ducts through the use of a contrast medium.

Indications: To detect obstruction of bile ducts, tumors, cysts of common bile duct, biliary sclerosis, and sclerosing cholangitis; to evaluate between obstructive and nonobstructive jaundice. There are three types:

- *Percutaneous transhepatic cholangiogram:* Contrast dye is injected directly into the bile duct. It is performed in jaundiced clients since they cannot process dye given orally or intravenously.
- *Operative cholangiogram:* It is done while client is undergoing a cholecystectomy to check common bile duct for stones.
- *T-Tube cholangiogram:* Dye is injected through the T-tube to check for patency of the common bile duct prior to removal of the T-tube.

Preparation: Low fat diet 24 hours before procedure, NPO 8 hours before, laxative evening before, and enema the morning of examination; obtain signed informed consent; preprocedure medication may include a sedative, analgesic, and antibiotic if ordered. Coagulation studies need to be within normal limits.

Procedure: For the percutaneous transhepatic cholangiogram, the client is placed supine on a tilting X-ray table, right upper abdomen is cleansed with povidone-iodine solution and surgically draped. With fluoroscopy guidance, needle is inserted into liver; placement in bile duct is confirmed by return flow of bile; contrast medium is injected; X-rays taken with client in various positions; dry sterile dressing to puncture site, may use sand bag to apply pressure.

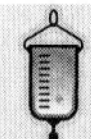

Clinical Alert

Contraindicated in clients with iodine or shellfish allergies, with prolonged clotting time, cholangitis, when client cannot remain still, and pregnant women.

Nursing Process Elements

- Assess vital signs before and after procedure
- Monitor for bleeding, increased pulse and decreased blood pressure
- bile extravasation, sepsis, and bacteremia after procedure
- Maintain NPO for a few hours after examination and bedrest for several hours
- Instruct to immediately report any adverse reactions to contrast as nausea, vomiting, headache, dizziness, or urticaria
- Inform client when diet can be resumed
- Teach to report signs of bleeding abdominal discomfort, drainage from puncture site or fever and chills
- Instruct to increase fluid intake to help excrete dye

Endoscopic GI Procedures: Direct visualization of upper GI tract with a flexible fiberoptic scope

- *Esophagogastroduodenoscopy (EGD)/Gastroscopy:* Visualizes esophagus, stomach, and upper duodenum
- *Sigmoidoscopy:* Visualizes anus, rectum, and sigmoid colon
- *Colonoscopy:* Visualizes entire large intestine

Indications:

- *EGD:* To view organ linings, aspirate fluid, removal foreign bodies, obtain tissue biopsies, and control bleeding
- *Sigmoidoscopy:* Can be diagnostic or therapeutic; detects polyps, ulcerative colitis, diverticular disease, granulomas or irritable bowel syndrome; used as screening test for colon cancer
- *Colonoscopy:* To detect tumors; to detect and remove polyps; to diagnose inflammatory bowel disease; to obtain biopsies; to dilate strictures; used as screening test for colon cancer

Preparation:

- *EGD:* Obtain signed informed consent. Fasting for 8–12 hours. Remove dentures. Preoperative medication includes an anticholinergic (atropine) to decrease secretions and a medication (such as midazolam) for sedation and relief of anxiety.
- *Sigmoidoscopy:* Usually clear fluids 24 hours before procedure, oral cathartics such as fleets phosphate soda, given on evening of examination and an enema in the morning.
- *Colonoscopy:* Clear liquid diet for 1–3 days and NPO for 8 hours; laxatives 1–3 days before and enemas night before or saline cathartic or 1 gallon Golytely or Colyte taken as an 8-oz glass every 10 minutes.

Procedure:

- *EGD:* Topical anesthetic applied to the pharynx to numb the gag reflex, a flexible scope is passed through the mouth to esophagus, air is insufflated to distend the area to clearly view GI organs, may take a biopsy or brushings for cytological specimens or remove polyps.
- *Sigmoidoscopy:* Client is sedated; positioned in left lateral or knee chest or lithotomy position; a flexible scope is placed into rectum up to about 25 inches, air is insufflated to aid with visualization; polyps may be removed or a biopsy taken
- *Colonoscopy:* Client is sedated, positioned in left lateral position. a flexible scope is placed into rectum and advanced to the ileocecal valve. Air is insufflated to aid with visualization; polyps may be removed or a biopsy taken

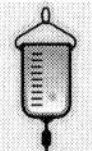

Clinical Alert

Complications

- *EGD:* Bleeding, cardiac arrhythmias, pulmonary aspiration or perforation
- *Sigmoidoscopy:* Bleeding from colon or rectum due to biopsy or polyp removal, perforation, cardiac arrhythmias, peritonitis
- *Colonoscopy:* Rectal bleeding, perforation

Nursing Process Elements

Special Considerations

- *EGD:* Monitor vital signs until fully awake. Inform client to resume eating once the gag reflex returns; instruct to use a soothing mouthwash for sore throat; call physician for any difficulty breathing or abdominal pain.
- *Sigmoidoscopy:* Monitor vital signs until fully awake. Inform client that slight bleeding may occur if biopsy taken or polyp removed. Instruct client to report bleeding, elevated temperature and abdominal pain to physician. Explain about occurrence of gas pains and flatulence after procedure.
- *Colonoscopy:* Monitor vital signs until fully awake. Observe for rectal bleeding if biopsy or polypectomy done. Assess for signs of perforation (malaise, abdominal distention, and tenesmus). Inform client that abdominal cramping may occur.

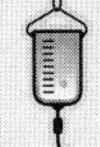

Clinical Alert

Colonoscopy is contraindicated for clients with acute diverticulitis, peritonitis, ischemic bowel disease, or fulminant ulcerative colitis and suspected perforation of the colon.

Liver Biopsy

- Sampling of liver tissue for histopathologic evaluation

Indications: To aid in diagnosis of cirrhosis, hepatitis, neoplasm; to monitor course of liver disease

Preparation: Check coagulation status (PT, clotting, or bleeding time). Check for type and x-match. Obtain signed informed consent. Obtain baseline vital signs. Explain position and breathing. NPO for 6 hours prior to the test.

Procedure: Puncture site is cleansed and local anesthetic is administered. Conscious sedation may be used. Client lies supine with right arm over head. He/she exhales fully and holds breath; needle is inserted between anterior right 6 and 7 or 8 and 9 ribs, and sample of liver tissue is aspirated.

Complications: Bile peritonitis, shock, pneumothorax

Nursing Process Elements

Monitor vital signs q 15 minutes ×2, q 30 minutes ×4, q1 hour ×4; position client on right side to keep pressure on area of needle insertion for minimum of 2 hours; keep flat for 12–14 hours.

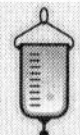

Clinical Alert

Generally contraindicated for clients with bleeding disorders, decreased platelet count, platelet dysfunction, extrahepatic obstruction, infection, and when there is difficulty locating the liver due to ascites or obesity.

NEUROLOGICAL SYSTEM

Cerebral Angiography

Traditional method

- It uses injected contrast medium and X-ray to visualize the cerebral, carotid and vertebral circulation.

Indications: To identify AV malformations, aneurysms, and blocked or leaking vessels

Preparation: NPO for 8–12 hours; preprocedure sedative, analgesic or hypnotic

Procedure: Head will be immobilized and client must lie still, contrast medium injected and serial X-rays taken

Complications: Allergic reaction; vasospasm which can be severe enough to occlude blood flow and cause permanent effects such as paresis or paralysis depending on the area of the brain affected.

Nursing Process Elements

- Tell client to expect a sensation of heat when the contrast media is injected.
- Administer antihistamines before and/or after if prescribed for clients with allergies.
- Check for allergy to iodine, shellfish, and contrast media.
- Obtain baseline vital signs and neurological assessment.
- After the procedure monitor vital signs and neurological signs every 15 minutes for first hour and then at increasing intervals.
- Monitor neurovascular signs in extremity distal to the site of contrast media injection (ability to feel and move, color, temperature, pulse, and capillary refill).
- Maintain bedrest for several hours with injected extremity straight and immobilized.
- Monitor injection site for bleeding.
- Encourage fluids when allowed to aid excretion of contrast material over next 24 hours.

Digital subtraction method

- It is less invasive and involves less risk of vasospasm.
- Angiocatheter is threaded into the brachial vein and into the superior vena cava near the right atrium; an initial reference X-ray is taken and loaded into a computer. The contrast medium is then injected. Subsequent pictures are computer compared to the original.
- There is no fluid restriction, but food restricted for 2 hours.
- There is no activity restriction postprocedure; otherwise care same as in traditional method.

Computerized Tomography (CT) Scan

- May be done with or without contrast medium
- Food withheld for 4 hours if contrast used; no fluid restriction

Indications: To identify tumors, infarctions, hemorrhage, hydrocephalus, and bone malformations

Nursing Process Elements

- Ensure wigs, hairpins, and the like are removed.
- Monitor for delayed allergic reaction if contrast used.

Magnetic Resonance Imaging (MRI)

- May use noniodine contrast substance, gadolinium
- No special preparation or follow up care.
- Contraindicated for confused, agitated, or pregnant clients and those with unstable vital signs or implanted ferromagnetic devices or tattoos. Also contraindicated for those on continuous life support.

Positron Emission Computed Tomography Scan (PET)

- It is different from CT scan and MRI because it shows function (glucose and oxygen metabolism and cerebral blood flow), not structure.

- Deoxyglucose tagged with a radioisotope is injected intravenously and is taken up in varying amounts by different areas of the brain depending on their activity. The greater the activity, the greater is the amount taken up. Areas with different amounts show different colors on the resultant films.
- Allows areas of metabolic alteration to be identified that are associated with seizure, dementia, etc.
- Client may wear earplugs and be blindfolded during the test.
- Client will be asked to perform different mental functions during the test to show activity in different areas of the brain.

Nursing Process Elements

- Keep client NPO for 6–12 hours before the test.
- Hold insulin, glucose solutions or any other drugs that alter glucose metabolism.
- Encourage fluids after the procedure; the isotope is excreted in urine but no special precautions are needed.

Lumbar Puncture

Insertion of a spinal needle between the third and fourth or fourth and fifth lumbar vertebrae into the subarachnoid space.

Indications: To obtain CSF for laboratory analysis; to obtain pressure readings; to check for obstruction; or inject medications

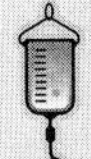

Clinical Alert

LP is generally contraindicated for clients with signs of increased ICP because of the risk of herniation of brain tissue through the uncus if the pressure is suddenly decreased and also for those with infection near the entry site because of the risk of introducing pathogens into the CSF.

Procedure: Once the needle is in place, pressure readings are obtained and samples collected and numbered sequentially.

Nursing Process Elements

- Have client empty bladder.
- Assist into side lying fetal position (chin on chest, back flexed, knees flexed on trunk and held in place with arms and hands) at side of bed or table.
- Hold client in place with hands behind knees and neck.
- After the procedure, maintain bedrest in a flat position if ordered for up to 4–8 hours.
- Encourage increased fluid intake up to 3000 ml/day for 2 days to encourage production of replacement CSF.
- Give analgesics for headache, which may be severe and throbbing as a result of the decrease in CSF.
- Monitor for complications: CSF leakage, infection and hematoma formation.

Electroencephalography

Indications:

- Determine general activity of the cerebral cortex; identify origin of seizure activity; monitor brain activity during anesthesia; diagnose sleep problems; diagnose brain death.
- May be done as a sleep deprived test; client is awakened at 2 or 3 a.m. and kept awake until after the test.
- Withhold CNS stimulant or depressant foods or medications for 24 hours before test.
- Test is done in a stimulus free environment
- Hair needs to be washed before test and after to remove gel.
- Client may be asked to hyperventilate; may be exposed to bright light; or may be put to sleep.

GENITOURINARY SYSTEM

KUB Plain Film

- Plain radiographic visualization of the abdomen (kidneys, ureters, and bladder).

Indications: To delineate size, shape, and position of kidneys; to aid in diagnosis of hydronephrosis, cysts, tumors, or displacement; to identify intra-abdominal diseases such as intestinal obstruction, masses, ruptured organs, abnormal gas accumulation, and ascites

Preparation: It should precede intravenous pyelogram (IVP) or other GI diagnostic studies. Remove all metal from X-ray field. Client teaching: Hold breath as instructed when images are taken.

Procedure: With client supine on examination table, abdominal X-ray films are obtained. For portable examination, head of bed is elevated to a high Fowler's position.

Nursing Process Elements

Reinforce information given regarding further testing, treatment, or referral.

Pyelogram

- Radiographic visualization of the kidney, ureters, bladder, and renal pelvis using contrast medium.

Indications: To aid in diagnosis of renovascular hypertension, determine cause of hematuria, assess for presence of renal calculi, cyst, tumor, or ureteral obstruction; to evaluate urinary tract function, congenital anomalies, or trauma

Preparation: Obtain signed informed consent, complete history and physical conditions (rule out pregnancy, dehydration, renal insufficiency, multiple myeloma, perforation of ureters or bladder, and allergy to shellfish and iodinated dye), baseline BUN and creatinine, pretest laxative, fasting for 8 hours, steroid/antihistamine prep for known iodine allergy; remove all metal from X-ray field.

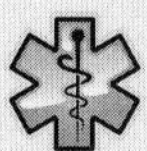

Nursing Intervention Alert

Clients who are taking metformin should discontinue the medication 2 days prior to the pyelogram to avoid the possibility of lactic acidosis occurring. After the procedure, renal function should be assessed for adequacy prior to resuming the medication.

Procedure: Radiopaque contrast medium administered intravenously (IVP or excretory urogram) or through ureteral catheters, which have been passed into the renal pelvis by cystoscopic manipulation (retrograde pyelogram). X-ray exposures made at 1, 5, 10, 15, 20, and 30 minutes and postvoiding to follow course and timing of contrast medium through urinary system.

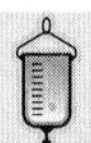

Clinical Alert

Complications include renal failure, IV or catheter related infections, allergic reaction.

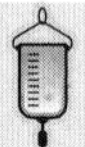

Clinical Alert

Failure to discontinue Glucophage may result in lactic acidosis.

Nursing Process Elements

Monitor for decreased urinary output, S&S of allergic response. Resume diet, medications, and activity (see alert regarding metformin). Increase fluid intake to assist with excretion of dye.

Renal Ultrasound

- Use of ultrasound to produce an image of an organ or tissue.

Indications: To evaluate size, shape, and position of kidney; to aid in diagnosis of tumors, malformations, or obstructions; to guide renal biopsy or nephrostomy tube insertion

Preparation: Client teaching: The client may be asked to inhale deeply and hold breath during examination.

Procedure: With client supine, conduction gel is applied to the skin and a transducer passes high frequency sound waves into the body, which are reflected back, electronically processed, and displayed as an image.

Nursing Process Elements

Test should precede CT or endoscopic examinations. There should be no barium studies for 2 days prior to ultrasound.

Renal Scan

- Assesses flow and rate of radionuclide through kidney. Does not use iodinated contrast medium, therefore, procedure considered safe for clients with allergy or compromised renal function.

Indications: To aid in diagnosis of renal artery disease, to detect renal infection or inflammatory diseases, abscess, trauma, calculi, obstructive uropathy, tumors, or congenital disorders

Preparation: Obtain signed informed consent. No fasting is required. Client needs to be well hydrated.

Procedure: Radioisotopes injected intravenously. Gamma camera detects emitted rays, tracks the rate of flow, plots the times on a graph, and stores the information in a computer. Delayed images are taken at 2–24 hours (may leave the nuclear medicine department and return later for delayed imaging)

Nursing Process Elements

Wear gloves when discarding urine. Wash gloved hands with soap and water before removing, then wash again after gloves removed. Radionuclide excreted within 6–24 hours.

Cystoscopy

- Direct endoscopic visualization of the bladder and urethra.

Indications: To aid in diagnosis of tumor, stone, ulcer, and obstruction; to allow insertion of ureteral catheters, removal of calculi, electrocautery of bleeding sites, dilation of urethra, and attainment of biopsy specimen

Preparation: Obtain signed, informed consent. No fasting is required if local anesthesia is to be used; 8-hour fast if general anesthesia planned. Client teaching: The client may be told that he/she may experience an urge to urinate during the procedure.

Procedure: Urethra cleansed, local anesthetic applied, and rigid or flexible cystoscope inserted through urethra into the bladder. Optical lens system provides magnified, illuminated view; water or saline inserted via the scope's attached irrigation system to aid in bladder visualization.

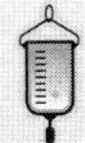

Clinical Alert

Complications include bleeding, infection, post-catheter urinary retention, and bladder rupture.

Nursing Process Elements

Monitor for UTI, urinary retention, or hemorrhage. Anticipate blood-tinged urine. Warm sitz bath and mild analgesics may relieve discomfort. Report burning on voiding, heavy bleeding, or decreased urine output; force fluids.

Cystourethrogram

- Radiographic visualization of the urethra and bladder during urination using contrast medium.

Indications: To identify injuries, tumors, strictures, vesicoureteric reflux, neurogenic bladder, or structural abnormalities; to evaluate emptying problems or incontinence.

Preparation: Obtain signed informed consent, steroid/antihistamine prep for known iodine allergy. Client teaching: The client may be told that he/she may experience pressure and an urge to urinate during procedure.

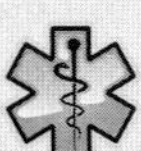

Nursing Intervention Alert

Cystourethrogram should be completed prior to any tests involving barium

Procedure: With client supine, urinary catheter inserted, radiopaque contrast medium injected and catheter clamped. X-ray images taken in various positions with the bladder full of contrast and while the bladder is being emptied.

Complications: Renal failure, catheter related UTI, and allergic reaction.

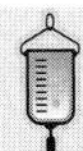

Clinical Alert

Failure to discontinue Glucophage may result in lactic acidosis.

Nursing Process Elements

Monitor for decreased urinary output, allergic reactions, infection, bleeding, or urinary retention. Resume diet and medications. Force fluids. Report fever, chills, urinary difficulty, or bleeding.

Cystometrogram

- Manometric study measuring bladder pressure and volume characteristics during filling and storage.

Indications: To evaluate motor and sensory causes of incontinence and monitor effects of treatment

Preparation: Obtain signed informed consent. No fasting is needed. Inform client that the urge to void may be felt as fluid or gas fills the bladder. Instruct client to report sensations during procedure.

Procedure: Client is observed during pretest voiding and the following data is recorded: start time, force and continuity of stream, volume voided, presence of dribbling, straining, or hesitancy, and stop time. With client supine, a urinary catheter is inserted and residual urine measured. The catheter is connected to a cystometer and pressure and volume readings are recorded and graphed for response to heat, full bladder, urge to void, and ability to inhibit voiding.

Complications: UTI and bleeding

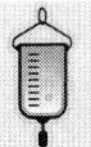

Clinical Alert

Procedure is contraindicated if UTI is present or patient is experiencing diarrhea.

Nursing Process Elements

Monitor for infection, bleeding, and urinary retention. Encourage client to increase fluid intake. Administer analgesics and antibiotics as ordered. Warm tub baths may aid in comfort. Instruct client to report pain, frank bleeding, and dysuria.

Renal Biopsy

- Excision of tissue sample from the kidney for microscopic analysis

Indications: To confirm diagnosis of cancer or renal disease; to determine extent of involvement in systemic lupus erythematous; to monitor progression of nephrotic syndrome; to monitor renal function after transplantation

Preparation: Obtain signed informed consent, obtain baseline chest X-ray and coagulation studies. NPO for 8 hours, withhold anticoagulant therapy for 7 days prior to test.

Procedure: Sandbag placed under abdomen with client in prone position. Following local anesthesia, client instructed to take a deep breath, exhale forcefully, and hold breath while percutaneous needle inserted through renal tissue with ultrasound guidance and rotated to obtain renal tissue.

May also be performed by open biopsy through a small flank incision under general anesthesia.

Complications: Bleeding, infection, and delayed allergic response

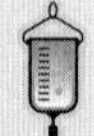

Clinical Alert

Obesity and spinal deformities make percutaneous approach impossible.

Nursing Process Elements

Client assisted to supine position. Bedrest for 24 hours. Monitor vital signs and dressing. Encourage fluid intake. Monitor output and observe for frank bleeding. Strenuous activity should be avoided for 2 weeks.

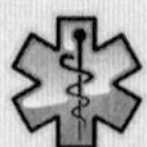

Nursing Intervention Alert

Observe for indications of hemorrhage (vital sign changes, back, flank or shoulder pain, lightheadedness). Observe for signs of punctured bowel or liver (abdominal pain/tenderness, decreased bowel sounds, and abdominal rigidity)

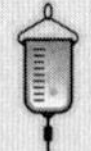

Clinical Alert

Generally contraindicated in clients with renal tumors, hydronephrosis, abscess, advanced renal failure, urinary tract infection, or if have only one kidney.

REPRODUCTIVE SYSTEM

Mammogram

- Radiographic imaging of the breast

Indications: To detect nonpalpable lesions and assist in diagnosing palpable masses; to evaluate nipple discharge, breast pain, nipple retraction, and dimpling of skin of breast

Preparation: Explain to client the need to avoid use of powders, lotions, or deodorant prior to examination as they may interfere with results

Procedure: Two views are taken of each breast; a craniocaudal view and a mediolateral oblique view; the breast is compressed from top to bottom and from side to side; the procedure takes about 20 minutes.

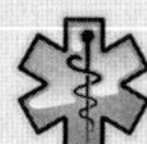

Nursing Intervention Alert

Inform clients of screening guidelines from the American Cancer Society which recommend a mammogram each year after reaching the age 40; screening for women who are high-risk is to begin 10 years before the age of the diagnosis of breast cancer in a family member.

Nursing Process Elements

Explain that there is a false-positive rate ranging between 5 and 10%, generally greater in younger women with greater breast density tissue

Colposcopy

- Direct visualization of the cervix and vagina via a colposcope

Indications: To identify area of cellular dysplasia following abnormal cervical Pap results

Preparation: Instruct client to avoid douching and sexual intercourse for 24 hours prior to the test. Obtain a signed informed consent.

Procedure: The client empties her bladder and is assisted into lithotomy position. External genitalia are cleansed and a vaginal speculum is inserted. The cervix is swabbed with 3% acetic acid solution to remove secretions/medications and to highlight abnormal areas. The areas are illuminated by the colposcope and biopsies taken of suspicious areas. The vagina is rinsed with sterile saline or water to remove the acetic acid.

Nursing Process Elements

Inform client that mild cramping, vaginal discomfort, and vaginal discharge may occur following the procedure. Discharge may continue for 1 week. Instruct client to avoid strenuous exercise for 24 hours. Tampons, douching, and intercourse should be avoided for 2 weeks. Instruct client to report abdominal pain, fever or frank vaginal bleeding, or if bleeding lasts for more than 2 weeks.

Pelvic Ultrasound

- Ultrasound imaging of structures in the pelvic region

Indications: To identify stones, tumors, and other disorders in urinary bladder; to evaluate ovaries, uterus, cervix, and fallopian tubes of women; to assess fetal development; to evaluate prostate, seminal vesicles, and bladder in men

Preparation: No fasting is required. A full bladder is needed during the examination. Instruct the client to drink 1 liter of water 1 hour before the test.

Procedure: The client is assisted to a supine position. A water-based gel is applied to the abdominal and pelvic area and a transducer is placed on the skin and moved as needed to provide good images. The examination can also be done transvaginally for women (bladder is emptied prior to this examination) and transrectally for men

Nursing Process Elements

Special Consideration

- Allow the client to void immediately after the examination is completed.

Nonstress Test (NST)

- A noninvasive test used to evaluate the status of the fetus

Indications: Used with pregnant clients who have diabetes or hypertension, when fetal development is abnormal, and in postterm pregnancy

Preparation: Instruct client to eat prior to the test to ensure a high maternal serum glucose level, which enhances fetal activity.

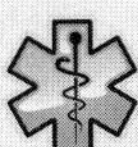

Nursing Intervention Alert

Explain to client that a nonreactive NST does not mean there is a problem with the fetus. The fetus may have been in a sleep cycle during the test.

Procedure: The client voids and is then assisted into a Sims' position. An external fetal monitor is applied. The client is instructed to push a button whenever fetal movement is felt. This is then correlated to fetal heart rate. If there is no fetal movement in 20 minutes, external stimulation is done (rubbing the abdomen or producing loud noise near abdomen).

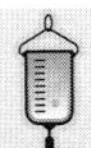

Clinical Alert

If there is no fetal movement for 40 minutes, the test is nonreactive, and the client is scheduled for a contraction stress test.

Amniocentesis

- An invasive diagnostic procedure involving transabdominal needle aspiration of amniotic fluid

Indications: To detect chromosomal abnormalities, to determine fetal maturity, and to detect Rh incompatibility

Preparation: No fasting is required. Obtain a signed informed consent. If client has full bladder due to having ultrasound prior to the amniocentesis, the client needs to void prior to the amniocentesis to avoid accidental puncture.

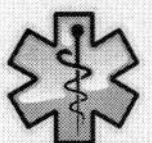

Nursing Intervention Alert

If the mother's blood is Rh negative and that of the fetus is Rh positive, obtain order for RhoGAM to be administered.

Procedure: The client is assisted to a supine position. The skin of the lower abdomen is cleansed, draped, and anesthetized. A spinal needle is inserted into the amniotic cavity and a fluid sample is aspirated. The needle is withdrawn and a dressing is applied. The sample is protected from light and transported to the laboratory.

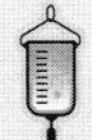

Clinical Alert

Possible complications include amniotic fluid embolism, fetal injury, hemorrhage, infection, premature labor, Rh sensitization, and spontaneous abortion.

Nursing Process Elements

Special Considerations

- Monitor fetal heart rate and maternal vital signs every 15 minutes until stable
- Monitor dressing for drainage
- Instruct client to report abdominal pain, cramping, chills, fever, vaginal bleeding, fetal hyperactivity, or lethargy

Hysterosalpingography

- An X-ray of the uterus and Fallopian tubes using fluoroscopy and a contrast medium

Indications: Used primarily as part of infertility workup to detect blocked fallopian tubes and uterine abnormalities

Preparation: Best performed 1 week after menstruation but before ovulation to make sure client is not pregnant. No fasting is required. Client may be asked to take a laxative or an enema to empty her bowels so that the uterus and surrounding structures can be seen clearly. Antibiotics and sedative may be given. Client needs to inform physician of any allergies and/or reactions, especially to contrast material.

Procedure: The client voids and is assisted into lithotomy position. A plain abdominal X-ray may be done to ensure adequacy of bowel prep. A vaginal speculum is inserted. The cervix is cleansed and a cannula is inserted into the cervix.

Contrast dye is injected through the cannula, and the flow of the dye is viewed fluoroscopically. Films are taken throughout the procedure.

Nursing Process Elements

Inform client that she may experience minor discomfort during and after the procedure but it should not last long. Shoulder pain may be experienced as the contrast medium leaks into the peritoneal cavity and irritates the diaphragm. Observe for allergic reaction to dye. Inform client bloody discharge may be present for 1–2 days. Client should report any fever, chills, abdominal pain, or frank bleeding.

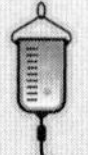

Clinical Alert

Possible complications include allergic reaction, infection, and uterine perforation. The test is contraindicated in clients who are pregnant, in their menses, with undiagnosed vaginal bleeding, or with pelvic inflammatory disease or untreated sexually transmitted disease.

MUSCULOSKELETAL SYSTEM

Arthrogram

- Visualization of joints of the elbow, knee, wrist, hip, and temporomandibular area

Indications: To aid in diagnosis of tears of the menisci, ligament disruption, and synovial cysts

Preparation: Assess the client for allergies to iodine, seafood, or local anesthetics. Obtain signed informed content.

Procedure: Skin is injected with local anesthetic. Needle is inserted into the joint space. Fluid may be aspirated for analysis prior to injecting radiopaque dye, air or both into the joint cavity. The needle is removed and the joint is manipulated to disperse the dye throughout the joint. X-rays are taken with the joint in various positions.

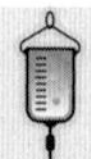

Clinical Alert

Clients who are or may be pregnant should not have this procedure due to the risk of radiation exposure.

Nursing Process Elements

- Observe for allergic reaction to dye.
- Apply ice and elastic wrap and administer analgesics. Encourage rest of injected joint for 12 hours. Teach client to report edema, redness, or unusual pain following the procedure.

Arthrocentesis (Synovial Fluid Aspiration)

- Removal of fluid from the joint for analysis.

Indications: To relieve edema and provide joint fluid sample for diagnosing gout, infection, or rheumatoid arthritis

Preparation: Obtain signed informed consent.

Procedure: With skin cleansed and anesthetized, sterile needle is inserted into the joint and fluid is aspirated.

Nursing Process Elements

Client teaching: Apply ice on joint for 20–30 minutes every 3–4 hours to relieve pain; take medication to relieve pain as prescribed by physician; avoid stressing the joint; apply an elastic bandage to support joint.

Bone Scan

- Visualization of abnormalities in bone or joint through the use of radioisotope

Indications: To aid in diagnosis of metastatic disease, tumors, osteomyelitis, trauma, arthritis, metabolic diseases, bone marrow hyperplasia, and Paget's disease

Preparation: No fasting is required. Obtain a signed informed consent. Radioisotope is injected intravenously 2 hours prior to the scan being performed. The client is to drink 4–6 glasses of water during the time between injection and scanning to help clear body of excess radionuclide.

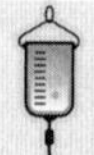

Clinical Alert

Clients who are or may be pregnant should not have this procedure due to the risk of radiation exposure.

Procedure: Client voids and is then assisted to supine position. Client lies quietly on examination table during scanning, which may take 1 hour.

Nursing Process Elements

Encourage increased fluid intake following examination to ensure excretion of isotope. No other radionuclide tests should be scheduled for 24–48 hours.

PULMONARY SYSTEM

Arterial Blood Gases

- Measure the pH (acidity), oxygen content, and carbon dioxide content of the blood.

LABORATORY VALUES

Tables 16-1 to 16-7 summarize important information about the major laboratory tests used in the assessment of each body system. Table 16-8 lists laboratory tests and values that are identified in the NCLEX-RN test plan as those the nurse "must know" or "must recognize when deviating from normal."

Table 16–1 Cardiovascular System

Test	Description/Definition	Use	Normal Values	Interpretation	Nursing Alerts
Creatinine Kinase (CK) Creatinine Phosphokinase	Enzyme found in higher concentrations in the heart and skeletal muscle and in the brain.	To identify injury to heart and skeletal muscle and the brain	50–325 mU/ml	With MI it begins to rise in 4–6 hrs, peaks in 24 and returns to normal in 48–72 hrs	Decreased values have no diagnostic meaning
(CPK) CK-MB (CK-MB_2)	Isoenzyme specific for cardiac muscle.	To identify cardiac injury	0–6%	With MI it rises within 3–8 hrs, peaks in 18–24 hrs	Serial blood samples are drawn every 6–8 hrs, three times
Aspartate Transaminase (AST)	Enzyme present in tissues of high metabolic activity.	To identify liver and heart muscle damage	7–40%	With MI it rises and peaks in 24 hrs	AST curve in MI parallels that of CK
Lactate Dehydrogenase (LDH)	Enzyme that is widely distributed in the tissues of the body.	Useful in diagnosis of MI when viewed in relation to other laboratory tests	140–280 U/l	Elevates in 36–55 hrs after an MI	
LDH_1	One of five isoenzyme of fractions of LDH. It is present in cardiac tissues.	Useful in diagnosis of cardiac damage	17–27% of total LDH	Released into the blood stream when cardiac tissue necrosis (MI) occurs	
LDH_2	One of five isoenzyme of fractions of LDH. It is present in cardiac tissues.	Useful in diagnosis of cardiac damage	29–39% of total LDH	Released into the blood stream when cardiac tissue necrosis (MI) occurs. LDH flip is very helpful in diagnosing MI	LDH flip occurs when LDH_1 levels are higher than LDH_2
Troponin I	Protein found only in cardiac muscle.	Useful in diagnosis of cardiac damage	<0.35 ng/ml	Rises with in 3–6 hrs of cardiac damage Peaks 12–16 hrs	
Cardiac troponin T	Protein which displays significant amino acid differences in cardiac and skeletal tissue.	Useful in diagnosis of cardiac damage	<0.2 ng/ml	Rises with in 4–8 hrs of cardiac damage Peaks 12–48 hrs	
Ischemia modified albumin (IMA)	Is a sensitive marker of myocardial ischemia, Acute Coronary Syndrome.	It was found that ischemia modified albumin rises so rapidly that it is present in the blood within 6–10 min after the ischemic episode.		It occurs more rapidly than any other indicator. It also clears fairly rapidly, in about 6 hrs from the blood	Must be used in conjunction with other cardiac markers (e.g., troponin).
High density lipoprotein cholesterol (HDL-C) "the good cholesterol"	Lipoprotein which removes cholesterol from the arteries and transports it to the liver.	Used to assess CAD risk	Men: >40 mg/dl Women: >50 mg/dl	Decreased levels of HDL-C are considered atherogenic	Requires a 9–12-hr fast before the test and no alcohol for 24 hrs before test

(continued on next page)

Table 16–1 *(continued from previous page)*

Test	Description/Definition	Use	Normal Values	Interpretation	Nursing Alerts
Low-Density Lipoprotein (LDL) "the bad cholesterol"	Lipoprotein which carries cholesterol to the arteries.	Used to assess CAD risk	Desirable <130 mg/dl Borderline high risk >140–159 High risk >160 mg/dl	Increased levels are considered atherogenic	Requires a 9–12-hr fast before the test and no alcohol for 24 hrs before test
Very low density lipoprotein (VLDL)	Lipoprotein which is a major carrier of triglycerides in the blood. VLDL degradation is a major source of HDL.	Used to assess CAD risk	10–15% of total cholesterol	Increased levels are considered atherogenic	
High sensitivity c-reactive protein-hs (CRP)	A specific abnormal protein that appears in the blood during an inflammatory process.	Used to determine risk for coronary event	Normal: <0.8 mg/dl	The higher the value the greater the risk of a coronary event	Requires a 9–12-hr fast before the test and no alcohol for 24 hrs before test
Apolipoprotein B (Apo B) plaque	Measures the level of lipoprotein phospholipase A2 (Lp-PLA2). Lp-PLA2 generates oxidized molecules within the blood vessel wall that are more prone to lead to both atherosclerosis and irritability of the atherosclerotic plaque.	Used to determine risk for coronary event	Normal 50–100 mg/dl	High levels of Apo B are indicative of increased risk for heart attack and stroke even when LDL is not in the high-risk range	Requires a 12-hr fast
Brain natriuretic peptide (BNP) test	Measures the amount of the BNP in the blood and is a marker for ventricular dysfunction.	Used to diagnose CHF	Normal <100 ng/l	Elevated levels indicate worsening of CHF. Decreased levels indicate improvement of CHF	Requires a 12-hr fast

Table 16–2 Hematologic/Immunologic System

Test	Description/Definition	Use	Normal Values	Interpretation	Nursing Alerts
Complete Blood Count (CBC)					
Red blood cell (RBC) count	RBCs are produced in the bone marrow and live 80–120 d.	Important for oxygen carried on Hgb molecules	Female 4.2 × 10^6/mm^3 to 5.4 × 10^6/mm^3 Male 4.7 × 10^6/mm^3 to 6.1 × 10^6/mm^3	Decreased in anemia, leukemia, and renal disease Increased in polycythemia	
Hemoglobin (Hgb)	Hgb is composed of *heme* (containing iron and porphyrin) and *globin* (protein).	Measures oxygen-carrying capacity of blood	Female 12–16 g/dl Male 13–18 g/dl	Decreased in anemia, leukemia, and renal disease Increased in polycythemia	
Hematocrit (Hct)	Proportion of RBCs to plasma within a sample of blood.	Assesses the extent of a client's blood loss	Female 37–48% Male 42–52%	A drop of 3% in Hct equals approx. 1 unit of blood	With normal hydration, RBC count and Hgb, the Hct is normally 3 times the Hgb
Mean corpuscular volume (MCV)	Measurement of average RBC size.	Aids in diagnosis of type of anemia	86–98 mm^3	Elevated = macrocytic anemia Decreased = microcytic anemia	Microcytic/ hypochromic anemia = Iron deficiency anemia

(continued on next page)

Table 16–2 *(continued from previous page)*

Test	Description/Definition	Use	Normal Values	Interpretation	Nursing Alerts
Mean corpuscular hemoglobin concentration (MCHC)	Hemoglobin content relative to the size of the RBC.	Aids in diagnosis of type of anemia	32–36 g/dl	Increased = hyperchromic Decreased = hypochromic	Macrocytic/ hyperchromic anemia = Folic acid and Vitamin B12 deficiencies
Platelet count	Formed in the bone marrow, lifespan of 8–12 d, removed from circulation by spleen.	Assesses hemostasis and blood clotting	150,000–400,000/mm^3	Increased = thrombocytosis Decreased = thrombocytopenia	Spontaneous bleeding occurs with platelet count < 20,000/mm^3 Concern of clot formation with extremely high platelet count
Blood Smear					
Heinz body test	Heinz bodies are intraerythrocytic insoluble inclusions of hemoglobin.	Used to detect hemolytic disorders associated with Heinz body formation.	Zero	Increased in G6PD deficiency, Homozygous B-Thalassemia	
Sickle cell test	Abnormality of hemoglobin. RBC have a crescent shape.	Used to diagnose sickle cell trait and sickle cell disease	None	A positive test means a number of erythrocytes have assume the typical sickle cell shape.	A positive test must be confirmed by electrophoresis
White Blood Cell (WBC) Count and Differential					
White blood cell (WBC) count	WBCs protect the body from threat of foreign agents such as bacteria.	Aids in determining type and severity of infection	4500–10,500/ mm^3	Increased = leukocytosis	WBC counts are lower in a.m. and higher in p.m.
Neutrophil	First WBC to arrive at area of inflammation; mature neutrophils = "segmented"; immature neutrophils = "bands."		Segs 40–60% Bands 0–3%	Decreased = leukopenia Increased in acute pyogenic infections	Percentages in the differential count total 100%. Thus, an increase in one type leads to a decrease in others.
Lymphocyte	Immune WBCs; integral part in the antibody response to antigens.		20–40%	Increased in viral infections (mono)	With low neutrophil count (neutropenia), client may require reverse isolation.
Monocyte	When move out of circulation and into tissue, mature into macrophages, which are phagocytic cells.		2–8%	Increased in chronic inflammatory disorders	
Eosinophil	Role in defense against parasitic infections, phagocytize cell debris in later stages of inflammation.		1–4%	Increased in parasitic infections	

(continued on next page)

Table 16–2 *(continued from previous page)*

Test	Description/Definition	Use	Normal Values	Interpretation	Nursing Alerts
Basophil	Release histamine, bradykinin, and serotonin when activated by injury or infection.		0.5–1%	May be increased in chronic conditions such as ulcerative colitis	
Coagulation Studies					
Prothrombin time (Protime, INR)	Useful for detecting bleeding disorders caused by problems in the extrinsic system (factors I, II, V, VII, and X).	Monitors anticoagulant therapy with warfarin	8.8–11.6 sec	Increased in DIC, factor deficiency, liver disease, and warfarin use	Standardized through use of international normalized ratio (INR). Target INR for DVT and afib treatment: 2.0–3.0 Target INR for mechanical heart valve: 2.5–3.5
Partial thromboplastin time (PTT)	Useful for detecting bleeding disorders caused by problems in the intrinsic system (factors I, II, V, VIII, IX, X, XI, and XII).	Monitors anticoagulant therapy with heparin	PTT: 60–90 sec APTT: 25–35 sec	Increased in DIC, factor deficiency, liver disease, and heparin use	Chemicals can be added to standardize results, a test known as APTT (activated PTT)
Bleeding time	Measures duration of bleeding after a standardized skin incision has been made. Detects disorders involving platelet function.	Screens for preoperative clients and those with personal or family history of bleeding tendencies	1–9 min	Increased in DIC, factor deficiency, hypocalcemia, bone marrow disorder, liver and renal disease, and thrombocytopenia	Prolonged bleeding time with normal platelet count indicates a qualitative platelet disorder
Electrolytes					
Sodium	Major cation in extracellular fluid Role in acid-base balance and neuromuscular functioning Inverse relationship with potassium	Assesses fluid balance of the body	135–145 mEq/l	Increased (hypernatremia) in: dehydration, diabetes insipidus, and impaired renal function Decreased (hyponatremia) in: diaphoresis, diarrhea, vomiting, GI suctioning, inadequate sodium intake, overhydration, and overdiuresis	Hypernatremia: dry mucous membranes, fever, thirst, and restlessness. Hyponatremia: lethargy, confusion, abdominal cramping, apprehension, oliguria, rapid weak pulse, headache, tremors, seizures, and coma
Potassium	Major cation in intracellular fluid. Responsible for acid-base balance, cellular osmotic pressure, electrical conduction in muscle cells (especially cardiac and skeletal).	Evaluates clients with cardiac and renal problems, confusion, GI distress	3.5–5.0 mEq/l	Increased (hyperkalemia) in acidosis, acute renal failure, diabetes, and hypoaldosteronism Decreased (hypokalemia) in alkalosis, diarrhea, hyperaldosteronism, liver disease, malabsorption, and vomiting	Hyperkalemia: S&S include weakness, malaise, nausea, diarrhea, muscle irritability, oliguria, and bradycardia. Hypokalemia: confusion, anorexia, muscle weakness, paresthesias, hypotension, cardiac dysrhythmias, and decreased reflexes.

(continued on next page)

Table 16–2 *(continued from previous page)*

Test	Description/Definition	Use	Normal Values	Interpretation	Nursing Alerts
Calcium	50% of calcium in blood is in free state; 50% is bound to albumin. Role in muscle contraction, heart function, transmission of nerve impulses, and clotting of blood. Release of calcium from bones into bloodstream controlled by parathyroid gland.	Measures parathyroid gland function and calcium metabolism	8.5–10.5 mg/dl	Increased (hypercalcemia) in hyperparathyroidism, hyperthyroidism, various cancers, and Paget's disease Decreased (hypocalcemia) in chronic renal disease, hypoparathyroidism, and malabsorption	Clients with hypercalcemia: deep bone pain, renal calculi, and muscle hypotonicity. With hypocalcemia: paresthesias, muscle twitching, cardiac dysrhythmias, convulsions
Magnesium	Primarily an ion of intracellular fluid. Essential for proper neuromuscular functioning, energy production, blood clotting. Majority found in bones combined with calcium and phosphorus.	Used in monitoring renal, GI, and cardiac conditions	1.5–2.0 mEq/l	Levels controlled by absorption from the intestines and excretion or absorption by the kidneys. Many causes of abnormal magnesium levels involve GI and renal problems	Increased serum magnesium levels: lethargy, flushing, hypotension, bradycardia, and weak reflexes Decreased levels: muscle twitching, tremors, tetany, cardiac dysrhythmias, and hyperactive reflexes
Phosphorus/ phosphate	Most phosphorus is combined with calcium in the bones. About 15% exists in blood; main anion in the intracellular fluid. Role in glucose and lipid metabolism, energy storage, acid-base balance. Levels controlled by parathyroid gland.	Measures parathyroid gland function	2.4–4.1 mg/dl	Increased phosphorus with decreased calcium: hypoparathyroidism, and renal disease Decreased phosphorus with increased calcium: hyperparathyroidism Decreased phosphorus and calcium: malabsorption, Vitamin D deficiency	Calcium and phosphorus in inverse relationship: excess in the serum of one results in kidneys excreting the other
Other					
Blood culture	Performed to detect infection due to bacteria or fungi in the blood (bacteremia).	Identifies cause of blood infections	Negative	The culture specifies the bacteria; the sensitivity identify antibiotics to which organism is susceptible or resistant	Specimen collection should occur prior to beginning antibiotic therapy
Therapeutic drug monitoring (digoxin, lithium, aminoglycosides)	Used to manage client drug therapy for drugs in which there is a narrow margin of safety between therapeutic drug effect and drug toxicity.	Monitors drug levels of medication	Varies with drug	Increased with toxic drug levels; decreased with Subtherapeutic drug levels	Drug levels are drawn at peak and trough times for aminoglycosides (antibiotics which are nephrotoxic and ototoxic)

(continued on next page)

Table 16–2 *(continued from previous page)*

Test	Description/Definition	Use	Normal Values	Interpretation	Nursing Alerts
Wound culture	In suspected wound infection, the interior of the wound is swabbed. Open wounds are cultured using aerobic culture tube; anaerobic tubes used if fluid aspirated from closed wound.	Identifies bacteria responsible for wound infection	Negative	The culture specifies the bacteria; the sensitivity identify antibiotics to which organism is susceptible or resistant	Specimen collection should occur prior to beginning antibiotic therapy

Indications: To determine changes in the acid–base status of the client due to problems involving the pulmonary, cardiovascular, renal, and gastrointestinal systems, or administration of certain medications

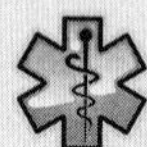

Nursing Intervention Alert

- Allen test should be performed before test is done
- Direct pressure should be applied for 2–5 minutes to the puncture site
- Note if client is receiving oxygen when the test is being done
- Rotate the blood in the test tube to be sure it has mixed with the heparin
- Place the sample on ice and take it to be analyzed

Urinalysis

Description/Definition: Urinalysis involves testing using two methods. A urine dipstick is used to test for numerous components, with a microscopic evaluation done to further investigate abnormalities.

Table 16–3 Respiratory System

Component	Description/Definition	Normal Values	Interpretation
Partial pressure of oxygen (PaO_2)	Indicates how well oxygen is able to move from the lungs into the blood.	70–100 mm Hg	If <70 then hypoxemia
Partial pressure of carbon dioxide ($PaCO_2$) pH	Indicates how well carbon dioxide is able to move from the blood into the lungs and then expired. Is a measure of hydrogen ion (H+) in blood which indicates the acid or base (alkaline) nature of blood.	35–45 mm Hg 7.35–7.45	Respiratory contribution to acid-base balance pH of less than 7.35 is acidic, and a pH greater than 7.45 is called alkaline.
Bicarbonate (HCO_3)	Is a chemical buffering substance that keeps the pH of blood within a normal range.	22–26 mEq/l	Metabolic (nonrespiratory) contribution to acid-base balance
Oxygen saturation (O_2Sat)	Provides information about the amount of oxygen in the blood.	95–100%	Measure of the amount of oxygen bound to hemoglobin

Table 16–4 Gastrointestinal System

Test	Description/Definition	Use	Normal Values	Interpretation	Nursing Alerts
Total serum protein	The total amount of albumin and globulin in serum, produce antibodies, steroids, thyroid hormones, transport blood components, preserve chromosomes.	Monitors protein levels, evaluate problems related to protein deficit, differentiate between albumin and globulin	Adult: 6.0–8.0 g/dl Child: 4.3–7.6 g/dl	Elevated levels found in liver disease, renal disease, multiple myeloma, and dehydration due to hemoconcentration. Low levels found with malnutrition, low protein diet, acute cholecystitis, Hodgkin's disease, malabsorption syndrome, and severe hepatic disease.	When albumin is low, assess for edema in lower extremities. Hyperglycemia may cause levels to appear greater than actual level. Check for albumin or protein in urine. Protein levels affected by recent dialysis. Client should avoid high fat foods 24 hrs before test. Encourage protein intake (eggs, meat, cheese) if levels are low.
Serum protein electrophoresis	A process that separates different protein fractions into albumin, alpha-1, alpha-2, globulin, beta globulin and gamma globulin. Results are determined by use of an electrical field: proteins separate by electrical charge and molecular shape and size.	Evaluates and fractions serum proteins to monitor causes of diseases; differentiates between protein fractions	Total protein: 6.0–8.0 g/dl Albumin: 3.3–5.0 g/dl Alpha 1 Globulin: 0.1–0.4 g/dl Alpha 2 Globulin: 0.5–1.0 g/dl Beta Globulin: 0.7–1.2 g/dl Gamma Globulin: 0.8–1.6 g/dl	Albumin Increased with dehydration and exercise. Decreased with liver disease third space losses, inflammatory disease, pregnancy, malnutrition, and malabsorption. *Alpha-1 globulin* Increased with inflammatory disease, burns. Decreased in a client with a genetic disease or without this enzyme. *Alpha-2 globulin* Increased with inflammatory disease, nephrotic syndrome. Decreased with hyperthyroidism, hemolysis, and hepatic disease. *Beta globulin* Increased with iron deficiency anemia, biliary cirrhosis. Decreased with malnutrition, malabsorption, and hepatic disease. *Gamma globulin* Increased with acute and chronic infection, cirrhosis, and malignancy arthritis. Decreased with genetic immune disorders, lymphocytic leukemia, and lymphosarcoma.	Test may be performed on serum or plasma. To detect changes with this test about a 30% drop in albumin is required. When protein electrophoresis value is abnormal, an immunofixation electrophoresis, (IFE) is performed.
Serum albumin	Functions to maintain oncotic pressure in vascular system and in the transportation of	Identifies abnormal levels of albumin caused by disease processes (see interpretation)	Adult: 3.5–5 g/dl Age above 60 yr: 3.4–4.8 g/dl	Elevated levels found with dehydration, Hodgkin's Disease, stress, pneumonia, RA, neoplasms,	Check for albumin in urine. Low serum albumin may require a 24-hr urine collection to measure protein loss.

(continued on next page)

Table 16–4 *(continued from previous page)*

Test	Description/Definition	Use	Normal Values	Interpretation	Nursing Alerts
	bilirubin, one of the two main protein factors in blood, the smallest amount of protein molecules, makes up largest percentage of total protein value.			exercise, diarrhea, and vomiting. Low levels found in malnutrition, leukemia, malabsorption syndrome, chronic renal failure, severe burns, CHF, toxemia of pregnancy, and chronic liver disease.	When serum albumin is below normal, the total serum calcium is decreased. A lack of albumin in serum allows fluids to leak out of interstitial spaces and into peritoneal cavity (causing ascites).
Serum globulin	Refers to nonalbumin portion of serum protein, made up of a complex group of serum proteins, five times as large as albumin molecules, but not as effective as albumin in maintaining osmotic pressure, forms the main transport system for substances and constitutes the antibody and clotting systems.	Measures globulins produced by liver and lymphoid tissue, evaluates presence of abnormal levels	2.3–3.5 g/dl	Elevated values with acute and chronic infection, malignancies, allergies, RA, iron deficiency anemia, biliary cirrhosis. Decreased levels found in hepatitis, asthma, and lupus erythematosus.	Electrophoresis divides globulins into alpha, beta, and gamma factors; medications that alter results: growth hormone, acetaminophen, estrogen, corticosteroids, niacin, and elevated serum lipid levels may cause abnormal results.
Liver Function Tests					
Alanine aminotransfer ase (ALT) (formerly SGPT)	Enzyme found primarily in liver and in some body fluids, injury to liver causes release of this enzyme into the bloodstream, elevating ALT levels.	Diagnoses hepatocellular destruction; monitors liver problems related to hepatotoxic medications and response to treatment of liver disease and routine screening for hepatitis in donor blood samples; differentiates between hemolytic jaundice and jaundice	4–36 IU/l	Elevated levels seen with hepatitis, cirrhosis, CHF, hepatic damage, hepatic cancer; and hepatotoxic drugs. Low levels seen with weight loss, hepatitis C, and exercise.	Medications that interfere with test should be held for 12 hr before and alcohol for 24 hr before test. With liver damage ALT elevates up to 50 times normal. ALT levels may be slightly elevated with myocardial infarction.
Alkaline phosphatase	Enzyme produced primarily in the liver and bone and in intestine, placenta, and kidneys; functions best at a pH of 9.	Diagnoses and monitors hepatic and bone diseases	Female: 30–100 IU/l Male: 45–115 IU/l Infant/ Child: 1–2 times of adult level	Elevated levels with bone or liver disease, obstructive jaundice, hyperparathyroidism, Paget's Disease, normal pregnancy, RA, MI, medications: antibiotics, Indocin, INH, allopurinol, and albumin made from placental tissue. Decreased levels with malnutrition, pernicious anemia, hypoparathyroidism, celiac disease, cystic fibrosis, scurvy, and placenta insufficiency. Medications: fluorides, phosphates, propranolol, and oxalates.	Alkaline phosphatase isoenzymes should be measured if alkaline phosphatase level is elevated. Levels increase during periods of bone growth. Benign hyperphosphatemia occurs mostly in young children and in a few adults, other enzyme tests may be ordered to verify client's diagnosis.

(continued on next page)

Table 16–4 *(continued from previous page)*

Test	Description/Definition	Use	Normal Values	Interpretation	Nursing Alerts
Aspartate Aminotransferase (AST) (formerly SGOT)	Increased AST levels occur when there is a serious damage to cells, related to disease or injury, AST is released into the blood stream; this enzyme is found primarily in heart, liver, and muscle tissue and in moderate amounts in pancreas and kidney.	Detects presence of AST, evaluates coronary artery disease or hepatocellular diseases, diagnoses an MI by comparing AST levels with CK and LDH	8–38 IU/l Newborn: four times of normal adult	Elevated values with an acute MI, alcoholism, cirrhosis, diabetes mellitus, severe burns, musculoskeletal disease, acute pancreatitis, strenuous exercise, IM injections. Decreased levels with diabetic ketoacidosis, pregnancy, uremia, liver disease, and beriberi.	AST levels are often compared with ALT levels. Do not administer IM injection before taking this blood test. Assess for symptoms of an MI. Increased levels are seen with cardiac catheterization, angioplasty, or surgery.
Bilirubin, blood	Bilirubin is formed in the liver, spleen, and bone marrow, and as a result of hemoglobin breakdown (RBC destruction). Direct (conjugated) bilirubin is excreted by the GI tract, with minimal amounts entering bloodstream. Indirect (unconjugated) bilirubin is normally in the bloodstream.	Used to differentiate causes of jaundice	Direct: 0–0.4 mg/dl Indirect: 0.1–1.0 mg/dl Total: 0.3–1.0 mg/dl	Direct bilirubin rises when obstructive jaundice (as from gallstones) or hepatic jaundice occurs. Indirect bilirubin rises in cases of hemolytic jaundice (breakdown of hemoglobin) and in cases of hepatocellular dysfunction (as with hepatitis)	Testing with contrast medium within 24 hr will alter test results. Exposure of blood sample to sunlight or artificial light will decrease bilirubin content of sample.
Gamma glutamyl transpeptidase (GGTP)	A biliary excretion enzyme that assists with transfer of peptides and amino acids across cellular membranes, primarily found in the liver, biliary tract, kidney, prostate, and spleen and heart muscle.	Detects hepatobiliary disease, monitors alcohol abuse and drug toxicity	Female: 3–31 IU/l Male: 4–23 IU/l	Elevated values with liver disease, biliary obstruction, and damage to liver from alcohol, alcoholism, renal cancer, acute pancreatitis or cholecystitis, CHF, MI. Medications: phenobarbital, warfarin, aminoglycosides, phenytoin, 5FU, and alcohol; decreased levels are not clinically significant	During late pregnancy, values are low. Encourage client with an alcohol problem to join AA. Document any client medications that interfere with test results on laboratory form
Lactic dehydrogenase (LDH)	Intracellular enzyme released as a result of injury to body tissue, found in liver, heart, brain, skeletal muscle, kidneys, and RBCs. Made up of various formations of isoenzymes as: LDH 1: cardiac and RBC; LDH 2: cardiac and RBC; LDH 3: pulmonary, liver, and spleen; LDH 4: hepatic and skeletal; LDH 5: hepatic and skeletal.	Diagnoses myocardial or skeletal muscle damage, compares results with other cardiac enzyme tests, detects organ involvement with LDH isoenzymes	100–190 IU/l *Isoenzymes* LDH 1: 25–36%, LDH 2: 35–46%, LDH 3: 13–26% LDH 4: 3–10%, LDH 5: 2–9%	Elevated levels with acute MI, leukemia, liver damage, shock/trauma, placental problems, pulmonary disease, skeletal muscle disease, stroke, and hepatitis. Medications: narcotics, anesthetics, aspirin, and alcohol; decreased results caused by ascorbic acid	Strenuous exercise may lead to increased LDH 1,2 and 5 levels. IM injections can increase results. Cancer or megaloblastic anemia result in very high LDH levels

(continued on next page)

Table 16–4 *(continued from previous page)*

Test	Description/Definition	Use	Normal Values	Interpretation	Nursing Alerts
5'-Nucleotidase	A specific liver isoenzyme, damage to hepatobiliary tissues leads to leakage of this isoenzyme into the blood resulting in elevated values.	Confirms diagnosis of hepatic/biliary obstructive disease, diagnoses a liver disorder by comparing test results with other liver enzyme tests, differentiates between a diagnosis of liver and bone cancer, 5'-Nucleotidase is rarely elevated in bone cancer	0–1.6 u at 37 °C 0.3–3.2 Bodansky units Children's values are lower than adults	Elevated values with hepatitis, cirrhosis, cholestasis, bile duct obstruction, alcoholism, sickle cell anemia, and metastasis to liver. Medications: aspirin, narcotics, phenytoin, phenothiazine, and acetaminophen	Other liver enzyme results such as ALP, GGT, and alkaline phosphatase should be evaluated along with this test to evaluate and diagnose liver function/disorders. Encourage client to eat well-balanced meals, especially with cancer of the liver and cirrhosis. Inform client about possible tendency towards bleeding.
Other GI-related Tests					
Ammonia	Waste product that forms as a result of nitrogen breakdown during intestinal protein metabolism and from digestion of blood from the GI tract. Normally converted into urea by the liver and excreted by the kidneys. If disorder prevents this conversion, ammonia accumulates in blood, leading to hepatic encephalopathy.	Evaluates confusion and coma. Monitors effectiveness of treatment for liver disease	Adult: 15–45 mcg/dl Children: 40–80 mcg/dl Newborn: 90–150 mcg/dl	Increased with azotemia, cirrhosis, GI bleeding, hemolytic disease of the newborn, hepatic failure, and renal failure	Fasting for 8 hrs is required for this test (water is permitted). The client should avoid strenuous exercise and smoking just prior to the test.
Fecal occult blood testing (FOBT)	FOBT is used as a screening tool for colon cancer. It detects the presence of blood in the stool, but does not differentiate the location of the blood loss (upper GI vs. colon). Samples of stool are placed on specially treated cards. A developing solution is applied, with blue coloration indicating the presence of blood.	Detects blood loss into the stool	Negative	Positive test results may be due to colon polyp, diverticulitis, esophageal varices, gastritis, GI cancer, GI trauma/surgery, hemorrhoids, inflammatory bowel disease, and ulcer.	Red meats and foods with high peroxidase activity (beets, broccoli, cantaloupe, cauliflower, horseradish, and parsnips, turnips) cause *false-positive* results with guaiac-based FOBT ASA and NSAIDs should be avoided for 2 d before the test
Helicobacter pylori (H pylori)	Antibody test, determines presence of H Pylori with use of serological testing or urea breath test Transmission of H Pylori can occur with use of contaminated endoscopic equipment.	Detects presence of organism, H Pylori, causing recurrent gastrointestinal disorders	Not present	Positive result indicates presence of this gram-negative bacilli, causing gastritis, gastric ulcers, duodenal ulcers or inflammation, peptic ulcers, and gastric cancer	Most duodenal ulcers are caused by H Pylori. When detected and treated, ulcers usually heal. Breath test contraindicated in pregnant clients and children due to use of radioactive carbon
Hepatitis associated antigens (HAA)	Tests performed to evaluate inflammation of the liver due to Hepatitis viruses A, B,	Group of tests used to detect major types and current status of Hepatitis. Positive	Negative	*Hepatitis A antibody* IgM identifies the acute phase of infection, IgG identifies past infection or immunity.	Maintain standard precautions, client is considered infected until serology tests

(continued on next page)

Table 16–4 *(continued from previous page)*

Test	Description/Definition	Use	Normal Values	Interpretation	Nursing Alerts
	C, and D. HEV, rarely seen in the United States, has no antigen or antibody tests available to identify virus at this time.	results indicate the specific type of Hepatitis that has infected the client		*Hepatitis B surface antigen (HBsAB)* Identifies active hepatitis, acute or chronic *Hepatitis B surface antibody (HBsAg)* Appears after disappearance of surface antigen, indicates end of acute infection phase. *HBe antigen (HBe Ag)* Detects presence of antigen in blood and development of chronic HBV infection. *HBe antibody (HBeAB)* Indicates resolution of acute infection. *HB core antibody (HBcAb)* Indicates increased level during time between disappearance of HBsAg and appearance of HbsAb. *Anti-HCV antibodies* Identified with the enzyme immunoassay (EIA) test, detects antibodies within 4 wk of infection; *Hepatitis delta antibody (HDV)* Detects presence within a few days after infection	indicate they are not, Hepatitis A, B, C (non-A, non-B), D, E, exist in acute, chronic, chronic active, and carrier phases.
Stool culture	Exposure to enteric pathogens may occur through foreign travel or contaminated food or water. GI symptoms can also occur if antibiotic therapy has suppressed normal intestinal flora, allowing remaining bacteria to become pathogenic.	Isolates and identifies organisms which might be causing GI symptoms	Normal flora present Negative for pathogens	Positive results occur with bacterial, parasitic, or protozoal enterocolitis	Follow-up stool analysis may be done if symptoms persist or to ensure pathogen is no longer present in stool

Use: A screening test used in the diagnosis of urinary tract infections and in the diagnosis of diseases unrelated to the urinary system.

Normal values and interpretation:

- Appearance: clear to slightly hazy
  - —Cloudy urine may be due to presence of WBCs, RBCs, bacteria
  - —Smoky urine may be due to presence of blood
- Color: light yellow to amber
  - —Many medications change the urine color
- Odor: aromatic
  - —Sweet/fruity urine due to ketonuria
  - —Fish/foul-smelling urine due to urinary tract infection
- Specific gravity (measure of urine concentration compared to water): 1.005–1.030
  - —Indication of kidneys' ability to concentrate and excrete urine

Table 16–5 Neuromusculoskeletal System

Test	Description/Definition	Use	Normal Values	Interpretation	Nursing Alerts
Erythrocyte sedimentation rate (ESR)	In the case of inflammation, necrosis, or physiologic stress (such as pregnancy), there is a change in blood proteins, which leads to a clumping of RBCs. The ESR measures the speed with which RBCs settle in a tube of blood. Clumped cells fall faster, resulting in a higher ESR (measured in mm/hr).	A nonspecific test for inflammatory and necrotic conditions	Male: <15 mm/hr Female: <20 mm/hr Elderly: slightly increased Child: 3–13 mm/hr Newborn: 0–2 mm/hr	Increased levels are seen in inflammatory bowel disease, infection, inflammation, malignancies, myocardial infarction, rheumatoid arthritis, temporal arteritis, tissue injury, and use of oral contraceptives. Aspirin and steroids decrease ESR levels.	Serial ESR measurements can be use to monitor effectiveness of steroids in treating conditions such as temporal arteritis.

—Increased in renal disease, congestive heart failure, dehydration, diabetes mellitus, excessive fluid loss (diarrhea, vomiting), increased secretion of ADH, liver disease

—Decreased in ADH deficiency, use of diuretics, high fluid intake

- pH: 4.6–8.0 with a mean of 5.0–6.0

—Provides information regarding acid-base status of the client

—Increased (alkaline) with chronic renal failure, urinary tract infection

—Decreased (acidic) with dehydration, diabetes mellitus, diarrhea

- Leukocyte esterase: Negative

—Tests presence of enzyme released from WBCs when bacteria are present in the urine

—False negative findings are extremely rare, but can occur when there is ascorbic acid or protein in the urine

—False positive results may occur if the urine sample is contaminated with vaginal secretions.

—Positive findings should be verified by a urine culture

- Nitrites: Negative

—Nitrate, normally found in the urine, is converted to nitrite when gram-negative bacteria are present in the urine.

—Some types of bacteria do not lead to a positive nitrite.

—Most accurate if done on first morning specimen

- Protein (albumin): Negative

—With normal renal function, there is no protein in the urine because the glomerular filtrate membrane of the kidney does not allow large protein molecules to pass through.

—Protein may be positive in diabetes mellitus, exercise, glomerulonephritis, preeclampsia, pyelonephritis, lupus

—False-positive results may occur if the urine is highly alkaline due to standing too long before being tested, if urine is highly concentrated, and after receiving contrast dye.

—False-negative results may occur if the urine is very dilute.

- Glucose: Negative

—If the serum glucose level is higher than the renal threshold for glucose, glucose will be excreted by the kidney

—Glucose may be present in acromegaly, Cushing's syndrome, diabetes mellitus, gestational diabetes, infection, and proximal tubular dysfunction

—Positive results should be followed by further testing to determine presence of diabetes mellitus.

- Ketones: Negative

—With uncontrolled diabetes mellitus, the body, unable to use glucose as an energy source, breaks down fatty acids for energy. This results in ketone bodies being formed and excreted in the urine.

—Positive results with alcoholism, anorexia, diabetes mellitus, diarrhea, fasting, high protein diet, hyperthyroidism, pregnancy, and vomiting.

- Urobilinogen: Negative or 0.1–1.0 Ehrlich units/dl

—Bilirubin is converted to urobilinogen by intestinal bacteria. Normally a very small amount of urobilinogen is present in the urine. This increases in the case of hepatic dysfunction or a hemolytic process

Table 16–6 Endocrine System

Test	Description/Definition	Use	Normal Values	Interpretation	Nursing Alerts
Fasting plasma glucose (FPG) Also known as fasting blood sugar (FBS)	Glucose is a primary source of energy within cells. It is formed from the metabolism of ingested carbohydrates and from the conversion of glycogen to glucose in the liver. Normal blood glucose is dependent upon proper functioning of glucagon and insulin.	Detects problems with glucose metabolism.	<100 mg/dl	Increased with brain trauma, burns, Cushing's syndrome, diabetes mellitus, hyperthyroidism, liver disease, pancreatic dysfunction, pituitary tumors, and medications such as beta-blockers, corticosteroids, diuretics, and estrogens. Decreased with Addison's disease, excessive exercise, hypothyroidism, insulinoma, islet cell carcinoma of the pancreas, malabsorption, stress, and intake of insulin	FPG of 100–125 mg/dl is considered "Impaired fasting glucose". A provisional diagnosis of diabetes mellitus is made with FPG of ≥126 mg/dl, but the diagnosis must be confirmed.
Glucose tolerance test (GTT)	After intake of a meal, the blood sugar peaks in 1 hr and then returns to premeal levels within 2–3 hrs. The GTT is used to evaluate the rate at which glucose is removed from the bloodstream following administration of an oral glucose load.	Measures glucose levels after giving client an oral carbohydrate challenge, confirms diagnosis of diabetes mellitus when persons have a high or slightly elevated blood glucose level, used for those with a family history of, women who have babies weighing more than 10 lbs	Fasting: <110 mg/dl After 30 min: <200 mg/dl	Elevated levels seen with diabetes mellitus, gestational diabetes, acute pancreatitis, liver disease, infections, burns, Cushing's Syndrome, hyperthyroidism, stress, and chronic renal failure; medications as corticosteroids, estrogens, and diuretics, salicylates; low levels are seen with hyperinsulinism, hypoparathyroidism, malabsorption, protein malnutrition, alcoholism, and Addison's disease	Insulin production is decreased due to aging, causing higher glucose levels; client with an FBS greater than 150mg/dl may not need GTT to confirm diabetes; obesity can increase glucose levels.
Hemoglobin A1C	One type of hemoglobin, Hemoglobin A1C, absorbs glucose. This glucose remains in the A1C for the lifespan of the RBC (120 d).	Used to monitor long-term diabetic control (2–3 mo average)	Nondiabetic 2.2–5% Diabetic <7%	Increased in hyperglycemia, newly diagnosed diabetes mellitus, poor diabetic control, and after alcohol consumption. Decreased with chronic loss of blood, chronic renal failure, hemolytic anemia, pregnancy, and splenectomy.	The use of testing for Hgb A1C is not recommended for diagnosis of diabetes mellitus.

(continued on next page)

Table 16–6 *(continued from previous page)*

Test	Description/Definition	Use	Normal Values	Interpretation	Nursing Alerts
Thyroid simulating hormone (TSH)	TSH stimulates the thyroid to release T3 and T4. When the levels of T3/T4 are elevated, the thyroid does not need to release more, so TSH levels decrease.	Used to diagnose and monitor client response to treatment for thyroid disease	0.4–4.0 μU/ml	Increased with Hashimoto's thyroiditis, Hyperpituitarism, pituitary adenoma, primary hypothyroidism, subtotal thyroidectomy, and medications such as amiodarone, lithium, and sulfa drugs. Decreased with hyperthyroidism, multinodular thyroid gland, and pituitary hypofunction.	Recent testing with radioactive isotope may affect test results. TSH levels are lowest around 10 a.m. and highest around 10 p.m.

Table 16–7 Genitourinary System

Test	Description/Definition	Use	Normal Values	Interpretation	Nursing Alerts
Blood urea nitrogen (BUN)	Urea nitrogen is produced by the liver as a result of protein metabolism. It is normally excreted by the kidneys. In renal disease, this excretion decreases, resulting in higher levels in the blood.	Test of renal function, specifically of glomerular function	Adult: 7–20 mg/dl Elderly: slightly increased	Increased in congestive heart failure, diabetes mellitus, GI bleeding, high-protein diet, renal disease and use of medications such as ACE-inhibitors, aminoglycosides, diuretics, NSAIDs, and contrast dye. Decreased in celiac disease, inadequate protein intake, liver failure, and pregnancy.	Nephrotoxic drugs must be used cautiously if BUN is increased. BUN and creatinine are to be assessed before contrast dye is administered to clients aged above 60 yrs, or those with renal disease, diabetes mellitus, or lupus.
Creatinine	Creatinine is a waste product of creatine phosphate, found in skeletal muscle tissue. It is excreted entirely by the kidneys. Normally it remains at constant level, even with aging.	Test of renal function.	Female 0.6–1.2 mg/dl Male 0.8–1.4 mg/dl Children 0.2–1.0 mg/dl	Increased levels indicate a slowing of the glomerular filtration rate. Seen in CHF, dehydration, diabetes mellitus, renal disease, lupus, urinary obstruction. Decreased levels occur in pregnancy and with muscle atrophy	BUN and creatinine are to be assessed before contrast dye is administered to clients age 60+, or those with renal disease, diabetes mellitus, or lupus Creatinine must be monitored at least every 12 mo for clients taking metformin for diabetes mellitus.
Prostate-specific antigen (PSA)	PSA is a glycoprotein found only in the epithelium of the prostate.	Screens for prostate cancer. Used to monitor disease progression and response to treatment.	<4 ng/ml	Increased levels with benign prostatic hypertrophy, cirrhosis, prostate cancer, prostate inflammation/trauma/manipulation, prostatitis, urinary retention, urinary tract infection	Falsely elevated levels can occur after urinary catheterization, cystoscopy, transrectal ultrasound or prostate biopsy

Table 16–8 Laboratory Values Essential to Basic Nursing Practice

Test	Value
Laboratory values about which the NCLEX-RN test plan states the test taker will "know"	
Arterial blood gases	
pH	7.35–7.45
PaO_2	70–100 mm Hg
$PaCO_2$	35–45 mm Hg
SaO_2	95–100%
HCO_3	22–26 mEq/l
Total cholesterol	160–200 mg/dl
Glucose (FBS)	<100 mg/dl
Hematocrit	Male: 42–52% Female: 37–48%
Hemoglobin	Male: 13–18 g/dl Female: 12–16 g/dl
HbA1C	Nondiabetic: 2.2–5% Diabetic: <7%
Platelets	150,000–400,000/mm^3
Serum potassium (K+)	3.5–5.0 mEq/l
Red blood cell count	Male: 4.7–6.1 × $10^6/mm^3$ Female: 4.2–5.4 × $10^6/mm^3$
Serum sodium (Na+)	135–145 mEq/l
Urine specific gravity	1.005–1.030
White blood cell count	4,500–10,500/mm^3
Laboratory values about which the NCLEX-RN test plan states the test taker will "recognize deviations from normal"	
ALT	4–36 IU/l
AST	8–38 IU/l
Bilirubin	Direct: 0–0.4 mg/dl Indirect: 0.1–1.0 mg/dl Total: 0.3–1.0 mg/dl
Bleeding time	1–9 min
Total calcium	8.5–10.5 mg/dl
High density lipoprotein cholesterol HDL-C)	Men: >40 mg/dl Women: >50 mg/dl
Low density lipoprotein (LDL)	Desirable: <130 mg/dl Borderline high risk: >140–159

Test	Value
Laboratory values about which the NCLEX-RN test plan states the test taker will "recognize deviations from normal"	
Creatinine	High risk: >10 mg/dl Male: 0.8–1.4 mg/dl Female: 0.6–1.2 mg/dl
Digoxin	0.2–1.0 mg/dl Therapeutic range: 0.9–1.2 ng/ml
Erythrocyte sedimentation rate (ESR)	Male: <15 mm/hr Female: <20 mm/hr SI increased elderly Child: 3–13 mm/hr Neonate: 0–2 mm/hr
Lithium	<1.5 mEq/l (serum level to avoid serious dose related side effects) Therapeutic range: 0.5–1.2 mEq/l
Magnesium	1.5–2.0 mEq/l
Partial thromboplastin time (PTT)	60–90 sec
Activated Partial thromboplastin time (APTT)	25–35 sec
International normalized ratio (INR)	0.7–1.8 (when used to monitor warfarin therapy, maintain between 2.0–3.0)
Phosphorus/phosphate	2.4–4.1 mg/dl
Total protein	Adult: 6.0–8.0 g/dl Child: 4.3–7.6 g/dl
Prothrombin time (PT)	8.8–11.6 sec
Urine albumin	Negative
Urine pH	4.6–8.0
Differential	Neutrophils: segs 40–60% Bands 0–3% Lymphocytes: 20–40% Monocyte: 2–8% Eosinophil: 1–4% Basophil: 0.5–1%

—Positive/increased with acute hepatitis, cirrhosis, cholangitis, hemolytic anemia, severe ecchymosis.

—Decreased with biliary obstruction, inflammatory disease, renal insufficiency, severe diarrhea.

- Bilirubin: Negative (no more than 0.2 mg/dl)

—Bilirubin is normally converted to urobilinogen in the intestine. If jaundice occurs due to obstruction or liver disease, direct bilirubin is unable to reach the GI tract and instead enters the bloodstream and is then excreted in the urine.

—Positive/increased in cirrhosis of the liver, hepatitis, and obstructive jaundice.

- Microscopic examination of urine

—Bacteria: Negative

—Casts: None

—Crystals: New

—RBCs: 0–2/hpf

—WBCs: 4–5/hpf

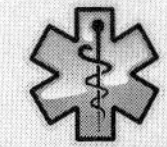

Nursing Intervention Alert

Most accurate results occur with first morning voiding. Specimen should be "clean catch," with the client carefully cleansing the area around the urethral meatus to avoid contamination of the specimen. The specimen should be taken to the laboratory as soon as possible for processing.

THERAPEUTIC PROCEDURES

INTRA-AORTIC BALLOON PUMP (IABP)

- A counter-pulsation mechanical aid to the circulatory function of the heart
- Improves coronary blood flow and systemic circulation
  —Increases perfusion of coronary arteries
  —Decreases cardiac workload
  —Decreases cardiac oxygen demand and consumption

Indications: To assess cardiogenic shock, unstable angina resistant to drug therapy, refractory ventricular dysrhythmias, ventricular septal rupture, and left ventricular failure after cardiac surgery

Preparation: Prepare the client and the family for the procedure. The client will be in a CCU or ICU setting with specially trained nurses or personnel to monitor the console and interpret the recordings. Obtain signed informed consent.

Procedure: An intra-aortic balloon and catheter is inserted percutaneously through the femoral artery and advanced to the descending aorta. This procedure is done in surgery, the cardiac catheterization laboratory or the critical care unit. The catheter is then connected to the console and pumping begins.

Nursing Process Elements

- Provide client education concerning IABP functioning and monitoring
- Make sure the catheter is secure and dry sterile occlusive dressing is in place
- Inspect site for signs of infection and complications
- Perform dressing change per protocol
- Change lines per protocol
- Assess vital signs, pulse oximetry, laboratory values, and hemodynamic parameters
- Assess peripheral perfusion by checking extremity for color, temperature, sensation, pulses, and movement
- Know procedures for immediate treatment if complications occur
- Maintain the head of the bed no higher than 45 degree elevation in order to prevent kinking of the catheter due to hip flexion
- Provide emotional support to client and family

Complications: Infection, embolism, thromboembolism, hemorrhage, dysrhythmias, peripheral ischemia, balloon perforation, inability to wean from IABP

Oxygen Therapy

- Provision of supplemental oxygen to restore the balance between oxygen taken in and carbon dioxide released
- Use results in reduced cardiac workload, decreased dyspnea, improved sleep, and exercise tolerance

Indications:

- Short-term use during recovery from acute lung disorder such as pneumonia, acute exacerbation of chronic obstructive pulmonary disease (COPD), or to decrease cardiac workload during congestive heart failure, angina, or acute myocardial infarction
- Long-term use for those with chronic lung diseases in which oxygen levels are consistently low, such as emphysema, occupational lung disease, lung cancer, cystic fibrosis, and nocturnal hypoxemia

Preparation:

- Need for oxygen therapy usually determined through oximetry or arterial blood gas analysis
- Prescription for oxygen therapy is needed, including oxygen flow rate in l/min, when to use the oxygen (such as while exercising or only while sleeping), how many hours to use the oxygen (some may need continuously), and the delivery system to be used.

Procedure:

- Oxygen can be supplied through three types of systems
  —Concentrators are devices that take oxygen from the room air and concentrate it for provision to the client. These devices are not available for portable use.
  —Compressed gas systems are available in metal cylinder tanks, which vary in size from large home-based tanks to small portable tanks.
  —Liquid gas systems include a large container of liquid oxygen and a portable unit, which can be refilled from the large container.
- Oxygen is delivered to the client from one of the above systems through the use of a nasal cannula, a mask, or a transtracheal catheter.
- During oxygen therapy, oximetry can be used to monitor oxygen saturation levels, with adjustments in oxygen flow settings made as needed.

You should never smoke while using oxygen. Warn visitors not to smoke near you when you are using oxygen. Put up no-smoking signs in your home where you most often use the oxygen. When you go to a restaurant with your portable oxygen source, ask to be seated in the nonsmoking section. Stay at least 5 feet away from gas stoves, candles, lighted fireplaces, or other heat sources. Do not use any flammable products like cleaning fluid, paint thinner, or aerosol sprays while using your oxygen.

If you use an oxygen cylinder, make sure it is secured to some fixed object or in a stand. If you use liquid oxygen, make sure the vessel is kept upright to keep the oxygen from pouring out; the liquid oxygen is so cold it can hurt your skin. Keep a fire extinguisher close by, and let your fire department know that you have oxygen in your home. If you use an oxygen concentrator, notify your electric company so you will be given priority if there is a power failure. Also, avoid using extension cords if possible.

Complications:

- Although side effects are rare, oxygen overuse can result in oxygen toxicity and atelectasis. Respiratory depression can occur if too high of flow rate is used in a client with COPD.
- Administration of high oxygen levels to premature infants can cause retinopathy of prematurity or contribute to occurrence of patent ductus arteriosus. Avoid PaO_2 (partial pressure of oxygen) levels greater than 80 mm Hg.
- Problems related to equipment include perforation of the nasal septum from use of nasal cannulas without humidification, and bacterial infections from contamination of humidification systems.

Nursing Process Elements

- Clients should be monitored for S&S of inadequate oxygenation including, restlessness, confusion, anxiety, cyanosis, drowsiness, or dyspnea.
- Monitor oxygen saturation levels through use of oximetry while at rest and with activity.
- Ensure proper use and cleaning of equipment.
  —Gauze may be placed under tubing to prevent skin irritation.
- Provide client with information on home oxygen equipment suppliers.

Client teaching for self-care

- Do not change the flow rate of oxygen unless directed to do so by the physician.
- Avoid use of alcohol or other central nervous system depressants, which depress the respiratory rate.
- Have no open flames, combustible products, including petroleum jelly, oils, and aerosol sprays, or equipment which might produce a spark.
  —If client requires lubricant on lips or nostrils, use water-based lubricants.
- Have a smoke detector and fire extinguisher in the home.
- Clean the oxygen delivery equipment as instructed.
- Keep oxygen cylinder in safe location where it will not fall over or become heated (avoid placement near flames or in trunk of car).
- Contact medical supplier early for additional oxygen supplies.

CHEST TUBE

- A tube inserted through the chest wall to remove air or fluid from the pleural space

Indications: To treat pneumothorax or hemothorax, to drain blood from the mediastinum after open-heart surgery

Preparation: Perform a baseline cardiopulmonary assessment. Explain the procedure to the client. Place the client in high Fowler's or semi-Fowler position. Obtain signed informed consent. Administer sedation as ordered.

Procedure: The skin is cleansed and injected with a local anesthetic. A 1-inch skin incision is made and a hemostat is used to enter the pleural space. The tube is inserted and attached to a drainage device and to wall suction.

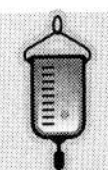

Clinical Alert

A postinsertion chest X-ray is done to ensure proper placement of the chest tube.

Nursing Process Elements

Routine Care

- Cardiopulmonary assessments are done at least every 4 hours.
- Monitor chest tube drainage every 2–4 hours.
- Dressing changes are done per hospital protocol
- Encourage client to cough and deep breathe, and to change positions every 2 hours.

Nursing Process Elements

Special Considerations

- Check chest drainage system for air leak.
  —Bubbling in the water seal chamber or air leak meter indicates the presence of an air leak.
  —If there is no leak, the water level in this chamber will oscillate with client respiration. This oscillation reflects normal pressure changes in the pleural cavity.
- Monitor chest tube drainage
  —Increased drainage suggests new or increased bleeding
  —Expect little drainage if the client has a pneumothorax (tube is draining air)
  —Check tube for blockage and kinks
- Maintain chest tube to water-seal drainage
  —Prevents air from entering the chest tube when client inhales.
  —Have the client take several deep breaths to fully inflate the lung and help push pleural air out through the tube.
  —Palpate the chest around the tube for subcutaneous emphysema and notify the MD if it increases.
  —Assess the function of the tube and describe and record amount of drainage.
- Care of the dislodged chest tube:
  —Cover the chest wall opening immediately with petroleum gauze.

—Apply pressure to prevent negative inspiratory pressure from sucking into the client's chest space.
—Call the physician and continue to keep the opening closed.
—Prepare/assist the physician to reinsert another chest tube
—If the drainage chamber is broken, change to a new chamber.

Complications: Inflammation, infection, subcutaneous emphysema

THORACENTESIS

- Insertion of needle through the chest wall in to the pleural space.

Indications: To obtain pleural fluid for analysis, to relieve lung compression

Preparation:

- Obtain signed informed consent
- No fasting is required
- Advise client not to move, cough, or deep breathe during the procedure
- A preprocedure chest X-ray is done

Procedure:

- The client leans forward with the arms resting on an overbed table
- The puncture site is cleansed and anesthetized
- A large needle is inserted and fluid withdrawn

Nursing Process Elements

- Assess vital signs, breath sounds
- Assist client to lie on unaffected side for 1 hour (to allow for lung expansion)
- Observe for S&S of pneumothorax, shock, leakage at puncture site
- Postprocedure chest X-ray may be done

TRACHEOSTOMY

- Incision into the trachea to form an opening called a stoma. The opening may be temporary or permanent.

Indications: Laryngectomy, severe infection, subglottic stenosis, congenital abnormalities of the airway, severe neck or mouth injuries, foreign body obstruction, tumors, need for prolonged respiratory support, chest wall injury, diaphragmatic dysfunction, neuromuscular disease, aspiration, cervical vertebral fractures, and coma

Preparation: Most tracheostomy procedures are done nonemergent, allowing time for client and family education regarding the procedure.

Procedure: Usually performed in the ICU or operating room. Client is monitored by EKG and pulse oximetry and receives IV sedation. A local anesthetic is given at the incisional area, located low in the neck below the larynx. A temporary tracheostomy tube is placed at the time of surgery. This is changed to a new tube 10–14 days post-op.

Complications: Respiratory distress, tube obstruction, bleeding, infection, tracheal stenosis, tracheoesophageal fistula, granuloma, and pressure necrosis

Nursing Process Elements

Special Considerations

- Monitor vital signs and respiratory status frequently
- Provide care for the tracheal site to prevent infection and skin breakdown (done daily or more frequently if on ventilator)
- Provide suction of the tracheal tube every 4–6 hours and as needed to remove mucus from the tube and trachea
- Change the tube every 1–4 weeks
  —Always have two people present for changing the tracheal tube
- Have emergency equipment available
- Ensure adequate environmental humidity (at least 50%)
- Prevent any substance or object from entering the tracheal tube
  —Avoid water, sand, dust, powder, talc, aerosol sprays, perfumes, ammonia, bleach, chalk dust, necklaces, fuzzy or fur clothing, and animal dander
  —Avoid smoke
- Avoid clothing that blocks the tracheal tube
- Ensure the client is up-to-date on all immunizations, including yearly flu shot

Client teaching for self-care

Before the client leaves the hospital, the client/family should demonstrate proficiency in care of the tracheal tube/site, including:

- Equipment functions
- Cleaning of equipment, especially inner cannula
- How to use a suction machine
- Observations to make/report (bleeding, infection, subcutaneous emphysema, tube obstruction, respiratory difficulty)
- Humidification of airway
- Dealing with tracheal ties
- Dealing with aspiration
- CPR

MECHANICAL VENTILATION

- Uses: To correct life-threatening alterations in blood gases; to reduce work of breathing allowing the respiratory muscles to rest; and to maintain ventilation during bronchoactive therapy

Invasive Mechanical Ventilation

- Uses an invasive airway (endotracheal tube or tracheostomy if long term)

Common ventilator modes

Determine whether breathing is client-controlled or ventilator-controlled and in what fashion and to what extent.

- *Assist/Control mode*: In ventilator-controlled mode, when client starts to inhale, the ventilator delivers a breath; if the client does not start to inhale to trigger the ventilator, the ventilator delivers breaths in accord with a preset number per minute (20–24 is standard) and a preset tidal volume thus providing continuous mechanical ventilation.
- *Synchronized intermittent mandatory ventilation (SIMV) mode*: Ventilator delivers breaths intermittently in synchronization with client's spontaneous breaths so client can take more breaths than the number per minute set for the ventilator; number of ventilator breaths can be gradually decreased until client is breathing entirely on his/her own.
- *CPAP*: One constant level of pressure is delivered during inspiration and expiration; respiratory rate and other parameters of respiration are controlled by the client
- *BiPAP*: It allows different levels of pressure during inspiration and expiration

Common types of ventilators

- Volume cycled: Positive pressure is applied during inspiration to deliver a constant volume of air; amount of pressure varies according to how much is required to deliver the preset volume of air
- Pressure cycled: Preset amount of positive pressure is used on each inspiration and so the volume of air delivered varies with airway conditions.

Noninvasive Positive-Pressure Ventilation (NPPV)

- Uses a tight fitting face or nasal mask with a volume- or pressure-cycled ventilator or continuous positive airway pressure (CPAP) or bilevel positive airway pressure (BiPAP) device
- Client must be alert, cooperative, free of excessive secretions, and stable hemodynamically
- May be used for up to 7 days
- Advantages: Mask may be removed for short intervals allowing client to speak, drink, use nebulizer; fewer complications
- Disadvantages: Risk for aspiration and local skin breakdown; some clients are unable to tolerate the mask

Nursing Process Elements

- Verify ventilator settings according to agency policy which is usually hourly.
- Respond to ventilator alarms: check for problem in systematic fashion starting at the client and working outward toward the ventilator
- Disconnect client and ventilate with an Ambu bag if respiratory distress occurs and problem cannot be corrected immediately
- Use closed system suctioning: Use ventilator to hyperoxygenate and inflate lungs then insert suction catheter and apply suction for not more than 10 seconds as the catheter is withdrawn
- Use meticulous sterile technique: Pneumonia is a major risk associated with prolonged mechanical ventilation
- Prepare for weaning according to agency protocol

Weaning: Initiated when client meets physiologic criteria related to hematocrit, ABGs and respiratory function, electrolyte balance and nutritional status.

Common methods

- T-piece weaning: With client sitting up, the ventilator is disconnected and a T-piece is attached to the endotracheal cuff through which oxygenated, humidified air is given. Ventilator is reconnected when fatigue or respiratory distress occurs. Time off the ventilator with the T-piece is gradually increased.
- SIMV weaning: client remains connected to the ventilator but the number of ventilator delivered breaths is gradually decreased until the client is breathing on his/her own.
- PSV weaning: Client remains connected to the ventilator and the level of preset positive pressure during weaning is gradually decreased until client is breathing independently.

Nursing Process Elements

Weaning:

- Promote good nutritional status in preparation for weaning.
  - —1500–2500 calories per day with 1–1.5 mg/kg or protein
- Avoid extra carbohydrates and calories because they can result in increased CO_2 production and, therefore, increased ventilatory demand.
- Explain the process noting several attempts may be required.
- Instruct in slow, deep breathing with a long exhalation phase.
- Obtain baseline vital signs, tidal volume, and vital capacity at start of weaning attempt.
- Coach in breathing.
- Assess for increased blood pressure, pulse or respiratory rate, dysrhythmias, diaphoresis, agitation or increasing somnolence which are signs of hypoxemia and hypercapnia.
- After weaning, monitor for increased work of breathing and respiratory distress.

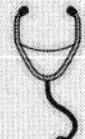

Assessment Alert

Respiratory distress is indicated by

- respiratory rate less than 8 or over 30 per minute or increase of 10 breaths per minute over baseline.
- pulse rate increased or decreased by 10 or more beats/minute.
- blood pressure increased or decreased by 20 or more mm Hg
- PaO_2 decrease or $PaCO_2$ increase.
- pH < 7.35.

Reproduced with permission from Monahan FD, Sands JK, Neighbors M, et al: *Phipps Medical Surgical Nursing: Health and Illness Perspectives,* 8ed. Elsevier, 2007, p. 704.

NEUROLOGICAL PROCEDURES

ECT Therapy

- Common mental illnesses include Alzheimer's disease, bipolar disorder, borderline personality disorder, depression, and schizophrenia. See Table 16-7 for the symptoms, treatment, and nursing interventions for these illnesses.
- An effective treatment for depression is electroconvulsive therapy (ECT). ECT is also used in the treatment of severe catatonia, mania, and schizophrenia.
  —ECT is used in clients who cannot tolerate side effects of antidepressants and in clients who are at risk for fluid and electrolyte imbalances secondary to the inability to eat or drink as a result of severe depression. ECT is also used in clients who experience major mood disorder; acute suicidal thoughts and behaviors; and melancholic, delusional, and psychotic depression.
  —Contraindications to ECT are increased intracranial pressure, recent myocardial infarction, aneurysms, acute respiratory infection, cardiac arrhythmias, thrombophlebitis, narrow-angle glaucoma, drug dependence, personality disorder, reactive depression, and paranoid schizophrenia.
  —The nurse obtains an informed consent from the client after the client, family, and significant others have been thoroughly educated regarding the purpose of treatment, proposed number of treatments, and risk factors associated with the procedure. Baseline tests—CBC, SMA, urinalysis, ECG, and physical examination—are performed prior to the procedure.
  —Clients scheduled for ECT fast overnight (NPO). Prior to the procedure, clients are asked to empty the bladder and remove jewelry, nail polish, eyeglasses, hearing aids, and dental work.
  —Thirty minutes prior to the procedure, the nurse administers 0.5 mg of atropine by intramuscular injection to reduce secretions.
  —The nurse ensures the procedure room is equipped with oxygen, suction equipment, and a cardiac arrest cart.
  —Appropriate staff includes a psychiatrist, anesthetist, and nurse. The anesthetist administers a short-acting anesthetic and muscle relaxant to decrease client injury. The nurse administers a mouth guard and oxygen.
  —The ECT electrodes are replaced after the client is anesthetized.
  —A brief electrical stimulus is administered (total duration of less than 2 seconds). The client's body does not move, and the seizure is confirmed by EEG monitoring.
  —After the client wakes, oxygen is discontinued, and the client is monitored for respiratory distress.
  —The nurse monitors the client for 1–3 hours. The client is discharged when vital signs are stable and the client is alert, oriented, and ambulatory.
  —Side effects associated with ECT are headache, memory loss, and fatigue. A mild analgesic and bedrest are usually offered after the procedure.
  —The nurse continues to teach and support the client, family, and significant others.
  —The nurse supports the client who experiences memory loss by providing orientation cues and an environment to express fears and anxiety.

GASTROINTESTINAL PROCEDURES

GI DECOMPRESSION AND DRAINAGE

- Insertion of a short nasogastric or long intestinal tube to remove fluids or gases by suction or gravity drainage

Indications: To protect suture lines after GI surgery; to remove GI contents when peristalsis and normal absorption is impaired such as after anesthesia or with obstruction; to remove toxic substances such as in drug overdose or accidental poisoning

Preparation: Estimate length of tube to be inserted: distance from tip of nose to ear lobe to xiphoid process for stomach tube; add 5 cm for intestine. Note distance marking on tube. Check for patency of nares.

Procedure: Place client in Fowler's position. Lubricate tube according to package directions. Apply water-soluble lubricant or wet with water. Insert tube into nare. Aid passage of tube by asking client to lower head a bit, swallow, and if permitted sip water when tube reaches pharynx. Check placement when estimated length of tube is passed. Most accurate method is X-ray. Less reliable options for gastric placement are: using a 50-ml syringe to aspirate gastric juice; instilling 10–20 ml of air into the tube; auscultating just left of the xiphoid tip for a "swoosh" as it exits the tube into the stomach; and measuring pH of aspirate.

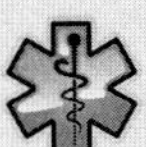

Nursing Intervention Alert

Placing end of tube in water to check for bubbling is not acceptable practice for checking tube placement.

Anchor gastric tubes and mark tube at level of exit with indelible pen to allow checking for tube movement. Do not anchor intestinal tubes at time of insertion as they must progress to desired location with peristalsis. Position client on right side until intestinal tube passes pyloric sphincter.

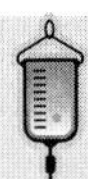

Clinical Alert

Signs that a GI tube is entering the trachea and must be withdrawn and reinserted are coughing, choking, and inability to talk or hum in an otherwise unimpaired client.

Nursing Process Elements

- Maintain suction at no greater than 25 mm Hg.
- Assess function q4 hour: Assessment should include: check drainage, note color, note amount, check consistency; note there is no c/o fullness or nausea; note there is no abdominal distention; check patency by irrigating with N/S as ordered.
- Check for passage of flatus or stool and report if it occurs; it indicates peristalsis so tube may no longer be needed.
- Assess for fluid, electrolyte or acid-base imbalance: monitor skin turgor, body weight, and serum electrolytes.
- Do not give ice chips, sips of water, etc. without orders because these are a source of hypotonic fluid, which can contribute to F&E imbalance.
- Record I&O; include irrigating solution instilled and returned.
- If tube is protecting a suture line, use strict sterile technique to irrigate.
- Assess for sore nares or throat from pressure of tube.
- Good mouth care because most intubated clients mouth breathe.
- Cleanse nares area and apply water-soluble lubricant.
- Prevent pull on tube and keep firmly anchored to prevent dislodgment.

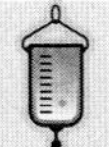

Clinical Alert

A clogged tube can lead to gastric distention and shock.

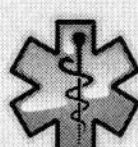

Nursing Intervention Alert

When peristalsis fully returns, a tube used for decompression and drainage is ready to be removed as indicated by presence of bowel sounds, absence of abdominal distention, tolerance of ice chips and/or clamping of the tube, decreased volume of drainage, and passage of flatus or feces.

Removal: Place client in semi-Fowler's position. Flush tube with 10 ml of N/S to cleanse and move away from mucosa to prevent damage; clamp; tell client to take deep breath; remove during exhalation; give mouth care. Gagging, sneezing, or nasal discomfort may occur. After removal of the tube, monitor for nausea, vomiting, and abdominal distention.

OSTOMY (GI)

- Surgical opening through the abdominal wall into the intestine. May enter ileum (ileostomy) or colon (colostomy). May be temporary (and be reversed) or permanent.

Indications: To aid in treatment of cancer, diverticulitis, Hirschsprung's disease, trauma, and perforated bowel

Preparation: Involve ostomy specialist prior to surgery to assist with client teaching and determination of stoma placement during surgery. Obtain signed informed consent. NPO at least 8 hours prior to surgery. Bowel prep as ordered. Preoperative sedation.

Nursing Process Elements

Special Considerations

- Monitor vital signs frequently postoperatively
- Keep skin around stoma clean and dry; monitor for leakage
- Assess pouching system for proper fit
- Empty and clean ostomy bag as needed

- Monitor amount of drainage from ostomy
- If ileostomy, bowel movements move through body more quickly than usual. Medications may need to be changed from "sustained release" formulation to more frequent dosing.

Client teaching for self-care

- Reinforce to the client that having an ostomy does not affect work, sexual function, or other activities
- Client should avoid very heavy lifting
- Application and cleaning of ostomy bag
- Irrigation of colostomy (if applicable)
- What to report (abdominal pain, vomiting, weakness, bleeding, and lack of ostomy output)
- Ostomy support group
- When traveling, carry supplies on person, not in luggage that might be lost
- With ileostomy, stools are liquid; client needs to maintain fluid intake to avoid dehydration (6–8 glasses per day)

DIALYSIS

- Life saving method of removing toxic substances from the blood when the kidneys are unable to do so.

Hemodialysis

- Removal of waste products and excess fluid from the blood by passing it through a machine outside of the body (dialyzer) with a semipermeable membrane and then returning the filtered blood, without the waste products and fluid, to the client through one of several types of access devices.
- Uses a combination of osmosis, diffusion, and filtration to remove by-products of protein metabolism, creatinine, and excess water thereby restoring acid-base and electrolyte balance and preventing complications associated with uremia.
- Performed three times per week for 3–4 hours per session, often in outpatient settings

Indications: To treat uremia or quickly remove drugs or poisons in acute situations

Preparation: Temporary or permanent access is established.

- Temporary access involves placing Y-shaped catheters in large veins (subclavian, internal jugular, or femoral) with one port for carrying blood to the dialyzer and the other port for returning filtered blood to circulation.
- Permanent access involves surgically connecting an artery and vein (arteriovenous fistula or AVF) or surgically placing a tube to join an artery and vein (arteriovenous graft or AVG) in an arm or leg.

AVF is typically allowed to mature for 3 months before being used; AVG may be used once the swelling subsides, usually 10–14 days. A temporary catheter is used in the interim.

Dry weight/target weight (the amount a client would weigh after urinating if renal function was not impaired) is established to determine the amount of fluid to be removed with each dialysis session.

Nursing Process Elements

Special Considerations

- Explain the purpose of hemodialysis and describe what to expect before, during, and after the procedure
- Monitor laboratory values including BUN/Creatinine, H&H, and Potassium
- Monitor weight, vital signs, and intake and output
- Assess circulation at the access site by auscultating for the presence of bruits and palpating for thrills lack of these may indicate a blood clot requiring immediate surgical attention
- Make sure the extremity used for vascular access is not used for intravenous therapy, blood pressure monitoring, or venipuncture
- Follow institution-specific protocols for care of temporary dialysis catheters
- Monitor for possible dialysis-related complications including bleeding, hypotension, nausea, vomiting, leg cramps, light-headedness, back pain, headache, chest pain, pruritus, infection, thrombosis, stricture, or aneurysm
- Only during emergency situations, should dialysis access devices be used for purposes other than dialysis
- Refer client and family for appropriate counseling and support

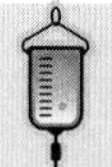

Clinical Alert

Life-threatening complications rarely occur, but include air embolism, acute hemolysis, and anaphylaxis

Client teaching for self-care

- Keep incision clean and dry
- Report pain, swelling, redness, or drainage in the accessed arm
- Use a stethoscope to auscultate for bruits
- Refuse treatment or procedures on the accessed arm, including blood pressure monitoring or needle punctures
- Avoid constriction of the accessed arm, such as wearing tight clothing, lying on it, or lifting heavy objects
- Avoid showering, bathing, or swimming for several hours after dialysis
- Take medications as prescribed; adhere to dietary restrictions and treatment plan

Peritoneal Dialysis (PD)

- Removes waste products and fluids without removing the blood from the body by using the peritoneal lining of the abdomen as a semipermeable dialyzing membrane
- A two-way catheter is placed in the abdomen and allows access for fluid exchanges
- May be continuous ambulatory peritoneal dialysis (CAPD) or continuous cyclical peritoneal dialysis (CCPD)
  —CAPD: Performed four times daily and involves filling the peritoneum with dialysate through tubing connected to the two-way catheter; dialysate remains for 3–6 hours; during this "dwell" time, fluid and waste products cross the peritoneal membrane through osmosis and diffusion; the dialysate containing the waste products is then exchanged for fresh fluid.
  —CCPD: Performed once daily over 8–12 hours, commonly while the client sleeps, and involves connecting a machine to the two-way catheter to move fluid in and out of the peritoneum.

Indications: PD offers some advantages over hemodialysis, including not having to travel to a dialysis center several times per week for therapy; fewer dietary and fluid restrictions, due to treatments being done daily; performed by client in own home environment

Preparation: Two-way catheter is surgically placed in the abdomen (Tenckhoff (most common), Toronto-Western Hospital (TWH), or Swan-neck).

Nursing Process Elements

Special Considerations

- Explain the purpose of PD and describe what to expect before, during, and after procedure
- Use sterile technique to change the catheter dressing daily
- Use sterile technique to open catheter for use
- Monitor for complications including peritonitis and catheter site infection

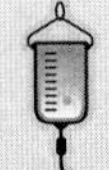

Clinical Alert

Dialysate must be present in the abdomen at all times with peritoneal dialysis to ensue adequate cleansing of the blood.

Client teaching for self-care

- Follow plan for frequency, duration, and timing of treatments
- Participate in a training program before performing independently
- Wear medical identification bracelet with contact information
- Report fever, persistent abdominal pain and cramping, slow or cloudy dialysis drainage, and swelling and tenderness around the catheter
- Follow up with doctor and dialysis team to evaluate success of treatment and detect any problems

PESSARY

- A device placed in the vagina to help support pelvic structures; used when surgery is contraindicated (can be temporary or permanent form of treatment)

Nursing Process Elements

- Explain to client the indications and use of the pessary
- Instruct client on how to remove, clean, and reinsert pessary
- Reinforce with client that pessary must be inspected and changed regularly to prevent ulceration, fistula formation, stool impaction, and infection
- Vaginal estrogen cream may help improve a woman's tolerance of the pessary
- Encourage lifestyle modifications including maintaining a healthy weight, practicing Kegel exercises to strengthen pelvic floor muscles, controlling coughing, and avoiding heavy lifting or straining
- Occasionally, a pessary may interfere with intercourse

PELVIC EXERCISES (KEGELS)

- Pelvic exercises used to strengthen and maintain the tone of the pubococcygeal muscle which supports the pelvic organs; involves the conscious contracting and relaxing of the pelvic muscles; also use is encouraged to reduce or prevent stress incontinence and uterine prolapse; enhance sensation during sexual intercourse, and hasten postpartum healing

Nursing Process Elements

- Explain the significance of performing Kegel exercises to client
- Instruct client to properly do exercises using the perivaginal muscles and anal sphincter while avoiding contracting the abdominal, buttock, or inner thigh muscles
- Measures that help reduce the symptoms of pelvic relaxation should be encouraged such as lying down with the legs elevated several times a day; encourage client to eat a healthy, well-balanced diet to avoid constipation and straining upon defecation

CATHETER DRAINAGE

- Removal of urine through a catheter inserted into the bladder.

Indications: To drain bladder; to relieve retention associated with neurogenic bladder, to temporarily manage incontinence

Preparation: Strict asepsis observed during catheter insertion.

Procedures:

- *Indwelling urethral*: Female client—The client is positioned supine with knees bent, hips flexed, and feet resting on bed about 2 feet apart. Labia minora separated, urethra meatus prepped with cotton pads saturated three times with iodine or hibiclens using downward strokes from anterior to posterior and discarding cotton pad after single use. Well-lubricated catheter, preconnected to a closed drainage system is inserted into urethral meatus using strict aseptic technique and advanced until urine flow is seen then advanced 2 inches further. Balloon inflated and catheter slightly withdrawn. Male client—Same procedure except positioned supine, meatus cleaned with circular motion, catheter advanced almost to its bifurcation before balloon inflated.
- *Suprapubic*: With the client in supine position, skin is prepped and local anesthetic is injected. Physician introduces catheter into bladder percutaneously via a guide wire through a small stab wound and catheter is advanced until flange is against the skin and secured with sutures.
- *Clean intermittent self catheterization (CISC):* Intermittent, self-placement of a catheter to drain the bladder. Client is taught to assemble equipment (catheter, lubricant, and drainage receptacle), wash hands with soap and water, lubricate catheter, clean around meatus, insert catheter and gently advance (upward insertion in females; penis held perpendicular to body in males), drain urine into receptacle, then withdraw catheter. Procedure is considered "clean" not sterile.

Complications: Urinary tract or kidney infections, septicemia, urethral injury, skin breakdown, bladder stones, and hematuria. After many years of catheter use, bladder cancer may also develop.

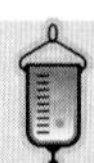

Clinical Alert

Catheterization intervals should be frequent enough to prevent the bladder from becoming over-distended with > 500 ml urine.

Nursing Process Elements

- Maintain unobstructed, downhill flow of urine.
- Empty bag at regular intervals, making sure the drainage valve is not contaminated.
- Wash hands before and after handling the catheter and drainage system and also between clients.
- Provide daily and as needed catheter care with mild soap and water; avoid pulling on catheter during cleaning; avoid using powders and sprays.
- Secure indwelling urethral catheter to thigh using tape, strap, or adhesive anchor; allow some slack for movement.
- Maintain asepsis during daily suprapubic catheter dressing changes.
- Assess color, consistency, and amount of drainage; record accurate I&O
- Monitor for fever, dysuria, pain, redness, swelling, or drainage around insertion.
- If a "trial of voiding" is requested, the suprapubic catheter is clamped for 4 hours, client voids, catheter unclamped and drained to measure residual volume.
- Follow institutional policy on obtaining urine specimens from catheters; label specimen as "catheterized specimen."
- Teach proper procedure for intermittent self-catheterization.

Client teaching for self-care

- Drink 8–12 glasses of fluid daily; increase intake if urine becomes dark and concentrated.
- Keep drainage bag at a lower level than the bladder.
- Wipe all connecting junctions with alcohol before changing from leg-bag drainage to overnight drainage bag.
- Discard disposable CISC catheters immediately after use. Wash reusable catheters with mild soap and water and store in a clean, closed container. Soak catheter in half strength vinegar solution overnight once a week.
- Report foul smelling or bloody urine, pain, fever, or diminished output.

ASSISTIVE DEVICES (WHEELCHAIRS, CANE, CRUTCHES, PROSTHESES)

- Devices used to aid a client in performing activities of daily living, including mobility

Wheelchairs

Uses: self-mobility, transportation

Nursing Process Elements

- Assess functionality of wheelchair
- Maintain cleanliness of multiuse wheelchairs
- Assure breaks are locked prior to transferring client to or from wheelchair

Client teaching for self-care

- Transfer from bed or chair to wheelchair
- Propelling nonmotorized wheelchairs
- Use of controls on motorized wheelchairs

Canes

- Several types are available: Straight-legged cane, quad cane (has four legs)

Uses: provides support while walking

Nursing Process Elements

- Assess ability to walk with cane; may encourage use of two canes

Client teaching for self-care

- Elbow should be flexed slightly when using cane
- Use cane on the unaffected side.

Crutches

Uses: Self-mobility, transportation

Nursing Process Elements

Teach client regarding correct use of crutches

- Weight should be placed on hand grips, not on axillary area
- Crutches always move with the affected leg
  - —When going up stairs, the unaffected leg goes first, followed by affected leg and crutches
  - —When going down stairs, the affected leg and crutches go first, followed by the unaffected leg

Prosthesis

- An artificial limb or part that replaces an injured, missing or malformed, or diseased body part, such as an arm, hand, or leg.

Uses: Joint replacement, limb replacement, breast augmentation, hearing (cochlear implant)

Nursing Process Elements

- Assess psychosocial response to prosthesis
- Assist the client through the grieving process
- Assess ability to attach prosthesis
- Encourage client involvement in the rehabilitative process
- Maintain cleanliness of prosthesis
- Assess skin integrity beneath applied prostheses
- Provide appropriate skin care as needed

Client teaching for self-care

- Teach the use of walker or crutches
- Teach how to propel nonmotorized wheelchairs
- Involve family in educational process

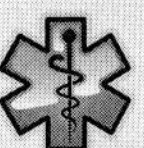

Nursing Intervention Alert

In the case of a total hip replacement, to prevent the prosthesis from dislocating after surgery, the hip is maintained in abduction through use of an abduction pillow.

CASTS

- A mold over a portion of the body using plaster or synthetic material

Uses: Maintain proper alignment and immobilization of a body part during healing.

Preparation: Cleanse skin; inspect skin for potential areas of infection or breakdown; bony prominences are padded with sheet wadding or felt

Nursing Process Elements

Special Considerations

- Monitor neurovascular status of the affected extremity
- Facilitate drying of plaster cast
- Petal rough edges

Client teaching for self-care

- Keep cast dry. When taking a shower cover it with a plastic bag and secure the bag to your skin with waterproof tape. If the cast gets wet, dry it thoroughly, including the cast padding inside the cast, with a blow dryer on low temperature to avoid burning yourself.
- Do not insert anything inside of the cast, such as additional padding or any device to scratch.
- Frequently move fingers or toes to prevent swelling and stiff joints.
- Elevate extremity to relieve swelling and reduce pain.
- Place padding under your cast to prevent scratching or damaging your furniture if you are resting the cast on a piece of furniture.
- Contact your physician if the edges of the cast become ragged, so that the physician can trim the cast.
- Contact your physician if the following occur: Persistent pain, cast feels too tight or loose, the cast becomes broken or cracked, if you feel painful rubbing under the cast, there is discoloration of the fingers or toes, or an unusual odor or drainage.

BUCK'S EXTENSION TRACTION

Simple skin traction using counter traction

Uses: Provides straight pull on the extremity for immobilization or to relieve muscle spasms

Preparation: Shave hair off extremity if an adhesive is being applied and apply tincture of benzoin to protect skin

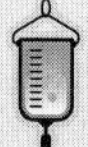

Clinical Alert

Contraindicated for clients with stasis dermatitis, arteriosclerosis, allergy to adhesive tape, severe varicosities of varicose veins, diabetic gangrene, or marked overriding bone fragments.

Postapplication Course:

- Maintain 8–10 pounds of traction
- Maintain foot of bed elevated to provide counter traction

Nursing Process Elements

Special Considerations

- Monitor neurovascular status of the affected extremity
- Maintain body in alignment
- Apply and maintain TED hose to nonaffected extremity
- Assess bony prominences for alteration in skin integrity, such as pressure ulcer
- Assess muscle strength, range of motion, and ability to perform ADLs

Client teaching for self-care

- Demonstrate how to move in bed without altering the traction

RUSSELL TRACTION

- Skin traction that provides a double pull by using a knee sling

Uses: To treat intertrochanteric fracture of femur prior to or without surgical repair

Nursing Process Elements

Special Considerations

- Maintain foot of bed slightly elevated
- Monitor neurovascular status of the affected extremity
- Maintain body in alignment
- Apply and maintain TED hose to nonaffected extremity
- Assess bony prominences for alteration in skin integrity, such as pressure ulcer

Client teaching for self-care

- Demonstrate how to move in bed without altering the traction

CERVICAL TRACTION

- Skin traction to the head

Uses: Used to treat muscle spasm, strain, or spasm by holding head in extension

Preparation: Applied with head halter, elastic bandages, or adhesive

Nursing Process Elements

Special Considerations

- Apply powder to ears to prevent friction rub
- Maintain head of bed elevated 30–40 degrees
- Maintain weights to pulley over the head of the bed
- Maintain body in alignment; when in side position, place a full length bath blanket roll behind client and pillow between the knees
- Apply and maintain TED hose
- Assess bony prominences for alteration in skin integrity, such as pressure ulcer
- Turn client by log rolling
- Align the client's head with the pull of the traction to maintain counter traction

Client teaching for self-care

- Demonstrate how to move in bed without altering the traction

PELVIC TRACTION

- Skin traction to the pelvis

Uses: Reduce muscle spasms and relieve low back, hip, or leg pain

Preparation: Apply the traction snugly over the pelvis and iliac crest and attach to weights

Nursing Process Elements

Special Considerations

- Assess for pressure and skin irritation under device
- Maintain weights hanging freely
- Maintain proper bed position for counter traction
- Maintain ropes in proper position
- Maintain body in alignment
- Apply and maintain TED hose

Client teaching for self-care

- Demonstrate how to move in bed without altering the traction

MONITORING CONSCIOUS SEDATION

CONSCIOUS SEDATION

- Minimally depressed level of consciousness in which the client retains the ability to maintain an airway and respond appropriately to verbal commands and physical stimuli but emotionally and physically accepts a painful procedure
- Associated with a low level of risk to client
- Typically achieved with sedative-hypnotics and/or opioids

Indications: To relax and/or relieve pain during procedures of short duration such as biopsy, radiologic imaging, endoscopic procedure, radiation therapy, bone marrow aspiration, painful dressing changes, wound packing, bedside wire or drain removals, or wherever client anxiety is likely to hinder necessary care. It is also commonly used as an adjunct to local or regional anesthesia for larger procedures such as dental surgeries, appliance removals, wound suturing, and other short but highly stimulating procedures.

Preparation:

- Assess client for any history of adverse reactions to the proposed medications or severe cardiopulmonary disease.
- Obtain informed consent for procedure and sedation.
- Verify plan for discharge, including a driver.
- Establish a working intravenous line.
- Connect monitors: Pulse oximeter, blood pressure monitor, three-lead ECG.
- Ensure availability of functioning wall or tank oxygen and delivery system.
- Ensure immediate access to emergency resuscitation equipment and medications.
- Ensure availability of medications to be used and reversal agents if any. Conscious sedation is usually accomplished through use of a short-acting benzodiazepine such as midazolam and a narcotic such as fentanyl (reversal agent for fentanyl is naloxone).
- Reassure the client that the medication (midazolam) has an amnesiac effect so there will be little or no memory of the procedure.
- Obtain baseline vital signs and oxygen saturation.

Procedure:

- The client is kept in the direct vision of a trained and licensed health care professional who is not involved in performing or assisting with the procedure.
- Medications are administered intravenously.
- Vital signs and oxygen saturation are measured every 5 minutes during the procedure.
- Sedation level is monitored throughout by conversation or ability to follow commands if client is unable to speak during the procedure.

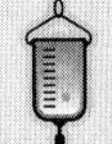

Clinical Alert

The oxygen saturation is the most sensitive parameter affected during the increased levels of conscious sedation.

- Common side effects of the sedation are: dizziness, nausea, amnesia, sleepiness, cardiovascular depression, respiratory depression, and pain or itching on injection.

Postsedation Care:

- Continue to monitor the client for at least 30 minutes, more if the amount of sedation was large or the procedure lengthy or complicated.
- Discharge when vital signs remain stable and client appears to have resumed preprocedure status.
- Provide all necessary instructions for self-care and follow up medical care.

WORKSHEET

TRUE & FALSE QUESTIONS

1. Glucophage should not be discontinued prior to a radiographic examination using contrast medium. ___ T ___ F
2. Start time for a 24-hour urine collection begins when the first urine sample is voided and saved. ___ T ___ F

(continued)

3. Only a sample of a 24-hour urine collection needs to be sent to the laboratory as long the total volume voided is accurately documented. ___ T ___ F

4. Serum BUN levels are decreased with kidney disease and acute renal failure. ___ T ___ F

FILL IN THE BLANKS

Fill in the blank space with the correct word or phrase to complete each statement.

1. What serum creatinine level indicates the need for renal dosing of medications excreted by the kidneys? ____________.
2. What should a client be instructed to avoid for 24 hours prior to a creatinine clearance test? ____________________.
3. What is the single most important indicator of fluid status? ____________.
4. What test needs to be done before arterial blood gases are drawn? ____________.
5. What is the most sensitive parameter affected during increased levels of conscious sedation? ____________.
6. When performing an electrocardiogram, where is the grounding electrode placed? ______.
7. If bronchospasm occurs during an exercise stress test using adenosine, what medication is used to reverse it? __________.
8. What is the range of normal oxygen saturation? __________.
9. What is the range normal specific gravity of urine? __________.
10. The normal volume of air inspired/expired during normal respiration is known as what?__________.
11. A chest X-ray would be contraindicated in what type of client? __________.
12. A postprocedure chest X-ray is done after a thoracentesis to check for what complication?__________.
13. For an upper GI series, the client drinks what substance? __________.
14. If the barium used in a lower GI series is not expelled within 2–3 days, what complication might occur? __________.
15. Why is a fat free meal taken the night before an oral cholecystogram? __________.
16. Why is a T-tube cholangiogram done? __________.
17. An EGD visualizes what parts of the GI tract? __________.
18. A client scheduled for a colonoscopy is to drink Colyte as the bowel prep. How is Colyte taken? __________.
19. What types of blood tests are especially important to obtain prior to a liver biopsy? __________.
20. After a liver biopsy, the client is placed in what position? __________.

21. What can a client do to relieve discomfort after a cystoscopy? ____________.

22. What substance is applied to the cervix during a colposcopy to highlight abnormal areas? ____________.

23. A pregnant woman should be instructed to do what before a nonstress test to enhance fetal activity? ____________.

24. What test should not be performed if the client has pelvic inflammatory disease? ____________.

25. If a woman undergoing an amniocentesis has Rh negative blood and her fetus is Rh positive, what medication should the woman receive? ____________.

26. What cholesterol is known as the "good" cholesterol? ____________.

27. A test useful in diagnosing congestive heart failure is what? ____________.

28. A protein found only in cardiac muscle with rises within 3–6 hours of cardiac damage is what? ____________.

29. A test used to assess for skeletal muscle damage is what? ____________.

30. Normal values of hemoglobin for a female are what? ____________.

31. Spontaneous bleeding occurs with platelet counts below what level? ____________.

32. Total red blood cell count is increased in what condition? ____________.

33. What type of white blood cell is involved in antibody responses to antigens? ____________.

34. What is the range of normal WBC count? ____________.

35. What test is used to monitor anticoagulant therapy with heparin? ____________.

36. What is the major cation in intracellular fluid responsible for electrical conduction in cardiac muscle cells? ____________.

37. The levels of what substances are controlled by the parathyroid gland? ____________.

38. Open wounds are cultured with what type of culture tube? ____________.

39. What is the normal range for arterial blood gas pH? ____________.

40. A test used to differentiate causes of jaundice is what? ____________.

41. What medications should be avoided for 2 days before fecal occult blood testing is done? ____________.

42. What is the nonspecific test for inflammatory conditions? ____________.

43. What is the counter-pulsation mechanical device used to aid the circulatory function of the heart? ____________.

44. What is used to determine the amount of fluid to be removed with each dialysis session? ____________.

45. What can a client do to decrease risk of infection which a urinary catheter is in place? ____________.

46. On which side of the body is a cane used? ____________.

APPLICATION QUESTIONS

1. Which of the following is a good indicator of the glomerular filtration rate (GFR)?
   a. BUN
   b. Bence-Jones
   c. Creatinine
   d. Urine cytology
2. Which of the following is a measurement of the kidney's ability to concentrate urine?
   a. Urine osmolality
   b. Creatinine clearance
   c. Specific gravity
   d. Urine cytology
3. Which of the following examinations requires a serum sample and 24-hour urine sample?
   a. Urine cytology
   b. Creatinine clearance
   c. Bicarbonate
   d. BUN
4. A 69-year-old client with diabetes mellitus type 2 is to undergo a CT scan using contrast media. Which laboratory test(s) should be performed prior to the CT scan?
   a. Liver function tests
   b. Electrolytes
   c. BUN and creatinine
   d. Fasting blood sugar
5. Which test can a pregnant woman undergo without concern for causing harm to the fetus?
   a. CT scan of the brain
   b. Chest X-ray
   c. CT scan of the abdomen
   d. Ultrasound of the gallbladder
6. Immediate postprocedure care of the client who has undergone a bronchoscopy includes all of the following except:
   a. monitoring vital signs
   b. ensuring siderails are up
   c. pushing fluids
   d. assessing breath sounds
7. You are monitoring a client who is receiving conscious sedation while undergoing a colonoscopy. Medications used are midazolam and fentanyl. You notice that the client is experiencing respiratory depression. You should:
   a. increase the intravenous infusion rate.
   b. administer naloxone.
   c. administer CPR.
   d. recheck the vital signs in 15 minutes.
8. A PPD test is administered to a healthy 23-year-old nurse who is starting employment at a local hospital. Which of the following measurements would be considered a "positive" reading for this individual?
   a. 10 mm of erythema
   b. 5 mm of induration
   c. 10 mm of induration
   d. 15 mm of induration
9. Which of the following procedures would be contraindicated in a client with a bleeding disorder?
   a. Intravenous pyelogram
   b. Liver biopsy
   c. Renal scan
   d. CT scan of the brain
10. A client with diabetes mellitus self monitors blood sugar at home. His primary care provider wants to assess the client's average blood sugar over a 3 month period. The best test for this would be:
    a. fasting plasma glucose
    b. urine dipstick for glucose
    c. glucose tolerance test
    d. hemoglobin A1C
11. A pregnant client is undergoing a nonstress test. Which of the following would be considered a "nonreactive" test?
    a. There is fetal movement only after she rubs her abdomen.
    b. There is no fetal movement in 20 minutes.
    c. There is fetal movement at 30 minutes only after a loud noise is placed near the abdomen.
    d. There is no fetal movement in 40 minutes.
12. A client has a severe bacterial infection. Which of the following would be expected on the client's complete blood count (CBC) with differential?
    a. WBC 8,500, lymphocytes 45%
    b. WBC 15,000, segmented neutrophils 50%
    c. WBC 25,000, band neutrophils 20%
    d. WBC 20,000, segmented neutrophils 58%
13. A client with atrial fibrillation is receiving warfarin (Coumadin) 5 mg each day. His INR today is

2.4. What is the expected change in medication dosage?
a. His INR is too low. His warfarin dose needs to be increased.
b. His INR is too high. His warfarin dose needs to be decreased.
c. His INR is too high. His warfarin dose needs to be increased.
d. His INR is within desired range. No change in warfarin dose is needed.

14. A client is experiencing cardiac dysrhythmias, confusion, and weakness. An abnormal level of which of the following would most likely be the cause?
a. Phosphorus
b. Calcium
c. Potassium
d. Sodium

15. For which of the following medications should a client undergo therapeutic drug monitoring?
a. Penicillin (antibiotic)
b. Propranolol (beta-blocker)
c. Furosemide (diuretic)
d. Digoxin (cardiac glycoside)

16. A client has acute hepatitis. Which of the following would most likely be elevated?
a. Serum protein electrophoresis
b. Alanine aminotransferase (ALT)
c. Ammonia
d. Troponin

17. You note that your client with chronic renal failure has a urine specific gravity (SG) of 1.035. You explain to the client that:
a. this specific gravity is normal.
b. this specific gravity indicates very concentrated urine and you recommend increased fluid intake.
c. this specific gravity is high and indicates the presence of a urinary tract infection.
d. this specific gravity indicates dilute urine due to the kidneys' lack of ability to concentrate urine.

18. Which of the following findings from a urinalysis would most likely indicate renal dysfunction?
a. Positive leukocyte esterase
b. Positive urobilinogen
c. Positive protein
d. Positive nitrites

19. Which of the following is a normal finding for the client with a chest tube?
a. New pockets of air are palpated under the skin
b. Bubbling is present in the water seal chamber
c. Drainage from the chest tube increases each day
d. The water level in the water seal chamber oscillates with the client's respirations

20. Which of the following is the most accurate method of determining proper placement of a nasogastric tube?
a. Using a 50-ml syringe to aspirate gastric contents
b. Instilling air into the tube and auscultating for a swooshing sound
c. Obtaining a chest X-ray
d. Placing the end of the tube in water to check for bubbling

21. A client is to undergo three tests: upper GI series, lower GI series (barium enema), and renal ultrasound. In what order should these tests be performed?
a. Lower GI series, then upper GI series, then renal ultrasound
b. Upper GI series, then renal ultrasound, then lower GI series
c. Renal ultrasound, then lower GI series, then upper GI series
d. It does not matter in what order these tests are performed

22. Colonoscopy is contraindicated for clients with which of the following disorders?
a. Polyps
b. Hemorrhoids
c. Diarrhea
d. Acute diverticulitis

23. Your client is a 32-year-old healthy female whose maternal grandmother had breast cancer at age 45. Your client is asking your guidance as to when she should have a mammogram. According to the American Cancer Society, she should begin screening at age:
a. 32
b. 35
c. 40
d. 50

24. Your client is to undergo an amniocentesis. Which of the following should be included in your care of this client?
a. The client should have a full bladder for the procedure.

(continued)

b. The client should be reassured that the procedure is risk-free.
c. The client should be instructed to report abdominal pain, cramping, chills, fever, vaginal bleeding, fetal hyperactivity, or lethargy.
d. Explanation that the procedure involves obtaining a sample of amniotic fluid through the cervical os.

25. A client is diagnosed with a wound infection which is quite painful. Which of the following is true?
a. An antibiotic should be started immediately. The client can return for a wound culture when the wound is less painful.
b. Antibiotic therapy will be withheld until the culture and sensitivity report is available.
c. A wound culture is obtained first, after which a broad spectrum antibiotic is started.
d. The culture report will identify the correct antibiotic to use to treat the infection.

ANSWERS & RATIONALES

TRUE & FALSE ANSWERS

1. Glucophage should not be discontinued prior to a radiographic examination using contrast medium. *False*
Failure to discontinue Glucophage on the day of test and for 48 hours following may result in lactic acidosis.

2. Start time for a 24-hour urine collection begins when the first urine sample is voided and saved. *False*
The timing begins with the first voiding, but the first sample of urine is discarded.

3. Only a sample of a 24-hour urine collection needs to be sent to the laboratory as long the total volume voided is accurately documented. *False*
Failure to collect and send to the laboratory ALL urine voided in the 24 hour period invalidates the test.

4. Serum BUN levels are decreased with kidney disease and acute renal failure. *False*
BUN measures urea and nitrogen levels in a blood sample and are elevated when kidney function is impaired and alters the excretion of these metabolic end products.

ANSWERS FOR FILL IN THE BLANKS

1. What serum creatinine level indicates the need for renal dosing of medications excreted by the kidneys? Answer: Level > 2.

2. What should a client be instructed to avoid for 24 hours prior to a creatinine clearance test? Answer: Consumption of meat, stress, and strenuous exercise.

3. What is the single most important indicator of fluid status? Answer: Daily weight.

4. What test needs to be done before arterial blood gases are drawn? Answer: Allen test.

5. What is the most sensitive parameter affected during increased levels of conscious sedation? Answer: Oxygen saturation.

6. When performing an electrocardiogram, where is the grounding electrode placed? Answer: On the right leg.

7. If bronchospasm occurs during an exercise stress test using adenosine, what medication is used to reverse it? Answer: aminophylline.

8. What is the range of normal oxygen saturation? Answer: 95–100%.

9. What is the range of normal specific gravity of urine? Answer: 1.005–1.030.

10. The normal volume of air inspired/expired during normal respiration is known as what? Answer: Tidal volume.

11. A chest X-ray would be contraindicated in what type of client? Answer: A pregnant client.

12. A postprocedure chest X-ray is done after a thoracentesis to check for what complication? Answer: Pneumothorax.

13. For an upper GI series, the client drinks what substance? Answer: Barium sulfate.

14. If the barium used in a lower GI series is not expelled within 2–3 days, what complication might occur? Answer: Intestinal obstruction.

15. Why is a fat free meal taken the night before an oral cholecystogram? Answer: It prevents contraction of the gallbladder and allows dye to accumulate in the gallbladder.

16. Why is a T-tube cholangiogram done? Answer: To check for patency of the common bile duct prior to removal of the T-tube after a cholecystectomy.

17. An EGD visualizes what parts of the GI tract? Answer: Esophagus, stomach, and upper duodenum (EGD stands for esophagogastroduodenoscopy).

18. A client scheduled for a colonoscopy is to drink Colyte as the bowel prep. How is Colyte taken? Answer: An 8-oz glass every 10 minutes until 1 gallon has been taken.

19. What types of blood tests are especially important to obtain prior to a liver biopsy? Answer: Coagulation studies (PT, bleeding time).

20. After a liver biopsy, the client is placed in what position? Answer: On the right side to keep pressure on area of needle insertion.

21. What can a client do to relieve discomfort after a cystoscopy? Answer: Warm sitz bath, mild analgesics.

22. What substance is applied to the cervix during a colposcopy to highlight abnormal areas? Answer: 3% acetic acid.

23. A pregnant woman should be instructed to do what before a nonstress test to enhance fetal activity? Answer: Eat a meal to ensure a high maternal serum glucose level.

24. What test should not be performed if the client has pelvic inflammatory disease? Answer: Hysterosalpingography.

25. If a woman undergoing an amniocentesis has Rh negative blood and her fetus is Rh positive, what medication should the woman receive? Answer: RhoGAM.

26. What cholesterol is known as the "good" cholesterol? Answer: High density lipoprotein cholesterol (HDL).

27. A test useful in diagnosing congestive heart failure is what? Answer: Brain Natriuretic Peptide (BNP).

28. A protein found only in cardiac muscle with rises within 3–6 hours of cardiac damage is what? Answer: Troponin.

(continued)

29. A test used to assess for skeletal muscle damage is what? Answer: Creatine kinase (CK).

30. Normal values of hemoglobin for a female are what? Answer: 12–16 g/dl.

31. Spontaneous bleeding occurs with platelet counts below what level? Answer: 20,000/mm^3.

32. Total red blood cell count is increased in what condition? Answer: Polycythemia.

33. What type of white blood cell is involved in antibody responses to antigens? Answer: Lymphocyte.

34. What is the range of normal WBC count? Answer: 4,500–10,500/mm^3.

35. What test is used to monitor anticoagulant therapy with heparin? Answer: PTT (partial thromboplastin time).

36. What is the major cation in intracellular fluid responsible for electrical conduction in cardiac muscle cells? Answer: Potassium.

37. The levels of what substances are controlled by the parathyroid gland? Answer: Calcium and phosphorus.

38. Open wounds are cultured with what type of culture tube? Answer: Aerobic.

39. What is the normal range for arterial blood gas pH? Answer: 7.35–7.45.

40. A test used to differentiate causes of jaundice is what? Answer: Bilirubin.

41. What medications should be avoided for 2 days before fecal occult blood testing is done? Answer: Aspirin and NSAIDs.

42. What is the nonspecific test for inflammatory conditions? Answer: Erythrocyte sedimentation rate.

43. What is the counter-pulsation mechanical device used to aid the circulatory function of the heart? Answer: Intra-aortic balloon pump.

44. What is used to determine the amount of fluid to be removed with each dialysis session? Answer: Dry weight/target weight.

45. What can a client do to decrease risk of infection which a urinary catheter is in place? Answer: Drink 8–12 glasses of fluid daily, keep drainage bag at a level lower than the bladder.

46. On which side of the body is a cane used? Answer: On the unaffected side.

APPLICATION ANSWERS

1. Which of the following is a good indicator of the glomerular filtration rate (GFR)?
   a. BUN
   b. Bence-Jones
   c. Creatinine
   d. Urine cytology

Rationale

Correct answer: c.

Creatinine is formed and excreted at a constant rate and is the ideal substance for measuring renal clearance. Incorrect answers: BUN reflects the balance between production and excretion of urea; Bence-Jones proteins are positive for multiple myeloma; urine cytology detects urinary inflammatory diseases.

2. Which of the following is a measurement of the kidney's ability to concentrate urine?

a. Urine osmolality
b. Creatinine clearance
c. Specific gravity
d. Urine cytology

Rationale
Correct answer: c.
Incorrect answers: a, b, and d—urine osmolality identifies the osmotic concentration; creatinine clearance determines the glomerular filtration rate; urine cytology detects urinary inflammatory diseases.

3. Which of the following examinations requires a serum sample and 24-hour urine sample?
   a. Urine cytology
   b. Creatinine clearance
   c. Bicarbonate
   d. BUN

Rationale
Correct answer: b.
Midway through the 24-hour urine collection, a serum creatinine level is collected to help calculate the rate at which kidneys are clearing creatinine from the blood.
Incorrect answers: a, c, and d—urine cytology requires a urine sample only; bicarbonate levels can be done on either serum or urine samples; BUN requires a serum sample.

4. A 69-year-old client with diabetes mellitus type 2 is to undergo a CT scan using contrast media. What laboratory test(s) should be performed prior to the CT scan?
   a. Liver function tests
   b. Electrolytes
   c. BUN and creatinine
   d. Fasting blood sugar

Rationale
Correct answer: c.
Clients undergoing CT scans using contrast media need adequate renal function to process the media. Elderly clients and clients with diabetes mellitus are at risk due to decreased renal function.
Incorrect answers: a, b, and d—Abnormal liver function, electrolyte, or blood sugar tests do not typically prevent a client from having a CT scan.

5. Which test can a pregnant woman undergo without concern for causing harm to the fetus?
   a. CT scan of the brain
   b. Chest X-ray
   c. CT scan of the abdomen
   d. Ultrasound of the gallbladder

Rationale
Correct answer: d.
An ultrasound of the gallbladder involves only sound waves, not radiation.
Incorrect answers: a, b, and c—CT scans and X-rays involve exposure of the fetus to radiation.

6. Immediate postprocedure care of the client who has undergone a bronchoscopy includes all of the following except:
   a. monitoring vital signs
   b. ensuring siderails are up
   c. pushing fluids
   d. assessing breath sounds

Rationale
Correct answer: c.
The client is not to have fluids until the nurse is certain the gag reflex is intact.
Incorrect answers: a, b, and d—After a bronchoscopy the nurse is to periodically monitor the vital signs and breath sounds to assess for development of complications such as pneumothorax. Due to receipt of sedation during the procedure, the client is to remain in bed with the siderails up until fully conscious.

7. You are monitoring a client who is receiving conscious sedation while undergoing a colonoscopy. Medications used are midazolam and fentanyl. You notice that the client is experiencing respiratory depression. You should:
   a. increase the intravenous infusion rate.
   b. administer naloxone.
   c. administer CPR.
   d. recheck the vital signs in 15 minutes.

Rationale
Correct answer: b.
The client is most likely experiencing respiratory depression from the narcotic fentanyl. The antidote for fentanyl overdose is naloxone.
Incorrect answers: a, c, and d—Increasing the IV rate will not affect the respiratory depression. CPR is not needed since the client is still breathing. Vital signs are to be monitored every 5 minutes during conscious sedation.

8. A PPD test is administered to a healthy 23-year-old nurse who is starting employment at a local hospital. Which of the following measurements would be considered a "positive" reading for this individual?
   a. 10 mm of erythema
   b. 5 mm of induration
   c. 10 mm of induration
   d. 15 mm of induration

(continued)

Rationale

Correct answer: c.

For health care workers, 10 mm and above of induration is considered positive.

Incorrect answers: a—Erythema is not considered as positive; b—5 mm of induration is positive if the person is immunocompromised; d—15 mm of induration is positive for persons with no known risk factors.

9. Which of the following procedures would be contraindicated in a client with a bleeding disorder?
   a. Intravenous pyelogram
   b. Liver biopsy
   c. Renal scan
   d. CT scan of the brain

Rationale

Correct answer: b.

Liver biopsy is contraindicated in clients with bleeding disorders due to the risk of bleeding from the biopsy site.

Incorrect answers: a, c, and d—A client with a bleeding disorder can safely undergo an intravenous pyelogram, renal scan, or CT scan of the brain since, other than a venipuncture for administration of contrast dye or radioisotope, they are noninvasive.

10. A client with diabetes mellitus self monitors blood sugar at home. Now the primary care provider wants to assess the client's average blood sugar over a 3 month period. The best test for this would be:
    a. fasting plasma glucose
    b. urine dipstick for glucose
    c. glucose tolerance test
    d. hemoglobin A1C

Rationale

Correct answer: d.

Hemoglobin A1C absorbs glucose and holds it for the lifespan of the red blood cell (up to 120 days).

Incorrect answers: a, b, and d—The fasting plasma glucose, urine dipstick for glucose, and glucose tolerance test provide information on glucose levels at one point in time.

11. A pregnant client is undergoing a nonstress test. Which of the following would be considered a "nonreactive" test?
    a. There is fetal movement only after she rubs her abdomen.
    b. There is no fetal movement in 20 minutes.
    c. There is fetal movement at 30 minutes only after a loud noise is placed near the abdomen.
    d. There is no fetal movement in 40 minutes.

Rationale

Correct answer: d.

The NST is considered nonreactive if there is no fetal movement in 40 minutes. A contraction stress test is then scheduled.

Incorrect answers: a, b, c—Any fetal movement in less than 40 minutes is considered normal, even if external stimulation, such as rubbing the abdomen or a loud noise, is needed to stimulate the fetus.

12. A client has a severe bacterial infection. Which of the following would be expected on the client's complete blood count (CBC) with differential?
    a. WBC 8,500, lymphocytes 45%
    b. WBC 15,000, segmented neutrophils 50%
    c. WBC 25,000, band neutrophils 20%
    d. WBC 20,000, segmented neutrophils 58%

Rationale

Correct answer: c.

With a severe bacterial infection, the total white blood cell count would be above normal. Band neutrophils would be elevated because the body is trying to quickly fight the infection; so quickly, that the neutrophils are being released into the circulation before they are mature cells.

Incorrect answer: a—WBC count is normal with elevated lymphocytes, indicating viral infection; b—WBC count is above normal but segs are normal, thus indicating the infection is not severe; d—although the WBC count is elevated, the segs are still within normal limits, again indicating the infection is not severe.

13. A client with atrial fibrillation is receiving warfarin (Coumadin) 5 mg each day. His INR today is 2.4. What is the expected change in medication dosage?
    a. His INR is too low. His warfarin dose needs to be increased.
    b. His INR is too high. His warfarin dose needs to be decreased.
    c. His INR is too high. His warfarin dose needs to be increased.
    d. His INR is within desired range. No change in warfarin dose is needed.

Rationale

Correct answer: d.

Target INR for clients with afib is 2.0–3.0. This client's INR is within this range.

Incorrect answers: a, b, and c—the client's INR is not too low or high.

14. A client is experiencing cardiac dysrhythmias, confusion, and weakness. An abnormal level of which of the following would most likely be the cause?
    a. Phosphorus
    b. Calcium

c. Potassium

d. Sodium

Rationale

Correct answer: c.

Low potassium levels (hypokalemia) cause confusion, anorexia, muscle weakness, paresthesias, hypotension, cardiac dysrhythmias, and decreased reflexes.

Incorrect answers: a, b, and d—Abnormal levels of phosphorus, calcium, and sodium do not result in the triad of dysrhythmias, confusion, and weakness.

15. For which of the following medications should a client undergo therapeutic drug monitoring?
    a. Penicillin (antibiotic)
    b. Propranolol (beta-blocker)
    c. Furosemide (diuretic)
    d. Digoxin (cardiac glycoside)

Rationale

Correct answer: d.

There is a narrow margin of safety between therapeutic drug effect and drug toxicity with digoxin.

Incorrect answers: a, b, and c—there is a wide margin of safety with penicillin, propranolol, and furosemide, so therapeutic drug monitoring is not needed.

16. A client has acute hepatitis. Which of the following would most likely be elevated?
    a. Serum protein electrophoresis
    b. Alanine aminotransferase (ALT)
    c. Ammonia
    d. Troponin

Rationale

Correct answer: b.

ALT, an enzyme found primarily in the liver, is elevated in clients with hepatitis.

Incorrect answers: a—serum protein electrophoresis is decreased in hepatitis; c—ammonia is not elevated until there is liver damage from long-term liver problems; d—troponin is a protein used in the diagnosis of cardiac damage.

17. You note that your client with chronic renal failure has a urine specific gravity (SG) of 1.035. You explain to the client that:
    a. this specific gravity is normal.
    b. this specific gravity indicates very concentrated urine and you recommend increased fluid intake.
    c. this specific gravity is high and indicates the presence of a urinary tract infection.
    d. this specific gravity indicates dilute urine due to the kidneys' lack of ability to concentrate urine.

Rationale

Correct answer: d.

Clients with renal disease lose the ability to concentrate urine.

Incorrect answers: a—normal specific gravity is 1.005–1.030, this client's SG is above normal; b—an increased SG indicates dilute, not concentrated urine; c—urinary tract infection does not typically cause this increase in SG.

18. Which of the following findings from a urinalysis would most likely indicate renal dysfunction?
    a. Positive leukocyte esterase
    b. Positive urobilinogen
    c. Positive protein
    d. Positive nitrites

Rationale

Correct answer: c.

With renal dysfunction, the glomerular filtrate membrane "leaks", allowing large protein molecules to pass through into the urine.

Incorrect answers: a, b, and d—positive leukocyte esterase and nitrites are indicative of urinary tract infection. Positive urobilinogen occurs with liver dysfunction.

19. Which of the following is a normal finding for the client with a chest tube?
    a. New pockets of air are palpated under the skin
    b. Bubbling is present in the water seal chamber
    c. Drainage from the chest tube increases each day
    d. The water level in the water seal chamber oscillates with the client's respirations

Rationale

Correct answer: d.

If there is no air leak, the water level in the water seal chamber will oscillate with the client's respirations.

Incorrect answers: a—pockets of air represent subcutaneous emphysema, the physician should be notified if it increases; b—bubbling in the water seal chamber indicates the presence of an air leak; c—increased drainage suggests new or increased bleeding and needs to be reported.

20. Which of the following is the most accurate method of determining proper placement of a nasogastric tube?
    a. Using a 50-ml syringe to aspirate gastric contents
    b. Instilling air into the tube and auscultating for a swooshing sound
    c. Obtaining a chest X-ray
    d. Placing the end of the tube in water to check for bubbling

Rationale

Correct answer: c.

A chest X-ray is the most accurate method.

Incorrect answers: a, and b—both of these methods are less reliable options; d—this option is not acceptable practice.

(continued)

21. A client is to undergo three tests: upper GI series, lower GI series (barium enema), and renal ultrasound. In what order should these tests be performed?
    a. Lower GI series, then upper GI series, then renal ultrasound
    b. Upper GI series, then renal ultrasound, then lower GI series
    c. Renal ultrasound, then lower GI series, then upper GI series
    d. It does not matter in what order these tests are performed

Rationale

Correct answer: c.

The renal ultrasound is done before any studies involving barium. Then the lower GI series is done so that barium from the upper GI series does not obscure the lower GI images.

Incorrect answers: a, b, and d—lower GI series is done before the upper GI series; renal ultrasound cannot be done within 2 days of barium studies, so it is best to complete this first.

22. Colonoscopy is contraindicated for clients with which of the following disorders?
    a. Polyps
    b. Hemorrhoids
    c. Diarrhea
    d. Acute diverticulitis

Rationale

Correct answer: d.

Performing a colonoscopy in the presence of acute diverticulitis increases the risk of perforation of the colon wall during the procedure.

Incorrect answers: a, b, and c—none of these problems would prevent the client from having a colonoscopy.

23. Your client is a 32-year-old healthy female whose maternal grandmother had breast cancer at age 45. Your client is asking your guidance as to when she should have a mammogram. According to the American Cancer Society, she should begin screening at age:
    a. 32
    b. 35
    c. 40
    d. 50

Rationale

Correct answer: b.

Screening for women who are high-risk is to begin 10 years before the age of the diagnosis of breast cancer in a family member.

Incorrect answers: a, b, and c—32 is her current age; age 40 is initial screening for those women with no personal or family history of breast cancer; age 50 is too late for initial screening to begin.

24. Your client is to undergo an amniocentesis. Which of the following should be included in your care of this client?
    a. The client should have a full bladder for the procedure.
    b. The client should be reassured that the procedure is risk-free.
    c. The client should be instructed to report abdominal pain, cramping, chills, fever, vaginal bleeding, fetal hyperactivity, or lethargy.
    d. Explanation that the procedure involves obtaining a sample of amniotic fluid through the cervical os.

Rationale

Correct answer: c.

These signs are all indicators of possible complications and need to be reported immediately.

Incorrect answers: a—the client should empty her bladder prior to the procedure to avoid accidental puncture during the amniocentesis; b—there are numerous possible complications of the procedure, including hemorrhage, infection, premature labor, and spontaneous abortion; d—the procedure involves transabdominal needle aspiration of amniotic fluid.

25. A client is diagnosed with a wound infection which is quite painful. Which of the following is true?
    a. An antibiotic should be started immediately. The client can return for a wound culture when the wound is less painful.
    b. Antibiotic therapy will be withheld until the culture and sensitivity report is available.
    c. A wound culture is obtained first, after which a broad spectrum antibiotic is started.
    d. The culture report will identify the correct antibiotic to use to treat the infection.

Rationale

Correct answer: c.

Specimen collection should occur prior to beginning antibiotic therapy.

Incorrect answers: a—treatment with antibiotics before obtaining the culture may produce false-negative results; b—the client is started on a broad spectrum antibiotic while awaiting the culture and sensitivity report. If the bacteria are found to be resistant to the prescribed antibiotic, the medication will be changed; d—the *sensitivity* report identifies the antibiotics to which the bacteria are susceptible.

CHAPTER 17

Test Plan Category:

Physiological Integrity

Sub-category: Reduction of Risk Potential—Part 2

Topics: Vital Signs
System Specific Assessments
Potential for Alteration in Body Systems

VITAL SIGNS (VS)

- Traditional four VS are temperature, pulse, respirations, and BP.
- Pain is now considered the fifth vital sign.
- Change in VS can indicate a problem before other more obvious and specific S&S occur.
- Baseline VS are taken on admission; in addition, VS should always be taken before and after any invasive procedure, when new S&S occur; before and after any interventions that could affect them such as getting a client out of bed postoperatively; or before and/or after administering a medication with desired effects or side effects affecting cardiovascular or respiratory function.

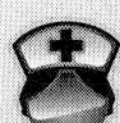

Practice Alert

VS can be delegated provided the clients have been assessed by the nurse as stable; therefore, the VS for those clients are routine.

TEMPERATURE

- Temperature is the balance between heat produced and heat lost.
- Heat is produced by
  —metabolism: the higher the basal metabolic rate, the higher the heat produced;
  —muscular activity including shivering and raising of goose bumps (piloerection);
  —increased cellular metabolism through increased thyroxine, action of epinephrine, norepinephrine sympathetic stimulation, and fever.
- Heat is lost by
  —radiation: transfer of heat from one surface to another without actual contact;
  —conduction: loss of heat from a warm molecule to a colder one, e.g., cooling by taking a cold shower;
  —convection: loss of heat by movement of air currents around the body, e.g., cooling by use of a fan;

—vaporization: continuous evaporation of moisture (insensible water loss) from skin, mucous membranes of mouth, and respiratory tract.

Temperature Control

- Core temperature, i.e., temperature deep in the tissues is relatively stable.
- Surface temperature, i.e., temperature of skin, subcutaneous tissue, and fat varies with environment.
- Core temperature is controlled by a center in the hypothalamus, which initiates heat loss mechanisms when the body temperature is too high and heat generating/conserving measures when it is too cold.
  —Heat loss measures are peripheral vasodilation and sweating.
  —Heat generating/conserving measures, e.g., shivering and piloerection, vasoconstriction, release of epinephrine to increase cellular metabolism.
- Factors influencing body temperature are
  —age: young and old do not regulate temperature as effectively as other age groups and are more vulnerable to negative effects from high or low environmental temperature;
  —time of day: temperature has a diurnal rhythm being highest between 8 p.m. and midnight and lowest between 4 and 6 a.m., with the variation being as high as 1.8°F;
  —exercise: hard work or strenuous exercise can raise temperature;
  —stress: raises temperature through release of epinephrine and norepinephrine and their effects on cellular metabolism;
  —hormones: progesterone raises temperature at the time of ovulation;
  —environmental temperature: extremes can raise or lower temperature once compensatory capacity has been exceeded.

Body Temperature Measurement

- Oral
  —If the client has been eating, drinking, or smoking, wait for 20 minutes before taking an oral temperature.
  —Instruct client to keep the lips shut; not to talk and not to bite down.
  —Contraindicated for confused or disoriented clients or anyone who cannot follow directions; those who cannot breathe through their noses because of packing or other problems; those with oral surgery/disease or those receiving oxygen.
- Rectal
  —Generally avoided in infants because of the risk of rectal perforation.
  —Children should be positioned prone across one's lap or on the side with knees flexed when a rectal temperature is taken.
  —Contraindicated for clients with rectal surgery, diarrhea, severe hemorrhoids, other rectal disease, and for those who are immunosuppressed or have a clotting disorder.
- Ear (tympanic)
  —For infants, position supine with head stabilized and pull the pinna straight back and slightly down; insert probe tip far enough to seal canal.
  —For children over age 3, pull pinna straight back and upward.
  —Do not use in the presence of active ear infection or tympanic membrane drainage tubes.
- Axillary
  —Preferred site in newborns because it eliminates risk of rectal perforation.

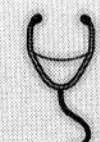

Assessment Alert

Temperature sensitive strips/chemical dots—if one of these is used to measure temperature and it indicates a fever, measurement should be repeated with a thermometer to obtain a more accurate reading.

Altered Body Temperature

Hyperthermia (pyrexia or fever: elevated body temperature)

- Cause: hypothalamic thermostat is set higher than normal temperature by tissue destruction, dehydration, or pyrogenic substances.

S&S:

—Fever onset
- S&S reflect body's attempt to generate heat and prevent heat loss in order to raise temperature.
- Cool, pale skin resulting from vasoconstriction and the absence of sweating; shivering and appearance of goose flesh, increased pulse and respiratory rates, complaints of feeling cold.

—Fever course
- When higher temperature is reached, heat generating mechanisms cease.
- Client is glassy-eyed, sensitive to light, thirsty, somewhat dehydrated, and may be drowsy, restless, delirious, or may seize; skin is warm; pulse and respirations are increased; and malaise, muscle aches, weakness, and fever blisters (herpetic lesions) may develop.

—Fever break
- Signs reflect body's attempt to lose heat.
- Skin is flushed and warm due to vasodilation and sweating.

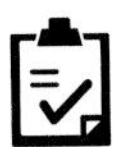

Nursing Process Elements

- Aid heat production and loss by adding clothing/blankets or removing them. Further heat loss by tepid sponge baths and reducing activity
- Provide 2500–3000 ml of fluid per day to prevent dehydration
- Provide nutrition to meet increased metabolic need
- Monitor VS and for signs of dehydration and infection
- Maintain comfort through mouth care, provision of clean dry linens

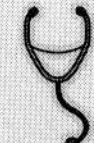

Assessment Alert

Fever is not always a good indication of the seriousness of a problem especially in older people who often have only a low-grade fever with pneumonia or a UTI.

Hypothermia

Low body temperature

- Cause: excessive heat loss as from a cold environment or immersion in cold water, insufficient heat production, or impaired hypothalamic control

S&S: Low body temperature, pulse and respiratory rates and BP; shivering and feelings of cold; pale, cool, waxy skin; low urinary output; lack of coordination, disorientation; drowsiness progressing to coma.

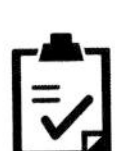

Nursing Process Elements

- Provide dry clothing, warm environment, blankets, or warming pads
- Keep limbs close to the body and cover head with a cap or turban
- Give warm oral or IV fluids

PULSE

- Palpable waves of blood flow are pumped by the heart into the arterial system
- Reflects stroke volume or amount of blood pumped into the arteries with each contraction of the ventricle
- Felt wherever an artery lies close to the surface of the body and can be compressed against firm, dense tissue or bone
- Assessing the pulse provides information about the function of the heart and the blood flow to an area of the body
- Rate, rhythm, and quality of the pulse are assessed when taking the pulse

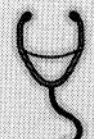

Assessment Alert

When the purpose of taking a pulse is to assess blood flow to a part, the same pulse on each side of the body must be compared.

Common sites for obtaining the pulse are

- temporal artery,
- carotid artery: indicates blood flow to the brain; used during CPR,

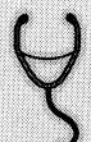

Assessment Alert

Never palpate both carotid arteries at the same time.

- brachial artery: used during cardiac arrest in infants,
- radial artery,
- femoral artery,
- popliteal artery,
- posterior tibial artery,
- dorsalis pedis artery, and
- apex of the heart (apical pulse).
  - —Auscultated with a stethoscope placed over point of maximal impulse (PMI)
  - —Located at about the left, fifth intercostal space at the midclavicular line and slightly more left in children
  - —Uses
    - Routine pulses in children up to age 3
    - Adults with cardiac, pulmonary, or renal disease or taking medications with a cardiac effect
  - —Lub-dub equals one heartbeat
    - Lub is the first heart sound (S1) heard when the atrioventricular valves close at the end of ventricular filling.
    - Dub is the second heart sound (S2) heard when the semilunar valves close after ventricular emptying.

Pulse Rate

- Number of bpm
- Normal pulse rate varies with age
  - —Infants: 120–160 bpm
  - —Toddlers: 90–140 bpm

—Preschoolers: 80–110 bpm
—School-agers: 75–100 bpm
—Adolescents: 60–90 bpm
—Adults: 60–100 bpm

- Tachycardia: pulse rate higher than the top of the range for the client's age.
- Bradycardia: pulse rate lower than the bottom of the range for the client's age. Athletic persons may have normal bradycardia.
- Factors affecting pulse rate are
  —exercise: pulse rate increases with activity;
  —temperature: pulse rate increases with fever;
  —emotion/stress: sympathetic stimulation increases rate and force of cardiac contraction;
  —medications: depending on the medication, either raises or lowers pulse rate;
  —trauma/hemorrhage: hypovolemia causes an increase in pulse rate as a compensatory mechanism to maintain BP in the face of low volume;
  —postural changes: with pooling of blood in the extremities, pulse increases to maintain BP despite the decreased venous return;
  —pulmonary conditions: if oxygenation is impaired, pulse rate increases in an attempt to supply adequate amounts of oxygen to the tissues.
- Always count an irregular pulse for a full minute.
- After activity, allow client to rest for 10–15 minutes before taking pulse to allow it to return to its resting rate.
- Most accurate rate is the apical.
- Pulse deficit: radial pulse rate is lower than the apical rate.
  —Occurs when some ventricular contractions are so weak that the resultant pulse wave does not reach the periphery or that pathology in or around the artery is preventing the passage of blood.
  —To measure a pulse deficit, two nurses are needed: one who counts the apical pulse and one who counts the radial pulse. They use one watch/clock and start and stop at a predetermined time.

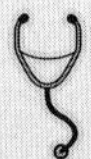

Assessment Alert

A peripheral pulse rate can never be higher than the apical rate because the heart generates the pulse wave.

Rhythm

Rhythm is the pattern of pulse waves or heartbeats.

- Regular rhythm: pulse waves or beats occur at evenly spaced intervals.
- Regularly irregular: pattern is irregular but consistent, e.g., skips every fifth beat.
- Irregular irregularity: no discernible pattern exists.

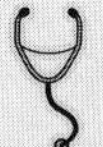

Assessment Alert

When an irregular pulse is detected, an apical pulse which is always counted for a full minute, should be obtained.

Quality

- Strength of the pulse wave
  —A full or strong pulse that is easily palpated is normal.
  —A bounding pulse is stronger than normal.
  —A weak or thready pulse is easily obliterated by pressure of the examiner's fingers.
- Quality depends on
  —stroke volume, which is the amount of blood ejected from the left ventricle with each contraction; normal for an adult is about 70 ml;
  —elasticity of the arteries;
  —adequacy of local blood flow.

Equality

- Equality is the comparison of corresponding pulses on the right and left sides of the body.
- Normally, pulse characteristics in an artery on right side of body should be equal to pulse characteristics in same artery on the left side.

DOPPLER DEVICE

- Doppler device detects movement of red blood cells through an artery; therefore, it eliminates environmental nose interference and produces audible sound.
- It is used to determine adequacy of blood flow when peripheral pulses cannot be palpated due to obesity, presence of occlusive vascular disease, cardiopulmonary collapse with vasoconstriction, postoperatively when peripheral blood flow may be compromised.

RESPIRATION

- Respiration is a process by which oxygen and carbon dioxide are transferred between the atmosphere and the blood and the blood and the cells.

- External respiration refers to the movement of oxygen and carbon dioxide between the alveoli of the lungs and the pulmonary blood.
- Internal respiration refers to the movement of oxygen and carbon dioxide between the circulating blood and the cells throughout the body.
- Ventilation is movement of air in and out of the lungs, i.e., inhalation and exhalation (breathing).

BREATHING

- Breathing is an automatic and involuntary process requiring functioning lungs, chest wall, respiratory muscles, respiratory center in the medulla oblongata, and functioning nerve tracts connecting brain to muscles.
- One breath is composed of one inspiration and one expiration.
- Inspiration is active; expiration is passive.
- Stimulus to breathe in healthy persons is an increase in CO_2 pressure in the arterial blood; the resultant increase in rate and depth of breathing removes the excess CO_2.
- Chemoreceptors located in the aorta and carotid arteries are sensitive to CO_2, pH, and low levels of O_2. If O_2 decreases, stimulus is sent to respiratory center.
- Cerebral cortex also exerts voluntary control over breathing allowing one to "hold the breath." The CO_2 stimulus to the respiratory center is stronger than the control.
- Basic types of breathing
  —Costal (thoracic) breathing
  - uses external intercostal muscles and other accessory muscles such as the sternocleidomastoids;
  - chest moves up and out.

  —Diaphragmatic (abdominal) breathing
  - uses the diaphragm;
  - abdomen moves in and out.
  - Young children are diaphragmatic breathers.
- Factors that influence breathing are
  —age: normal range of respiratory rates varies with age;
  —medications: narcotics and sedatives can decrease rate and depth;
  —stress/anxiety: increases rate and depth through action of fight or flight hormones;
  —exercise: increases rate and depth to meet cells' increased demand for oxygen and removal of carbon dioxide;
  —altitude: increases rate to compensate for decreased atmospheric oxygen;
  —gender;
  —body position: can inhibit or facilitate chest expansion;
  —environmental temperature: high temperature increases the respiratory rate and low temperature decreases the respiratory rate;
  —fever: increases respiratory rate as a result of increased metabolism;
  —presence of pain;
  —smoking;
  —neurological injury: increased ICP associated with decreased respiratory rate;
  —hemoglobin abnormalities.
- Respiratory characteristics to be assessed are rate and rhythm.

Rate

- Number of breaths per minute
- Resting normal respiratory rate ranges for different age groups are
  —newborn: 30–60 rpm
  —infant: 30–50 rpm
  —toddler: 25–32 rpm
  —child: 20–30 rpm
  —adolescent: 16–19 rpm
  —adult: 12–20 rpm
- Eupnea—normal rate and depth
- Tachypnea—abnormally fast respiratory rate
- Bradypnea—abnormally slow respiratory rate
- Apnea—absence of respiration, described in terms of length of time between respirations, e.g., apnea × 15 seconds; continuous apnea is respiratory arrest

Rhythm

- Rhythm is a pattern of inspiration and expiration.
- Normally, pattern is regular with expiration twice as long as inspiration.

Depth

- Depth is described as shallow, deep, or normal.
- Normal tidal volume (amount of air taken in and let out during a normal respiration) in an adult is 500 ml or 6–8 l/min.
- Hyperventilation is very deep, rapid respiration.
- Hypoventilation is shallow respiration.

Quality

- Normal is quiet and effortless or easy.
- Abnormal is labored and/or noisy.
  —Dyspnea: labored breathing
  —Orthopnea: needs to be in an upright sitting or standing position to breathe
  —Wheeze: continuous, high-pitched musical sound resulting from air passing through obstructed airways; may be expiratory and/or inspiratory

—Gurgles: bubbling sounds heard as air passes through wet secretions
—Stridor: harsh shrill sound heard on inspiration when larynx is obstructed
—Stertor: snoring sound heard as air passes through a partially obstructed upper airway

BLOOD PRESSURE

- Blood pressure is the force of blood against the arterial walls.
- Determinants of BP are cardiac output, peripheral vascular resistance (size of the arterioles and capillaries and arterial elasticity), blood volume, and blood viscosity.
- Pressure when ventricle is contracting is the systolic; pressure when heart is at rest is the diastolic.
- Pulse pressure is the difference between diastolic and systolic pressure.
- Factors influencing BP are
  —age: increases from birth to puberty; declines somewhat and then tends to increase again with age-related loss of elasticity of arterial walls;
  —time of day: lowest in early morning and peaks late afternoon or evening;
  —stress/emotion;
  —gender and race: females tend to have lower BP than men at least until menopause when it tends to rise; black males are more likely to have hypertension than any other group;
  —medications;
  —family history;
  —environment;
  —extremity on which measured: same extremity should be used to obtain consistent and comparable measurements;
  —vasodilation/vasoconstriction;
  —head injury;
  —changes in blood volume, exercise, or body position.

Measuring Blood Pressure

- Use correct-size cuff.
  —The short side of the cuff bladder should be 40% the diameter of the extremity where it will be placed; the long side should be 60% of the diameter of the extremity where it will be placed.
  —Too narrow a cuff gives a false high reading; too wide a cuff gives a false low reading.
- Support the limb at heart level and allow the client to rest before taking.
  —If the limb is unsupported or above the level of the heart or the client has insufficient rest prior to measurement, the BP will be falsely high. If the limb is below heart level, the pressure is falsely low.
- Wrap cuff smoothly and tightly.
  —If it is uneven or too loose, BP will be falsely high.
- Deflate cuff at a rate of 2–3 mm Hg/sec.
  —If the cuff is deflated too slowly, the diastolic pressure may be falsely high.
  —If the cuff is deflated too quickly, the systolic reading may be falsely low and the diastolic falsely high.
- Wait for 1–2 minutes before repeating the procedure.
  —If redone immediately systolic reading can be falsely high and diastolic falsely low.

Measuring BP when client has just eaten, is in pain, or is smoking can result in falsely high readings.

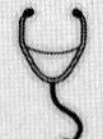

Assessment Alert

Do not take BP in an arm with an IV, cast, or dialysis shunt; that has recently been used to draw blood samples; is on the side with a mastectomy or the side affected by a stroke.

Orthostatic Hypotension

- Orthostatic hypotension is the drop in BP that occurs when the client assumes a sitting or standing position.
- Assess for orthostatic hypotension by
  —taking pulse and BP after client has been in a supine position for 2–3 minutes;
  —assist client to sit or stand for at least 1 minute and then repeat measures using same locations.
- Increase of 40 bpm in pulse rate or a drop of 30 mm Hg or more in BP indicates orthostatic abnormality.

PAIN

- Pain is what the client says it is: it is subjective and only the client knows what he or she feels.
- Reaction to pain is in part a learned experience and as such is influenced by the individual's life and background.
- Clients do not/cannot always describe pain accurately; therefore, careful assessment is necessary.
- Clients do not always use the term pain; soreness, pressure, heaviness, and other words may be used.
- Clients have a right to pain relief.
- Pain is a complex experience and multiple approaches may be needed for pain relief to be effective.

Types of Pain

- Cutaneous
  - —Cutaneous pain originates in skin and subcutaneous tissue.
  - —It is short, sharp, sometimes burning, and well-localized pain.
- Deep somatic
  - —Deep somatic pain originates in ligaments, tendons, bones, blood vessels, and nerves.
  - —It is diffuse, longer lasting, feeling of burning, aching, or pressure.
- Visceral
  - —Visceral pain originates in cranial, thoracic, or abdominal cavities.
  - —It is often diffuse and difficult to localize, may be crampy, sharp or like deep somatic a feeling of burning, aching, or pressure.
  - —It results from stretching of tissues, ischemia, or muscle spasm.
- Radiating pain: felt at site of problem but also in surrounding areas.
- Referred pain: pain felt in an area distant from the source of the problem.
- Intractable pain: pain that is very difficult to relieve.
- Neuropathic pain: results from damage to the nervous system.
  - —It is sharp, spasmatic pain along the path of a nerve.
  - —It is severe, burning pain from damage to a peripheral nerve in the extremities.
  - —Phantom pain: perception of pain in an amputated or paralyzed part of the body.

Acute Versus Chronic Pain

- Acute pain
  - —Duration of the pain is limited to the time it takes for healing to occur.
  - —Pain is not referred to as acute because of its intensity or abruptness of onset.
  - —Acute pain usually has not as a known cause such as trauma (accidental or therapeutic), infection, or inflammation.
  - —Sympathetic nervous system responses predominate: elevated VS, sweating, pupil dilation; client reports pain; manifests signs of pain such as restlessness, anxiety, crying, guarding, or holding affected area.
- Chronic pain
  - —Its duration is of 3 months or longer.
  - —It accompanies progressive diseases such as cancer and sickle cell disease, may be due to a neuropathic pain syndrome such as postherpetic neuralgia or the cause may be unknown.
  - —Parasympathetic nervous system predominates: normal VS, warm, dry skin, normal or constricted pupils; appears depressed or withdrawn, does not report pain unless asked, pain behaviors absent.

Factors Influencing Response to and Tolerance of Pain

- Culture: attitudes of stoicism
- Age
- Environment
- Support systems
- Past experience with pain
- Meaning of pain: something to be endured for a good outcome such as cure or delivery of a baby or something indicating loss of function or injury
- Psychological factors such as anxiety, stress, depression, and boredom decrease pain tolerance; faith and belief increase it
- Fatigue decreases tolerance to pain

Pain Management

- Analgesics
  - —Opioids
    - Alter perception of pain by action in the CNS.
    - Classified as strong, e.g., morphine and weak, e.g., codeine based on the strength of effect.
    - Relieve moderate to severe pain but must be taken regularly to maintain relief.
    - Tolerance, the need for larger doses to obtain the same analgesic effect, develops in some clients but doses can be increased to maintain analgesia, because no dosage ceiling exists.
    - Constipation is most common side effect.
    - Naloxone (Narcan) is the antidote for respiratory depression induced by opioids.
  - —Non-opioids
    - Block pain impulses at the periphery and if an NSAID decrease pain from inflammation due to an anti-inflammatory effect.
    - Effective for mild to moderate pain.
    - Most common: acetaminophen and NSAIDs.
    - NSAIDs in combination with opioids reduce the dose of opioids needed and provide better pain relief than either type of drug alone.
  - —Adjuvant analgesic drugs
    - Diazepam (Valium), chlorpromazine (Thorazine), hydroxyzine (Vistaril), and amitriptyline (Elavil).
    - Drugs not developed as analgesics but found to support pain relief.

- Nonpharmacological treatments for pain relief
  - —Electrical stimulation
    - By externally (Transcutaneous Electrical Nerve Stimulation [TENS] unit) or internally placed electrodes (spinal cord stimulators)
    - Works by using the electrical stimulus to block or change the pain stimulus
  - —Acupuncture
  - —Behavior modification
  - —Biofeedback
  - —Hypnosis

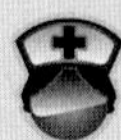

Practice Alert

Drugs, dosages, and time intervals for administration of analgesics need to be tailored to the needs of the individual client and very often a combination of drugs is needed for effective pain control.

Equianalgesic Dosing

- Equianalgesic dosing applies when clients are being switched from one opioid analgesic to another.
- Reasons for such a switch include occurrence of adverse effects or need for change of route of administration.
- Equianalgesic dosing refers to giving a dose of the new opioid that is equivalent to the previous opioid in its ability to provide pain relief.

Nursing Process Elements

- Treat clients in accord with Joint Commission directives regarding pain
  - —Tell client as part of the initial discussion of care that pain relief is an important part of care and that caretakers will act quickly to provide relief measures when pain is reported
  - —Assess pain each time VS or other assessments are made
  - —Use client's report of presence, quality, and intensity of pain as the primary guide to the need for pain relief
  - —Develop a goal and plan of care related to pain relief in collaboration with the client and other members of the health care team

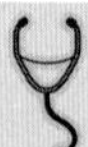

Assessment Alert

When assessing VS, always compare findings to baseline data.

- Obtain a pain history
  - —Location: have client point to area of pain or mark on diagram of body
  - —Quality: what does it feel like?
  - —Severity: use a pain intensity scale
    - Most scales ask client to rate pain intensity on a scale of 0–5 or 0–10 where 0 is no pain and the highest number is the most severe pain imaginable
    - Scales also may have word modifiers such as moderate or very severe pain
    - Scales that show faces with differing expressions along with the numbers may be used with children and adults who cannot communicate verbally due to developmental stage, cognitive impairment, or language barrier

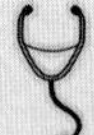

Assessment Alert

A pain rating of three or higher requires intervention.

- Onset of pain: abrupt or gradual
- Pattern of pain: constant or intermittent; if intermittent, what is the duration, duration of time between periods of pain
- Associated symptoms might include nausea and vomiting, abdominal distention, diarrhea, dizziness, visual changes, and weakness
- Precipitating or Aggravating factors might include eating, exercising, exposure to heat or cold, positioning, or emotionally stressful experience
- Relieving factors: restriction of movement, rubbing, positioning, decreased light, hot liquids, rest, meditation, prayer, herbs, medications
- Treatments tried that were ineffective
- When pain is chronic, also determine
  - —effect of pain on daily life;
  - —prior pain experiences;
  - —meaning of pain to the client;
  - —coping strategies used to deal with the pain;
  - —emotional reaction to the pain.
- Suggest use of a daily pain diary for persons with chronic pain if needed to help identify and clarify the above information
- Assess for physical manifestations of pain
  - —Facial grimacing
  - —Moaning, groaning, crying, or screaming
  - —Guarding/limiting movement of painful area
  - —Rhythmic body movements

—Restless, purposeless movements

—Early in pain experience signs of sympathetic nervous stimulation: elevated pulse, and respiratory rates, elevated BP, pallor, diaphoresis, and dilation

- Assess and manage common side effects of opioids: constipation, sedation, respiratory depression, nausea, postural hypotension, and pruritus
  - —Monitor bowel movements
  - —Ensure adequate fluid intake
  - —Encourage increase in dietary fiber
  - —Administer stool softeners and stimulants as prescribed

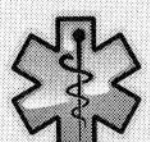

Nursing Intervention Alert

Stool softeners alone will not prevent constipation; they must be used in conjunction with a stimulant laxative.

- —Monitor sedation level especially during the first 12–24 hours of opioid therapy. Note if client is sleeping but arousable, awake, and alert; somewhat drowsy but easily aroused; frequently drowsy, drifting off to sleep during conversations but arousable; somnolent with minimal or no response to physical stimulation. If sedative effects last beyond 2–3 days required to build up tolerance, dosage and/or drug regimen needs revision
- —Monitor respiratory status especially during the first 12–24 hours that opioids are taken; make certain naloxone (Narcan) is available
- —Administer antiemetic for nausea on a scheduled basis; if nausea persists beyond the 2–3 days needed to develop tolerance, change the opioid
- —Encourage self-care activities, deep breathing, and use of incentive spirometer to decrease depressant effect on respirations
- —Encourage client to change position slowly and provide assistance when moving from a lying or sitting to standing position because of the risk of dizziness and falling due to orthostatic hypotension
- —Administer antihistamines as prescribed for pruritus; support effectiveness with cool compresses, lotion, and diversional activities
- —Reassure client that pruritus should disappear as tolerance is developed

- Assess for adverse effects of NSAIDs
  - —Monitor for signs of GI or other bleeding
  - —Monitor serum levels of NSAIDs and for signs of hepatic or renal toxicity in older adults with renal impairment
- Assess for signs of hepatotoxicity in clients taking acetaminophen and be certain that the maximum daily dose is not exceeded
- Promote effectiveness of analgesics or other pain-relief modalities through use of guided imagery; relaxation exercises; distraction or in some cases provision of a quiet, darkened environment; application of heat or cold, rubbing/massage

Client teaching for self-care

- Prevent constipation if taking opioids; adequate fluid and fiber intake; taking a mild laxative regularly in the evening; using a rectal suppository in the morning if needed in addition
- Take NSAIDs with food and full glass of fluid
- Report any signs of bleeding
- Do not mix alcohol with NSAIDs; and do not mix different NSAIDs
- Proper use of TENS
  - —Do not place electrodes over hair, broken skin areas, the carotid sinus (may induce bradycardia), throat (may induce laryngeal or pharyngeal spasms), or pregnant uterus
  - —Use prep pad to wipe the skin before applying the conductor pad
  - —Remove and wash both electrodes and underlying skin every day
  - —Expect to feel numbness or tingling during use; if not, check battery
- Proper application of heat and cold
  - —Apply over painful area when possible; otherwise apply on the opposite side of the body over an acupuncture point located between the pain and the CNS
  - —Use a towel or other cover to protect skin from direct contact with source of heat or cold
  - —Apply ice for a maximum of 10 minutes at a time and heat for 20–30 minutes and never so cold or hot that it hurts
  - —Use heat or cold when pain starts; don't wait for it to worsen

Think Smart/Test Smart

If the limb needs to be supported at heart level for an accurate BP measurement then if a BP must be taken in the lower extremity the client must be positioned in a prone or supine position.

Common system specific assessment measures used in nursing practice are presented in Table 17-1.

Table 17–1 System Specific Assessments

System/Function to be Assessed	How to Assess	When to Assess
Bowel function/ peristalsis	Auscultate for bowel sounds. Check for passage of flatus. Determine if defecation has occurred. Check for abdominal distention or crampy pain. Assess frequency and consistency of bowel movements.	Post general or spinal anesthesia After barium studies; during opioid therapy
Bladder/urethral function	Monitor time and amount of voiding.	After cystoscopy or other urethral/bladder instrumentation or surgery; post prostatectomy; after vaginal childbirth During opioid therapy With BPH or prostate cancer
Kidney function	Monitor I&O.	After general or spinal anesthesia; when disease exists that is associated with decreased renal blood flow
Respiratory status	Check breath sounds. Assess rate and depth of respirations.	Before and after coughing, deep breathing, use of incentive spirometer or other respiratory therapy During opioid therapy or magnesium sulfate therapy
Cardiac status	Assess apical pulse.	If radial pulse is irregular; prior to administering medications such as digoxin that act on the heart
Arterial blood flow to an extremity	Assess pedal pulses for blood flow to feet; popliteal for blood flow to lower leg; femoral for blood flow to thigh; brachial for blood flow to forearm and radial and ulnar for blood flow to the respective sides of the hand.	After vascular surgery involving the extremity; in clients presenting with a cold or cyanotic extremity or with intermittent claudication; after insertion of a dialysis shunt.
Neurovascular status of an extremity	Assess most distal pulse; check for normal color, warm temperature, normal capillary refill, and ability to move part and perceive touch.	After application of a cast or other potentially constricting device or garment.
Venous and lymphatic flow in an extremity	Assess for peripheral edema.	With kidney disease; after dissection or removal of area lymph nodes as with mastectomy.
Neurological function	Assess orientation to time, place, and person. Assess PERRLA. Assess lifts and grips.	Following head trauma or intracranial surgery; after CVA; in the presence of degenerative neurological disease, meningitis, encephalitis, space occupying intracranial lesions, post seizure.
Swallowing	Assess swallow reflex.	Before initiating oral feeding in clients with CVAs, Parkinson's disease.
Gagging	Assess gag reflex.	Post general anesthesia

(continued on next page)

Table 17–1 *(continued from previous page)*

System/Function to be Assessed	How to Assess	When to Assess
Wound healing	Assess for approximation, redness, warmth, swelling, drainage in wounds healing by primary intention. Assess for granulation tissue in wounds healing by second intention Assess for adherence to wound bed, color, signs of epithelialization, vascularization and new granulation in grafts.	
Reproductive system	Obtain a pregnancy test. Assess height and contraction of the fundus.	Clients who present with undiagnosed abdominal pain; prior to administration of category X drugs; prior to an abortion. Postpartum

SYSTEM SPECIFIC ASSESSMENTS

CONFUSION/DELIRIUM/AGITATION

- *Confusion*—Impairment of memory, cognitive function, perception, emotional function; disorientation; reduced level of consciousness
- *Delirium*—acute onset (hours or days) with fluctuation over the course of the day of impaired cognition, perception, speech and memory; sleep disturbance; exaggerated emotions with displays of aggression, paranoia, or terror. May be hyperactive or hypoactive delirium.
- *Agitation*—result of confusion or delirium; may manifest as abusive behaviors (physical or verbal), hiding or hoarding behaviors, or repetitive actions such as pacing, dressing, and undressing, etc.

Etiology: Medications such as opioids, phenothiazines, benzodiaszepines, anticholinergics, beta-blockers, diuretics, dopaminergics, steroids, atropine, phenytoin, H2 antagonists, toxic level of digoxin; unrelieved pain; full bladder or bowel; infection such as UTI, respiratory, septicemia; brain pathology; cardiac or respiratory failure; nicotine, alcohol, or drug withdrawal; metabolic problem such as increased BUN; fever; sleep deprivation; or extreme anxiety.

Rx: Determined by etiology, e.g., treat infection, discontinue medication, hydrate.

Nursing Process Elements

Assessment: Use standardized tool to confirm and identify degree of confusion or delirium; assess for etiology, e.g., palpate for full bladder, check for history of drug use, check medications.

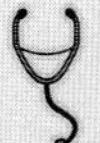

Assessment Alert

If the client is confused or delirious, always assess for client safety.

Intervention:

- Provide consistent, repeated reorientation to client as tolerated and needed for care
- Institute safety measures
- Support family and explain expected response to intervention

PRURITUS (ITCH)

Etiology: Dry or wet, macerated skin; contact dermatitis; drugs such as morphine, phenothiazines, or antibiotics; fungal infections or infestations with lice, scabies, fleas, bed bugs; renal failure; jaundice; infiltration of tumors into subcutaneous tissues.

Complications: break in skin integrity with or without infection.

Rx: See below for nonpharmacologic measures and Table 17–2 "Pharmacologic Interventions for the Management of

Table 17–2 Pharmacologic Interventions for the Management of Pruritus

Medication	Use
Antihistamines Topical corticosteroids	Acute, localized itch only; not for chronic or generalized itch
Ondansetron	Opioid, uremia, or jaundice associated itch
Antifungal creams	Itch associated with Candida infection
Systemic corticosteroids	Itch associated with inflammatory and neoplastic conditions
Bile acid sequestrants	End-stage liver disease itch
Anesthetics	Intractable itch

Pruritus" for pharmacologic measures. TENS may also be used for localized pruritus.

Nursing Process Elements

Assessment: Onset, duration, severity, location, condition of skin including integrity, rash, or other lesion; aggravating or relieving factors; review of history for precipitating or associated factors.

Client teaching for self-care

- Avoid measures that cause excessive drying of the skin such as frequent baths and use of hot water, deodorant soaps, alcohol, and other irritants. Use tepid water, neutral pH cleansers, and apply skin moisturizer/lubricant
- Wear loose, light clothing and keep environment cool to prevent sweating and increased moisture on the skin
- Take cool starch baths or use cool compresses to decrease itch
- Avoid alcohol, caffeine, and theophylline all of which can increase itch

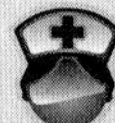

Practice Alert

Do not apply cool compresses to extremities if peripheral vascular compromise is present.

ANOREXIA

Etiology: Nausea & vomiting; constipation; pain; oral problems such as dry mouth or mucositis; dental problems such as pain or ill-fitting dentures; change in taste or smell of foods; impaired gastric emptying; depression; confusion; dementia; anxiety; fatigue; medications such as opioids and antibiotics; radiation; chemotherapy; symptom of disease such as mononucleosis.

Rx: Treat problems contributing to the anorexia. See Table 7-3 for pharmacologic interventions for the management of anorexia.

Nursing Process Elements

Assessment: History of anorexia; condition of mouth and teeth; signs of bowel function including bowel sounds; food likes and dislikes.

Assess for symptoms of problems that can cause anorexia.

Interventions:

- Provide food that the client likes and at time of request.
- Provide frequent meals with small portions attractively served.
- Avoid very hot or very cold food and those with strong odors.
- Give nutritional supplements as tolerated.
- Refer to dietician.

Client teaching for self-care

- Eat small, frequent meals
- Avoid very hot or very cold food and those with strong odors

CONSTIPATION

- Constipation is characterized by abnormally infrequent defecation and/or passage of abnormally hard stool.
- Colon absorbs water from GI contents; therefore, the longer stool stays in rectum, the drier it becomes and the harder to pass.

Table 17–3 Pharmacologic Interventions for the Management of Anorexia

Medication	Use
Gastrokinetic agents	Control nausea and early satiety
Corticosteroids	Short term improvement of appetite
Progesterone analogs	Improve appetite; decrease n&v; reduce taste and odor changes; promote weight gain
Cannabinoids	Stimulate appetite
Alcohol (beer or sherry before meals)	Improve appetite and morale
Vitamins	Reported to improve appetite

Adapted with permission from Waller, A. Caroline NL: *Handbook of Palliative Care in Cancer,* 2nd ed. Elsevier, 2000, p. 87.

- The gastrocolic reflex in which food entering stomach initiates the urge to defecate. If urge is suppressed feces will remain in the bowel and become increasingly dry as more water is absorbed. The urge may not recur for 24 hours as it is strongest after breakfast.
- Occasional constipation is basically a universal experience; more common experience in the elderly.

Etiology: Factors that cause decreased bowel motility or retention of stool include endocrine and neurological diseases such as diabetes mellitus, hypothyroidism, Parkinson's disease, multiple sclerosis, side effect of drugs including opioids, anticholinergics, anticonvulsants, and calcium channel blockers. Lifestyle factors such as physical inactivity, stress, dietary changes, inadequate dietary bulk or fluids, and ignoring urge to defecate.

Complications: Hemorrhoids from repeated straining, impaction, primary symptoms of which are pain and bleeding on defecation. External hemorrhoids appear as lumps of pink or red tissue around the anus and often itch.

Rx: Diet and fluid, fiber supplements, increased activity, regular fluid modifications, stool softeners, and laxatives.

Nursing Process Elements

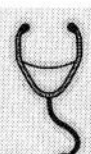

Assessment Alert

Abnormal refers to variance from what is normal for the individual. Normal patterns of defecation vary widely from person to person ranging from three times per day to once every three or more days.

Client teaching for self-care

- High-fiber diet
- 2000 ml of fluid daily
- Regular exercise
- Planned daily time for defecation
- Bulk forming rather than harsh laxatives for occasional constipation

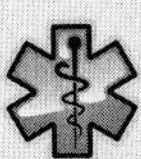

Nursing Intervention Alert

Institution of measures to prevent constipation in clients at risk is more effective and easier than treating constipation that has developed. Clients at great risk are those on opiates for pain, confused, immobilized clients.

HICCOUGHS (SINGULTUS)

- Hiccoughs are characterized by involuntary contraction of the diaphragm followed by rapid closure of the glottis.

Etiology: Gastric distention related to impaired motility or excessive gas, esophagitis, gastritis, peptic ulcer disease, gastric or pancreatic cancer, gall bladder disease, bowel obstruction; irritation of the vagus or phrenic nerve as seen for example with an enlarged spleen or a grossly distended urinary bladder; mediastinal, cervical or lung tumors; thoracic surgery or trauma, uremia, hypocalcemia, hyponatremia; renal or hepatic problems; respiratory problems such as COPD, TB, pneumonia; pulmonary edema; malaria, herpes zoster, influenza, sepsis; CNS tumors, stroke, MS, hydrocephalus, ventriculoperitoneal shunts, AV malformations, head trauma; general anesthesia; IV corticosteroids, barbiturates, benzodiazepines, diazepam; stress, grief reaction, personality disorders, and anorexia.

Rx: Treat underlying cause.

Nursing Process Elements

Assessment:

- Severity of the problem (frequency, duration, degree of discomfort)
- S&S of any causative problems
- History of causative factors such as medications, relationship to sleep (gone at night suggests psych)
- Relief measures

Interventions:

- Promote symptomatic relief by instructing client to
  —hold breath or hyperventilate;
  —rebreathe into a paper bag;
  —coughing;
  —gargle with water;
  —bite a lemon;
  —swallow crushed ice or a teaspoon of table sugar.
- Recommend hypnosis or acupuncture because these can also be effective.

BLADDER SPASMS

- Intermittent, painful contractions of the detrusor muscle accompanied by pain and a sense of urgency.

Etiology: Indwelling catheter, UTI, pressure of tumor, radiation, or chemotherapy cystitis, urethral obstruction by clots or tumor, stroke, spinal cord lesions, MS.

Rx: Antispasmodic medications (oxybutynin, NSAIDS, B&O suppositories).

Nursing Process Elements

Assessment: Appropriate catheter size, placement and function, signs of UTI or other disease problem, hematuria, adequacy of fluid intake, fecal impaction.

Interventions:

- Assist to void every 4 hours, sitting or standing
- Teach relaxation techniques

INCREASED INTRACRANIAL PRESSURE (IICP)

- Normally, intracranial pressure (ICP) varies continually within a range of 80–180 mm of H_2O or 0–15 mm Hg.
- ICP is temporarily increased by actions such as bending, coughing, sneezing, and straining at stool, which increase intrathoracic or intra-abdominal pressure.
- ICP is lower when sitting or standing.

Etiology: Obstruction of CSF flow, tumors, intracranial hemorrhage, inflammation with edema as in meningitis, encephalitis, or abscess.

Rx:

- Treat underlying problem
- Osmotic diuretics such as mannitol given IV to draw fluid from brain tissue into vascular system; have short-term effect but useful during surgery or as an emergency measure
- Steroids such as dexamethasone (Decadron) to decrease inflammation and edema
- Analgesics for headache
- Anticonvulsants to prevent seizures

Nursing Process Elements

Assessment: Signs of increasing ICP: new headache, vomiting, slow irregular respirations, which may ultimately become Cheyne–Stokes respirations, altered mental status, decreased motor function, increased restlessness, agitation, blurred vision, and widening pulse pressure.

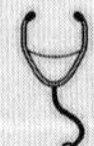

Assessment Alert

Change in level of consciousness (early changes include restlessness, irritability, drowsiness, confusion, apathy, difficulty or hesitation in following simple directions or in verbalizing) is the most sensitive sign of increasing ICP.

Fixed, dilated pupils are a late sign of increased ICP because these result from compression of the oculomotor nerve due to herniation of the cerebral brain tissue through the uncus onto the brain stem.

Interventions:

- Maintain semi-Fowler's position to promote venous return and decrease cerebral blood volume.
- Provide darkened, quiet environment.
- If diuretic is given, monitor urinary output to evaluate its effectiveness.
- If glucocorticoids are given, monitor for GI bleeding, infection, and hyperglycemia.

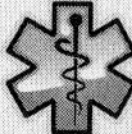

Nursing Intervention Alert

Opioids can contribute to ICP because of their vasodilation and respiratory depression effects. Tramadol is contraindicated with ICP because it can lower seizure threshold.

OTALGIA

Ear pain

Etiology:

- Infection
- Trauma
- Pressure change in the Eustachian tubes
- Temporomandibular joint disease
- Pressure from a tumor in the head or neck

Rx: Treat underlying problem.

Nursing Process Elements

Assessment: One or both ears affected; constant or intermittent type of pain; feeling of fullness, pressure, throbbing, or pounding.

OTORRHEA

Drainage from the ear

Etiology:

- Trauma such as skull fracture can cause hemorrhage with bloody drainage leakage of CSF that presents as clear, watery drainage or a combination of the two.

- Infection of the external or middle ear can cause thick, yellow, foul smelling, purulent sometimes bloody drainage.
- Tumors can cause bloody or serosanguineous drainage.

Rx: Treat underlying problem.

TINNITUS

Ringing or buzzing in one or both ears

Etiology:

- Most commonly associated with aspirin toxicity
- Accompanies some sensorineural hearing loss
- Chronic ear infection
- Labyrinthitis
- Systemic diseases such as arteriosclerosis, hypertension, anemia, and hypothyroidism
- Temporomandibular joint disease

Rx:

- Treat underlying problem when possible
- Masking
  —Use a hearing aid-like device, which produces low level white noise that blocks perception of tinnitus.
  —Residual inhibition: masking of tinnitus occurs for a short time after masking device is removed.
- Alternative treatments (none are proven effective)
  —Magnesium, zinc, Ginkgo biloba, or vitamin B supplements, acupuncture, magnets, hyperbaric oxygen, hypnosis, craniosacral therapy
- Hearing aid
  —Hearing aid is most likely to help if hearing loss is in the same frequency range as the tinnitus because hearing aids allow ambient sound to be heard that covers up the ringing.
- Biofeedback to control stress
- Cognitive therapy
  —Cognitive therapy is designed to change perception of tinnitus and the emotional reaction to it by promoting identification of negative behaviors and thoughts and then altering them.
- Drug therapy
  —Antianxiety drugs like Xanax, antidepressants like nortriptyline, antihistamines, and anticonvulsants
- Tinnitus retraining therapy (TRT)
  —TRT combines low-level, steady background sounds produced by an in-the-ear generator for a minimum of 8 hr/d with one-on-one client/clinician directive counseling
  —In 1–2 years, clients habituate to the tinnitus and no longer need the sound generator to make them unaware of the tinnitus.

Nursing Process Elements

Assessment: Ask about use of products containing aspirin; how often and how much. Explore carefully because many OTC products contain aspirin although aspirin is not in their name and often clients are unaware of its presence.

Interventions:

- Provide information about available treatment approaches
- Provide referrals as needed

BLURRED VISION

Etiology: Most often results from refractive error. Other intraocular causes are cataracts, glaucoma, and inflammation. Systemic causes include diabetes mellitus, hypertension, and kidney disease. Can be related to use of tobacco, phenothiazines, sulfonamides, and beta-blockers.

Rx: Treat underlying cause.

Nursing Process Elements

Assessment: Date of last eye examination, history of eye disease or of systemic diseases known to cause blurred vision, S&S of eye or systemic diseases; use of tobacco, phenothiazines, sulfonamides, and beta-blockers.

Interventions:

- Caution to take regarding risk for injury while vision is blurred

DIPLOPIA

Double vision: may be horizontal (two images side by side) or vertical (one image above the other)

Etiology: Weakness or paralysis of an extraocular muscle associated with problems such as TIA, myasthenia gravis, trauma, or use of alcohol or drugs such as imipramine, diazepam (Valium), and nitrofurantoin (Macrodantin).

Rx: Treat underlying cause.

Nursing Process Elements

- Insitute/teach safety measures

FLOATERS

Tiny, moving dots or squiggles in the visual field

Etiology: Most common in near-sighted persons and in the older population especially when tired or worried. Many floaters occasionally result from a retinal detachment but most often floaters do not indicate a problem.

Rx: No treatment unless related to retinal detachment.

PHOTOPHOBIA

Photophobia is sensitivity to ultraviolet light.

Etiology:

- Occupation/lifestyle exposure to bright, intense sunlight, snow dazzle, constant darkness, or fine, close work
- Use of contact lenses
- Eye disease: keratitis, corneal abrasion, iritis, and foreign bodies
- Systemic disease: migraine headache, meningitis, Rocky Mountain spotted fever
- Drugs: Cholinergic-blocking agents, antimalarial drugs, MAO inhibitors, vidarabine and idoxuridine, and rabies vaccines.

Nursing Process Elements

- Instruct in use of dark glasses

EDEMA

- Excess fluid in intercellular tissues (Also see ascites and superior vena cava syndrome)

Peripheral (Extremities) Edema

Etiology: Obstruction of venous return, e.g., CHF, DVT, constricting bandages, clothing, etc; renal failure.

Rx: Treat underlying problem; diuretics if lung crackles also present, good skin care.

Nursing Process Elements

Assessment: Pitting, nonpitting, severity (amount), increasing or decreasing, duration, new, recurrent, temperature, and perfusion of skin in involved area, presence or absence of fluid leaking through skin, S&S of underlying problem

Interventions:

- Promote venous return by
  —use of compression stockings;
  —active or passive exercise;
  —elevation of extremities above heart level.
- Prevent skin breakdown

SUPERIOR VENA CAVA SYNDROME (SVCS)

- Upper body edema
- Oncologic emergency

Etiology: Obstruction of the superior vena cava caused by lung cancer or other primary or metastatic tumor in the mediastinal or paratracheal lymph nodes.

S&S: Dyspnea, facial and neck swelling, chest pain, cough, dysphagia, and ruddy facial coloration.

Rx: Palliative radiation with or without steroids. Diuretics have no effect.

Nursing Process Elements

Assessment: Presence and severity of S&S: papilledema, facial edema, distended neck veins, arms, dyspnea, headache, chest pain, dry cough, visual or mental status changes, dizziness, vertigo.

ASCITES

- Ascites is the accumulation of excess fluid in the peritoneal cavity.

Etiology: Obstruction of portal vessels with resultant fluid leak into peritoneal cavity as in cirrhosis, CHF, hepatic, gastric, ovarian, endometrial, breast, colon, or pancreatic cancer or lymphoma; decreased plasma albumin in nephritic syndrome and malnutrition, lymphatic obstruction, pancreatitis, TB, and bowel perforation.

Rx: Symptomatic: spironolactone, paracentesis, analgesics for pain, fluid restriction to 500–1000 mg/d and sodium 200–1000 mg/d, paracentesis, administration of albumin to replace that lost from blood into body fluid. Diuretics are generally ineffective.

Nursing Process Elements

Assessment: S&S of underlying problems, weight gain, tachycardia, dyspnea, orthopnea, unable to bend or sit straight, abdominal pressure, abdominal girth measure (in cms at standard location), tenderness, distention, fluid wave, abdominal striae, distended abdominal veins, anorexia, and early satiety.

Interventions:

- Monitor I&O.
- Restrict fluids and sodium as ordered

DIARRHEA

Diarrhea is the passage of abnormally liquid feces and/or abnormal frequency of defecation.

Etiology:

- Increased water in intestinal contents
  - —Impaired absorption occurs due to disorders of the intestinal wall cells.
  - —Increased secretion of water into intestine occurs as a reaction to presence of bacteria, toxins, and hormones.
  - —Presence of solutes such as bran, which pulls water into intestine by osmosis.
- Increased intestinal motility from inflammation, abnormal bowel contents, or intrinsic irritability, which results in inadequate absorption time
  - —Enteritis
  - —Ulcerative colitis and Crohn's disease
  - —Irritable bowel syndrome

Accompanying S&S: Abdominal cramping, urgency, tenesmus, perianal discomfort, presence of mucus, blood, or fat in unformed stool.

Complications: Dehydration and electrolyte imbalance, metabolic acidosis, malnutrition, skin breakdown in anal area.

Rx: Treatment of underlying cause; fluid and electrolyte replacement.

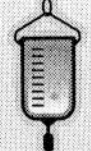

Clinical Alert

Potassium is not added to IV fluids until renal function is confirmed.

Nursing Process Elements

- Monitor I&O
- Obtain daily weight
- Monitor stool; measure liquid stool and count as output
- Administer IV fluids as ordered
- Limit oral intake because of its stimulating effect on peristalsis: NPO then small amounts of clear liquids and thin-cooked cereal; add low residue, bland foods as tolerated
- Avoid cold liquids, caffeine, spicy foods, and concentrated sweets
- Protect skin in rectal area by regular cleansing and use of protective salves; Sitz baths for irritation

DYSPHAGIA

Difficulty swallowing

Etiology: Motility disorders of the esophagus such as achalasia, laryngeal cancer, chemotherapy, radiation therapy, neuromuscular disorders, occasionally occurs with mitral stenosis.

Rx: Treat underlying problems.

Nursing Process Elements

Client teaching for self-care

- Sit up straight; keep head upright but tilted slightly forward
- Eat slowly; do not rush
- Take small bites of food and small sips of liquid
- Eat a soft or blenderized diet
- Avoid sticky foods
- Avoid spicy, highly seasoned and very hot or cold foods
- May need thickened liquids

DYSPNEA

Dyspnea is characterized by labored or difficult breathing. Its symptoms include distressful feeling of breathlessness or suffocation.

Etiology: COPD, CHF, pulmonary embolism, pleural effusion, anemia, pneumothorax, lung tumor, ascites, and CNS disease.

S&S: Rapid, audible, labored breathing, use of accessory muscles of respiration, gasping, cyanosis, dilated nostrils, tachycardia, and anxious facies.

Rx: Oxygen, palliative thoracentesis.

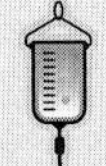

Clinical Alert

For terminal client—cannula not mask, value of O_2 based on relief of dyspnea not pulse oximetry, opioids for bronchodilation, high dose steroids for obstructive or inflammatory problems, bronchodilators, anticholinergics, and anxiety control.

Nursing Process Elements

Assessment: Onset, respiratory rate and depth, use of accessory muscles, lung sounds, constant or intermittent, triggers, and alleviating measures.

Interventions:

- High Fowler's position

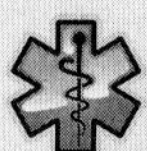

Nursing Intervention Alert

COPD client is relieved leaning forward with upper arms supported on a table.

- Encourage pursed-lip breathing in COPD clients
- Maintain a cool environment with fan blowing on client
- Use of guided imagery or relaxation techniques

COUGH

Etiology: Infection, inflammation, left HF, pleural effusion, bronchospasm, bronchogenic cancer, ACE inhibitors, environmental respiratory pollutants including smoking, allergies, and GERD.

Rx: Nonproductive cough: non-opioid or opioid antitussives; productive cough: may use humidifier or expectorants to facilitate raising sputum; treat underlying disorder.

Nursing Process Elements

Assessment: Productive, nonproductive, paroxysmal (periodic, spasmodic); sputum amount color, consistency; fever; effect on quality of life; fatigue, lethargy, and weakness.

Interventions:

- Productive cough: encourage expectoration and proper disposal of tissues; increased fluid intake to liquefy mucus; good mouth care; for pain or muscle ache on coughing demonstrate splinting

FATIGUE

Etiology: COPD, CHF, hypothyroidism, uremia, hypercalcemia, advanced malignancy, sepsis, anemia, chronic pain, dyspnea, nausea, vomiting, etc, radiation therapy, chemotherapy, medications such as beta-blockers, antihistamines, benzodiazepines, phenothiazines, zidovudine, and nutritional deficiencies.

Rx: Treat underlying cause. If medication-induced, taper, change, or alter administration schedule.

Nursing Process Elements

Assessment: Degree of fatigue, constant or intermittent; effect on quality of life, and functional status; S&S of underlying problems; type and dose of medications used; presence of uncontrolled debilitating symptoms, e.g., dyspnea, pain, vomiting, sleep and rest patterns, stress, and anxiety level.

Interventions:

- Balance activity and rest throughout the day
- Use equipment designed to decrease exertion—use of bedside commode or electric bed
- Set realistic goals for ADLs
- Set priorities for activities
- Caution against prolonged bed rest or inactivity

HYPOXIA/HYPOXEMIA

- Hypoxia is a lack of sufficient oxygen in the tissues of the body.
- Hypoxemia is the decreased oxygen in the blood as indicated by a decreased PaO_2.

Etiology: Ventilation/perfusion mismatch, high altitude, anemia or abnormal hemoglobin, and circulatory dysfunction.

S&S: The symptoms of hypoxia include restlessness, tachycardia, tachypnea, irritability, apprehension, clumsiness, poor judgment, headache, and ultimately decreased level of consciousness. Chronic hypoxia causes fatigue, apathy, drowsiness, and muscle twitches.

Rx: Treatment of underlying disorder; oxygen.

Nursing Process Elements

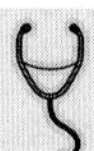

Assessment Alert

Monitor respirations of clients with chronic hypoxemia closely if oxygen is administered because with chronic hypoxemia the stimulus to breathe becomes a decrease in oxygen as opposed to the increase in CO_2, which is the normal stimulus. Because of this administration of high levels of oxygen can result in the client ceasing to breathe.

HYPERCAPNIA

Hypercapnia is an excess of CO_2 in the arterial blood.

Etiology: Respiratory depression, pneumonia, pulmonary edema, and COPD.

S&S: Tachycardia, hypertension, dizziness, headache, mental clouding, and acidosis.

HYPOCAPNIA

Hypocapnia is the presence of too little CO_2 in the arterial blood.

Etiology: Hyperventilation secondary to anxiety, fever, anemia, salicylate poisoning, and incorrect mechanical ventilation.

S&S: Light-headedness, fatigue, tingling, muscle twitching, inability to concentrate, irritability and change in level of consciousness.

INTERMITTENT CLAUDICATION

- Intermittent Claudication is severe aching or cramping pain in the lower extremities precipitated by walking or muscular contraction and relieved by rest.
- It is usually bilateral.

Etiology: Arterial insufficiency is usually due to a block in the femoral arteries.

Dx: After pain has disappeared with rest, it can be re-elicited by walking the same distance again.

Rx: Femoral–popliteal bypass.

NAUSEA

- Nausea is accompanied by autonomic nervous system changes: increased salivation, diaphoresis, dizziness, faintness, pallor, and tachycardia.
- Nausea usually precedes vomiting.

Etiology: Pregnancy, GI dysfunction, cholecystitis, radiation illness, spinal anesthesia, motion sickness, food poisoning, chemotherapy, drugs such as opioid analgesics.

Rx: Treatment of underlying cause; antiemetic drugs: anticholinergics, antihistamines, serotonin blockers.

Nursing Process Elements

Assessment:

- Frequency, duration, association with emesis, presence of pain, and appetite.
- Precipitating factors.

Interventions:

- Keep environment quiet and free of stimuli likely to induce nausea
- Encourage deep breathing when feeling nauseated
- Provide oral hygiene and comfort measures
- Give small amounts of clear liquids such as ginger ale as tolerated and gradually progress to small, frequent meals of bland, nonirritating foods

VOMITING

- Vomiting occurs when the vomiting center in the brain is stimulated.
- The vomiting center can be stimulated in the following three ways:
  —by pressure when ICP is increased;
  —by autonomic nervous system stimulation that occurs as the result of factors such as gastric distention, irritation or toxins; pain, injury to abdominal viscera, and even emotion;
  —by stimulation from the chemoreceptor trigger zone, an area which is stimulated by emetic drugs such as morphine and ergot as well as metabolic products resulting from radiation, uremia, and infection, and which in turn causes vomiting by impulses sent to the vomiting center.

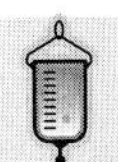

Clinical Alert

Projectile vomiting is associated with increased ICP and pyloric obstruction.

Rx:

- Treatment of both underlying cause and precipitating factors, e.g., N/G tube for gastric distention; suction to remove irritating gastric contents.
- Antiemetic drugs decrease sensitivity of the CRTZ.

Complications:

- Fluid and electrolyte imbalance: dehydration, metabolic alkalosis, and hypokalemia.
- Aspiration causing asphyxia, atelectasis, pneumonitis.

Nursing Process Elements

Assessment:

- Characteristics of emesis: color, consistency, odor, amount and frequency (coffee ground, bile colored, undigested food, or hematemesis).

- Precipitating factors/causes as: GI disorders, intestinal obstruction, food poisoning, medication side effects, pregnancy, motion sickness, neurological disorders as migraines.

Interventions:

- Keep environment quiet and free of stimuli likely to induce vomiting.
- Encourage deep breathing when feeling nauseated.
- Position client on the side or in a sitting position to decrease risk of aspiration.
- Remove false teeth.
- Give mouth care after every episode of emesis.
- Maintain record of I&O; measure and include all emesis.
- When oral intake is resumed, give small amounts of clear fluids such as ginger ale as tolerated and gradually progress to small, frequent meals of bland, nonirritating foods.
- Drink fluids an hour before or after meals to avoid over distending the stomach and causing vomiting.
- Offer mouth care and comfort measures.
- Maintain fluid and electrolyte balance.
- Administer medications as antiemetics, anticholinergics, antihistamines, and serotonin blockers.

ALTERED LEVEL OF CONSCIOUSNESS

- Content of consciousness: ability to think, communicate and feel; functions of cerebral cortex
- Arousal: state of wakefulness; function of the reticular activating system and brain stem
- Full consciousness: awake, alert, oriented to time, place, and person; appropriate in communication
- Unconsciousness: unable to interact with environment; unable to open eyes, obey commands; speak

Terms used to describe levels of consciousness between these extremes include confusion, delirium, stupor, and semicomatose.

Nursing Process Elements

Assessment:

- Assess status using Glasgow Coma Scale that scores the client on eye opening, motor and verbal response. Each of the three parameters is scored for a maximum possible score of 15 and a minimum possible score of 3. The fully conscious client scores the maximum 15; the totally unconscious client scores the minimum 3.

Parameter	Response	Score
Opens eyes	Spontaneously	4
	On verbal command	3
	In response to pain	2
	Do not open	1
Best motor response	Obeys verbal command	6
	Localizes pain	5
	Normal flexion withdrawal	4
	Abnormal flexion	3
	Extension	2
	Does not respond	1
Best verbal response	Oriented and carries on conversation	5
	Confused and converses	4
	Uses inappropriate words	3
	Makes incomprehensible sounds	2
	Does not respond	1

- Check PERRLA and the corneal reflex.
- Assess patency of airway and rate, rhythm, and depth of respirations.
- Auscultate for adventitious breath sounds.
- Check circulatory status by taking pulse and BP and checking color, temperature, and capillary refill in extremities.
- Monitor rectal temperature for elevation which may be the first sign of a drug reaction or a urinary tract, respiratory tract, wound, or other infection.
- Monitor skin for signs of breakdown.

Interventions:

- Maintain a patent airway.
  - —Turn client at least every 2 hours to prevent pooling of secretions in the lungs.
  - —Do not position supine because of the risk of tongue falling back and obstructing the airway.
  - —Have suction equipment quickly available and use to remove pooled secretions from the oro or nasopharynx.
  - —If suctioning a tracheostomy, preoxygenate and suction no longer than 15 seconds to avoid hypercapnia and increase in ICP.
- Maintain skin integrity.
  - —Turn a minimum of every 2 hours to relieve pressure on skin; utilize other pressure-relieving devices as needed.
- Keep skin clean, dry, and free from friction and irritating substances such as urine and feces.
- Position to minimize pressure on bony prominences and to maintain good alignment.
- Maintain NPO status because of absence of swallowing and gag reflexes.
- If the blink reflex is absent, apply an eye patch being careful not to let it touch the cornea, or tape the eyes

shut. Apply saline drops or artificial tears four times per day.

- Record I&O; notify physician if urinary output drops below 30 ml/hr.
- Monitor for signs of UTI if an indwelling catheter is in place: odor, cloudy appearance, and hematuria.
- Record occurrence of bowel movements and their characteristics.
- Palpate abdomen to detect distention.
- Auscultate bowel sounds to confirm peristalsis.
- Perform passive range of motion to maintain joint mobility.
- Use a foot board or high-top sneakers to prevent foot drop.
- Support limbs at heart level to prevent dependent edema.

SPINAL CORD COMPRESSION

Signs: Sudden loss of sensation, motor function of lower extremities with or without loss of bladder or bowel control

- Warning signs of impending compression: escalating back pain with or without bladder changes and before lower extremity weakness, worse when lying down, improved with standing.

Rx: Steroids and if ambulatory palliative radiation.

Nursing Process Elements

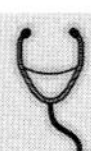

Assessment Alert

Early recognition and treatment is critical because the amount of impairment at time of treatment is generally permanent.

GASTROINTESTINAL BLEEDING

Occult Blood

Presence of unseen blood in the stool.

Etiology: Bleeding associated with GI disease such as colon cancer or peptic ulcer disease or from medications as aspirin, iron–potassium preparations, thiazide diuretics.

Dx: Occult blood test (Guaiac test)

Rx:

- Treatment of condition causing blood in stool
- Elimination of medications causing occult blood

Melena

Black, tarry stool with a distinctive foul odor as a result of the presence of digested blood

Etiology: Bleeding from esophagus, stomach, or small intestine.

Rx: Control of bleeding and treatment of underlying cause.

Think Smart/Test Smart

Do not assume that black, sticky stool indicates the presence of digested blood. Other factors such as oral iron and ingestion of black licorice can produce similar effects.

HEMATEMESIS

Vomiting of blood: may be frank blood or, if bleeding is slow or has stopped and gastric juices have acted on the blood, have the appearance of coffee grounds.

Etiology: Gastric or duodenal ulcers, esophageal varices, and esophagitis.

Rx: Management of underlying problem; transfusions; IV fluids; proton pump inhibitors or H-2 receptor antagonist.

Nursing Process Elements

Assessment:

- Consistency and character of emesis: fluid, mixed with food, light red, coffee ground if bleeding slowed or stopped
- Amount
- Frequency
- Clotting
- S&S of underlying problem

Intervention:

- Position client to prevent aspiration
- Monitor I&O

FLATUS

Flatus is the gas passed through the rectum.

Nursing Process Elements

Assessments:

- Auscultate for presence and frequency of bowel sounds
- Abdominal distention

- Type of diet, foods eaten as beans, cabbage, lentils, carbonated beverages; assess if client eats large amounts of fruits, sugars, and proteins (increase flatus)
- Pain

Interventions:

- Enemas to relieve gas.
- Encourage ambulation to increase peristalsis
- Turning in bed, when on bedrest

Client teaching for self-care

- Avoid gas-forming foods
- Use of antiflatulent medications and simethicone

JAUNDICE

Jaundice is characterized by the yellow discoloration of the skin, sclerae, and mucous membranes as a result of excessive amounts of bilirubin in the blood.

Etiology:

- Hemolytic jaundice: result of destruction of red blood cells with release of bilirubin which is occurring more rapidly than the liver can remove the bilirubin from the blood; occurs in pernicious anemia, sickle cell anemia, and transfusion reactions.
- Hepatocellular jaundice: result of liver cells being unable to metabolize bilirubin due to infection such as hepatitis, drug or chemical injury as with cirrhosis, or necrosis as in liver cancer.
- Obstructive jaundice: results from obstruction of bile flow in the ductules of the liver or in the common bile duct; can be due to inflammation or tumor.

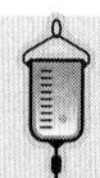

Clinical Alert

Physiological jaundice is jaundice that occurs in the newborn as a result of the normal breakdown of red blood cells, which occurs with entry into extrauterine life exceeding the ability of the immature liver to metabolize the hemoglobin. This is a transient phenomenon but a potentially dangerous one because bilirubin can cross the blood–brain barrier of the newborn and result in kernicterus.

Associated S&S: Light-colored stool because bile is not emptied into intestine in normal amounts.

- Deep orange, tea-like urine that foams when shaken because bile is excreted through the kidney.
- Pruritus because irritating bile salts are deposited in the skin.

Rx: Treatment of underlying cause.

Nursing Process Elements

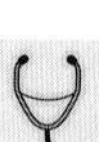

Assessment Alert

In light-skinned individuals, jaundice is generally first apparent in the sclerae; in dark-skinned individuals, jaundice is best identified in the hard palate because the sclerae often have a normal yellow tinge.

- Initiate measures to relieve pruritus (see section on pruritus).
- Maintain skin integrity.

AMENORRHEA

Amenorrhea is characterized by the absence of menstruation.

- Physiologic amenorrhea: normal absence of menses before puberty, during pregnancy, and after menopause.
- Primary amenorrhea: menses never began.
- Secondary amenorrhea: occurs after menses has been established.

Etiology:

- Hypothalamic, pituitary, ovarian, adrenal, pancreatic or thyroid disorders; congenital defects of uterus, vagina or hymen; cirrhosis, nephritis and other chronic illness; anorexia nervosa or bulimia.
- Temporary secondary amenorrhea: stress, strenuous exercise, low body weight, severe illness, use of phenothiazides and oral contraceptives.

ABNORMAL UTERINE BLEEDING

Patterns of abnormal bleeding are

- infrequent or scant bleeding;
- frequent but regular bleeding;
- excessive bleeding at regular intervals (menorrhagia);
- normal amount of bleeding occurring irregularly (metrorrhagia);
- excessive bleeding occurring at irregular but frequent intervals (menometrorrhagia).

Etiology: Endocrine or organic

- Menorrhagia: at puberty, usually the result of low estrogen levels; later associated with ovarian tumors, uterine fibroids, polyps, endometritis, and PID.
- OB Metrorrhagia: occurs with ectopic pregnancy, threatened abortion, and hydatidiform mole disease.
- Bleeding outside menstrual cycle in a perimenopausal woman or bleeding after menopause is often the first indication of endometrial or cervical cancer.
- Medications causing abnormal bleeding include androgens, estrogens or corticosteroids; thiazide diuretics; digoxin; anticholinergics, and phenothiazines.

LEUKORRHEA

Leukorrhea is a vaginal discharge other than blood.

Etiology:

- Over secretion of Bartholin's glands or the cervical glands whose normal function is to moisturize and lubricate the mucous membrane of the vagina and external genitalia.
- Vaginal or cervical infection in which case the discharge is purulent or mucopurulent and may be foul smelling.
- Infected or necrotic uterine polyps or tumors.

WORKSHEET

FILL IN THE BLANKS

Fill in the blank spaces with the correct word or phrase to complete each statement.

1. Normal pulse pressure in adult is about _______ mm Hg.
2. Pulse pressure >_______ mm Hg or <_______ is abnormal.
3. Adult systolic pressure as measured in the popliteal artery is _______ to _______ mm Hg higher than in the brachial artery because of the larger cuff bladder.
4. Fluid intake for clients with a fever should be between _______ and _______ ml/d unless contraindicated by a coexisting condition.
5. The diurnal variation in temperature can be as high as _______ °F.
6. The normal pulse rate for a toddler is between _______ and _______ bpm.
7. After activity, allow client to rest for _______ minutes before taking pulse to allow it to return to its resting rate.
8. The apical pulse in an adult is found at the level of the _______ intercostal space.
9. The normal respiratory rate of a newborn is between _______ and _______ rpm.
10. The stimulus to breathe in the healthy client is the pressure of _______ in the arterial blood.
11. Normal tidal volume (amount of air taken in and let out during a normal respiration) in an adult is _______ ml or _______ l/min.
12. The short side of the cuff bladder should be _______ the diameter of the extremity where it will be placed; the long side should be _______ of the diameter of the extremity where it will be placed.
13. When measuring BP, the cuff should be deflated at a rate of 2–3 mm Hg/sec.
14. A _______ occurs when some ventricular contractions are so weak that the resultant pulse wave does not reach the periphery or when pathology in or around the artery is preventing the passage of blood.

(continued)

15. When assessing for orthostatic hypotension, take pulse and BP after client has been in a supine position for _______ to _______ minutes.

16. A rating of pain of _______ or more on a 0–10 pain scale requires intervention.

17. For clients taking opioids, sedation level must be monitored especially during the first _______ to _______ hours of opioid therapy.

18. The drug used to counteract opioid-induced respiratory depression is _______.

19. Nausea associated with the start of opioid therapy should disappear in _______ to _______ days.

20. Fluid restriction to _______ to _______ ml/d is typically part of the protocol for managing ascites.

TRUE & FALSE QUESTIONS

Mark each of the following statements True or False. Correct all false statements in the space provided.

1. A UTI in an elderly person may be the cause of confusion. ___ T ___ F
2. Phenothiazines, opioids, and antibiotics can cause generalized pruritus. ___ T ___ F
3. If a BP cuff is inflated, deflated, and immediately reinflated, the resulting BP reading is likely to be incorrect with the systolic reading falsely low and diastolic falsely high. ___ T ___ F
4. Hypovolemia causes an increase in pulse rate as a compensatory mechanism to maintain BP in the face of low volume. ___ T ___ F
5. Under age three, the carotid artery is used routinely to obtain the pulse rate. ___ T ___ F
6. Phantom pain refers to perceived pain in an amputated or paralyzed part of the body. ___ T ___ F
7. Measuring BP when the client has just eaten, is in pain, or is smoking can result in falsely high readings. ___ T ___ F
8. NSAIDs in combination with opioids, reduce the dose of opioids needed and provide better pain relief than either type of drug alone. ___ T ___ F
9. Females tend to have lower BP then men at least until menopause when it tends to rise. ___ T ___ F
10. The client's report of presence, quality, and intensity of pain should be used as the primary guide to the need for pain relief. ___ T ___ F
11. If a TENS unit is functioning correctly, the client feels nothing during use. ___ T ___ F
12. Vomiting of black, coffee ground like material occurs when bleeding has occurred into the stomach and the blood has begun to be digested before being vomited. ___ T ___ F
13. Streaks of red blood on the stool indicates bleeding somewhere between the ileum and the rectum. ___ T ___ F

14. For the terminally ill client, administration of oxygen is guided by pulse oximetry readings. ___ T ___ F
15. Joint deformity is a symptom of rheumatoid arthritis. ___ T ___ F
16. Leukorrhea is a pathological event indicative of inflammation or infection of the vagina. ___ T ___ F
17. Gastrokinetic agents are given to anorexic clients to control nausea and early satiety. ___ T ___ F
18. Agitation may manifest as verbally or physically abusive behaviors. ___ T ___ F
19. Setting priorities for activities is an important aspect of managing fatigue. ___ T ___ F
20. Menstrual bleeding that occurs with abnormal frequency; is excessive in amount; or lasts an abnormal amount of time is referred to as dysfunctional bleeding. ___ T ___ F
21. Hepatotoxicity is a major risk associated with overdose of acetaminophen. ___ T ___ F
22. The management of ascites includes daily administration of diuretics. ___ T ___ F
23. Stridor is a snoring sound heard as air passes through a partially obstructed upper airway. ___ T ___ F
24. Vomiting from increased ICP differs from most other types of vomiting in that it is sudden, forceful, and spews away from the body. ___ T ___ F
25. Chronic hypoxia causes fatigue, apathy, drowsiness, and muscle twitches. ___ T ___ F
26. Metabolic alkalosis is a complication of diarrhea. ___ T ___ F
27. Breath sounds should be auscultated before and after use of an incentive spirometer. ___ T ___ F
28. Floaters indicate free blood in the aqueous humor and require immediate evaluation. ___ T ___ F
29. Melena is indicative of colon bleeding. ___ T ___ F
30. Diuretics are effective in relieving edema associated with superior vena cava syndrome. ___ T ___ F

APPLICATION QUESTIONS

1. The nurse should plan to obtain an apical pulse on which client?
   a. The client with a tachy dysrhythmia.
   b. The client who is less than 12 hours postoperative.
   c. The client with orthostatic hypotension.
   d. The client who is unconscious.

2. When assessing the progression of ascites, which parameter would the nurse assess?
   a. Serum albumin
   b. Intake and output
   c. Lung sounds
   d. Abdominal girth

3. Which assessment finding would indicate to the nurse that an antitussive medication administered to a client with bronchogenic cancer is having the desired effect?
   a. Dyspnea is relieved.
   b. Coughing is decreased.
   c. Expectoration is increased.
   d. Wheezes and gurgles have diminished.

(continued)

4. When caring for a client with pruritus related to jaundice, which intervention is appropriate for the nurse to recommend?
   a. Apply skin moisturizer
   b. Dab alcohol onto the itchy areas
   c. Take frequent, warm baths
   d. Drink tea

5. A client complains of constipation. In assessing this complaint, which is the most important question for the nurse to ask?
   a. What is the consistency of the stool?
   b. How often do you normally move your bowels?
   c. When did you move your bowels last?
   d. Do you strain when you move your bowels?

6. What direction should the nurse give to a male client with bladder spasms related to pressure from a tumor?
   a. Always sit to void.
   b. Empty the bladder at least every 4 hours.
   c. Limit fluid intake to 1500 ml/d.
   d. Use the Crede technique to ensure that the bladder is empty.

7. When assessing a client admitted with a traumatic head injury, how should the nurse interpret a gradually increasing systolic BP accompanied by a gradually decreasing diastolic pressure?
   a. Precursor of seizure activity
   b. Expected response as cranial blood flow stabilizes
   c. Indicative of developing hypovolemic shock
   d. Suggestive of increasing ICP

8. When evaluating the effect of a progesterone analog given to a client with metastatic cancer, which data would the nurse collect? Mark all that apply.
   a. ___ Weight
   b. ___ Presence or absence of mouth sores
   c. ___ Food intake
   d. ___ Occurrence of N&V
   e. ___ Ability to swallow
   f. ___ Presence of abnormal taste

9. Which type of medication would the nurse expect to administer for control of pruritus associated with neoplastic infiltration of subcutaneous tissues?
   a. Ondansetron
   b. Antifungal cream
   c. Systemic corticosteroid
   d. Bile acid sequester

10. Which assessment finding should the nurse interpret as indicative of impending spinal cord compression in a client with metastatic prostate cancer?
   a. Increasing back pain, which is worse when standing than when lying down
   b. Lower extremity weakness and/or paresthesias
   c. Urgency accompanied by bladder spasms
   d. Lower extremity muscle cramping

11. The nurse is giving instructions regarding taking morning temperatures to an unlicensed assistant. Which clients would not be on the list of those to have an oral temperature taken?
   Mark all that apply.
   a. ____ An alert 80-year old with a cardiac dysrhythmia
   b. ____ A 64-year old with delirium tremens
   c. ____ A 21-year old with nasal packing
   d. ____ A 55-year old with a tracheostomy
   e. ____ A 10-year old with a seizure disorder

12. When taking a tympanic temperature on a 2-year old, how does the nurse position the ear for insertion of the probe?
   a. Pull the ear lobe straight down
   b. Pull pinna straight back and upward
   c. Pull pinna straight back and slightly down
   d. Pull the pinna forward

13. Which instructions would the nurse give to a mother regarding the care of her 9-year-old child with a fever?
   a. Encourage fluids to between 2500 and 3000 ml/d
   b. Keep child warmly covered
   c. Limit food intake to small amounts of light — CHO foods like toast
   d. Call physician if child exhibits sensitivity to light

14. Which action would be contraindicated as part of the immediate care for a client with hypothermia?
   a. ___ Remove wet clothing
   b. ___ Cover the head snugly and warmly
   c. ___ Place in a tepid bath
   d. ___ Give warm fluids

15. To ease dyspnea in a terminally ill client, which intervention is most appropriate?
   a. Administer oxygen by mask rather than cannula
   b. Coach in slow, deep rhythmic breathing
   c. Have a fan blowing across the client
   d. Maintain a warm, humidified environment

16. When giving medication instructions to a client who is to take Tylenol for pain following an out-client surgical procedure, the nurse stresses the importance of not taking more than ___ mg in a 24-hour period because of the danger of liver damage.

    Answer is _______ mg.

17. Following a knee replacement, a client receives OxyContin for pain control in accord with an established protocol. The side effects of N&V develop and on the fourth postoperative day, still persist. Which is an appropriate nursing intervention?
    a. Withhold the medication and see if the N&V are relieved.
    b. Move the client to a private room because an intestinal virus is likely the cause of the symptoms.
    c. Request a change in medication order to another opioid.
    d. Notify the physician that the client apparently is allergic to the OxyContin.

18. Which statement made by the caretaker of a client with severe fatigue indicates the need for further teaching regarding client care?
    a. "I will get a bedside commode so she doesn't have to walk to the bathroom since she has to go so frequently."
    b. "I will have her rest quietly before meals so she can have more energy to eat."
    c. "I will investigate getting an electric bed so she can change position easily."
    d. "I will try to anticipate her needs so she has to move as little as possible."

19. Which nursing intervention is appropriate for a client with increased ICP?
    a. Position supine with head elevated no more than 30 degrees
    b. Keep room darkened
    c. Avoid rectal treatments
    d. Keep radio or TV on to provide meaningful sound

20. Which is the priority goal of nursing care for a client with ankles that swell by the end of the day and return to normal overnight?
    a. Increase venous return
    b. Promote urinary output
    c. Protect against infection
    d. Maintain skin integrity

21. When delegating BP measurement to an unlicensed assistant, the nurse cautions that correct technique must be used to avoid obtaining falsely low pressures. Which errors in technique should be identified as the potential causes of falsely low pressures? Mark all that apply.
    a. ___ Taking the BP on an extremity positioned below heart level
    b. ___ Using a cuff that is too wide
    c. ___ Deflating the cuff too rapidly
    d. ___ Applying the cuff unevenly to the arm

22. A decrease in pulse rate of ____ bpm or more between the pulse taken after the client has been supine for 3 minutes and the pulse taken after the client arises and stands for a minute is indicative of orthostatic hypotension.

    Answer is _______ .

23. Why is monitoring respiratory status a nursing priority when a client with COPD is receiving oxygen?
    a. Hyperventilation leading to respiratory alkalosis and loss of consciousness is a risk.
    b. Sudden increase in arterial oxygen can precipitate diaphragmatic spasm.
    c. Decreased arterial oxygen is the stimulus for breathing in a client with COPD.
    d. Oxygen administration can trigger reflex bronchospasm.

24. To prevent an increase in ICP, tracheostomy suctioning should be limited to no more than ___ seconds following each preoxygenation.

25. When assessing a client with a head injury, which finding should the nurse interpret as an early sign of increasing ICP?
    a. Widening pulse pressure
    b. Fixed dilated pupils
    c. Confusion
    d. Cheyne–Stokes respirations

ANSWERS & RATIONALES

ANSWERS FOR FILL IN THE BLANKS

Fill in the blank spaces with the correct word or phrase to complete each statement.

1. Normal pulse pressure in adult is about __40__ mm Hg.
2. Pulse pressure >__50__ mm Hg or <__30__ is abnormal.
3. Adult systolic pressure as measured in the popliteal artery is __20__ to __30__ mm Hg higher than in the brachial artery because of the larger cuff bladder.
4. Fluid intake for clients with a fever should be between __2500__ and __3000__ ml/d unless contraindicated by a coexisting condition.
5. The diurnal variation in temperature can be as high as __1.8__ °F.
6. The normal pulse rate for a toddler is between __90__ and __140__ bpm.
7. After activity, allow client to rest for __10–15__ minutes before taking pulse to allow it to return to its resting rate.
8. The apical pulse in an adult is found at the level of the __fifth__ intercostal space.
9. The normal respiratory rate of a newborn is between __30__ and __60__ rpm.
10. The stimulus to breathe in the healthy client is the pressure of __CO_2__ in the arterial blood.
11. Normal tidal volume (amount of air taken in and let out during a normal respiration) in an adult is __500__ ml or __6–8__ l/min.
12. The short side of the cuff bladder should be __40%__ the diameter of the extremity where it will be placed; the long side should be __60%__ of the diameter of the extremity where it will be placed.
13. When measuring BP, the cuff should be deflated at a rate of 2–3 mm Hg/sec.
14. A _____ pulse deficit _____ occurs when some ventricular contractions are so weak that the resultant pulse wave does not reach the periphery or when pathology in or around the artery is preventing the passage of blood.
15. When assessing for orthostatic hypotension take pulse and BP after client has been in a supine position for __2__ to __3__ minutes.
16. A rating of pain of __3__ or more on a 0–10 pain scale requires intervention.
17. For clients taking opioids, sedation level must be monitored especially during the first __12__ to __24__ hr of opioid therapy.
18. The drug used to counteract opioid induced respiratory depression is __naloxen (Narcan)__.
19. Nausea associated with the start of opioid therapy should disappear in __1__ to __2__ days.
20. Fluid restriction to __500__ to __1000__ ml/d is typically part of the protocol for managing ascites.

TRUE OR FALSE ANSWERS

Mark each of the following statements True or False. Correct all false statements in the space provided.

1. A UTI in an elderly person may be the cause of confusion. *True*

2. Phenothiazines, opioids, and antibiotics can cause generalized pruritus. *True*

3. If a BP cuff is inflated, deflated, and immediately reinflated, the resulting BP reading is likely to be incorrect with the systolic reading falsely low and diastolic falsely high. *False*
   If a BP cuff is inflated, deflated, and immediately reinflated, the resulting BP reading is likely to be incorrect with the systolic reading falsely high and diastolic falsely low.

4. Hypovolemia causes an increase in pulse rate as a compensatory mechanism to maintain BP in the face of low volume. *True*

5. Under age three, the carotid artery is used routinely to obtain the pulse rate. *False*

6. Phantom pain refers to perceived pain in an amputated or paralyzed part of the body. *True*

7. Measuring BP when the client has just eaten, is in pain, or is smoking can result in falsely high readings. *True*

8. NSAIDs in combination with opioids, reduce the dose of opioids needed and provide better pain relief than either type of drug alone. *True*

9. Females tend to have lower BP than men at least until menopause when it tends to rise. *True*

10. The client's report of presence, quality, and intensity of pain should be used as the primary guide to the need for pain relief. *True*

11. If a TENS unit is functioning correctly, the client feels nothing during use. *False*
    If a TENS unit is functioning correctly, the client should feel numbness or tingling during use.

12. Vomiting of black, coffee ground like material occurs when bleeding has occurred into the stomach and the blood has begun to be digested before being vomited. *True*

13. Streaks of red blood on the stool is indicates bleeding somewhere between the ileum and the rectum. *False*
    Stool with streaks of red blood on it occurs with colon or rectal bleeding; bleeding in the ileum causes red blood mixed in with the stool.

14. For the terminally ill client, administration of oxygen is guided by pulse oximetry readings. *False*
    For the terminally ill client, use of oxygen is guided by the relief of dyspnea, not by pulse oximetry readings.

15. Joint deformity is a symptom of rheumatoid arthritis. *True*

16. Leukorrhea is a pathological event indicative of inflammation or infection of the vagina. *False*
    Leukorrhea may be the result of a normal increase in vaginal secretions in response to the increased estrogen levels of pregnancy.

17. Gastrokinetic agents are given to anorexic clients to control nausea and early satiety. *True*

18. Agitation may manifest as verbally or physically abusive behaviors. *True*

(continued)

19. Setting priorities for activities is an important aspect of managing fatigue. *True*

20. Menstrual bleeding that occurs with abnormal frequency; is excessive in amount; or lasts an abnormal amount of time is referred to as dysfunctional bleeding. *True*

21. Hepatotoxicity is a major risk associated with overdose of acetaminophen *True*

22. The management of ascites includes daily administration of diuretics. *False*
Diuretics are generally ineffective in the treatment of ascites.

23. Stridor is a snoring sound heard as air passes through a partially obstructed upper airway. *False*
Stertor is a snoring sound heard as air passes through a partially obstructed upper airway.

24. Vomiting from increased ICP differs from most other types of vomiting in that it is sudden, forceful, and spews away from the body. *True*

25. Chronic hypoxia causes fatigue, apathy, drowsiness, and muscle twitches. *True*

26. Metabolic alkalosis is a complication of diarrhea. *False*
Metabolic acidosis is a complication of diarrhea.

27. Breath sounds should be auscultated before and after use of an incentive spirometer. *True*

28. Floaters indicate free blood in the aqueous humor and require immediate evaluation. *False*
Floaters on can occur with a retinal detachment but the vast majority of the time they are clinically insignificant and do not require treatment.

29. Melena is indicative of colon bleeding. *False*
Melena is indicative of bleeding higher up in the GI tract; bleeding in the colon presents as red blood as it is unaffected by the digestive enzymes.

30. Diuretics are effective in relieving edema associated with superior vena cava syndrome. *False*
Diuretics are not effective in relieving edema associated with superior vena cava syndrome because the cause of the edema is obstruction of the lymphatic drainage by tumor and diuretics work on the kidney to increase fluid output.

APPLICATION ANSWERS

1. The nurse should plan to obtain an apical pulse on which client?
   a. The client with a tachy dysrhythmia.
   b. The client who is less than 12 hours postoperative.
   c. The client with orthostatic hypotension.
   d. The client who is unconscious.

Rationale

Correct answer: a.

An apical pulse should be obtained on any client with an irregular heartbeat because the strength of myocardial contractions may vary and not all may be of sufficient strength to generate a pulse wave that can be felt in a peripheral artery. Being newly postoperative, unconscious or having orthostatic hypertension does not necessitate taking an apical pulse.

2. When assessing the progression of ascites, which parameter would the nurse assess?
   a. Serum albumin
   b. Intake and output
   c. Lung sounds
   d. Abdominal girth

Rationale

Correct answer: d.

Ascites is the accumulation of excess fluid in the peritoneal cavity. This fluid distends the abdomen and so abdominal girth increases as more fluid collects. Decreased plasma albumin that occurs with nephritic syndrome and malnutrition is a cause of ascites. Restricted fluid and sodium intake may be prescribed in the management of ascites but I&O measurement is not a measure of progression of ascites. Lung sounds are unrelated to ascites although ascites may cause dyspnea.

3. Which assessment finding would indicate to the nurse that an antitussive medication administered to a client with bronchogenic cancer is having the desired effect?
   a. Dyspnea is relieved.
   b. Coughing is decreased.
   c. Expectoration is increased.
   d. Wheezes and gurgles have diminished.

Rationale

Correct answer: b.

An antitussive stops coughing. Antitussives are used for nonproductive coughs and to prevent exhaustion from coughing. Antitussives are not typically used for productive coughs because the secretions need to be raised. Secretions that are not raised will be pulled by gravity deep into the lung where the warm, dark, moist environment is supportive of bacterial growth. Antitussives do not relieve dyspnea. Antitussives do not increase expectoration rather they decrease it because they suppress coughing. Wheezes and gurgles are caused by narrowed airways and presence of secretions. Since antitussives do not act on either of these problems, their decrease is not reflective of the desired effect of an antitussive.

4. When caring for a client with pruritus related to jaundice, which intervention is appropriate for the nurse to recommend?
   a. Apply skin moisturizer
   b. Dab alcohol onto the itchy areas
   c. Take frequent, warm baths
   d. Drink tea

Rationale

Correct answer: a.

Application of moisturizers to prevent drying helps limit pruritus. Alcohol is drying so it aggravates the itch. Cool baths can soothe itch; warm baths increase it. Drinking tea is contraindicated because it contains caffeine and theophylline, which increase itch.

5. A client complains of constipation. In assessing this complaint, which is the most important question for the nurse to ask?
   a. What is the consistency of the stool?
   b. How often do you normally move your bowels?
   c. When did you move your bowels last?
   d. Do you strain when you move your bowels?

Rationale

Correct answer: a.

Abnormally hard stool is always an indication of constipation so determining the consistency of the stool is the most important question to determine the validity of the client's complaint. Frequency of defecation varies significantly among different people so what constitutes an abnormally infrequent defecation for a person can only be determined by asking about what is normal and when he or she defecated last. Thus, these are pertinent assessment questions but they do not define constipation as well as the question about consistency. Straining generally accompanies constipation but does not define it.

6. What direction should the nurse give to a male client with bladder spasms related to pressure from a tumor?
   a. Always sit to void
   b. Empty the bladder at least every 4 hours
   c. Limit fluid intake to 1500 ml/d
   d. Use the Crede technique to ensure that the bladder is empty

Rationale

Correct answer: b.

Clients with bladder spasms should empty the bladder at least every 4 hours and can either sit or stand to void. Fluid intake should not be limited and the Crede techniques should not be used.

7. When assessing a client admitted with a traumatic head injury, how should the nurse interpret a gradually increasing systolic BP accompanied by a gradually decreasing diastolic pressure?
   a. Precursor of seizure activity
   b. Expected response as cranial blood flow stabilizes
   c. Indicative of developing hypovolemic shock
   d. Suggestive of increasing ICP

Rationale

Correct answer: d.

Widening pulse pressure (systolic minus diastolic pressure) is a sign of increased ICP. Other signs of increased ICP are new headache, vomiting, change in respirations, altered mental status, decreased motor function, increased restlessness, agitation, and blurred vision. Tramadol is contraindicated in the presence of ICP because it can lower the seizure threshold but widening of the pulse pressure is not indicative of the onset of seizure activity.

8. When evaluating the effect of a progesterone analog given to a client with metastatic cancer, which data would the nurse collect? Mark all that apply.
   a. ___ Weight
   b. ___ Presence or absence of mouth sores

(continued)

c. ___ Food intake
d. ___ Occurrence of N&V
e. ___ Ability to swallow
f. ___ Presence of abnormal taste

Rationale

Correct answers: a, c, d, and f.
Progesterone analogs are used to improve appetite; decrease N&V; reduce taste and odor changes; and promote weight gain. They are not used for problems related to mouth sores or ability to swallow; therefore, these factors are unrelated to their effectiveness.

9. Which type of medication would the nurse expect to administer for control of pruritus associated with neoplastic infiltration of subcutaneous tissues?
   a. Ondansetron
   b. Antifungal cream
   c. Systemic corticosteroid
   d. Bile acid sequester

Rationale

Correct answer: c.
Systemic corticosteroids are used for pruritus associated with inflammatory or neoplastic conditions. Ondansetron is used for pruritus related to opioid use, uremia, or jaundice. Antifungal cream is used for Candida-associated itch. Bile acid sequesters are used for itch related to end-stage liver disease.

10. Which assessment finding should the nurse interpret as indicative of impending spinal cord compression in a client with metastatic prostate cancer?
   a. Increasing back pain, which is worse when standing than when lying down
   b. Lower extremity weakness and/or paresthesias
   c. Urgency accompanied by bladder spasms
   d. Lower extremity muscle cramping

Rationale

Correct answer: a.
Escalating back pain with or without bladder symptoms, worse on lying down and improved on standing is the warning sign of impending spinal cord compression. Sudden loss of sensation and motor function in the lower extremities occurs with compression. Loss of bowel or bladder control may or may not occur.

11. The nurse is giving instructions regarding taking morning temperatures to an unlicensed assistant. Which clients would not be on the list of those to have an oral temperature taken?
   Mark all that apply.
   a. ____ An alert 80-year old with a cardiac dysrhythmia
   b. ____ A 64-year old with delirium tremens
   c. ____ A 21-year old with nasal packing
   d. ____ A 55-year old with a tracheostomy
   e. ____ A 10-year old with a seizure disorder

Rationale

Correct answers: b, c, and e.
Oral temperatures are contraindicated for clients who are unable to close their mouths tightly or follow directions to keep their mouth shut and not bite down; for clients unable to breathe through their noses; and for clients with surgery or mouth disease that could be painful, disrupted, or otherwise worsened by the insertion of the thermometer. Therefore, clients with delirium tremens, nasal packing, or seizures are among those for whom oral temperatures are contraindicated.

12. When taking a tympanic temperature on a 2-year old, how does the nurse position the ear for insertion of the probe?
   a. Pull the ear lobe straight down
   b. Pull pinna straight back and upward
   c. Pull pinna straight back and slightly down
   d. Pull the pinna forward

Rationale

Correct answer: c.
The pinna is pulled straight back and slightly downward prior to inserting the tympanic probe when taking temperatures on children under the age of three. Over the age of three, the pinna is pulled straight back or upward. The ear lobe is never pulled straight down nor is the pinna pulled forward for a tympanic temperature.

13. Which instructions would the nurse give to a mother regarding the care of her 9-year-old child with a fever?
   a. Encourage fluids to between 2500 and 3000 ml/d
   b. Keep child warmly covered
   c. Limit food intake to small amounts of light -CHO foods like toast
   d. Call physician if child exhibits sensitivity to light

Rationale

Correct answer: a.
Fluids in the amounts of 2500–3000 ml/d are needed to prevent dehydration. The child should be kept warmly covered to aid heat production during the period when temperature is rising but child should be uncovered to aid heat loss when temperature is falling. Foods should be given according to child's appetite and tolerance. Fever increases metabolic need for food stuffs and so efforts should be made to encourage intake not discourage it. Sensitivity to light is an expected symptom during the course of a fever and the client often appears glassy-eyed. This does not warrant notifying the physician.

14. Which action would be contraindicated as part of the immediate care for a client with hypothermia?
   a. ___ Remove wet clothing
   b. ___ Cover the head snugly and warmly
   c. ___ Place in a tepid bath
   d. ___ Give warm fluids

Rationale

Correct answer: c.

The client would not be placed in a tepid bath rather dry clothing, a warm environment and blankets or warming pads are provided. Wet clothing is removed, the head is covered with a cap or turban and warm oral or IV fluids are given. In addition, the limbs are kept close to the body to conserve heat.

15. To ease dyspnea in a terminally ill client, which intervention is most appropriate?
   a. Administer oxygen by mask rather than cannula
   b. Coach in slow, deep rhythmic breathing
   c. Have a fan blowing across the client
   d. Maintain a warm, humidified environment

Rationale

Correct answer: c.

Air blowing across the client is successful in relieving dyspnea in the terminally ill client. Oxygen should be administered via cannula rather than mask because the mask can create a feeling of suffocation. Coaching in slow, deep breathing is not identified as an effective intervention and the environment should be cool not warm.

16. When giving medication instructions to a client who is to take Tylenol for pain following an out-client surgical procedure, the nurse stresses the importance of not taking more than ___ mg in a 24-hour period because of the danger of liver damage.

Rationale

Correct answer: 4 grams/4000 mg.

17. Following a knee replacement, a client receives OxyContin for pain control in accord with an established protocol. The side effects of N&V develop and on the fourth postoperative day, still persist. Which is an appropriate nursing intervention?
   a. Withhold the medication and see if the N&V are relieved.
   b. Move the client to a private room because an intestinal virus is likely the cause of the symptoms.
   c. Request a change in medication order to another opioid.
   d. Notify the physician that the client apparently is allergic to the OxyContin.

Rationale

Correct answer: c.

N&V is a common response to opioids in the client who has not taken them before and developed tolerance. However, tolerance should develop and N&V disappear by day three. If this does not occur, a different opioid should be ordered for pain. Pain medication would not be withheld in order to determine the effect on the N&V because severe pain follows a knee replacement and pain interferes with healing. Further, clients have a right to pain relief. Although an intestinal virus can cause N&V, it is not the most likely cause since opioids also cause N&V and the client is receiving them. Therefore, it is not appropriate to move the client to a private room because of the likelihood of an intestinal virus. Allergic reactions involve rash, itch, hives, difficulty breathing, and outright anaphylactic shock. N&V are not signs of an allergic reaction.

18. Which statement made by the caretaker of a client with severe fatigue indicates the need for further teaching regarding client care?
   a. "I will get a bedside commode so she doesn't have to walk to the bathroom since she has to go so frequently."
   b. "I will have her rest quietly before meals so she can have more energy to eat."
   c. "I will investigate getting an electric bed so she can change position easily."
   d. "I will try to anticipate her needs so she has to move as little as possible."

Rationale

Correct answer: d.

Prolonged inactivity and bedrest places the client at risk for all the hazards of immobility. When a client has severe fatigue, it is beneficial to use equipment which requires the least exertion such as a bedside commode and an electric bed. It is also important to space activities such as eating and bathing with periods of rest. However, caution must be taken not to limit activity to the point where the negative effects of immobility occur.

19. Which nursing intervention is appropriate for a client with increased ICP?
   a. Position supine with head elevated no more than 30 degrees
   b. Keep room darkened
   c. Avoid rectal treatments
   d. Keep radio or TV on to provide meaningful sound

Rationale

Correct answer: b.

Unnecessary stimuli should be avoided so the room should be kept dark and quiet. The client should be maintained in semi-Fowler's position. Rectal treatments are not contraindicated by ICP.

(continued)

20. Which is the priority goal of nursing care for a client with ankles that swell by the end of the day and return to normal overnight?
   a. Increase venous return
   b. Promote urinary output
   c. Protect against infection
   d. Maintain skin integrity

Rationale

Correct answer: a.

The cause of peripheral edema that occurs during the day when sitting and standing and resolves overnight when lying down is impaired venous return. When sitting and standing, venous return must occur against the force of gravity; when lying down, the legs are on the same level as the heart so the force of gravity is not a significant factor. Because impaired venous return is the causative factor, the goal of nursing interventions is to improve it. Interventions to meet this goal include encouraging use of compression stockings, active or passive exercise of the lower extremities, elevating the legs at specified intervals throughout the day and whenever sitting down, and avoiding constricting clothing or bandages. Skin that is edematous is at risk for breakdown so maintenance of skin integrity is a nursing goal; however, it is not the primary goal because if the venous return problem is corrected the risk for skin breakdown of edematous tissue will also be resolved. Promoting urinary output does not impact edema from impaired venous return. Protection against infection is not a primary goal.

21. When delegating BP measurement to an unlicensed assistant, the nurse cautions that correct technique must be used to avoid obtaining falsely low pressures. Which errors in technique should be identified as the potential causes of falsely low pressures? Mark all that apply.
   a. ___ Taking the BP on an extremity positioned below heart level
   b. ___ Using a cuff that is too wide
   c. ___ Deflating the cuff too rapidly
   d. ___ Applying the cuff unevenly to the arm

Rationale

Correct answers: a, b, and c.

Taking the BP on an extremity positioned below heart level; using a cuff that is too wide; and deflating the cuff too rapidly all can cause falsely low BP. Applying the cuff unevenly to the arm can cause a falsely high BP.

22. A decrease in pulse rate of ____ bpm or more between the pulse taken after the client has been supine for 3 minutes and the pulse taken after the client arises and stands for a minute is indicative of orthostatic hypotension.

Rationale

Correct answer: 40 bpm.

23. Why is monitoring respiratory status a nursing priority when a client with COPD is receiving oxygen?
   a. Hyperventilation leading to respiratory alkalosis and loss of consciousness is a risk.
   b. Sudden increase in arterial oxygen can precipitate diaphragmatic spasm.
   c. Decreased arterial oxygen is the stimulus for breathing in a client with COPD.
   d. Oxygen administration can trigger reflex bronchospasm.

Rationale

Correct answer: c.

Decreased oxygen in the blood is the stimulus for breathing in a client with COPD. Therefore, if oxygen is administered there is the risk that respiratory arrest will occur because high oxygen saturation levels in the blood eliminate the stimulus for breathing. This is a particular risk with the administration of 100% oxygen. The normal stimulus to breathe is an increase in CO_2 in the blood but the client with COPD has become insensitive to CO_2 because of long-term elevated levels associated with the COPD. Oxygen administration does not cause hyperventilation; nor does it precipitate diaphragmatic spasm or bronchospasm.

24. To prevent an increase in ICP, tracheostomy suctioning should be limited to no more than ___ seconds following each preoxygenation.

Rationale

Correct answer: 15.

Fifteen seconds is the length of time that can elapse without oxygen before pulse rate and BP increase in response to a decrease in oxygen in the brain. Increased pulse and BP increases cerebral blood flow, which in turn occupies more space in the bony cranium and thereby causes an increase in ICP.

25. When assessing a client with a head injury, which finding should the nurse interpret as an early sign of increasing ICP?
   a. Widening pulse pressure
   b. Fixed dilated pupils
   c. Confusion
   d. Cheyne–Stokes respirations

Rationale

Correct answer: c.

Change in level of consciousness, the early signs of which include restlessness, irritability, drowsiness, confusion, apathy, difficulty or hesitation in following simple directions or in verbalizing, is the most sensitive indicator of increasing ICP. Widening pulse pressure and Cheyne–Stokes respirations are considered late signs and fixed dilated pupils are late signs and indicate that pressure has increased to the degree that a portion of cerebral cortex has slipped under the tentorium through the uncus and is compressing the area of the brainstem where the oculomotor nerve exits.

Test Plan Category:

Physiological Integrity

Sub-category: Reduction of Risk Potential—Part 3

Topic: Potential for Complications from Surgical Procedures and Health Alterations

PERIOPERATIVE CARE

PREOPERATIVE CARE

Nursing responsibilities preoperatively:

- Physical assessment:
  - —Cardiovascular system
    - Compare BP bilaterally.
    - Assess for hypoxia by checking for clubbing and capillary refill.

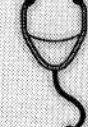

Assessment Alert

Notify physician if there is a difference of more than 15 mm Hg in either the systolic or diastolic pressure between the right and left extremity.

—Respiratory system
- Assess lung sounds.
- Assess respiratory rate and pattern.
- Assess symmetry of chest expansion and use of accessory muscles.
- Review medical history for disease processes that place client at increased risk for pulmonary aspiration.
  - Gastric esophageal reflux disease
  - Hiatal hernia
  - Gastric motility disorders
  - Pregnancy
  - Bowel obstruction
  - Diabetes
  - Obesity
- Identify risk factors related to higher incidence of postoperative pulmonary complications.
  - Smoking
  - Chronic obstructive pulmonary disease
  - Respiratory infection
  - Skeletal deformities

—GI system
- Inspect contour and symmetry of abdomen.
- Auscultate bowel sounds.
- Palpate abdomen for tenderness or distension.

—GU system
- Inspect and palpate the suprapubic area for distension.
- Obtain sample for urinalysis, if ordered.

—Neurological system
- Assess orientation to person, place, and time.
- Assess pupils for uniformity in size and shape and reaction to light.
- Assess speech pattern.

—Psychological system
- Assess client's understanding of the surgical procedure and postoperative care.
- Encourage client to talk about anxiety related to surgery.

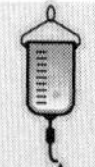

Clinical Alert

Risk factors for surgical complications need to be identified preoperatively to allow the nurse to provide appropriate preoperative teaching and postoperative management. Risk factors include:

- Hypovolemia
- Dehydration, electrolyte imbalance
- Nutritional deficits (serum albumin <3.5 mg/dl)
- Extremes of age and weight
- Infection, sepsis
- Toxic conditions
- Immunological abnormalities
- Pulmonary disease (obstructive disease, restrictive disorder, respiratory infection)
- Renal or urinary tract disease (decreased renal function, urinary tract infection, obstruction)
- Pregnancy
- Cardiovascular disease (coronary artery disease, previous myocardial infarction, cardiac failure, dysrhythmias, hypertension, prosthetic heart valve, thromboembolism, hemorrhagic disorders, cerebrovascular disease)
- Endocrine dysfunction (diabetes mellitus, adrenal disorders, thyroid malfunction)
- Hepatic disease (cirrhosis, hepatitis)
- Preexisting mental or physical disability

- Review medication list for prescribed and over-the-counter drugs

—Instruct client on the possible interaction of prescribed medications with anesthetic agents
- Corticosteroids: may potentiate cardiovascular collapse if stopped suddenly.
- Diuretics: may cause excessive respiratory depression during surgery from an associated electrolyte imbalance.
- Phenothiazines: may increase hypotensive action of anesthetics.
- Tranquilizers: may cause anxiety, tension, and seizures with sudden withdrawal of medication.
- Insulin: may interact with anesthetics.
- Antibiotics: may cause interruption in nerve transmission when combined with curariform muscle relaxants resulting in apnea from respiratory paralysis.
- Anticoagulants: can increase possibility of bleeding intraoperatively and postoperatively.
  - Instruct client that use of aspirin will increase likelihood of bleeding intraoperatively and postoperatively.
- Antiseizure medication: will need to have IV dose during surgery to prevent seizure activity.
- Monoamine oxidase (MAO) inhibitors: may increase hypotensive action of anesthetics.

—Instruct client on the possible interaction of over-the-counter medications with anesthetic agents

- Echinacea angustifolia: There is a risk of hepatotoxicity; may decrease effectiveness of corticosteroids.
- Tanacetum parthenium (Feverfew) may inhibit platelet aggregation and increase bleeding time.
- Allium sativum (Garlic) inhibits platelet aggregation, potentiates warfarin, increases INR and PT, and decreases blood glucose levels.
- Zingiber officinale (Ginger) has an anticoagulant action, large doses will cause bleeding and dysrhythmias.
- Panax ginseng (Ginseng root) causes tachycardia and hypertension; inhibits platelet aggregation; decreases effectiveness of warfarin; decreases INR and PT; lowers blood glucose; potentiates effects of digoxin.
- Gingko Bilboa inhibits platelet-activating factor; prolongs bleeding time; increases effects of anticoagulants.
- Piper methysticum (Kava-kava) potentiates central nervous system depressants, anesthetics, and alcohol; increases hypertension and edema; neutralizes antibiotics; potentiates corticosteroids.
- Hypericum perforatum (St. John's wort) prolongs sedative effects of anesthesia and opioids; possible interactions with warfarin, steroids, benzodiazepines, and calcium channel blockers, and protease inhibitors.
- Valeriana officinalis (Valerian) causes hepatotoxicity with other herbs; prolongs sedative effects of anesthesia; potentiate actions of barbiturates and alcohol.

—Inform anesthesiologist of client's use of herbal medications that may interact with anesthetic agents

Client teaching for self-care

- Assess learning needs.
- Provide explanations for diagnostic tests that may be required prior to the surgical procedure.
- Discuss anesthesia that might be used for the particular procedure.
  —Contact anesthesia department for specific questions that client may have.
- Discuss nutritional requirements prior to surgical procedure.
  —Importance of nutrition prior to surgical procedure
  —Importance of not eating or drinking starting at 8 hours prior to the scheduled surgery
- Review operating procedure.
  —Explain to client and family that there will be a short period of time in which client will be in the holding area.
  —Described the surgical garb that the nurses and doctors will be wearing in the operating room.
  —Describe the operating room setting, including cool temperature of the rooms.
  —Describe the equipment that will be used to provide anesthesia and monitor client during surgery.
- Review postanesthesia care unit (PACU).
  —Describe to client the typical equipment used (oxygen via nasal canula, sequential compression device, pain control) and sensations that might be experienced as anesthesia is wearing off, such as feeling chilled.
- Instruct on leg exercises.
  —Straight leg raises: leg is lifted off bed straight, repeat five times at least four times per day on each leg.
    - Do not have client perform this exercise if having abdominal surgery or has existing back problems.
  —Quad sets: tighten thigh muscles and hold for 5 seconds, repeat five times each hour.
  —Ankle pumps: point toes up and down (moving ankle) and then circle ankles, repeat 10 times each hour.
  —Gluteal tightening: tighten buttock muscles and hold for 5 seconds then relax, repeat five times each hour.

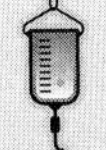

Clinical Note

Client may initially have sequential compression devices on both legs to stimulate the movement of blood through the lower extremities.

  —Instruct on respiratory hygiene exercises.
    - Deep breathe and coughing (three deep breaths and forceful cough)
    - Splinting incisional area to decrease pain when coughing
    - Incentive spirometry
    - Blow bottle
- Perform preoperative preparation appropriate for surgical procedure.
  —Cleanse skin using an antiseptic solution the evening or morning before surgery.
    - Shaving of the surgical site will typically be done in the operating room.
  —Bowel prep will depend on the surgical procedure and can include antibiotics to decrease intestinal flora, enemas, and/or laxatives.
  —Preoperative medications are administered 45 minutes to 1 hour prior to induction of anesthesia
    - Decrease anxiety: diazepam (Valium), hydroxyzine hydrochloride (Vistaril, Atarax)
    - Permit a smoother induction of the anesthetic agent: pentobarbital sodium

- Decrease the amount of anesthetic required (meperidine hydrochloride, morphine sulfate, fentanyl citrate (Sublimaze, Duragesic)
- Provide amnesia for the events preceding the surgical procedure: midazolam hydrochloride (Versed)
- Decrease pharyngeal, respiratory, and gastric secretions: atropine sulfate, glycopyrrolate (Robinul), scopolamine hydrobromide (Hyoscine), ranitidine, metoclopramide
- Provide sedation and impairs memory of perioperative events: lorazepam (Ativan)

• Review preoperative checklist

—Surgical consent is signed and understood by client

—Identification of client using two sources of information

—Verification of reports on chart

- X-rays: chest
- 12-lead electrocardiogram
- Pulmonary function test, if ordered
- Laboratory reports
  - CBC with differential
  - Basic metabolic panel: BUN, creatinine, glucose, potassium, sodium, chloride, and CO_2
  - Liver enzymes
  - Coagulation studies: prothrombin time (PT), partial prothroboplastic time (PTT), international normalized ratio (INR)
  - Beta-human chorionic gonadotropin
  - Urinalysis

—Completion of nursing physical assessment

—VS.

PEDS **Pediatric considerations:**

- Use of play, books, films, tours, rehearsals, and other age appropriate orientation activities familiarize the child with the perioperative procedures and help to decrease the stress of the surgical experience.
- Having the parent with the child during induction or leaving a favorite possession with the child and reuniting parent and child as soon as possible after surgery decreases stress.

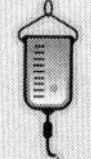

Clinical Alert

Infants should not be without fluids for an extended time prior to surgery because of the risk of dehydration and glycogen depletion.

- Children should be encouraged to drink fluids prior to being NPO to ensure hydration and decrease later thirst.
- Preoperative medications should be given orally (e.g., oral transmucosal fentanyl or fentanyl Oralet) or by existing IV (e.g., Versed) to avoid unnecessary stress.

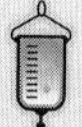

Clinical Alert GERI

Physiological changes related to aging place older clients at greater perioperative complications.

- Cardiovascular: hypotension, dysrhythmia, congestive heart failure, thrombi, hypervolemia, and delayed stress response
- Gastrointestinal: aspiration, paralytic ileus, constipation, and altered drug metabolism
- Immunologic: reduced ability to protect against microorganisms
- Integumentary: pressure ulcer, impaired healing, delayed recovery from anesthetics due to storage in adipose tissue, and hypothermia
- Metabolic: decreased inflammatory response, altered fluid dynamics, increased cardiac workload, delayed shivering, and delayed recovery from anesthetics
- Musculoskeletal: deep vein thrombosis, positioning difficulty, pathological fracture, and falls
- Neurologic: delirium, falls, and increased anxiety
- Renal: prolonged response to anesthesia, overhydration, delirium, and urinary retention
- Respiratory: difficult intubation, aspiration, decreased gas exchange, ineffective cough, and difficulty maintaining airway

POSTOPERATIVE CARE

Nursing responsibilities postoperatively:

• PACU

—Maintain airway.

- Provide oxygen therapy until client is breathing on his/her own.
  - Shivering increases oxygenation needs.
  - Use oxygen cautiously with clients with a history of COPD.
- Encourage client to deep breathe.
- Elevate head of bed unless contraindicated.

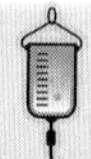

Clinical Alert

Common causes of airway obstruction include: tongue blocking the airway, hypoxemia ($PO_2 < 60$ mm Hg, atelectasis, pulmonary edema), bronchospasm, hypoventilation (decreased respiratory rate, hypoxemia, increased $PaCO_2$).

—Assess client every 10–15 minutes dependent on client condition and wakefulness for VS, oxygen saturation level, lung sounds, level of consciousness, neurological status, capillary refill, and color of skin and mucous membranes.

—Maintain cardiovascular stability.

- Monitor for S&S of hypotension and shock.
  - Pallor
  - Cool, moist skin
  - Rapid breathing
  - Cyanosis (lips, gums, tongue)
  - Rapid, weak, thready pulse
  - Decreasing pulse pressure
  - Decreasing BP
  - Concentrated urine
- Monitor for hemorrhage.
  - Pulse rate increased
  - Restless, apprehensive, thirsty
  - Skin is cold, moist, and pale
  - Low hemoglobin level
  - Decreased cardiac output
- Monitor for hypertension and dysrhythmia.

—Monitor intake (IV fluids) and output (all drains, including urinary output).

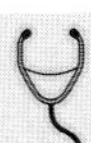

Assessment Alert

Encourage client without a Foley catheter to use bedpan or urinal to empty bladder, thereby preventing the possible development of a urinary tract infection secondary to urinary stasis.

—Assess all tubes and drains for insertion site, drainage, and security to body.

—Assess surgical dressing.

—Provide warm blanket(s) to decrease hypothermia.

—Administer medications per physician's order (i.e., narcotic, antiemetic, antihypertensive agent).

—Assess for potential reaction to the administration of anticholinesterase (neostigmine, pyridostigmine) to reverse nondepolarizing anesthetic agents.

—Administer naloxone (Narcan) to reverse opioids.

—Provide pain management.

—Provide antiemetics as needed to relieve N&V.

- Phenothiazines: promethazine, prochlorperazine
- Butyrophenones: haloperidol, droperidol
- Antihistamines: hydroxyzine, diphenhydramine
- Anticholinergics: transdermal scopolamine, atropine
- Benzamides: metoclopramide, domperidone
- Serotonin antagonists: ondansetron, dolasetron, granisetron
- Corticosteroids: dexamethasone, betamethasone

—Determine client's readiness for discharge from PACU.

- Stable VS
- Oriented to person, place, time
- Pulmonary function not impaired
- Pulse oximetry is 92% or greater
- Urine output greater than 30 ml/hr
- N&V is absent or under control
- Minimal pain

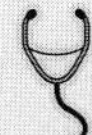

Assessment Alert

There is the potential for the client to experience respiratory depression.

- Nursing Unit

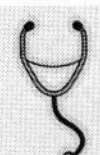

Assessment Alert

The client returning to the surgical unit will need to be assessed frequently. The frequency of assessing VS or other body systems can be as often as every 15 minutes until the client is stable. Most often once the client has been discharged from PACU VS and body systems are assessed every 4 hours, which is the minimum frequency of assessment to assure client safety.

—Respiratory system

- Assess lung sounds.
- Assess respiratory rate and pattern.
- Assess symmetry of chest expansion and use of accessory muscles.
- Encourage respiratory hygiene activities.
- Assess for hypoxia (oxygen saturation level, capillary refill).

—Cardiovascular

- Assess heart rate.
- Assess BP; notify physician if the systolic is greater than 15% of the client's baseline value.

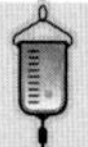

Clinical Alert

An irregular heart rate can be an effect of anesthesia or a preexisting arrhythmia, such as atrial fibrillation.

—GU
- Monitor urinary output (normal output should be 0.5–1 ml/kg/hr)
- Assess for difficulty voiding if the client does not have a Foley catheter

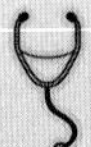

Assessment Alert

Causes of postoperative urinary retention include: medication, such as atropine and opioids, administered to manage pain which can decrease parasympathetic stimulation; epidural anesthesia, recumbent position, abdominal surgery (pelvic, perineal, and bowel), prolonged immobility, and sympathetic nerve stimulation due to pain, anxiety, or fear.

—GI
- Assess bowel sounds (peristalsis should be present within 6 hours postoperatively with normal bowel sounds present within 24–48 hours).
- Assess for distension and rigidity.
- Assess for Cullen's sign (bluish tinge around the umbilicus that is an indicator of intra-abdominal or peritoneal bleeding).
- Encourage ambulation to promote peristalsis.
- Administer stool softener if prescribed.

—Neurological
- Assess orientation to person, place, and time.
- Assess pupils for uniformity in size and shape and reaction to light.
- Assess speech pattern.

—Surgical site
- Monitor postoperative dressing, including type of dressing and any drainage if present.
- Change per physician's order.
- Monitor and maintain patency of drains.
- Assess surgical incision and periwound skin.
- Remove sutures and/or staples per physician's order, typical 7–10 days postoperatively.

—Ostomy care
- Describe and monitor output of a bowel diversion (ileostomy, ascending colostomy, transverse colostomy, descending colostomy, or sigmoid colostomy) and/or urinary diversion (ileal conduit).
- Consult the ostomy nurse (WOCN).
- Monitor stoma for circulatory problems, such as gray color or darkening of mucosa.

—Assess for potential infection.
- Monitor temperature and other vital signs.

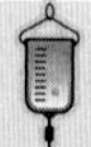

Clinical Alert

Typical changes in VS with infection include an elevated temperature, tachycardia, and either an elevation of BP or hypotension. The client may also experience a decrease in urinary output.

- Monitor urinary output.
- Monitor wound and drain sites.
- Monitor laboratory values (i.e., WBC).
- Assess for changes in mentation.

—Monitor and record I&O.
- Monitor IV fluids.
- Record output from all tubes and drains (i.e., nasogastric tube, HemoVac, or Jackson Pratt drain (JP drain).
- Monitor nutritional intake.

—Encourage mobility and ambulation, if appropriate.

—Provide comfort.
- Offer ice chips if client has bowel sounds.
- Reposition.
- Offer distraction activities, such as television, radio.
- Offer a back rub, if appropriate based on surgical site.

—Pain management
- Encourage client to splint surgical site when coughing.
- Encourage use of PCA pump.
- Offer and provide nonanalgesic pain measures.
  - Imagery
  - Relaxation
  - Heat/cold, if prescribed by physician
  - Distraction, such as TV, radio
  - Back rub
  - Noncontact therapeutic touch

—Monitor nutrition.

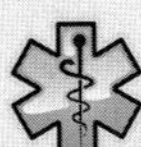

Nursing Intervention Alert

Surgery increases the basal metabolic rate requiring more calories than is usually consumed by the client.

- Administer supplemental protein if client is protein deficient (serum albumin level < 3.5 g/dl) or immunocompromised.
- Consult nutritionist if client is only receiving IV fluids for 3 or more days.
- Encourage client to consume meals provided to get adequate calories needed to spare protein and replace lost body mass from the catabolic phase that follows stress.
- Determine special nutritional needs to promote wound healing:
  - Vitamin C (needed for capillary and antibody formation)
  - Vitamin K (needed for blood clotting)
  - Vitamin A (needed for tissue synthesis, reverses the suppression of immune response created by the stress of surgery)
  - Iron (replaces iron lost from blood loss associated with surgery)
  - Zinc (needed for protein synthesis and wound healing)

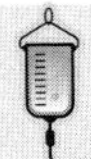

Clinical Alert

Protein stores will deplete within 3–5 days without adequate calorie and protein intake. Some clients may require total parenteral nutrition (TPN).

—Perform nursing interventions to prevent postoperative complications.
- Turn and position every 2 hours, unless contraindicated by physician's orders, to promote circulation and decrease alteration in skin integrity.
- Encourage deep breathing and coughing.
- Encourage calf muscle exercises, if client does not have sequential compression devices or TED stockings in place.
- Promote ambulation.
- Perform either active or passive range of motion.
- Monitor for hypovolemia.

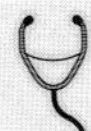

Assessment Alert

The most common postoperative complications include pressure ulcer, paralytic ileus, pulmonary emboli, fat emboli, hypostatic pneumonia, hematoma, deep vein thrombosis, infection, and wound dehiscence and evisceration.

- Managing postoperative complications

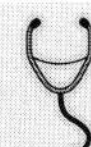

Assessment Alert

Common risk factors for DVT include: orthopedic surgery (hip, knee, and lower extremities), transurethral prostatectomy, general surgery and gynecological/obstetric client over 40 years old, and neurosurgical clients.

—Wound dehiscence and evisceration
- Use moist wound healing products (i.e., hydrogel, alginate) to manage dehisced surgical incision.
- Apply abdominal binder to prevent evisceration.

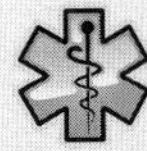

Nursing Intervention Alert

Immediate action is to be taken when bowel eviscerates through a dehisced surgical wound.

- Position client in low-Fowler's.
- Instruct client to lie quietly.
- Cover exposed intestine with a moist sterile saline dressing.
- Notify surgeon.

—Paralytic ileus
- Insertion of nasogastric tube to decompress intestine

—Urinary retention
- Insert straight catheter to empty bladder.
- Encourage fluid intake, if not NPO.

—Pulmonary emboli

—Fat emboli

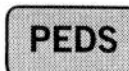 **Pediatric considerations:**

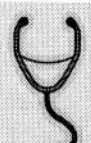

Assessment Alert

Monitor for malignant hyperthermia, a genetic myopathy characterized by hypermetabolism, and muscle destruction, which may occur during or after surgery. Symptoms include: tachycardia, tachypnea, rising BP, mottled skin, muscle rigidity, and ultimately high fever.

During the preoperative assessment, questions should be asked to determine if any family members had problems with anesthesia suggestive of this disorder.

- Use age-appropriate techniques (drawing, story telling, play) to discover child's ideas and reactions to the surgery and support or correct perceptions to alleviate sources of continuing stress.

CARDIOVASCULAR SURGERY

VALVULOPLASTY

- Valvuloplasty involves repair or reconstruction of a stenosed or regurgitant cardiac valve.
- Type of valvuloplasty depends on the cause and type of valve dysfunction.
    - —Commissurotomy is performed to separate the thickened, adherent leaves of a stenosed valve. The site where leaflets meet is called a commissure.
        - Closed commissurotomies do not require cardiopulmonary bypass and the valve is not directly visualized.
            - Percutaneous balloon valvuloplasty is a nonsurgical invasive technique in which a balloon is positioned across the stenosed valve and inflated.
            - A midsternal incision is made and a dilator is used to break open the commissure.
        - Open commissurotomy is a direct visualization of the valve and requires cardiopulmonary bypass.
            - Annuloplasty involves repair of a narrowed or enlarged valve annulus, the supporting ring of the valve.
            - Chordoplasty involves repair of the chordae tendineae and most generally involves the mitral valve. The chordae tendineae can be shortened, reattached to the leaflet, or lengthened.
            - Leaflet repair is for leaflets that have been damaged as a result of stretching, shortening, or tearing.

Valve Replacement

- Complete replacement of the valve.
    - —Two types
        - Mechanical valves are considered to be more durable and longer lasting. Often used for younger clients. Thromboemboli are a significant complication and thus, clients require lifetime anticoagulation with warfarin (Coumadin).
        - Tissue or biologic valves are not as durable as mechanical valves and require replacement more frequently but are less likely to cause thromboemboli and the client does not require long-term anticoagulation therapy.
            - Three types: Xenograft (also known as heterograft) valves are from animals generally pigs or cows. Homografts (also known as allografts) are from human cadavers. And autografts are excised from the client's own pulmonic valve.

Nursing Process Elements

- Assess VS and hemodynamic parameters.
- Assess for clinical manifestations of decreased cardiac output.
- Monitor I&O and note any weight gain greater than 3–5 lb/24 hrs.
- Administer medications as ordered.
- Assess and treat pain.
- Assess laboratory values—CBC, APPT, PT, and ABGs.
- Provide emotional support.
- Provide wound care if open procedure was used.
- Implement bleeding precautions if client is on anticoagulant therapy.
- Provide client education following surgical interventions.
- Alternate periods of rest and activity.

Client teaching for self-care

- Schedule rest periods to prevent fatigue.
- Resume usual activities gradually.
- Report S&S of CHF including weight gain, increased pulse rate, and difficulty breathing.
- Know S&S of strep throat and seek treatment immediately.
- Adhere to routine for prophylactic antibiotic treatment prior to dental work and invasive procedures, if required.
- If on anticoagulant therapy
  —Use bleeding precautions including using a soft-bristled tooth brush and electric razor.
  —Report signs of bleeding immediately: joint pain, black or tarry stools, blood in urine, and bleeding gums.
  —Adhere to laboratory schedule for hematocrit (Hct) and hemoglobin (Hgb), Prothrombin time, and bleeding times.
  —Know dose and side effects of warfarin (Coumadin).
  —Know to avoid medications such as aspirin or foods such as dark green, leafy vegetables that may increase bleeding times or that interfere with vitamin K production.
- If an open procedure was used
  —Know wound care.
  —Know S&S of infection including redness, warmth, edema, exudate at incisional site.
  —Know follow-up routine care schedule.
- If a valve replacement was done
  —Know how long the usual life of the replacement valve should be.
  —Report immediately S&S of valve failure: decreased BP, increased pulse rate, dyspnea, and weight gain.

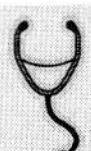

Assessment Alert

Clinical manifestations of infective endocarditis include: murmur, cough, fever, chills, petechiae, splinter hemorrhages, and Osler's nodes.

Dynamic Cardiomyoplasty

- The client's own latissimus dorsi muscle is used as a graft, wrapped around the heart, and then is stimulated in synchrony with cardiac systole
- It is a muscle-powered cardiac assist procedure
- Dynamic cardiomyoplasty decreases myocardial wall stress and myocardial oxygen demand
- It requires insertion of an epicardial pacing wire and implanted pace maker
- Two incisions are needed: a thoracotomy to dissect the latissimus muscle and a mediastinal incision in order to wrap the muscle around the heart.

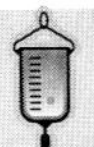

Clinical Alert

Hypertrophic cardiomyopathy is considered a contraindication.

Use: Generally used for Class III NYHA heart failure clients who are deteriorating despite maximal medical therapy.

Preparation: Usual preoperative care for cardiac surgery including physical, emotional, and psychosocial assessment; preoperative teaching of client and family concerning postoperative care; and close monitoring of the client's condition.

Postoperative course: similar to client's undergoing open heart surgery. Pacing is not started for 2–3 weeks following surgery and takes up to 3 months for full function to be achieved.

Nursing Process Elements

- Monitor hemodynamic measures.
- Assess cardiac monitoring.
- Measure and record I&O hourly.
- Assess pain level.
- Administer medications as ordered.
- Provide emotional support to client and family.
- Evaluate respiratory status.
- Assess incisions for presence of infection and drainage.
- Assess for S&S of complications.

Client teaching for self-care

- Schedule rest periods to prevent fatigue.
- Resume usual activities gradually.
- Report S&S of CHF including weight gain, increased pulse rate, and difficulty breathing.
- Know follow-up routine and when cardiac conditioning will be maximized.
- Understand cardiac pacing and how to check heart rate and pacing effectiveness.
- Understand that procedure is palliative.
- Follow low-fat cardiac diet
- Adhere to medical regime.

MYOTOMY/MYECTOMY

- The dissection or cutting of a muscle (myotomy)
- The excision of all or part of the muscle (myectomy)

Use: Hypertrophic Cardiomyopathy, used with severe symptomatic clients to remove a portion of the thickened muscle of the upper portion of the cardiac ventricular septum to relieve outflow obstruction.

Preparation: Usual preoperative care for client undergoing open heart surgery including physical, emotional, and psychosocial assessment; preoperative teaching of client and family concerning postoperative care including respiratory support, sensory stimuli, monitoring equipment; and close monitoring of the client's condition.

Postoperative course: As for clients undergoing open heart surgery, client will be in an intensive care unit for 1–3 days and will be discharged home after a total hospital stay of 7–10 days.

Nursing Process Elements

- Monitor hemodynamic measures.
- Assess cardiac monitoring.
- Measure and record I&O hourly including chest tube drainage.
- Monitor laboratory values especially Hct & Hgb, ABGs, CBC, and APPT.
- Keep temporary pacemaker at bedside.
- Assess for S&S of cardiac tamponade: increased heart rate, decreased BP, increased CVP, decreased UOP, and distant heart sounds.
- Monitor core body temperature and keep temperature above 96.8°F (36°C)
- Assess pain level.
- Administer medications as ordered.
- Note ETT placement and ventilator settings.
- Provide emotional support to client and family.
- Evaluate respiratory status.
- Assess incisions for presence of infection and drainage.
- Assess for S&S of complications.

Client teaching for self-care

- Schedule rest periods to prevent fatigue.
- Resume usual activities gradually.
- Report S&S of CHF including weight gain, increased pulse rate, and difficulty breathing.
- Know follow-up routine.
- Know wound care.
- Understand that procedure is palliative.
- Follow low-fat cardiac diet.
- Adhere to medical regime.

PERICARDECTOMY

- Pericardectomy-operation to remove the pericardium

Use: In cases of pericardial disease, it may be necessary to remove or partially remove the pericardial sac to remove scarred and inflexible areas of the pericardium or to prevent recurrent pericarditis. Requires a sternotomy and thoracotomy.

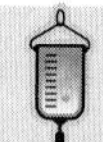

Clinical Alert

Even though the pericardium helps to support and protect the heart, its removal does not cause any harm. The heart can function without it.

Preparation: Usual preoperative care for client undergoing open heart surgery including physical, emotional, and psychosocial assessment; client education concerning the anatomy and physiology of the heart and the surgical procedure, pain management and emotional support, sensory stimuli, and monitoring equipment; and the need for close monitoring of the client's condition.

Postoperative course: As for clients undergoing open heart surgery. Client will be in an intensive care unit for 1–2 days and will be discharged home after a total hospital stay of 5–7 days.

Nursing Process Elements

- Monitor hemodynamic measures.
- Assess cardiac monitoring.
- Measure and record I&O hourly including chest tube drainage.
- Monitor laboratory values especially Hct & Hgb, ABGs, CBC, and APPT.
- Keep temporary pacemaker at bedside.
- Assess for S&S of cardiac tamponade: increased heart rate, decreased BP, increased CVP, decreased UOP and distant heart sounds.
- Monitor core body temperature and keep temperature above 96.8°F (36°C).
- Assess pain level.
- Administer medications as ordered.
- Note Endotracheal tube placement and ventilator settings.
- Provide emotional support to client and family.
- Evaluate respiratory status.
- Assess incisions for presence of infection and drainage.
- Assess for S&S of complications.

Client teaching for self-care

- Schedule rest periods to prevent fatigue.
- Resume usual activities gradually.

- Report S&S of CHF including weight gain, increased pulse rate, and difficulty breathing.
- Know follow-up routine.
- Know wound care.
- Understand that procedure is palliative.
- Follow low-fat cardiac diet.
- Adhere to medical regime.

PERICARDIOSTOMY

- Surgical construction of an opening into the pericardium

Use: For pericardiocentesis (procedure to remove fluid from the pericardial sac) and pericardial decompression (cardiac tamponade)

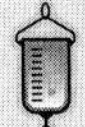

Clinical Alert

Cardiac tamponade is a life-threatening event and requires emergency treatment.

Preparation: Gather supplies: pericardiocentesis tray, ECG machine and patches, emergency cart and defibrillator; provide client support; be sure permit is signed.

Postprocedure: Monitor client; send samples to laboratory; record amount of fluid removed; if chest tube was inserted during procedure, assure the patency of the tube and system.

Nursing Process Elements

- Monitor hemodynamic measures.
- Assess cardiac monitoring.
- Assess for S&S of cardiac tamponade: increased heart rate, decreased BP, increased CVP, decreased UOP, and distant heart sounds.
- Assess pain level.
- Administer medications as ordered.
- Provide emotional support to client and family.
- Evaluate respiratory status.
- Assess incisions for presence of infection and drainage.
- Assess for S&S of complications.

Client teaching for self-care

- Resume usual activities gradually.
- Report S&S of complications or recurring symptoms.
- Know follow-up routine.
- Know wound care.
- Adhere to medical regime.

MINIMALLY INVASIVE DIRECT CORONARY ARTERY BYPASS GRAFT (MICAB)

- MICAB is an alternative to traditional CABG.
- A small anterior thoracotomy incision is used.
- It does not require cardiopulmonary bypass.
- A chest wall artery is grafted to the affected heart area while the heart continues to beat

Uses: For low risk clients who have a single anterior lesion and for high risk clients who are not candidates for conventional bypass surgery.

Preparation: Usual preoperative care for client undergoing heart surgery including physical, emotional and psychosocial assessment; preoperative teaching of client and family concerning postoperative care and close monitoring of the client's condition.

Postoperative course: Client will be admitted to PACU for recovery from anesthesia and then to a telemetry unit for 1–3 days.

Nursing Process Elements

- Monitor hemodynamic measures.
- Assess cardiac monitoring.
- Assess pain level.
- Administer medications as ordered.
- Evaluate respiratory status (especially if the lung was collapsed for the surgery in which case may have a chest tube in place).
- Assess incisions for presence of infection and drainage.
- Assess for S&S of complications.

Client teaching for self-care

- Schedule rest periods to prevent fatigue.
- Resume usual activities gradually.
- Report S&S of angina.
- Know follow-up routine.
- Know wound care.
- Understand that procedure is palliative.
- Follow low-fat cardiac diet.
- Adhere to medical regime.

CORONARY ARTERY BYPASS GRAFT (CABG) AND OFF PUMP CORONARY ARTERY BYPASS (OPCAB)

- A blood vessel from another part of the body is used to bypass the obstructed coronary artery. Attachment is made from the aorta or if using the internal mammary artery, the proximal end remains attached to the subclavian artery, and the other end of the vessel is attached to the distal portion of the obstructed coronary artery thus, providing revascularization of the heart.
- CABG is performed on a stopped heart and requires the use of extracorporeal circulation by the cardiopulmonary bypass pump.
- OPCAB is similar to conventional CABG but cardiopulmonary bypass pump is not used; a median sternotomy approach is used.

Uses: For clients with severe CAD, clients with blockages greater than 70% of two or three coronary arteries, left main coronary artery lesions greater than 60%, unstable angina, angina which cannot be controlled by medical therapy or when complications have developed from percutaneous coronary intervention (PCI).

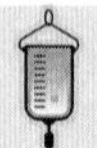

Clinical Alert

When using cardiopulmonary bypass pump, the client receives Heparin to prevent thrombus formation and hypothermia is maintained to decrease the body's metabolic needs.

Preparation: Usual preoperative care for client undergoing open heart surgery including physical, emotional, and psychosocial assessment; provide emotional support; client education concerning the anatomy and physiology of the heart and the surgical procedure, postoperative procedures and equipment including hemodynamic monitoring equipment, ventilator, endotracheal tube, pacing wires, chest tubes, and nasogastric tube, ICU policies and visiting hours, possible complications and treatments, pain management, and sensory stimuli and sensory overload.

Postoperative course: As for clients undergoing open heart surgery, client will be in an intensive care unit for 1–2 days and will be discharged home after a total hospital stay of 5–7 days.

Nursing Process Elements

- Monitor hemodynamic measures.
- Assess cardiac monitoring.
- Assess peripheral pulses.
- Assess bowel sounds and measure abdominal girth every 8 hours.
- Measure and record I&O hourly including chest tube and NG drainage.
- Monitor laboratory values especially Hct and Hgb, ABGs, CBC, APPT, and electrolytes.
- Keep temporary pacemaker at bedside.
- Monitor core body temperature and keep temperature above 96.8°F (36°C).
- Assess pain level.
- Administer medications as ordered.
- Note ETT placement and ventilator settings.
- Provide emotional support to client and family.
- Evaluate respiratory status.
- Assess incisions for presence of infection and drainage.
- Turn and have client deep breathe.
- Assess for S&S of complications including thrombophlebitis, pulmonary embolism, CHF, and cardiac tamponade.

Client teaching for self-care

- Schedule rest periods to prevent fatigue.
- Resume usual activities gradually.
- Report S&S of CHF including weight gain, increased pulse rate, and difficulty breathing.
- Know follow-up routine.
- Know wound care.
- Understand that procedure is palliative: risk factor modification.
- Follow low-fat cardiac diet.
- Adhere to medical regime.
- Can resume sexual intercourse in 3–4 weeks.
- Avoid heavy lifting and excessive arm movements for 6–8 weeks.
- No driving for 6–8 weeks.

PERCUTANEOUS TRANSLUMINAL CORONARY ANGIOPLASTY (PTCA)

- Alternative to CABG for some clients.
- Insertion of a balloon-tipped catheter to dilate a stenotic artery and revascularize the myocardium.
- Performed in the cardiac catheterization laboratory.

Uses: For clients who have CAD in one or more vessels, have recurrent chest pain unresponsive to medical interventions, poor surgical candidates.

Preparation: Similar to client undergoing cardiac catheterization. Preoperative teaching concerning the procedure and recovery; NPO for several hours prior to procedure; client will be awake during the procedure and may be asked to take deep breaths, cough, describe pain, etc; anticoagulants, antiplatelets, and/or vasodilators may be given preprocedure.

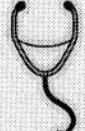

Assessment Alert

Ask client if he/she is allergic to dye or shellfish because contrast may be given during the procedure.

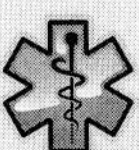

Nursing Intervention Alert

Warn clients that they may feel warm, flushed, or get a metallic taste when contrast is injected and they may feel intense chest pain when balloon is inflated.

Postoperative course: Sheath will be removed in 2–4 hours and client will be discharged 6–8 hours later.

Nursing Process Elements

- Observe catheter insertion site for bleeding, hematoma, and pseudoaneurysm.
- Check peripheral pulses for color, pulses, sensation according to hospital protocol.

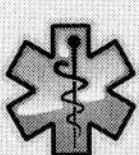

Nursing Intervention Alert

Remember "P's of circulatory checks": pain, paresthesia, paralysis, pulse, pallor, poikilothermia (cold)

- Continuously monitor cardiac rhythm.
- Obtain 12-lead ECG if signs of cardiac ischemia or client complains of chest pain.
- If leg used, maintain client, according to hospital protocol, on complete bed rest with head elevated no higher than 30 degrees and cannulated extremity straight.
- Monitor I&O.

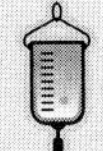

Clinical Alert

Contrast dyes cause osmotic diuresis and can cause renal damage.

- Monitor laboratory values especially electrolytes, BUN, CBC, creatinine, PTT, and cardiac enzymes.
- Observe for signs of decreased cardiac output.
- Assess client for pain and anxiety.
- Medicate as prescribed.
- Have emergency drugs on hand.
- Observe client for S&S of vasovagal reaction when sheath is removed-hypotension, light-headedness, and bradycardia.

Client teaching for self-care

- Schedule rest periods to prevent fatigue.
- Resume usual activities gradually.
- Report S&S of angina, CHF, and vessel reocclusion.
- Know follow-up routine.
- Know puncture site care.
- Understand that procedure is palliative: risk factor modification
- Follow low-fat cardiac diet.
- Adhere to medical regime.

EMBOLECTOMY

- A surgical incision into an artery for the removal of an embolus or thrombi.
- An embolectomy catheter may be inserted to extract the embolus.

Uses: For acute artery occlusion due to thrombi or embolus which may include an accumulation of air, fat, bacteria, amniotic fluid, or other material. Arterial emboli are often associated with MI, atrial fibrillation, left-sided heart failure, pericarditis, or endocarditis.

S&S:

- Pain in affected area
- Paralysis
- Pulselessness
- Pallor
- Paresthesia
- Numbness
- Poikilothermia (cool)

Preparation: Usual preoperative teaching and preparation. Since this is often emergency surgery, the client and family may be quite anxious. Nursing measures should focus on gaining the client's trust and decreasing the client's and family's anxiety. The client is usually on bed rest with the affected extremity kept level of slightly dependent.

Postoperative course: Generally discharged within 1–2 days.

Nursing Process Elements

- Observe incisional site for bleeding, hematoma, and infection
- Check extremities for color, pulses, and sensation according to hospital protocol.
- Maintain fluid volume.
- Monitor laboratory values especially APTT if client is on heparin.
- Assess client for pain and anxiety.
- Medicate as prescribed.
- Discourage activities that decrease circulation to extremities such as knee gatch, crossed legs, and pillow under the knees.
- Keep client warm to increase circulation.

Client teaching for self-care

- Resume usual activities gradually.
- Report S&S of reocclusion or infection.
- Know follow-up routine.
- Know incisional site care.
- Understand risk factor modification.
- Adhere to medical regime.

ENDARTERECTOMY

- Surgical incision is made in an artery and atheromatous material is removed.

Uses: To remove plaque accumulation from an artery.

Preparation: Usual preoperative teaching and care.

Postoperative course: Generally discharged within 1–2 days.

Nursing Process Elements

- Observe incisional site for bleeding, hematoma, and infection.
- Check peripheral pulses for color, pulses, and sensation according to hospital protocol.
- Maintain fluid volume.
- Monitor laboratory values especially APTT if client is on heparin.
- Assess client for pain and anxiety.
- Medicate as prescribed.
- Discourage activities that decrease circulation to extremities such as knee gatch in use, crossed legs, pillow under the knees, and neck not in alignment.
- Keep client warm to increase circulation.

Client teaching for self-care

- Resume usual activities gradually.
- Report S&S of reocclusion or infection.
- Know follow-up routine.
- Know incisional site care.
- Understand risk factor modification.
- Adhere to medical regime.

VASCULAR GRAFTS

- Grafts may be used to reroute the blood flow around an occluded area.
- Grafts may be autologous (using client's own vein) or synthetic.

Uses: Revascularization of occluded vessels

Preparation: Usual preoperative teaching and care

Postoperative course: Generally discharged within 2–3 days.

Nursing Process Elements

- Assessment of graft patency.
- Observe incisional site for bleeding, hematoma, and infection.
- Check extremities for color, pulses, and sensation according to hospital protocol.
- Maintain fluid volume.
- Assess ankle-brachial index (ABI) every 8 hours for first 24 hours then everyday.
- Monitor laboratory values especially APTT if client is on heparin and BUN and creatinine if graft was above renal arteries.
- Assess client for pain and anxiety.
- Medicate as prescribed.
- Discourage activities that decrease circulation to extremities such as knee gatch in use, crossed legs, pillow under the knees, neck not in alignment, and hip flexion.
- Keep client warm to increase circulation.
- Prevent skin breakdown, sheepskin, foot cradle, frequent repositioning.

Client teaching for self-care

- Resume usual activities gradually.
- Report S&S of reocclusion or infection.

- Know follow-up routine.
- Know incisional site care.
- Understand risk factor modification and life style changes.
- Adhere to medical regime.

SPLENECTOMY

- Splenectomy is the removal of the spleen.
- It may be done through an upper left quadrant abdominal incision or by laparoscope.

Use: Control hemorrhage or remove a spleen ruptured by traumatic injury; treatment of idiopathic thrombocytopenia purpura, hemolytic anemia, thrombosis of splenic vessels, portal hypertension, hereditary spherocytosis (splenectomy is only treatment since the fragile blood cells are injured passing through the spleen), or significant splenomegaly associated with leukemia or lymphoma.

Preparation: If performed as an elective procedure,
- client is vaccinated against pneumococcal pneumonia and meningitis about a month before surgery;
- any infection is treated; and
- attempts are made to return blood parameters to normal.

Postoperative course:
- If performed as an emergency procedure, vaccines are given postoperatively.
- PEDS Children receive long-term antibiotic therapy as prophylaxis against sepsis.
- Healing complete in 4–6 weeks.

Complications:
- Postsplenectomy syndrome characterized by elevated platelet count with risk of thrombosis, erythrocyte destruction, and increased susceptibility to infection
- Pancreatitis

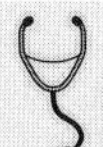

Assessment Alert

PEDS Children have the greatest risk of postsplenectomy sepsis. Older adults also have increased risk of both infection and thrombosis.

Nursing Process Elements

- Assess for pain in the left shoulder, which can be an indication of hemorrhage due to stimulation of the phrenic nerve as a result of pressure from the accumulation of blood in the operative area, which is just beneath the diaphragm.

Client teaching for self-care

- See health care provider if any signs or type of infection occur; this includes otherwise benign infections such as sinusitis, sore throat, or ear ache.
- Avoid travel to areas with endemic infections such as malaria.
- Get booster of pneumococcal vaccine in 5–10 years.

RESPIRATORY SURGERY

TONSILLECTOMY

Tonsillectomy is the removal of the palatine tonsils; bleeding areas are cauterized and sutured; it can be combined with an adenoidectomy—removal of the adenoids; most common surgery for children

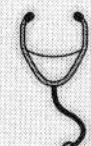

Assessment Alert

Contraindicated with bleeding disorders, presence of acute infections at time of surgery, systemic diseases that are not under control as diabetes, cardiac or renal disease.

Use: Tonsillectomy treats recurrent tonsillitis, peritonsillar abscess, hypertrophy of tonsils causing swallowing difficulty, difficult breathing; adenoidectomy relieves persistent otitis media, breathing and swallowing difficulty, sleep apnea, and speech distortion.

Preparation: NPO, IV, check temperature; child needs to be without a fever and without a sore throat; no respiratory infection for about 2 weeks before surgery; no aspirin or ibuprofen for 2 weeks before surgery; assess for loose teeth; ask if child has been given herbal medication.

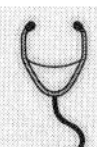

Assessment Alert

Check for bleeding tendencies in child and family.

Postoperative course:

- Monitor VS frequently, also for airway obstruction, and respiratory distress.
- Check for signs of hemorrhage: increased pulse, low BP, restlessness, and frequent swallowing.
- Begin diet with ice chips and, flavored ice pops but nothing brown or red which may cause emesis to look like old or new blood.
- Low-grade fever and earache are common postoperative symptoms.

Nursing Process Elements

- Assess for complications as hemorrhage, injury to upper airway, and aspiration pneumonia.
- Place on side or abdomen until completely awake.
- Administer acetaminophen and apply ice collar to neck for pain relief.
- Encourage fluids.
- Discourage coughing and clearing throat.
- Encourage to chew gum, to relieve muscle spasms around the throat.

Client teaching for self-care

- Encourage rest and quiet activities.
- Include soft foods, cool liquids and nothing irritating in diet.
- Teach to take analgesics and antibiotics as ordered; do not take aspirin
- Report any signs of bleeding.
- Report an elevated temperature more than 102°F or 38.8°C to the surgeon

LARYNGECTOMY

Removal of all or part of the larynx.

- Partial laryngectomy involves removal of a section of the larynx, a vocal cord and tumor; airway remains intact; there is no difficulty in swallowing but the voice quality is changed.
- Hemilaryngectomy is the removal of one half the larynx and a portion of the vocal chord along with the tumor; airway and swallowing remain intact but the voice may be hoarse with limited projection.
- Supraglottic laryngectomy involves removal of the hyoid bone, glottis, and false vocal cords.
- Total laryngectomy involves the removal of the larynx, epiglottis, thyroid cartilage, three tracheal rings, hyoid bone, and vocal chords; speech is lost, and a permanent tracheostomy is created, which may be in place permanently or removed leaving a natural stoma.

Use: Treatment of cancer of the larynx

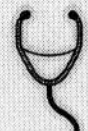

Assessment Alert

An advantage of the supraglottic is that the vocal chords are intact and the voice is preserved, although the voice quality may change.

Preparation: Encourage discussion with the client and significant others about their fears and anxiety related to surgery. Review procedures to expect after surgery such as IV fluids, suctioning, humidification, NG tubes feedings, and a laryngectomy tube. Additional treatment may include chemotherapy and radiation. Reinforce teaching about loss of normal speech and breathing through a hole in the neck. Plan for immediate postoperative communication using a pad and pencil or pictures. Arrange a meeting with a speech pathologist about changes in means of communication with use of esophageal speech, external voice boxes, or an artificial larynx.

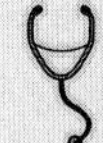

Assessment Alert

If metastasis to cervical lymph nodes is detected, a radical neck dissection may be performed.

Postoperative course:

- Monitor for respiratory complications, check rate, effort, and ABG values.
- Elevate head of bed 30–40 degrees, this promotes ventilation and decreases edema.
- Support client's feelings and encourage discussion about loss of voice and altered body image.
- Need to assess wound for bleeding, edema, infection, and poor wound healing.
- Cleanse incision with one-half strength hydrogen peroxide.
- Promote adequate pain relief.
- Maintain sterile technique during tracheostomy care and suctioning; suction as needed.
- Introduce speech rehabilitation.

Nursing Process Elements

- Refer to a laryngectomy support group; arrange a visit by a postlaryngectomy client.
- Teach need to report symptoms that require special medical attention.
- Encourage to follow speech therapist's recommendations.
- Give information about devices used to produce speech, this information may be obtained from the American

Cancer Society or the International Association of Laryngectomies.
- Maintain adequate intake as IV fluids; provide nutrition by NG feeding; and initiate oral intake of soft foods.

Client teaching for self-care

- Self care of tracheostomy or stoma; offer guidance and opportunities to practice.
- Protect site with a shield during a shower.
- Use a special device for swimming to prevent drowning.
- Use a humidifier to add humidity to the air to maintain moist mucous membranes and secretions.
- Purchase an ID alert bracelet, chain, or card.

PNEUMONECTOMY

- Pneumonectomy involves removal of an entire lung usually through a posterolateral incision.
- It is done only when disease involves entire lung.

Use: Treatment of lung cancer, lung abscess, bronchiectasis, extensive unilateral tuberculosis

Preparation:

- Chest X-rays, lung scan, and EKG to determine cardiorespiratory status and ability to tolerate the surgery
- Pulmonary function tests to determine if lung tissue that will remain after surgery is adequate to support client and ADLs.
- ABGs to provide another measure of pulmonary reserve and a baseline for postoperative assessment
- Exercise tolerance test
- Clients who smoke are encouraged to stop or cut down to improve oxygen saturation and reduce secretions
- Any existing infection treated with antibiotics
- Postural drainage to remove secretions if needed

Postoperative course:

- No chest tube inserted for pneumonectomy: diaphragm is paralyzed in an elevated position and remaining space is left to fill with serosanguineous fluid, which ultimately solidifies.
- Severe shoulder and chest pain causes guarding, which predisposes to hypoventilation and atelectasis is expected and must be treated.
- Pain control may be aided by long-acting local anesthetic nerve block at end of surgery.
- Breathing exercises and passive shoulder range of motion begun immediately after recovery from anesthesia.
- Oxygen for 24 hours.
- Temperature is maintained between 98°F and 102°F because hypothermia or hyperthermia causes change in metabolism and respiratory demand.

Think Smart/Test Smart

Every implication of every fact cannot be identified in a text. Therefore, it is important as you review to think about not just what the fact is but what does it mean for the nurse in practice. It is also important to think about how questions can be asked about the practice implications of the fact. For example, if temperature needs to be maintained within certain range then temperature must be monitored at regular intervals to determine if it is within the desired range. If it is outside the range, then an action must be taken to return it to within the acceptable range. If a corrective action is an independent nursing intervention such as applying blankets for hypothermia or if it is a dependent action such as giving an antipyretic for hyperthermia but an order is already written for it, then the nurse implements the action and evaluates its effectiveness. If there is no order for a dependent intervention or if an independent intervention is not effective, the nurse must notify the physician. Thus, questions that could be asked based on the knowledge that temperature affects demand on the respiratory system and, therefore, needs to be maintained between 98°F and 102°F include how often temperature needs to be monitored following a pneumonectomy; for what reasons is it important to monitor temperature; what is the appropriate action for the nurse to take if the client's temperature is either lower or higher than the specified range; and which situation/finding requires that the physician be notified.

- Dangled evening of surgery; ambulated next day.
- Oral fluids begun when alert and bowel sounds are present.

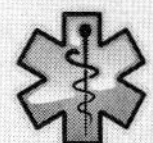

Nursing Intervention Alert

Rate of IV infusion may be as low as 10 ml/hr because of risk of pulmonary edema as a result of a decrease in the pulmonary vascular bed.

- Scant serous/serosanguineous drainage is normal.
- Weakness and easy fatigue expected for 3–4 weeks.
- Altered sensation, numbness, or tenderness may persist for months in area around incision.

Complications:

- Atelectasis most often due to retained bronchial secretions
- Pneumonia
- Hemorrhage
- Cardiac dysrhythmia
- Pulmonary edema due to overinfusion of fluids and loss of pulmonary vascular bed
- Empyema:
  —pus in the pleural cavity
  —S&S: pleuritic pain, fever, dullness to percussion over affected area
  —Rx: chest drainage and antibiotics
- Bronchopleural fistula
  —Abnormal opening between a bronchus and a pleural space
  —S&S: hemoptysis, fever, subcutaneous emphysema, and severe air leak
  —Occurs in first postoperative week
  —Rx: surgery to reclose bronchial stump
- Persistent air leak
  —Openings in lung tissue fail to close within 72 hours after surgery
  —S&S: bubbling in water seal compartment of chest drainage system
  —Rx: injection of a sclerosing agent into pleural cavity or surgery
- Subcutaneous emphysema
  —Presence of air under the skin as a result of escape from the respiratory tract from a persistent air leak or a blocked chest tube
  —S&S: Puffiness and crepitation (crackling sound) on palpation
- Respiratory failure
- Hypotension
- Mediastinal shift
  —Movement of the mediastinum including the heart, trachea, esophagus and great vessels to one side of the thorax

Nursing Process Elements

- Assess respiratory status. Monitor for slow, rapid, shallow, or irregular respirations; use of accessory muscles; duskiness or cyanosis; restlessness, irritability, confusion, somnolence, decreased or absent breath sounds over remaining lung tissue, and changes in ABGs.
- Assess cardiovascular status.

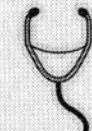

Assessment Alert

After pneumonectomy, clients are at particular risk for:

- dysrhythmias especially atrial fibrillation and atrial flutter
- pulmonary edema—severe dyspnea, tachycardia, dull percussion note over unoperated areas, adventitious breath sounds, persistent cough with frothy, blood tinged sputum, cyanosis, and apprehension.
- mediastinal shift—severe dyspnea, restlessness, agitation, rapid or irregular pulse, cyanosis, displacement of the trachea from the midline, and change in location of point of maximum impulse (PMI).

  —Monitor fluid and electrolyte status: CVP below the normal range of 5–12 cm of water is indicative of hypovolemia and above the normal range of hypervolemia.
- Position client on back or with unoperated side up to aid maximal expansion of remaining lung.
- Turn every 2 hours to reduce pooling of secretions in a dependent area of the remaining lung.
- Encourage client to splint incision and to cough and deep breathe every 1–2 hours to prevent atelectasis: Use palm of hands or a pillow or folded sheet or towel as a splint; sit client upright or on side with hip and knees flexed; direct client to take 2–3 short breaths and then a deep one; contract the abdominal muscles; and cough forcefully with the mouth open.
- Assess breath sounds before and after coughing and deep breathing.
- Encourage huffing if client is unable to cough: take a deep breath and exhale forcefully in a rapid huff.

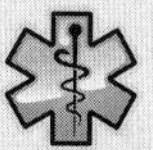

Nursing Intervention Alert

Postural drainage, percussion, and vibration may be ordered to aid removal of copious secretions. Never percuss or vibrate over operative site.

- Space nursing care activities to allow rest periods.
- Support affected arm on pillows or with a sling to decrease pull on transected muscles.
- Put affected shoulder through passive range of motion at least two times every 4 hours for the first 24 hours postoperatively; then guide in active ROM 10–20 times every 2 hours.

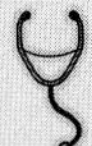

Assessment Alert

Report immediately if sputum is excessive or contains bright red blood.

Client teaching for self-care

- Continue breathing exercises at home as directed, usually about 3 weeks.
- Continue arm and shoulder exercises (10–20 of each) five times per day.
- Use a mirror to check if posture is erect: if the affected side is being favored, practise standing straight with shoulders even in front of the mirror.
- Apply hot soaks or a heating pad for chest or shoulder soreness, which is expected for several weeks.
- Avoid lifting more than 20 lb for 3 months when muscles of chest will be completely healed.
- Stop any activity that causes dyspnea, chest pain, or excessive fatigue.
- Avoid exposure to respiratory irritants and to persons with respiratory infections.
- Obtain influenza and pneumonia vaccine.
- Report signs of respiratory infection (fever, cough, and increased sputum), shortness of breath, decreased mobility, or increased discomfort in chest or shoulder.

LOBECTOMY

- Removal of a lobe of the lung
- May be done by open thoracotomy or by thoroscopic surgery.
- Chest tubes used to drain air and fluid from chest cavity and allow reexpansion of remaining lobes. When two chest tubes are placed, the upper tube drains air and the lower one drains fluid.

Use: Manage disease such as lung cancer or bronchiectasis limited to a single lobe of the lung.

Preparation and postoperative course:

- Similar to pneumonectomy if an open thoracotomy is done.
- After thoracoscopic lobectomy:
  —Pain is slight and managed with an analgesic such as acetaminophen.
  —Clients ambulate on the day of surgery and resume normal activity thereafter.
  —Shower as soon as chest tube(s) is/are removed.

Nursing Process Elements

- Monitor chest drainage every 15 minutes and then at progressively longer intervals.
- Maintain drainage system below level of client's chest; keep free of leaks, dependent loops, and external pressure.
- Place rolled towel under chest tube when client is lying on affected side to keep body weight from compressing it.

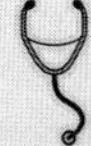

Assessment Alert

Report persistent chest drainage of more than 200 ml/hr.

Care is otherwise similar to that of postpneumonectomy.

Client teaching for self-care

- After open lobectomy, teaching is the same as after pneumonectomy. See above.
- After thorascopic lobectomy:
  —Continue to cough and deep breathe while awake.
  —Exercise arm on affected side by lifting arm up over the head and doing arm circles.
  —Wash incisions daily; shower at will.
  —Avoid heavy lifting for a month.
  —Report any shortness of breath, temperature over 101°F, incisional swelling, redness, or drainage.

NEUROLOGICAL SURGERY

INTRACRANIAL SURGERY

- Supratentorial: surgery performed on the cerebral hemispheres
- Infratentorial: surgery performed on the brain stem or cerebellar region below the cortex

STEREOTACTIC SURGERY

- Refers to targeting the operative area of the brain by using three-dimensional coordinates determined by CT or MRI.
- Preciseness of approach limits damage to healthy brain tissue
- Used for biopsy, removal of an area of tissue by dissection, or destruction of tissue by radiosurgery.
- It is done under local or general anesthesia.
- Craniotomy is done to allow entry of instruments: probe, biopsy needles etc.

CRANIOTOMY

- Location depends on area of brain that needs to be reached: frontal, parietal, occipital, temporal, or a combination.
- Burr holes are drilled; bone between holes is sawed to create a flap that is removed and then wired or sutured back in place when the surgical procedure is completed.
- Drains may be placed to remove blood and fluid.

Uses: Access the brain and meninges for removal of tumors, management of bleeding or vascular defects, treatment of infection/ abscesses, repair damage from trauma

Preparation:
- Routine preoperative preparation
- Include in teaching:
  —Head will be shaved when under anesthesia; hair will grow back at about ¾ in./mo; wigs, hats, and turbans can be used.
  —Client will be on positioning restriction postoperatively (see under "Nursing Process Elements")

Postoperative course:
- ICU until stable: Usually 24–48 hours because this is the time frame in which maximal swelling of the operative area occurs
- Dressing in place 3–5 days (when no dressing, OR cap is used to cover area)
- Protocols for incision care vary: Scalp may be washed with antiseptic soap once dressing is removed; incision may be cleansed with antiseptic and an antibiotic ointment applied; or no special treatment is ordered unless signs of infection develop.
- By time of discharge, client can usually shampoo with a mild soap and blow dry on a warm to cool setting
- Without complications and depending on reason for and type of surgery, discharge may be in as few as 2–3 days
- Rehabilitation may be needed for residual deficits: Help with mobility and ADLs, communication, and job retraining

Nursing Process Elements

- Obtain a baseline preoperative neurological assessment.
- Postoperative assessment: As for ICP (See Chapter 16).
- Primary goal: Prevent increased ICP.
- Maintain prescribed position:
  —Flat or 10–15 degree head elevation and no neck flexion for posterior fossa incisions.
  —30–45 degree head elevation for anterior or middle fossa incisions.
  —Do not position on operative side if craniectomy (removal of bone flap) was done.
  —Assess dressing for drainage; when dressing removed assess incision: A boggy feeling to the tissue around the incision indicates fluid accumulation.

GAMMA KNIFE SURGERY

- Gamma knife surgery is a type of sterotactic radiosurgery.
- Stereotactic radiosurgery uses ionizing radiation targeted by means of a guiding device through the closed skull to destroy an intracranial lesion.
- Gamma knife usually uses cobalt 60 radiation in either a single high dose or fractionated over several treatments.
- CT or MRI scans done to target area; cerebral angiograms also done if blood vessels are involved such as in repair of an arteriovenous malformation.
- Three dimensional frame attached to client's head using four burr holes and metal pins.
- Procedure done under general anesthesia on children. Teens and others are lightly sedated.
- Helmet with over 200 separate ports for radiation beams is placed over head frame: individual beams are too weak to damage tissue but they converge at the site of the lesion and destroy it.
- Each treatment takes 2–15 minutes.
- Most effective for lesions of 3 cm or less.

Nursing Process Elements

Client teaching for self-care

- Head does not need to be shaved.
- No unusual sounds or sensations are experienced during treatments.
- Staff can see and talk to client and client can talk to staff.
- Helmet is removed when treatment is completed.
- Pin site care: Remove four dressings morning after frame is removed; wash daily with mild soap and water; apply bacitracin ointment if ordered; observe for signs of infection.
- Shampoo day after surgery.
- Have someone stay with you for 24 hours after discharge.
- Do not drive or ingest alcohol for 24 hours after discharge because of the sedation.
- Avoid heavy lifting (>5 lbs) for 24 hours after discharge, then resume normal activity.
- Contact surgeon if seizures, numbness, tingling, paresis, paralysis, loss of coordination, prolonged N&V, change in speech, hearing, taste, smell or vision, temperature over 100.5 for 24 hours, or signs of pin infection occur.

SURGERY OF THE EYE AND EAR

OPHTHALMIC SURGERY

General care considerations:

- Approach from unaffected side decreases risk of startle.
- Provide constant description and reinforcement.
- Test corneal reflexes and PERRLA.

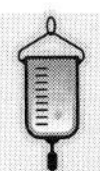

Clinical Alert

Mydriatic and cycloplegic drugs are contraindicated in narrow angle glaucoma.

- Pledgets soaked in a mixture of mydriatic/cycloplegic eye drops (may also add antibiotic and local anesthetic) which stay in the eye 15–20 minutes may be used in place of traditional eye drop preoperative routine which takes an hour
- Dressing depends on procedure: sterile eye pad secured with nonallergic tape; eye shield if protection from external pressure is needed, gauze roller bandage over sterile eye pad if compression needed. May just use collagen corneal shield rather than traditional ointment and dressing.

CATARACT REMOVAL

Use: Restore vision impaired by a clouded or opaque lens (cataract) at the point at which the impairment interferes with daily activities—no longer wait until the cataract is "ripe"

Preparation: Face scrub and instillation of cycloplegic dilating drop in the operative eye

Procedure:

- Extracapsular cataract extraction, most common, usually with phacoemulsification (ultrasonic vibration to break up the lens for removal)
- Local anesthesia
- Intraocular lens implant (IOL) placed behind iris: Restores vision to near 20/20; no loss of depth vision
- Often no dressing needed if a collagen corneal shield is used

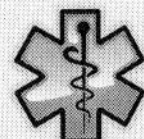

Nursing Intervention Alert

Most clients need glasses for reading after cataract removal because the implanted lens cannot accommodate but an accurate prescription cannot be made until vision stabilizes 8–12 weeks after surgery. Bifocal and multifocal lens implants are available which can eliminate the need for glasses.

Complications: Infection, bleeding, and elevated IOP

Nursing Process Elements

Client teaching for self-care

- Plan for transportation to/from ambulatory surgical site.
- Plan for help at home during first few postoperative days.

- Postoperatively, report promptly drainage, excessive tearing, redness, swelling, decline in visual acuity, or acute, unrelieved eye pain, or severe headache.
- Keep dressing on eye as directed, usually 1–2 days, and wear eye shield at night for 2–3 weeks to avoid accidental trauma to the eye.
- Avoid use of OTC drugs unless first approved by MD.
- Avoid activities that increase IOP.
- Do not do strenuous exercise.
- Sleep on unaffected side.
- Wear dark glasses for photophobia.
- Do not rub or squeeze eyes shut.

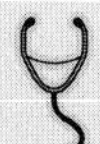

Assessment Alert

Severe, acute unrelieved pain after cataract surgery is typically indicative of increased IOP, which requires immediate intervention to prevent loss of vision.

- Avoid touching eye or getting soap, water, hairspray or other foreign matter in it.
- Resume normal activities as feels comfortable but exercise in moderation and avoid heavy lifting. Resume sexual activity and driving when approved by MD.
- Wash hands before instilling eye medications; wait 2–5 minutes between different medications; use eye ointments last.
- Wear sunglasses to protect against dazzle from bright light or color.
- Note: No limitation on bending is required unless an unusually large incision was necessary.

Glaucoma Surgery

- Goal: Create path for outflow of aqueous humor from the anterior chamber of the eye thereby lowering IOP
- Common Types:
  —Argon laser trabeculoplasty (ALT): Uses laser beam to create a surface burn on the trabecular meshwork thereby increasing its tension and allowing increased outflow of aqueous humor.
  —Trabeculectomy: Typically used when ALT is not successful. Fistula is created at limbus under a thin flap of sclera through which aqueous humor can flow into the subconjunctival spaces.
    - Complications of trabeculectomy: fibrosis at site of flap with increase in IOP
    - Postoperative care: sitting position to have any hyphema in dependent location; use of cycloplegics and combination steroids and antibiotics; monitoring of IOP and condition of bleb

Retinal Reattachment Surgery

Use: Treat retinal detachment

Preparation: If large detachment or macula is threatened, client is encouraged not to make any abrupt, jerky movement that might further the detachment; otherwise normal activities are permitted.

Postoperative course:
- Eye is patched in immediate postoperative period.
- Position face down using pillows and head supports to maintain intraocular gas bubble in place against the repair.
- Avoid coughing, sneezing, and vomiting because of risk of raising IOP. Medicate PRN to prevent.
- Moderate eye pain is expected, treat with analgesics.
- Give cycloplegic ophthalmic drops to rest iris.
- Administer alpha agonist to prevent increase IOP.
- Provide corticosteroid and antibiotic combination eye drop to prevent infection and decrease inflammation.

Nursing Process Elements

Client teaching for self-care
- Use cold compresses to reduce edema.
- Use dim lights and dark glasses to prevent discomfort from light sensitivity.
- Wear eye shield for sleep for 2 weeks.
- Report acute eye pain, increased discharge, or symptoms of retinal detachment.
- Positioning restrictions: lying prone; sitting with face down supported on a table; walking with head down but not bent at waist may be in place from 4 to 30 days if applicable
- Activity restrictions will vary with location and severity of detachment and the corrective procedure used.

EAR SURGERY

Common types of procedures:
- Tympanoplasty: repair or replacement of some or all of the conductive mechanism of the middle ear; various types of prostheses used which may consist of bone, cartilage, or other material.
- Myringoplasty: simple repair of the tympanic membrane; graft used in repair held in place with Gelfoam or similar substance.
- Myringotomy: incision into the tympanic membrane to remove fluid and relieve pressure when antibiotics and

decongestants have not been successful and there is acute infection with bulging of the membrane. Drainage tubes may be inserted which eject themselves with time.

- Mastoidectomy: removal of the mastoid bone to treat infection, remove cholesteatoma or treat other inner ear problems.

Nursing Process Elements

Client teaching for self-care

- Avoid rapid head movements, bending over for 3 weeks.
- Blow nose or cough gently.
- Avoid drinking with a straw. Open mouth if sneezing is unavoidable.
- Avoid vomiting.
- Do not drive for 7 days.
- Avoid swimming or diving for 4 weeks; longer for certain procedures such as insertion of myringotomy tubes.
- Avoid air travel for 1–4 weeks varies with procedure.
- Contact surgeon in event of URI, foul smelling drainage from ear, increased pain in operated ear, fever, bleeding or clear otorrhea or rhinorrhea, and vertigo.

MUSCULOSKELETAL SURGERY

AMPUTATION

Removal of a body part, such as hand or leg, by trauma or surgery

Uses: To control pain or a disease process that is affecting the limb, such as cancer, ischemia, or gangrene

Preparation: Food and fluid restrictions, possible antibiotics

Postoperative course:

- Phantom limb pain that may be represented as an itch, ache or the felling that the limb is moving.
- Most clients are fitted with a prosthesis.

Nursing Process Elements

- Elevate stump on pillow for first 24–28 hours to decrease swelling. Keep joint, such as the knee, straight.
- Wrap stump in 2 in., 3 in., or 4 in. ace wraps to keep surgical dressing in place and reduce swelling. The ace wrap should be removed every 4–6 hours or sooner if the bandage becomes loose. Assess the stump for drainage and note the color, temperature, and most proximal pulse before rewrapping the stump.
- Prevent development of flexion contractures of lower extremity by not placing a pillow under hip or knee of residual limb.
- Support client through grieving process for lost limb.

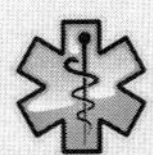

Nursing Intervention Alert

Keep a tourniquet at the bedside and apply immediately if hemorrhage occurs and contact physician.

Client teaching for self-care

- Inspect stump incision daily for redness, swelling, warmth, pain to touch, drainage or an opening in the incision.
- Clean stump daily with mild soap and water, rinse and pat dry. Apply lotion to stump if skin gets too dry.
  —Gentle massage to the stump (residual limb) decreases sensitivity and increases tolerance to pressure in preparation for use of a prosthetic device.
  —Provide information on phantom limb pain and management of pain.

External Fixation

Also known as external fixators

Uses: Manage open fractures with soft tissue damage.

Preparation: Food and fluid restriction

Postoperative course: Remains in place for approximately 6 weeks, though can remain in place for longer periods of time dependent on the type and severity of fracture.

Nursing Process Elements

- Provide pain management.
- Assess for neurovascular impairment every 2–4 hours.
- Assess pin sites for redness, drainage, tenderness, pain, and loosening of pin.
- Perform pin care tid using NS on cotton tip applicator.
- Skin assessment with appropriate skin care.

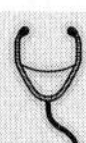

Assessment Alert

Completion of skin risk assessment tool, such as Braden or Norton Scale for clients that are on prolonged bed rest.

Client teaching for self-care

- Take diet adequate in protein, minerals, and vitamins, particularly calcium, zinc, phosphorous, and vitamins C and D.
- Avoid smoking.
- Limit alcohol consumption.
- Maintain optimum body weight or lose weight as is appropriate.
- Maintain mobility as is permitted, including range of motion exercises.
- Learn skin and/or pin care.
- Understand medication use.
- Know about signs of complications, such as infection and neurovascular compromise.
- Use assistive devices, if appropriate.
- Safety measures including fall prevention, if appropriate

Internal Fixation

Uses: Stabilization of fractures using pins, nails, rods, or screw plates.

Preparation: Food and fluid restriction

Postoperative course: Weight bearing limitations

Nursing Process Elements

- Provide pain management.
- Assess for neurovascular impairment.
- Skin assessment with appropriate skin care.

Client teaching for self-care

- Diet adequate in protein, minerals, and vitamins, particularly calcium, zinc, phosphorous, and vitamins C and D.
- Avoid smoking.
- Limit alcohol consumption.
- Maintain optimum body weight or lose weight as is appropriate.
- Maintain mobility as is permitted, including range of motion exercises.
- Learn skin and/or wound care
- Learn medication use
- Report signs of complications, such as infection and neurovascular compromise.
- Use of assistive devices, if appropriate.
- Observe safety measures including fall prevention, if appropriate.

TOTAL JOINT REPLACEMENT (HIP, KNEE)

Uses: Replacement of a joint with a synthetic prosthesis to restore mobility, stability, and relieve pain.

Preparation: NPO after midnight or as ordered by physician, education of client and family regarding expected postoperative regime (possible bed rest for up to 48 hours, range of motion exercises, physical therapy).

Postoperative course: Hip precautions if appropriate.

Nursing Process Elements

- Continuous passive motion (CPM) device for knee replacement
- Turn and reposition every 2 hours while on bed rest
- Hip precautions for hip surgery
- Maintain affected joint in proper body alignment
- Administer analgesics
- Monitor for complications, such as hypovolemic shock, fat emboli (S&S include apprehension, diaphoresis, fever, dyspnea, pulmonary effusion, tachycardia, seizure, decreased level of consciousness, petechia on chest and shoulders), infection, dislocation of hip replacement (S&S will include sudden severe pain, shortening or internal/external rotation of surgical leg)
- Assist client in performing range of motion exercises as appropriate

Client teaching for self-care

- Report S&S of infection
- Report to health care provider a sudden increase in pain (possible dislocation of prosthetic device
- Continue exercise regime to promote function of joint replacement
- Follow limitations described by physician based on surgical procedure
  —Total hip precautions: do not cross legs or adduct operative leg beyond midline of body, avoid flexing hips more than 90 degrees when rising from bed or chair,

avoid turning affected leg inward, use high-seated chairs and raised toilet seat, do not flex hip to put on clothing

—Total knee replacement: avoid bending or lifting, excessive stair climbing, sitting for prolonged periods, overuse of replaced joint

DISKECTOMY/LAMINECTOMY

Uses: Relieve pressure on the spinal cord or nerve roots due to a herniated disc (herniated nucleus pulposus)

Preparation: NPO after midnight or when indicated by physician, baseline assessment of motor function and sensation, demonstrate logrolling

Postoperative course: Cervical discectomy: a cervical collar is worn for approximately 6 weeks. Laminectomy: gradually increase activity over a 6-week period and avoid heavy work for 2–3 months; may need to wear a back brace or corset if pain continues.

Nursing Process Elements

- Bed rest as ordered by the physician
- Maintain head of bed flat for first 24 hours with client in supine position
- Maintain body alignment when in side-lying position with knees flexed to chest and pillow between knees
- Assess neurovascular status
- Logrolling to maintain body alignment
- Administration of analgesics

Client teaching for self-care

- S&S of surgical site infection
- Gradual resumption of activities as directed by physician
- Maintain and use proper body mechanics
- Sleep on firm surface

SPINAL FUSION

Uses: Grafting of bone chips between vertebral spaces to stabilize the spine.

Preparation: NPO after midnight or when indicated by physician, baseline assessment of motor function and sensation.

Postoperative course: Activity restrictions including prolonged sitting, lifting heavy objects, bending over, and climbing long flights of stairs.

Nursing Process Elements

- Bed rest as ordered by the physician
- Maintain head of bed flat for first 24 hours with client in supine position
- Maintain body alignment when in side-lying position with knees flexed to chest and pillow between knees
- Assess neurovascular status
- Logrolling to maintain body alignment
- Administration of analgesics

Client teaching for self-care

- S&S of surgical site infection
- Gradual resumption of activities as directed by physician
- Maintain and use proper body mechanics
- Sleep on firm surface

GASTROINTESTINAL (GI) SURGERY

General considerations:

- Clients having GI surgery are at particular risk for
  —Infection
    - abdominal wall—very susceptible to infection
    - GI tract not sterile
    - risk greater with intestinal as opposed to gastric surgery

  —Wound dehiscence
    - Predisposing factors: stress from breathing, coughing, moving, defecating; nutritional deficits, and postoperative abdominal distention

- Prevention: careful nutritional and F&E assessment and replacement preoperatively; protein and vitamin C for wound healing, NG tube for decompression postoperative.

—Ileus

—Atelectasis

—Urinary retention

Nursing Process Elements

- Monitor for signs of peritoneal irritation caused by leaking of the suture line
- Assess for return of peristalsis: check for bowel sounds, passage of flatus, and feces
- Check for presence of bowel sounds and a soft, nondistended abdomen, which indicate that oral intake can be resumed.
- Teach client to splint abdomen with pillows when coughing,
- When surgery will involve an upper abdominal incision, preoperative respiratory assessment and instruction on coughing and deep-breathing techniques is critical because the location of the incision near the diaphragm tends to limit respiratory excursion. Postoperatively, respiratory status should be checked initially every hour, then at least q 4 hour. Look for shallow or guarded breathing, weak cough, decreased or adventitious breath sounds.
- Injury to the suture line can occur if GI suction is not functioning correctly. Nausea and abdominal distention are signs of malfunction. Measure girth to check for developing distention.
- Fever occurring 4–7 days postoperative suggests a leak at the anastomosis or a wound abscess

GASTRECTOMY

- Total or subtotal: excision of all or part of the stomach
  - —Total: esophagus sutured to duodenum or jejunum
  - —Subtotal: Billroth I/II
    - Billroth I: pyloric portion of stomach is removed; remaining stomach sutured to duodenum (gastroduodenostomy)
    - Billroth II: pyloric portion of the stomach is removed; end of duodenum is sutured closed, and a gastrojejunostomy is done.

Uses: Removal of tumors or chronic ulcers; stop bleeding from a perforated ulcer.

Preparation:

- Fluid diet ×24 hours then NPO after MN before surgery.
- Parenteral nutrition for protein replacement PRN
- Vitamin K and C supplementation PRN

Postoperative course: NPO on IV therapy until BS return and NG tube removed, then clear fluids progressed to six small, bland meals with 120 ml fluid between.

Nursing Process Elements

- Assess preoperative nutritional status: dietary history, weight loss or gain, signs of dehydration, serum electrolyte, and albumin levels
- Assess amount and character of NG tube drainage: expect it to be bloody for 24 hours, then changing to brown-tinged, and then to yellow or clear. Fecal odor indicates regurgitation of large intestine contents into operative area

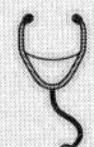

Assessment Alert

NG drainage decreases as peristalsis returns and is less after total than after partial gastrectomy.

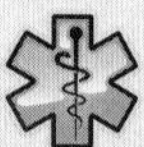

Nursing Intervention Alert

Measure abdominal girth to check for development of abdominal distention; notify surgeon if it occurs.

- Assess for bowel sounds, flatus, and defecation
- Assess tolerance of fluids and foods when oral intake resumed
- Assess for signs of dumping syndrome: N&V and diarrhea
- Do not give fluids with meals to prevent early satiety

Client teaching for self-care

- Decrease S&S of dumping syndrome by
  - —eating six small meals per day of dry foods;
  - —not drinking fluids with meals;
  - —avoiding concentrated carbohydrates;
  - —lying down for 30–60 minutes after eating;
  - —avoiding very hot or very cold foods; and
  - —taking prescribed anticholinergic drugs 30 minutes before meals as prescribed.
- Control postprandial hypoglycemia by
  - —eating frequent meals low in sugar and
  - —ingesting sugar or hard candy when symptoms occur.
- Report persistent fatigue which could indicate iron or B12 deficiency

FUNDOPLICATION

- Fundoplication is an antireflux procedure in which the gastric fundus is wrapped around the LES to stabilize it. It may be done laparoscopically or via open chest or abdomen.

Nursing Process Elements

Prevention of respiratory complications is primary concern.

INTESTINAL RESECTION

Intestinal resection is excision of part of the small or large bowel; with anastomosis, intestine is rejoined and function is normal; without anastomosis, an ostomy is created.

Uses: Removal of neoplasms, areas of obstruction, inflammatory bowel disease, ischemic or traumatic injury or perforated diverticulum.

Preparation:

- Extensive bowel cleansing: Low residue diet followed by liquid diet for 24 hours before surgery so stool does not collect; liquid preparations and/or series of enemas to empty bowel; nonabsorbable antiinfective such as neomycin, kanamycin sulfate, or succinylsulfathiazole to disinfect the bowel.
- Fluid electrolytes, vitamins C and K for wound healing and clotting, and PRN for protein as needed to make up preoperative deficiencies/losses.
- Insertion of NG or intestinal tube to remove secretions and prevent vomiting until peristalsis returns.
- Insertion of an indwelling urinary catheter because urinary retention is common after intestinal surgery, especially if on the colon or rectum.

Postoperative course: IV fluids, PRN, tube for low intermittent suction until bowel sounds return and suture lines begin to heal; when tube removed, clear fluids progressing to regular diet as tolerated.

Nursing Process Elements

- Assess NG or intestinal tube for patency and amount and color of drainage q 4 hours (drainage may be bloody for 24 hours, then turns brown tinged, to yellow or clear and should decrease in 24–48 hours), S&S of fluid imbalance, serum electrolyte values, and I&O
- Measure abdominal girth to check for developing distention
- Semi-Fowler's position to relieve stress on the suture line
- Ambulate and use of rectal tube to promote peristalsis and relieve gas pains

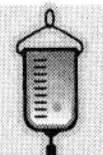

Clinical Alert

Jejunal resection results in malabsorption of fluids, electrolytes, fat, and fat-soluble vitamins (A, D, E, K).

Ileal resection results in malabsorption of fat and vitamin B12.

Resections involving the ileocecal valve frequently result in diarrhea.

Weight loss expected after almost all bowel resections; regained over a period of months.

ILEOSTOMY

- Surgically created opening between the ileum and the abdominal wall.
- Ileum is brought to the surface of the abdomen and formed into a stoma through which fecal material exits the body.
- Abdominal perineal resection: Ileostomy is created and remaining colon, rectum and anus are removed and the anal canal is closed.
- Continent or Kock ileostomy: A reservoir with a nipple to prevent leakage, is constructed from the ileum to hold fecal material until it is drained by the insertion of a catheter through the nipple.

Use: To treat recurrent or advanced inflammatory bowel disease (considered a cure for ulcerative colitis: sometimes used to treat Crohn's disease) and cancer of the colon.

Preparation:

- Emotional support including arranging for a visit with an ostomate if desired
- Referral to an enterostomal specialist for stoma site selection
- Bowel preparation that includes a variety of cathartics, enemas, and intestinal antibiotics; a low-fiber diet several days prior to surgery; a clear fluid diet the day before surgery

Postoperative course:

IV fluids; NPO with NG tube to low suction; frequent stoma care; monitoring of fluid and electrolytes; assessment of bowel sounds; pain management; wound care; progressive diet; and activity.

Nursing Process Elements

- Assess stoma: should be pink or red, moist and protrude 2 cm from the abdominal wall

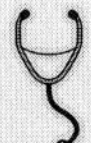

Assessment Alert

A dusky, dark brown, black, or white stoma indicates a lack of circulation.

- Expect stoma drainage to be serosanguineous and contain mucus at first with fecal drainage beginning between days 2 and 4
- Take regular measurements of stoma size and cut the opening of the appliance so that it is no more than one-eighth of an inch bigger than the stoma; size changes as edema subsides starting between days 5 and 7 and reaching final size by week 8
- Empty the pouch when it is one-third full to prevent excessive pulling on the skin
- Record I&O, including output from the stoma
- Assess for fluid and electrolyte imbalances: large amounts of water, sodium, and potassium can be lost in the initial postoperative period in the fecal discharge
- Protect peristomal skin from contact with fecal drainage
- Cleanse skin with warm water and skin cleanser and pat dry
- Apply skin sealants under pouch adhesives and skin barrier paste around the stoma base
- If an abdominoperineal resection, provide care for perineal wound that may be either packed or sutured: may take Sitz baths after packing is removed

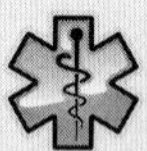

Nursing Intervention Alert

No rectal procedures, including, temperatures are possible with an abdominal perineal resection because the anal canal is closed.

Client teaching for self-care

- How to assess stoma and peristomal skin; empty, change, and apply ostomy appliances
- Encourage adequate fluid and salt intake, especially if perspiring
- Consume foods high in potassium (bananas, melons, oranges, avocados, yogurt, and potatoes) because of potassium loss through ileostomy drainage
- Recognize signs of fluid and electrolyte imbalances:
  —Decreased urine output
  —Excessive thirst
  —Weakness, dizziness, and light-headedness
  —Muscle and abdominal cramps
  —N&V
- Avoid gas-producing foods, as well as foods that may cause blockage such as popcorn, raw fruits, and vegetables with or without skins, nuts, or seeds
- Chew all foods thoroughly
- Avoid eating large meals close to bedtime because food passes through an ileostomy in 4–6 hours
- Recognize signs of obstruction: decreased fecal drainage or crampy abdominal pain
- Use warm shower/tub bath, peristomal massage, knee–chest position, pouch change to treat obstruction; seek medical attention if unrelieved.
- Assist client to achieve a positive self-concept:
  —Encourage verbalizations about stoma
  —Facilitate contact with the local chapter of the United Ostomy Association if not done preoperatively
  —Assure clients they can resume all regular activites

COLOSTOMY

- Surgically created opening between the colon and the wall of the abdomen named for the part of the colon from which they are formed: ascending colostomy, transverse colostomy, descending colostomy or sigmoid colostomy.
- Colon is brought to the surface of the abdomen and formed into a stoma through which fecal material exits the body.
- Consistency of fecal matter varies with location of colostomy: the closer the colostomy to the rectum, the more of the water-absorbing function of the colon is conserved so the less liquid is the fecal matter. With a descending colon colostomy, a bag is sometimes not needed because predictable elimination through the colostomy can be obtained with diet regulation and/or irrigation.
- May be temporary or permanent; if temporary, once the inflammation or trauma to the bowel has been resolved, the ends of the colon are reanastomosed and placed back into the abdominal cavity.
- May be single barreled (one stoma formed from end of bowel proximal to the incision: [fecal matter] exits the GI tract through this stoma because the proximal bowel is the section that remains continuous with the upper GI tract through which food enters) or double barreled (two stomas, one being the end of the proximal section of bowel and one being the end of the distal section of the bowel, which connects to the rectum).
- Due to placement of the colostomy in the large bowel, clients usually do not have the fluid and electrolyte problems associated with ileostomies.

Use: To treat cancer of the colon/rectum; bowel obstruction; bowel inflammation; and intestinal trauma.

Preparation and postoperative course: See "Ileostomy."

Nursing Process Elements

- Stoma and skin care as for ileostomy
- If the colostomy is double barreled, expect the proximal stoma to drain feces and the distal stoma to drain mucus
- Other activities as for ileostomy

Client teaching for self-care

- How to assess stoma and peristomal skin and empty, change, and apply ostomy appliances
- Dietary guidelines
- Dietary adjustments vary from individual to individual and in fact, no alteration may be needed
- To limit gas, avoid gas-forming foods: beans, cabbage, eggs, peas, carbonated drinks, broccoli, cauliflower, dairy products; also avoid gas-producing behaviors: gum chewing, skipping meals, and smoking.
- To improve consistency of stool, avoid foods that loosen stool: fried foods, spicy foods, chocolate, raw fruits, and vegetables.
- To limit odor, avoid foods that increase fecal odor: garlic, onions, eggs, cabbage, asparagus, fish, etc.
- Irrigate the colostomy to achieve regularity if so directed: instillation of water into the colostomy stimulates peristalsis and results in the movement of fecal material.

APPENDECTOMY

Appendectomy is the removal of appendix under either local or general anesthesia; it may be done laparoscopically if uncomplicated.

Use: Usual treatment of appendicitis.

Preparation: Usual preoperative care, prophylactic IV antibiotics, NG tube inserted if ileus suspected

Postoperative course: Fluids when alert progressing to regular diet as tolerated; activity as tolerated as soon as alert; discharge may be same day or in 1–3 days.

Nursing Process Elements

- Place client in Fowler's position when recovered from anesthesia.
- Recognize that client/family may be anxious and need information because of limited preoperative teaching due to emergency nature of the surgery.
- Assess for return of bowel sounds and tolerance of p.o. intake when resumed.
- Assess for S&S of complications.

Client teaching for self-care

- Wash incision with soap and warm water daily; Steri-Strips if present will fall off by themselves.
- Avoid clothing such as bikini underwear that puts pressure on incision.
- Inspect incision daily and report increased redness, swelling, or drainage.
- Resume normal activities gradually over 2–3 weeks and avoid strenuous exercise and heavy lifting.
- Eat small, frequent high-calorie meals and increase as tolerated.
- Report chills, fever, or increased pain.

HERNIORRHAPHY

- Herniorrhaphy is permanent surgical reduction of a hernia sometimes with mesh reinforcement; it may be done laparoscopically; intestinal resection is necessary if herniated intestine is necrotic.
- It is as an emergency procedure in cases of incarceration and strangulation.

Use: Repair hernia to relieve or prevent strangulation.

Complications: Infection, hemorrhage, compromise of the vas deferens.

Nursing Process Elements

- Assess for respiratory infection, chronic cough, or allergies since postoperative coughing and sneezing can disrupt the repair. Surgery may be delayed or antihistamines ordered.
- Urination may be difficult after surgery especially during the first 8 hours after an inguinal repair—measure I&O; observe and palpate suprapubic area for bladder distention; report distention.
- Assess for pain and scrotal swelling that usually last 24–48 hours.
- Discourage coughing but encourage turning and deep breathing.
- Elevate scrotum and apply ice packs when in bed; scrotal support when OOB.
- Instruct to splint incision with hands or pillow if must cough or sneeze; also sneeze with mouth open. Avoid straining at stool to avoid pull on suture line.

Client teaching for self-care

- Report difficulty urinating.

- Resume nonstrenuous activities gradually over 5–7 days.
- Avoid heavy lifting or sexual activity for 6–8 weeks or as specified by surgeon.
- Avoid straining at stool: eat a high-residue diet; drink at least 2000 cc/d of fluid; take stool softeners as ordered.
- Wear scrotal support if ordered.

BARIACTRIC SURGERY

Bariactric surgery is a surgical procedure designed to aid weight loss. It can be done through an open abdominal incision or laparoscopically. Lifestyle changes are necessary in addition to the surgery for weight loss goals to be reached.

Use: To assist with weight loss in clients who have Body Mass Index (BMI) of 40 or greater or BMI of 35 and a serious medical condition related to obesity.

Other desirable characteristics of candidates for bariactric surgery are

- history of obesity for at least 5 years with serious, but unsuccessful attempts to lose weight using other approaches;
- no history of alcohol abuse, depression, or other major emotional disorder; and
- age between 18 and 65 years.

RESTRICTIVE OPERATIONS

- Restrictive operations lead to decrease in the size of the stomach resulting in a sense of fullness after eating less food to limit the amount of food and number of calories consumed.
  —Stomach stapling (vertical banded gastroplasty)
  —Surgical staples and a plastic band are used to make a small pouch at the top of the stomach, which holds only half to one cup of food before an uncomfortable feeling of fullness occurs
  —Gastric banding: Small band around the upper stomach creates a pouch like that in stapling but the band can be inflated or deflated to change the size of the opening between the pouch and the stomach depending on the need of the client

Postoperative course: Studies estimate that about 80% of clients lose some weight and about 30% drop to normal weight; a significant number regain the lost weight in 3–5 years.

Complications: Infection in the incision or peritonitis from a leak of gastric contents into the abdominal cavity; pulmonary embolism; development of gallstones or anemia or osteoporosis from malnutrition. Second surgery may be needed if stomal stenosis causing N&V or esophageal reflux occurs or if staples loosen, or bands slip.

Client teaching for self-care

- Resume normal activities within 3–5 weeks.
- Chew food well and stop eating when you feel full which will be after eating only a cup or less of food.
- N&V or other discomfort will develop if too much food is eaten or it is not chewed well.
- Repeated overeating can stretch the pouch, eliminating any benefit from the surgery.
- Nutritional problems can develop and you may need to take vitamins or other supplements.
- Liquids and foods that contain little or no fiber can pass through the pouch more quickly than meats, fruits, and vegetables so drinking high-calorie liquid such as soda or milk shakes or eating a diet high in highly refined foods can limit weight loss or cause weight to be regained.

GASTRIC BYPASS PROCEDURES

- Gastric bypass procedures involve construction of a gastric pouch to restrict food intake along with a bypass of the lower stomach and upper small intestine so fewer nutrients and, therefore, fewer calories are absorbed.
- This creates a state of malabsorption.

ROUX-EN-Y GASTRIC BYPASS (RGB)

After the stomach is stapled or banded to form a gastric pouch, a Y-shaped section of the small intestine is attached to the pouch to allow food to bypass the duodenum as well as the first portion of the jejunum.

BILIOPANCREATIC DIVERSION

After the stomach is stapled or banded to form a gastric pouch, remainder of the stomach is removed and the pouch is connected directly to the ileum, completely bypassing both the duodenum and jejunum.

Complications:

- Bypass surgery has the same complications as the restrictive procedures but the risk of nutritional deficiency (B12 and iron in particular) is increased, with the greatest risk associated with biliopancreatic bypass.
- May cause "dumping syndrome," with its symptoms of nausea, weakness, sweating, faintness, and, occasionally, diarrhea after eating and the inability to tolerate high-carbohydrate foods.

Nursing Process Elements

Client teaching for self-care

See Restrictive procedures above. Also refer to section on GI surgery.

HEPATIC AND BILIARY TRACT SURGERY

CHOLECYSTECTOMY

Cholecystectomy is the removal of gall bladder; most done laparoscopically, open done if acute inflammation or adhesions are present; T tube is placed into common bile duct if duct is explored.

Use: Treat cholelithiasis and cholecystitis

Preparation: Food and fluid restriction, cleansing enemas, NG tube and urinary catheter before laparoscopic procedures to decompress stomach and bladder and decrease the risk of accidental perforation.

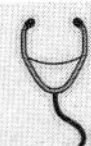

Assessment Alert

Check PT of clients with obstructive jaundice. vitamin K may be needed before surgery.

Postoperative course: Laparoscopic: minimal pain

Open:

- Serosanguinous drainage with small amount of bile expected from Penrose drain in first 24 hours; drain removed in 48 hours
- T-tube drainage of 500 ml in first 24 hours, decreasing to about 200 ml/24 hours for next 3–4 days; initially bloody then green–brown
- Diet progressed as tolerated, dietary fat may be limited temporarily
- Excess bile drainage may be returned to client via NG tube to prevent electrolyte imbalance or synthetic bile salts given

Nursing Process Elements

Laparoscopic cholecystectomy:

- Assess for pain referred to the right shoulder secondary to pressure on the phrenic nerve from carbon dioxide insufflated into the abdomen during the procedure.
- Position in left Sims' for comfort.
- Encourage ambulation to promote CO_2 absorption.

Client teaching for self-care

- Take oral analgesics as prescribed for pain.
- Resume usual activities gradually over 3 days; avoid heavy lifting for 10.
- Report increased redness, swelling, or the appearance of bile-colored drainage at the puncture sites.

Nursing Process Elements

Open cholecystectomy:

- Medicate for pain; Demerol is generally drug of choice; opiates can increase biliary duct spasm.
- Assess respiratory status.
- Coach in deep breathing; because of pain secondary to location of incision near the diaphragm, breathing tends to be shallow.
- Position in semi-Fowler's or on side; turn frequently.
- Splint incision when moving, coughing, or deep breathing.
- Monitor I&O; include T tube drainage in output measurement every shift.
- Monitor for displacement of T tube: bile drainage at tube exit site may indicate displacement.
- Check T-tube patency and amount and character of drainage.
- Maintain closed gravity T-tube drainage system.
- Keep drainage bag below level of T tube.
- Keep tubing free of pressure, tension, and kinks.
- Monitor skin around drain(s) and cleanse often since bile extremely irritating.
- Monitor stool and urine color. Expect light stools while bile is exiting T tube; color darkens as T-tube drainage decreases.
- Assess for signs of peritonitis.

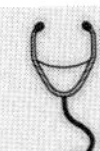

Assessment Alert

A sudden increase in T-tube drainage after it has diminished can indicate an obstruction below the T tube. Report immediately.

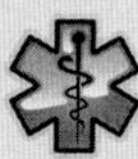

Nursing Intervention Alert

Never irrigate, aspirate, or clamp a T tube; back pressure may disrupt suture line. Exception: T tube may be ordered to be clamped 1 hour ac and pc to check client's tolerance to elimination of external drainage. Immediately unclamp tube and notify surgeon if distress occurs.

Client teaching for self-care

- If discharged with a T tube, instruct in care of tube as stated above with the following additional directions:
  - —Avoid tight-fitting clothing, which can irritate wound and put pressure on tube.
  - —Wear clothing that can be washed in a solution of detergent, bleach and baking soda if bile staining occurs.
  - —Drain the bile bag at the same time each day and record amount of drainage.
  - —Take showers, not baths, to minimize bacterial contamination of the wound.
- Resume normal activities gradually; avoid heavy lifting for at least 6 weeks.
- Report signs of complications: fever, pain, foul drainage, N&V, jaundice, dark urine, and pale stools.

ENDOCRINE SURGERY

HYPOPHYSECTOMY

- Hypophysectomy involves removal of the pituitary gland.
- It is used for treatment of pituitary adenoma.
- It may be total or subtotal.
  - —Total hypophysectomy
    - Used if adenoma has spread outside sella turcica.
    - Performed through a transfrontal craniotomy.
    - Results in panhypopituitarism requiring lifelong hormone replacement due to the absence of ACTH, thyrotropin, and the gonadotropins.
  - —Subtotal hypophysectomy
    - Uses transsphenoidal microsurgery with entry of instruments through an incision in the mouth at the junction of the gum and the upper lip or may be through the nose.
    - Dura mater may be patched with fascia or muscle from leg to prevent leakage of CSF.
    - Nose is packed to absorb drainage and a gauze dressing or sling is placed under the nose.

Complications: Transient diabetes insipidus from damage to the posterior pituitary is most common; also can be ICP, cerebrospinal fluid leak, visual impairment, and other hormonal dysfunction.

Preparation: Antibiotic therapy as prophylaxis against meningitis

Postoperative course:

- Pain similar to a headache occurs and is controlled with low dose narcotics.
- Nasal packing removed in 24 hours.
- Dura mater should seal in 72 hours.
- Prophylactic antibiotic therapy is given.

Nursing Process Elements

- Assess neurological status to detect early signs of increased pressure from cerebral edema: monitor for restlessness, lethargy, confusion, bradycardia, widening pulse pressure, dilated pupils, double or blurred vision, and weakening of lifts and grips.
- Elevate head of bed 30 degrees to reduce cerebral edema.
- Assess for signs of CSF leak: frequent swallowing, complaints of a postnasal drip, or rapid saturation of gauze under nose.
- Test any nasal drainage for glucose: presence of glucose is indicative of CSF because nasal secretions do not contain glucose.
- Coach the client in taking five deep breaths every half hour postoperatively to support ventilation but caution not to cough.
- Medicate promptly for nausea because if vomiting occurs, ICP is raised.
- Measure I&O to detect onset of diabetes insipidus.

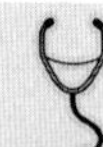

Assessment Alert

If output is more than 100 ml/hr, notify the physician.

- Change pad under nostrils as soon as soiled to eliminate medium for bacterial growth.
- Provide frequent oral hygiene using mouthwash or a foam toothette (no bristles because of risk of mechanical trauma to incision line) to keep the incision line clean.
- Assess changes in S&S related to endocrine function.
- Assess for signs of meningitis such as nuchal rigidity and severe headache.

Client teaching for self-care

Avoid all activities that increase ICP such as bending, sneezing, coughing, or vigorous hair brushing because increased ICP can cause leaking of CSF.

THYROIDECTOMY

- Removal of the thyroid gland; may be total or subtotal
  - —Total thyroidectomy requires lifelong thyroid hormone replacement therapy
  - —Subtotal thyroidectomy: enough gland is left to produce needed thyroid hormone without replacement therapy; in cases of thyroid cancer, lifelong thyroid hormone replacement may be used to suppress thyroid function and decrease risk of recurrence

Use: Treat thyroid cancer, or relieve dyspnea or dysphagia resulting from pressure on the esophagus or trachea from an enlarged thyroid gland.

Preparation: Restore a euthyroid state to the extent possible.

- Antithyroid medications to reduce hormone levels
- Iodine preparations to decrease size and vascularity of the gland thereby reducing the risk of hemorrhage associated with surgery

Postoperative course:

- Temporary hoarseness may occur due to placement of the endotracheal tube or edema; permanent hoarseness can result from injury to the laryngeal nerve
- Humidification provided to facilitate respiration
- Risk of hemorrhage greatest in first 12–24 hours postoperatively
- Tetany may occur 1–7 days after surgery if parathyroid glands were removed inadvertently or injured

Complications: Recurrent laryngeal nerve injury, hemorrhage, transient hypocalcemia, and respiratory obstruction.

Nursing Process Elements

- Monitor for respiratory distress that can occur if edema or bleeding compresses the trachea and blocks airflow; if laryngeal spasm occurs due to hypocalcemic tetany secondary to injury or removal of the parathyroid glands; or vocal cord spasm secondary to laryngeal nerve damage.

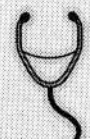

Assessment Alert

Onset of tetany from injury to the parathyroid glands is typically in 24–48 hours.

- Assess for hoarseness, which may simply indicate temporary irritation form intubation or may be the first sign of recurrent laryngeal nerve damage, which can lead to spasm of the vocal cords and respiratory distress.

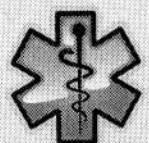

Nursing Intervention Alert

Keep a tracheostomy set, oxygen and suction equipment immediately available to the bedside.

- Monitor pulse and BP for signs of hypovolemic shock.
- Assess for bleeding: check dressing and under the client's neck and shoulders because blood may pool there as a result of gravity.
- Check tightness of dressing: dressing may become too tight as a result of bleeding in the operative area.

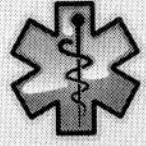

Nursing Intervention Alert

If hemorrhage causes compression of the trachea and respiratory distress, loosen the dressing immediately. If distress is not relieved, notify surgeon immediately as sutures or clips may need to be removed.

- Ask the client to speak out loud and note changes in quality or tone from preoperative assessment.
- Monitor for hypocalcemia and onset of tetany: check serum calcium levels and assess for numbness and tingling in the extremities, muscle twitching, positive Chvostek's and Trousseau's signs.

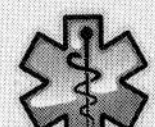

Nursing Intervention Alert

Make certain IV calcium gluconate or calcium chloride is immediately available to the bedside.

- Position in semi-Fowler's with head and neck supported with pillows to reduce strain on suture line.

Client teaching for self-care

- Preoperative teaching: How to decrease strain on the suture line when moving, sitting up in bed, or coughing by placing both hands behind the neck.
- Reassure client that scar will heal to a thin line, which can be covered with a collar, scarf, or piece of jewelry.
- If hypocalcemia has occurred, reinforce need to take oral calcium supplements until parathyroid function has returned.

PARATHYROIDECTOMY

- Parathyroidectomy is the removal of one or more abnormally enlarged parathyroid glands through a 5–6-cm transverse incision in the neck under general anesthesia.
- When multiple glands are removed, some of the excised parathyroid tissue excised is autotransplanted in the client's forearm.

Use: Treatment of primary hyperparathyroidism.

Preparation: Parathyroid hormone levels are determined.

Postoperative course:

- Parathyroid hormone levels are drawn in the operating room to confirm the abnormal glands have been removed
- Presence of an incisional drain is common
- Serum ionized calcium levels decrease to near normal levels 24–48 hours postoperatively
- Transient tetany may occur due to sudden drop in calcium concentration and the rapid absorption of serum calcium by the demineralized bone
- 1–2 days' hospitalization
- If all the glands are removed, high-calcium diet and calcium and vitamin D supplements are prescribed for several months until bone recalcification stabilizes
- Renal damage that occurred prior to surgery may be irreversible
- Bony deformities are permanent
- Complications: airway obstruction, paralysis of vocal cords, temporary or permanent hoarseness due to injury or inflammation of the vocal nerve, or hypocalcemia

Nursing Process Elements

- Monitor serum calcium levels: should drop to near normal in 24–48 hours.
- Assess for symptoms of tetany: tingling and spasms of the extremities. Positive Chvostek's and Trousseau's signs.
- Keep tracheostomy set immediately available at bedside.
- If parathyroid tissue autotransplanted, be certain to check condition of both the cervical incision and the site of transplant.

Client teaching for self-care

- Increase fluid intake before being NPO to decrease risk of renal calculi.
- Dressing changes and care of the incision.
- Inspect the incision daily.
- Report occurrence of any of the following symptoms:
  —Tingling and spasms of the extremities
  —Fever
  —Warmth, redness, or swelling around the incision
  —Drainage
- Resume normal activities after 1–2 weeks of rest

ADRENALECTOMY

- Surgical removal of one or both adrenal glands.
- Performed under general anesthesia using an open incision or laparoscopic approach.

Use: Cancer of the adrenal; benign tumors such as aldosterone-secreting adenoma and pheochromocytoma or idiopathic hyperplasia, which excrete hormones causing severe Cushing's syndrome. Also an option for pituitary-dependent Cushing's syndrome (Cushing's disease) when transsphenoidal hypophysectomy is contraindicated.

Postoperative course:

- Continuous hemodynamic monitoring (CVP, BP, P, and sometimes pulmonary capillary wedge pressure) to guide maintenance of fluid and electrolyte balance
- Fluids usually include saline–dextrose solutions
- IV cortisol replacement for 24–48 hours
- On postoperative day 2, mineralocorticoid replacement is begun
- Lifelong glucocorticoid and mineralocorticoid replacement is required after bilateral adrenalectomy
- After unilateral adrenalectomy, temporary physiologic cortisol replacement may be needed because of suppression of the normal ACTH-adrenal axis. Cortisol doses are gradually tapered off but replacement may be needed for 6 months to 2 years
- 4–5-days' hospitalization with an open adrenalectomy and 2–3 days with a laparoscopic adrenalectomy
- Generally, no restrictions after a laparoscopic adrenalectomy

Complications: Adrenal crisis, hypo or hypertension, high or low blood glucose, fluid and electrolyte imbalance.

Nursing Process Elements

- Maintain invasive hemodynamic monitoring.
- Monitor serum electrolytes daily.
- Monitor blood glucose every 4 hours.
- Keep hourly I&O record.
- Weigh client daily.
- Assess for signs that glucocorticoid dosage need to be increased: marked weakness, anorexia, N&V
- Maintain strict aseptic technique during wound care and avoid exposure to sources of contagion because infection is a significant risk due to excess cortisol.
- Alternate care activities with rest periods because the client may have significant activity intolerance.
- Protect from effects of orthostatic hypotension: change position slowly, assist with ambulation, and apply elastic stockings.
- Assist with ambulation until BP stabilizes.

Client teaching for self-care

- Protocol for prescribed hormone replacement therapy.
- Keep bandages clean and dry.
- After laparoscopic adrenalectomy, return to normal activities such as showering, driving, walking up stairs, light lifting, and work as soon as you feel comfortable.
- Avoid heavy lifting or straining for 6–8 weeks after open surgery.
- Do not drive if taking narcotic medications for pain.
- Notify the surgeon if any of the following symptoms occur.
- Fever.
- Worsening pain.
- Redness, swelling, or warmth to the touch around the incision.
- Drainage from the incision.
- Follow dietary guidelines that often include restriction of calories, sodium, lipids, and cholesterol.
- Keep follow-up appointment 2 weeks after the procedure.

URINARY SURGERY

NEPHRECTOMY

Nephrectomy is the removal of kidney either laparoscopically through three small incisions in the abdomen and flank, or open (radical) through a larger transabdominal, flank, or extraperitoneal incision. Radical nephrectomy, performed to prevent metastasis, includes removal of the kidney, adrenal gland, proximal ureter, renal artery and vein, and surrounding fascia.

Use: Remove cancerous or diseased kidney; remove healthy kidney for donation.

Preparation: Informed consent, preoperative laboratory and diagnostic screening, food and fluid restriction, cleansing enema, surgical skin prep.

Postoperative course:

- Serosanguineous drainage expected; JP drain removed when decreased to less than 30 ml/d
- Fluid and electrolytes balanced through IV therapy, and monitoring of I&O, daily weight, hematocrit, hemoglobin, and electrolyte levels
- Incisional pain managed with opioid analgesics
- Diet progressed as tolerated
- Sutures/staples removed when healing by primary intention occurs (~7–10 days)
- Deep breathing, coughing, and incentive spirometry exercises reduce risk for postoperative pneumonia
- Sequential compression devices (SCDs), prophylactic anticoagulation with low molecular weight heparin (LMWH), and early ambulation decrease risk of DVT

Nursing Process Elements

- Assess BP, fluid and electrolyte balances carefully as these functions are controlled in part by the kidney.
- Medicate for pain.
- Assess cardiovascular and respiratory status.
- Coach in deep breathing exercises.
- Assess incision for evidence of wound healing.
- Monitor for S&S of infection.
- Keep JP drain compressed and empty when half full.
- Monitor urinary catheter drainage and perform routine catheter care.
- Teach about home care; refer for support as appropriate.

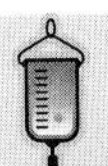

Clinical Alert

If both kidneys removed or remaining kidney functioning is impaired, renal replacement will be necessary with dialysis or kidney transplantation.

Client teaching for self-care

- Take oral analgesics as prescribed for pain.
- Splint incision when moving, coughing, or deep breathing.
- Resume usual activity gradually; avoid strenuous activity for 6 weeks.
- Report incisional redness, swelling, or drainage, unrelieved pain, or temperature ≥101°F.
- Keep appointments for postoperative follow-up.

CYSTECTOMY

Cystectomy is the removal of all (radical) or part (segmental) of the bladder. Transurethral resection may be used for a partial cystectomy. Radical cystectomy requires a large abdominal incision and involves removing the entire bladder, nearby lymph nodes, part of the urethra, and establishing a urinary diversion. In males, radical cystectomy may also include removal of the prostate and seminal vesicles; in females, it may include removal of the anterior vaginal wall, uterus, cervix, fallopian tubes, and ovaries.

Use: Treat cancer that has invaded the bladder wall.

Preparation: Informed consent, preoperative laboratory and diagnostic screening, food and fluid restriction, cleansing enema, surgical skin prep, autologous blood donation.

Postoperative course:

- Fluid and electrolytes balanced through IV therapy, and monitoring of I&O, daily weight, hematocrit, hemoglobin, and electrolyte levels
- Transfusion may be required for significant perioperative blood loss
- Incisional pain managed with opioid analgesics
- Diet progressed as tolerated
- Activity increased gradually
- Serosanguineous drainage expected; JP drain removed when decreased to less than 30 ml/d
- Urine pink initially, but changes to clear by the third postoperative day
- Beefy red and edematous stoma expected; mucous discharge may be present
- Intermittent catheterization required for continent urostomy
- Sutures/staples removed when healing by primary intention occurs (~7–10 days)
- Surgical treatment often complemented with radiation and chemotherapy

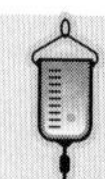

Clinical Alert

In the immediate postoperative period following a partial cystectomy, bladder capacity is usually less than 60 ml. Over several months time, elastic tissue of the bladder regenerates and capacity increases up to 400 ml.

Nursing Process Elements

- Encourage deep breathing exercises and promote early ambulation.
- Monitor patency and output of urinary catheters and surgical drains.
- Monitor for bright red blood on dressings or in urine.
- Administer analgesics to control pain.
- Provide opportunity to grieve and begin to cope with changes in body image and function.
- Assess for potential postoperative complications including infection, fistula formation, bowel obstruction, rectal injury, or sexual dysfunction.
- Arrange home care supplies.
- Refer to enterostomal therapy nurse and ostomy support group if urinary diversion created.

Client teaching for self-care

- Take oral analgesics as prescribed for pain.
- Splint incision when moving, coughing, or deep breathing.
- Resume usual activity gradually; avoid strenuous activity for 6 weeks.
- Report incisional redness, swelling, or drainage, unrelieved pain, temperature ≥101°F, bloody urine, or decreased output.
- Assess stoma and surrounding skin daily.
- Follow instructions for ostomy management.
- Keep appointments for postoperative follow-up.

ILEAL CONDUIT

Ileal conduit is the most common urinary diversion procedure whereby the ureters are excised from the bladder and transplanted into a segment of resected ileum brought through the abdominal wall to the skin surface creating a stoma and allowing the ileal segment to function as a passageway for urine. The intestinal segment of the resection is then anastomosed and GI function returns to normal after healing.

Use: Divert urine postradical cystectomy or irreparable trauma to the bladder.

Preparation: Informed consent, preoperative laboratory and diagnostic screening, food and fluid restriction, bowel prep and intestinal antibiotics, surgical skin prep.

Postoperative course:

- Visualization of stoma, stents, and sutures created by transparent pouch
- Beefy red and edematous stoma expected; mucous discharge may also be present
- Urine pink initially, but changes to clear by the third postoperative day
- Pouch changed within 24–48 hours after surgery to allow greater visualization and assessment of stoma and peristomal skin
- Pouch positioned to drain to the side of the bed and valve opened for continuous drainage
- Pain managed with opioid analgesics
- Diet progressed as tolerated
- Activity increased gradually
- Fluid and electrolytes balanced through IV therapy, and monitoring of I&O, daily weight, hematocrit, hemoglobin, and electrolyte levels

Nursing Process Elements

- Encourage deep breathing exercises and promote early ambulation.
- Monitor patency and output of urinary catheters and surgical drains.
- Monitor for bright red blood on dressings or in urine.
- Restrict food and oral fluids if bowel sounds absent.
- Administer analgesics to control pain.
- Assess for potential complications including breakdown or leakage of the anastomosis, paralytic ileus, mucocutaneous separation, stomal necrosis, retraction, hernia, UTI, and peristomal skin irritation.
- Assist client to master self-care before discharge.
- Refer to enterostomal therapy nurse and ostomy support group.

Client teaching for self-care

- Increase oral fluid intake to 3 l/d.
- Keep urine acidic with cranberry juice and vitamin C.
- Uncover stoma during showering or bathing and pat gently, but do not scrub as tiny capillaries in the highly vascular stoma may cause it to bleed easily.
- Report any noticeable changes in color, texture, contour, or general appearance of stoma and surrounding skin.
- Wash and air-dry peristomal skin daily. Use prescribed cleaners and ointments as directed
- Use mirror to help center faceplate on the stoma.
- Empty bag every 2 hours; leg bags can be used for extra capacity.
- Report flank/back pain, fever, unusually strong smelling urine, dark urine, or reduction in output
- Keep a spare ostomy appliance available at all times in a clean drawer or box.
- Keep appointments for follow-up.

NEPHROSTOMY

Surgically created passageway maintained by a tube, stent, or catheter that perforates the skin, passes through the renal parenchyma, and terminates in the renal pelvis or calyx. The procedure is performed under fluoroscopy, ultrasonographic or CT scan guidance, or open surgery.

Use: Provides urinary drainage when ureter obstructed (renal stones, ureteral tumors, postoperative and radiation strictures, anatomical anomalies), and provides access to upper urinary tract for certain diagnostic or therapeutic procedures such as stone removal, radiography, or chemotherapy.

Preparation: Informed consent, preoperative laboratory and diagnostic screening, food and fluid restriction, surgical skin prep. Often performed as outpatient procedure.

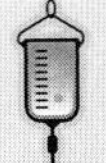

Clinical Alert

Tight control of blood pressure is an essential preparation as uncontrolled hypertension increases the risk for developing perirenal hematoma or hemorrhage.

Postoperative course:

- Postobstructive diuresis can occur
- Urine pink initially, but changes to clear by the second postoperative day
- Asepsis maintained when changing nephrostomy dressing
- Pain managed with opioid analgesics

Nursing Process Elements

- Maintain hydration and voiding schedule.
- Maintain patency and dependent position of nephrostomy tube.
- Monitor patency and output of urinary catheters and perform routine catheter care.
- Strain urine for calculi and send specimen for analysis.
- Administer antibiotics and analgesics as prescribed.
- Assist client to master self-care before discharge.
- Monitor for complications including acute bleeding, pneumothorax, infection, impaired urinary elimination, or return of calculi.

Client teaching for self-care

- Increase oral fluid intake (up to 3 l/d).
- Take medication as directed.
- Strain urine as directed.
- Avoid bathing, swimming, strenuous activity, and sports until nephrostomy tube is removed.
- Keep dressing clean and dry; protect when showering.
- Change dressing daily as directed.
- Rinse external drainage bag and clean once a week with soap and warm water.
- Report redness, tenderness, or drainage at nephrostomy site, fever, urinary frequency or urgency, incontinence, painful or bloody urination, or recurrence of costovertebral pain.
- Keep appointments for follow-up.

URETEROSIGMOIDOSTOMY

In ureterosigmoidostomy, ureters are detached from the bladder and implanted into the sigmoid colon to drain urine, eliminating the need for an outside stoma.

Use: Uncommonly used urinary diversion procedure except in parts of the world where adhesive devices are unavailable or not practical because of tropical heat.

Preparation: Informed consent, preoperative laboratory and diagnostic screening, food and fluid restriction, bowel prep, and surgical skin prep.

Postoperative course:

- Pain managed with opioid analgesics
- Diet progressed as tolerated
- Activity increased gradually
- Fluid and electrolytes balanced through IV therapy, and monitoring of I&O, daily weight, hematocrit, hemoglobin, and electrolyte levels.

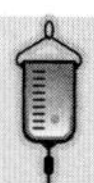

Clinical Alert

Neoplasia occurs at the anastomosis of the ureters and colon in 24% of clients with any urinary diversion that mixes urine and stool at 20 years of follow-up. An annual flexible sigmoidoscopy is recommended starting 10 years after surgery.

Nursing Process Elements

- Assess surgical incision for signs of healing or evidence of infection.
- Administer analgesics for pain as needed.
- Evaluate fluid and electrolyte status frequently.
- Report abnormal blood chemistry results.
- Monitor for potential complications including kidney infections from reflux of feces and biochemical blood changes.

Client teaching for self-care

- Take oral analgesics as prescribed for pain.
- Splint incision when moving, coughing, or deep breathing.
- Resume usual activity gradually; avoid strenuous activity for 6 weeks.
- Report incisional redness, swelling, or drainage, unrelieved pain, temperature ≥101°F, costovertebral pain, significant changes in color, consistency, or amount of output.
- Keep appointments for postoperative follow-up.

CUTANEOUS URETEROSTOMY

In cutaneous ureterostomy, one (single ureterostomy) or both (bilateral ureterostomy) ureters are detached from the bladder and brought to the surface of the abdomen with the formation of a stoma to allow passage of urine. A double-barrel ureterostomy brings both ureters to the same side of the abdominal surface and a transuretero ureterostomy (TUU) brings both ureters through the same stoma.

Use: Urinary diversion postcystectomy or irreparable bladder damage.

Preparation: Informed consent, preoperative laboratory and diagnostic screening, food and fluid restriction, bowel prep, and surgical skin prep.

Postoperative course:

- Visualization of stoma and sutures created by transparent pouch
- Beefy red and edematous stoma expected; mucous discharge may also be present
- Urine pink initially, but changes to clear by the third postoperative day
- Pouch changed within 24–48 hours after surgery to allow greater visualization and assessment of stoma and peristomal skin
- Pouch positioned to drain to the side of the bed and valve opened for continuous drainage
- Pain managed with opioid analgesics
- Diet progressed as tolerated
- Activity increased gradually

- Fluid and electrolytes balanced through IV therapy, and monitoring of I&O, daily weight, hematocrit, hemoglobin, and electrolyte levels

Nursing Process Elements

- Assess surgical incision for signs of healing or evidence of infection.
- Assess color and appearance of the stoma and surrounding skin.
- Assess client and family's response to stoma and readiness to learn about stoma care
- Monitor fluid and electrolyte status.
- Monitor for potential complications including infection and anastomotic leaking.
- Assist client to master self-care before discharge.
- Refer to enterostomal therapy nurse and ostomy support group.

Client teaching for self-care

- Increase oral fluid intake to 3 l/d
- Keep urine acidic with cranberry juice and vitamin C.
- Uncover stoma during showering or bathing and pat gently, but do not scrub as tiny capillaries in the highly vascular stoma may cause it to bleed easily.
- Report any noticeable changes in color, texture, contour, or general appearance of stoma and surrounding skin.
- Wash and air-dry peristomal skin daily. Use prescribed cleaners and ointments as directed
- Use mirror to help center faceplate on the stoma.
- Use bag fitted with antireflux valve to prevent urine backflow.
- Empty bag every 2 hours; leg bags can be used for extra capacity.
- Report flank/back pain, fever, unusually strong smelling urine, dark urine, or reduction in output.
- Keep a spare ostomy appliance available at all times in a clean drawer or box.
- Keep appointments for follow-up.

PROSTATECTOMY

Prostatectomy is the removal of all or part of the prostate gland through a transurethral resection (TURP) or lower abdominal incision (open surgery).

Use: Treatment of Benign Prostatic Hypertrophy (BPH) or prostate cancer.

Preparation: Informed consent, preoperative laboratory and diagnostic screening, food and fluid restriction, cessation of medications that impair clotting, surgical skin prep, preoperative teaching about procedure's effects on urinary elimination, sexual functioning and fertility, and the expected postoperative course.

Postoperative course:

- A 3-way urinary catheter (urethral or suprapubic) and bladder irrigation with sterile normal saline keeps urine pink-tinged
- Urine becomes clear by third postoperative day
- Catheter may be left in place for several weeks following open surgery
- Bladder spasms treated with antispasmodics
- Pain managed with opioid analgesics
- Diet progressed as tolerated
- Activity increased gradually
- Fluid and electrolytes balanced through IV therapy, and monitoring of I&O, daily weight, hematocrit, hemoglobin, and electrolyte levels
- Constipation prevented with stool softener, mild laxatives, and adequate hydration

Nursing Process Elements

- Monitor flow of irrigation solution.
- Monitor fluid and electrolyte status closely.
- Encourage hydration and voiding schedules.
- Monitor for potential complications including blood clots that interfere with urinary drainage, infection, infertility, impotence, and incontinence.
- Provide opportunity to express anxiety and begin to cope with changes in body image and function.
- Assess for S&S of embarrassment with female care provider; if necessary and possible, assign client to male nurse.
- Assist client to master self-care before discharge.
- Refer to support group.

Client teaching for self-care

- Take medication as prescribed.
- Increase oral fluid intake (up to 3 l/d).
- Void at regular intervals.
- Empty and measure urinary catheter every 8 hours.
- Keep drainage bag in dependent position to prevent reflux.
- Wash around catheter insertion site daily with mild soap and water.
- Avoid heavy lifting, climbing, driving, and sexual activity for 3 weeks.
- Avoid alcoholic beverages.

- Avoid antihistamines that increase risk for urinary retention.
- Report fever ≥ 101°F, symptoms of cloudy, foul-smelling, bloody, painful urination, or changes in urine stream.
- Anticipate ejaculate fluid to be projected into the bladder instead of through the penis.
- Keep appointments for follow-up care.

DERMATOLOGIC SURGERY

BIOPSIES

- Shave biopsy: Scalpel is used to shave lesion to depth of mid-dermis.
- Excision biopsy: Entire lesion is removed.
- Curettage: Lesion is scraped off the surface of skin.

  In addition to biopsy, it is used to remove superficial skin lesions such as keratoses and nevi.

  Heal by second intention.
- Punch biopsy: Punch devices removes a circle of tissue containing the lesion down to the level of the subcutaneous tissues
  —Removes deep lesions up to 10 mm in diameter
  —Allows for histological study
  —Requires sutures or healing by secondary intention

Cryosurgery: destruction of tissue takes place by topical application of a freezing substance such as liquid nitrogen.

- Used to remove a variety of benign and malignant lesions
- Depth of tissue destruction depends on degree of freeze
- Tingling pain occurs when freezing substance applied
- Tissue necrosis occurs in first 24 hours after surgery and a bulla forms; serous exudate during first week is followed by crust, which drops off in 3–4 weeks.
- Topical antibiotic applied to prevent infection
- No inflammation or bleeding usually occurs but hypopigmentation may result

Electrosurgery: destruction of tissue occurs with a high-frequency alternating current.

- Electrodessication
  —Superficial skin destruction
  —Used to remove surface lesions such as warts and angiomas
- Electrocoagulation
  —Deep skin destruction
  —Used to remove lesions such as superficial skin cancers other than melanoma and telangiectases
- Delayed bleeding may occur but is easily controlled with direct pressure
- Wound left exposed for air-drying or covered with dressing to protect from trauma

LASER SURGERY

Laser surgery is used to treat many skin lesions including port wine stains and telangiectases.

CHEMICAL DESTRUCTION OR PEELING

- Topical application of a chemical that destroys or peels lesions
- Crust forms overtreated area, sloughs in about a week
- Used to remove benign and premalignant lesions; cosmetic chemical peel done to smooth, firm, and remove wrinkles from skin

Nursing Process Elements

Client teaching for self-care

Skin surgery

- Need for aseptic technique including good hand washing when caring for wound.
- How and when to change dressings if used.
- Keep wound dry; do not remove any crust.
- Protect site from trauma and irritation.
- Cleanse gently as directed with pH neutral mild soap-like agent.
- Apply alcohol to promote drying if directed.
- Whether covering with makeup is permissible.
- Report signs of bleeding or infection (redness, edema, or pain).
- Avoid aspirin and other drugs affecting clotting for 7 days before and after surgery.

REPRODUCTIVE TRACT SURGERY

MASTECTOMY

- Mastectomy is the removal of breast.
- Total (simple) mastectomy: All breast tissue is removed but all or most axillary of the lymph nodes and chest muscles remain intact.
- Modified radical mastectomy: Entire breast, some or most lymph nodes, and sometimes the pectoralis minor chest muscles are removed. Major chest muscles are left intact.
- Radical (Halsted's) mastectomy: Rarely performed removal of the entire breast, skin, major and minor pectoral muscles, axillary lymph nodes, and sometimes internal mammary or supraclavicular lymph nodes.
- Mastectomy may be done with or without breast reconstruction.

Use: Treatment of breast cancer; occasionally prophylaxis for breast cancer in genetically positive women.

Preparation: Psychological: allow time for client to verbalize fears and anxieties; assess support systems and involve significant others as determined by client.

Postoperative course:

- IV fluids, strict I&Os, Foley catheter, elastic compression stockings while on bed rest, drain(s), incentive spirometer, diet progression as tolerated

Nursing Process Elements

- Keep arm on affected side moderately elevated to relieve discomfort, prevent tension on surgical site, and prevent venous congestion.
- Prepare client to look at the incision at the first dressing change by describing the incision.
- Empty drain regularly; recording amount each shift; noting the color and consistency.
- Start limited postoperative arm exercises within 24 hours after surgery.
- Encourage use of the affected arm for activities that do not require that the arm be abducted or raised above shoulder height until the drains are removed.

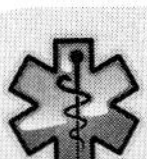

Nursing Intervention Alert

Place a sign on the woman's bed warning that no BP readings, injections, IV lines, or blood sampling should be performed on the arm on the operative side.

Client teaching for self-care

- Begin teaching wound care to client with first dressing change; have client demonstrate care of the drain and wound prior to discharge.
- Explain it is normal to have decreased sensation in the surgical area or to have phantom breast pain.
- Wear loose-fitting clothing.
- Gently massage healed incision with emollients.
- Hold affected arm appropriately—no dangling or swinging; place arm above heart level when sitting/lying down.
- Maintain well-balanced, nutritious meals and adequate fluid intake to promote healing.
- Gradually resume normal activities; schedule alternating rest and activity periods during day, especially when sitting/standing is prolonged.
- Continue exercise program for at least 1 year.
- Protect affected hand and arm from injury and infection: wear long sleeves and gloves when gardening, be cautious sewing and doing dishes, use potholders when handling hot items, avoid lifting or moving heavy objects, and do not carry purse or wear jewelry/wristwatch on affected side.
- Never allow BP to be taken, blood withdrawn, immunizations or medications injected, or IV fluids administered on the affected side.
- Seek medical evaluation for S&S of breast or arm infection: redness, warmth, edema, purulent wound drainage, fever/chills.
- Use positions for sex that avoid pressure on the chest wall; explore alternative forms of sexual expression such as cuddling, touching, and massage.
- Perform regular self-breast exam on unaffected breast; follow recommended schedule for mammography.
- Keep regular medical follow-up appointments.

LUMPECTOMY

- Lumpectomy is the removal of a cancerous mass from the breast along with some normal tissue for clean margins.
- An initial excisional biopsy may be the lumpectomy.
- Reexcision may be needed of the margins that are not clean in the original biopsy.

Use: Treatment of breast cancer.

Nursing Process Elements

- Assess for pain and medicate with mild analgesic as prescribed.
- Assess dressing for bleeding or drainage.
- Prepare client for wound by describing it to her before she views it.

Client teaching for self-care

- Wound care.
- Take oral analgesics as prescribed for pain.
- S&S of infection, hematoma formation, and over the long term, recurrence of breast cancer in the incision.
- Resume usual activities gradually over 3 days; avoid heavy lifting for 10 days.
- Keep follow-up appointment with health care provider for assessment of wound healing and review of pathology reports; discuss further treatment options as necessary.

VULVECTOMY

- Vulvectomy is the removal of abnormal tissue of the vulva, through procedures such as the skinning technique, local wide excision, or a simple or radical vulvectomy.
- *Simple vulvectomy:* removal of the labia majora, labia minora, and sometimes the glans.
- *Radical vulvectomy:* excision of tissue from the anus to a few centimeters below the symphysis pubis (skin, labia majora, labia minora, and clitoris); bilateral dissection of groin lymph.
- Nodes, superficial groin and deep inguinal, femoral, iliac, hypogastric, obturator, may also be done.

Use: Treatment of vulvar carcinoma.

Preparation: Psychosocial support; extensive counseling on what the procedure will entail and what to expect postoperatively; sexual counseling; NPO after midnight the night before procedure; shave of the perineal, pubic, and inguinal areas; vulva cleansing with hexachlorophene or povidone-iodine shower or scrub; enema to evacuate intestinal tract before surgery; Foley catheter insertion on the morning of the procedure

Postoperative course: IV fluids, drains with suction (Hemovac), compression stockings, Foley catheter, low-dose anticoagulant therapy, diet progression as tolerated, and analgesics.

Nursing Process Elements

- Assess for pain and medicate as prescribed.
- Monitor VS.
- Record I&O.
- Maintain low-Fowler's position to promote comfort and reduce tension on sutures.
- Change dressing frequently to keep wound clean and dry.
- Monitor drains and/or tubes for amount and color of drainage.
- Keep compression stockings on while on bed rest.
- Encourage early ambulation.
- Prevent straining with defecation by providing a low-residue diet initially with stool softeners.
- Maintain patency of urinary catheter and administer frequent peri-care.
- Give frequent Sitz baths, including after bowel movements.
- Encourage client to ventilate feelings about sexual mutilation.
- Help client explore alternate methods of sexual intimacy and encourage her to discuss feelings with her partner.
- Encourage sexual counseling.

Client teaching for self-care

- Teach client to do frequent dressing changes.
- Perform frequent peri-care, including Sitz baths, including after bowel movements.
- Maintain patency of Foley catheter that usually remains in place for 7–14 days or until healing is adequate.
- Avoid sitting with the legs dependent, standing, and crossing the legs.
- Keep follow-up visits for additional therapy if needed.
- Seek care/early evaluation of any suspicious lesions, bleeding, or discharge.
- Obtain regular health checkups and screening for cancer and other age-related illness.

HYSTERECTOMY

- Hysterectomy is the removal of the uterus.
- It can be done abdominally or vaginally depending on the underlying disease process.

Use: Treatment of uterine cancer and nonmalignant conditions such as endometriosis, fibroid tumors, pelvic relaxation with uterine prolapse; to control life-threatening bleeding/hemorrhage and in the event of intractable pelvic infection or irreparable rupture of the uterus.

Abdominal hysterectomy types: Subtotal (partial): body of the uterus is removed, cervical stump remains.
Total: removal of the uterus and cervix.

Total with bilateral salpingo-oophorectomy: Removal of the uterus, cervix, fallopian tubes, and ovaries is the treatment of choice for invasive cancer, fibroid tumors that are rapidly growing or produce severe abnormal bleeding, and endometriosis invading other pelvic organs.

Total pelvic exenteration (TPE): Total hysterectomy with dissection of pelvic lymph nodes and bilateral salpingo-oophorectomy, total cystectomy, and abdominoperineal resection of the rectum. Colostomy and/or urinary conduit may or may not be performed.

Vaginal hysterectomy types:

Vaginal hysterectomy or laparoscopically assisted vaginal hysterectomy (LAVH): Performed for certain conditions, such as uterine prolapse, cystocele/rectocele, carcinoma in situ, and when high-risk obesity exists.

Preparation: Lower half of the abdomen and the pubic and perineal regions are cleansed with soap and water and may be shaved; intestinal tract emptied and Foley catheter inserted to prevent contamination and injury to the bladder and intestinal tract; enema and antiseptic douche may be prescribed the evening before surgery.

Postoperative course:

- IV fluids, fluid and food restriction for 1 or 2 days, until bowel sounds and peristalsis returns; may have a NG tube
- Foley catheter
- Elastic compression stockings when on bed rest
- Rectal tube for abdominal distension
- Wound care
- Strict I&O

Nursing Process Elements

- Administer analgesics as prescribed.
- Allow client to verbalize her concerns about the effects of surgery: change in body image and reproductive ability; and feelings of loss.
- Monitor abdominal dressings for drainage (abdominal hysterectomy).
- Monitor VS.
- Assess bleeding and extent of saturation of perineal pads.
- Assess for signs of deep vein thrombosis or phlebitis: leg pain, warmth, redness, positive Homan's sign.
- Monitor for signs of pulmonary embolism: chest pain, dyspnea, and tachycardia.
- Encourage and assist client in changing positions often when in bed with pressure under knees avoided; discourage crossing of legs and ankles, encourage to exercise legs and ankles.
- Encourage early ambulation.
- Monitor CBCs for blood count and WBCs.
- Monitor abdominal girth for distension.

Client teaching for self-care

- Take oral analgesics for pain as prescribed.
- Check surgical incision daily for redness or discharge.
- Report elevated temperature to health care provider.
- Although periods are now over, monitor for bleeding; some light bleeding/discharge is normal postsurgery for a few days; if persistent, notify health care provider immediately.
- Report vaginal discharge and/or foul odor to health care provider.
- Consume diet and fluid intake adequate for healing, bowel and bladder function.
- Resume activities gradually.
- Take stool softeners as prescribed and empty bladder frequently.
- Avoid prolonged sitting with pressure behind knees, crossing legs/ankles, and inactivity.
- Expect postoperative fatigue, which should gradually decrease.
- Seek out counseling and/or support groups for self and family.
- Keep follow-up appointment with health care provider.

OVARIECTOMY (OOPHORECTOMY)

Ovariectomy is the removal of one or both ovaries.

Use: To remove tumors of the ovaries.

Preparation: Surgical staging of the tumor is essential in guiding treatment. Preoperative workup includes a barium enema or colonoscopy, upper GI series, chest X-rays, and IV urography. CT scans and immunoscintigraphy, the use of radioactive antibodies, may be used preoperatively to rule out intra-abdominal metastasis.

Postoperative course: IV fluid, I&Os, Foley catheter, wound care, compression stockings, drainage tubes; diet progressed as bowel sounds/peristalsis returns.

Nursing Process Elements

- Monitor VS.
- Assess for pain and medicate as prescribed.
- Monitor CBC blood counts and WBCs.
- Assess dressing for bleeding/drainage.
- Maintain strict I&O.
- Assess for signs of deep vein thrombosis or phlebitis.
- Encourage frequent position changes.
- Encourage early ambulation.
- Manage any drainage tubes.
- Assess for S&S of pleural effusion: shortness of breath, hypoxia, cough, and pleuritic chest pain.

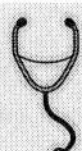

Assessment Alert

Clients with advanced ovarian cancer may develop ascites and pleural effusion.

- Provide small, frequent meals.
- Decrease fluid intake.
- Administer diuretic agents as prescribed.
- Provide frequent rest periods.
- Monitor for side effects of chemotherapy and treat as appropriate.

Client teaching for self-care

- Take oral analgesics for pain as ordered.
- Check surgical incision daily for redness or discharge.
- Report elevated temperature to health care provider.
- Report vaginal discharge and/or foul odor to health care provider.
- Maintain diet and fluid intake adequate for healing, and bowel and bladder function.
- Resume activities gradually.
- Maintain bowel and bladder function (stool softener as prescribed and emptying bladder frequently.
- Avoid prolonged sitting with pressure behind knees, crossing legs/ankles, and inactivity.
- Expect postoperative fatigue, which should gradually decrease.
- Seek out counseling and/or support groups for self and family.
- Keep follow-up appointment with health care provider.

SALPINGECTOMY

Salpingectomy is the removal of one or both of the fallopian tubes.

Use: Management of tubal pregnancies, infected tube, or as part of the surgical treatment of tubal cancer. Commonly done in conjunction as part of a "complete" hysterectomy, or salpingo-oophorectomy where the uterus and both ovaries and fallopian tubes are removed at the same time.

Preparation: NPO night before procedure if not an emergency situation; Foley catheter; premedication for anxiety.

Postoperative course: IV fluid, I&O, Foley catheter, wound care; diet progressed as bowel sounds/peristalsis return.

Nursing Process Elements

Similar to hysterectomy and oophorectomy.

VASECTOMY

Vasectomy is the ligation and transection of the vas deferens, with or without removal of a segment of the vas deferens.

Use: Male sterilization

Nursing Process Elements

Client teaching for self-care

- Apply ice packs, intermittently for several hours, to the scrotum to decrease edema and pain.
- Wear cotton jockey-type brief for added comfort and support.
- Reassure client that procedure has no effect on sexual potency, erection, ejaculation, or production of male hormones.
- Use another form of contraception until infertility is confirmed by examination of the ejaculate; some physicians examine ejaculate 1 month after surgery and again in a month; other physicians consider clients to be sterile after 36 ejaculations.

PENECTOMY

Penectomy is the removal of part or all of the penis with or without removal of groin tissue and lymph nodes.

Use: Treatment of penile cancer.

Nursing Process Elements

- Refer to cancer support groups.
- Refer to therapists who work with couples experiencing changes in their sex lives to teach new ways of arousing and satisfying each other.

PENILE IMPLANT

Penile implant is the insertion of a penile prosthesis used in clients with erectile dysfunction secondary to organic causes.

Nursing Process Elements

Refer client and partner for counseling because this is usually needed to help in adapting to the prosthesis.

TRANSPLANT SURGERY

Use: Tissue and organ transplants are typically done when an organ is no longer able to function despite medical intervention, as a result of traumatic injury such as burns, or disease has rendered it nonfunctional.

Types of grafts:

- Autograft—transplantation of tissue from one area of the body to another
- Heterograft—transplantation of tissue from two different species. Most commonly done in skin grafts with pig skin and is usually temporary
- Allograft—transplantation of tissue between the same species using either live or cadaver donors

Common transplants:

- Cornea
- Bone
- Bone Marrow
- Kidney
- Liver
- Heart
- Lung
- Pancreas
- Skin

Once the client has been deemed an eligible recipient, the client's name is entered into the United Network for Organ Sharing (UNOS) computer database. This organization is responsible for ensuring available organs are distributed in an equitable and nondiscriminatory manner.

Legal requirements of donation and transplantation

- Uniform Anatomical Gift Act (UAGA)—authorizes donation of all or part of the human body. This act provides
  - —guidelines for who can donate, how donation can occur, and who can receive donation
  - —for the organ donor card
  - —liability protection for health care providers
- Required-Request Legislation—defines hospital responsibilities in identifying potential donors and requires information about the opportunity to donate be provided to families
- National Organ Transplant Act—established the National Organ Procurement and Transplantation Network, which creates national registries to track potential recipients and posttransplantation organ recipients. Also establishes national system to match organs with potential recipients. Prohibits the selling of organs and tissues
- Uniform Determination of Death Act—guideline for states to develop a legal definition of death

Types of donors:

- Live donor:
  - —Usually related to the client
  - —Primarily used in kidney transplants
  - —Used with segmental organ donation such as one lobe of lung or liver, usually a parent provides to a recipient child
- Cadaver donor:
  - —Organs removed after death, most commonly brain death
  - —Family required to give written consent prior to organ removal

Pretransplant considerations:

- General criteria for determining transplant need:
  - —End-stage organ failure
  - —Short life expectancy
  - —Severe functional disability
  - —No other serious health problems
  - —Psychological readiness
  - —Financial status
- Clinical status
  - —Immunologic
    - Histocompatibility is the ability of the transplanted tissue or organs to live without attack by the immune system. The closer the histocompatibility antigens match between donor and recipient, the less likely the immune system is to recognize transplanted tissue as nonself
    - Donor–Recipient compatibility testing
      - Tissue typing—determines the degree to which the donor and recipient tissue match
      - Cross-matching—tests the recipient for antidonor antibodies that may have developed from a prior organ transplant, blood transfusions, or pregnancy. Antidonor antibodies can cause rapid rejection including death
      - ABO Typing—blood group typing
  - —General laboratory studies
    - CBC with differential
    - Blood chemistries
    - Coagulation studies
    - Urinalysis
    - Viral titers

- Infection testing-blood cultures, urine cultures, etc
  - —Cardiac studies
    - ECG
    - Echocardiogram
  - —Radiographic
    - Chest X-ray
- Psychological status evaluation
- Financial status

Posttransplantation complications:
While each type of organ transplant has unique posttransplant complications, there are three major types of complications associated with transplantation in general.

- Technical complications are associated with the surgical procedure.
  - —Vascular thrombosis: blood clot in the vasculature of the transplanted organ or tissue, usually the major artery.
  - —Bleeding: usually occurs postoperatively and is managed similarly to other postsurgery clients, except with liver transplant clients.
  - —Anastomosis leakage: occurs at area where transplanted organ/tissue is joined to the client, usually occurs 1–3 weeks after transplant. Most often will require surgical intervention to repair.
- Graft rejection is an immune response by the body against the new tissue.
  - —Acute rejection: cell-mediated response; sudden onset, days or months following transplant.
  - —Hyperacute rejection: humoral, hypersensitivity response, occurs within minutes to hours of transplant, rare due to better donor–recipient screening
  - —Chronic rejection: humoral, can begin any time after transplant and take years to make the transplant nonfunctional
- Immunosuppressant-related problems are caused from the drugs given to prevent rejection.
  - —Infection: major problem following, transplant in clients, whose immune systems are suppressed, who are unable to mount the same type of response as an immunocompetent client.

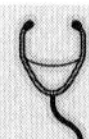

Assessment Alert

Monitor for fever posttransplant as it is the primary symptom of infection.

- Types of infection—bacterial, viral, fungal, and parasitic
- Lungs and urinary tract are most common sites of infection

—Organ dysfunction: frequently caused by nephrotoxicity and hepatotoxicity, which can occur with any organ transplant but is very serious if it involves transplanted kidney or liver

—Malignancy: common problem with long-term immunosuppressant therapy

—Steroid-induced problems: due to long-term steroid therapy and would include such things as hyperglycemia and weight gain

KIDNEY TRANSPLANT

- Kidney transplant is the oldest and most common type of transplant surgery.
- It is used to treat clients with End-Stage Renal Disease (ESRD).
- It reverses majority of pathophysiological changes associated with kidney failure.

Preoperative Care

A regular dialysis schedule should be maintained until the time of transplant if possible.

Client teaching for self-care

- Advise client that dialysis may be needed during the first few weeks postoperatively since there is a 20% chance that the transplanted kidney will not function immediately.
- Review rationale for immunosuppressant therapy and need to comply with treatment regimen.
- Stress importance of reducing the risk of infection after surgery.
- Maintain vascular access patency and clearly identify vascular access site
- Additional diagnostic testing:
  - —GI X-rays
  - —Abdominal ultrasound
  - —Voiding cystourethogram

Postoperative Care

- Care of the donor:
  - —Pain management
  - —Ambulation
  - —Respiratory care
- Care of the recipient:
  - —Maintain fluid and electrolyte balance
  - —Monitor I&O hourly
  - —Titrate IV fluids to replace output amount for the first 12–24 hours
  - —Monitor for hypokalemia
  - —Monitor for sudden decrease in urine output

—Monitor Foley catheter patency
—Monitor for signs of infection
—Monitor for hypertension

Client teaching for self-care

- Medications: oral and written instruction.
- S&S of infection or rejection:
  —Flank pain
  —Fever
  —Changes in urinary pattern
  —Sudden weight gain
  —Difficulty breathing
  —Edema
- Maintain any activity restrictions, which usually include
  —avoiding heavy lifting (more than 20 lb) for 6 weeks to allow time for the incision to heal and the scar gain strength;
  —no return to work for 6–12 weeks; and
  —refraining from sexual intercourse for 4–6 weeks.
- Weight and cholesterol monitoring: steroids increase appetite and increase risk of hyperlipidemia; cyclosporine also increases risk of lipidemia.
- Pregnancy prevention during first year if appropriate to establish good renal function and decrease dosage of immunosuppressant drugs.
- Follow-up appointments.

CORNEA TRANSPLANT

- Cornea transplant is a common type of transplant and is the most successful of all tissue transplants
- It is carried out for those clients who have corneal damage due to infection, injury, or hereditary condition that has resulted in vision loss
- It can be done as long as the retina is intact.
- It is usually done as an outpatient procedure.

Preoperative care:
- Prep client based on type of anesthesia to be administered
- Assess VS

Postoperative care:
- Ensure eye patch is in place
- Assess VS

Client teaching for self-care

- Eye protection.
- Activity restrictions.
- Medication use and compliance.
- Follow-up appointments.

LIVER TRANSPLANT

- Major transplant indicators:
  —Chronic irreversible liver disease
  —Primary malignant tumors of the liver and biliary tree
  —Fulminant hepatic failure
  —Biliary atresia

Preoperative care:
- Explain any special postoperative considerations: NG tube, IV fluids, ICU, etc
- Teach preventive postoperative exercises: deep breathing, leg exercises, use of rails for turning
- Additional diagnostic labs:
  —Liver function test
  —Portal vein sonogram & Doppler
  —Abdominal CT scan
  —Liver biopsy

Postoperative care:
- Promote oxygenation.
- Ensure fluid and electrolyte balance.
- Maintain GI tube patency.
- Maintain low-protein diet.
- Monitor for rejection.
- Monitor for S&S of infection.

Client teaching for self-care

- S&S of infection and rejection
- Medication use and compliance
- Changes in medication routine
- When to notify physician

HEART TRANSPLANT

- Major transplant indicators:
  —Cardiomyopathy
  —Valvular heart disease
  —Ventricular aneurysm
  —Viral myocarditis
  —Congenital malformations
  —Arteriosclerotic coronary artery disease

Preoperative care:
- Similar to other cardiac preoperative care

- Additional diagnostic labs:
  —Endomyocardial biopsy
  —ABG
  —Chest X-ray
  —Pulmonary function testing
  —Ventilation/perfusion scan
  —Chest CT scan
  —Echocardiogram
  —Doppler study
  —Duplex scan of legs
  —Cardiac catheterization

Postoperative care:

- Monitor cardiac function
- Maintain fluid and electrolyte balance
- Monitor renal function
- Monitor for S&S of infection
- Monitor for S&S of rejection

Client teaching for self-care

- Medication use and compliance.
- S&S of infection and rejection.
- Possible need for cardiac rehabilitation.
- Risk factor reduction.
- Required follow-up schedule.

BONE MARROW TRANSPLANT

- Bone marrow transplant is commonly used as a treatment for some types of leukemia and lymphoma.
- It is done during a remission phase.
- Goals:
  —Replace diseased marrow with healthy.
  —Save healthy bone marrow from treatment effect for implantation posttreatment.
  —Replace diseased stem cells with healthy stem cells.

Preoperative care:

- Intensive regimen of chemotherapy and total body irradiation for immunosuppression and to kill residual tumor cells.
- Maintain strict isolation to reduce risk of infection.
- Monitor for S&S of infection.

Client teaching for self-care

- Importance of following isolation procedures.
- Postoperative isolation expectations.
- Provide emotional support.

Postoperative care:

- Maintain strict isolation, usually for 2–4 weeks.
- Provide emotional support.
- Assess psychological status.
- Monitor closely for S&S of infection.
- Monitor for signs of rejection.
- Monitor for signs of bleeding.
- Reduce risk for injury by padding any sharp surfaces.
- Potentially fatal complications.
  —Graft versus host disease

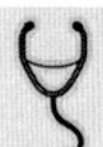

Assessment Alert

Monitor for skin erythema
—Interstitial pneumonia

PLASTIC SURGERY

Types of plastic surgery

- Cosmetic surgery
  —Reshapes normal structures of the body
  —Done to improve the client's appearance and self-esteem
- Reconstructive surgery
  —Performed on abnormal structures of the body, caused by birth defects, developmental abnormalities, trauma or injury, infection, tumors, or disease
  —Done to improve function or to create a normal appearance
  —Procedure performed is the lowest on the reconstructive ladder that will accomplish the goal: simple procedures such as wound closures are first rung and highly complex procedures such as microsurgery to reattach severed limbs occupy the top rung
  —May require complex planning and a number of procedures done in stages

—Children may need long-term follow-up and additional procedures to accommodate to changes caused by growth

Psychological considerations:

- Creates both physical changes and changes in self-esteem
- Insight into personal goals and why plastic surgery is desired is essential to good postoperative adjustment to the results
- Plastic surgery needs to be done for self not out of the desire to please or impress someone else
- Expectations need to be realistic
- Surgery should be planned when the client is free of personal stress, or physical or emotional burden and during the initial consultation questions will be asked not only about how the client feels about his or her appearance, how he or she believes others view him or her, and how he or she would like to look and feel but about potential sources of stress such as relationships, home life, and work. longer and more difficult recovery periods
- Clients who are obsessed with a very minor defect or those with serious mental illness exhibiting delusional or paranoid behavior are not appropriate candidates for plastic surgery.
- Consider the feelings of the child and the parents
- Feelings about self-image tend to change with maturity; therefore, cosmetic surgery should never be forced on a teenager

Postoperative considerations:

- Recuperation time after plastic surgery varies with the procedure and with the health status of the client
  —Generally, assistance is needed for the first 2 days; more, if small children need to be cared for
  —Slow-walking routine is usually begun on the second postoperative day
  —Regular aerobic and more vigorous activities are avoided during the first 2 weeks in order to decrease the risks of bleeding, swelling, and bruising
  —Weight lifting and contact sports typically are allowed at 1 month
- Feelings of "let-down," the "blues," or even depression are common starting about the third day after surgery and lasting a few days or several weeks. Many factors contribute to this but the stress of the postoperative appearance and the waiting for healing or for completion of a staged procedure plays a significant role
- Adjustment to the changed body appearance also takes time: the more dramatic the change, the longer the adjustment period. A sense of unfamiliarity with one's reflection is not uncommon.
- Brisk walks, light social activity, small outings, and a source of emotional support aid adjustment.

Complications:

Potential complications include infection; excessive bleeding such as hematomas, significant bruising and impaired wound healing; and problems related to anesthesia and surgery.

Smoking, connective tissue disease, skin damage from radiation therapy, decreased circulation to area of surgery, impaired immunity, and malnutrition increase the risk of complications.

AUGMENTATION MAMMAPLASTY

- Augmentation mammoplasty involves insertion of inflatable implants filled with saline to increase breast size.
- It is usually performed as an outpatient procedure under local anesthesia with sedation, or general anesthesia.

Postoperative course: Temporary soreness, swelling, change in nipple sensation, and bruising. Breast sensitive to stimulation for a few weeks.

Complications: May require removal or replacement

- Deflation
- Formation of scar tissue around the implant making the breast feel tight or hard
- Bleeding
- Infection
- Permanent increased or decreased sensation in nipples or breast

Nursing Process Elements

Client teaching for self-care

- Avoid physical contact with breasts for 3–4 weeks.
- Return to work in 2–3 days if not required to lift more than 15 lb.
- Report bleeding/drainage, increased swelling, redness, or pain.
- Expect scars to fade slowly over several months to a year or more.
- Inform technician that mammography requires a special technique.

MASTOPEXY

- Mastopexy is the elevation and reshaping of sagging breasts by removing excess skin and repositioning breast tissue and nipples.
- It is usually performed as an outpatient procedure under local anesthesia with sedation, or general anesthesia.

Postoperative course:

Temporary bruising, swelling, discomfort, numbness, dry breast skin.

Complications:

- Heavy scarring (keloid)
- skin loss
- infection
- Unevenly positioned nipples
- Permanent loss of feeling in nipples or breast

Nursing Process Elements

Client teaching for self-care

- Avoid strenuous activities for 4 weeks.
- Return to work in 7–14 days.
- Report bleeding/drainage, increased swelling, redness, or pain.
- Expect scars to fade slowly over several months to a year or more.
- Gravity, pregnancy, aging, and weight changes may cause new sagging.

CHEMICAL PEEL

- Solution of phenol or trichloroacetic acid (TCA) is used to peel away surface layers of the skin.
- It removes superficial wrinkles, blemishes, sun damage, and uneven pigment.
- It works best on fair, thin skin.
- It is usually done as an outpatient procedure without anesthesia though sedation and EKG monitoring is used in some cases. Hospital admission may be required for a full-face phenol peel.

Postoperative course: Temporary throbbing, tingling, swelling, redness; acute sensitivity to sun. New skin forms in 7–21 days after a phenol peel; 5–10 days with TCA. Permanent lightening of treated skin and loss of ability to tan also occur when phenol is used.

Complications:

- Tiny whiteheads (resolve with time)
- Infection
- Scarring
- Flare-up of skin allergies
- Fever blisters
- Cold sores
- Permanent abnormal color changes and rarely, cardiac arrhythmias with phenol

Nursing Process Elements

Client teaching for self-care

- Effects of phenol peels are permanent but new wrinkles can develop; effects of TCA are temporary.
- Resume normal activities in 2–4 weeks.
- Full healing and resolution of erythema takes 3–6 months.

COLLAGEN/FAT INJECTIONS

- Collagen/Fat injections are used to fill out facial creases, furrows or sunken areas, or to add fullness to lips or backs of hands.
- This method is most effective on thin, dry, light-colored skin.
- The effect lasts a few months to a year.
- It is an outpatient procedure; no anesthesia for collagen injections; local anesthesia for fat injections.
- Skin test to check for allergy is required prior to collagen injections.

Postoperative course: Temporary stinging, throbbing, or burning sensation; mild erythema; edema.

Complications:

- Irregular contour
- Infection
- Also with Collagen: allergic reaction including rash, hives, swelling, or flu-like symptoms; possible triggering of connective tissue or autoimmune diseases

DERMABRASION

- Dermabrasion is the removal of the surface layers of the skin by scraping with a high-speed rotary wheel.
- It is used to smooth out surface irregularities such as acne scars and fine wrinkles, especially around the mouth. It may require more than one session.
- It is usually done as an outpatient procedure with a numbing spray, local or general anesthesia.

Postoperative course: Temporary tingling, burning, itching, swelling, redness; acute sun sensitivity; lightening and loss of tanning capacity of treated skin.

Complications:

- Permanent color changes
- Tiny whiteheads (resolve with time)
- Infection
- Scarring
- Flare-up of skin allergies

- Fever blisters
- Cold sores

Nursing Process Elements

Client teaching for self-care

- Effects are permanent although new wrinkles can develop with aging.
- Return to work 2 weeks.
- Avoid strenuous activities for 4–6 weeks.
- Expect redness for about 3 months.
- Avoid sun exposure until pigmentation returns in 6–12 months.

OTOPLASTY

- Otoplasty involves setting prominent ears back closer to the head, or reducing the size of large ears. It is most often done on children between the ages of 4 and 14 years.
- It is an outpatient procedure done under general anesthesia on young children and under general or local anesthesia with sedation on older children or adults.

Postoperative course: Temporary throbbing, aching, swelling, redness, and numbness.

Complications:

- Infection of cartilage
- Excessive scarring
- Formation of a blood clot requiring drainage
- Mismatched or artificial-looking ears
- Recurrence of the protrusion

Nursing Process Elements

Client teaching for self-care

- Return to school in 5–7 days.
- Avoid strenuous activities and contact sports for 1–2 months.

BLEPHAROPLASTY

- Blepharoplasty is the removal of excess fat, skin, and muscle to correct drooping upper eyelids and puffy bags below the eyes.
- It is usually done as an outpatient procedure under local anesthesia with sedation; may be done under general anesthesia.

Postoperative course: Antibiotics may be applied to sutures. Sutures removed in 3–7 days. Temporary discomfort, tightness of lids, swelling, bruising. Temporary dryness, burning, itching of eyes. Excessive tearing, sensitivity to light for first few weeks. Independent activity by day 2. Wearing sunglasses, may feel comfortable going out in public as to the store by day 3–4, and with makeup able to return to work in 5–7 days.

Complications:

- Temporary blurred or double vision
- Infection
- Bleeding
- Swelling at the corners of the eyelids
- Dry eyes
- Formation of whiteheads
- Asymmetrical eyelids
- Scarring
- Difficulty in closing eyes completely (usually temporary)
- Pulling down of the lower lids (may require surgical correction)
- Blindness (extremely rare)

Nursing Process Elements

Client teaching for self-care

- Apply iced compresses to reduce swelling and discoloration.
- Do not read for 2–3 days.
- Do not wear contact lenses for 2 weeks or more.
- Return to work in 5–10 days; can use makeup to cover bruising.
- Avoid strenuous activities and use of alcohol for 3 weeks.
- Expect bruising and edema to persist for several weeks.

RHYTIDECTOMY

- Rhytidectomy is the removal of excess fat, tightening of muscles, and redraping of the skin to reduce sagging facial skin, jowls, and loose neck skin.
- It is usually done as an outpatient procedure under local anesthesia with sedation; sometimes under general anesthesia and occasionally admission for 1–2 days.

Postoperative course:

- Bruising, swelling, numbness, and tenderness of skin for 2–3 weeks; tight feeling, dry skin

- Rest for 24 hours head elevated and without neck flexion to support circulation, decrease edema, and reduce risk of bleeding
- Independent activity resumed by day 2
- Dressings removed in 3–5 days; face cleansed of drainage; antibiotic ointment applied
- Generally, swelling decreased sufficiently in 5–7 days that the client is comfortable going out in public
- Men need to shave behind ears because beard-growing skin is repositioned there

Complications:

- Injury to the nerves that control facial muscles or feeling (usually temporary but may be permanent)
- Infection
- Bleeding
- Poor healing/excessive scarring
- Asymmetry or change in hairline

Nursing Process Elements

Client teaching for self-care

- Keep the head elevated and the neck straight when in bed.
- Rest for 48 hours then gradually resume activity.
- Return to work in 10–14 days; earlier if not in public view.
- Resume more strenuous activity such as lifting or bending in 2 weeks or more; these actions encourage edema and bleeding.
- Take nonnarcotic analgesics, but not any containing aspirin, as directed for discomfort.
- Drink nourishing liquids through a straw and gradually add soft foods and progress to a regular diet as chewing comfort allows.
- Do not shampoo hair until all sutures have been removed; use hair dryer on warm only because of the risk of burns because of decreased sensitivity of the skin/ears.
- Limit exposure to sun for several months.
- Effect typically lasts for 5–10 years.

FACIAL IMPLANTS

- Shaped implants are used to change the basic shape and balance of the face
- Can build up a receding chin, add prominence to cheekbones, or reshape the jawline.
- Usually an outpatient procedure performed under local anesthesia with sedation, or under general anesthesia; occasionally requires overnight admission.

Postoperative course: Temporary discomfort, swelling, bruising, numbness, and/or stiffness. After jaw surgery, the client cannot open mouth fully for several weeks. Appearance is normal in 2–4 weeks.

Complications:

- Shifting or malpositioned implant
- Infection which may require more surgery or removal
- Unnatural shape due to excessive tightening and hardening of scar tissue around an artificial implant

Nursing Process Elements

Client teaching for self-care

- Return to work in about a week.
- Avoid activity that could jar or bump face for 6 weeks or more.

FOREHEAD LIFT (BROWLIFT)

- Removal of excess tissue, adjustment of muscles and tightening the forehead skin to minimize forehead creases, drooping eyebrows, hooding over eyes, furrowed forehead and frown lines. Traditionally done by means of an incision across the top of the head just behind the hairline; may also be done endoscopically by means of three to five short incisions.
- Usually an outpatient procedure performed under local anesthesia with sedation; occasionally under general anesthesia.

Postoperative course: Temporary swelling, numbness, headaches, bruising. Possible itching and hair loss with traditional procedure. Bruising takes 2–3 weeks to abate.

Complications:

- Injury to facial nerve, causing loss of motion, muscle weakness, or asymmetrical look
- Infection
- Marked scarring

Nursing Process Elements

Client teaching for self-care

- Return to work in 7–10 days, usually sooner after an endoscopic forehead lift.
- Resume more strenuous activity in several weeks.
- Limit sun exposure for several months.
- Effect typically lasts for 5–10 years.

HAIR REPLACEMENT SURGERY

- Hair replacement surgery involves use of client's own hair to fill in balding areas.
- Techniques include scalp reduction, tissue expansion, strip grafts, scalp flaps, or clusters of punch grafts (plugs, mini plugs, and microplugs).
- It is most successful on men with male pattern baldness after hair loss has stopped.
- It may require multiple procedures over 18 months or more.
- It is usually an outpatient procedure performed under local anesthesia with sedation. Flaps and tissue expansion may be done with general anesthesia.

Postoperative course: Temporary achy, tight scalp. Unnatural look in early stages.

Complications:
- Unnatural look
- Infection
- Excessive scarring
- Failure to "take"
- Loss of scalp tissue and/or transplanted hair

Nursing Process Elements

Client teaching for self-care
- Return to work usually in 2–5 days.
- Resume more strenuous activities in 10 days to 3 weeks.
- Final result will not be apparent for up to 18 months depending on procedure.

LASER FACIAL RESURFACING

- Laser facial resurfacing uses a CO_2 laser to smooth the face and fine wrinkles, soften lines around the eyes and mouth, and minimize facial scars and unevenly pigmented areas.
- It may require more than one session.
- It is usually an outpatient procedure under local anesthesia with sedation.

Postoperative course: Temporary swelling and discomfort. Lightening of treated skin. Acute sun sensitivity. Increased sensitivity to makeup. Pinkness or redness in skin that may persist for up to 6 months. Pigmentation returns in 6–12 months.

Complications:
- Burns or injuries caused by laser heat
- Scarring
- Abnormal changes in skin color
- Flare-up of viral infections such as cold sores and rarely development of other infections

Nursing Process Elements

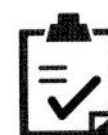

Client teaching for self-care
- Return to work in 2 weeks.
- Resume more strenuous activities in 4–6 weeks.
- Avoid sun exposure for 6–12 months and then only light exposure.
- Does not stop aging: New wrinkles/expression lines may form as skin ages.

LIPOSUCTION

- Liposuction is the removal of exercise-resistant fat deposits with a tube and vacuum suction device.
  - —Tumescent technique: Fat cells are infused with saline solution and a local anesthetic before suctioning to reduce postoperative bruising and swelling.
  - —Ultrasound-assisted lipoplasty (UAL): Fat is liquefied via an ultrasound probe inserted under the skin before suctioning is begun, used when large amounts of fat must be removed or when area is fibrous.
- Common sites for liposuction are chin, cheeks, neck, upper arms, above breasts, abdomen, buttocks, hips, thighs, knees, calves, ankles, etc.
- Local, epidural, or general anesthesia may be used.
- It is usually an outpatient procedure though extensive procedures may require short admission.

Postoperative course: Temporary bruising, swelling, numbness, soreness, and burning sensation.
- Drainage from incision sites with tumescent technique
- Compression garment or tape kept in place for 7–10 days
- Full recovery from swelling and bruising: 1–6 months or more. Use of tumescent technique or UAL may decrease postoperative bruising and swelling

Complications:
- Asymmetry
- Rippling or bagginess of skin
- Pigmentation changes
- Fluid retention
- Hypovolemic shock from excessive fluid loss
- Infection
- Thermal burn injury caused by the heat from the ultrasound device with UAL

Nursing Process Elements

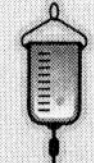

Clinical Alert

Anticoagulants are contraindicated for liposuction clients because of the risk of bleeding.

Client teaching for self-care

- Rest for 12 hours, then gradually resume activity.
- Apply ice packs to surgical area to decrease edema.
- Take nonaspirin, nonnarcotic pain relievers for discomfort.
- Return to work in 1–2 weeks.
- Resume more strenuous activity in 2–4 weeks.
- Full result of the surgery on the body contour may not be seen for 8–16 weeks because of edema.
- Eat a sensible diet and exercise to avoid weight gain, which can negate the effect of the surgery.

MALE BREAST REDUCTION

- Male breast reduction involves reduction of enlarged, female-like breast in men using liposuction and/or excision of excess glandular tissue.
- It is usually an outpatient procedure performed under general or local anesthesia.

Postoperative course: Temporary bruising, swelling, numbness, soreness, and burning sensation.

Complications:

- Infection
- Fluid accumulation
- Injury, rippling, or bagginess of the skin.
- Asymmetry
- Pigmentation changes that may become permanent if exposed to sun
- Excessive scarring if tissue was cut away

Nursing Process Elements

Client teaching for self-care

- Return to work in 3–7 days.
- Resume more strenuous activity in 2–3 weeks.
- Expect swelling and bruising for 3–6 months.

NOSE SURGERY (RHINOPLASTY)

- Nose surgery involves permanent reshaping of the nose by reducing or increasing size, removing hump, changing shape of tip or bridge, narrowing span of nostrils, or changing angle between nose and upper lip.
- It may also relieve some breathing problems.
- It is usually an outpatient procedure performed under local anesthesia with sedation, or under general anesthesia.

Postoperative course: Temporary swelling, bruising around eyes and nose, headaches, some bleeding, and stiffness.

Complications:

- Infection
- Small burst blood vessels resulting in tiny, permanent red spots
- Incomplete improvement requiring additional surgery

Nursing Process Elements

Client teaching for self-care

- Resume work in 1–2 weeks.
- Resume more strenuous activities in 2–3 weeks.
- Avoid hitting or sunburning the nose for 8 weeks. Final appearance: 1 year or more.

ABDOMINOPLASTY (TUMMY TUCK)

- Abdominoplasty is the removal of excess fat and skin and tightening muscles of abdominal wall to flatten the abdomen.
- Depending on extent of procedure either in or outpatient with either general anesthesia, or local anesthesia with sedation.

Postoperative course: Temporary pain, swelling, soreness, numbness of abdominal skin, bruising, and tiredness for several weeks or months. Generally takes 2–4 days before clients can move around independently.

Complications:

- Blood clots
- Infection
- Bleeding under the skin flap
- Poor healing with conspicuous scarring or skin loss

Nursing Process Elements

Client teaching for self-care

- Return to work in 2–4 weeks; desk job as early as 5–10 days.

- Avoid more strenuous activity for 4–6 weeks or more. Fading and flattening of scars: 3 months to 2 years.

BOTOX® INJECTION

- Botox injection is a form of botulinum toxin.
- It is used to temporarily reduce or eliminate frown lines, forehead creases, crows feet near the eyes, and thick bands in the neck.
- It works by blocking nerve impulses causing temporary paralysis of the muscles that cause wrinkles.
- It is effective in relieving migraine headaches, excessive sweating, and muscle spasms in the neck and eyes.

WOUND CLOSURE

- Direct closure: used for skin-surface wounds that have straight edges.
- Skin grafts: used for wide wounds that cannot be directly closed.
  —Split-thickness skin graft: consists of surface layers of skin usually taken from anterior thigh; commonly used to treat burn wounds; revascularizes quickly but is susceptible to trauma, lacks sensation, tends to contract; has impaired sweating ability, and a poor cosmetic appearance; called a mesh graft when many tiny slits are cut in it to allow stretching to cover a large area.
  —Full-thickness skin graft: entire area of skin removed from donor site which then is closed with sutures; used for deep, large burn wounds or to cover jointed areas where maximum skin elasticity and movement are needed.
  —Composite graft: consists of skin, fat and sometimes cartilage; used when the wound needs underlying support.
  —Autograft: tissue transferred from donor site to wound site on same person.
    - Location of the donor site is determined in part by the size and color of the skin patch needed.
    - Donor sites are covered with a transparent dressing for moist healing or single layer, nonadherent gauze for dry healing with a pressure dressing in place for 24–48 hours to control bleeding.
    - Donor sites heal in about 2 weeks and can be used over and over again.
    - New skin at donor site of a split-thickness graft has less pigment than the original skin.
  —Allograft (homograft): graft tissue comes from a different person; sloughs off after 3–10 weeks.
  —Heterograft (xenograft): tissue used is from an animal; sloughs in 3–7 days and then is replaced until wound is healed or otherwise grafted; used to limit fluid loss, control temperature, and decrease risk of infection.
  —For a graft to take, it must have a good blood supply and be immobilized so that newly forming capillaries are not destroyed.
  —Petrolatum-impregnated dressings used to prevent graft from drying out and not "taking."
  —Pressure dressing used for 24–48 hours to control bleeding on both graft and donor sites.
  —Successful graft appears pink and is attached to wound bed at time of first dressing change in about 3 days.

Think Smart/Test Smart

A successful graft appears pink and is attached to the wound bed. This means that the nurse must regularly assess the color and attachment of the graft. The graft appears pink because it has a good blood supply; if the blood supply is not good, the graft will be pale. There are many ways understanding of these concepts can be tested. A question might ask which S&S indicates that a graft has taken—pink color would be a correct answer. On the other hand, the question might ask which assessment finding indicates a grafting procedure is unsuccessful. In this case, pallor could be the correct answer. Other related questions could ask what assessments would be part of the plan of care for a client with a graft or how should the nurse interpret an assessment finding of pink coloration of a graft placed 4 days ago. Answers to these questions are color and adherence to the wound bed for the first question; and successful graft, the graft has taken, the graft has a good blood supply or revascularization has occurred are possible answers to the second question.

- Tissue expansion
  —An expander (balloon-like device) is inserted under the skin near the area to be repaired and then gradually filled with salt water over time, causing the skin to stretch and grow.
  —Time involved varies with size of area to be repaired and characteristics of the client.
  —Provides a near-perfect match of skin color, sensation, and texture.

—Decreases risk of tissue loss because the skin remains connected to its original blood and nerve supply.

—Scars are less apparent than those in flaps or grafts.

- Flap Surgery/Microsurgery
  - —Microsurgery allows reattachment of amputated parts.
  - —Flaps allow transplantation of large sections of tissue, muscle, or bone from one area of the body to another with the original blood supply intact.
  - —A flap is a section of living tissue with its own blood supply.
    - Random-pattern flaps: blood supply is from random vessels
    - Axial-pattern flaps: have identifiable arterial and venous vessels
    - Local flap
      - Piece of skin and underlying tissue that lies adjacent to the wound.
      - Flap remains attached at one end so it maintains its original blood supply, and is repositioned over the wounded area.
    - Regional flap
      - Section of tissue moved to a new site that is attached by a specific blood vessel to its original site.
      - Pedicle: name given to the tissue that houses the blood vessels going to a flap.
      - Pedicles are tunneled under other tissues, e.g., for breast reconstruction, the pedicle may be in the abdomen or in the axilla depending on whether the graft is taken from the abdomen or the back.
    - Musculocutaneous flap (muscle and skin flap)
      - Used when the area to be covered needs more bulk and a greater blood supply, e.g., in breast reconstruction
    - Microvascular free flap
      - Section of tissue and skin that is completely detached from its original site and reattached to its new site by hooking up all the tiny blood vessels.
      - Free flaps do not have a pedicle because a new blood supply has been created.

Nursing Process Elements

- Assess graft for adherence to wound bed, color, and signs of epithelialization, vascularization, and new granulation. Also assess for signs of infection: redness including redness of skin surrounding the graft, foul odor, and purulent drainage.
- Check circulation peripheral to the graft.
- Inspect any splints or other immobilization devices for proper application and placement.
- Assess donor sites for healing or signs of infection.
- Maintain immobility of grafted area and ensure dressing does not move.
- Elevate graft site if possible to promote drainage and prevent damage to new capillaries from increased intravascular pressure.
- Keep flap and area of pedicle free of pressure to prevent interference with blood supply and resultant flap necrosis.
- Use bed cradle or other device to keep bed linens off graft and donor sites.
- Prevent shearing of graft because this destroys any ingrowth of capillaries.
- Use strict aseptic technique during graft care until graft as taken.
- Medicate for pain; donor sites are more painful than graft sites.

Client teaching for self-care

After direct wound closure

- Keep wound dry and covered for 24 hours.

After grafting

- Wear pressure garments as prescribed over graft area.
- If grafting involves an extremity, keep it elevated.
- Dress in layers to prevent injury from cold.
- When healed, massage graft/donor site with lanolin or cocoa butter at least once per day for 8 weeks to a year and a half to decrease itch, increase blood flow, and soften skin.
- Take care to protect graft site from trauma including sunburn because of its loss of feeling.

COMPLICATIONS RELATED TO COMMON HEALTH ALTERATIONS

Complications of common health alterations are listed in Table 18–1.

Table 18–1 Complications from Health Alterations

Primary Problem	Potential Complications	Clinical Notes
Pericarditis	Pericardial effusion	Abnormal collection of fluid between pericardial tissue layers: rapid increase in fluid compresses heart and causes pericardial tamponade. Slow increase causes distant heart sounds, cough, mild dyspnea.
	Cardiac tamponade	Compression of heart due to collection of fluid in pericardial sac causes critical drop in cardiac output due to interference with ventricular filling and pumping. Major indicator of tamponade: pulsus paradoxus—pulse that markedly decreases in amplitude during inspiration: Diminished or absent carotid or femoral pulse during inspiration; drop in systolic BP of 10 mm Hg or more during inspiration.
Infective endocarditis	Heart failure Infarction of other organs Abscess Aneurysm	 Due to embolization of vegetative fragments Due to infiltration of arterial wall by infective organisms
Heart failure	Cardiogenic shock Pulmonary edema GI problems	 Due to congestion and enlargement of liver and spleen with increased intra-abdominal pressure and ascites.
	Impaired liver function Dysrhythmias	From prolonged right heart failure. From myocardial distention.
Aortic aneurysm	Rupture and hemorrhage.	Risk is associated with both abdominal and thoracic aneurysms.
	Embolus to lower extremities.	Occurs with abdominal aortic aneurysms. Occurs with dissecting aortic aneurysms.
	Hemorrhage, renal failure, MI, HF, cardiac tamponade, sepsis, weakness, or paralysis of lower extremities.	
Peripheral atherosclerosis	Gangrene and amputation of an extremity. Infection and sepsis Pulmonary embolism.	
Deep vein thrombosis Anemia Leukemia	CHF. Neurologic: subarachnoid hemorrhage, retinal hemorrhage, seizures, coma. Pulmonary bleeding. Renal insufficiency or failure. CV: hemorrhage, thrombophlebitis. DIC. Immunologic: abscesses, septicemia. Chronic venous insufficiency.	
Sinusitis	Extension of infection into tissue or bone of the orbit; intracranial spread resulting in meningitis, epidural, subdural or brain abscess, or venous sinus thrombosis.	
Pulmonary tuberculosis	Emphysema Bronchopleural fistula Pneumothorax	From rupture of a tuberculosis lesion. From air escape at point of rupture.

(continued on next page)

Table 18–1 *(continued from previous page)*

Primary Problem	Potential Complications	Clinical Notes
Asthma	Respiratory failure	S&S: Inaudible breath sounds, decreased wheeze, ineffective cough Assessment Alert: Can be mistaken for improvement because symptoms seem to be relieved.
	Status asthmaticus	Severe, prolonged attack unresponsive to standard therapy; can lead to respiratory failure.
	Dehydration Respiratory infection Atelectasis Pneumothorax Cor pulmonale	
Pneumococcal pneumonia	Pleuritis	Most common complication although bacteremia can result in meningitis, endocarditis, or peritonitis.
Ruptured intracranial aneurysm	Rebleeding	Risk greatest in first 24 hours after initial bleed and on days 7–10 when clot dissolves. S&S: Sudden, severe headache, N&V, change in LOC, new neurologic deficits.
	Vasospasm	Occurs 3–10 days after subarachnoid hemorrhage Causes ischemia and tissue damage in areas affected; if global causes loss of consciousness.
	Hydrocephalus	Accumulation of CSF in ventricles; increases ICP.
Staphylococcus aureus and gram-negative pneumonia	Parenchymal necrosis, lung abscess, emphysema	
Multiple sclerosis	Urinary: recurrent UTI, incontinence Neuro: seizures, dementia Blindness	
Myasthenia gravis	Pneumonia, aspiration	Dependent on degree of muscle weakness and specific muscles involved.
	Myasthenic crisis	From missed doses of medication, under medication, infection. Sudden worsening of motor weakness, tachypnea, tachycardia, severe respiratory distress, dysphagia, restlessness, impaired speech, and anxiety.
	Cholinergic crisis	From overdose of cholinergic drugs: S&S: Severe muscle weakness, vertigo, respiratory distress, GI symptoms. Differentiated from myasthenic crisis by absence of response to Tensilon.
Gastroenteritis	Dehydration, hypovolemia	May progress to hypovolemic shock.
Anorexia nervosa	Fluid, electrolyte and acid–base imbalance	
	Low cardiac output, dysrhythmias	Decreased cardiac muscle mass.
	Anemia Hypoglycemia Increased uric acid levels Osteoporosis Liver dysfunction	
Bulimia nervosa	Stomatitis Fluid, electrolyte and acid–base imbalance. Dysrhythmias Esophageal tears, stomach rupture	
	Metabolic acidosis	If diarrhea predominates.
	Metabolic alkalosis	If vomiting predominates.
	Hypokalemia	With both vomiting and diarrhea.

(continued on next page)

Table 18–1 *(continued from previous page)*

Primary Problem	Potential Complications	Clinical Notes
GERD	Esophageal stricture. Barrett's esophagus	Causes dysphagia. Changes in cells with increased risk of esophageal cancer.
Peptic ulcer disease	Hemorrhage Obstruction Perforation	Most frequent complication in older adult.
Gastrectomy	Dumping syndrome	5–30 minutes after eating: nausea, may vomit, epigastric pain, borborygmi, diarrhea due to hyperosmolar chyme rapidly entering small intestine; rapid increase in blood glucose triggering release of large amount of insulin. 2-3 hours after eating: hypoglycemia Lasts 6-12 months postoperative.
	Pernicious anemia Folic acid deficiency Deficiency of vitamin D and calcium	Lack of intrinsic factor needed for absorption of B12. Impaired absorption. Impaired absorption.
Intestinal obstruction	Hypovolemia and shock Impaired respiration Strangulation	Leads to varied organ dysfunction including renal failure. Abdominal distention elevates diaphragm and inhibits ventilation. Impairs blood flow causing gangrene with bleeding and eventually perforation, peritonitis, septic shock.
Appendicitis Peritonitis	Perforation, peritonitis, abscess Hypovolemic shock Abscess formation Adhesions in abdominal cavity	S&S: Increased pain, high fever. From fluid loss into abdominal cavity. Abscess limits effectiveness of immune response and access by antibiotics. Late complication; can cause obstruction.
Crohn's disease	Intestinal obstruction Abscess Fistula	Due to repeated inflammation and scarring. Small bowel to small bowel: asymptomatic Small bowel to large bowel: increased diarrhea, weight loss, malnutrition Small bowel to bladder: recurrent UTI.
Ulcerative colitis	Hemorrhage Toxic megacolon	Can occur with severe attacks. Acute paralysis and dilation of all or part of the colon: may be precipitated by electrolyte imbalance of narcotic medication S&S: fever, tachycardia, hypotension, dehydration, abdominal tenderness and cramping, change in defecation.
	Perforation Increased risk of colorectal cancer	Toxic megacolon increases risk.
Colorectal cancer	Bowel obstruction Perforation of the bowel wall	From occlusion of the lumen by the tumor mass. From infiltration by the tumor.
Cholelithiasis	Common bile duct obstruction	May lead to jaundice and liver damage or pancreatitis.
Cholecystitis	Gangrene and perforation of gallbladder with peritonitis. Empyema Fistula formation Gallstone ileus	Collection of infected fluid within the gall bladder. Between gall bladder and stomach, duodenum or colon. Blockage of the small intestine with a large gallstone.

(continued on next page)

Table 18–1 *(continued from previous page)*

Primary Problem	Potential Complications	Clinical Notes
Acute pancreatitis	Intravascular volume depletion with acute tubular necrosis and renal failure ARDS Pancreatic necrosis Pancreatic abscess Pancreatic pseudocyst Pancreatic ascites	Usually occurs within 24 hours. Usually develops 3-7 days after onset of pancreatitis; most common in clients with severe volume depletion. Causes an inflammatory mass, may lead to infection, shock , and multiorgan failure. Tends to form 6 or more weeks after onset of acute pancreatitis S&S: tender epigastric mass. Encapsulated collection of fluid; may rupture and cause peritonitis S&S; increasing abdominal girth, elevated serum amylase, absence of abdominal pain.
Cirrhosis	Diabetes Primary hepatic cancer DIC Ruptured Esophageal varices	Distended esophageal vessels are so thin, eating rough foods may cause rupture.
Fractures (Limb Fractures)	Compartment syndrome	From pressure of edema or hemorrhage in a space enclosed by a fascia resulting in lack of blood flow to muscles and nerves within the space. Most often occurs within 48 hours after injury; arterial pulses may be normal even though circulation is compromised sufficiently to cause tissue damage. S&S: pain becoming severe particularly on passive flexion; paresthesias, paresis, cyanosis, kidney failure from release of myoglobin from damaged muscle. Volkmann's contracture following elbow fractures can result from compartment syndrome.
(Long bone fractures)	Fat embolism syndrome	Fat globules from the bone marrow enter and travel through the blood stream causing ischemia in tissues beyond point at which they lodge. Occurs within hours to weeks after injury. S&S: Neurologic changes e.g., confusion, altered LOC; respiratory distress e.g., pulmonary edema, atelectasis, ARDS; petechiae on chest, upper arms and axilla from thrombocytopenia. Prevention: early stabilization of long bone fractures. Rx: rapid identification and intervention to prevent hypoxemia, corticosteroids to reduce inflammatory response.
Fractures	Deep vein thrombosis Infection Delayed union, nonunion Delayed healing Chronic stump pain Phantom pain Contractures	Greatest risk with open fractures; any decrease in circulation also increases risk of infection. Risk factors: infection, impaired circulation, electrolyte imbalances, malnutrition, vasoconstriction from smoking, venous thrombosis, decreased CO. Burning pain from neuroma formation. Painful sensation in missing part. Abnormal flexion and fixation of joint above amputation occurs from lack of extension and ROM. Prolonged sitting after BK amputation leads to hip contracture. Postural exercises required for upper extremity amputation to prevent hunching to one side because of weight loss.

(continued on next page)

Table 18–1 *(continued from previous page)*

Primary Problem	Potential Complications	Clinical Notes
Osteoporosis Gout	Fractures Joint pain, deformity, restricted movement Kidney disease Renal calculi	 From deposition of urate crystals (tophi). Occurs with untreated gout especially in hypertensive clients. Uric acid crystals precipitate out.
Systemic lupus erythematosus	Nephrotic syndrome, renal failure CVA; organic brain syndrome	 OBS: memory loss, impaired cognitive function, personality changes, disorientation.
Chronic pancreatitis	Malabsorption and malnutrition Diabetes mellitus Pancreatic abscess, pseudocyst, stricture of the common bile duct. Increased risk of pancreatic cancer.	
Urinary calculi	Obstruction of urinary tract Hydronephrosis Infection	Slowly developing: may be asymptomatic Acute onset: severe symptoms which depend on location, extent, and duration of obstruction. Distention of renal pelvis and calyces resulting from back up of urine due to obstruction Slow onset: dull back or flank ache/pain Rapid onset: sharp, colicky pain often radiating to groin, N&V, abdominal pain Fever, hematuria, pyuria may accompany either. Secondary to urinary stasis.
Uremia	GI: peptic ulcer, bleeding Neuro: seizures, decreased LOC, coma CV: pericarditis, pericardial effusion, cerebrovascular disease, Heart failure Spontaneous abortion Spontaneous bone fracture Secondary to osteomalacia and osteoporosis.	Pericarditis occurs irritation of the pericardial sac by retained toxins; less likely if dialysis started early.
Radiation therapy for prostate cancer	Erectile dysfunction Urethral stricture Rectal/anal stricture Cystitis Diarrhea Proctitis Rectal ulcer Bowel obstruction Urinary incontinence	Delayed complications: develops months or years after treatment. Develops months or years after treatment.
Gonorrhea	PID in women Epididymitis and prostatitis in men Infection of blood and joints Blindness, sepsis, joint infection in neonate Increased susceptibility to HIV and increased risk of transmission.	Can result in chronic pain, abscesses, ectopic pregnancy, infertility. Can result in dysuria and infertility. If contracted during delivery.
Herpes zoster	Postherpetic neuralgia Permanent loss of vision	More common in older clients. Risk when lesions involve ophthalmic division of the trigeminal nerve.

(continued on next page)

Table 18–1 *(continued from previous page)*

Primary Problem	Potential Complications	Clinical Notes
Diabetes mellitus	Hyperglycemia, Diabetic ketoacidosis, Hyperglycemic hyperosmolar nonketotic coma. Hypoglycemia Neuro: Paresthesias, pain, loss of sensation, loss of fine motor control. Eye: diabetic retinopathy, cataracts, glaucoma. CV: orthostatic hypotension, accelerated atherosclerosis, CVA, MI, PVD, platelet disorders. Renal: hypertension, albuminuria, edema, chronic renal failure. Joint contractures Foot ulcers, gangrene of feet Atrophy of skin Increased susceptibility to infection. Periodontal disease	From imbalance among amount of insulin, amount of physical activity, and CHO intake, e.g., too much insulin taken, excessive work/exercise, missing a meal. Also can be due to alcohol intake and drugs such as Coumadin MAO inhibitors and salicylates. Polyneuropathies: bilateral sensory problems starting in toes and feet and moving upward are most common Hypertension, hyperlipidemia, obesity and smoking further increase risk of CV problems. Microcirculatory changes primarily affect eye and kidney. Microalbuminuria-(small amount) – first sign of nephropathy. Usually begin as a superficial lesion; diabetics at risk for foot trauma because of lack of sensation so don't feel pressure, pain as from shoes that don't fit correctly or an ingrown nail. Tb more common in diabetics. Not more frequent in diabetics but more rapidly progressive.
Burns	Infection Fluid volume deficit Electrolyte imbalance ARDS Renal, GI or hepatic dysfunction	
Chemical skin peel	Bleaching of skin	From removal of melanocytes.

WORKSHEET

FILL IN THE BLANKS

Fill in the blank spaces with the correct word or phrase to complete each statement.

1. Surgical removal of one or more of the fallopian tubes is referred to as a ____________________.

2. A ____________________ may be performed to control life-threatening bleeding/hemorrhage and in the event of intractable pelvic infection.

3. After a vasectomy, applying ____________________ to the scrotum intermittently for several hours will help to reduce swelling and relieve discomfort.

4. The client on a cardiopulmonary bypass pump is maintained in a state of hypothermia in order to ____________________.

5. Postoperatively, the client who has had a CABG procedure usually is instructed to avoid excessive arm movements for ____________________ weeks.

6. What piece of equipment must be kept at the bedside of postoperative amputees? ____________________.

7. To check for development of abdominal distention, the nurse measures ____________________.

8. When caring for a client who had a kidney removed, the nurse would expect the Jackson–Pratt drain to be removed when drainage has decreased to less than ____________________ ml/d.

9. The client who has had a craniotomy is at greatest risk for ICP during the first ____________________ hours after surgery because this is the time during which edema peaks.

10. The client with a middle fossa craniotomy should be positioned with the head of the bed elevated ____________________ degrees.

11. Transplantation from one part of the body to another is called a(n) ____________________.

12. The live donor is primarily used in ____________________ transplants.

13. ____________________ transplant is the only type of transplant done as outpatient surgery.

14. A major indicator for heart transplant is ____________________.

15. Graft rejection, immunosuppressant related, and ____________________ are the three major types of transplant-associated complications.

16. The ____________________ transplant client must be weighed daily.

17. In addition to loss of vision, bleeding and infection, a complication associated with eye surgery is ____________________.

18. The two greatest risk associated with inner ear surgery are infection and ____________________.

19. A life-threatening complication of a long bone fracture is a ____________________.

20. Infection most often occurs when an amputation is ____________________.

21. List four categories of medication that interact with anesthetic agents.
    a. ____________________
    b. ____________________
    c. ____________________
    d. ____________________

22. Identify three causes of airway obstruction following a surgical procedure.
    a. ____________________
    b. ____________________
    c. ____________________

(continued)

23. List four symptoms of hemorrhage.
    a. ______
    b. ______
    c. ______
    d. ______

24. Identify two types of exercises a client can be taught to perform to decrease the postoperative complication deep vein thrombosis.
    a. ______
    b. ______

25. The medication commonly used to reverse the effects of opioids is ______.

26. Hypoxia can be assessed by performing ______ and ______.

27. Normal bowel sounds following a surgical procedure generally are audible within ______ hours.

28. Identify 3 examples of nonnarcotic pain management.
    a. ______
    b. ______
    c. ______

29. A herbal medicine that neutralizes antibiotics is ______.

30. Arthritic changes of the cervical spine can result in ______.

31. A bluish tinge around the umbilicus that is an indicator of either intra-abdominal bleeding peritoneal bleeding is called ______.

32. List three causes of urinary retention in a postoperative client.
    a. ______
    b. ______

TRUE & FALSE QUESTIONS

Mark each of the following statements True or False. Correct all false statements in the space provided.

1. Dilation and curettage may be necessary for a woman with dysfunctional bleeding. ___ T ___ F
2. An advantage to use of a biologic heart valve for valve replacement is that it lasts longer than a mechanical valve. ___ T ___ F
3. Dynamic cardiomyoplasty is performed to correct hypertrophic cardiomyopathy. ___ T ___ F
4. The pericardium can be removed without any significant harmful effects on the client. ___ T ___ F

	T	F
5. Speech is lost with a supraglottic laryngectomy.	T	F
6. Tracheostomy suctioning is a clean procedure.	T	F
7. Clients with a tracheostomy cannot swim.	T	F
8. A pillow is placed under the stump of an above the knee amputation (AK) to support it in an elevated position.	T	F
9. Nasogastric drainage decreases as peristalsis returns after gastric surgery.	T	F
10. A client with an ileal conduit should take a shower with the urine collection bag in place.	T	F
11. Clients having a skin lesion removed by cryosurgery should be told that they will feel a tingling sensation when the freezing substance is applied.	T	F
12. Phantom breast pain can occur following a mastectomy.	T	F
13. Reducing tension on the suture lines is an important part of the care for a client with a vulvectomy.	T	F
14. Surgically induced menopause occurs in premenopausal women who have a bilateral salpingo-oophorectomy.	T	F
15. The goal of surgery done to treat glaucoma is to lower IOP.	T	F
16. The United Network for Organ Sharing (UNOS) is responsible for ensuring available organs are distributed equitably.	T	F
17. The National Organ Transplant Act established the organ donor card system.	T	F
18. Before organs can be harvested, the family must give written consent.	T	F
19. Psychological readiness and severe functional disability are not criteria for determining transplant need.	T	F
20. A complication of breast augmentation is the formation of scar tissue around the implant, which makes the breast feel tight or hard.	T	F
21. Preoperative preparation of the operative site includes shaving the site prior to the client going to the operating room.	T	F
22. Shivering during the immediate postoperative patient is indicative of a need for continued use of oxygen.	T	F
23. Hypoxemia is defined as a PO_2 level less than 65 mm Hg.	T	F
24. Clients in the PACU are usually assessed every 15 minutes.	T	F
25. A client whose skin that is cool, moist, and pale is experiencing hypotension.	T	F
26. Warm blankets are provided to clients in PACU to reduce hypothermia.	T	F

(continued)

27. The basal metabolic rate of a client increases during surgery. ___ T ___ F

28. Gynecological surgery places a client at risk for deep vein thrombosis. ___ T ___ F

29. Only the use of sequential compression devices can prevent the development of deep vein thrombosis. ___ T ___ F

30. A client with skeletal deformities has a higher risk of postoperative pulmonary complications. ___ T ___ F

31. Antiseizure medications should not be administered during surgery even for the client who routinely takes this category of medication. ___ T ___ F

32. Nurses are not to provide education on what a client should expect to see in the operating room. ___ T ___ F

33. Clients do not need to ambulate in order for peristalsis to return following a surgical procedure. ___ T ___ F

34. A change in the color of a stoma, such as a colostomy, from bright red to pale gray is not unusual. ___ T ___ F

35. Surgical clients should receive total parenteral nutrition if they are not able to take in nutrients for more than 3 days. ___ T ___ F

MATCHING QUESTIONS

Match the following:

1. ____ Endarterectomy	a. Antireflux procedure
2. ____ Partial laryngectomy	b. Removal of the urinary bladder
3. ____ Cystectomy	c. Removal of the vocal cord and a section of the larynx
4. ____ Fundoplication	d. Procedure done for glaucoma
5. ____ Salpingectomy	e. Removal of the Fallopian tubes
6. ____ Trabeculectomy	f. Urinary diversion procedure
7. ____ Supraglottic laryngectomy	g. Incision into the ear drum
8. ____ Myringotomy	h. Incision into an artery with removal of atheromatous material
9. ____ Ileal conduit	i. Procedure used for pancreatic cancer
10. ____ Whipple procedure	j. Removal of the hyoid bone, glottis and false vocal cords

Medication	Used for
11. ____ Atropine sulfate	a. Permits smoother induction of anesthetic
12. ____ Hydroxyzine hydrochloride	b. Decreases amount of anesthetic needed
13. ____ Midazolam hydrochloride	c. Provides amnesia
14. ____ Morphine sulfate	d. Decreases respiratory and gastric secretions
15. ____ Panax ginseng	e. Decreases anxiety
16. ____ Pentobarbital sodium	f. Prolongs sedative effects of anesthesia
17. ____ Valeriana officinalis	g. Inhibits platelet aggregation

Medical Problem	Description
18. ____ Paralytic ileus	a. Absent bowel sounds
19. ____ Cullen's sign	b. Separation of approximated wound edges
20. ____ Dehiscence	c. Bowel protruding from a surgical incision
21. ____ Evisceration	d. An indication of intraabdominal bleeding

Interaction that may result when anesthetic is administered	Medication Category
22. ____ Anxiety and seizures occur with sudden withdrawal	a. Anticoagulant
23. ____ Increase hypotensive action of anesthetics	b. Phenothiazines
24. ____ Can induce electrolyte imbalance	c. Corticosteroids
25. ____ Increase bleeding intra- and postoperatively	d. Tranquilizers
26. ____ If stopped suddenly potentiate cardiovascular collapse	e. Diuretics

Nutrient	Role in wound healing
27. ____ Vitamin C	a. Tissue synthesis
28. ____ Vitamin K	b. Replaces elements from blood loss
29. ____ Vitamin A	c. Capillary formation
30. ____ Iron	d. Protein synthesis
31. ____ Zinc	e. Clot formation

(continued)

Disease Process	Resulting postoperative complication
32. ____ Diabetes mellitus	a. Wound dehiscence
33. ____ Gastric esophageal reflux disease	b. Airway obstruction
34. ____ Obesity	c. Impaired wound healing
35. ____ Bronchospasms	d. Pulmonary aspiration

APPLICATION QUESTIONS

1. The nurse goes in to meet and assess her client who had a vulvectomy 2 days ago. The client is dozing in bed in Fowler's position but states she is uncomfortable, when asked. Which action should the nurse take first?
   a. Call the physician
   b. Reposition the client in semi-Fowler's
   c. Administer pain medication
   d. Explain it is normal to be uncomfortable after the surgery.

2. The nurse should interpret a weight gain of 5.5 lb over 24 hours in a client with a biologic cardiac valve replacement as a sign of the development of which problem?
   a. Graft rejection
   b. Pericarditis
   c. Congestive heart failure
   d. Pyelonephritis

3. After which surgical procedure would the nurse plan to monitor the client's ankle-brachial index (ABI)?
   a. Off pump coronary artery bypass
   b. Dynamic cardiomyoplasty
   c. Carotid endarterectomy
   d. Femoral-popliteal bypass

4. The evening nurse goes in to care for a client who had a modified mastectomy that morning. Which fact is essential for the nurse to know to provide safe care?
   a. The involved arm should be wearing an elastic sleeve.
   b. The involved arm should not be used for BP measurement.
   c. The involved arm should be not be exercised for 10 days.
   d. The involved arm should be maintained at the level of the heart.

5. Which assessment finding(s) on a client who had a transurethral resection of the prostate for BPH 4 hours ago would indicate the need to notify the physician?
   a. Red bloody urine with small clots
   b. BP of 110/50 mm Hg, pulse 130 bpm
   c. Urinary output of 200 ml. greater than intake
   d. Pain related to bladder spasms

6. The nurse should interpret a complaint of joint pain from a client with a mechanical heart valve as potentially indicative of which problem?
   a. Streptococcal infection
   b. Vegetative embolus
   c. Bleeding
   d. Hypoxemia

7. A client with atrial fibrillation suddenly complains of acute, severe pain in the left arm. On assessment the nurse finds the arm to be cold, pale, and without palpable pulses. Which problem should the nurse suspect?
   a. Myocardial infarction
   b. Compartment syndrome
   c. Arterial embolus
   d. Hypovolemic shock

8. When caring for a postoperative client who has had a thyroidectomy, which medication should the nurse ensure is immediately available at the bedside?
   a. Calcium gluconate
   b. Propylthiouracil
   c. SSKI
   d. Synthroid

9. A client having surgery for glaucoma asks the nurse how the doctor will know if the surgery is successful. Which would be an appropriate response for the nurse to make?
   a. IOP will decrease
   b. Ability to read small print will improve
   c. Pupil will remain permanently dilated
   d. Peripheral vision will increase

10. Which advice would be appropriate for the nurse to give to a client with dumping syndrome?
    a. Take a drink after every four to five bites of food at a meal
    b. Eat several small meals per day of wet foods
    c. Remain in an upright position for 30–60 minutes after eating
    d. Avoid foods that are concentrated carbohydrates

11. When caring for a client who has had a kidney transplant, the nurse assesses for signs of rejection. For which S&S would the nurse observe? Mark all that apply.
    a. Change in urinary output
    b. Flank pain
    c. Edema
    d. Sudden weight gain

12. After which procedure would the nurse be expected to titrate IV fluids to replace output during the first 24 hours?
    a. Liver transplant
    b. Heart transplant
    c. Kidney transplant
    d. Lung transplant

13. Which action should the nurse take when during assessment, he/she finds the client who is 2 days post a liver transplant has a temperature persistent of 101.5°F, pulse 95, and respiratory rate of 18?
    a. Reposition the client
    b. Administer oxygen
    c. Administer pain medication
    d. Call the physician

14. When conducting discharge teaching for a transplant client, the nurse must make sure the client and family understand the importance of which self-care activities? Mark all that apply.
    a. Medication compliance
    b. Reporting of S&S etc.
    c. Keeping follow-up appointments
    d. Establishing a set sleep/wake routine

15. Which directions would the nurse give to a client who is being prepared for discharge following a pneumonectomy? Mark all that apply.
    a. Continue breathing exercises at home.
    b. Exercise arm and shoulder five times per day.
    c. Practice standing straight with shoulders even in front of the mirror.
    d. Do not lift more than 20 lb for at least a month.
    e. Stop any activity that causes dyspnea, chest pain, or excessive fatigue.
    f. Obtain influenza and pneumonia vaccines.
    g. Expect an intermittent cough with increased sputum.

16. A client with which problem needs careful assessment for the development of ARDS?
    a. Pericarditis
    b. Anemia
    c. Acute pancreatitis
    d. Pyelonephritis

17. A client having cryosurgery for removal of a squamous cell carcinoma asks if the procedure will hurt. Which is the correct answer for the nurse to give?
    a. "You will not feel anything."
    b. "There will be a brief tingling pain."
    c. "There will be no pain but you may experience a slight odd smell."
    d. "There will be a momentary, stabbing pain."

18. When planning for the postoperative care of clients having a thyroidectomy, which piece of equipment is most essential for the nurse to have available at the bedside?
    a. Suction machine
    b. Tracheostomy set
    c. Cardiac monitor
    d. Humidifier

19. Which S&S occurring in a client 48 hours postadrenalectomy indicate that glucocorticoid dosage needs to be increased?
    a. Marked weakness, anorexia, nausea or vomiting.
    b. Severe dyspnea, tachycardia, apprehension
    c. Paresthesias, numbness and tingling in the extremities, muscle spasms
    d. Orthostatic hypotension, depressed reflexes, slow mentation.

20. A visitor with an obvious upper respiratory infection arrives to see a client 24 hours postoperative from an adrenalectomy. The nurse explains that it is very important that the client not be exposed to anyone

(continued)

with a contagious illness. The visitor asks why. Which fact should be the basis of the nurse's answer?

a. The client is unable to fight infection because of loss of stress hormones.

b. Fluid and electrolyte fluctuations create an environment in which infective organisms can thrive.

c. Risk of infection is greatly increased because of excess cortisol.

d. The immune system is suppressed as part of the preparation for surgery and it takes 3–4 weeks for it to regain normal function.

21. When teaching self-care to a client who has had abdominal liposuction, which information should the nurse include?

a. Wear the compression garment when up for 2 weeks

b. Take aspirin as needed for discomfort

c. Expect asymmetry in the first few weeks after which it will taper off.

d. Avoid weight gain so effect of surgery is not negated.

22. Which statement made by a client who has had a blepharoplasty indicates the need for further teaching?

a. "I will avoid reading for 2–3 days."

b. "I will not be able to wear my contact lenses for at least 2 weeks."

c. "I will apply warm compresses to control swelling."

d. "I need to avoid alcohol for 3 weeks."

23. A client scheduled for a nephrectomy asks during the preoperative teaching session when the drain in the wound will be removed. Which is the best reply for the nurse to give?

a. At the same time the sutures are removed.

b. Not until urinary output is clear and at least 600 ml/24 hours.

c. After narcotics are no longer required for pain relief.

d. When drainage has decreased to less than 30 ml/d.

24. Which problem places a client scheduled for a nephrostomy at the greatest risk for postoperative hemorrhage?

a. Diabetes mellitus

b. History of urinary tract infections

c. Uncontrolled hypertension

d. Pernicious anemia

25. Which information should be included in the teaching plan for a client who has had a ureterosigmoidostomy?

a. Lifelong prophylactic antibiotics will be needed.

b. Annual sigmoidoscopy should be obtained starting 10 years after surgery.

c. Fluid intake should not exceed 1200 ml/d.

d. Diet should be high in fiber and low in fat

ANSWERS & RATIONALES

ANSWERS FOR FILL IN THE BLANKS

1. Surgical removal of one or more of the fallopian tubes is referred to as a salpingectomy.

2. A hysterectomy may be performed to control life-threatening bleeding/hemorrhage and in the event of intractable pelvic infection.

3. After a vasectomy, applying ice to the scrotum intermittently for several hours will help to reduce swelling and relieve discomfort.

4. The client on a cardiopulmonary bypass pump is maintained in a state of hypothermia in order to decrease metabolic needs.

5. Postoperatively, the client who has had a CABG procedure usually is instructed to avoid excessive arm movements for 6–8 weeks.

6. What piece of equipment must be kept at the bedside of postoperative amputees? Answer: tourniquet.

7. To check for development of abdominal distention, the nurse measures abdominal girth.

8. When caring for a client who had a kidney removed, the nurse would expect the Jackson–Pratt drain to be removed when drainage has decreased to less than 30 ml/d.

9. The client who has had a craniotomy is at greatest risk for ICP during the first 24–48 hours after surgery because this is the time during which edema peaks.

10. The client with a middle fossa craniotomy should be positioned with the head of the bed elevated 30–40 degrees.

11. Transplantation from one part of the body to another is called a(n) autograft.

12. The live donor is primarily used in kidney transplants.

13. Cornea transplant is the only type of transplant done as outpatient surgery.

14. A major indicator for heart transplant is cardiomyopathy.

15. Graft rejection, immunosuppressant related, and technical are the three major types of transplant-associated complications.

16. The kidney client must be weighed daily.

17. In addition to loss of vision, bleeding and infection, a complication associated with eye surgery is increased IOP.

18. The two greatest risk associated with inner ear surgery are infection and leakage of CSF.

19. A life-threatening complication of a long bone fracture is a fat embolism.

20. Infection most often occurs when an amputation is traumatic.

21. List four categories of medication that interact with anesthetic agents.
    a. ____________________
    b. ____________________
    c. ____________________
    d. ____________________
    Answers may include corticosteroids, diuretics, phenothiazines, tranquilizers, insulin, antibiotics, antiseizure medication, and monoamine oxidase inhibitors.

22. Identify three causes of airway obstruction following a surgical procedure.
    a. ____________________
    b. ____________________
    c. ____________________
    Answers may include tongue blocking the airway, hypoxemia, bronchospasm, and hypoventilation.

(continued)

23. List four symptoms of hemorrhage.

a. ______

b. ______

c. ______

d. ______

Answers may include increased pulse rate, restlessness, cold moist skin, low hemoglobin level, and decreased cardiac output.

24. Identify two types of exercises a client can be taught to perform to decrease the postoperative complication deep vein thrombosis.

a. ______

b. ______

Answers may include straight leg raises, quadriceps sets, gluteal tightening, and ankle pumps.

25. The medication commonly used to reverse the effects of opioids is ______.

Answer: Narcan (It is a narcotic antagonist and blocks opiate receptor sites.)

26. Hypoxia can be assessed by performing ______ and ______.

Answer: Oxygen saturation level and capillary refill.

27. Normal bowel sounds following a surgical procedure generally are audible within ______ hours.

Answer: 24–48 hours. (Peristalsis should begin about 6 hours after the surgical procedure, but can take up to 24 hours to be considered normal bowel sounds.)

28. Identify three examples of nonnarcotic pain management.

a. ______

b. ______

c. ______

Answers may include: Imagery, relaxation, heat/cold, distraction, back rub, and noncontact therapeutic touch.

29. A herbal medicine that neutralizes antibiotics is ______.

Answer: Kava-kava, which also potentiates central nervous system depressants, anesthetics, alcohol, and corticosteroids.

30. Arthritic changes of the cervical spine can result in ______.

Answer: difficult intubation.

31. A bluish tinge around the umbilicus that is an indicator of either intra-abdominal bleeding peritoneal bleeding is called ______.

Answer: Cullen's sign.

32. List three causes of urinary retention in a postoperative client.

a. ______

b. ______

c. ______

Correct answers may include: medication (opioids, atropine), epidural anesthesia, recumbent position, abdominal surgery, prolonged immobility, sympathetic nerve stimulation due to pain, anxiety, and fear.

TRUE & FALSE ANSWERS

Mark each of the following statements True or False. Correct all false statements in the space provided.

1. Dilation and curettage may be necessary for a woman with dysfunctional bleeding. *True.*

2. An advantage to use of a biologic heart valve for valve replacement is that it lasts longer than a mechanical valve. *False*
   Biological valves do not last as long as mechanical valves but they have the advantage of being less likely to cause thromboemboli.

3. Dynamic cardiomyoplasty is performed to correct hypertrophic cardiomyopathy. *False*
   Hypertrophic cardiomyopathy is a contraindication to dynamic cardiomyoplasty.

4. The pericardium can be removed without any significant harmful effects on the client. *True*

5. Speech is lost with a supraglottic laryngectomy. *False*
   Voice quality is changed with a supraglottic laryngectomy; it is only lost with a total laryngectomy.

6. Tracheostomy suctioning is a clean procedure. *False*
   Tracheostomy care and suctioning requires use of sterile technique.

7. Clients with a tracheostomy cannot swim. *False*
   Clients with a tracheostomy can swim but only with a special device to prevent water from entering the respiratory tract.

8. A pillow is placed under the stump of an above the knee amputation (AK) to support it in an elevated position. *False*
   The stump is kept in an extended position to avoid development of a contracture at the hip.

9. Nasogastric drainage decreases as peristalsis returns after gastric surgery. *True*

10. A client with an ileal conduit should take a shower with the urine collection bag in place. *False*
    The stoma should be uncovered during showering or bathing but should be patted, not rubbed, to cleanse and dry it.

11. Clients having a skin lesion removed by cryosurgery should be told that they will feel a tingling sensation when the freezing substance is applied. *True*

12. Phantom breast pain can occur following a mastectomy *True*

13. Reducing tension on the suture lines is an important part of the care for a client with a vulvectomy. *True*

14. Surgically induced menopause occurs in premenopausal women who have a bilateral salpingo-oophorectomy. *True*

15. The goal of surgery done to treat glaucoma is to lower IOP. *True.*

16. The United Network for Organ Sharing (UNOS) is responsible for ensuring available organs are distributed equitably. *True*

17. The National Organ Transplant Act established the organ donor card system. *False*
    The Uniform Anatomical Gift Act established the organ donor card system.

18. Before organs can be harvested, the family must give written consent. *True*

19. Psychological readiness and severe functional disability are not criteria for determining transplant need. *False*
    Criteria for determining transplant need are end-stage organ failure, short life expectancy, severe functional disability, absence of other serious health problems, psychological readiness and financial status.

(continued)

20. A complication of breast augmentation is the formation of scar tissue around the implant, which makes the breast feel tight or hard. *True*

21. Preoperative preparation of the operative site includes shaving the site prior to the client going to the operating room. *False*
Shaving in of the surgical site occurs in the operating room.

22. Shivering during the immediate postoperative patient is indicative of a need for continued use of oxygen. *True*
Shivering increases the oxygenation needs of the client due to the expenditure of energy.

23. Hypoxemia is defined as a PO_2 level less than 65 mm Hg. *False*
Hypoxemia is a PO_2 level <60 mm Hg.

24. Clients in the PACU are usually assessed every 15 minutes. *True*
An assessment is performed every 10–15 minutes of the clients' condition, which includes VS.

25. A client whose skin that is cool, moist, and pale is experiencing hypotension. *False*
Though cool, moist skin is a symptom of hypotension and shock when the skin becomes pale the client is hemorrhaging.

26. Warm blankets are provided to clients in PACU to reduce hypothermia. *True*
During surgery client's experience hypothermia both due to the coldness of the room and administration of anesthetic agents.

27. The basal metabolic rate of a client increases during surgery. *True*
During surgery the client's basal metabolic rate increases, which requires use of more calories than client typically consumes.

28. Gynecological surgery places a client at risk for deep vein thrombosis. *True*

29. Only the use of sequential compression devices can prevent the development of deep vein thrombosis. *False*
Lower leg and ankle exercises performed by the client and use of TEDS can assist in preventing deep vein thrombosis.

30. A client with skeletal deformities has a higher risk of postoperative pulmonary complications. *True*
Other diseases and behaviors that increase the postoperative risk of pulmonary complications include smoking, chronic obstructive pulmonary disease, and respiratory infection.

31. Antiseizure medications should not be administered during surgery even for the client who routinely takes this category of medication. *False*
Antiseizure medications will be administered intravenously during surgery to prevent the occurrence of seizure activity.

32. Nurses are not to provide education on what a client should expect to see in the operating room. *False*
It is important to instruct the client on the general environment of the operating room to decrease their preoperative anxiety and to decrease the number of unknowns.

33. Clients do not need to ambulate in order for peristalsis to return following a surgical procedure. *False*
Ambulation facilitates the return of peristalsis.

34. A change in the color of a stoma, such as a colostomy, from bright red to pale gray is not unusual. *False*
A stoma with adequate circulation is always bright red. Any change in color is indicative of loss of circulation to the bowel.

35. Surgical clients should receive total parenteral nutrition if they are not able to take in nutrients for more than 3 days. *True*
Surgical clients will deplete their protein stores within 3–5 days if the only nutrition being given is IV fluids.

MATCHING ANSWERS

1. __h__ Endarterectomy	a. Antireflux procedure
2. __c__ Partial laryngectomy	b. Removal of the urinary bladder
3. __b__ Cystectomy	c. Removal of the vocal cord and a section of the larynx
4. __a__ Fundoplication	d. Procedure done for glaucoma
5. __e__ Salpingectomy	e. Removal of the Fallopian tubes
6. __d__ Trabeculectomy	f. Urinary diversion procedure
7. __j__ Supraglottic laryngectomy	g. Incision into the ear drum
8. __g__ Myringotomy	h. Incision into an artery with removal of atheromatous material
9. __f__ Ileal conduit	i. Procedure used for pancreatic cancer
10. __i__ Whipple procedure	j. Removal of the hyoid bone, glottis and false vocal cords

Medication	Used for
11. __d__ Atropine sulfate	a. Permits smoother induction of anesthetic
12. __e__ Hydroxyzine hydrochloride	b. Decreases amount of anesthetic needed
13. __c__ Midazolam hydrochloride	c. Provides amnesia
14. __b__ Morphine sulfate	d. Decreases respiratory and gastric secretions
15. __g__ Panax ginseng	e. Decreases anxiety
16. __a__ Pentobarbital sodium	f. Prolongs sedative effects of anesthesia
17. __f__ Valeriana officinalis	g. Inhibits platelet aggregation

Medical Problem	Description
18. __a__ Paralytic ileus	a. Absent bowel sounds
19. __d__ Cullen's sign	b. Separation of approximated wound edges
20. __b__ Dehiscence	c. Bowel protruding from a surgical incision
21. __c__ Evisceration	d. An indication of intraabdominal bleeding

Interaction that may result when anesthetic is administered	Medication Category
22. __d__ Anxiety and seizures occur with sudden withdrawal	a. Anticoagulant

(continued)

23. __b__	Increase hypotensive action of anesthetics	b. Phenothiazines
24. __e__	Can induce electrolyte imbalance	c. Corticosteroids
25. __a__	Increases bleeding intra- and postoperatively	d. Tranquilizers
26. __c__	If stopped suddenly potentiate cardiovascular collapse	e. Diuretics

Nutrient		Role in wound healing
27. __c__	Vitamin C	a. Tissue synthesis
28. __e__	Vitamin K	b. Replaces elements from blood loss
29. __a__	Vitamin A	c. Capillary formation
30. __b__	Iron	d. Protein synthesis
31. __d__	Zinc	e. Clot formation

Disease Process		Resulting postoperative complication
32. __c__	Diabetes mellitus	a. Wound dehiscence
33. __d__	Gastric esophageal reflux disease	b. Airway obstruction
34. __a*__	Obesity	c. Impaired wound healing
35. __b__	Bronchospasms	d. Pulmonary aspiration

*The correct answer is a. Though obesity can also be a cause of pulmonary aspiration, the more likely postoperative complication is wound dehiscence.

APPLICATION ANSWERS

1. The nurse goes in to meet and assess her client who had a vulvectomy 2 days ago. The client is dozing in bed in Fowler's position but states she is uncomfortable, when asked. Which action should the nurse take first?
   a. Call the physician
   b. Reposition the client in semi-Fowler's
   c. Administer pain medication
   d. Explain it is normal to be uncomfortable after the surgery

Rationale

Correct answer: b.

Change client's position to semi-Fowler's to alleviate discomfort and tension on suture line; sitting in a Fowler's position puts direct pressure on suture line(s) and causes discomfort. Pain medication cannot be administered without first checking for an order and determining when it was last given. In addition, change in position that may relieve the discomfort can be done immediately while the nurse is at the bedside, so it is the first action the nurse should take. Explaining discomfort is normal may relieve anxiety but client's have a right to pain relief whether pain is expected or not.

2. The nurse should interpret a weight gain of 5.5 lb over 24 hours in a client with a biologic cardiac valve replacement as a sign of the development of which problem?
   a. Graft rejection
   b. Pericarditis
   c. Congestive heart failure
   d. Pyelonephritis

Rationale

Correct answer: c.

Weight gain, dyspnea, and tachycardia are symptoms of CHF, which can occur with graft failure. Hyperacute graft rejection is almost exclusively limited to transplanted kidneys and is a rare event because of careful cross matching before transplant. Symptoms of pericarditis include severe precordial pain, which is worse when lying supine and reduced when sitting up, fever, tachycardia, and myalgia. Symptoms of pyelonephritis include fever, chills, flank pain, costovertebral angle tenderness, and signs of lower UTI.

3. After which surgical procedure would the nurse plan to monitor the client's ankle-brachial index (ABI)?
   a. Off pump coronary artery bypass
   b. Dynamic cardiomyoplasty
   c. Carotid endarterectomy
   d. Femoral-popliteal bypass

Rationale

Correct answer: d.

Ankle-brachial index is a test of arterial status in the lower extremity. Normal arteries in the foot (dorsalis pedis and posterior tibial) have an index of 1.0–1.2. An index below 1.0 indicates arterial obstruction. After a bypass graft procedure in the leg, ABI is measured every 8 hours for the first 24 hours and then once a day. Peripheral pulses, color, and sensation in the extremity are also monitored. Arterial status of the foot is not a major concern after off pump coronary artery bypass, dynamic cardiomyoplasty, or carotid endarterectomy.

4. The evening nurse goes in to care for a client who had a modified mastectomy that morning. Which fact is essential for the nurse to know to provide safe care?
   a. The involved arm should be wearing an elastic sleeve.
   b. The involved arm should not be used for BP measurement.
   c. The involved arm should be not be exercised for 10 days.
   d. The involved arm should be maintained at the level of the heart.

Rationale

Correct answer: b.

BP should not be measured on the arm on the operative side because the procedure interferes with circulation and can cause venous congestion in the affected extremity. Elastic sleeves are used in the management of lymphedema after a mastectomy. Limited exercises of the affected arm are started on the evening of surgery. The involved arm should not be kept in a dependent position for an extended length of time and if edema is present, it should be elevated as much time as possible.

5. Which assessment finding(s) on a client who had a transurethral resection of the prostate for BPH 4 hours ago would indicate the need to notify the physician?
   a. Red bloody urine with small clots
   b. BP of 110/50 mmHg, pulse 130 bpm
   c. Urinary output of 200 ml greater than intake
   d. Pain related to bladder spasms

Rationale

Correct answer: b.

A rapid pulse with a low BP is a potential sign of excessive blood loss and physician should be notified based on this finding. Some hematuria is usual for several days after surgery. A urinary output of 200 ml or greater than intake is adequate. Bladder spasms are expected to occur following surgery.

6. The nurse should interpret a complaint of joint pain from a client with a mechanical heart valve as potentially indicative of which problem?
   a. Streptococcal infection
   b. Vegetative embolus
   c. Bleeding
   d. Hypoxemia

Rationale

Correct answer: c.

Mechanical valves require that a client be on anticoagulant therapy for life because of the risk of thromboemboli. Therefore, the client is at risk for bleeding associated with anticoagulation, signs of which are joint pain, black or tarry stools, blood in the urine, and bleeding gums. Streptococcal infection occurs anywhere in the body and symptoms depend in part on location of the infection. Osteomyelitis may be streptococcal in origin and bone pain occurs but not necessarily joint pain. A vegetative embolus is a complication of infective endocarditis in which a piece of the platelet fibrin bacteria mass called vegetation which

(continued)

forms on the heart valves breaks off and travels in the blood stream. Symptoms of an embolus depend on where it lodges in the body and to what extent blood flow to the tissues is disrupted. Hypoxemia refers to decreased oxygen in the blood defined as a below normal PaO2; hypoxia is oxygen lack at the tissue level. Joint pain due to hypoxia is seen in vasoocclusive crisis in sickle cell disease.

7. A client with atrial fibrillation suddenly complains of acute, severe pain in the left arm. On assessment the nurse finds the arm to be cold, pale, and without palpable pulses. Which problem should the nurse suspect?
   a. Myocardial infarction
   b. Compartment syndrome
   c. Arterial embolus
   d. Hypovolemic shock

Rationale

Correct answer: c.

Arterial emboli are often associated with atrial fibrillation and often cause acute arterial occlusion the S&S of which are pain in the affected area, paralysis, absence of pulses, pallor, paresthesias, numbness and coolness. MI can cause an arterial embolus but an MI itself does not cause these symptoms. Compartment syndrome occurs when pressure, usually from edema, bleeding, or restrictive dressing, increases in a limited anatomic space and compromises circulation and function of tissues within the space. It is not caused by atrial fibrillation and symptoms are unrelenting pain, pallor, pulselessness, and paresthesias. Symptoms of hypovolemic shock are systemic, not limited to one extremity.

8. When caring for a postoperative client who has had a thyroidectomy, which medication should the nurse ensure is immediately available at the bedside?
   a. Calcium gluconate
   b. Propylthiouracil
   c. SSKI
   d. Synthroid

Rationale

Correct answer: a.

Calcium gluconate should be immediately available at the bedside of a client who has had a thyroidectomy because of the risk of hypocalcemic tetany. Propylthiouracil, an antithyroid drug, blocks synthesis of thyroid hormone and is used in the treatment of hyperthyroidism. SSKI decreases blood flow to the thyroid gland. Synthroid is a thyroid hormone replacement drug and is used in the treatment of hypothyroidism.

9. A client having surgery for glaucoma asks the nurse how the doctor will know if the surgery is successful. Which would be an appropriate response for the nurse to make?
   a. IOP will decrease
   b. Ability to read small print will improve
   c. Pupil will remain permanently dilated
   d. Peripheral vision will increase

Rationale

Correct answer: a.

The reason surgery is done for glaucoma is to lower IOP because increased IOP causes progressive loss of vision. Surgery is done when medication is ineffective. Damage done by increased IOP is permanent; therefore, ability to read is not improved. The pupil is not affected by the surgery so contraction and dilation occur normally. Glaucoma causes loss of peripheral vision before loss of central vision and this loss is irreversible.

10. Which advice would be appropriate for the nurse to give to a client with dumping syndrome?
    a. Take a drink after every four to five bites of food at a meal
    b. Eat several small meals per day of wet foods
    c. Remain in an upright position for 30–60 minutes after eating
    d. Avoid foods that are concentrated carbohydrates

Rationale

Correct answer: d.

Foods that are concentrated carbohydrates should be avoided. Dumping syndrome has vasomotor (tachycardia, diaphoresis, flushing, weakness, palpitations, and anxiety) and GI symptoms (distention, nausea, vomiting, and diarrhea) and occurs when there is a rapid entry of boluses of hyperosmolar food directly into the small intestine. To decrease the symptoms of dumping syndrome, a client also should eat six small meals per day of dry foods and should not drink fluids with meals; avoid very hot or cold foods; and lie down for 30–60 minutes after eating.

11. When caring for a client who has had a kidney transplant, the nurse assesses for signs of rejection. For which S&S would the nurse observe? Mark all that apply.
    a. Change in urinary output
    b. Flank pain
    c. Edema
    d. Sudden weight gain

Rationale

Correct answers: a, b, c, and d.

Change in urinary output, flank pain, edema, and sudden weight gain that is reflective of edema because water has weight are all symptoms of rejection of a kidney transplant.

12. After which procedure would the nurse be expected to titrate IV fluids to replace output during the first 24 hours?
    a. Liver transplant
    b. Heart transplant
    c. Kidney transplant
    d. Lung transplant

Rationale

Correct answer: c.

Maintenance of fluid and electrolyte status is a key aspect of care following liver, heart, kidney, and lung transplants. However, it is only following a kidney transplant that I&O is checked hourly and IV fluids are titrated to replace output for the first 12–24 hours.

13. Which action should the nurse take when during assessment, he/she finds the client who is 2 days post a liver transplant has a temperature persistent of 101.5°F, pulse 95, and respiratory rate of 18?
    a. Reposition the client
    b. Administer oxygen
    c. Administer pain medication
    d. Call the physician

Rationale

Correct answer: d.

Because immunosuppressed clients do not have as robust an immune response to infection and symptoms will be more subtle such as a temperature of 101.5°F, tachycardia, and tachypnea. Infection and its treatment are the critical concerns in this situation for this client and none of the other options address these.

14. When conducting discharge teaching for a transplant client, the nurse must make sure the client and family understand the importance of which self care activities? Mark all that apply.
    a. Medication compliance
    b. Reporting of S&S etc.
    c. Keeping follow-up appointments
    d. Establishing a set sleep/wake routine

Rationale

Correct answers: a, b, and c.

Establishing a set sleep/wake routine is not essential for the transplant client and is not a part of routine discharge teaching for these clients.

15. Which directions would the nurse give to a client who is being prepared for discharge following a pneumonectomy? Mark all that apply.
    a. Continue breathing exercises at home.
    b. Exercise arm and shoulder five times per day.
    c. Practice standing straight with shoulders even in front of the mirror.
    d. Do not lift more than 20 lb for at least a month.
    e. Stop any activity that causes dyspnea, chest pain, or excessive fatigue.
    f. Obtain influenza and pneumonia vaccines.
    g. Expect an intermittent cough with increased sputum.

Rationale

Correct answers: a, b, c, e, and f.

Breathing exercises need to be continued usually for about 3 weeks. Arm and shoulder exercises need to be continued five times a day with 10–20 repetitions each time. Clients need to practice standing straight with shoulders even because the shoulder on the affected side will tend to be lower due to the transection of muscles and natural tendency to guard sore areas. Looking in the mirror is the best way to see how the shoulder needs to be held for posture to be correct. Any activity that causes dyspnea, chest pain, or excessive fatigue should be stopped; these are signs of exceeding the ability of the remaining lung to meet the demand for oxygen. Chest pain may indicate inadequate oxygen reaching the myocardium. Obtaining the pneumonia and influenza vaccines is important because with only one remaining lung there is almost no respiratory reserve and so the ability to cope with a respiratory infection is severely compromised.

It is incorrect to tell the client not to lift more than 20 lb for at least a month because heavy lifting must be avoided for 3–6 months. An intermittent cough with increased sputum is not expected. In fact if this occurs, it should be reported immediately.

16. A client with which problem needs careful assessment for the development of ARDS?
    a. Pericarditis
    b. Anemia
    c. Acute pancreatitis
    d. Pyelonephritis

Rationale

Correct answer: c.

ARDS is a complication of acute pancreatitis usually developing 3–7 days after the onset of the pancreatitis. It is most common in clients with severe volume depletion. The complication associated with pericarditis is pericardial effusion, with anemia the risk is for congestive heart failure. With pyelonephritis, intractable infection that may require surgery, even nephrectomy, to eradicate it.

(continued)

17. A client having cryosurgery for removal of a squamous cell carcinoma asks if the procedure will hurt. Which is the correct answer for the nurse to give?
    a. "You will not feel anything."
    b. "There will be a brief tingling pain."
    c. "There will be no pain but you may experience a slight odd smell."
    d. "There will be a momentary, stabbing pain."

Rationale

Correct answer: b.

A brief tingling pain is felt with cryosurgery. An unpleasant odor can occur when electrocautery is used to burn abnormal tissue as in cases of cervical dysplasia or genital warts.

18. When planning for the postoperative care of clients having a thyroidectomy, which piece of equipment is most essential for the nurse to have available at the bedside?
    a. Suction machine
    b. Tracheostomy set
    c. Cardiac monitor
    d. Humidifier

Rationale

Correct answer: b.

A tracheostomy set is needed at the bedside because of the risk of respiratory distress from compression of the trachea from bleeding or edema, laryngeal spasm from hypocalcemic tetany, or vocal cord spasm secondary to laryngeal nerve damage.

19. Which S&S occurring in a client 48 hours postadrenalectomy indicate that glucocorticoid dosage needs to be increased?
    a. Marked weakness, anorexia, nausea, or vomiting.
    b. Severe dyspnea, tachycardia, apprehension
    c. Paresthesias, numbness and tingling in the extremities, muscle spasms
    d. Orthostatic hypotension, depressed reflexes, slow mentation.

Rationale

Correct answer: a.

Marked weakness, anorexia, nausea, or vomiting are S&S indicating that the dose of glucocorticoids needs to be increased. Severe dyspnea, tachycardia, and apprehension are S&S of respiratory/cardiovascular problems such as pulmonary edema. Paresthesias, numbness, tingling in the extremities, and muscle spasms are symptoms of hypocalcemic tetany. Orthostatic hypotension occurs postadrenalectomy but does not indicate a need for increased glucocorticoids nor do depressed reflexes and slow mentation.

20. A visitor with an obvious upper respiratory infection arrives to see a client 24 hours postoperative from an adrenalectomy. The nurse explains that it is very important that the client not be exposed to anyone with a contagious illness. The visitor asks why. Which fact should be the basis of the nurse's answer?
    a. The client is unable to fight infection because of loss of stress hormones.
    b. Fluid and electrolyte fluctuations create an environment in which infective organisms can thrive.
    c. Risk of infection is greatly increased because of excess cortisol.
    d. The immune system is suppressed as part of the preparation for surgery and it takes 3–4 weeks for it to regain normal function.

Rationale

Correct answer: c.

Excess cortisol increases the risk of infection because it decreases the inflammatory response. Loss of epinephrine and norepinephrine are not the important factors in the increased risk of infection. Fluid and electrolyte fluctuations do not create an environment in which infective organisms can thrive. The immune system is not suppressed in preparation for surgery.

21. When teaching self-care to a client who has had abdominal liposuction, which information should the nurse include?
    a. Wear the compression garment when up for 2 weeks
    b. Take aspirin as needed for discomfort
    c. Expect asymmetry in the first few weeks after which it will taper off.
    d. Avoid weight gain so effect of surgery is not negated.

Rationale

Correct answer: d.

Weight gain will negate the effect of the surgery. The compression garment must be worn for 7–10 days. Aspirin, as well as all anticoagulants, must be avoided because of the risk of bleeding. Asymmetry is a complication of the liposuction, it is not expected.

22. Which statement made by a client who has had a blepharoplasty indicates the need for further teaching?
    a. "I will avoid reading for 2–3 days."
    b. "I will not be able to wear my contact lenses for at least 2 weeks."
    c. "I will apply warm compresses to control swelling."
    d. "I need to avoid alcohol for 3 weeks."

Rationale

Correct answer: c.

Iced compresses are used to control swelling and discoloration. All other statements correctly apply to the client who has had a blepharoplasty.

23. A client scheduled for a nephrectomy asks during the preoperative teaching session when the drain in the wound will be removed. Which is the best reply for the nurse to give?
    a. At the same time the sutures are removed.
    b. Not until urinary output is clear and at least 600 ml/24 hr.
    c. After narcotics are no longer required for pain relief.
    d. When drainage has decreased to less than 30 ml/d

Rationale

Correct answer: d.

The Jackson–Pratt drain is removed when there is less than 30 ml of drainage in 24 hours. Sutures are removed in 7–10 days when the incision has healed. Urinary output is via the remaining kidney and has no relationship to the need for a drain in the operative area. Incisional pain is managed with opioid analgesics but pain is unrelated to drainage and the need for a drain.

24. Which problem places a client scheduled for a nephrostomy at the greatest risk for postoperative hemorrhage?
    a. Diabetes mellitus
    b. History of urinary tract infections
    c. Uncontrolled hypertension
    d. Pernicious anemia

Rationale

Correct answer: c.

BP needs to be tightly controlled in clients undergoing a nephrostomy because of the risk of hemorrhage. Diabetes mellitus, prior urinary tract infections, or pernicious anemia do not increase the risk of hemorrhage from the procedure.

25. Which information should be included in the teaching plan for a client who has had a ureterosigmoidostomy?
    a. Lifelong prophylactic antibiotics will be needed.
    b. Annual sigmoidoscopy should be obtained starting 10 years after surgery.
    c. Fluid intake should not exceed 1200 ml/d.
    d. Diet should be high in fiber and low in fat.

Rationale

Correct answer: b.

An annual sigmoidoscopy is recommended starting 10 years after surgery because of the increased risk of neoplasia developing in the sigmoid colon at the site of anastomosis of the ureters. Prophylactic antibiotics are not given, however, because there is the risk of kidney infection from reflux of feces, any temperature of 101°F or more, costovertebral angle pain, or significant changes in color, consistency, or amount of output should be reported to the health care provider. There is no limitation on fluid intake and no dietary restrictions.

CHAPTER 19

Test Plan Category:

Physiological Integrity

Sub-category: Physiological Adaptation—Part 1

Topics: Alterations in Body Systems
Illness Management
Section 1: Cardiovascular Problems

CARDIOVASCULAR PROBLEMS

PERICARDITIS

- Pericarditis refers to the inflammation of the layers of the pericardium.
- It may involve the diaphragm.
- It may be primary or secondary to other diseases.
- It is a frequent complication of end-stage renal disease.

Etiology: It may result from bacterial, viral, or fungal infections, immunologic disorders, connective tissue diseases, neoplasms, renal failure, myocardial infarction (MI), myocardial injury, radiation, or drugs.

Precipitating factors: Clients with conditions that leave them immunocompromised as noted above.

S&S:

- Chest pain that worsens when deep breathing or lying in a supine position and improves when sitting up taking shallow breaths (this is one means to discriminate from acute MI since chest pain in MI is usually not effected by change in position)
- Dyspnea
- Malaise
- Fever
- Cough
- Elevated ESR and WBC
- Pericardial friction rub heard most commonly on expiration

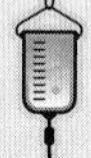

Clinical Alert

Pericardial effusion with the potential for cardiac tamponade is a rare but life-threatening complication.

Dx: Presence of pericardial friction rub upon auscultation of lung sounds, ECG reveals diffuse ST segment elevation and PR segment depression, abnormal CBC, changes to cardiac enzymes in response to inflammatory processes, positive blood cultures, ESR, echocardiography shows thickening and calcification of pericardium, hemodynamic monitoring, CXR, CT scan, and MRI

Rx: Treat underlying cause and initiate measures to relieve symptoms, treat pain with NSAIDs, and treat with antibiotics or antivirals as needed

Nursing Process Elements

- Monitor vital signs (VS) and heart sounds
- Administer pain medication to treat malaise and other flu-like symptoms
- Administer NSAIDs as ordered
- Allow for rest periods
- Monitor for signs of decreased cardiac output
- Provide comfort measures such as increased fluids, rest periods, and distraction techniques

Client teaching for self-care

Teach client to

- know the nature of the disease and ways to prevent recurrence
- adhere to medication schedule
- adopt ways to modify lifestyle to conserve energy and reduce fatigue during acute episode of illness
- recognize signs of recurrence such as chest pain, fever, and malaise

MYOCARDITIS

- Myocarditis refers to the inflammation of the myocardium.
- This inflammatory process causes edema and damage to the cells of the heart.
- It results in weakening of the heart muscle and decreased contractility.

Etiology: Infectious agents such as bacteria, viruses, protozoa, or helminths, toxins, systemic disease, radiation, and selective drugs.

Precipitating factors: Most common are viral infections especially for immunocompromised individuals (i.e., HIV).

S&S:

- Initially may be asymptomatic
- Tachycardia and dysrhythmia
- Unexplained heart failure
- Fever and chills
- Pleuritic chest pain with presence of friction rub
- Fatigue
- Dyspnea
- Palpitations
- Rales

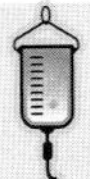

Clinical Alert

Presentation of myocarditis is often subacute and, if left untreated, can become a chronic condition that ultimately leads to dysrhythmias, congestive heart failure (CHF), or death.

Dx: Elevated viral titers and ESR, increased serum cardiac enzymes, nonspecific ST–T wave changes on ECG. Definitive diagnosis established with positive endomyocardial biopsy

Rx: IV antibiotics or antiviral, antipyretics, treat for signs of heart failure or dysrhythmias (medications to improve cardiac output or to treat dysrhythmias), monitor for complications such as cardiac tamponade or pneumothorax or bleeding postbiopsy

Nursing Process Elements

- Modify ADLs to respond to fatigue
- Address anxiety
- Provide emotional support
- Monitor VS and heart sounds
- Be alert for signs of heart failure
- Maintain bed rest or limited activity to decrease demands on cardiac function
- Place client in semi-Fowler's position to facilitate gas exchange
- Administer antibiotics or antivirals as well as other medications as needed

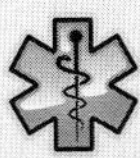

Nursing Assessment Alert

Monitor for digitalis toxicity since clients with myocarditis have increased sensitivity to digitalis.

Client teaching for self-care

Teach client to

- conserve energy
- plan activities throughout the day to allow for rest periods
- avoid NSAIDs since these have been found to increase myocardial damage
- follow a heart-healthy diet
- adhere to medication regimen
- know early signs of heart failure such as dyspnea and peripheral edema to avoid recurrence or complications

ENDOCARDITIS

- Endocarditis refers to the infection of the endocardial surface (lining) of the heart including the valves.
- The inflammatory process allows the formation of clots or vegetations to form on the heart valves and these areas become an area to which bacteria migrate and multiply.
- The presence of the vegetation fosters bacterial growth.
- It has acute and subacute classifications.

Etiology: Rheumatic heart disease, clients with prosthetic heart valves, IV drug use, mitral valve prolapse (very common cause), and infection-causing organisms usually bacteria (*Streptococci*, *Enterococci*, or *Staphylococcus aureous*).

Precipitating factors: Underlying cardiac conditions, dental, surgical, or invasive procedures, or urological procedures. There must be some mechanism to allow entrance of bacteria to the bloodstream.

S&S:

- Malaise
- Anorexia
- Fever
- Fatigue
- Weight loss
- Night sweats
- Heart murmurs
- Elevated ESR and WBC

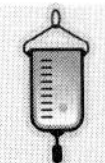

Clinical Alert

Infective endocarditis has a 20–30% mortality rate.

Dx: Positive blood cultures, laboratory work reflecting an infectious or inflammatory process, and presence of valvular vegetations on echocardiogram

Rx: Prolonged course of antibiotics to eliminate all microorganisms from the vegetative growth (4–6 weeks in duration) and to prevent complications. Clients with valve damage may require surgical repair or replacement of damaged valves

Nursing Process Elements

- Monitor VS and heart sounds (assess for presence of murmurs)

- Administer IV antibiotics and monitor for side effects such as renal or ototoxicity associated with high doses or prolonged therapy
- Monitor for signs of heart failure
- Assess for signs of embolic event or dysrhythmias
- Provide adequate rest periods

Client teaching for self-care

Teach client

- ways to avoid recurrence of infection such as use of antibiotic prophylaxis for dental or urological procedures
- ways to modify lifestyle so as to avoid excessive fatigue and to stop activities that result in chest pain, faintness, or dyspnea
- about the importance of completing medication schedule for antibiotics and to not stop therapy prematurely since this may lead to recurrence or complications
- about the side effects of medications

RHEUMATIC FEVER

- Rheumatic fever is a systemic inflammatory autoimmune disease.
- It usually follows a group A beta-hemolytic streptococcal infection.
- It can involve the heart, joints, skin, and brain.

Etiology: It is a delayed illness of an upper respiratory infection caused by a group A beta-hemolytic streptococcal infection.

Precipitating factors: An upper respiratory infection, such as strep throat, scarlet fever, tonsillitis, pharyngitis, approximately 2–6 weeks prior.

S&S:

- Fever
- Joint pain, migratory polyarthritis
- Joint swelling; redness, or warmth
- Abdominal pain
- Skin rash (erythema marginatum)
- Aschoff bodies, inflammatory hemorrhagic bullous lesions located on the myocardium usually found on autopsy
- Sydenham's chorea also called St.Vitus Dance—emotional instability, muscular weakness and rapid, uncoordinated jerky movements affecting primarily the face, feet, and hands
- Epistaxis (nosebleeds)
- Carditis
- Subcutaneous nodules located on extensor surfaces of knees, elbows, and knuckles
- Cardiac murmur

Dx: Based on clinical presentation with signs and symptoms of carditis, polyarthritis, chorea, characteristic rash, and subcutaneous nodules being major manifestations.

Rx: Anti-inflammatory medications such as aspirin or corticosteroids; antibiotic therapy (penicillin, erythromycin), includes the continuous use of low dose antibiotics to prevent recurrence; supportive therapy for other symptoms

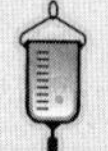

Clinical Alert

Salicylates are avoided until the diagnosis is confirmed or denied as they may mask some symptoms of rheumatic fever.

Nursing Process Elements

- Assess for risk factors
- Monitor VS
- Assess laboratory values for elevated erythrocyte sedimentation rate, C-reactive protein
- Monitor heart sounds and ECG
- Medicate as prescribed for pain
- Implement comfort measures
- Administer antibiotics as prescribed
- Maintain bed rest during acute stage
- Maintain fluid balance
- Provide emotional support
- Provide client and family education with respect to prophylactic antibiotic therapy to reduce the risk of recurrent rheumatic fever
- Instruct client and family in proper and prompt treatment of strep throat and scarlet fever
- Provide client and family education on the course and recurrence of rheumatic fever

CARDIAC DYSRHYTHMIA

- Cardiac dysrhythmias refers to any disturbance or abnormality in the cardiac conduction system causing an alteration in cardiac rate or rhythm.
- Normal conduction goes from the Sinoatrial (SA) Node → Atrioventricular (AV) Node → bundle of His → bundle branches → Purkinje fibers.

- Dysrhythmias may be benign or lethal.
- The terms "arrhythmia" and "dysrhythmia" are used interchangeably.
- Normal ECG interpretation:
  —Heart rate is 60–100 bpm.
  —Rhythm is regular.
  —P wave is present and there is one in front of every QRS.
  —PR interval is 0.12–0.20 seconds.
  —QRS is 0.06–0.10 seconds.

Etiology: There are two major categories of dysrhythmias:

- Alteration in impulse formation
  —Rate: tachycardia (over 100 bpm) or bradycardia (under 60 bpm)
  —Rhythm: regular or irregular
  —Ectopic: impulse starts outside the SA node, may be in the atria, junction, or ventricles
- Alteration in conductivity
  —Heart blocks
  —Reentry phenomena: activation of the muscle twice for one impluse

Precipitating factors: Ischemia, electrolyte disturbances, fever, acidosis, stress, exercise, pain, hypoxia, anemia, hypovolemia, cardiac and systemic diseases, atherosclerosis, medications, trauma, metabolic disorders, caffeine, alcohol, and aging.

S&S:

- May be asymptomatic
- Dizziness, angina, disorientation, hypotension, syncope, palpitations, diaphoresis, fatigue, shortness of breath, changes in pulse rate or rhythm
- Lethal dysrhythmias may progress to absence of pulse, heart sounds, blood pressure, and consciousness. Pupils can become dilated and cyanosis and seizures can develop leading to death

Dx: 12-lead ECG, continuous ECG monitoring, intermittent ECG recording, stress test, electrophysiology studies, history and physical examination. Diagnostic studies to help determine cause of dysrhythmias may include blood chemistry, chest X-ray, and echocardiogram

Rx: Depends on the dysrhythmia

SINUS TACHYCARDIA

In sinus tachycardia,

- pacemaker site is SA node,
- heart rate is between 101 bpm and 160 bpm,
- rhythm is regular,
- P waves present and one in front of every QRS,
- PRI is normal, and
- QRS is normal.

Etiology: Usually a symptom of an underlying condition which causes a compensatory response that enhances automaticity. There is either an increase in sympathetic nervous system response or a decrease in parasympathetic nervous system response. Increases cardiac workload and oxygen use.

Precipitating factors: Fever, exercise, fear, strong emotions, stress, alcohol, caffeine, nicotine, stimulants, thyrotoxicosis, myocardial ischemia, shock, hemorrhage, and anemia.

S&S:

- Often asymptomatic
- Increased pulse rate, palpitations, dyspnea, syncope, angina, disorientation, and anxiety
- Can produce pulmonary edema if prolonged and severe

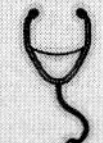

Assessment Alert

Reduced diastolic filling time may lead to decreased cardiac output with syncope and hypotension. It can be an early sign of cardiac dysfunction.

Dx: 12-lead ECG

Rx: Treat or eliminate underlying cause

- May need no intervention if client is asymptomatic
- Treat heart rate if unable to find or treat cause or symptoms persist
- Give oxygen at 2–4 lpm (liters per minute), if oxygen saturation decreases
- Beta blockers, verapamil, digoxin, or adenosine may be used to slow heart rate

Nursing Process Elements

- Monitor VS and cardiac rhythm
- Assess for underlying cause
- Treat underlying cause
  —Medicate for fever
  —Provide emotional support
  —Treat pain
  —Stop exercise
  —Eliminate caffeine and stimulants
  —Follow medical regime
- Assess S&S for developing complications

- Provide client education
- Administer medications as prescribed

Client teaching for self-care

Teach client

- to make necessary lifestyle changes
  - —eliminate stimulants
  - —reduce anxiety
  - —exercise in moderation
- about the causes and treatments for sinus tachycardia
- about when to seek medical care
- about the medication regime
  - —the side effect of medication
  - —how to take pulse
- to monitor pulse and blood pressure

SINUS BRADYCARDIA

In sinus bradycardia,

- pacemaker site is SA node,
- heart rate is less than 60 bpm,
- rhythm is regular,
- P waves present and one in front of every QRS,
- PRI is normal, and
- QRS is normal.

Etiology: It may be a result of increased vagal activity or decreased automaticity due to injury or ischemia of the sinus node.

Precipitating factors: Normally seen in well-trained athletes and often when people are sleeping. Other causes include vagal stimulation (severe pain, vomiting, bearing down during defecation, carotid massage), medications (digoxin, beta blockers, calcium channel blockers), increased intracranial pressure, metabolic disorders, hypothermia, ischemia of the sinus node, and inferior wall MI.

S&S:

- Often asymptomatic
- Decreased heart rate
- May cause hemodynamic instability such as syncope, dyspnea, hypotension, angina, decreased level of consciousness, ST-segment changes

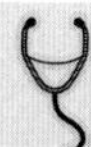

Assessment Alert

Always assess the client for hemodynamic instability before treating dysrhythmia.

Dx: 12-lead ECG, history and physical examination

Rx: None if client is asymptomatic. If client is becoming hemodynamically unstable, treat the cause and raise the heart rate.

- Stop or prevent further vagal stimulation
- Stop or decrease medications as ordered
- Decrease intracranial pressure
- Treat underlying conditions
- Decrease cardiac workload
- Give oxygen 2–4 lpm, if oxygen saturation is decreased
- Give medication to increase heart rate: Atropine 0.5–1.0 mg IVP
- Start emergency transcutaneous pacing if necessary

Nursing Process Elements

- Assess client for hemodynamic instability
- Monitor VS and cardiac rhythm
- Assess for underlying cause
- Treat underlying cause
  - —Decrease or stop medications (beta blockers, digoxin) as ordered
  - —Provide emotional support
  - —Decrease cardiac workload
  - —Maintain client safety
  - —Prepare for emergency treatment
  - —Follow medical regime
- Assess S&S for developing complications
- Provide client education
- Administer medications as prescribed

Client teaching for self-care

Instruct client

- about the causes and treatments for sinus bradycardia
- about when to seek medical care
- about the medication regime
  - —the side effect of medication
  - —how to take pulse
- to monitor pulse and blood pressure

PREMATURE ATRIAL CONTRACTIONS

In premature atrial contractions (PAC),

- pacemaker site is atrial tissue,
- rate is variable but underlying rate is normal,

- rhythm is irregular with normal rhythm being interrupted with an early beat,
- P waves are present for each QRS, but P wave for early beat will look different from sinus P waves and the P wave may be hidden in the previous T wave,
- PRI will be 0.12–0.20 seconds but may be shorter or longer for the early beat, and
- QRS is normal.

Etiology: Irritable foci in the atria assume the pacemaker function for a single beat. Irritable foci is often due to hypoxia.

Precipitating factors: Can occur in people with normal hearts. Causes include increase in stimulants such as caffeine or nicotine, stress, alcohol, stretched myocardium, hypoxemia, hypokalemia, hypermetabolic state, or atrial ischemia.

S&S:

- Often asymptomatic
- May feel heart "skip a beat"
- A pulse deficit (difference between apical and radial pulse) may exist
- May feel a pause when taking the pulse

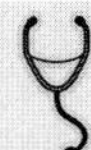

Assessment Alert

The most common cause for a pause in the heartbeat is a PAC.

Dx: 12-lead ECG

Rx: If infrequent, no treatment is necessary. If increasing in frequency and causing symptoms, treatment is focused on treating and/or eliminating the cause

- Decrease or stop stimulants
- Stress reduction
- Decrease or stop alcohol intake
- Treat CHF or underlying medical conditions
- Give oxygen 2–4 lpm as prescribed
- Treat electrolyte imbalances

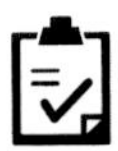

Nursing Process Elements

- Monitor VS and cardiac rhythm
- Assess for underlying cause
- Treat underlying cause
  —Provide emotional support
  —Treat underlying medical condition
  —Give oxygen
  —Treat electrolyte imbalance
  —Eliminate caffeine and stimulants
  —Follow medical regime
- Assess S&S for developing complications
- Provide client education
- Administer medications as prescribed

Client teaching for self-care

Teach client

- to make necessary lifestyle changes
  —eliminate stimulants
  —reduce anxiety
  —reduce alcohol intake
- about the causes and treatments for premature atrial contractions
- about when to seek medical care
- about the medication regime
  —the side effect of medication
  —how to take pulse
- to monitor pulse and blood pressure

ATRIAL TACHYCARDIA

In case of atrial tachycardia,

- pacemaker site is atrial tissue,
- rate is 101–250 bpm,
- rhythm is regular,
- P waves may or may not be present for each QRS. If present the P waves will look different from sinus P waves. P wave may be hidden in the previous T wave,
- PRI may or may not be measurable depending on the rate, and
- QRS is normal.

Etiology: Irritable foci in the atria assumes the pacemaker function which is rapid and sustained. Reentry phenomenon or abnormal automaticity.

Precipitating factors: Basically the same causes as PAC but atrial tachycardia is clinically more significant because the rate is prolonged and more rapid. Causes include increase in stimulants such as caffeine or nicotine, stress, alcohol, stretched myocardium, fever, sepsis, hypoxemia, hypokalemia, hypermetabolic state, atrial ischemia, and heart disease.

S&S:

- May be asymptomatic if rate is slower
- May feel heart "racing," palpitations
- A pulse deficit (difference between apical and radial pulse) may exist

- Dizziness, dyspnea, anxiety, diaphoresis, angina, fatigue, and polyuria
- If sustained may lead to angina, heart failure, and MI

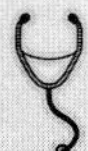

Assessment Alert

The more rapid the rate, the more likely a client is to experience symptoms since there is a decrease in diastolic filling time, increase in myocardial oxygen consumption, decrease in oxygen supply and decrease in cardiac output.

Dx: 12-lead ECG, continuous ECG monitoring, intermittent ECG recording if required, stress test, electrophysiology studies, history and physical examination

Rx: Decrease heart rate; stop reentry phenomenon

- Vagal stimulation
  —Have client "bear down" like having a bowel movement
  —Carotid sinus massage on one side at a time by a physician
- Treat CHF or underlying medical conditions
- Give oxygen 2–4 lpm as prescribed
- Medications to decrease heart rate:
  —Adenosine (Adenocard) 6-mg IV bolus followed with 20-ml saline flush; repeat with 12-mg bolus if necessary (contraindicated with people with severe asthma)
  —Amiodarone, diltizam, and digoxin
- Electrical synchronized cardioversion

Nursing Process Elements

- Assess client for hemodynamic instability
- Monitor VS and cardiac rhythm
- Assess for underlying cause
- Treat underlying cause
  —Provide emotional support
  —Treat underlying medical condition
  —Give oxygen
  —Treat electrolyte imbalance
  —Eliminate caffeine and stimulants
  —Follow medical regime
- Assess S&S for developing complications
- Provide client education
- Administer medications as prescribed
- Prepare for emergency electrical synchronized cardioversion

Client teaching for self-care

Instruct client

- to make necessary lifestyle changes
  —eliminate stimulants
  —reduce anxiety
- to reduce alcohol intake
- about the causes and treatments for atrial tachycardia
- about when to seek medical care
- about the medication regime
  —the side effect of medication
  —how to take pulse
- to monitor pulse and blood pressure

ATRIAL FLUTTER

In the case of atrial flutter,

- there are multiple pacemaker sites in the atrial tissue,
- atrial rate is between 250 bpm and 400 bpm; ventricular rate depends on AV conduction and is usually 75–150 bpm,
- atrial rhythm is regular, ventricular may be regular or irregular,
- P waves are saw-toothed and are called flutter or F waves,
- PRI is not measurable. Conduction ratio of atrial to ventricular may be 2:1, 3:1, 4:1,5:1, 6:1, or variable, and
- QRS is normal.

Etiology: Intra-atrial reentry mechanism which causes a rapid and regular atrial rhythm.

Precipitating factors: Preexisting cardiac disease such as CHF, coronary artery disease (CAD), MI, cardiomyopathy; pulmonary embolism, thyrotoxicosis, abnormal conduction syndromes, and conditions that stimulate the sympathetic nervous system such as anxiety, caffeine, stress, and alcohol intake.

S&S:

- May be asymptomatic if ventricular rate is slower
- May feel heart "fluttering," palpitations
- A pulse deficit may exist
- Dizziness, dyspnea, anxiety, diaphoresis, angina, fatigue, and decreased urinary output
- If sustained may lead to angina, heart failure, and MI

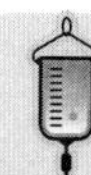

Clinical Alert

May lose the benefit of the atrial kick, which causes a further decrease in cardiac output.

Dx: 12-lead ECG

Rx: Decrease heart rate; stop reentry phenomenon

- Vagal stimulation may be used to help slow down rate to accurately identify rhythm
  - —Have client "bear down" like having a bowel movement
  - —Carotid sinus massage on one side at a time by a physician
- Treat underlying medical conditions
- Give oxygen 2–4 lpm as prescribed
- Medication to convert rhythm
  - —first line ibutilide (Corvert)
  - —second line flecainide, propafenone, procainamide, and amiodarone
- Medications to slow conduction via AV node
  - —Calcium channel blockers, beta blockers, and digoxin
- Electrical synchronized cardioversion
- Atrial overdrive pacing
- Radiofrequency ablation (RFA)

Nursing Process Elements

- Assess client for hemodynamic instability
- Monitor VS and cardiac rhythm
- Assess for underlying cause
- Treat underlying cause
  - —Provide emotional support
  - —Treat underlying medical condition
  - —Treat electrolyte imbalance
  - —Eliminate caffeine and stimulants
  - —Follow medical regime
- Start oxygen at 2–4 lpm if ordered
- Assess S&S for developing complications
- Provide client education
- Administer medications as prescribed
- Prepare for emergency elective cardioversion or surgery

Client teaching for self-care

Instruct client

- to make necessary lifestyle changes
  - —eliminate stimulants
  - —reduce anxiety
  - —reduce alcohol intake
- about the causes and treatments for atrial flutter
- about when to seek medical care
- about the medication regime
  - —the side effect of medication
  - —how to take pulse
- to monitor pulse and blood pressure

ATRIAL FIBRILLATION

In the case of atrial fibrillation,

- pacemaker sites are multiple reentry circuits in the atrial tissue,
- atrial rate is between 300 bpm and 600 bpm; ventricular rate depends on AV conduction and is usually 100–180 bpm,
- rhythm is irregularly irregular; irregular R-to-R intervals,
- P waves not identifiable, presence of chaotic fibrillatory wavelets,
- PRI is not measurable, and
- QRS is normal.

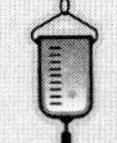

Clinical Alert

It is the most frequently encountered dysrhythmia in United States.

Etiology: Several intra-atrial reentry circuits which cause atria to quiver rather than contract.

Precipitating factors: Preexisting cardiac disease such as left ventricular hypertrophy, CHF, valvular heart disease, acute MI, myocarditis, and pericarditis; pulmonary embolism, hypertension, thyrotoxicosis, pneumonia, abnormal conduction syndromes, and conditions that stimulate the sympathetic nervous system such as anxiety, caffeine, stress, and alcohol intake.

S&S:

- May be asymptomatic if ventricular rate is slower
- May feel heart "fluttering," palpitations
- A pulse deficit may exist
- Dizziness, dyspnea, anxiety, diaphoresis, angina, fatigue, and decreased urinary output
- If sustained may lead to angina, heart failure, thrombus formation, stroke, and MI

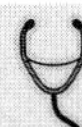

Assessment Alert

Loses the benefit of the atrial kick, which causes a further decrease in cardiac output.

Peripheral pulses are irregular and of variable strength.

Dx: 12-lead ECG

Rx: Stop reentry phenomenon and convert to NSR; control ventricular rate

- Treat underlying medical conditions
- Give oxygen 2–4 lpm as prescribed
- Medication to convert rhythm
  —Emergency drugs IV ibutilide (Corvert), amiodarone
  —Long term medications to maintain client in NSR include amiodarone, disopyramide, flecainide, and moricizine
- Medications to slow conduction via AV node
  —Calcium channel blockers, beta blockers, and digoxin
- Anticoagulants
- Electrical synchronized cardioversion
- Atrial pacing
- Cox-Maze III surgical procedure

Nursing Process Elements

- Assess client for hemodynamic stability
- Monitor VS and cardiac rhythm
- Assess for underlying cause
- Treat underlying cause
  —Provide emotional support
  —Treat underlying medical condition
  —Eliminate caffeine and stimulants
  —Follow medical regime
- Start oxygen at 2–4 lpm if ordered
- Assess S&S for developing complications
- Provide client education
- Administer medications as prescribed
- Prepare for emergency elective cardioversion or surgery

Client teaching for self-care

Teach client

- to make necessary lifestyle changes
  —eliminate stimulants
  —reduce anxiety
  —reduce alcohol intake
- about the causes and treatments for atrial flutter
- about when to seek medical care
- about the medication regime
  —the side effect of medication
  —how to take pulse
- to monitor pulse and blood pressure

PREMATURE VENTRICULAR CONTRACTIONS

In the case of premature ventricular contractions (PVC),

- pacemaker site is an irritable foci in the ventricular tissue,
- the normal rate is 60–100 bpm,
- the rhythm is irregular: PVC interrupts normal rhythm; it has a full compensatory pause,
- P wave is not present,
- PRI is absent, and
- QRS is wide and bizarre (>0.12 seconds).

Etiology: Irritable foci in the ventricle assumes the pacemaker function for one beat. Reentry phenomenon or abnormal automaticity may also be causes.

Precipitating factors: Acute ischemia, preexisting cardiac diseases such as CHF, CAD, mitral valve prolapse, or acute MI, metabolic abnormalities such as hypokalemia, hypoxemia, acidosis, digitalis toxicity, sympathomimetic drugs, and conditions that stimulate the sympathetic nervous system such as anxiety, caffeine, stress, and alcohol intake.

S&S:

- May be asymptomatic
- May feel heart "skip a beat," palpitations
- Depends on frequency of PVCs and on concomitant factors

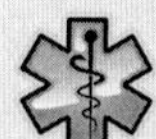

Nursing Intervention Alert

Treatment is indicated only when symptoms of decreased CO exist.

Dx: 12-lead ECG, continuous ECG monitoring, intermittent ECG recording if intermittent, stress test, electrophysiology studies, history and physical examination

Rx: Treat if client is experiencing symptoms

- Treat underlying medical conditions
- Check electrolytes
- Give oxygen 2–4 lpm as prescribed
- Eliminate stimulants
- Check for digitalis toxicity
- Monitor drugs for proarrhythmic effect
- Beta blockers may be given to reduce response to sympathetic stimulation

Nursing Process Elements

- Assess client for hemodynamic instability
- Monitor VS and cardiac rhythm

- Assess for underlying cause
- Monitor electrolytes
- Treat underlying cause
  —Provide emotional support
  —Treat underlying medical condition
  —Eliminate caffeine and stimulants
  —Follow medical regime
- Start oxygen at 2–4 lpm if ordered
- Assess S&S for developing complications
- Provide client education
- Administer medications as prescribed

Client teaching for self-care

Teach client

- to make necessary lifestyle changes
  —eliminate stimulants
  —reduce anxiety
  —reduce alcohol intake
  —stop tobacco use
- about the causes and treatments for PVCs
- about when to seek medical care
- about the medication regime
  —the side effect of medication
  —how to take pulse
- to monitor pulse and blood pressure

VENTRICULAR TACHYCARDIA

In the case of ventricular tachycardia (VT),

- pacemaker site is an irritable foci in the ventricular tissue which takes over as pacemaker for three or more consecutive beats,
- the atrial rate is indeterminable while the ventricular rate is 101–250 bpm,
- the rhythm is usually regular but may be slightly irregular,
- P wave is usually buried in the preceding QRS complex,
- PRI is indeterminable, and
- QRS is wide and bizarre (>0.12 seconds).

Etiology: Irritable foci in the ventricle assume the pacemaker function for three or more consecutive beats usually as a result of a reentry phenomenon.

Precipitating factors: Acute ischemia, preexisting cardiac diseases such as CHF, CAD, mitral valve prolapse, or acute MI and metabolic abnormalities such as hypokalemia, hypoxemia, acidosis, digitalis toxicity, and proarrhythmic effect of certain antidysrhythmic medications.

S&S:

- May feel heart "skip a beat," palpitations
- Depends on frequency of PVCs and on concomitant factors

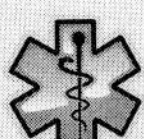

Nursing Intervention Alert

Pulseless VT is a serious dysrhythmia and must be treated immediately.

Dx: 12-lead ECG, continuous ECG monitoring, intermittent ECG recording if intermittent, stress test, electrophysiology studies, history and physical examination

Rx: Treat if client is experiencing symptoms

- Cardiac monitoring
- Treat underlying medical conditions
- Check electrolytes
- Give oxygen 2–4 lpm as prescribed
- Check for digitalis toxicity
- Monitor drugs for proarrhythmic effect
- Pulseless VT—treat with defibrillation
- Stable VT with rate <100—monitor client
- Stable VT with rate >100—treat
  —Pharmacologically: amiodarone, beta blockers, and lidocaine
  —Overdrive pacing
  —Synchronized cardioversion
  —Implantable cardioverter defibrillator (ICD)

Nursing Process Elements

- Assess client for hemodynamic instability
- Monitor VS and cardiac rhythm
- Assess for underlying cause
- Monitor electrolytes
- Treat underlying cause
- Provide emotional support
- Give oxygen
- Follow medical regime
- Assess S&S for developing complications
- Provide client education
- Administer medications as prescribed
- Prepare for emergency interventions

Client teaching for self-care

- Teach client
  —about the causes and treatments for VT

- —about when to seek medical care
- —about the medication regime
  - the side effects of medication
  - how to take pulse
- —to monitor pulse and blood pressure
- —about the emergency treatments
- —about the use of implanted cardioverters
- —to understand how AED works
- Ensure family members know CPR

VENTRICULAR FIBRILLATION

In the case of ventricular fibrillation (VF),

- pacemaker site is chaotic electrical activity in the ventricles with multiple foci,
- the rate cannot be determined,
- the rhythm is grossly irregular,
- there is no P wave,
- PRI is indeterminable, and
- QRS consists of bizarre undulating waves.

Etiology: Multiple irritable foci in the ventricles cause rapid, ineffective, and disorganized depolarization of the ventricles. Ventricles quiver.

Precipitating factors: Acute ischemia, preexisting cardiac disease such as CHF, CAD, or acute MI; hyperkalemia, hypoxemia, acidosis, digitalis toxicity, proarrhythmic effect of certain antidysrhythmic medications, and electrical shock.

S&S:

- No pulse
- Loss of consciousness
- No blood pressure
- No respirations

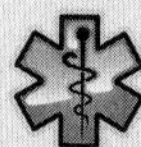

Nursing Intervention Alert

Medical emergency. Clinically VF is indistinguishable from asystole.

Dx: 12-lead ECG

Rx:

- Defibrillation
- CPR
- Antidysrhythmic drugs if initial attempts at defibrillation are not successful
  - —Amiodarone
- Advanced life support

Nursing Process Elements

- Assess client for hemodynamic instability
- Monitor VS and cardiac rhythm
- Assess for underlying cause
- Monitor electrolytes
- Treat underlying cause
- Administer medications as prescribed
- Prepare for emergency interventions

Client teaching for self-care

Teach client to

- know what are the causes and treatments for VF
- know when to seek medical care
- understand medication regime
  - —know the side effects of medication
  - —know how to take pulse
- monitor pulse and blood pressure
- understand emergency treatments
- understand the use of implanted defibrillators
- prepare a living will and a medical power of attorney

HEART FAILURE

- Heart failure (HF) is also referred to as congestive heart failure (CHF).
- Its onset can be chronic or acute heart failure (pulmonary edema or cardiogenic shock).
- It refers to the inability of the heart to pump sufficient blood to meet the needs of tissues for oxygen and nutrients.
- The incidence and prevalence of CHF increase with age.

Etiology: Damage to the heart, regardless of the cause, leads to decreased cardiac output and decreased tissue perfusion. Fluid overload or inadequate tissue perfusion results in altered ventricular filling and emptying.

- Types:
  - —Left-sided heart failure

    Left ventricle is unable to pump blood effectively into systemic circulation and thus blood returns back into pulmonary circulation
  - —Right-sided heart failure

    Right ventricle is unable to effectively pump blood into pulmonary circulation and blood returns back into systemic circulation

Think Smart/Test Smart

When thinking about heart failure remember: the *Ls go together and the Rs go together.* In *L*eft-sided failure, there is a backup of blood/pressure in the *L*ung. In *R*ight-sided failure, there is a backup of blood/pressure in the *R*est of the body.

—High-output failure Cardiac output is adequate but exceeded by metabolic needs of the tissues
—Biventricular failure Both ventricles fail to function adequately

- Classification according to New York Heart Association criteria:
  —Class I Normal activity does not initiate symptoms
  —Class II Normal activity does initiate symptoms but symptoms subside with rest
  —Class III Minimal activity initiates symptoms but symptoms subside with rest
  —Class IV Any activity initiates symptoms and symptoms are present at rest

Precipitating factors: Underlying cardiac disease, pulmonary disease, hyperthyroidism, anemia, or pregnancy.

S&S:

- Left heart failure (pulmonary symptoms remember "Left and Lung")—tachypnea, tachycardia, cough, bibasilar crackles, gallop rhythm, increased pulmonary artery pressure, hemoptysis, fatigue, cyanosis, dyspnea, orthopnea, nocturia, and paroxysmal nocturnal dyspnea (PND)
- Right heart failure (systemic symptoms remember "Right and Rest of the body")—peripheral edema, hepatomegally, splenomegaly, ascites, jugular vein distension (JVD), increased central venous pressure, weakness, anorexia, nausea, indigestion, weight gain, mental changes, bounding pulses, oliguria, and cool extremities
- Biventricular failure—symptoms of both right and left heart failure

Clinical Alert

OB CHF is progressive over time—early intervention and management enhances quality and length of life.

Woman who become pregnant and have been classified as having Class I or Class II of heart disease according to the New York Heart Association Classification (1994) usually experience a normal pregnancy without complications. Women in Classes III and IV may have difficulty achieving a pregnancy and are at risk for complications including fetal demise and heart failure. All women with existing heart disease will require vigilant monitoring during pregnancy because of the risk of heart failure. The workload of the heart peaks at the end of the second trimester or the beginning of the third trimester. The greatest risk for the development of heart failure would be as the woman reaches this period of gestation. If the cardiac condition allows, the woman will be allowed to enter labor spontaneously, although induction may be necessary due to cardiac difficulty. A low forceps delivery with adequate pain management usually produces the least cardiac stress.

Dx: Clinical manifestations, chest X-ray, echocardiogram, increased CVP, increased pulmonary artery pressure, ABG analysis, and liver function test

Rx: Reduce oxygen demands of the myocardium by eliminating and managing contributing factors. Decrease cardiac workload by decreasing afterload and preload, improve contractility, and manage symptoms

Think Smart/Test Smart

Remember the terms "preload" and "afterload" refer to the ventricles, primarily used in reference to the left ventricle.

Preload refers to the amount of blood sitting in the left ventricle "ready to go" when the ventricle contracts. The more blood in the ventricle, the more the ventricular wall is stretched; the greater the stretch, the greater the contractility, and the greater the cardiac output.

Afterload refers to the amount of pressure beyond the left ventricle, i.e., the pressure in the aorta and arterial system. The greater the afterload, the smaller is the cardiac output. Therefore, if the afterload is decreased, the cardiac output will increase.

- Low-sodium diet
- Medications include angiotensin-converting enzyme (ACE) inhibitors, diuretics, digitalis, beta blockers, nitrates, antihypertensives, positive inotropes (dopamine, dobutamine), direct vasodilators, and morphine sulfate
- Physical and psychological rest

- Oxygen
- If medical intervention is unsuccessful then mechanical assist devices (intra-aortic balloon pump [IABP], left ventricular assist devices), and heart transplant

Nursing Process Elements

- Monitor I&O
- Check weight daily
- Assess for signs of fluid overload
- Monitor level of consciousness
- Assess VS, heart and lung sounds
- Monitor for cardiac dysrhythmias
- Maintain bed rest with HOB elevated
- Instruct client to avoid valsalva maneuver
- Assess and record abdominal girth
- Monitor ABGs
- Oxygen as prescribed
- Provide emotional rest
- Monitor electrolytes
- Administer medications as ordered
- Provide client teaching
- Provide low-sodium diet as ordered

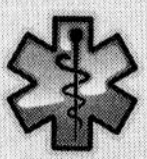

Nursing Alert

Monitor for hypokalemia with potassium depleting diuretics

Client teaching for self-care

Instruct client

- to perform activity without adding to fatigue, so he/she should pace and prioritize daily activities
- to avoid extremes in temperature that would tax cardiac function
- to stop activity if experiencing lightheadedness or shortness of breath
- to plan for periods of rest alternating with periods of activity
- to maintain a low-sodium diet
- to take potassium replacement if taking a potassium depleting diuretic and/or include foods high in potassium in the diet, e.g., orange and tomato juice, bananas, raisins, figs, prunes, apricots, spinach, cauliflower, and potatoes
- to take diuretics at times that allow for uninterrupted sleep
- to adhere to medical regime
- to weigh self daily and report to physician a greater than 3-lb weight gain
- how to take pulse and report to physician if pulse is <60 bpm or >120 bpm
- to know S&S of complications or worsening of HF

HYPERTENSION

- Hypertension is a disorder characterized by BP readings greater than 140 mm Hg systolic and/or 90 mm Hg diastolic, noted on the averaged results of at least two readings, several weeks apart.
- BP is the product of cardiac output and peripheral resistance.
- Approximately one-fourth of the adult population in the United States has hypertension.
- It develops most commonly between the age of 25 and 55 years.
- There is an increased incidence in the African American population.
- It can be a sign, a risk factor, or a disease.

Etiology: 90–95% of all cases are *primary* (also called *essential* or *idiopathic*) hypertension where there is no known cause but there is an alteration in one or more of the factors affecting cardiac output and/or peripheral resistance. The remaining cases are called *secondary* hypertension and a specific cause can be identified: such conditions include adrenal disorders, renal disorders, pregnancy-induced hypertension, and medications.

- Hypertensive crisis
  —Hypertensive emergency: BP must be lowered immediately (MI, dissecting abdominal aneurysm, and intracranial hemorrhage)
  —Hypertensive urgency: BP must be lowered within a few hours

Precipitating: factors for primary hypertension: Hyperlipidemia, obesity, physical inactivity, positive family history, stress, age, ethnicity, high sodium intake, cigarette smoking, and excessive alcohol intake.

S&S:

- Often asymptomatic, is called "the silent killer"
- Sustained elevated BP readings
- Occipital morning headaches, blurred vision, vertigo, fatigue, dyspnea on exertion, palpitations, retinal changes, epistaxis, pain in calf muscles, angina, polyuria, weight gain, edema, nocturia, and diminished or absent peripheral pulses
- Symptoms may occur as target organs develop vascular damage

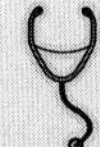

Assessment Alert

A rise in systolic BP when a client moves from a supine to standing position is indicative of essential hypertension.

Dx: Consistently elevated BP readings above 140/90 mmHg. History to identify risk factors and physical examination. Diagnostic tests may include blood chemistry, urinalysis, kidney function tests, ECG, chest X-ray, and echocardiogram

Rx: Controlling hypertension and preventing complications.

- A stepwise approach is recommended starting with modification to lifestyle, which includes
  - —managing weight
  - —limiting alcohol intake
  - —increasing aerobic physical activity
  - —reducing sodium intake to no more than 2.4 g/d
  - —giving up smoking
  - —reducing stress
  - —consuming a diet high in fruits, vegetables, whole grains, and nonfat dairy products
- Medications are then added as needed
  - —No specific medication is recommended
  - —Diuretics (Thiazide, Loop, and Potassium sparing) and beta blockers or both are initial drug choices starting with low doses and then increasing the doses as needed
  - —Other drugs to use include ACE inhibitors, angiotensin II receptor blockers, alpha blockers, and calcium antagonists

Nursing Process Elements

- Monitor blood pressure lying, sitting, and standing, in both arms
- Assess for risk factors
- Assess for S&S of developing complications (CHF, renal involvement, and neurovascular)
- Monitor laboratory tests (BUN, creatinine, and electrolytes)
- Use cardiac monitoring when starting a client on cardiac meds (beta blockers, calcium antagonists)
- Accurately measure daily I&O
- Weigh the client daily before breakfast
- Administer medications as prescribed and monitor closely
- Provide client education to maintain a healthy lifestyle
- Collaborate with dietary to establish an appropriate diet

Client teaching for self-care

Teach client

- to make necessary lifestyle changes including modification of risk factors
  - —maintain blood pressure <140 mmHg systolic and <90 mmHg diastolic
  - —maintain ideal weight
  - —keep total cholesterol <200 mg/dL
  - —stop all forms of tobacco use
  - —eat a diet low in sodium, saturated fats, excess calories, and processed foods, but high in fruits, vegetables, and nonfat dairy products
  - —increase physical activity
  - —use relaxation techniques
- about hypertension and its complications
- about medication regime
  - —supplement potassium if on Loop diuretic
  - —know side effects of medications including S&S of hypotension
  - —know to report S&S of CHF (weight gain, orthopnea, edema, especially if on a beta blocker)
  - —change position slowly to prevent dizziness due to orthostatic hypotension
  - —not take over-the-counter cold medications or nasal decongestants
  - —not suddenly stop taking medications (may cause rebound hypertension)
- how to take and monitor blood pressure and apical pulse
- about the need for adherence to medical regime and that treatment is palliative and not curative

ATHEROSCLEROSIS

- Atherosclerosis refers to the chronic form of arteriosclerosis. There is thickening and hardening of large and medium arteries, which supply blood to the heart, brain, kidneys, extremities, and internal viscera.
- In atherosclerosis, injury to the vessel wall and deposits of lipids, cholesterol, cellular waste, and fibrin interfere with blood flow through the arteries producing ischemia to the tissues and organs.
- It develops slowly, insidiously, and progressively over a lifetime.
- It is the most common cause of MI.

Etiology: Precipitated by an unknown factor which leads to the development of fatty streaks which gradually build to atheromas.

Precipitating factors: Hypertension, hyperlipidemia, obesity, elevated serum triglyceride level, smoking, genetic predisposition, high-fat diets, physical inactivity, stress, age, gender, disease processes such as diabetes mellitus, hormone status and use of oral contraceptives, elevated serum iron levels, and toxic substances in the environment.

S&S:

- Asymptomatic until there is 75% or more impaired blood flow to tissues or organs
- Tissue hypoxia leads to acidosis, cellular damage and when severe enough, can cause necrosis
- Depends on the degree of ischemia to affected tissues or organ: pain, diminished pulses, systolic bruits, and pallor

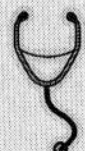

Assessment Alert

The best treatment is the identification of risk factors. Look for xanthomas, which are lipid-containing nodules of the skin.

Dx: Often based on symptoms and history of risk factors

Rx: Prevention and elimination of modifiable risk factors. Control of chronic diseases especially diabetes mellitus, obesity, hypertension and hyperlipidemia through lifestyle changes and compliance to medical regime. Medications to reduce hyperlipidemia include HMG-CoA reductase inhibitors (simvastatin [Zocor]), bile acid-sequestering resins (cholestyramine [Questran]), nicotinic acid (Niacin), fibric-acid derivatives (gemfibrozil [Lopid]), and Omega-3 fish oils

Nursing Process Elements

- Assess for risk factors
- Assess for S&S
- Assess laboratory tests for elevated cholesterol, homocysteine, triglycerides, and iron levels
- Provide client education to maintain a healthy lifestyle
- Support client in adhering to medical regime

Client teaching for self-care

Instruct client

- to maintain blood pressure <90 mmHg diastolic and <140 mmHg systolic
- to maintain ideal weight
- to keep total cholesterol <200 mg, LDL <100 mg, HDL >40 mg
- to stop all forms of tobacco use
- to eat a low-fat, high-fiber diet. The American Heart Association recommends <30% of daily calories from fat, 55% from CHO, and 15% from protein; dietary cholesterol <300 mg and limit sodium to <3000 mg, decrease intake of processed foods
- to follow regular exercise routine
- about stress management and stress reduction
- about the importance of adherence to medical regime for chronic illnesses
- that drug therapy is palliative and not curative

CORONARY ARTERY DISEASE

- Coronary artery disease (CAD) refers to the narrowing of the coronary arteries obstructing blood flow to the myocardium producing ischemia.
- Atherosclerosis is the most common cause of CAD.
- Highest incidence of CAD is found in the Western world.
- It is the leading cause of death in the United States for both men and women.
- Women are at greater risk of CAD after menopause.

Etiology: Narrowing of the artery walls by atherosclerosis producing ischemia to the myocardium. Begins in childhood and generally manifests in adulthood.

Precipitating factors: Hypertension, hyperlipidemia, obesity, elevated serum triglyceride level, smoking, genetic predisposition, high-fat diets, physical inactivity, stress, age, gender, disease processes such as diabetes mellitus, hormone status and use of oral contraceptives, elevated serum iron levels, and toxic substances in the environment.

S&S:

- Generally asymptomatic until 75% or more of a coronary artery is occluded
- Approximately 15% of individuals remain asymptomatic even with advanced CAD
- S&S are dependent on the degree of arterial narrowing and resulting ischemia
- May present as angina pectoris or MI
- Pain, heaviness, or tightness located in chest, arms, jaw, and shoulders when ischemia is severe
- Pain often develops when there is a decrease in blood flow to the myocardium or an increase in myocardial oxygen demand brought on by exercise, stress, cold temperatures, anemia, hyperthyroidism, and substance abuse
- Dyspnea on exertion

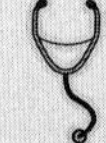

Assessment Alert

Pain lasts no longer than 3 minutes and is relieved with rest.

Dx: Often based on symptoms and history of risk factors and tests including cholesterol panel, triglyceride level, homocysteine levels, CBC, exercise stress test, ECG, cardiac radionuclear scan, echocardiogram, coronary angiography, and cardiac catheterization

Rx: Prevention and elimination of modifiable risk factors.

- Control of chronic diseases especially diabetes mellitus, obesity, hypertension, and hyperlipidemia through lifestyle changes and compliance to medical regime
- Medications to reduce hyperlipidemia include HMG-CoA reductase inhibitors (simvastatin [Zocor]), bile acid-sequestering resins (cholestyramine [Questran]), nicotinic acid (Niacin), fibric-acid derivatives (gemfibrozil [Lopid]) and Omega-3 fish oils

- Drugs that reduce oxygen demand or increase oxygen supply to the myocardium include nitrates, beta blockers, calcium channel blockers, antihypertensives, and antiplatelet agents such as low-dose aspirin
- Revascularization procedures such as transluminal coronary angioplasty, laser angioplasty, coronary atherectomy, intracoronary stents and surgical interventions including coronary artery bypass grafting (CABG), minimally invasive coronary bypass (MIDCAB), and transmyocardial laser revascularization (TMLR)

Nursing Process Elements

- Assess for risk factors
- Assess for S&S
- Assess laboratory tests for elevated cholesterol, homocysteine, triglycerides, and iron levels
- Provide client education to maintain a healthy lifestyle
- Support client in adhering to medical regime
- Provide client teaching for drug therapies
- Provide client teaching pre- and postrevascularization procedure
  - —Client will be awake during coronary angiogram or cardiac catheterization
  - —Client may experience a hot flash and metallic taste as dye is injected
  - —Client will be on bed rest with affected extremity immobilized following procedure to decrease risk of bleeding
- Provide client teaching pre- and postrevascularization surgery
- Postrevascularization Nursing Process Elements
  - —Observe for bleeding from surgical site
  - —Monitor for ECG changes: T-wave changes, ST segment elevation, dysrhythmias
  - —Monitor for chest pain
  - —Monitor VS
  - —Monitor I&O; if dye was used, have client drink large amounts of fluid to decrease renal toxicity

Client teaching for self-care

Instruct client

- to maintain blood pressure <90 mmHg diastolic and <140 mmHg systolic
- to maintain ideal weight
- to keep total cholesterol <200 mg, LDL <100 mg, HDL >40 mg
- to stop all forms of tobacco use
- to eat a low-fat, high-fiber diet. The American Heart Association recommends <30% of daily calories from fat, 55% from CHO, and 15% from protein; keep dietary cholesterol <300 mg and limit sodium to <3000 mg; decrease intake of processed foods
- to follow a regular exercise routine
- how to take pulse rate and alert doctor if pulse is <60 or >120
- about stress management and stress reduction
- about the importance of adherence to medical regime for chronic illnesses
- understand that drug and medical therapies are palliative and not curative
- to stop and rest at onset of chest discomfort

ANGINA PECTORIS

- Angina pectoris is also known as acute coronary syndrome.
- It refers to the chest pain brought on by myocardial ischemia.
- It is caused due to an imbalance of coronary blood supply and demand.
- The most common cause is atherosclerosis.

Etiology: Reduction of coronary blood flow or increased oxygen demand to the myocardium producing ischemia. Decreased oxygen supply causes cells to switch from aerobic to anaerobic metabolism. Lactic acid builds up. Cell membrane permeability is affected and histamine, bradykinins, and enzymes are released which stimulate nerve fibers.

- Types of angina:
  - —Stable Consistent pattern with exertion and pain relieved with rest
  - —Unstable Increase in frequency, duration, and severity of pain
  - —Prinzmetal's or variant Pain at rest and usual cause is coronary artery vasospasm

Precipitating factors: Hypertension, hyperlipidemia, obesity, elevated serum triglyceride level, smoking, genetic predisposition, high-fat diets, physical inactivity, stress, age, gender, disease processes such as diabetes mellitus, hormone status and use of oral contraceptives, elevated serum iron levels, and toxic substances in the environment.

S&S:

- Generally asymptomatic until 75% or more of a coronary artery is occluded
- S&S are dependent on the degree of arterial narrowing and resulting ischemia and the location
- Pain, heaviness, or tightness located in chest (often substernal or retrosternal), arms, jaw, shoulders, back, or abdomen
- Pain develops when there is a decrease in blood flow to the myocardium or an increase in myocardial oxygen

demand brought on by exercise, stress, cold temperatures, anemia, hyperthyroidism, and substance abuse (cocaine)

- Pain may be accompanied by nausea, vomiting, weakness, dyspnea, indigestion, dizziness, anxiety, diaphoresis, pallor, hypotension, and pulse changes
- Women often present with atypical symptoms such as GI distress
- Elderly and diabetic clients may present with dyspnea or weakness without pain

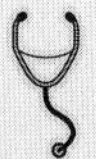

Assessment Alert

Pain lasts for less than 15 minutes and is relieved with rest and/or nitroglycerine.

Dx: Based on symptoms, history of risk factors, and tests including cardiac enzymes (CPK-MB, troponin, and myoglobin), cholesterol panel, triglyceride level, CBC, exercise stress test, ECG (T wave inversion, ST segment depression), cardiac radionuclear scan, echocardiogram, coronary angiography, and cardiac catheterization

Rx: To decrease myocardial oxygen consumption and increase myocardial oxygen supply

- Stop activity and rest in semi-Fowler's position
- Take nitroglycerine sublingually
- Administer oxygen 2–4 lpm via nasal cannula
- Thrombolytic therapy if thrombi is the cause
- Prevention and elimination of modifiable risk factors
- Control of chronic diseases especially diabetes mellitus, obesity, hypertension, and hyperlipidemia through lifestyle changes and compliance to medical regime
- Medications to reduce hyperlipidemia include HMG-CoA reductase inhibitors (simvastatin [Zocor]), bile acid-sequestering resins (cholestyramine [Questran]), nicotinic acid (Niacin), fibric acid derivatives (gemfibrozil [Lopid]), and Omega-3 fish oils
- Drugs that reduce oxygen demand or increase oxygen supply to the myocardium include nitrates, beta blockers, calcium channel blockers, antihypertensives, and antiplatelet agents such as low-dose aspirin
- Revascularization procedures such as transluminal coronary angioplasty, laser angioplasty, coronary atherectomy, intracoronary stents and surgical interventions including CABG, MIDCAB, and TMLR (see Chapter 18.)

Nursing Process Elements

- Have client stop activity and rest in semi-Fowler's position
- Give client nitroglycerine sublingually
- Administer oxygen 2–4 lpm via nasal cannula
- Assess PQRST of pain where P—position, Q—quality and quantity, R—radiation and relief, S—severity and symptoms, and T—timing
- Assess for risk factors
- Assess for S&S
- Assess laboratory tests for elevated cardiac enzymes, cholesterol, triglycerides, and iron levels
- Assess 12-lead ECG for ST-wave changes
- Provide emotional support
- Provide client education to maintain a healthy lifestyle
- Support client in adhering to medical regime
- Provide client teaching for drug therapies
- Provide client teaching pre- and postrevascularization procedure
  - —Client will be awake during coronary angiogram or cardiac catheterization
  - —Client may experience a hot flash and metallic taste as dye is injected
  - —Client will be on bed rest with affected extremity immobilized following procedure to decrease risk of bleeding
- Provide client teaching pre- and postrevascularization surgery
- Postrevascularization Nursing Process Elements
  - —Observe for bleeding from surgical site
  - —Monitor for ECG changes: T-wave changes, ST segment elevation, and dysrhythmias
  - —Monitor for chest pain
  - —Monitor VS
  - —Monitor I&O; if dye was used, have client drink large amounts of fluid to decrease renal toxicity

Client teaching for self-care

Instruct client

- to reduce the risks of angina by balancing oxygen supply and demand
- to stop activity or stress and take Nitroglycerine when pain occurs
- about the proper use of nitroglycerine
  - —Go to hospital if no pain relief after nitroglycerine
  - —Know the side effects: headache and hypotension
  - —Keep in original bottle
  - —Keep with you at all times
  - —Replace every 3 months
- to maintain blood pressure <90 mm Hg diastolic and <140 mm Hg systolic
- to maintain ideal weight
- to keep total cholesterol <200 mg, LDL <100 mg, HDL >40 mg
- to stop all forms of tobacco use

- to eat a low-fat, high-fiber diet. The American Heart Association recommends <30% of daily calories from fat, 55% from CHO, and 15% from protein; keep dietary cholesterol <300 mg and limit sodium to <3000 mg; decrease intake of processed foods
- to follow a regular exercise routine
- how to take pulse rate and alert doctor if pulse is <60 or >120
- about stress management and stress reduction
- about the importance of adherence to medical regime for chronic illnesses
- that drug and medical therapies are palliative and not curative

MYOCARDIAL INFARCTION

- Myocardial infarction (MI) is also known as Acute Coronary Syndrome.
- It refers to the chest pain brought on by acute obstruction of coronary blood flow.
- MI occurs suddenly.
- It results in imbalance of myocardial oxygen supply and demand.
- It causes the death of myocardial cells.

Think Smart/Test Smart

Remember the three *I*s of the progression of pathophysiology of an MI: *I*schemic tissue progresses to *I*njured tissue, which in turn progresses to *I*nfarcted or dead tissue.

Etiology: Obstruction of coronary blood flow due to thrombus, emboli, or vasospasm. May also result if oxygen supply is diminished such as with acute hypovolemia or if oxygen demand is increased as with tachycardia.

Precipitating factors: Hypertension, hyperlipidemia, obesity, elevated serum triglyceride level, smoking, genetic predisposition, high-fat diets, physical inactivity, stress, age, gender, disease processes such as diabetes mellitus, hormone status and use of oral contraceptives, elevated serum iron levels, toxic substances in the environment.

S&S:

- Acute substernal pain described as crushing which may radiate to back or jaw
- Feeling of impending doom
- Shortness of breath
- Shocked, pale, and anxious
- Nausea and vomiting

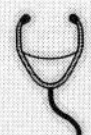

Assessment Alert

Pain lasts more than 20 minutes and is not relieved with rest and/or nitroglycerine.

Dx: Based on presenting symptoms, history of risk factors, ECG (T-wave inversion, ST-segment elevation, and abnormal Q wave), and serum cardiac enzyme values (CK-MB, Myoglobin, and Troponin)

Rx: Goal is to minimize myocardial damage and preserve function

Think Smart/Test Smart

Remember MONA for the care of the client with an MI in the Emergency Room: Morphine sulfate, Oxygen, Nitroglycerine, Aspirin.

- Have client stop activity and rest in semi-Fowler's position
- Administer oxygen
- Reperfuse area of damage with thrombolytic medication
  —Goal is to give within 30 minutes of arrival in ER
  —Make certain no absolute contraindications are present (e.g., active bleeding, hemorrhagic CVA within 2 months, severe uncontrolled hypertension, recent major surgery or trauma, pregnancy; if giving streptokinase, history of allergic reaction to streptokinase, recent streptococcal infection)
- Analgesics, generally morphine sulfate given IV bolus
- Drugs that reduce oxygen demand or increase oxygen supply to the myocardium include nitrates, beta blockers, ACE inhibitors, calcium channel blockers, antihypertensives, and antiplatelet agents such as low-dose aspirin
- Revascularization procedures such as transluminal coronary angioplasty, laser angioplasty, coronary atherectomy, intracoronary stents and surgical interventions including CABG), MIDCAB, and TMLR

Think Smart/Test Smart

When answering questions about treatment of an MI, remember "Time is muscle." The faster reperfusion of cardiac muscle is established following an MI, the less muscle is lost. Conversely, the longer cardiac muscle goes without oxygenated blood, the more muscle is lost. Therefore, speed of treatment is critical.

Nursing Process Elements

- Maintain bed rest with semi-Fowler's position
- Administer oxygen 2–4 lpm via nasal cannula
- Establish IV access
- Provide pain relief
- Assess for S&S
- Assess laboratory tests for elevated cardiac enzymes, elevated WBC, increased ESR, and elevated cholesterol level
- Assess 12-lead ECG for T-wave, ST-segment, and Q-wave changes
- Monitor for dysrhythmias
- Monitor VS, oxygen saturation, urinary output, and hemodynamic parameters
- Provide emotional support
- If thrombolytics are given
  —Have two to three IV sites established prior to infusion
  —Handle client gently, no IM injections
  —Observe for signs of active bleeding
  —Monitor for allergic or anaphylactic reaction with streptokinase
  —Have antidote to streptokinase which is aminocaproic acid (Amicar) available
- Progress diet from NPO, to clear liquids, etc.
- Administer stool softener as ordered
- Provide client education for cardiac rehabilitation and to maintain a healthy lifestyle
- Support client in adhering to medical regime
- Provide client teaching for drug therapies
- Provide client teaching pre- and postrevascularization procedure
  —Client will be awake during coronary angiogram or cardiac catheterization
  —Client may experience a hot flash and metallic taste as dye is injected
  —Client will be on bed rest with affected extremity immobilized following procedure to decrease risk of bleeding
- Provide client teaching pre- and postrevascularization surgery
- Postrevascularization Nursing Process Elements
  —Observe for bleeding from surgical site
  —Monitor for ECG changes: T wave changes, ST segment elevation, dysrhythmias
  —Monitor for chest pain
  —Monitor VS
  —Monitor I&O; if dye was used, have client drink large amounts of fluid to decrease renal toxicity

Client teaching for self-care

Instruct client

- to reduce the risks of MI by balancing oxygen supply and demand
- about the cause, process, and treatment of MI
- about the medication regimen
- to make necessary lifestyle changes including modification of risk factors
  —maintain blood pressure <90 mm Hg diastolic and <140 mm Hg systolic
  —maintain ideal weight
  —keep total cholesterol <200 mg, LDL <100 mg, HDL >40 mg
  —stop all forms of tobacco use
  —eat a low-fat, high-fiber diet. The American Heart Association recommends <30% of daily calories from fat, 55% from CHO, and 15% from protein; keep dietary cholesterol <300 mg and limit sodium to <3000 mg; decrease intake of processed foods
- to enroll in cardiac rehabilitation program
- how to take pulse rate and alert doctor if pulse is <60 or >120
- about stress management and stress reduction
- about the importance of adherence to medical regime
- to understand that drug and medical therapies are palliative and not curative
- about S&S of MI. Get to ER if chest pain lasts longer than 15 minutes and is not relieved with rest and nitroglycerine

VALVULAR HEART DISEASE

- Valvular heart disease refers to a disease or condition that interferes with the unidirectional blood flow of the heart.
- It can affect all four valves in the heart: aortic, pulmonic, mitral, and tricuspid.

Etiology: Can be a result of acquired valvular disorders or congenital heart defects resulting in stenosis which impedes the forward flow of blood through a valve or regurgitation which causes a backward flow of blood through a valve.

Precipitating factors: Rheumatic Fever, endocarditis, MI, calcium deposits, congenital defects, and syphilis.

S&S:

- Asymptomatic at first
- Pulmonary congestion, dyspnea, and pulmonary hypertension
- Decreased cardiac output, S3 or S4 heart sounds, murmur, tachycardia, and angina
- Fatigue and S&S of CHF

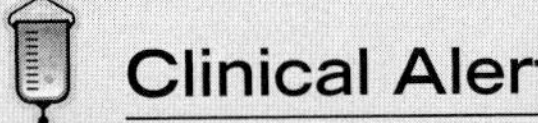

Clinical Alert

OB With valvular heart disease, hemodynamic changes occur both in front of and behind the affected valve. Blood flow and pressures are reduced in front of the affected valve and pressures are increased behind the affected valve.

During pregnancy, there is an increased volume of blood as well as the need for increased cardiac output. These factors can lead a pregnant woman with valvular disease to develop heart failure. The greatest risk occurs as the woman approaches the third trimester of pregnancy.

At the time of labor, prophylactic antibiotics are recommended to prevent bacterial endocaritis in the woman with symptomatic valvular disease.

Dx: Client history and physical examination, cardiac catheterization, CXR, ECG, and echocardiogram

Rx:

- Pharmacological interventions include digitalis glycosides (Digoxin) to increase force of the contraction of the heart, diuretics, and ACE inhibitors to reduce preload and afterload
- Antibiotics are prescribed prior to any dental work or invasive procedures to decrease the risk of endocarditis
- Surgery to repair or replace a diseased valve provides definitive treatment for valve repair
- Repair rather than replacement of diseased valve is the preferred treatment because it provides a lower risk of complications and mortality

(See cardiac surgery in Chapter 18 for Nursing Process Special Considerations.)

PEDS CONGENITAL HEART DEFECTS

- A congenital heart defect is a structural defect of the heart and/or great vessels present at birth or shortly thereafter.
- Congenital heart defects are categorized as acyanotic (increased pulmonary blood flow) and cyanotic (blood flow bypasses the lungs).
  —Acyanotic defects include defects that cause oxygenated blood to recirculate through the lungs and heart and defects that obstruct blood flow from the heart. Acyanotic heart defects that recirculate the blood are often termed "left to right" as blood flows from the oxygenated left side through a defect into the unoxygenated right side.
    - Atrial septal defect (ASD)
    - Ventricular septal defect (VSD)
    - Patent ductus arteriosus
    - Coarctation of the aorta

  —Cyanotic defects involve a shunt that bypasses the lungs and delivers venous (deoxygenated) blood from the right side of the heart into the arterial circulation. These defects are frequently called "right to left" shunts.
    - Transposition of the great vessels
    - Truncus arteriosus
    - Tetralogy of Fallot
- They are a major cause of death in children during the first year of life.
- They occur in about 8–10 of 1000 live births.

Acyanotic Heart Defects

Septal defects

- Atrial septal defect (ASD)
  —In ASD, there is an opening between the right and left atria.
  —Shunting of blood occurs from the left atrium (slightly higher pressure) oxygen-rich blood to the right atrium (lower pressure) increasing the amount of blood to the right ventricle and then to the lungs.

Etiology: Cause is generally unknown.

Precipitating factors: Rubella during pregnancy, chromosomal abnormalities, maternal age over 40 years, alcoholism, and type I diabetes.

S&S:

—Often asymptomatic, if the defect is small. Defect may close on its own within 12–18 months
—When defect is large, may cause CHF (shortness of breath, easy fatigability, or poor growth pattern), respiratory infections, and cardiac enlargement
—Murmur
—S&S may not begin to develop until 4–6 weeks after birth

Rx:

—Small ASDs may close on their own by 12–18 months
—If ASD does not close and defect is not too large, it may be closed by placement of a device called an Amplatzer Septal Occluder during a cardiac catheterization
—If ASD is large, open heart surgery is needed
—If CHF develops, especially with VSD, client may be managed medically with diuretics and digoxin

Postoperative course: Same as for clients undergoing open heart surgery. Client will be in an ICU for 1–2 days and will be discharged home after a total hospital stay of 5–7 days.

Nursing Process Elements

See VSD

Client teaching for self-care

See VSD

- Ventricular septal defect
  - —In VSD, there is an opening between the right and left ventricle.
  - —Shunting of blood occurs from the left ventricle (high pressure) oxygen-rich blood to the right ventricle (low pressure) increasing the amount of blood to the lungs.
  - —It is the most common congenital defect

Etiology: Cause is generally unknown.

Precipitating factors: Rubella during pregnancy, chromosomal abnormalities, maternal age over 40 years, alcoholism, and type I diabetes.

S&S:

—CHF is common

—Shortness of breath, easy fatigability, or poor growth pattern, respiratory infections, and cardiac enlargement

—Murmur

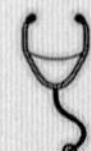

Assessment Alert

Systolic murmur heard over the pulmonary valve area which is caused from the large volume of blood going through the pulmonary valve.

Dx: Physical examination, echocardiogram, ECG, and chest X-ray

Rx:

—CHF is managed medically with diuretics and digoxin

—Palliative surgery (including pulmonary artery banding) may be done to improve the child's condition and promote growth prior to corrective surgery

—Corrective open heart surgery

Postoperative Course: Same as for clients undergoing open heart surgery. Client will be in an ICU for 1–2 days and will be discharged home after a total hospital stay of 5–7 days.

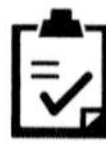

Nursing Process Elements

Preoperatively

—Provide emotional support for client and family

—Provide information about the anatomy and physiology of the heart and the surgical procedure, postoperative procedures and equipment including equipment for hemodynamic monitoring, ventilator, endotracheal tube, pacing wires, chest tube and nasogastric tube, ICU policies and visiting hours, possible complications and treatments, pain management, and sensory stimuli and overload

Postoperatively

—Monitor hemodynamic measures

—Assess cardiac monitoring

—Assess peripheral pulses

—Assess bowel sounds and measure abdominal girth every 8 hours

—Measure and record I&O hourly including chest tube and NG drainage

—Monitor laboratory values especially Hct and Hgb, ABGs, CBC, APPT, and electrolytes

—Keep temporary pacemaker at bedside

—Monitor core body temperature and keep temperature above 96.8°F (36°C)

—Assess pain level

—Administer medications as ordered

—Note ETT placement and ventilator settings

—Provide emotional support to client and family

—Evaluate respiratory status

—Assess incisions for presence of infection and drainage

—Turn client and have client take a deep breath

—Assess for S&S of complications including thrombophlebitis, pulmonary embolism, CHF, and cardiac tamponade

Client teaching for self-care

Instruct client

—to schedule rest periods to prevent fatigue

—to resume usual activities gradually

—to report S&S of CHF including weight gain, increased pulse rate, and difficulty in breathing

—about follow-up routine with cardiologist

—about wound care

—that following closure there should be no further treatment required or activity restrictions

Patent ductus arteriosus

The ductus arteriosus is a fetal structure that allows blood going from the right ventricle to bypass the lungs and enter the aorta. Since the blood is oxygenated by the placenta, this blood is oxygen rich. As the fetal lungs are not used for respiration, a minimal amount of blood is needed to feed the lung tissue. When the ductus arteriosus fails to close shortly after birth, the infant is diagnosed as having a patent ductus arteriosus (PDA).

- PDA is an acyanotic heart defect.
- It is a common anomaly in the preterm infant.

Etiology: Unknown. Associated with preterm deliveries and respiratory involvement in the neonate.

Precipitating factors: Prematurity and respiratory distress in the neonate.

S&S:

- Murmur
- Recurrent apnea, increased $PaCO_2$, and decreased PaO_2
- CHF

Dx: Assessment of signs and symptoms with confirmation by echocardiogram

Rx: Respiratory care, diuretics. Indomethacin, a prostaglandin synthetase inhibitor may precipitate closure. If unsuccessful, surgical ligation will be required

Nursing Process Elements

- Monitor all newborns for signs of respiratory congestion, murmur, and apnea
- When indomethacin is administered, monitor the infant for bleeding and renal function
- Preoperative and postoperative care is focused on promoting respiratory function, monitoring for infection, renal function, and promoting growth
- The infant should be monitored for necrotizing enterocolitis, NEC, a complication of respiratory distress during the newborn period. Monitor for regurgitation or feeding residual, abdominal distress, and positive guaiac

Client teaching for self-care

Explain to parents

- the causes and signs and symptoms of PDA
- surgical procedures and medications used in treatment

Coarctation of the aorta

- Coarctation of the aorta is an obstructive congenital heart defect where there is narrowing of the aorta restricting outflow.
- In this defect, the left ventricle has to work harder to force blood through a narrowed vessel.

Etiology: Cause is generally unknown but seems to be linked to chromosomal abnormalities such as Turner's syndrome.

Precipitating factors: Rubella during pregnancy, chromosomal abnormalities, maternal age over 40 years, alcoholism, and type I diabetes.

S&S: Depends on the degree of narrowing of the aorta

- If severe, infants will have significant changes within several hours to days after birth and closure of the ductus arteriosus
  —High blood pressure and bounding pulses in the arms
  —Decreased or absent pulses in the groin and legs
  —CHF
  —Cool lower extremities
- If less severe, it may not be detected for several years
  —Headache
  —Dizziness
  —Epistaxis
  —High blood pressure in the arms
  —Diminished lower extremity pulses
  —Murmur

Dx: Echocardiogram, MRI, CT scan, and ECG

Rx: For infants with severe coarctation, urgent open heart surgery is preformed to repair the narrowing. In older children with less narrowing, a cardiac catheterization with balloon dilatation may be an option or open heart surgery for repair

Postoperative course: Same as for clients undergoing heart surgery. Client will be in an ICU for 1–2 days and will be discharged home after a total hospital stay of 5–7 days.

Nursing Process Elements

Preoperatively

- Provide emotional support for client and family
- Provide information about the anatomy and physiology of the heart and the surgical procedure, postoperative procedures and equipment including equipment for hemodynamic monitoring, ventilator, endotracheal, tube, pacing wires, chest tube and nasogastric tube, ICU policies and visiting hours, possible complications and treatments, pain management, and sensory stimuli and overload

Postoperatively

- Monitor hemodynamic measures
- Assess cardiac monitoring
- Assess peripheral pulses
- Assess bowel sounds and measure abdominal girth every 8 hours
- Measure and record I&O hourly including chest tube and NG drainage
- Monitor laboratory values especially H&H, ABGs, CBC, APPT, and electrolytes
- Keep temporary pacemaker at bedside
- Monitor core body temperature and keep temperature above 96.8°F (36°C)
- Assess pain level
- Administer medications as ordered
- Note ETT placement and ventilator settings
- Provide emotional support to client and family
- Evaluate respiratory status
- Assess incisions for presence of infection and drainage
- Turn client and have client take a deep breath
- Assess for S&S of complications including thrombophlebitis, pulmonary embolism, CHF, and cardiac tamponade

Client teaching for self-care

Instruct parents/caregiver

- to schedule rest periods to prevent fatigue
- to resume usual activities gradually
- to report S&S of CHF including weight gain, increased pulse rate, and difficulty in breathing
- to have knowledge of long-term follow-up routine with cardiologist
- about wound care

Cyanotic Heart Defects

Tetralogy of Fallot

- Tetralogy of Fallot is a congenital heart defect that includes four structural anomalies:
  —VSD
  —Juxtaposition of the aorta (aorta overrides the septum and receives blood from both the right and left ventricles)
  —Right ventricular hypertrophy
  —Pulmonary stenosis
- It involves a right to left shunt which mixes unoxygenated and oxygenated blood into the systemic circulation.

Etiology: Cause is generally unknown.

Precipitating factors: Rubella during pregnancy, chromosomal abnormalities, maternal age over 40 years, alcoholism, and type I diabetes.

S&S:

- Cyanosis—The extent of cyanosis is dependent on the amount of narrowing of the pulmonary valve and right ventricular outflow tract
- Dyspnea, tachypnea
- Fatigue
- Loud and harsh heart murmur
- Clubbing of the fingers and toes
- Poor growth pattern
- Polycythemia

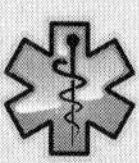

Nursing Intervention Alert

The arterial oxygen saturation of babies with Tetralogy of Fallot can suddenly drop, especially when the baby is crying or stressed. This phenomenon is called a "tet spell" or "blue spell." A tet spell can sometimes be treated by comforting the infant and flexing the knees forward and upward or else the child may squat down. Most often, however, immediate medical attention is necessary.

Dx: Hyperoxia test where the cyanosis does not improve with supplemental oxygen, echocardiogram, cardiac catheterization

Rx: Depends on the degree of hypoxia. If oxygen levels are critically low soon after birth, a prostaglandin infusion is usually initiated to keep the ductus arteriosus open. These infants usually require open heart surgery in the neonatal period. Palliative surgery is often used as a temporary measure to improve the physical condition of the child to allow growth. Complete repair is usually performed in the first year of life.

Postoperative course: Same as for clients undergoing open heart surgery. Client will be in an ICU for 1–2 days and will be discharged home after a total hospital stay of 5–7 days.

Nursing Process Elements

Preoperatively

- Provide emotional support for client and family
- Provide information about the anatomy and physiology of the heart and the surgical procedure, postoperative procedures and equipment including equipment for hemodynamic monitoring, ventilator, endotracheal tube, pacing wires, chest tube and nasogastric tube, ICU policies and visiting hours, possible complications and treatments, pain management, and sensory stimuli and overload

Postoperatively

- Monitor hemodynamic measures
- Assess cardiac monitoring
- Assess peripheral pulses
- Assess bowel sounds and measure abdominal girth every 8 hours
- Measure and record I&O hourly including chest tube and NG drainage
- Monitor laboratory values especially H&H, ABGs, CBC, APPT, and electrolytes
- Keep temporary pacemaker at bedside
- Monitor core body temperature and keep temperature above 96.8°F (36°C)
- Assess pain level
- Administer medications as ordered
- Note ETT placement and ventilator settings
- Provide emotional support to client and family
- Evaluate respiratory status
- Assess incisions for presence of infection and drainage
- Turn client and have client deep breath
- Assess for S&S of complications including thrombophlebitis, pulmonary embolism, CHF, cardiac tamponade

Client teaching for self-care

Instruct family/caregiver

- to schedule rest periods to prevent fatigue
- to resume usual activities gradually

- to report S&S of CHF including weight gain, increased pulse rate, and difficulty in breathing
- to have knowledge of long-term follow-up routine with cardiologist
- about wound care
- about available resources

Transposition of the great vessels

- Transposition of the great vessels is a congenital heart defect where the pulmonary artery exits from the left ventricle and the aorta exits from the right ventricle.
- There are two separate and parallel systems, thus there is no communication between the pulmonary and systemic circulations.
- This condition is not compatible with life unless there is a large ASD or VSD that allows the oxygenated and unoxygenated blood to mix.

Etiology: Cause is generally unknown.

Precipitating factors: Rubella during pregnancy, chromosomal abnormalities, maternal age over 40 years, alcoholism, and type I diabetes.

S&S: The baby

- is blue at birth and cyanosis does not improve with oxygen supply
- is very lethargic and depressed
- has a very poor Apgar score

Dx: Clinical presentation with no improvement with oxygen; echocardiogram

Rx: Prostaglandin is started intravenously to maintain the small connection (the ductus arteriosus) between the pulmonary and systemic circulations. If an ASD is not present or is small, an ASD may be created or enlarged by balloon septostomy. Open heart surgery to adjust the vessels may be required shortly after birth

Pre- and postoperative care: If open heart surgery is needed, the usual preoperative care for a client undergoing open heart surgery will be needed including physical, emotional, and psychosocial assessment; provide emotional support for client and family, client education concerning the anatomy and physiology of the heart and the surgical procedure, postoperative procedures and equipments including hemodynamic monitoring equipment, ventilator, endotracheal tube, pacing wires, chest tubes, nasogastric tube, ICU policies and visiting hours, possible complications and treatments, pain management and sensory stimuli and sensory overload.

Postoperative course: Baby will be in NICU for many weeks depending on the severity of the situation, if palliative surgery is performed, and when corrective surgery is performed.

Nursing Process Elements

- Monitor hemodynamic measures
- Assess cardiac monitoring
- Assess peripheral pulses
- Assess bowel sounds and measure abdominal girth every 8 hours
- Measure and record I&O hourly including chest tube and NG drainage
- Monitor laboratory values especially H&H, ABGs, CBC, APPT, and electrolytes
- Keep temporary pacemaker at bedside
- Monitor core body temperature and keep temperature above 96.8 F (36 C)
- Assess pain level
- Administer medications as ordered
- Note ETT placement and ventilator settings
- Provide emotional support to client and family
- Evaluate respiratory status
- Assess incisions for presence of infection and drainage
- Turn client and have client take a deep breath
- Assess for S&S of complications including thrombophlebitis, pulmonary embolism, CHF, cardiac tamponade, and dysrhythmias
- Refer family to appropriate agencies and support services

Client teaching for self-care

Teach parents or caregiver to:

- Schedule rest periods to prevent fatigue
- Resume usual activities gradually
- Report S&S of CHF and complications
- About long-term follow-up routine with cardiologist
- About wound care
- About appropriate community and support agencies

ANEURYSMS

- Aneurysm refers to a localized dilatation, weakness, or outpouching of the wall of a blood vessel.
- Most commonly, aneurysms occur in the abdominal aorta and peripheral arteries because of the high blood flow pressure in these vessels.
- It may involve one or all of the layers of the vessel wall.
- Classification
  - —Fusiform: Uniform, spindle-shaped, large aneurysm involving the entire circumference of the vessel.
  - —Saccular: An outpouching on one side only of a vessel, for example, berry aneurysm.
  - —Dissecting: A separation of the arterial wall layers to form a cavity that fills with blood.
  - —True: Affects all three layers of the vessel wall and occurs over a long time usually as a result of atherosclerosis and hypertension.
  - —False: Usually a result from a traumatic break in the vessel wall rather than progressive weakening of the vessel wall.

- It occurs most often in men aged 50–70 years.
- The type of aneurysm is determined by its location.

Etiology: Risk factors that weaken the vessel wall combine with high blood flow pressures to gradually dilate the vessel.

Precipitating factors: Atherosclerosis, hypertension, trauma, infection, syphilis, and connective tissue diseases.

S&S:

- Generally asymptomatic until aneurysm becomes large enough to press on other structures or the aneurysm starts to leak or rupture.
  —Thoracic aortic aneurysm: deep, diffuse chest pain, hoarseness, dysphagia, dyspnea, brassy cough
  —Abdominal aortic aneurysm: palpable pulsating mass, systolic bruit, abdominal or back pain, cool extremities, diminished femoral pulses
  —Dissecting abdominal aortic aneurysm: sudden, severe tearing or ripping pain in the back or anterior chest, pallor, diaphoresis, tachycardia, initially elevated blood pressure, undetectable peripheral pulses, shock

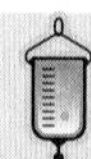

Clinical Alert

Half of all aneurysms greater than 6 cm in size will rupture within 1 year.

Dx: Based on history and physical examination, CXR, aortography, ultrasonogram, CT scan, MRI, renal function studies

Rx: Prevention of aneurysm rupture by control of blood pressure and smoking cessation, surgical resection of the aneurysm, and graft replacement

Nursing Process Elements

- Preoperative care
  —Assess risk factors
  —Assess for S&S of complications
  —Regulate blood pressure and pulse according to parameters
  —Assess peripheral circulation: capillary refill, pulses, LOC, pulse oximetry, temperature, sensation, neurochecks
  —Monitor laboratory values
  —Assist in pain management
  —Decrease client's anxiety
  —Provide pre- and postoperative teaching
- Postoperative care
  —Monitor hourly circulation checks, urine output, neurochecks
  —Monitor hemodynamic parameters, VS, CVP, PAP, PCWP
  —Assess for complications: presence of back pain (may indicate retroperitoneal hemorrhage), respiratory distress, paralytic ileus, graft occlusion, cardiac dysrhythmias, hypovolemia, shock, paralysis, and renal failure
  —Maintain client flat in bed without sharp flexion
  —Prevent thrombophlebitis: sequential boots, turning, dorsiflexion of feet
  —Assist in pain management
  —Assist in wound management
  —Provide postoperative teaching to client

Client teaching for self-care

Instruct client to

- report S&S of complications
- observe limited lifting for 4–6 weeks
- monitor incision for bleeding or infection
- ensure proper wound care
- maintain blood pressure <90 mm Hg diastolic and <140 mm Hg systolic
- avoid constipation and straining
- keep total cholesterol <200 mg, LDL <100 mg, HDL >40 mg
- stop all forms of tobacco use
- eat a low-cholesterol, low-saturated-fat diet
- develop a gradual progressive exercise routine
- take pulse rate and alert doctor if pulse is <60 or >120
- ensure stress management and stress reduction
- Adhere to medical regime

PERIPHERAL VASCULAR DISEASE

- Peripheral vascular disease (PVD) refers to an abnormal condition that causes interference with blood flow to or from the extremities.
- It can be arterial or venous.
- It may be acute or chronic.

Etiology: Pooling of blood or decrease in blood supply and nutrients to extremity leads to hypoxia and tissue damage.

- Arterial—Vessel compression, vasospasm, or structural defect.
- Venous—Occlusive disorders or ineffective blood return.

Precipitating factors: Arteriosclerosis, atherosclerosis, hypertension, obesity, diabetes mellitus, smoking, stress, immobility, heart disease, pregnancy, hypercoagulability, trauma, and sedentary occupations.

S&S:

- Arterial
  —intermittent claudication
  —burning sensation in the extremities
  —cool, numb extremities

—pallor when extremity elevated
—rubor when extremity in dependent position
—skin is thin and shiny with hair loss and discoloration
—thickened toenails
—decreased or absent peripheral pulses
—ulcers or skin breakdown often on toes

- Venous
  —aching relieved with elevation of extremity
  —tenderness in the extremity
  —normal temperature
  —discoloration of the lower extremity, brawny
  —skin is thick and tough
  —edema
  —positive Homan's sign
  —present peripheral pulses
  —ulcers often around ankles

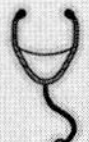

Assessment Alert

Pain that occurs in the foot at rest and is relieved when the foot is in a dependent position is a sign of more advanced disease.

Dx: History and physical examination, digital subtraction angiography, Doppler ultrasound, angiography, plethysmography, arteriogram, stress testing, oscillometry, coagulation studies, cholesterol and lipid studies

Rx: Goals are to provide adequate tissue perfusion, relieve discomfort and prevent complications.

- Medications: Aspirin, pentoxifylline (Trental), cilostazol (Pletal), vasodilator, prostaglandins, anticoagulants
- Medical treatment: Regular walking program where the client walks to the point of intermittent claudication then stops and rests for 3 minutes before continuing; weight reduction; smoking cessation
- Surgical treatment: Angioplasty, bypass grafting, endarterectomy, thrombectomy

Nursing Process Elements

- Assess pain and provide pain relief
- Assess circulation—check pedal pulses, sensation, capillary refill, edema, and temperature
- Assess skin integrity
- Elevate legs above heart to decrease edema
- Measure circumference of ankle and calf daily
- Provide pre- and postoperative care instructions

Client teaching for self-care

Instruct client to

- inspect skin for breakdown
- protect extremities from injury
- maintain a daily walking program
- elevate legs above heart for a fixed period of time each day
- avoid flexing and crossing legs
- not stand or sit for long periods of time
- avoid wearing constricting clothing
- stop smoking
- maintain ideal weight

BUERGER'S DISEASE (THROMBOANGITIS OBLITERANS)

- Buerger's disease is an inflammatory occlusive vascular condition in which the small and medium arteries and veins become thrombotic.
- It may occur in the upper or lower extremities but occurs usually in the leg or foot.
- It occurs most often in males between the age of 25 and 40 years.
- It involves periods of exacerbation and remission.

Etiology: Cause is unknown. Inflammation occurs in the adventitia leading to thrombi formation, abscesses, vasospasms, and vessel occlusion.

Precipitating factors: Genetic predisposition, cigarette smoking, chewing tobacco, autoimmune reaction.

S&S:

- Burning, numbness, or tingling of the extremity
- Intermittent claudication
- Pain at rest
- Smoking, cold temperatures, or emotional distress may trigger symptoms
- Intolerance to cold
- Decreased distal pulses
- Involved digits or extremity pale or cyanotic
- Skin shiny and thin
- Nails are thick and malformed
- Ulceration and gangrene in later stages

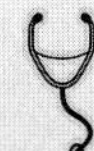

Assessment Alert

Small, red, tender vascular cords may be palpable in the affected extremity.

Dx: Based on client history and symptoms. Doppler studies, angiography, and MRI may be used to determine location and extent of disease

Rx:

- Stop smoking and tobacco use
- Keep extremity warm
- Decrease stress
- Protect extremity from injury
- Perform Buerger-Allen exercises
- Medications include analgesics, steroids, antibiotics to decrease pain and inflammation; calcium channel blockers (Cardizem) to decrease vasospasms; antiplatelets (Trental) to decrease blood viscosity, and vasodilators
- Surgery—Arterial bypass grafting, sympathectomy, and amputation

Nursing Process Elements

- Assess pain and provide pain relief
- Assess circulation—check pedal pulses, sensation, capillary refill, edema, temperature
- Assess skin integrity
- Measure circumference of ankle and calf daily
- Promote Buerger-Allen exercises
- Provide pre- and postoperative care instructions

Client teaching for self-care

Instruct client to

- inspect skin for breakdown
- keep extremity warm
- protect extremities from injury
- maintain a daily walking program
- avoid restricting clothing
- do Burger-Allen exercises
- elevate legs above heart for a period of time each day
- avoid flexing and crossing legs
- not stand or sit for long periods of time
- stop smoking
- identify and alleviate precipitating factors that increase pain
- engage in a weight reduction progam if needed

RAYNAUD'S DISEASE

- Raynaud's disease involves intermittent episodes of arterial spasms of the fingers, toes, ears, or nose.
- It occurs most frequently in women between the age of 15 and 45 years.

Etiology: Arterial spasms limit arterial blood flow to the digits, ears, or nose. Unknown etiology.

Precipitating factors: Autoimmune disorders such as systemic lupus erythematous, and rheumatoid arthritis, genetic predisposition, stress, cold temperatures, caffeine, and tobacco use.

S&S:

- Intermittent color changes of the involved digits or areas
- Absence or decrease in pulse during spasms
- Coldness, numbness, tingling in one or more digits often brought on by cold temperatures or emotional upsets
- Pain increases as disease progresses
- Nails may become thick and brittle
- Ulceration and gangrene are serious complications

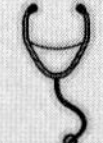

Assessment Alert

Triphasic color changes—involved areas become white (ischemia) then blue (collection of deoxygenated blood) and then red (spasms stop and circulation continues).

Dx: Based on symptoms and confirmed by arteriogram. Called Raynaud's phenomenon early-on when involvement is unilateral and limited generally to one or two digits. Considered Raynaud's Disease after 2–3 years by when symptoms have progressed to bilateral and increased involvement

Rx: Treatment of underlying disease, elimination of precipitating factors. Medications include analgesics, vasodilators, calcium channel blockers, sympathectomy

Nursing Process Elements

- Assess symptoms
- Determine presence of precipitating factors
- Assess extremities for complications including edema, ulcerations, and gangrene
- Teach client ways to eliminate precipitating factors: stop tobacco use, protect extremities from cold and injury, reduce stress

Client teaching for self-care

Instruct client to

- inspect skin for breakdown
- keep involved areas warm by the use of gloves, hats, wool socks, and comfortable shoes. May need to wear gloves when working with cold foods and in an air-conditioned environment

- ensure proper stress management
- protect extremities from injury
- avoid restricting clothing
- avoid flexing and crossing legs
- not stand or sit for long periods of time
- stop smoking
- identify and alleviate precipitating factors that increase pain

ARTERIOSCLEROSIS OBLITERANS

- Arteriosclerosis obliterans refers to a gradual narrowing of arteries leading to occlusion of the artery due to thrombosis and injury to the intima.
- It most often affects the abdominal aorta or the lower extremities.
- It occurs most frequently in men between the age of 50 and 60 years.

Etiology: Caused by arteriosclerosis.

Precipitating factors: Hypertension, diabetes mellitus, hyperlipidemia, obesity, elevated serum triglyceride level, smoking, genetic predisposition, high-fat diets, physical inactivity, stress, and gender.

S&S:

- Decreased or absent peripheral pulses in the lower extremities
- Skin on lower legs is shiny and thin with hair loss
- Pain and paresthesias
- Pallor when legs are elevated for 1–2 minutes and rubor when legs are in a dependent position

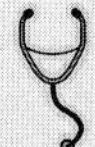

Assessment Alert

Pain may be both intermittent claudication and occur at rest.

Dx: History and physical examination, angiography, Doppler studies, and oscillometry

Rx: Prevention and elimination of risk factors, Buerger-Allen exercises, control of chronic diseases, medications to reduce hyperlipidemia, vasodilators, analgesics, and anticoagulants, surgery—bypass graft, endarterectomy, sympathectomy, angioplasty, and amputation

Nursing Process Elements

- Assess symptoms
- Determine presence of precipitating factors
- Assess extremities for complications including edema, ulcerations, and gangrene
- Assist client with Buerger-Allen exercises
- Encourage client to do a slow progressive walking program
- Provide pre- and postoperative teaching

Client teaching for self-care

Instruct client to

- inspect skin for breakdown
- ensure stress management
- protect extremities from injury
- avoid restricting clothing
- avoid flexing and crossing legs
- not stand or sit for long periods of time
- stop smoking
- identify and alleviate precipitating factors that increase pain
- do Buerger-Allen exercises
- eat a low-fat diet
- maintain good foot care

THROMBOPHLEBITIS

- Thrombophlebitis refers to thrombus formation on the wall of a vein with resulting inflammation.
- It may occur in superficial (SVT—generally in the upper extremities) or deep (DVT—generally in the lower extremities) veins.
- The most commonly affected veins are the saphenous, femoral, and popliteal.

Etiology: Precipitated by Virchow's triad factors— stasis of blood, injury to the vessel wall, and hypercoagulability of the blood. As a thrombus increases in size, it causes partial to complete occlusion of the vessel.

Precipitating factors: Bed rest, intravenous catheters, obesity, immobilization, pregnancy, childbirth, oral contraception, MI, CHF, malignancies, altered coagulability states, atherosclerosis, varicosities, multiple sclerosis, pelvic and abdominal surgeries, atrial fibrillation, and cigarette smoking.

S&S:

- Vary depending on thrombus size, location, and adequacy of collateral circulation. May be asymptomatic
- SVT—Tenderness, redness, palpable cord-like vein, increased warmth over involved vein
- DVT—Unilateral edema, tenderness over involved vein, warm skin, elevated temperature, cyanosis of affected extremity, general malaise

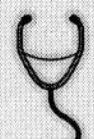

Assessment Alert

Homan's sign is no longer considered the classic manifestation of DVT because less than 20% of clients with DVT actually have a positive Homan's sign.

Dx: Ascending phlebography (injection of contrast medium into a vein), Doppler ultrasound, plethysmography (measures changes in fluid volume passing through a vessel), blood cultures, WBC, ESR, venous pressure measurement (high in affected limb until collateral circulation is developed)

Rx:

- SVT—relief of symptoms and reversal of inflammation process
  - —Warm moist heat application
  - —Anti-inflammatory medications
  - —Antibiotic therapy
  - —Anticoagulants if condition is progressing
- DVT
  - —Anticoagulant therapy with heparin (APTT at 1.5–2 times the control) or with low molecular weight heparin (LMWH) such as enoxaparin (Lovenox) which is prescribed according to weight 1 mg/kg subcutaneously every 12 hours
  - —Bed rest with leg elevated
  - —Oral anticoagulation with warfarin (Coumadin) is initiated along with heparin and LMWH. Therapeutic international normalized ratio (INR) is 2.0–3.0
  - —Thrombolytic therapy with streptokinase, urokinase, or tissue plasminogen activator
  - —Surgical intervention: venous thrombectomy, transvenous filtration devise placed in the inferior vena cava

Nursing Process Elements

- Assess for risk factors
- Asses pain level
- Provide bed rest with elevation of affected extremity
- Apply continuous warm moist compresses if ordered
- Administer medications
  - —Heparin
    - Use infusion pump to administer IV heparin
    - Inject heparin into fatty layer of abdomen above iliac crest and 2 inches away from umbilicus
    - Insert needle at 90 degree angle
    - Do not aspirate
    - Apply pressure after injection but do not massage
    - Assess for S&S of bleeding: petechiae, epistaxis, bleeding gums
    - Have antidote protamine sulfate available
  - —Warfarin
    - Instruct client to use soft tooth brush and to maintain bleeding precautions
    - Have antidote vitamin K available
    - Instruct client on factors that may affect anticoagulant response
- Monitor laboratory values
- Apply antiembolic stockings if ordered
- Monitor for possible complications like pulmonary emboli
- Measure involved extremity daily
- Provide client teaching

Client teaching for self-care

Teach client

- to adhere to medical regime
- about the importance of maintaining hydration
- to avoid standing and sitting for long periods or crossing legs
- to not wear constrictive clothing
- to not use tobacco
- to not use oral contraceptives
- about using antiembolism hose
- to maintain bleeding precautions when on Coumadin
- to avoid food which contains high levels of vitamin K like green leafy vegetables
- to follow drug regime and laboratory schedule
- to wear medic-alert bracelet
- to adhere to a progressive exercise regime
- about the S&S to report

PULMONARY EMBOLISM

- In pulmonary embolism (PE), a thrombus dislodges and travels through the venous circulation to the right side of the heart and lodges in a pulmonary artery.
- Most pulmonary emboli arise from detached venous thrombus originating in the deep veins of the legs, the right side of the heart, or the pelvic area.
- PE can manifest itself as one large clot, several tiny clots, or a shower of clots in the lungs.

Etiology: Obstruction of pulmonary artery by blood clot or other emboli (fatty or air); usually resulting from DVT that breaks loose and travels to pulmonary vasculature; characterized by VQ inequality (ventilation greater than perfusion)

Precipitating factors: DVT following orthopedic or abdominal surgery, use of oral contraceptives, pregnancy, prolonged immobility, any conditions characterized by venous stasis, hypercoagulability, and vein wall damage (Virchow's triad).

S&S:

- Dyspnea, tachypnea, crackles (rales), and wheezing
- Tachycardia and sharp, localized chest pain
- Restlessness and anxiety
- Hypoxemia
- Hemoptysis
- Hypotension
- If DVT is present there will be calf swelling, warmth at site, and mild fever

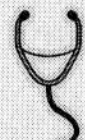

Assessment Alert

PE is difficult to diagnosis; therefore, the nurse needs to monitor in S&S for any client at risk.

Dx: VQ scan demonstrates a ventilation/perfusion mismatch, pulmonary angiography, ABGs, and CXR

Rx: For acute episode, IV heparin and thrombolytic agents (urokinase, streptokinase) to inhibit coagulation and prevent further clots; proactive treatment of clients at risk for DVT with low-dose SQ heparin and then oral anticoagulants; if heparin contraindicated may insert inferior vena cava filter, very rarely pulmonary embolectomy

Nursing Process Elements

- Elevate head of bed
- Maintain bed rest
- Administer oxygen
- Promote controlled breathing technique
- Monitor VS, LOC, and respiratory status
- Auscultate heart and lung sounds
- Do not massage legs
- Maintain hydration
- Apply elastic stockings (antiembolic) and pneumatic compression devices
- Monitor laboratory work for effectiveness of anticoagulant therapy
- Administer pain medications as needed
- Reduce anxiety

Client teaching for self-care

- Instruct client to avoid risk factors for further DVT
- Provide teaching related to anticoagulant therapy to avoid unnecessary bleeding
- Teach the importance of follow-up care

VARICOSE VEINS

- Varicose veins are irregular, dilated, tortuous veins with incompetent valves.
- Any veins may be involved but most commonly affects the veins of the lower body.
- Saphenous veins of the leg are the most affected.
- Varicose veins of the rectum are called hemorrhoids.
- Varicose veins of the esophagus are called varices.
- They are more common in women over the age of 35 years.

Etiology: Sustained stretching of the vein due to increased intravenous pressure prevents the valves from closing properly. As the amount of blood increases in the vein, there is increased venous stasis, the vein continues to stretch, the pressure increases, and the valves become increasingly incompetent.

- Primary varicose veins—no involvement of deep veins.
- Secondary varicose veins—caused by the obstruction of deep veins.

Precipitating factors: Prolonged standing, obesity, pregnancy, family predisposition, trauma to vein or valve, congenital weakness, and thrombophlebitis.

S&S:

- May be asymptomatic
- Pain in leg
- Leg fatigue
- Leg heaviness
- Visible dilated veins
- Feeling of heat in the leg
- Edema
- Itching over affected area
- Stasis ulcers
- Discoloration of the skin above the ankles

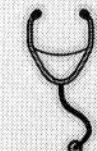

Assessment Alert

Positive Trendelenburg test to check for valve competency. Client is placed in supine position with legs elevated. As the client sits up and dangles legs, veins normally fill from the distal end. If the veins fill from the proximal end, there are varicosities.

Dx: Visual presence of varicosities and client history. Diagnostic tests include the tourniquet test, Doppler ultrasonic flow, angiographic studies, and plethysmography

Rx: There are no cures. Goals are to improve venous circulation, prevent skin breakdown, and provide pain relief.

Treatment is palliative: antiembolism stockings, walking, elevating legs throughout the day, compression sclerotherapy, and vein stripping

Nursing Process Elements

- Assess pain and provide pain relief
- Assess circulation—check pedal pulses, sensation, capillary refill, edema, and temperature
- Promote a regular exercise routine
- Apply antiembolism stockings and remove every 8 hours for short periods and reapply
- Assess skin integrity
- Elevate legs above heart to decrease edema
- Measure circumference of ankle and calf daily
- Teach client to not wear restrictive clothing or cross legs and to avoid prolonged periods of sitting or standing
- Provide pre- and postoperative care
  - —Sclerotherapy involves injecting a sclerosing agent into the vein; compression bandages are worn for up to 6-weeks postoperation
  - —Vein ligation: Postoperation, do hourly circulation checks, elevate extremity, and apply sequential compression hose

Client teaching for self-care

Instruct client to

- wear properly fitting antiembolism hose
- remove hose at least every day for an hour
- inspect skin for breakdown
- protect extremities from injury
- maintain a daily walking program
- elevate legs above heart for a fixed period of time each day
- avoid flexing and crossing legs

VENOUS STASIS ULCERS

- Venous stasis ulcer is a chronic disorder where the flow of blood through a vein is slowed or halted causing ischemia to the extremities and ulcer formation.
- More than 85% of leg ulcers are venous.

Etiology: When blood return from the legs is slowed either from valve incompetence or thrombosis, high pressure develops. Venous hypertension causes stretching of the veins and rupture of small veins and venules and further decrease in blood return. Eventually stasis causes edema and ulceration.

Precipitating factors: Thrombophlebitis, hypertension, varicose veins, trauma, pregnancy, obesity, and prolonged standing or sitting.

S&S:

- Brownish discoloration and leathery quality of the skin
- Edema of the extremity
- Pain that reduces when leg is elevated
- Moist ulcers are most often found around the malleolus

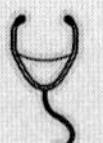

Assessment Alert

Pulses are palpable and extremity is warm.

Dx: History and physical examination

Rx: Compression wrap (Unna boot), elevation of extremity, bed rest, wound care (antibiotic or fungal therapy, hydrocortisone or zinc oxide as indicated), surgical or enzymatic debridement, and skin grafting

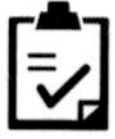

Nursing Process Elements

- Provide bed rest with legs elevated
- Provide wound care
- Give medications as prescribed
- Assess for risk factors
- Pre- and postoperative teaching

Client teaching for self-care

Teach client to

- inspect skin for breakdown
- protect extremities from injury
- avoid restricting clothing
- avoid flexing and crossing legs
- not stand or sit for long periods of time
- identify and alleviate precipitating factors that increase pain
- care of boot or compression bandage
- plan periods of rest with legs elevated
- use elastic stockings after ulcer heals
- adhere to medical regime since ulcers generally reoccur

PEDS KAWASAKI DISEASE

- Kawasaki disease (KD) is also called "mucocutaneous lymph node syndrome."
- It causes acute systemic vasculitis, i.e., inflammation of arterioles, venules, and capillaries.
- It may progress to coronary artery aneurysms and coronary thrombosis.

Etiology: Unknown. Because of seasonal outbreaks, an infectious etiology may be involved. KD does not spread from person to person contact as is typical in infectious diseases.

Precipitating factors: Occurs more frequently in children younger than 5 years of age.

S&S:

- High fever that does not respond to typical treatment
- Bilateral conjunctivitis
- Strawberry tongue and cracking of the lips
- Edema of the periphery
- Desquamation of the palms of the hands and soles of the feet

Dx: History and physical examination

Rx: Salicylate therapy, intravenous gamma globulin administration

Nursing Process Elements

- Monitor cardiac function, I&O, and daily weights
- Give medication as ordered, monitor for aspirin toxicity
- Administer IVIG per manufacturer's recommendation
- Promote comfort: oral care, skin care, oral hydration

Client teaching for self-care

Teach client

- about skin care: avoiding lotions and soaps
- about oral care for comfort
- Monitor temperature
- Safe salicylate administration
- Complications of IVIG

WORKSHEET

SHORT ANSWER QUESTIONS

1. The nurse places a client on cardiac telemetry and notices the following pattern. Identify the rate, rhythm, and the cardiac pattern.

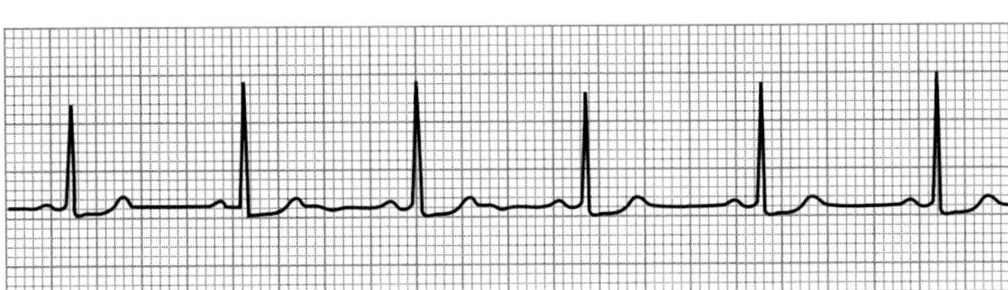

Rate _______________

Rhythm _______________

Pattern _______________

2. The nurse notices the following rhythm on the cardiac monitor. What would be the correct rate and rhythm interpretation?

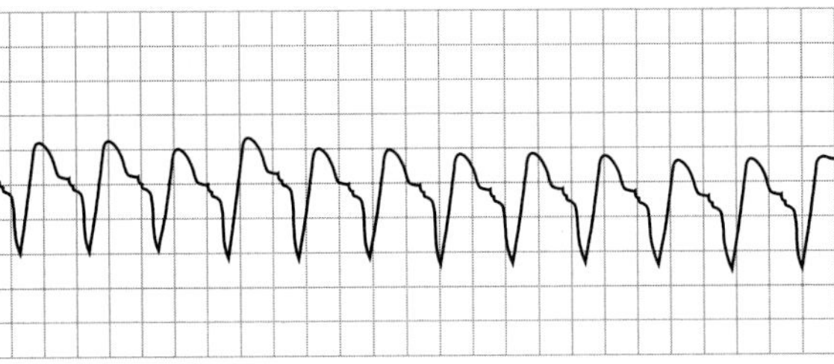

(continued)

3. Label the following: P wave, PR interval, QRS, and QT interval and state what each represents.

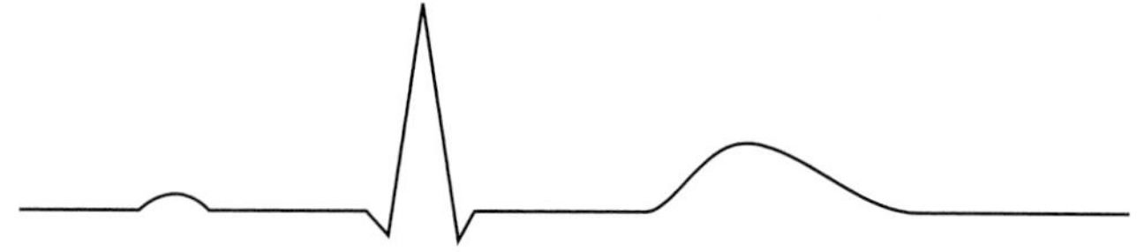

4. Briefly list the things a nurse should do before giving thrombolytics to a client suspected of having a myocardial infarction.

5. What are the three "I"s that describe the progression of pathophysiology when a patient has an MI?.

6. Discuss briefly the etiology and precipitating factors of endocarditis.

7. Discuss briefly why anticoagulant therapy is initiated for clients experiencing atrial fibrillation.

8. List 5 points of information to be included in a teaching plan for a client newly diagnosed with hypertension.

9. State what is meant by the PQRST of pain assessment for an MI patient.

10. Identify the Virchow's triad factors of thrombophlebitis.

11. The nurse is to give digoxin 1.25-mg IV push. The nurse has digoxin 0.5 mg per 2 ml. The nurse would give ______ ml.

12. A client who is being treated for congestive heart failure has lost 4 lbs so far. How much fluid has the client lost?

13. Identify the statements below as to whether they are true for Mechanical or Tissue (biologic) heart valves.
    a. ______ Considered to be more durable
    b. ______ Three basic types—xenografts, homografts, and autografts
    c. ______ Less likely to cause thromboemboli
    d. ______ Requires lifetime anticoagulant therapy
    e. ______ Often used for younger clients

APPLICATION QUESTIONS

1. The nurse realizes that more teaching is needed when the client on a cardiac low-cholesterol diet makes which choice from the menu?
    a. Stewed chicken, green beans, and noodles
    b. Liver and onions, salad with ranch dressing, and milk
    c. Ham and bean soup, salad with vinaigrette dressing, and cornbread
    d. Pork roast, brown rice, and beets

2. When taking a client's medical history, which are the precipitating factors for myocardial infarction? (Select all that apply.)
    a. Hypothyroidism
    b. Cigarette smoking
    c. Hyperlipidemia
    d. Rheumatic fever
    e. Elevated serum iron level
    f. High density lipids <40 mg
    g. Using oral contraceptives

3. When the nurse performs an admission assessment on a client, the nurse notes that the client has xanthomas present on both eyelids. The laboratory value that the nurse would want to check based on this assessment finding is
    a. triglyceride level
    b. homocystine level
    c. cardiac enzymes—CPK-MB, troponin, and myoglobin
    d. cholesterol panel

4. A client presents to the clinic with the following symptoms: a burning sensation in the lower extremities, thickened toe nails, and pain in legs when walking. The nurse would assess the client for which additional factor consistent with Burger's disease (thromboangitis obliterans)?
   a. Bounding peripheral pulses
   b. Rubor when the extremities are elevated
   c. Intolerance to heat
   d. Symptoms triggered by stress
5. A goal for a client with arteriosclerosis obliterans is to increase arterial blood supply to the extremities. Which of the following nursing interventions would be appropriate for this goal?
   a. Elevate the extremities above the level of the heart for 15 minutes four times a day.
   b. Have client perform Buerger-Allen exercises four times a day.
   c. Maintain client on bed rest with legs in a neutral position.
   d. Position client in high-Fowler's position with legs straight.
6. Which of the following assessment findings are consistent with the diagnosis of venous stasis?
   a. Absent or diminished peripheral pulses
   b. Hair loss on the extremity
   c. Moist ulcers around the malleolus
   d. Edema of the extremity
   e. Coolness of the extremity
   f. Leathery quality of the extremity
   g. Pallor of the extremity
7. A client is returned to the unit after having a repair of an abdominal aortic aneurysm. The nurse should place the client in which of the following positions?
   a. High-Fowler's
   b. Sims
   c. Semi-Fowler's
   d. Flat
8. The nurse is giving a client low molecular weight heparin, enoxaparin. The correct nursing interventions when administering this medication include all of the following except
   a. using a TB syringe
   b. injecting the medicine using Z-track method
   c. not rubbing the site postinjection
   d. administering the medicine in the anterolateral abdominal wall
9. In order to prevent the postoperative complication of thrombophlebitis in a client who has had mitral valve replacement, the nurse would have the client engage in which of the following activities?
   a. Perform dorsiflexion of the feet several times every hour while awake
   b. Cough and take deep breaths every hour while awake
   c. Sit up in a chair for several hours during the afternoon
   d. Eat a high-fiber, high-calorie diet
10. The nurse is caring for a client who has just arrived on the unit following a cardiac catheterization. Which of the following assessments would be most immediate?
    a. Heart and lung sounds
    b. Pain at the catheter insertion site
    c. Pulses distal to the insertion site
    d. Urine output
11. A client comes into the ER complaining of "his heart racing." Cardiac monitor shows atrial tachycardia with a ventricular rate of 190 bpm. The nurse anticipates that the physician will order adenosine (Adenocard) to be given. Prior to giving the medication the nurse should do which of the following?
    a. Determine when the client last ate
    b. Ask the laboratory to draw serum BUN and creatinine levels
    c. Ask the client if he/she has a history of asthma
    d. Have the client sign a consent
12. Metoprolol tartrate (Lopressor) is ordered for a client who has had a myocardial infarction. The nurse would expect which therapeutic result from administration of this drug?
    a. Increased urinary output
    b. Decreased coronary artery spasms
    c. Increased cardiac output
    d. Decreased resting heart rate
13. A client's cardiac monitor strip shows the following: HR 42/min, rhythm regular, PRI 0.16 seconds, QRS 0.06 seconds. The client is experiencing dizziness, nausea, and chest pain rated as 3 on a scale of 1–10 with 10 being the worst pain. The drug of choice to treat this dysrhythmia is
    a. Lidocaine (Xylocaine)
    b. Adenosine (Adenocard)
    c. Atropine sulfate
    d. Epinephrine (Adrenalin)
14. A client is admitted to the ER with new onset atrial fibrillation with a ventricular response of 110/min.

(continued)

The nurse would anticipate which of the following treatment options to be ordered. (Select all that apply.)
a. Defibrillation
b. Start oxygen at 2–4 lpm
c. Anticoagulant therapy
d. Medicate with beta blocker
e. Start Lidocaine drip
f. Atrial pacing

15. The nurse is assessing a newborn infant who is exhibiting the following signs and symptoms: elevated blood pressure, bounding brachial pulses, diminished pedal pulses, elevated Jugular venous distention (JVD), and cardiac murmur. Based on the assessment, the nurse would suspect that the client may have which of the following conditions?
a. Congestive heart failure
b. Coarctation of the aorta
c. Mitral valve prolapse
d. Transposition of the great vessels

16. The nurse has assessed a client and has determined that the client is exhibiting signs and symptoms of left heart failure. Identify which of the following are indicative of left heart failure.
a. Tachypnea, loss of appetite, ST elevation on the ECG
b. Hemoptysis, cogwheel murmur, midsternal chest pain
c. Ascites, oliguria, fatigue
d. Orthopnea, bibasilar crackles, gallop rhythm

17. The nurse is providing nutritional counseling for a client who is receiving a loop diuretic. Which meal plan would be most appropriate for this client?
a. Raisin bran cereal, tomato juice, whole grain toast
b. Boiled chicken, green beans, tossed salad
c. Vegetable soup, low-salt crackers, skim milk
d. Poached fish, beets, macaroni and cheese

18. The nurse is reading a 6-second cardiac rhythm strip and notes 9 QRS complexes in it. The client's heart rate is
a. 54
b. 63
c. 81
d. 90

19. A client has been diagnosed with pericardial effusion. The nurse would prepare the client for which of the following procedures?
a. Myotomy
b. Pericardiectomy
c. Pericardiostomy
d. Dynamic cardiomyoplasty

20. Which instruction would be inappropriate to give a client following coronary artery bypass graft surgery?
a. No driving for 6–8 weeks
b. Avoid smoking or tobacco use for 4–6 weeks
c. No heavy lifting for 6–8 weeks
d. Can resume sexual intercourse in 3–4 weeks

21. A nurse checks the client's arterial blood gas results which are as follows: pH, 7.38; PO_2, 88 mm Hg; PCO_2, 33 mm Hg; HCO_3, 24 mEq/l; and O_2 saturation, 96%. Which is the correct interpretation of these results?
a. Metabolic acidosis
b. Metabolic alkalosis
c. Normal values
d. Respiratory alkalosis

22. Which of the following instructions regarding a cardiac nuclear scan should a nurse give the client?
a. Avoid coffee, tea, and cocoa the morning of the test
b. Take a clear liquid diet for 24 hours before the test
c. Dress in comfortable clothing and walking shoes
d. Take all medications as prescribed prior to the test

23. Which assessment finding in a neonate should the nurse interpret as a sign of possible coarctation of the aorta?
a. Triphasic color changes in the upper extremities
b. Pulsating abdominal mass with a systolic bruit and cool lower extremities
c. Decreased distal pulses, thick, malformed nails, cyanotic upper extremity digits
d. Bounding pulses in the arms and absent pulses in the groin and legs

24. The nurse is administering a beta blocker to a client admitted with an MI. The client's wife asks what the medication will do. Which fact should be the foundation of the nurse's reply? The medication will:
a. reduce the amount of oxygen needed by the heart muscle
b. decrease the risk of a blood clot
c. enhance the affinity of oxygen for hemoglobin
d. increase the volume of blood in the coronary arteries

25. The nurse would expect to administer morphine sulfate, oxygen, nitroglycerine and aspirin to a client with which problem?
a. Raynaud's disease
b. Myocardial infarct
c. Valvular heart disease
d. Kawsaki disease

ANSWERS & RATIONALES

ANSWERS FOR SHORT ANSWER QUESTIONS

1. The nurse places a client on cardiac telemetry and notices the following pattern. Identify the rate, rhythm, and the cardiac pattern.

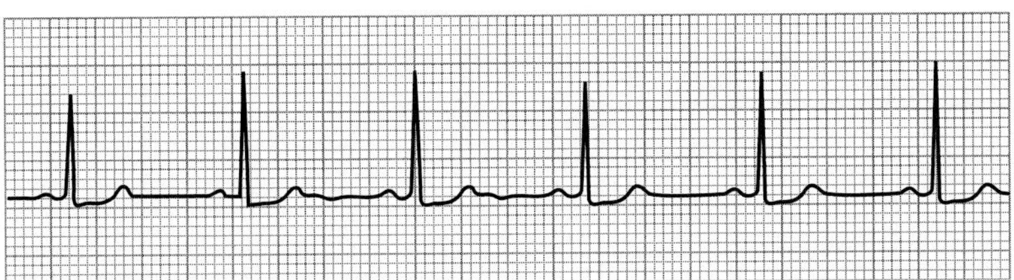

Answer
Rate 78 (1500 ÷ 19 = 78)
Rhythm regular
Pattern normal sinus rhythm

2. The nurse notices the following rhythm on the cardiac monitor. What would be the correct rate and rhythm interpretation?

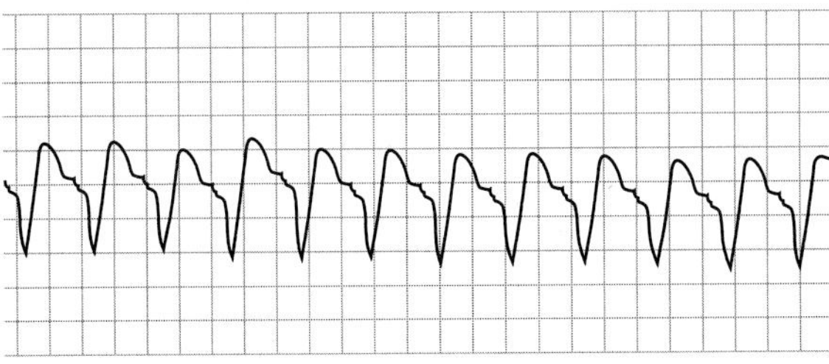

Answer
Ventricular rate 1500 ÷ 11 = 136
QRS wide and bizarre
Rhythm regular
Interpretation ventricular tachycardia

3. Label the following: P wave, PR interval, QRS, and QT interval and state what each represents.

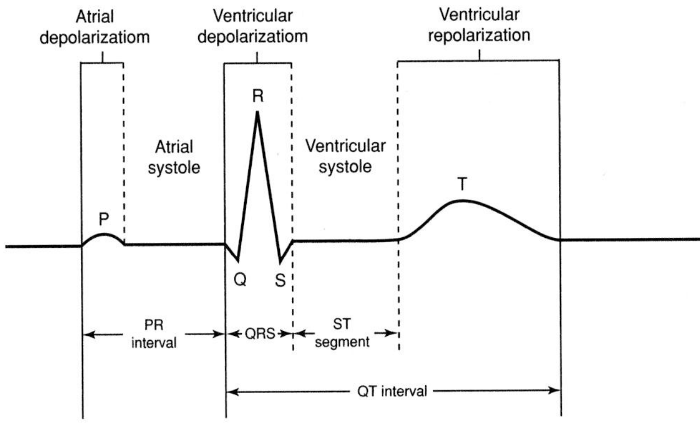

(continued)

4. Briefly list the things a nurse should do before giving thrombolytics to a client suspected of having a myocardial infarction.

Answer
Before giving a thrombolytic, the nurse should establish 2–3 IV sites, give no IM injections, assess for allergies especially if receiving streptokinase, handle the client gently, continuously monitor the client's cardiac pattern, assess laboratory values for bleeding times and elevation in cardiac enzymes, and provide emotional support.

5. What are the three "I"s that describe the progression of pathophysiology when a patient has an MI?

Answer
Ischemia progresses to injury progresses to infarction

6. Discuss briefly the etiology and precipitating factors of endocarditis.

Answer
Etiology: Rheumatic heart disease, clients with prosthetic heart valves, IV drug use, mitral valve prolapse (very common cause), and infectious organisms usually bacteria (*Streptococci*, *Enterococci*, or *Staphylococcus aureous*)

Precipitating factors: Underlying cardiac conditions, dental, surgical or invasive procedures, or urological procedures. There must be some mechanism to allow bacteria entrance to the bloodstream.

7. Discuss briefly why anticoagulant therapy is initiated for clients experiencing atrial fibrillation.

Answer
Since the atria are quivering and not squeezing, blood can pool in the atria and thrombus formation may occur. Anticoagulant therapy helps prevent thrombus formation.

8. List 5 points of information to be included in a teaching plan for a client newly diagnosed with hypertension..

Answer
a. Necessary lifestyle changes including modification of risk factors
b. Complications of hypertension
c. Medication regimen
d. Methods for monitoring blood pressure and apical pulse
e. Need for adherence to medical regime and that treatment is palliative and not curative

9. State what is meant by the PQRST of pain assessment for an MI patient.

Answer
P—position
Q—quality and quantity
R—radiation and relief
S—severity and symptoms
T—timing

10. Identify the Virchow's triad factors of thrombophlebitis.

Answer
a. Stasis of blood
b. Injury to the vessel wall
c. Hypercoagulability of the blood

11. The nurse is to give digoxin 1.25-mg IV push. The nurse has digoxin 0.5 mg per 2 ml. The nurse would give ______ ml.

Answer
The nurse is to give digoxin 1.25-mg IV push. The nurse has digoxin 0.5 mg per 2 ml. The nurse would give __0.5__ ml.

12. A client who is being treated for congestive heart failure has lost 4 lbs so far. How much fluid has the client lost?

Answer

One liter of fluid = 2.2 lbs. Thus, 4 ÷ 2.2 = 1.8.
The client has lost 1.8 liters of fluid so far.

13. Identify the statements below as to whether they are true for Mechanical or Tissue (biologic) heart valves.
    a. _____ Considered to be more durable
    b. _____ Three basic types—xenografts, homografts, and autografts
    c. _____ Less likely to cause thromboemboli
    d. _____ Requires lifetime anticoagulant therapy
    e. _____ Often used for younger clients

Answer

a. __Mechanical__ Considered to be more durable
b. __Tissue__ Three basic types- xenografts, homografts, and autografts
c. __Tissue__ Less likely to cause thromboemboli
d. __Mechanical__ Requires lifetime anticoagulant therapy
e. __Mechanical__ Often used for younger clients

APPLICATION ANSWERS

1. The nurse realizes that more teaching is needed when the client on a cardiac low-cholesterol diet makes which choice from the menu?
   a. Stewed chicken, green beans, and noodles
   b. Liver and onions, salad with ranch dressing, and milk
   c. Ham and bean soup, salad with vinaigrette dressing, and cornbread
   d. Pork roast, brown rice, and beets

Rationale

Correct answer: b.
The client should avoid liver because organ meat is high in cholesterol.

2. When taking a client's medical history, which are the precipitating factors for myocardial infarction? (Select all that apply.)
   a. Hypothyroidism
   b. Cigarette smoking
   c. Hyperlipidemia
   d. Rheumatic Fever
   e. Elevated serum iron level
   f. High density lipids <40 mg
   g. Using oral contraceptives

Rationale

Correct answers: b, c, e, f, and g.
Hypothyroidism is not a risk factor for MI. Rheumatic fever is a risk factor for valve disease.

3. When the nurse performs an admission assessment on a client, the nurse notes that the client has xanthomas present on both eyelids. The laboratory value the nurse would want to check based on this assessment finding is
   a. triglyceride level
   b. homocystine level
   c. cardiac enzymes—CPK-MB, troponin, and myoglobin
   d. cholesterol panel

Rationale

Correct answer: d.
Cholesterol accumulates in tumor nodules on the skin. Triglyceride level is a measure of fats in the blood stream. Elevated homocystine levels are considered an independent risk factor for atherosclerosis. Cardiac enzymes elevate with MI.

4. A client presents to the clinic with the following symptoms: a burning sensation in the lower extremities, thickened toe nails, and pain in legs when walking. The nurse would assess the client for which additional factor consistent with Burger's disease (thromboangitis obliterans)?

(continued)

a. Bounding peripheral pulses
b. Rubor when the extremities are elevated
c. Intolerance to heat
d. Symptoms triggered by stress

Rationale

Correct Answer: d.

Symptoms are triggered by stress.

5. A goal for a client with arteriosclerosis obliterans is to increase arterial blood supply to the extremities. Which of the following nursing interventions would be appropriate for this goal?
   a. Elevate the extremities above the level of the heart for 15 minutes four times a day.
   b. Have client perform Buerger-Allen exercises four times a day.
   c. Maintain client on bed rest with legs in a neutral position.
   d. Position client in high-Fowler's position with legs straight.

Rationale

Correct answer: b.

These exercises help drain static blood from the legs when elevated and then increase the amount of blood going to the legs when in a dependent position and when the legs are flat, the person exercises their ankles and feet increasing circulation. Answer "a" drains static blood from the legs and is used with varicose veins. Answers "c" and "d" do not drain stagnant blood from the legs and thus will not increase arterial blood flow to them.

6. Which of the following assessment findings are consistent with the diagnosis of venous stasis?
   a. Absent or diminished peripheral pulses
   b. Hair loss on the extremity
   c. Moist ulcers around the malleolus
   d. Edema of the extremity
   e. Coolness of the extremity
   f. Leathery quality of the extremity
   g. Pallor of the extremity

Rationale

Correct answers: c, d, and f.

Moist ulcers around the malleolus, leathery quality to the skin of the extremity, and edema of the extremity are signs of venous stasis. Absent pulses, coolness, pallor and hair loss are all signs of arterial insufficiency.

7. A client is returned to the unit after having a repair of an abdominal aortic aneurysm. The nurse should place the client in which of the following positions?
   a. High-Fowler's
   b. Sims
   c. Semi-Fowler's
   d. Flat

Rationale

Correct answer: d.

The client should be placed in a flat position so that flexion of the graft is prevented.

8. The nurse is giving a client low molecular weight heparin, enoxaparin. The correct nursing interventions when administering this medication include all of the following except
   a. using a TB syringe
   b. injecting the medicine using Z-track method
   c. not rubbing the site postinjection
   d. administering the medicine in the anterolateral abdominal wall

Rationale

Correct answer: b.

Z-track method is used for IM injections in order to trap medicine in the muscle.

9. In order to prevent the postoperative complication of thrombophlebitis in a client who has had mitral valve replacement, the nurse would have the client engage in which of the following activities?
   a. Perform dorsiflexion of the feet several times every hour while awake
   b. Cough and take deep breaths every hour while awake
   c. Sit up in a chair for several hours during the afternoon
   d. Eat a high-fiber, high-calorie diet

Rationale

Correct answer: a.

Performing dorsiflexion of the feet several times every hour while awake prevents venous stasis. Answers "b" and "c" help prevent pneumonia and answer "d" aids healing.

10. The nurse is caring for a client who has just arrived on the unit following a cardiac catheterization. Which of the following assessments would be most immediate?
    a. Heart and lung sounds
    b. Pain at the catheter insertion site
    c. Pulses distal to the insertion site
    d. Urine output

Rationale

Correct answer: c.

All assessments would need to be done but the risk of a clot-decreasing circulation is most important.

11. A client comes into the ER complaining of "his heart racing." Cardiac monitor shows atrial tachycardia with a ventricular rate of 190 bpm. The nurse anticipates that the physician will order adenosine (Adenocard) to be given. Prior to giving the medication the nurse should do which of the following?
    a. Determine when the client last ate
    b. Ask the laboratory to draw serum BUN and creatinine levels
    c. Ask the client if he/she has a history of asthma
    e. Have the client sign a consent

Rationale

Correct answer: c.

Adenosine (Adenocard) can cause bronchospasms in asthmatic clients.

12. Metoprolol tartrate (Lopressor) is ordered for a client who has had a myocardial infarction. The nurse would expect which therapeutic result from administration of this drug?
    a. Increased urinary output
    b. Decreased coronary artery spasms
    c. Increased cardiac output
    d. Decreased resting heart rate

Rationale

Correct answer: d.

It is a beta-adrenergic blocking agent, which slows the heart rate.

13. A client's cardiac monitor strip shows the following: HR 42/min, rhythm regular, PRI 0.16 seconds, QRS 0.06 seconds. The client is experiencing dizziness, nausea, and chest pain rated as 3 on a scale of 1–10 with 10 being the worst pain. The drug of choice to treat this dysrhythmia is
    a. Lidocaine (Xylocaine)
    b. Adenosine (Adenocard)
    c. Atropine Sulfate
    d. Epinephrine (Adrenalin)

Rationale

Correct answer: c.

Atropine sulfate blocks vagal impulses to the heart and increases heart rate. Lidocaine is used for control of ventricular dysrhythmias. Adenosine is used to restore NSR in clients with supraventricular tachycardia. Epinephrine is a catecholamine which acts on alpha and beta receptors and is used for anaphylactic reactions and relief of bronchospasms.

14. A client is admitted to the ER with new onset atrial fibrillation with a ventricular response of 110/min. The nurse would anticipate which of the following treatment options to be ordered. (Select all that apply.)
    a. Defibrillation
    b. Start oxygen at 2–4 lpm
    c. Anticoagulant therapy
    d. Medicate with beta blocker
    e. Start Lidocaine drip
    f. Atrial pacing

Rationale

Correct answers: b, c, d, and f.

Elective cardioversion and not defibrillation may be used. Lidocaine is used to treat ventricular dysrhythmias.

15. The nurse is assessing a newborn infant who is exhibiting the following signs and symptoms: elevated blood pressure, bounding brachial pulses, diminished pedal pulses, elevated Jugular venous distention (JVD), and cardiac murmur. Based on the assessment, the nurse would suspect that the client may have which of the following conditions?
    a. Congestive heart failure
    b. Coarctation of the aorta
    c. Mitral valve prolapse
    d. Transposition of the great vessels

Rationale

Correct answer: b.

There is narrowing of the aorta restricting outflow so that there is elevated pressure in the upper extremities and diminished outflow to the lower extremities.

16. The nurse has assessed a client and has determined that the client is exhibiting signs and symptoms of left heart failure. Identify which of the signs and symptoms are indicative of left heart failure.
    a. Tachypnea, loss of appetite, ST elevation on the ECG
    b. Hemoptysis, cogwheel murmur, midsternal chest pain
    c. Ascites, oliguria, fatigue
    d. Orthopnea, bibasilar crackles, gallop rhythm

Rationale

Correct answer: d.

Blood backs into the lungs causing congestion and respiratory symptoms and a gallop rhythm develops from increased blood flow across the valves. Answer "b" consists of signs and symptoms of pulmonary air embolism. Answer "c" consists of signs and symptoms of right heart failure.

(continued)

17. The nurse is providing nutritional counseling for a client who is receiving a loop diuretic. Which meal plan would be most appropriate for this client?
    a. Raisin bran cereal, tomato juice, whole grain toast
    b. Boiled chicken, green beans, tossed salad
    c. Vegetable soup, low-salt crackers, skim milk
    d. Poached fish, beets, macaroni and cheese

Rationale

Correct answer: a.

Tomato juice and raisins contain potassium, which is lost through loop diuretics.

18. The nurse is reading a 6-second cardiac rhythm strip and notes 9 QRS complexes in it. The client's heart rate is
    a. 54
    b. 63
    c. 81
    d. 90

Rationale

Correct answer: d.

$9 \times 10 = 90$

19. A client has been diagnosed with pericardial effusion. The nurse would prepare the client for which of the following procedures?
    a. Myotomy
    b. Pericardiectomy
    c. Pericardiostomy
    d. Dynamic cardiomyoplasty

Rationale

Correct answer: c.

Pericardiostomy is the creation of an opening into the pericardium. It is usually done to drain a pericardial effusion. Myotomy is the cutting into a muscle. Precardiectomy is the excision of a part of the pericardium. Dynamic cardiomyoplasty is a procedure done to improve the pumping action of the myocardium.

20. Which instruction would be inappropriate to give a client following coronary artery bypass graft surgery?
    a. No driving for 6–8 weeks
    b. Avoid smoking or tobacco use for 4–6 weeks
    c. No heavy lifting for 6–8 weeks
    d.Can resume sexual intercourse in 3–4 weeks

Rationale

Correct answer: b.

Smoking and use of tobacco should be stopped entirely not just for 4–6 weeks. All other instructions are appropriate for the client following coronary artery bypass graft surgery.

21. A nurse checks the client's arterial blood gas results which are as follows: pH, 7.38; PO_2, 88 mmHg; PCO_2, 33 mmHg; HCO_3, 24 mEq/l; and O_2 saturation 96%. Which is the correct interpretation of these results?
    a. Metabolic acidosis
    b. Metabolic alkalosis
    c. Normal values
    d. Respiratory alkalosis

Rationale

Correct answer: c.

The blood gas results listed are all in normal range so no acid-base imbalance is present.

22. Which of the following instructions regarding a cardiac nuclear scan should a nurse give the client?
    a. Avoid coffee, tea, and cocoa the morning of the test
    b. Take a clear liquid diet for 24 hours before the test
    c. Dress in comfortable clothing and walking shoes
    d. Take all medications as prescribed prior to the test

Rationale

Correct answer: c.

23. Which assessment finding in a neonate should the nurse interpret as a sign of possible coarctation of the aorta?
    a. Triphasic color changes in the upper extremities
    b. Pulsating abdominal mass with a systolic bruit and cool lower extremities.
    c. Decreased distal pulses, thick, malformed nails, cyanotic upper extremity digits
    d. Bounding pulses in the arms and absent pulses in the groin and legs

Rationale

Correct answer: d.

Bounding pulses in the upper extremities and decreased or absent pulses in the groin and legs occurring several hours to days after birth and the closure of the ductus arteriosus are signs of severe coarctation of the aorta.

Triphasic skin changes in the affected parts are characteristic of Raynaud's disease. A pulsating abdominal mass with a systolic bruit and cool lower extremities are signs of an abdominal aortic aneurysm. Decreased distal pulses, thick, malformed nails, cyanotic upper extremity digits are symptoms of thromboangitis obliterans (Buerger's disease).

24. The nurse is administering a beta blocker to a client admitted with an MI. The client's wife asks what the medication will do. Which fact should be the foundation of the nurse's reply? The medication will:

a. reduce the amount of oxygen needed by the heart muscle
b. decrease the risk of a blood clot
c. enhance the affinity of oxygen for hemoglobin
d. increase the volume of blood in the coronary arteries

Rationale

Correct answer: a.

Drugs that reduce oxygen demand or increase the oxygen supply to the myocardium are part of the immediate care of clients with an MI. These drugs include nitrates, beta blockers, calcium channel blockers, antihypertensives, and antiplatelet agents. Beta blockers reduce oxygen demand by the myocardium.

25. The nurse would expect to administer morphine sulfate, oxygen, nitroglycerine and aspirin to a client with which problem?

a. Raynaud's disease
b. Myocardial infarct
c. Valvular heart disease
d. Kawasaki disease

Rationale

Correct answer: b.

MONA (morphine sulfate, oxygen, nitroglycerine and aspirin are administered in the emergency rook to clients with myocardial infarcts. The treatment of Raynaud's consist of elimination of precipitating factors, medications such as analgesics, vasodilators, and calcium channel blockers, or sympathectomy. Treatment of valvular heart disease includes digitalis, diuretics, ACE inhibitors, antibiotics prior to dental work or invasive procedures to prevent endocarditis, and surgical repair or replacement. Salicyclate therapy and intravenous gamma globulin administration is the treatment for Kawasaki disease.

Test Plan Category:

Physiological Integrity

Sub-category: Physiological Adaptation—Part 1

Topics: Alterations in Body Systems
Illness Management
Section 2: Hematologic Problems

ANEMIA

Anemia is caused by a reduction in the number of circulating red blood cells (RBCs). Reduced RBCs can be due to:

- decrease in total blood volume,
- decreased production,
- impaired maturation, and
- increased destruction or hemolysis.

Anemias are classified and named based on the cause of the reduction in circulating red blood cells. Nursing management for prevention and risk factor reduction of anemia are:

- dietary teaching,
- awareness of exposure to environmental toxins,
- injury prevention,
- early and periodic screening for conditions that may cause blood loss,
- early detection of chronic bleeding disorders, and
- genetic counseling for hereditary anemic disorders.

Various types of anemia.

ACUTE HEMORRHAGIC ANEMIA

Caused by rapid or sudden loss of blood volume

Etiology: Trauma, surgery, platelet dysfunction, and coagulation disorders

S&S:

- Signs and symptoms are those of hypovolemia and hypoxemia
- Decreased hemoglobin and hematocrit are late signs
- Severity of symptoms correlates to amount of blood loss
- If not controlled, irreversible shock can occur

Nursing Process Elements

- Educate clients about the potential need for transfusion of blood products

- Monitor for signs and symptoms of transfusion reaction for any blood products given

CHRONIC ANEMIA

Due to gradual loss of blood

Etiology:

- Gastrointestinal: gastritis, peptic ulcers, hemorrhoids, esophageal ulcerations, or chronic use of aspirin or NSAIDs
- Vaginal: excessive menses, postpartum bleeding, reproductive hormone abnormalities, benign or malignant uterine lesions
- Malnourishment

S&S:

- Client may remain asymptomatic
- Common symptoms when present are fatigue, dyspnea, tachycardia
- Lab findings: decreased RBCs, Hgb, Hct, MCV, and MCHC

Nursing Process Elements

Client teaching for self-care

- Client education on diet and foods high in iron and vitamins, spacing of activities and frequent rest periods.
- Client education on compliance with routine screenings and blood tests.

APLASTIC ANEMIA

- Results from impaired erythrocyte production
- Characterized by a reduction or cessation of all blood-producing elements thus RBCs, platelets, and white blood cells are affected

Etiology:

- Fifty percent of clients have no knowledge of causative etiologic agent
- Aplastic anemia can be drug, chemical, or infection induced
- It can be congenital

S&S:

- Pallor of skin and mucous membranes
- Fatigue
- Palpitations
- Exertional dyspnea
- Infections of the skin and mucous membranes in severe cases
- Hemorrhagic: bleeding into skin and mucous membranes, spontaneous bleeding from nose, gums, vagina, or rectum
- Development of symptoms gradually over weeks or months

Dx:

- Initial diagnosis most often through laboratory analysis of blood
- Definitive diagnosis through bone marrow analysis

Nursing Process Elements

- Primary foci of nursing care: Monitor for signs of bleeding, which is a risk because of decreased platelets, and prevent infection, which is a risk because of immunosuppression.
- Monitor any puncture sites for bleeding and signs of infection
- Minimize any invasive procedures such as venipuncture, injections, bladder catheterization
- Avoid rectal temperatures, medications, or enemas
- Test urine and stool for occult blood
- Plan activities so that fatigue is prevented
- Monitor for excessive fatigue
- Assist client in developing coping strategies to deal with prolonged hospitalization

Client teaching for self-care

- Importance of strict hand washing for family and visitors
- Need for meticulous personal hygiene
- Ways to reduce risk of hemorrhage such as not using a toothbrush for oral care and padding any sharp corners on furniture
- Rationale for protective isolation if applicable

HEMOLYTIC ANEMIA

- Destruction of erythrocytes at a rate greater than bone marrow can compensate for the reduction.
- Two types of hemolysis
  - —Extravascular: premature removal of erythrocytes from circulation by the spleen
  - —Intravascular: erythrocytes lyse as a result of an enzyme deficiency in the cell membrane, or mechanical injury to the cell membrane

AUTOIMMUNE HEMOLYTIC ANEMIA

There are three classifications

- Warm-reacting
  - —Most often idiopathic
  - —More common in women
  - —May be associated with SLE, RA, chronic lymphocytic leukemia, and myeloma

—Pathophysiology: antibodies develop against own erythrocytes and combine more easily at body temperature hence the term warm-reacting

—Common signs and symptoms: jaundice, pallor, and splenomegaly

- Cold-reacting

—Less common, usually affecting older adults

—Raynaud's phenomenon is an example

—Associated with mononucleosis, mycoplasma pneumoniae, Epstein-Barr virus, mumps, and Legionnaires' disease

—Pathophysiology: immunoglobulin M antibodies react with antigens on the erythrocyte at temperatures below 88 °F causing red cells to clump in capillary beds

—Signs and Symptoms: cyanosis, pain, paresthesias, and hemoglobinuria

- Drug-induced

—Causes about a fifth of cases

—Most frequently caused by methyldopa, penicillin, quinine, and quinidine

—Pathophysiology: response is abnormal antibody production specific to the drug

Dx:

- Positive Coombs' test
- Decreased Hct, increased reticulocyte count
- Increased bilirubin

Rx: Determined by the severity of condition

Nursing Process Elements

Promote use of effective strategies to cope with a chronic condition

Client teaching for self-care

- Importance of compliance with drug therapy
- Avoidance of cold if applicable

HEREDITARY SPHEROCYTOSIS

Alteration in the erythrocyte shape leads to osmotic swelling of the RBC and vulnerability to destruction by the spleen due to the cell's inability to move through the spleen's microcirculation.

S&S: pallor, fatigue, exertional dyspnea, jaundice, and enlarged spleen, increased reticulocyte count, increased serum bilirubin

Rx: splenectomy often with cholecystectomy as well

Nursing Process Elements

- Plan care to conserve energy.
- Provide perioperative care as discussed in Chapter 18.

SICKLE CELL DISEASE

- Inherited hemoglobinopathies that cause abnormal sickle-shaped hemoglobin to partially or totally replace normally shaped hemoglobin
- Two most common forms are:

—sickle cell trait: Individuals who are heterozygous for the disease are said to have the "trait" and are carriers for the disease.

—sickle cell anemia: Individuals who are homozygous for the trait, have predominantly sickle hemoglobin, and are symptomatic.

- Affected person produces an abnormal form of hemoglobin called hemoglobin S

—Nonaffected individuals produce a form of hemoglobin call hemoglobin A (Adult hemoglobin)

—A fetal form of hemoglobin is found in all newborns. At approximately 4–6 months of age, the hemoglobin converts to an adult form of hemoglobin.

—Affected individuals are normal at birth but symptoms appear at 4–6 months of age.

- Under conditions of decreased oxygen tension in the blood, the hemoglobin S red blood cell, which has normal oxygen-carrying capacity, forms a sickle shape

—Sickled RBCs tend to clump together increasing blood viscosity and obstructing blood flow through small vessels resulting in tissue hypoxia.

—RBCs with hemoglobin S are more fragile than RBCs with hemoglobin A (the adult form of hemoglobin). Normal RBCs last approximately 120 days. RBCs with hemoglobin S have a life span of 10–20 days. Shortened life span leads to a chronic anemia.

—Amount of sickling correlates with the severity of symptoms: the more the sickling, the more severe the symptoms.

- Three forms of crisis are associated with sickle cell disease

—Vaso-occlusive crisis: When oxygen levels in the blood drop, the RBCs assume the sickle shape, clump together, and obstruct small blood vessels.

—Anemic crisis: An ongoing problem for the individual with sickle cell anemia.

—Sequestration crisis: A pooling of blood in the spleen of individuals with sickle cell anemia that leads to circulatory collapse. It tends to occur in children younger than 6 years of age. By the age of 7, the spleens of most children with the disease become nonfunctioning due to repeated infarcts and would no longer be susceptible to sequestration crisis.

Etiology:

- Inherited as autosomal recessive
  - —Both parents must be at least carriers
- Primarily affects blacks
  - —Also seen in individuals of Mediterranean and Hispanic descent

Risk Factors:

- Contributing factors for a vasoocclusive crisis include any condition that decreases oxygen in the blood, increases the uptake of oxygen from the blood, or slows the blood flow.
  - —High altitudes, flying in unpressurized planes, exercise, infection, fever, cold weather, and emotional stress can lead to a vasoocclusive crisis.

S&S:

- Vaso-occlusive crisis
  - —The major symptom of a vaso-occlusive crisis is pain due to ischemia; pain may be localized, migratory, or generalized
  - —Hand and foot syndrome: a self limiting vaso-occlusive crisis causing swelling and pain of the hands or feet
  - —Vaso-occlusive crisis involving the brain can lead to a cerebral vascular accident (stroke), blindness, and convulsions
  - —Acute chest syndrome is another serious vaso-occlusive crisis involving the lungs and causing cough, chest and abdominal pain, and fever
  - —Other symptoms depend upon the location of the vaso-occlusive crisis
- Sequestration crisis
  - —Sudden onset of paleness, hypovolemic shock
- Anemia
  - —Pallor, jaundice, delayed growth
- Other symptoms include cholelithiasis, which is not usually seen in children without the disease
- Chronic problems
  - —Leg ulcers
  - —Renal problems as a result of repeated infarctions
  - —Ocular problems as a result of repeated infarctions resulting in retinal detachment and blindness
  - —Musculoskeletal problems including necrosis and uneven growth
  - —Bacterial infection susceptibility from lack of spleen function
  - —Pulmonary problems can include pneumonia, fat embolism, and pulmonary hypertension
  - —Cardiac problems as a result of increased cardiac workload
  - —Priapism in males

Dx:

- Prenatal diagnosis can be made by chorionic villi sampling or amniocentesis
- Newborn screening is mandatory in most states
- Hemoglobin electrophoresis
- Screenings can include sickle turbidity test (Sickledex) which does not differentiate those with the trait (carriers) from those with the disease
- Reticulocyte count will be elevated due to fragility of RBCs

Rx:

- Therapeutic management involves promoting optimal oxygenation conditions
- Routine vaccinations plus pneumococcal, meningococcal, and yearly flu vaccines are recommended
- During crisis
  - —Intravenous fluids for hydration
  - —Narcotic analgesics
  - —Oxygen therapy
  - —Blood transfusions if vaso-occlusive crisis is in a critical area such as the brain

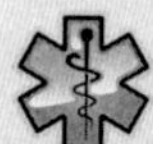

Nursing Intervention Alert

Meperidine (Demerol) should not be administered to children with sickle cell as they are particularly sensitive to the neurologic complications related to the buildup of meperidine metabolites.

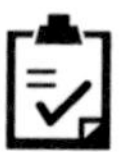

Nursing Process Elements

- During crisis
  - —Monitor vital signs and pulse oximetry
  - —Monitor for changes in mental status
  - —Assess respiratory function
  - —Promote rest to decrease oxygen utilization
  - —Encourage hydration with clear liquids
  - —Monitor pain and administer narcotics as needed
  - —Reduce emotional stress
  - —Administer blood as ordered
  - —Minimize exertion and promote rest periods
- Assess psychosocial status and provide referrals to support services and resources
- Provide client/family teaching on crisis triggers and activities necessary to reduce risk of crisis, behaviors that promote positive coping with a chronic illness, and importance of medical follow-up care

Client teaching for self-care

- General health practices to promote normal growth and development
  - —Nutrition to support RBC production: high protein, calcium, vitamins, and iron
  - —Immunizations
  - —Prevention of infection including importance of avoiding infectious individuals and good hand washing
- Information about the disease process
- Signs and symptoms of crisis
- Treatment of crisis

THALASSEMIA

- Most common inherited single-gene disorder
- Most often affects people of Mediterranean descent
- Characterized by decreased RBC production and chronic hemolytic anemia
- Two types
  - —Thalassemia minor: mild, usually asymptomatic anemia that does not require treatment
  - —Thalassemia major (aka Cooley's anemia): severe anemia resulting in growth failure and death between the ages of 17 and 30

Rx: Transfusion therapy is used for symptom alleviation or to maintain hemoglobin at a more normal level

Nursing Process Elements

- Monitor for transfusion reaction
- Provide supportive care
- Teach about disease process and progression

IRON DEFICIENCY ANEMIA

Inadequate amount of iron impairs formation of hemoglobin and RBCs and results in decreased ability of the blood to transport oxygen to the tissues.

Etiology:

- Chronic blood loss
- Poor nutrition (inadequate intake or absorption of iron)

S&S:

- Pallor
- Sensitivity to cold
- Fatigue
- Exertional dyspnea
- Severe deficiency symptoms include brittle spoon-shaped nails with longitudinal ridges, smooth shiny tongue, and cheilosis
- Decreased Hgb, Hct, iron ferritin, and reticulocytes

Rx:

- Identify cause and correct
- Iron rich diet with avoidance of teas and coffee (which reduce iron)
- Oral iron supplements, for example, ferrous sulfate (Feosol), iron dextran (DexFerrum)
- Transfusion if necessary

Nursing Process Elements

- Assess cardiovascular and respiratory status to detect decreased activity tolerance and dyspnea on exertion
- Monitor stool, urine, and emesis for occult blood
- Administer medications prescribed to replace iron stores
- Provide mouth and skin care
- Protect the client from falls caused by weakness and fatigue

Client teaching for self-care

- Correct method for taking iron supplements
- When to contact the physician
- Components of a proper diet and foods high in iron

VITAMIN B12 DEFICIENCY ANEMIA

- Chronic, progressive, macrocytic anemia
- Lack of B12 results in defective maturation of RBCs.

Etiology:

- Inadequate dietary intake of vitamin B12 which is a particular risk with strict vegetarian diets
- Prolonged iron deficiency, malabsorption secondary to intestinal disease or intestinal resection
- Lack of absorption as a result of deficiency of intrinsic factor resulting from autoimmune disease
- Gastric mucosal atrophy or gastric resection

Think Smart/Test Smart

Be sure to distinguish among the various types of vitamin B12 deficiency based on cause. When vitamin B12 deficiency anemia is caused by a lack of intrinsic factor, a substance normally secreted by the gastric mucosa, it is called pernicious anemia. Because vitamin B12 is absorbed in the ileum and intrinsic factor is required for its absorption, clients with pernicious anemia must receive lifelong injections of vitamin B12.

S&S:

- Pallor
- Anorexia and dyspepsia
- Weight loss
- Constipation or diarrhea
- Gait disturbances
- Paresthesias of the hands and feet
- Dyspnea
- Glossitis, sore mouth
- Scleral jaundice
- Bone marrow aspiration shows increased megaloblasts, few maturing erythrocytes, and defective leukocyte maturation
- Positive *Romberg* test and *Shilling* test

Rx:

- Increased dietary intake of vitamin B12: animal proteins especially organ meats, eggs and dairy products; dried beans, nuts, green leafy vegetables, and Brewer's yeast for deficiency due to inadequate intake.
- Vitamin B12 supplement if needed.
- Transfusion therapy if severely symptomatic.
- Weekly B12 injections for pernicious anemia and when B12 cannot be absorbed for reasons other than deficiency of intrinsic factor; may become monthly injections as disease is controlled.

Nursing Process Elements

- Assess cardiovascular status to detect signs of compromise as the heart works harder to compensate for the reduced oxygen-carrying capacity of the blood
- Administer prescribed medications
- Provide mouth care before and after meals for glossitis
- Prevent client from falling
- Monitor and record vital signs
- Maintain activity as tolerated
- Monitor lab values to detect effectiveness of therapy

Client teaching for self-care

- Foods high in vitamin B12 if dietary deficiency is the cause of the anemia
- Need for lifelong, monthly B12 injections if pernicious anemia or other inability to absorb vitamin B is the cause of the anemia

POLYCYTHEMIA VERA

- Bone marrow disorder characterized by an abnormal increase in RBCs (erythrocytosis) often accompanied by leukocytosis and thrombocytosis (abnormally high number of circulating platelets)
- Causes increased blood viscosity and platelet dysfunction (platelet dysfunction can increase susceptibility to bleeding problems)
- Despite the increased number of RBCs, generalized hypoxia exists because the abnormal cells have an impaired oxygen-carrying capacity
- Untreated survival time is 1–2 years; with treatment, 7–15 years

Etiology: Unknown

S&S:

- None in early disease
- With hypervolemia from increased blood viscosity: headache, vertigo, tinnitus, blurred vision, red appearing skin, thromboemboli (DVT, CVA, MI, pulmonary embolism, etc).
- Epistaxis, ecchymoses, and GI bleeding from platelet dysfunction

Rx: Periodic phlebotomy to remove RBCs and return Hct and Hgb to normal. Myelosuppressive therapy may also be used but carries the risk of leukemia transformation especially in younger clients.

Nursing Process Elements

Client teaching for self-care

- Attend to signs of thrombi or emboli and give importance to seeking immediate attention
- Provide interventions to decrease the risk of thrombus formation
- Drink adequate amounts of fluid (3 l/d) to decrease blood viscosity

- Avoid smoking and wearing of constricting clothing.
- Wear support hose when out of bed and elevate feet whenever sitting.
- Take anticoagulants as ordered and take precautions against bleeding.
- Exercise only as directed by health care provider.

NEUTROPENIA

- Neutrophil count of less than $2000/mm^3$
- Another name for agranulocytosis

Etiology: Primary or secondary to leukemia, aplastic anemia, hypersplenism, various chemicals, or drugs such as propylthiouracil and the sulfonamides

Rx: Treatment or removal of underlying cause

Nursing Process Elements

- Provide assessments and interventions aimed at preventing infection which may be life threatening
- Institute neutropenic precautions

LEUKEMIA

- Cancer of blood forming organs causing an uncontrolled production of white blood cells (leukocytes, myelocytes, and their precursors) by the bone marrow
- Stem cells of the bone marrow produce an immature WBC that is incapable of fighting infection
- Bone marrow fills with immature WBCs limiting the production of RBCs and platelets leading to the major symptoms of leukemia: infection, anemia, and bleeding episodes
- Four primary categories of leukemia according to the type of WBC involved and the rate of cell growth
  - —Acute lymphoblastic leukemia (ALL)
  - —Acute myelogenous leukemia (AML)
  - —Chronic lymphoblastic leukemia (CLL)
  - —Chronic myelogenous leukemia (CML)
    - Lymphoblastic denotes cancerous changes in lymphocytes
    - Myelogenous denotes cancerous changes in granulocytes and monocytes
    - Forms of leukemia other than ALL are often referred to under the generic term ANLL (acute nonlymphoblastic leukemia).

PEDS Most common pediatric leukemia is acute lymphoblastic (or lymphoid) leukemia

- Classified as acute or chronic based on cell differentiation progression, that is, maturity of the WBCs
  - —All leukemic cells are immature, but those involved in acute leukemia are more immature.
  - —Acute leukemia affects immature cells causing rapid onset and progression.

With the more mature WBC in the chronic form of leukemia, these cells can do a better job of fighting infection.

PEDS Most pediatric leukemias are the acute form.

Etiology: Although not fully understood, multiple factors have been associated with the development of leukemia.

- Genetic factor
  - —Identical twins have a higher incidence of concordance in the development of leukemia than fraternal twins.
  - —Selected chromosomal disorders including Down's syndrome and Fançoni's syndrome have been associated with a higher risk for leukemia.
- Infectious agents have been suspected of contributing to the development of leukemia. A virus has been documented in cats as a causative agent for feline leukemia
- Exposure to radiation and selected chemical toxins

S&S:

- Acute leukemia: rapid onset and progression of symptoms because immature cells are affected.
  - —Lack of normal WBCs results in numerous infections
  - —Early symptoms
    - Fever
    - Bruising
    - Lymphadenopathy
    - Pallor
    - Malaise
    - Fatigue due to anemia
    - WBC count may be normal, decreased, or increased
  - —Other symptoms
    - Bone pain (from bone marrow over crowding)
    - Increased abdominal girth
    - Hepatosplenomegaly
    - Dehydration

- DIC
- Nausea and vomiting
  - Headache
  - Blurred vision
- Chronic leukemia: insidious onset, slow progression over many years because mature cells are affected
  —WBC count is usually elevated
  —Usual disease presentation is nonspecific flu-like symptoms
  —Early symptoms
  - Fatigue
  - Weakness
  - Anorexia
  - Weight loss
  - Enlarged spleen and liver, which are palpable
  - Fever
  - Pallor, lethargy, and anorexia
  - Bruising, petechiae, and purpura
  - Bone pain (due to overcrowded bone marrow)

ACUTE LYMPHOBLASTIC LEUKEMIA

- PEDS Peak incidence occurs in children between 2 and 6 years of age
- Boys are affected more commonly that girls

Etiology: ALL is caused by a single lymphoid stem cell with abnormal maturation and accumulation of malignant cells in bone marrow.

Dx:

- Peripheral blood smear demonstrates immature WBCs. Total WBCs may be low or elevated at initial diagnosis. A low WBC count at the time of diagnosis is associated with a better prognosis; a high WBC with the greater number of immature cells, the worse the prognosis.
- Bone marrow aspiration provides definitive diagnosis. The iliac crest is the most frequent site for this test in children.
- Following diagnosis, a lumbar puncture may be performed to determine the presence of CNS involvement.

Rx:

- The goal of treatment is remission, that is, the absence of all leukemic symptoms including a bone marrow containing less than 5% blasts (normal bone marrow).
- Treatment includes chemotherapy and radiation.
- Chemotherapy involves several drugs used in combination to prevent the development of resistance. The particular combination of chemical agents is called the protocol and varies from institution to institution.
- Four phases of chemotherapy
  —Induction is the first phase of therapy with a goal of remission. This usually occurs during the first 4–6 weeks of treatment.
  —Consolidation is the second phase of treatment. Once the child is in remission, additional drugs will be administered to eradicate residual leukemic cells.
  —Intensification, the third phase, is designed to prevent the emergence of cells which are resistant to chemotherapy.
  —Maintenance therapy is the fourth phase which continues for several years to preserve the remission.
- Irradiation of the CNS or testes may be added if leukemic involvement has been noted in these areas.
- Relapse is the term given to reappearance of leukemic cells after a remission has been obtained. When remission occurs, the chemotherapy protocol is modified to include drugs not previously used.
- Hematopoietic stem cell transplant provides the best opportunity for cure but carries serious morbidity and mortality concerns. The source of the stem cells is an antigen-matched donor or from umbilical cord blood.

Nursing Process Elements

- Prior to diagnosis, provide the child and parents with information about the diagnostic process.
- Provide emotional support to the child and parents as they undergo the numerous invasive procedures involved in the diagnosis.
- Explain expected effects of chemotherapy that depresses the bone marrow leading to low WBCs, RBCs, and platelets.

  RBCs
  —The child will be tired.
  —Additional rest periods will be needed.
  —Blood transfusions may be required if the child's hemoglobin and hematocrit drop too low.

  Platelets
  —The child will be at risk for hemorrhage.
  —Care in handling the child is required to prevent or reduce bruising.
  —Soft toothbrush or gauze covered finger may be used for oral care if bleeding gums become problematic.
  —Increase in liquid intake and use of stool softeners will be needed to prevent constipation and straining with elimination.

  WBCs
  —The child's ability to fight infections will be diminished.
  —It is required to make certain that all persons in contact with the child wash hands scrupulously.
  —Good skin care will be needed to maintain a healthy first line of defense.

—Aseptic technique will be used for all invasive procedures.

—Fresh flowers and plants should be kept away from the child as they may harbor organisms.

—Live organism vaccinations should be avoided.

—All family members should to receive a flu shot.

—Exposure to a large number of visitors or anyone with any sign of contagious illness should be avoided.

—If the WBC count becomes extremely low, reverse or protective isolation may be instituted to reduce exposure.

—The child should be monitored for signs and symptoms of infection.

- Management of chemotherapy toxicity

—Control/reduce nausea and vomiting by the use of antiemetics.

  - Administer antiemetics prior to the chemotherapy rather than waiting until nausea occurs.
  - Maintain the environment free of nauseating stimuli, for example, keep the emesis basis handy but out of sight.
  - Odors may be problematic so keep the room fresh without perfumes and other strong odors.
  - Plan chemotherapy administration for other than around meal time whenever possible.

—Monitor intake and output

—Combat anorexia which is a symptom of the disease and a response to the chemotherapy, because a well nourished cell is more responsive to the chemotherapy so maintaining good nutrition is paramount to treatment success.

  - Provide small frequent feedings of bland foods.
  - Provide high protein and high calorie snacks.
  - Keep in mind that foods from home may be more acceptable to the hospitalized child than hospital food.

—Obtain daily weights.

—Treat mouth ulcers which are a painful complication of many chemotherapeutic agents.

  - Rinse the mouth with plain water several times a day to reduce development of oral ulcers.
  - Use a soft toothbrush for oral care.
  - Avoid the use of alcohol in mouthwashes.
  - Use local anesthetics as necessary.
  - Avoid spicy acidic food.

—If the child is to receive a drug that has alopecia as a known side effect, prepare the child for this side effect. The child may want to shave his or her head before the hair falls out or may chose to wear scarves and hats to cover the hair loss. If a child chooses to wear a wig, the wig should be selected prior to hair loss.

—If a chemotherapeutic agent is to be given that makes the skin more susceptible to sunlight, cover the skin and use sun blocks at all times since even a mild exposure can cause a severe burn.

Client teaching for self-care

- The family needs to know how to administer the chemotherapeutic agents the child receives at home.
- The child and family should be prepared for the specific side effects of the drugs that the child is receiving.
- Cytotoxic chemicals will be excreted from the child's body for up to 48 hours after administration and family members should be protected from exposure.

—Double flush the commode after the child uses it.

—Place a plastic liner over the mattress to prevent the mattress from absorbing chemicals excreted from the body.

—Wash the child's clothing and bed linens separately from the rest of the family laundry.

ACUTE MYELOGENOUS LEUKEMIA

- Primarily affects ages 12–20 and over age 55

Etiology: It is caused by a single myeloid stem cell resulting in immature myeloblasts to develop in bone marrow

Dx: Diagnosis is by bone marrow biopsy.

Rx:

- Bone marrow transplant: HLA identical allogeneic or autologous
- Autologous stem cell transplant: Client's own blood cells collected and centrifuged to remove malignant cells, then stored and reinfused after client's bone marrow is destroyed.
- Chemotherapy: Cytarabine and doxorubicin are commonly used.

Remission occurs in 50–70% of clients. Allogeneic bone marrow transplant use is increasing in frequency as a treatment option.

CHRONIC LYMPHOBLASTIC LEUKEMIA

- CLL primarily affects ages 50–70, found more commonly in men
- Proliferation of small abnormal mature B lymphocytes occurs
- Abnormal lymphocyte accumulation begins in the lymph nodes, spreading to other lymphatic tissue and the spleen

Dx: Diagnosis is through blood smear

S&S:

- Additional symptoms specific to CLL are pruritic vesicular skin lesions, anemia thrombocytopenia, and spleen enlargement

- Clotting episode may be the first manifestation of the disease due to increased blood viscosity

Rx: Treatment (alkylating agents such as chlorambucil or glucocorticoids) usually only occurs when symptoms present, no treatment is curative

Average lifespan after diagnosis is 4.5–5.5 years.

CHRONIC MYELOGENOUS LEUKEMIA

- Primarily affects ages 30–50
- CML is 14% of all leukemia cases.
- It commonly changes from a chronic phase to an accelerated or blastic phase progressing quickly to fulminant mirroring an acute leukemia with anemia and thrombocytopenia.
- During the blastic phase, blood vessels are blocked by the leukemic cells. Leukemic infiltrates into various tissues, epidural tumors which can cause spinal cord compression, and lytic bone lesions may occur.

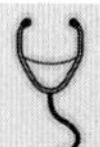

Assessment Alert

Adverse effects of interferon-alpha therapy

Early effects lasting about 2 weeks are: fever, chills, malaise, arthralgia, fatigue, and headache.

Late toxic effects are: hepatitis, proteinuria, hypothyroidism, depression and psychosis

Adverse effects of Imatinib are fluid retention which can cause sudden ascites, pulmonary edema, or pleural or pericardial effusion; gastrointestinal irritation and hematologic changes.

Etiology: CML results from an acquired injury (not inherited or present at birth) to a bone marrow stem cell's DNA leading to uncontrolled proliferation of granulocytes.

S&S: Classic symptoms of chronic leukemia are fatigue, weakness, anorexia, weight loss, and splenomegaly.

Dx: Diagnosis through blood smear which shows granulocytes in all stages of maturity, blasts to mature neutrophils

Rx: BMT done for early disease in otherwise healthy clients; hydroxyurea, which requires frequent blood checks because of its myelosuppressive effects, is used for chronic phase in other clients. In the blastic phase, anthracycline, cystosine arabinoside, or interferom alpha therapy are used but with very limited success.

- Overall survival rate is poor, with only 30% surviving 5 years after diagnosis
- Complications are usually treatment related

Nursing Process Elements

Client teaching for self-care

- Disease process and therapy effects
- Infection and bleeding prevention
- What symptoms need to be immediately reported
- Medications and side effects
- Need for good nutrition and fluid intake
- Stomatitis risk reduction through meticulous oral care
- Chemotherapy regimen and need for periodic blood counts
- Community resources and support groups
- Ongoing medical follow-up

HEMOPHILIA

- Bleeding disorder related to deficiency of a clotting factor
  - —The normal individual has more than 10 different clotting factors that work together to form a clot
  - —Clotting factors are produced by the liver and found in the plasma
- Two primary forms of hemophilia based on the deficient clotting factor
  - —Classic hemophilia or hemophilia A is a deficiency of Factor VIII, the antihemophilic factor
  - —Christmas disease, also called hemophilia B is a deficiency of Factor IX, plasma thromboplastin component
- Severity of the disease is based on the level of factor in the blood and can range from mild to severe. The severity of the disease runs in families.

Etiology: Both forms of hemophilia are inherited as sex linked recessive, carried by the female and primarily affecting males.

Risk Factors: The gene that controls the production of the involved clotting factors is located on the long arm of the X chromosome. Since women have two X chromosomes, each child of a carrier female has a 50/50 chance of receiving the affected X. Men have only one X chromosome. When the man reproduces, he gives his Y chromosome to the son who will not be affected, but his daughters will receive the affected X and can further transmit the disease.

S&S: Any injury can lead to a bleeding episode. The symptoms and severity of bleeding is dependent upon the type and site of injury and can include

- Ecchymoses (bruises)
- Epistaxis (nosebleed)
- Hematuria (blood in the urine)
- Hemarthrosis (bleeding into the joints)

Dx:

- It may be diagnosed in the newborn nursery after a circumcision that fails to clot or as a toddler learning to walk
- Partial prothrombin time (PTT) is delayed. Prothrombin time (PT), thrombin time (TT), and fibrinogen and platelet count are normal
- Carrier determination is possible in classic hemophilia with DNA testing
- It can be diagnosed by chorionic villi sampling or amniocentesis

Rx:

- IV administration of the missing factor (either factor VII or factor IX)
  —Administered at first evidence of a bleed
  —Dose is individualized based on child's degree of deficiency
  —Prophylactic factor is administered in the morning as it has a short half-life
- Factor is a blood product found in fresh or fresh frozen plasma
  —Factor is now available in a recombinant form (lab made) but may still be stabilized with the addition of albumin
  —Factor may be stored in the refrigerator in the client's home for ready use
- DDAVP (desmopressin acetate) may be administered to the child with mild hemophilia to increase factor VIII activity

Nursing Process Elements

- Controlling bleeding episodes
  —RICE—rest, ice, compression, and elevation
- Avoid any drug known to affect bleeding time including aspirin and ibuprofen
- With bleeding into joints, a goal of treatment is to avoid loss of joint function
  —Immobilization and elevation during an acute bleed
  —Range of motion, once the bleed is contained

Client teaching for self-care

- In addition to the pathophysiology of hemophilia, the need to recognize symptoms of a hemorrhage and preparation to implement appropriate first aid by the family and child.
- Safe and effective administration of the factor: Toddlers may have a subcutaneous venous port inserted to make intravenous insertion easier. Older children are taught to start their own intravenous line for the administration of the factor.
- Activities to promote growth and development while protecting the child from hemorrhages: Discuss with the parents and child, sports activities that are safe; contact sports must be avoided, but sports such as golf and swimming will allow for normal competition without placing the child in danger.
- Good oral hygiene: Avoiding dental care may lead to dental caries and loss of teeth which may cause a bleeding episode.
- In case surgery or tooth extraction is required, the need to keep the child in a controlled environment with prophylactic factor administration.

THROMBOCYTOPENIA

- Decreased number of circulating platelets
- Normal adult platelet count is 150,000 to 400,000/mm^3; below 60,000/mm^3 there is a risk of bleeding with trauma; below 20,000/mm^3, spontaneous, life-threatening hemorrhage can occur.

Etiology:

- Thrombocytopenia can result from decreased production, decreased survival time, increased destruction, and sequestration of blood in the spleen, loss from hemorrhage, or increased use.

- Most common type of thrombocytopenia is idiopathic thrombocytopenic purpura in which there is increased destruction.
  - —Acute ITP: self limiting with a duration of less than 6 months; typically follows a viral disease
  - —Chronic ITP: Autoimmune disease of young adulthood
  - —Drug induced ITP: Causative drugs include alcohol, digitoxin, thiazides, rifampin, aspirin and NSAIDs; lasts 1–2 weeks after drug is discontinued

S&S: Petechiae (occur only with thrombocytopenia), ecchymosis, purpura, bleeding (e.g., nose bleeds, bleeding gums, hypermenorrhea, hematuria)

Dx: Decreased platelet count; increased bleeding time

Rx: ITP: corticosteroid and immunosuppressive therapy to decrease antibody production; splenectomy since spleen is the organ where platelets are destroyed.

Platelet concentrate as a temporary measure to control bleeding.

Nursing Process Elements

- Monitor for bleeding
- Institute bleeding precautions if platelet count below 20,000/mm^3
  - —Test all urine and stool for blood
  - —No rectal treatments (temperatures, suppositories, enemas, etc.)
  - —No IM injections
  - —Put firm pressure on all venipuncture sites for 5 minutes and on arterial puncture sites for 10 minutes.

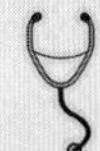

Assessment Alert

Assess effectiveness of any platelet transfusion by checking platelet count before transfusion and 1 hour after. If no change has occurred in the count, the transfusion was ineffective. Keep in mind that viability of platelets between collection and transfusion is only several days and viability after transfusion is 24–48 hours as opposed to the life of normal platelets which is 10 days.

Client teaching for self-care

Take precautions to prevent trauma and bleeding:

- Use a soft toothbrush, swab, or gauze covered finger for mouth care.
- Do not use dental floss.
- Shave with an electric razor to decrease the risk of accidental cuts.
- Put nothing in the rectum.
- Put firm, consistent pressure on any bleeding area for 5–10 minutes.
- Avoid aspirin containing products and any other medications or herbs with an anticoagulant effect.

VITAMIN K DEFICIENCY

Vitamin K is a fat soluble vitamin essential for synthesis of clotting factors II, VII, IX, and X.

Sources: diet from foods such as green leafy vegetables, produced by intestinal bacteria

Etiology:

- Decreased dietary intake
- Decreased intestinal production as a result of destruction of intestinal flora by broad spectrum antibiotic therapy
- Lack of absorption of the vitamin because of intestinal problems such as malabsorption syndrome, Crohn's disease and ulcerative colitis
- Impaired action of the vitamin by drugs such as coumarin, aspirin, and quinine

S&S: Bleeding

Dx: Prolonged PT and PTT

Rx:

- Correct underlying problem
- Menadione (water soluble vitamin K) PO or IV (works in 6–24 hours)
- Transfusion of fresh frozen plasma for immediate effect

PEDS At birth, the neonate is lacking vitamin K because the gut is sterile so vitamin K is not being produced. To cover the period of time between birth and when intestinal flora is established and begins to synthesize adequate amounts of vitamin K, aqueous menadione is administered as part of initial newborn care.

Nursing Process Elements

- Assess for bleeding: bruising, hematuria, bleeding gums, etc.
- Teach precautions related to preventing trauma and decreasing risk of bleeding

LYMPHEDEMA

Abnormal collection of lymphatic fluid in a part as a result of obstructed lymphatic flow

Etiology:

- Primary: results from abnormalities in development of the lymph system
- Secondary: results from injury to the lymph nodes from surgery, for example, lymph node dissection in diagnosis and management of cancer, radiation, or parasites

S&S:

- Soft, pitting edema, which changes over time to hard, nonpitting edema.
- Occurs more often in left lower extremity than in right and is aggravated by pregnancy, obesity, warm weather, menstruation, and prolonged standing.
- Severe enlargement of an extremity is called elephantiasis.

Complication: Infection

Rx: Diuretics, long term antibiotics, intermittent pneumatic compression stocking

Nursing Process Elements

- Assess for signs of infection
- Assess for skin breakdown

Client teaching for self-care

- Avoid constricting clothing or accessories.
- Elevate affected extremity.
- Use compression stocking/garment or pump as ordered.
- Exercise involved limb to stimulate lymph flow.
- If a lower extremity, avoid prolonged standing.
- Follow any prescribed medication and dietary guidelines.

HODGKIN'S DISEASE

- It is a malignant disorder of the lymph nodes.
- Reed Sternberg cell is the signature cell of the disease.
- Disease has a predictable pattern of spread.
- Prognosis depends heavily on stage of disease at time of diagnosis.
- Accurate staging is essential to determining the correct treatment protocol.

Etiology: Unknown but some association with the Epstein–Barr virus noted

S&S:

- Unexplained fever
- Night sweats
- Generalized pruritus
- Anorexia and weight loss
- Cough
- Hepatomegaly and splenomegaly
- Fatigue and weakness
- Malaise and lethargy
- Recurrent infection and fever
- Enlarged, nontender, firm and movable cervical, axillary, or inguinal lymph predictable pattern of spread

Dx: Lymph node biopsy is positive for Reed–Sternberg cells (Hodgkin's disease)

Rx:

- Radiation for stages IA, IB, IIA, IIB
- Chemotherapy for stages III and IV using MOPP regimen (mechlorethamine (nitrogen mustard), vincristine (Oncovin), prednisone and procarbazine)

Nursing Process Elements

- Decrease risk of skin injury and infection.

NON-HODGKIN'S LYMPHOMA

- It is also called malignant lymphoma.
- Tumors occur throughout lymphatic organs in an unpredictable pattern.

Etiology: Environmental or genetic factors

S&S:

- Anorexia and weight loss
- Unexplained fever
- Night sweats
- Cough
- Hepatomegaly and splenomegaly
- Malaise and lethargy
- Recurrent infection
- Prominent, painless, and generalized lymphadenopathy

Dx: Bone marrow aspiration and biopsy reveals small, diffuse lymphocytic cells (malignant lymphoma)

Rx:

- Radiation therapy
- Transfusion of packed RBCs
- Diet high in protein, calories, vitamins, minerals, iron, and calcium
- Chemotherapy: Cytoxan, Oncovin, and Adriamycin

Nursing Process Elements

- Monitor for bleeding, infection, jaundice, and electrolyte imbalance to detect the complications of lymphoma
- Assess and manage side effects of therapy
- Provide mouth and skin care
- Encourage fluids
- Administer medications as prescribed
- Administer transfusion therapy
- Encourage the client to express feelings

Client teaching for self-care

- Recognize early signs and symptoms of motor and sensory deficits that can indicate spinal cord compression.

WORKSHEET

MATCHING QUESTIONS

1. Acute lymphoblastic leukemia
2. Acute myelogenous leukemia
3. Chronic lymphoblastic leukemia
4. Chronic myelogenous leukemia
5. Aplastic anemia
6. Hemolytic anemia
7. Iron deficiency anemia
8. Pernicious anemia
9. Christmas disease
10. Non-Hodgkin's lymphoma
11. Thrombocytopenia
12. Classic hemophilia
13. Polycythemia vera
14. Hodgkin's disease
15. Thalassemia major

a. characterized by a reduction or cessation of all blood-producing elements

b. primarily affects children ages 2–4

c. brittle spoon-shaped nails with longitudinal ridges is a symptom

d. results from an acquired injury to a bone marrow stem cell DNA

e. proliferation of small abnormal mature B lymphocytes

f. primarily affects ages 12–20 and over age 55

g. Hereditary spherocytosis

h. Unpredictable pattern of malignant tumors throughout lymphatic organs

i. Related to absence of Intrinsic factor

j. Form of erythematosus

k. Below normal number of circulating platelets

l. Factor IX

m. Associated with the Reed Sternberg cell

n. Factor VIII

o. Most common inherited single-gene disorder

TRUE & FALSE QUESTIONS

		T	F
1.	Reduced hemoglobin and hematocrit would be seen early with acute hemorrhagic anemia.	___ T	___ F
2.	White blood cell count is usually elevated with chronic leukemias.	___ T	___ F
3.	Hemoglobin in sickle cell disease has abnormal oxygen-carrying capacity.	___ T	___ F
4.	Thalassemia most often affects African-Americans.	___ T	___ F
5.	DDAVP (desmopressin acetate) may be administered to the child with mild hemophilia to increase factor VIII activity.	___ T	___ F
6.	Each child of a female who is a carrier of hemophilia has a 50/50 chance of receiving the affected X chromosome.	___ T	___ F
7.	The major symptom of a vaso-occlusive crisis is pain due to ischemia.	___ T	___ F
8.	ALL commonly changes from a chronic phase to an accelerated phase progressing quickly to fulminant mirroring an acute leukemia.	___ T	___ F
9.	Severity of symptoms of sickle cell anemia varies with the degree of sickling.	___ T	___ F
10.	Failure of a circumcision to clot may be the first sign of hemophilia.	___ T	___ F
11.	A person who is heterozygous for the sickle cell trait is called a carrier.	___ T	___ F
12.	Symptoms of sickle cell anemia are present within a week after birth.	___ T	___ F
13.	Hemophilia varies from person to person in severity.	___ T	___ F
14.	Desmopressin acetate increases factor VIII activity.	___ T	___ F
15.	Priapism is a potential problem for males with sickle cell disease.	___ T	___ F
16.	Decreased hemoglobin and hematocrit are early signs of hemorrhagic anemia.	___ T	___ F
17.	Monitoring for signs of bleeding which is a risk because of decreased platelets and preventing infection which is a risk because of immunosuppression are the two primary nursing concerns related to the care of the client with aplastic anemia.	___ T	___ F
18.	The most common pediatric leukemia is acute myelogenous leukemia.	___ T	___ F
19.	Chronic leukemia typically begins with nonspecific flu-like symptoms.	___ T	___ F
20.	An elevated WBC count at the time of diagnosis of acute lymphoblastic leukemia is predictive of a good prognosis with a likelihood of cure.	___ T	___ F

FILL IN THE BLANKS

Fill in the blank space with the correct word or phrase to complete each statement.

1. For the client with sickle cell disease, traveling to an area of high altitude creates the risk of ___________.

2. Sequestration crisis occurs primarily in persons with sickle cell disease who are less than _____ years of age.

3. The normal platelet count in an adult ranges from _________ to _____________.

4. Severe enlargement of an extremity due to obstructed lymph flow is called ___________.

5. A client with neutropenia would have a neutrophil count of less than ___________.

6. Agranulocytosis is another name for ___________.

7. Prolonged PT and PTT are diagnostic of ___________ deficiency.

8. The major complication associated with lymphedema is ___________.

9. Life threatening spontaneous hemorrhage is a risk when the platelet count drops to ___________.

10. The most common type of thrombocytopenia is ___________.

11. The generic name for Oncovin is ___________.

12. Firm pressure should be maintained on any venipuncture site for ________ minutes when caring for a client with thrombocytopenia.

13. Cytotoxic chemicals used in the treatment of acute lymphoblastic leukemia will be excreted from the child's body for up to ______ hours after administration.

14. The life of transfused platelets is ____ to ____ days.

15. Acute idiopathic thrombocytic purpura has a duration of less than ________.

APPLICATION QUESTIONS

1. For the client in sickle cell crisis, the nurse should frequently assess for
   a. amount of fluid intake
   b. level of pain
   c. prolonged erection in males
   d. lower leg ulcers

2. How should the nurse interpret laboratory results consisting of a positive Coombs' test, decreased Hct, increased reticulocyte count, and increased bilirubin? These results are consistent with
   a. Hereditary spherocytosis
   b. Autoimmune hemolytic anemia
   c. Sickle cell disease
   d. Acute lymphocytic leukemia

3. When teaching the leukemia client and his family, which is the reason why the nurse stresses the importance of hand washing, reducing the number of visitors, and monitoring temperature?
   a. High risk of cross-contamination
   b. High risk for infection

c. Risk of poor hygiene

d. Risk of ineffective healing

4. When initiating care for a client in the emergency department with an estimated blood loss of 3 l from a chain saw injury, for which factor should the nurse assess first?
   a. Hypovolemia
   b. Pain
   c. Impaired cognition
   d. Peripheral paresthesias

5. Which information should the nurse give to a sickle cell client in regard to hand and foot syndrome?
   a. Without immediate treatment, necrosis and need for amputation can occur.
   b. Incidence of hand and foot syndrome declines with age.
   c. Prodromal signs of hand and foot disease are muscle spasms and mottling of the skin.
   d. Episodes of hand and foot syndrome are self limiting.

6. How should the nurse interpret sudden onset of paleness and symptoms of hypotension in clients with sickle cell disease?
   a. The client is bleeding.
   b. A vaso-occlusive crisis is beginning.
   c. The client is experiencing a sequestration crisis.
   d. Systemic vasodilation has occurred.

7. While doing health teaching with a client newly diagnosed with polycythemia vera, the client asks the nurse what causes blood clots to be such a problem with this disease. Which is the reason that should form the basis of the nurse's response?
   a. Viscosity is increased.
   b. Blood volume is decreased.
   c. Arterial diameter is narrowed.
   d. Platelet activity is decreased.

8. Which information should the nurse give to a client newly diagnosed with pernicious anemia?
   a. Symptoms will begin to disappear once you begin eating a diet high in iron.
   b. You should expect intermittent episodes of nausea and diaphoresis once therapy is started.
   c. Injections of vitamin B12 will be required for the rest of your life.
   d. It is important to avoid eating foods that cause increased peristalsis and loose stool.

9. During a home visit to a client with ITP who lives alone, which findings would suggest to the nurse that additional teaching related to self-care is required? Mark all that apply.
   a. ___ A bottle of aspirin in on the counter with the client's other medications.
   b. ___ There is an electric razor in the bathroom.
   c. ___ There is no dental floss with the client's dental care equipment
   d. ___ There is an appointment on the client's calendar with an oral surgeon.
   e. ___ There are golf clubs in the entry hall.

10. A client just diagnosed with thrombocytopenia related to a thiazide diuretic asks the nurse how long the condition will last. Which is the correct answer for the nurse to give?
    a. 1–2 weeks
    b. 2–4 weeks
    c. 1–6 months
    d. It is unpredictable

11. A client who has come to the clinic because of hypermenorrhea asks if this problem will make her anemic. The nurse's response should reflect understanding that the client is at risk for which type of anemia as a result of the hypermenorrhea? Mark all that apply.
    a. ___ Acute hemorrhagic anemia
    b. ___ Chronic hemorrhagic anemia
    c. ___ Iron deficiency anemia
    d. ___ Hemolytic anemia

12. Which symptoms reported by a client 3 days after starting on Interferon alpha therapy for the blastic phase of chronic myelogenous leukemia are expected adverse effects of the medication? Mark all that apply.
    a. __ Depression
    b. __ Chills
    c. __ Joint pain
    d. __ Ankle edema
    e. __ Headache

13. Which are the three major pathophysiological effects of leukemia that direct the plan of nursing care?
    a. — Infection
    b. — Bleeding
    c. — Neural excitability
    d. — Anemia
    e. — Decreased glomerular filtration
    f. — Impaired myocardial perfusion

(continued)

14. A child is scheduled for a bone marrow aspiration as part of the diagnostic evaluation for acute lymphocytic leukemia. The nurse's explanation of the procedure will be based on the knowledge that the procedure will be performed on which part of the body?
    a. Sternum
    b. Scapula
    c. Iliac crest
    d. Sacrum

15. Which is an appropriate nursing intervention for the client with a lymphocyte count of 19,000/mm^3?
    a. Institution of DVT precautions
    b. Institution of protective isolation
    c. Institution of bleeding precautions
    d. Institution of seizure precautions

16. For which adverse effects must the nurse monitor a client with leukemia who is receiving Imatinib? Mark all that apply.
    a. ___ Ascites
    b. ___ Hepatitis
    c. ___ Pulmonary edema
    d. ___ Hypothyroidism
    e. ___ Hyperparathyroidism

17. As part of a community health education event, a nurse is speaking about sickle cell anemia. A question that is asked is, "How early can sickle cell disease be diagnosed?" Which is the correct answer for the nurse to give?
    a. Prenatal detection is possible.
    b. It can be diagnosed within 48 hours of birth.
    c. It can be diagnosed between 4 and 6 months of age.
    d. It can be diagnosed whenever symptoms develop.

18. When planning care for a client with aplastic anemia, which nursing order should be included?
    a. Test urine and stool for occult blood.
    b. Monitor for signs of pulmonary edema.
    c. Encourage flossing after each meal.
    d. Prevent chilling.

19. Which instruction should the nurse give to the parents of a child receiving out-client chemotherapy for acute lymphoblastic leukemia? Mark all that apply.
    a. ___ Launder the child's clothing and linens separately.
    b. ___ Wear gloves when touching the child.
    c. ___ Limit contact with the child to no more than 10 minutes/hour.
    d. ___ Use a plastic mattress cover on the child's bed.
    e. ___ Double flush the toilet after the child uses it.
    f. ___ Use disposable eating utensils for the child.

20. Which direction would be given to the parent of a child with hemophilia?
    a. Administer prophylactic factor at bedtime.
    b. Store factor in the refrigerator.
    c. Give ibuprofen for joint pain.
    d. Plan frequent rest periods throughout the day.

21. Which statement made by the parent of a child with a diagnosis of thalassemia minor indicates the need for further explanation about the disease?
    a. Being of Mediterranean descent put my child at risk for the disease.
    b. My child will need lifelong treatment but will have a normal lifespan.
    c. My child will be anemic but won't have symptoms that require treatment.
    d. The problem is too few red blood cells are made and some get destroyed.

22. Which statement made by a client with sickle cell anemia indicates a correct understanding of an aspect of the disease?
    a. I inherited my disease from my father and his side of the family.
    b. Any children I have will also have the disease.
    c. If I had my spleen removed, my symptoms would basically disappear.
    d. My red blood cells only sickle when oxygen tension in my blood decreases.

23. Increase in which food would most appropriately be among the nurse's recommendations for the diet of a client with vitamin B12 deficiency as a result of inadequate intake?
    a. Yellow vegetables
    b. Red meats
    c. Poultry
    d. Dairy products

24. When assessing a client with sickle cell disease, the nurse should be alert for signs of which chronic problems that are related to the disease? Mark all that apply.
    a. ___ Vision loss
    b. ___ Gastrointestinal bleeding
    c. ___ Leg ulcers

d. ___ Osteoporosis

e. ___ Pulmonary hypertension

25. While reinforcing information about methods of preventing infection, the client with sickle cell disease asks the nurse why she is at risk for infection. Which fact should form the basis of the nurse's response?

a. The lack of a functioning spleen increases the risk of infection.
b. When the number of white blood cells is decreased, the risk of infection is increased.
c. Repeated infarctions in various body tissues increase the risk of infection.
d. Increased cardiac workload decreases the effectiveness of humoral immunity.

ANSWERS & RATIONALES

MATCHING ANSWERS

1. b Acute lymphoblastic leukemia
2. f Acute myelogenous leukemia
3. e Chronic lymphoblastic leukemia
4. d Chronic myelogenous leukemia
5. a Aplastic anemia
6. g Hemolytic anemia
7. c Iron deficiency anemia
8. i Pernicious anemia
9. l Christmas disease
10. h Non-Hodgkin's lymphoma
11. k Thrombocytopenia
12. n Classic hemophilia
13. j Polycythemia vera
14. m Hodgkin's disease
15. o Thalessemia major

a. characterized by a reduction or cessation of all blood-producing elements
b. primarily affects children ages 2–4
c. brittle spoon-shaped nails with longitudinal ridges is a symptom
d. results from an acquired injury to a bone marrow stem cell's DNA
e. proliferation of small abnormal mature B lymphocytes
f. primarily affects ages 12–20 and over age 55
g. hereditary spherocytosis
h. unpredictable pattern of malignant tumors throughout lymphatic organs
i. related to absence of Intrinsic factor
j. form of erythematosus
k. below normal number of circulating platelets
l. involves factor IX
m. associated with the Reed Sternberg cell
n. involves factor VIII
o. most common inherited single-gene disorder

TRUE & FALSE ANSWERS

1. Reduced hemoglobin and hematocrit would be seen early with acute hemorrhagic anemia. *False*
   Decreased hemoglobin and hematocrit are late signs of acute hemorrhagic anemia.
2. White blood cell count is usually elevated with chronic leukemias. *True*
3. Hemoglobin in sickle cell disease has abnormal oxygen-carrying capacity. *False*
   Hemoglobin in sickle cell disease has normal oxygen-carrying capacity.
4. Thalassemia most often affects African-Americans. *False*
   Thalassemia most often affects persons of Mediterranean descent.
5. DDAVP (Desmopressin acetate) may be administered to the child with mild hemophilia to increase factor VIII activity. *True*
6. Each child of a female who is a carrier of hemophilia has a 50/50 chance of receiving the affected X chromosome. *True*
7. The major symptom of a vaso-occlusive crisis is pain due to ischemia. *True*
8. ALL commonly changes from a chronic phase to an accelerated phase progressing quickly to fulminant mirroring an acute leukemia. *False*
   CML, not ALL, commonly changes from a chronic phase to an accelerated phase progressing quickly to fulminant mirroring an acute leukemia.
9. Severity of symptoms of sickle cell anemia varies with the degree of sickling. *True*
10. Failure of a circumcision to clot may be the first sign of hemophilia. *True*
11. A person who is heterozygous for the sickle cell trait is called a carrier. *False*
    A person who is homozygous for the sickle cell trait will have the disease; persons who are heterozygous for the trait are called carriers.
12. Symptoms of sickle cell anemia are present within a week after birth. *False*
    Symptoms of sickle cell anemia develop between 4–6 months of age when the fetal form of hemoglobin converts to an asult form.
13. Hemophilia varies from person to person in severity. *True*
14. Desmopressin acetate increases factor VIII activity. *True*
15. Priapism is a potential problem for males with sickle cell disease. *True*
16. Decreased hemoglobin and hematocrit are early signs of hemorrhagic anemia. *False*
    Decreased hemoglobin and hematocrit are late signs of hemorrhagic anemia.
17. Monitoring for signs of bleeding, which is a risk because of decreased platelets, and preventing infection, which is a risk because of immunosuppression are the two primary nursing concerns related to the care of the client with aplastic anemia. *True*
18. The most common pediatric leukemia is acute myelogenous leukemia. *False*
    The most common pediatric leukemia is acute lymphoblastic leukemia.
19. Chronic leukemia typically begins with nonspecific flu-like symptoms. *True*
20. An elevated WBC count at the time of diagnosis of acute lymphoblastic leukemia is predictive of a good prognosis with a likelihood of cure. *False*
    A high WBC with ALL means there is an increased number of immature white blood cells and this is associated with a poorer prognosis than if there are fewer immature white blood cells.

ANSWERS FOR FILL IN THE BLANKS

1. For the client with sickle cell disease, traveling to an area of high altitude creates the risk of vaso-occlusive crisis.
2. Sequestration crisis occurs primarily in persons with sickle cell disease who are less than 6 years of age.
3. The normal platelet count in an adult ranges from 150,000 to 400,000 /mm^3.
4. Severe enlargement of an extremity as a result of obstructed lymph flow is called elephantiasis.
5. A client with neutropenia would have a neutrophil count of less than 2000/mm^3.
6. Agranulocytosis is another name for neutropenia.
7. Prolonged PT and PTT are diagnostic of vitamin K deficiency.
8. The major complication associated with lymphedema is infection.
9. Life threatening spontaneous hemorrhage is a risk when the platelet count drops to 20,000 mm^3.
10. The most common type of thrombocytopenia is ITP (idiopathic thrombocytopenic purpura).
11. The generic name for Oncovin is vincristine.
12. Firm pressure should be maintained on any venipuncture site for 5 minutes when caring for a client with thrombocytopenia.
13. Cytotoxic chemicals used in the treatment of acute lymphoblastic leukemia will be excreted from the child's body for up to 48 hours after administration.
14. The life of transfused platelets is 1 to 2 days.
15. Acute idiopathic thrombocytic purpura has a duration of less than 6 months.

APPLICATION ANSWERS

1. For the client in sickle cell crisis, the nurse should frequently assess for
   a. amount of fluid intake
   b. level of pain
   c. prolonged erection in males
   d. lower leg ulcers

Rationale

Correct answer: b.

Pain is the primary symptom of sickle cell crisis. Prolonged erection and lower leg ulcers are chronic problems associated with sickle cell disease.

2. How should the nurse interpret laboratory results consisting of a positive Coombs' test, decreased Hct, increased reticulocyte count, and increased bilirubin? These results are consistent with
   a. Hereditary spherocytosis
   b. Autoimmune hemolytic anemia
   c. Sickle cell disease
   d. Acute lymphocytic leukemia

(continued)

Rationale

Correct answer: b.

A positive Coombs' test, decreased Hct, increased reticulocyte count, and increased bilirubin are indicative of autoimmune hemolytic anemia. Hereditary spherocytosis is associated with increased fragility of red blood cells, an elevated reticulocyte count and an elevated serum bilirubin along with the presence of spherocytes on a peripheral blood smear. The major laboratory findings related to sickle cell anemia are the large percentage of hemoglobin S present on electrophoresis and the percentage of irreversibly sickled red blood cells. In addition the hematocrit is decreased and the reticulocyte count and white blood cell count are usually increased. Laboratory findings associated with acute lymphocytic leukemia are decreased hemoglobin, hematocrit and platelet count and a white cell count that may be normal, low or elevated.

3. When teaching the leukemia client and his family, which is the reason why the nurse stresses the importance of hand washing, reducing the number of visitors, and monitoring temperature?
   a. High risk of cross-contamination
   b. High risk for infection
   c. Risk of poor hygiene
   d. Risk of ineffective healing

Rationale

Correct answer: b.

The client with leukemia has a high risk of infection because of the impaired immunity associated with the disease. High risk for cross contamination is incorrect because it presupposes that infection is present which can be transmitted. Risk for poor hygiene may exist but it is not the reason reducing the number of visitors and monitoring temperature is stressed. Risk of ineffective healing is not correct because it presupposes something to be healed and also hand washing, limiting visitors, and monitoring temperature do not directly affect healing.

4. When initiating care for a client in the emergency department with an estimated blood loss of 3 l from a chain saw injury, for which factor should the nurse assess first?
   a. Hypovolemia
   b. Pain
   c. Impaired cognition
   d. Peripheral paresthesias

Rationale

Correct answer: a.

Hypovolemia is a potentially life threatening condition which can result from hemorrhage. Because it can lead to shock and is potentially life threatening, it is the priority assessment because immediate intervention is needed. Pain level is important but not a life threatening issue. Impaired cognition and peripheral paresthesias are not pertinent.

5. Which information should the nurse give to a sickle cell client in regard to hand and foot syndrome?
   a. Without immediate treatment, necrosis and need for amputation can occur.
   b. Incidence of hand and foot syndrome declines with age.
   c. Prodromal signs of hand and foot disease are muscle spasms and mottling of the skin.
   d. Episodes of hand and foot syndrome are self limiting.

Rationale

Correct answer: d.

Hand and foot syndrome refers to a self limiting vaso-occlusive episode characterized by pain and edema in the hands and feet. It does not progress to necrosis and amputation of an extremity and incidence does not decline with age. Muscle spasms and mottling of the skin are unrelated to hand and foot syndrome.

6. How should the nurse interpret sudden onset of paleness and symptoms of hypotension in clients with sickle cell disease?
   a. The client is bleeding.
   b. A vaso-occlusive crisis is beginning.
   c. The client is experiencing a sequestration crisis.
   d. Systemic vasodilation has occurred.

Rationale

Correct answer: c.

Sudden onset of paleness and hypotension are signs of a sequestration crisis. These symptoms can indicate hemorrhage but in a client with known sickle cell disease, the more likely interpretation is sequestration crisis. Pain and edema are signs of vaso-occlusive crisis.

7. While doing health teaching with a client newly diagnosed with polycythemia vera, the client asks the nurse what causes blood clots to be such a problem with this disease. Which is the reason that should form the basis of the nurse's response?
   a. Viscosity is increased.
   b. Blood volume is decreased.
   c. Arterial diameter is narrowed.
   d. Platelet activity is decreased.

Rationale

Correct answer: a.

Increased numbers of red blood cells increase the viscosity of the blood and slow blood flow. These changes support clot formation. Blood volume is not decreased; it is increased because of the increased number of red blood cells. Arterial structure is unaffected by polycythemia vera. Platelet activity is not decreased. In many cases the number of platelets is increased concurrently with the erythrocytosis.

8. Which information should the nurse give to a client newly diagnosed with pernicious anemia?
   a. Symptoms will begin to disappear once you begin eating a diet high in iron.
   b. You should expect intermittent episodes of nausea and diaphoresis once therapy is started.
   c. Injections of vitamin B12 will be required for the rest of your life.
   d. It is important to avoid eating foods that cause increased peristalsis and loose stool.

Rationale

Correct answer: c.

Injections of vitamin B12 are required for the rest of the client's life because the problem is the inability to absorb the vitamin from the ileum and hence the GI tract must be bypassed in order to get the B12 into the system. In some cases oral vitamin B12 nasally administered vitamin B12 may also be prescribed. Eating a diet high in iron corrects symptoms of iron deficiency anemia. There are no side effects to B12 so nausea and diaphoresis do not occur. Degree of peristalsis and consistency of stool are unrelated to pernicious anemia.

9. During a home visit to a client with ITP who lives alone, which findings would suggest to the nurse that additional teaching related to self-care is required? Mark all that apply.
   a. ___ A bottle of aspirin in on the counter with the client's other medications.
   b. ___ There is an electric razor in the bathroom.
   c. ___ There is no dental floss with the client's dental care equipment
   d. ___ There is an appointment on the client's calendar with an oral surgeon.
   e. ___ There are golf clubs in the entry hall.

Rationale

Correct answers: a and d.

The client with thrombopenia needs to avoid increasing the risk of bleeding. Therefore aspirin should not be taken and elective surgery including tooth extraction need to be avoided. Seeing aspirin in the client's home and an appointment with an oral surgeon indicates the need for the nurse to gather information about these findings and reinforce teaching regarding the risk of bleeding and its prevention.

An electric razor should be used because there is less risk of cutting oneself. No dental floss should be used and the toothbrush should be soft or a swab should be used for mouth care. Contact sports should be avoided but sports like golfing, swimming and fishing are acceptable.

10. A client just diagnosed with thrombocytopenia related to a thiazide diuretic asks the nurse how long the condition will last. Which is the correct answer for the nurse to give?
    a. 1– 2 weeks
    b. 2– 4 weeks
    c. 1– 6 months
    d. It is unpredictable

Rationale

Correct answers: a.

Drug induced thrombocytopenia lasts 1–2 weeks after the drug is discontinued. Acute self limiting idiopathic thrombocytopenic purpura lasts less than months.

11. A client who has come to the clinic because of hypermenorrhea asks if this problem will make her anemic. The nurse's response should reflect understanding that the client is at risk for which type of anemia as a result of the hypermenorrhea? Mark all that apply.
    a. ___ Acute hemorrhagic anemia
    b. ___ Chronic hemorrhagic anemia
    c. ___ Iron deficiency anemia
    d. ___ Hemolytic anemia

Rationale

Correct answers: b and c.

Hypermenorrhea involves loss of blood gradually over time which is the defining characteristic of chronic hemorrhagic anemia. Acute hemorrhagic anemia is associated with sudden loss of blood volume. Iron deficiency anemia results from inadequate amounts of iron to meet the need for red blood cell production. The iron deficiency can stem from either too little dietary intake to meet normal need or chronic blood loss creating additional need. Hemolytic anemia results from destruction of red blood cells at a rate faster than which the bone marrow can replace them.

12. Which symptoms reported by a client 3 days after starting on Interferon alpha therapy for the blastic phase of chronic myelogenous leukemia are expected adverse effects of the medication?
    Mark all that apply.
    a. __ Depression
    b. __ Chills
    c. __ Joint pain
    d. __ Ankle edema
    e. __ Headache

Rationale

Correct answers: b, c, and e.

Chills, joint pain and headache as well as fever, malaise, and fatigue are adverse effects of interferon-alpha therapy

(continued)

which typically last about two weeks. Depression is a late toxic effect as are hepatitis, proteinuria, hypothyroidism, and psychosis. Edema is an adverse effect of Imatinib.

13. Which are the three major pathophysiological effects of leukemia that direct the plan of nursing care?
    a. ___ Infection
    b. ___ Bleeding
    c. ___ Neural excitability
    d. ___ Anemia
    e. ___ Decreased glomerular filtration
    f. ___ Impaired myocardial perfusion

Rationale

Correct answers: a, b, and d.

Leukemia is a disease of the white blood cells which impairs their ability to generate a normal immune response to bacteria and other pathogens. This results in a markedly increased risk of infection. Because the uncontrolled proliferation of white blood cells overcrowds the bone marrow, production of red blood cells and lymphocytes is impaired resulting in anemia and risk for bleeding.

14. A child is scheduled for a bone marrow aspiration as part of the diagnostic evaluation for acute lymphocytic leukemia. The nurse's explanation of the procedure will be based on the knowledge that the procedure will be performed on which part of the body?
    a. Sternum
    b. Scapula
    c. Iliac crest
    d. Sacrum

Rationale

Correct answer: c.

In a child, a bone marrow aspiration is performed on the iliac crest. In as adult it may be done on the iliac crest or the sternum.

15. Which is an appropriate nursing intervention for the client with a lymphocyte count of 19,000/mm^3?
    a. Institution of DVT precautions
    b. Institution of protective isolation
    c. Institution of bleeding precautions
    d. Institution of seizure precautions

Rationale

Correct answer: a.

Lymphocytes function in blood clotting. When the lymphocyte count falls below 20,000/mm^3, there is a risk of life threatening, spontaneous bleeding so bleeding precautions are instituted. Protective isolation is required for neutropenia because of the high risk of infection. Deep vein thrombosis and seizure precautions are not required because of a low lymphocyte count.

16. For which adverse effects must the nurse monitor a client with leukemia who is receiving Imatinib? Mark all that apply.
    a. ___ ascites
    b. ___ hepatitis
    c. ___ pulmonary edema
    d. ___ hypothyroidism
    e. ___ hyperparathyroidism

Rationale

Correct answers: a and c.

Fluid retention is a major adverse effect of Imatinib and it can be both sudden and severe. Therefore clients must be carefully monitored for ascites and pulmonary edema as well as pleural and pericardial effusions. Hepatitis and hypothyroidism are late toxic effects of interferon-alpha therapy. Hyperparathyroidism is unrelated.

17. As part of a community health education event, a nurse is speaking about sickle cell anemia. A question that is asked is, "How early can sickle cell disease be diagnosed?" Which is the correct answer for the nurse to give?
    a. Prenatal detection is possible.
    b. It can be diagnosed within 48 hours of birth.
    c. It can be diagnosed between 4 and 6 months of age.
    d. It can be diagnosed whenever symptoms develop.

Rationale

Correct answer: a.

Sickle cell disease can be diagnosed prenatally by amniocentesis or chorionic villous sampling. Symptoms develop between 4 and 6 months of age when fetal hemoglobin is replaced by the adult hemoglobin which is sickled.

18. When planning care for a client with aplastic anemia, which nursing order should be included?
    a. Test urine and stool for occult blood.
    b. Monitor for signs of pulmonary edema.
    c. Encouraging flossing after each meal.
    d. Prevent chilling.

Rationale

Correct answer: a.

Aplastic anemia is an impairment of red blood cell production. Because production of white blood cells and platelets is also affected the client is at risk for infection and bleeding. Testing urine and stool for occult blood is done to detect bleeding. Monitoring for pulmonary edema is essential if the client has heart failure but would not be part of a general care plan related to aplastic anemia. Dental flossing is contraindicated when a risk for bleeding exists. Chilling must be prevented for clients with cold induced autoimmune anemia.

19. Which instruction should the nurse give to the parents of a child receiving out-client chemotherapy for acute lymphoblastic leukemia? Mark all that apply.
   a. ___ Launder the child's clothing and linens separately.
   b. ___ Wear gloves when touching the child.
   c. ___ Limit contact with the child to no more than 10 minutes/hour.
   d. ___ Use a plastic mattress cover on the child's bed.
   e. ___ Double flush the toilet after the child uses it.
   f. ___ Use disposable eating utensils for the child.

Rationale

Correct answers: a, d, and e.

Cytotoxic chemicals are excreted for up to 48 hours after administration so precautions must be taken to protect the family from exposure. Clothing and linens need to be laundered separately; the mattress is covered with plastic to prevent it from absorbing excreted chemicals, and the toilet is double flushed after use. It is not necessary to wear gloves, limit contact to 10 minutes per hour, or use disposable dishes or other eating utensils.

20. Which direction would be given to the parent of a child with hemophilia?
   a. Administer prophylactic factor at bedtime.
   b. Store factor in the refrigerator.
   c. Give ibuprofen for joint pain.
   d. Plan frequent rest periods throughout the day.

Rationale

Correct answer: b.

Factor must be stored in the refrigerator to be on hand in case of need. Prophylactic factor is given in the morning because of its short life. Ibuprofen is not given to a client with hemophilia because it is an NSAID and increases bleeding. Frequent rest periods are not needed by a child with hemophilia any more than by a child without hemophilia. The child with hemophilia needs to be protected from trauma which may start a bleed.

21. Which statement made by the parent of a child with a diagnosis of thalassemia minor indicates the need for further explanation about the disease?
   a. Being of Mediterranean descent put my child at risk for the disease.
   b. My child will need lifelong treatment but will have a normal lifespan.
   c. My child will be anemic but won't have symptoms that require treatment.
   d. The problem is too few red blood cells are made and some get destroyed.

Rationale

Correct answer: b.

Thalassemia minor is generally asymptomatic and does not require treatment. It is an inherited disorder which most often affects persons of Mediterranean descent. The disease is characterized by decreased production of RBCs and chronic hemolytic anemia.

22. Which statement made by a client with sickle cell anemia indicates a correct understanding of an aspect of the disease?
   a. I inherited my disease from my father and his side of the family
   b. Any children I have will also have the disease.
   c. If I had my spleen removed, my symptoms would basically disappear.
   d. My red blood cells only sickle when oxygen tension in my blood decreases.

Rationale

Correct answer: d.

The hemoglobin S red blood cell, which has normal oxygen-carrying capacity, forms a sickle shape under conditions of decreased oxygen tension in the blood. The sickled cells tend to clump and block small blood vessels thereby causing tissue hypoxia. Sickle cell anemia is inherited as an autosomal recessive disorder which means a defective gene had to be inherited from both the mother and the father. Therefore, if a woman with sickle cell anemia has a child with a man who does not have the disease and is not a carrier; the child will be a carrier but will not have the disease itself. Splenectomy does not relieve the symptoms of sickle cell disease; it relieves the symptoms of hereditary spherocytosis.

23. Increase in which food would most appropriately be among the nurse's recommendations for the diet of a client with vitamin B12 deficiency as a result of inadequate intake?
   a. Yellow vegetables
   b. Red meats
   c. Poultry
   d. Dairy products

Rationale

Correct answer: d.

Dairy products are a good source of vitamin B12 along with organ meats, green leafy vegetables, dried beans, nuts, citrus fruits and Brewer's yeast.

24. When assessing a client with sickle cell disease, the nurse should be alert for signs of which chronic problems that are related to the disease? Mark all that apply.
   a. ___ Vision loss
   b. ___ Gastrointestinal bleeding
   c. ___ Leg ulcers

(continued)

d. ___ Osteoporosis
e. ___ Pulmonary hypertension

Rationale

Correct answers: a, c, and e.

Ocular problems such as retinal detachment and blindness occur as a result of repeated infarctions. Leg ulcers are common skin manifestations and pulmonary hypertension is a long term pulmonary complication. Gastrointestinal bleeding and osteoporosis are unrelated to sickle cell disease.

25. While reinforcing information about methods of preventing infection, the client with sickle cell disease asks the nurse why she is at risk for infection. Which fact should form the basis of the nurse's response?
    a. The lack of a functioning spleen increases the risk of infection.
    b. When the number of white blood cells is decreased, the risk of infection is increased.
    c. Repeated infarctions in various body tissues increase the risk of infection.
    d. Increased cardiac workload decreases the effectiveness of humoral immunity.

Rationale

Correct answer: a.

The spleen of a client with sickle cell anemia usually becomes nonfunctional by age 6 as a result of repeated infarctions. This leaves the client at increased risk of infection because the spleen plays a role in preventing bacterial infection. A decrease in white blood cells does increase the risk of infection but this is not the mechanism involved in sickle cell disease. Increased cardiac workload and humoral immunity are unrelated.

Test Plan Category:

Physiological Integrity

Sub-category: Physiological Adaptation—Part 1

Topics: Alterations in Body Systems
Illness Management
Section 3: Respiratory Problems

PEDS CROUP

- Croup or acute spasmodic laryngitis is an upper respiratory tract infection characterized by laryngeal obstruction resulting from the spasm of the larynx.
- Incidence is high among children of age 6 months to 3 years.

Etiology:

- Viral parainfluenza types 1 and 2 viruses are the most common agents.
- Influenza virus
- RSV
- Adenovirus

Precipitating/risk factors:

- Anxiety
- Allergy

S&S:

- Barking cough and inspiratory stridor with supra sternal and inspiratory retraction

- Insidious onset with hoarse voice
- Hoarseness and anxiety
- Cool skin
- Afebrile

Dx:

- Chest X-ray shows subglottic narrowing

Rx:

- Epinephrine
- Aerosol
- Systemic steroids
- Cool-moist therapy

Nursing Process Elements

Alert: Preventing laryngeal spasm is the major nursing goal.

- Apply cool-moist treatment as ordered
- Provide clear fluids
- Provide calm, quiet environment to the child
- Keep the child calm

Client teaching for self-care

- Instruct the parent or caregiver to take the child to a steamy bathroom during acute distress at home
- If the spasm does not subside, then take the child into the emergency room (ER)

TONSILLITIS

- Tonsillitis is an infection or inflammation of the palatine tonsils.
- Tonsils filter and protect the respiratory tract from invasion by pathogens.
- Infections can be acute, recurrent, or chronic.

Etiology: Bacteria (often group A beta-hemolytic streptococcus) or virus spread by droplet nuclei.

Precipitating/risk factors:
Often occurs with pharyngitis; strep infections develop often in cold locations in-between the fall and spring; viral tonsillitis can affect those living in crowded conditions and lead to an epidemic; more common in children and young adults.

S&S:

- Tonsils are red and enlarged
- White exudates may be observed on tonsils
- Child has difficulty swallowing and breathing
- Mouth breathing
- Sore throat
- Enlarged, tender cervical lymph nodes
- Malaise
- Muscle aching
- Fever

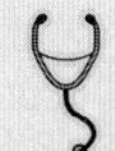

Assessment Alert

PEDS Assess adolescents for mononucleosis.

Dx: Based on symptoms and a visual assessment of the tonsils; throat cultures.

Rx: Provide supportive care; administer analgesics as ordered, acetaminophen for viral tonsillitis: treat symptoms, use humidification, and gargle with warm salt water; for bacterial tonsillitis: antibiotics are ordered such as penicillin, if child is allergic, erythromycin used. Tonsillectomy (See Chapter 18) for recurrent or chronic infections, when there is extensive hypertrophy that leads to difficult breathing and when a peritonsillar abscess closes off the pharynx.

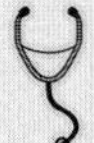

Assessment Alert

Complications of streptococcal tonsillitis are otitis media, rheumatic fever, and acute glomerulonephritis so monitor closely for S&S.

Nursing Process Elements

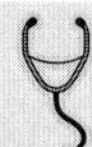

Assessment Alert

Tonsillar material grows rapidly during childhood and reaches adult size during early childhood. Thus, the presence of enlarged tonsils does not always indicate tonsillitis.

- Inquire about previous tonsil infections
- Provide comfort
- Administer antibiotics and analgesics as ordered, acetaminophen relieves fever and throat pain
- Check with parents if any herbal medications were given and report to the physician
- Prepare parents and child for surgery if required and provide perioperative care as described in Chapter 18.

Client teaching for self-care

- Instruct to take antibiotic for 10 days
- Stress need for adequate rest

- Use warm salt water gargle to provide comfort
- Offer a diet with nonirritating cool fluids, soft, bland foods and ice chips to prevent dehydration

PEDS EPIGLOTTITIS

- Acute epiglottitis is a life-threatening bacterial infection, which causes progressive swelling of the epiglottis and surrounding tissue.
- It may lead to respiratory arrest.
- It affects children of 3–7 years of age

Etiology: H. influenza type B

Precipitating/risk factors:
- Upper respiratory infection
- Influenza

S&S: Epiglottitis is an upper airway obstruction; therefore, it is an inspiratory problem.
- Drooling
- Fever
- Tachycardia
- Labored respirations with retractions
- Dysphagia
- Muffled voice
- Irritability and restlessness
- Anxious appearing but quiet

Dx:
- Increased WBC
- Neck X-ray

Rx:
- Respiratory support
- Antibiotics
- Antipyretics
- Intubation if needed

Nursing Process Elements

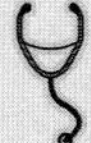

Assessment Alert

Direct examination of the epiglottis is never done unless the anesthesiologist is ready to intubate the client because it may precipitate spasm and obstruction.

- Provide mist tent oxygen as ordered
- Suction as needed
- Administer antibiotics as ordered

Client teaching for self-care

Discuss measures to prevent further upper respiratory attacks.

PEDS LARYNGOTRACHEOBRONCHITIS

- Viral infection most common in children under 5 years of age.
- Infection of the larynx extends to trachea and bronchi if not treated
- Unlike croup onset is more gradual (Usually several days) and it takes longer to resolve.

Etiology: Parainfluenza virus

Precipitating/risk factors:
- Upper respiratory infection
- Fever

S&S:

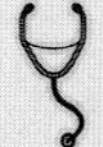

Assessment Alert

Laryngotracheobronchitis is the most common cause of stridor in children.

- Inspiratory stridor, fever, barking cough, and coryza
- Tachycardia, tachypnea, and retractions

Dx:
- Chest X-ray

Rx:
- Epinephrine in acute cases
- Antibiotics if infection is present
- Oxygen therapy
- IV fluids if dehydrated

Nursing Process Elements

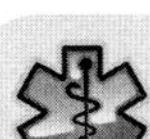

Nursing Intervention Alert

Providing respiratory support to minimize complications is the key nursing goal.

- Monitor VS, skin color, and respiratory status
- Maintain hydration
- Provide calm, quiet atmosphere
- Provide cool-moist vapor as ordered
- Provide emotional support

Client teaching for self-care

- Instruct the parent or caregiver to take the child into a steamy bathroom during acute distress at home
- Reassure the parent that vomiting large amounts of mucus posttherapy is normal

PEDS TRACHEOESOPHAGEAL DEFECT

- Tracheoesophageal defect is a serious, congenital condition in which there is an abnormal connection between the trachea and the esophagus; the esophagus ends before reaching the stomach and/or the esophagus develops as a pouch connected to the trachea by a fistula.
- Classified by American Academy of Pediatrics as
  - —Type A-esophageal atresia without fistula
  - —Type B-esophageal atresia with tracheoesophageal fistula to proximal segment
  - —Type C-esophageal atresia with fistula to distal segment
  - —Type D-esophageal fistula with fistula to both segments
  - —Type E-tracheoesophageal fistula without atresia
- It is associated with other anomalies affecting the heart, GU system, or anorectal areas

Etiology: Failure of embryonic trachea and esophagus to develop and separate correctly.

Risk Factors: Prematurity and polyhydramnios.

S&S:

- Excessive oral secretions
- Constant drooling
- Intolerance of feedings
- Regurgitation of feedings
- Periodic episodes of choking and cyanosis
- When fed, infant swallows but coughs, gags, and returns feeding through the nose and mouth
- Respiratory distress from aspiration of secretions
- Abdominal distention occurring soon after birth when air from the trachea enters esophagus and stomach through the fistula

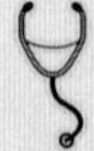

Assessment Alert

Assess for symptoms immediately after birth. Delay in assessment and treatment may be fatal due to fluids and secretions entering lungs; may develop pneumonia.

Dx: X-ray taken with radiopaque catheter placed in esophagus to check for obstruction; standard chest X- ray shows a dilated air-filled upper esophageal pouch and can demonstrate pneumonia; inability to pass a NG tube into stomach because it meets resistance; bronchoscopy visualizes fistula between trachea and esophagus; abdominal ultrasound; and an echocardiogram to check for cardiac abnormalities.

Rx:

Surgery:

- Usually an emergency, is performed as soon as infant is stable.
- Involves ligation of fistulas and anastamosis of esophagus to stomach.
- Completed in one procedure if possible or done as a staged repair.

Supportive care until surgery; IV antibiotics; GT inserted before surgery to decompress stomach.

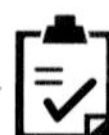

Nursing Process Elements

- Assess for symptoms immediately after birth
- Assess patency of esophagus before feeding or putting to breast
- Evaluate difficulty feeding, respiratory distress, excess drooling, choking, and coughing
- Assess lung sounds
- Use semi-Fowler's position to prevent reflux of gastric contents into trachea and to ease respiratory effort
- Monitor respiratory status closely
- Prevent aspiration
- Maintain fluid and electrolyte balance
- Administer IV fluids to prevent dehydration
- Provide emotional support and reassurance to parents
- Encourage parents to spend as much time with infant as possible
- Place in warm, humidified environment

Client teaching for self-care

- Involve parents in care of infant to facilitate bonding by means of touch and eye contact
- Offer information to parents about the defect, surgical repair, pre- and postoperative care and prognosis, and need for possible further surgery
- Teach parents how to administer gastrostomy feedings until esophagus heals

PEDS BRONCHIOLITIS

- Bronchiolitis is a viral infection, which causes increased mucus production, decreased diameter of the bronchi, hyperinflation, and atelectasis.
- It affects infants of 2–8 months.

Etiology:
- Respiratory syncytial virus (Virus invades epithelial cells of nasopharynx and spreads to lower respiratory tract causing increased mucus production, decreased diameter of the bronchi, and hyperinflation.)

Precipitating/risk factors:
- Preterm
- Congenital cardiac anomaly
- Diabetes
- Immunocompromised infant

S&S:
- Toxic appearance
- Fatigue
- Air-hunger/nasal flaring
- Tachycardia and tachypnea, severe dyspnea
- Increased wheezing and grunt sound
- Intercostal retraction
- Prolonged expiratory phase
- Harsh cough
- Moist rales

Dx:
- Chest X-ray
- WBC count may be normal

Rx:
- RSV—immunoglobulins given monthly for the high-risk babies to prevent infection
- Synagis—given monthly to prevent infection
- Humidified oxygen therapy
- Bronchodilators such as albuterol
- Antiviral treatment such as ribavirin

Nursing Process Elements

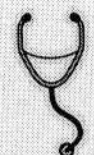

Assessment Alert

Bronchiolitis is a lower respiratory tract infection; therefore, must monitor for expiratory problems

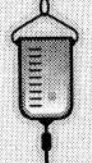

Clinical Alert

Prevention and maintenance of airway patency is the key nursing goal.

- Administer antibiotics as ordered to eradicate infection
- Administer antipyretic as ordered
- Increase fluid intake to loosen secretions
- Remove and control secretions
- Maintain a high humidity environment
- Administer humidified oxygen therapy.
- Offer small, frequent feedings

Client teaching for self-care
- Discuss with the parent the importance of high humidity environment (at home-take the child to the bathroom and open the hot water in a closed environment to provide humidity)
- Teach the parent the importance of getting the monthly synagis injection at the scheduled time

PNEUMONIA

- Pneumonia is an acute infection/inflammation of the lung parenchyma leading to consolidation of lung tissue as the alveoli fill with exudate that impairs gaseous exchange.
- Major pneumonias may be classified as community-acquired, hospital-acquired, aspiration, or pneumonias in an immunocompromised host.
- Community-acquired pneumonia (CAP) occurs in the community or within 48 hours of entering a hospital or other facility.
- Hospital-acquired pneumonia (HAP) has symptoms that occur more than 48 hours after admission to a hospital or other facility; also called nosocomial

Etiology: Pathogens (bacteria, viruses, mycobacteria, chlamydiae, mycoplasma, fungi, and parasites), irritants such as chemicals or aspirated material. Most common causes of bacterial pneumonia are *S. pneumoniae, S. aureus, E. coli, Pseudomonas aeruginosa, and H. influenzae*. Bacterial pneumonias are predominant during winter and early spring and mostly affect the elderly.

PEDS Viruses are the most common cause of pneumonia in infants and children.

Precipitating/risk factors:
- Atelectasis/aspiration
- Chronic illness and debilitation such as lung cancer
- Abdominal or thoracic surgery
- Colds and viral respiratory infection
- COPD, asthma bronchiectasis, and cystic fibrosis
- Smoking and alcoholism
- Malnutrition
- Sickle cell disease
- Tracheostomy
- Exposure to noxious gases
- Immunosuppressive therapy

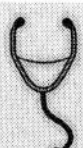

Assessment Alert

Elderly or debilitated clients, those receiving NGT feedings, as well as clients with an impaired gag reflex, poor oral hygiene, or decreased LOC are at high risk for aspiration pneumonia.

S&S:

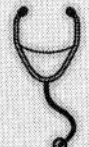

Assessment Alert

S&S vary with type of pneumonia. Four cardinal S&S of bacterial pneumonia are cough, sputum production, pleuritic chest pain, and fever.

- Greenish to rusty-colored sputum
- Rapid, shallow respirations with expiratory grunt, nasal flaring, intercostal rib retraction, and use of accessory muscles of respiration
- Fever, chills, chest pain, and weakness
- Tachycardia, cyanosis, profuse perspiration, and abdominal distention

Dx:
- Chest X-ray (shows consolidation over affected area)
- Increased WBC
- Decreased PaO_2
- Sputum culture determines the specific organism
- VQ scan identifies early *Pneumocystis carinii* pneumonia

Rx:
- Antimicrobial treatment (varies according to organism)
- Supportive measures include
  —humidified oxygen;
  —high-calorie diet with increased fluid intake to 2–3 l/d;
  —bed rest as indicated;
  —analgesics to relieve pleuritic chest pain;
  —mechanical ventilation for respiratory failure.

Nursing Process Elements

- Assess for changes in temperature and pulse, frequency and severity of cough, amount and color of sputum, degree of dyspnea, and changes in chest assessment findings
- Facilitate adequate ventilation
  —Oxygen administration
  — Semi-Fowler's position
  —Turn and reposition clients who are immobilized
  —Administer analgesics to relieve pain associated with breathing (avoid morphine that can depress respirations; codeine is the choice of medication)
  —Auscultate lung sounds and monitor ABGs
- Support removal of secretions
  —Deep breathing and coughing exercises, suction as needed, increase fluid intake to 2–3 l/d, expectorants as ordered, humidification of inhaled air, nebulizer treatment as ordered
  —Perform good oral hygiene after expectoration
- Provide adequate rest and pain relief
  —Limit physical activity
  —Limit visitors and conversation
  —Plan uninterrupted rest periods
  —Schedule nursing care in parts to ensure rest periods in-between
- Administer antibiotic, antipyretic medication as ordered; monitor client response to therapy and document
- Institute isolation precaution as per protocol
- Monitor for complications such as confusion from hypoxia, shock, respiratory failure, atelectasis, pleural effusion, and suprainfection

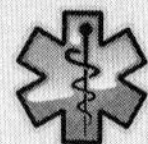

Nursing Intervention Alert

Nursing care focuses on facilitation of adequate ventilation, removal of secretions, comfort and rest, and medication administration.

Client teaching for self-care

- Antibiotic therapy regime and side effects to expect and/or report need to limit activity and obtain adequate rest
- Maintain increased fluid intake
- Continue with deep breathing and coughing exercises
- Importance of adequate nutrition
- Encourage annual influenza vaccine
- Need for reporting the S&S of upper respiratory tract infection to his/her health care provider especially when cystic fibrosis or immobility is a problem

LEGIONNAIRES' DISEASE

- Legionnaires disease is an acute bronchopneumonia in which the inflammation of the lung begins in the terminal bronchioles.
- It occurs epidemically or sporadically.
- The mortality is about 15%.

Etiology:
- *Legionella bacillus* (gram-negative) occurs in water and can be inhaled from aerosols in showers or water spray, or aspirated when drinking contaminated water. Exposure to

Legionella can occur in homes, workplace, hospitals, or other public places.

S&S:

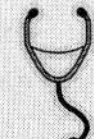

Assessment Alert

Major symptom of Legionnaires' pneumonia is cough: initially nonproductive eventually progressing to grayish, nonpurulent, and blood-streaked sputum.

- Fever
- Generalized weakness
- Malaise
- Recurrent chills

Dx:
- Chest X-ray shows patchy, localized infiltration, which progress to multilobar consolidation
- Fluorescent testing for antibody titer
- Sputum, urine and blood sample studies

Rx:
- Oxygen therapy
- Antibiotic treatment: most antibiotics are effective including levofloxacin, ciprofloxacin, azithromycin, and erythromycin
- Antipyretics
- Inotropic agents

Nursing Process Elements

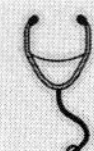

Assessment Alert

Maintenance of respiratory function is the key focus of nursing care. Closely monitor respiratory status, chest wall expansion, depth and pattern of respiration.

- Monitor VS including pulse oximetry and ABG values
- Provide mechanical ventilation as ordered
- Administer medication as prescribed

Client teaching for self-care

Teach the client S&S of Legionella infection

TUBERCULOSIS

Tuberculosis is an infectious, airborne, communicable disease primarily affecting the lung parenchyma.

Once inhaled, the organisms implant in the lung; start dividing slowly; and eventually lead to caseation (the conversion of necrotic tissue into a cheese-like material) and fibrosis. May be spread though lymph and circulatory system to kidney, bone, meninges, and lymph nodes.

Infection may be acute or chronic.

High-risk populations:
- People in inner-city neighborhoods
- People in over or densely populated areas
- Non-whites
- Socially and economically disadvantaged

Etiology:
- *Mycobacterium tuberculosis*

Precipitating/risk factors:
- Age 65 and over
- Overpopulation
- Immunocompromise
- Chemotherapy
- Radiation therapy
- HIV infection
- Malnutrition
- Leukemia
- Hodgkin's disease

S&S:
- Pulmonary symptoms
  —Productive cough, yellow mucoid sputum
  —Dyspnea
  —Pleurtic pain
  —Hemoptysis
  —Rales (crackles)
- Systemic symptoms
  —Fatigue
  —Weakness
  —Anorexia
  —Weight loss
  —Night sweats
  —Low-grade fever

Dx:
- Chest X-ray indicates presence and extent of disease process but cannot differentiate active or inactive tuberculosis
- PPD positive: area of induration of 10 mm or more after 48 hours. (Reading must be within 48–72 hours.)
- Sputum positive for acid-fast *Bacillus*
- Culture positive
- WBC and ESR increased.

Rx:
- Drug therapy
  —Antituberculosis: Initial treatment

—isoniazid (INH), rifampin (RIF), pyrazinamide, ethambutol, or streptomycin; daily dosing of all for 2 weeks. Subsequently, 6 weeks of twice weekly dosing and then 4 months of twice weekly doses of INH and RIF. Alternatively, daily dosing with all four for 8 weeks until drug resistance is ruled out, then 4 months of INH and RIF.

—INH preventative therapy (300 mg/d for 3–6 months) for persons with positive PPD and no clinical signs of disease who are at risk for progression of disease.

—Antibiotic: Streptomycin (usually for 9 months).

- Chest physiotherapy, postural drainage, and incentive spirometry
- Dietary changes, including high-carbohydrate, high-protein, vitamin B6, and vitamin C

Nursing Process Elements

- Maintain respiratory precautions. Client is not considered infectious 2–3 weeks after the initiation of medication
  —Teach the client methods to prevent spread of droplets when coughing
  —Client should be in a well-ventilated negative pressure room with door closed at all times
  —All visitors and staff should wear mask when in contact with client and discard before leaving the patient room
  —All specimens should be labeled AFB precautions.
  —Hand washing required after direct contact with the client
- Offer small frequent meals and nutritional supplement to promote nutritional intake.
- Weigh the client at least two times a week
- Prevent social isolation

Client teaching for self-care

- Prevent transmission of disease: cover mouth with tissue when coughing, sneezing, or laughing; dispose of used tissue safely in the garbage; and wash hand after coughing or sneezing
- Explain the medication regimen; prepare a sheet with medication name, dosage, time, and major side effects. This helps increase medication compliance
- Identify the signs of reoccurrence such as persistent cough, fever, weight loss; explain the importance of seeing a physician if these occur
- Reinforce the need for follow-up care including physical exam, sputum cultures, and chest X-ray
- Need for a high-protein, high-calorie, high-vitamin diet

PEDS Aspiration of Foreign Object in the Respiratory System:

- Aspiration of a foreign object in the respiratory system is a common problem among toddlers (children under 4 years of age).
- Symptoms and severity of symptoms depend on the type of object and its placement in the airway or the lung.

Precipitating/risk factors:

- Age: Toddler

S&S:

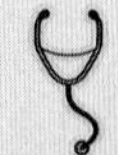

Assessment Alert

Symptoms depend on the type of object and its placement in the respiratory tract.

- If the object is in the upper airway: sudden onset of respiratory distress characterized by coughing, dyspnea, wheezing, stridor, and apnea
- If the object is in the lower airway: persistent respiratory infection/ pneumonia, cough, and mild respiratory distress

Dx:

- Chest X-ray
- Bronchoscopy
- Laryngoscopy

Rx:

- Immediate removal of the object if in the upper airway
- Surgical removal if it is the lower airway
- Symptomatic treatment such as antibiotics if there are signs of infection.

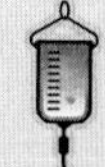

Clinical Alert

- If a foreign object is in the upper respiratory tract, it needs immediate removal; if the object is in the lower airway, it is less emergent.

Nursing Process Elements

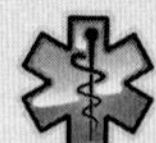

Nursing Intervention Alert

Two major nursing responsibilities are to perform Heimlich maneuver and prevent further damage.

- Reassure the child and parent
- Administer humidified oxygen as ordered
- Administer antibiotics as ordered

Client teaching for self-care

- Teach the parents about age-related expected behaviors and age-appropriate safety precautions

PEDS APNEA OF INFANCY

- Apnea is cessation of breathing.
  - —Central apnea results from the lack of respiratory effort.
  - —Obstructive apnea results from total airway obstruction.

Etiology:
- Prematurity
- Surgical therapy such as tonsillectomy

Precipitating/risk factors:
- Infection
- Anemia
- Hypoglycemia
- Delayed growth and development

S&S:
- Apneic spell
- Bradycardia
- Daytime sleepiness
- Loud snoring
- Night insomnia
- Mouth breathing
- Rapid onset with or without crying
- Polycythemia
- Cor pulmonale

Dx:
- CBC
- ABG

Rx:
- Symptomatic treatment
- Theophylline, caffeine, nasal CPAP, and intubation if needed
- Weight loss
- Tonsillectomy if enlarged and obstructive

Nursing Process Elements

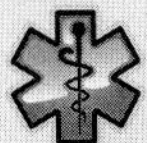

Nursing Intervention Alert

Nursing care is based on etiology.

- Respiratory support
- Avoid stress
- Place client on constant observation
- Administer medication as ordered

PEDS SUDDEN INFANT DEATH SYNDROME (SIDS)

- Sudden death of an infant that is unexpected by history and is without evidence of cause on postmortem examination.
- Incidence peaks at 3 months.
- Usually occurs during sleep.
- No evidence of struggle and death is silent.

Etiology: Unknown.

Precipitating/risk factors:
- Preterm infants, twins, triplets, low birth weight
- Abnormalities in respiration, feeding, or other neurological symptoms

S&S:

Two- to three-month-old infant found cyanotic, apneic, and pulseless in the bed.

Dx:
- Autopsy

Nursing Process Elements

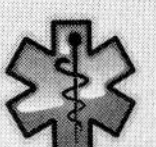

Nursing Intervention Alert

Support parent and family (parents tend to think it is their fault).

- Provide room to be alone if possible
- Let parent say good-bye to baby
- Allow parent to hold the baby
- Reinforce that death is not their fault
- Provide appropriate support, referrals, clergy, local SIDS program

Client teaching for self-care:

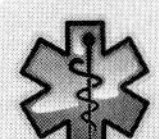

Nursing Intervention Alert

Teach prevention.

American Academy of Pediatrics Guidelines for Reducing SIDS Risk

- Always place a baby on his or her back during naps and at night; supine position decreases risk.

- Place babies on a firm sleep surface such as a safety-approved crib mattress that is covered with a fitted sheet.
- Do not smoke during pregnancy or near babies.
- Do not let a baby overheat during sleep.
- Always keep the head and face uncovered.
- Keep a baby's sleep area close to, but separate from, where parents and others sleep.
- Offer a clean, dry pacifier when placing a baby on his or her back to sleep. Do not reinsert it after the baby falls asleep.
- Reduce the chance that flat spot will develop on the baby's head by providing "tummy time" when the baby is awake and someone is watching.
- Do not use home respiratory or cardiac monitors to reduce SIDS risk.
- Keep soft objects, toys, sheepskins and loose bedding out of a baby's sleep area.
- Avoid products claiming to reduce SIDS risk.

PEDS REACTIVE AIRWAY DISEASE

- Reactive airway disease is a syndrome of wheezing and coughing that occurs in children when airways react to a stimulus with narrowing and mucus production.
- Precipitating factors include respiratory infection and inhalation of environmental pollutants.
- It may or may not lead to asthma; children with asthma in the family are at higher risk.

S&S: Rapid, shallow breathing; wheezing; dry cough; flaring nares; intercostal retractions.

Dx: Clinical presentation

Rx:

- Treat underlying problem
- Bronchodilators (aerosol or MDI)
- Steroids such as Prelone or Orapred for several days to reduce inflammation in the airways.

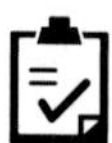

Nursing Process Elements

- Assess for signs and symptoms of the problem
- Monitor response to therapy

Client teaching for self-care

- Avoid exposure to cigarette smoke, perfume, and other fumes
- Use only prescribed medications: do not give child OTC medications unless directed to do so by health care provider
- Contact health care provider if:
  —child does not smile, play, or show interest in normal activity for at least a few minutes out of 4 hours;
  —wheezing or difficulty breathing worsens;
  —child complains of tightness in the chest;
  —breathing becomes markedly fast and shallow;
  —baby cannot suck and breathe simultaneously or chokes when sucking;
  —child cannot be calmed for at least a few minutes every hour;
  —persistent coughing occurs after medication is taken.
- Call 911 if any of the following develops:
  —severe lethargy (child barely responds)
  —severe dyspnea
  —inspiratory grunting
  —cyanotic lips, gums, and nail beds
  —inability to speak while trying to breathe
  —apnea of more than 5-seconds duration

ASTHMA

- Asthma is increased bronchial reactivity in the lower respiratory tract to various stimuli, which produces episodic bronchospasm and airway obstruction and inflammation.
- It is the most common respiratory disease in children. In younger children, it affects twice as many boys as girls and evens out by adolescence.
- Immunologic/allergic reaction results in histamine production causing edema of the mucus membrane, spasm of the smooth muscle of bronchi and bronchioles, and accumulation of secretions.
- Asthma can be intrinsic (allergen is not obvious) or extrinsic (results from sensitivity to specific external allergens).

Etiology:

- Extrinsic asthma: exposure to pollens, animal dander, house dust or mold, feather pillows, silky materials, food additives.
- Intrinsic asthma: irritants, emotional stress, fatigue, endocrine changes, temperature and humidity changes, and exposure to noxious fumes.

Precipitating/risk factors:

- Allergen
- Upper airway infection
- Sudden change in temperature or weather
- Exercise, anxiety, excessive coughing, or laughing

S&S:

- Sudden dyspnea, wheezing, and tightness in the chest
- Coughing that produces thick, clear, or yellow sputum
- Tachypnea and use of accessory respiratory muscles
- Rapid pulse, profuse perspiration, hyperresonant lung fields, diminished breath sounds
- Barrel chest appearance from chronic air trapping
- Irritability from hypoxia

Dx:

- Physical examination
- Chest X-ray: hyperinflated lungs with air trapping and local atelectasis during attacks, normal during remission

- Sputum: presence of Cruschmann's spirals (casts of airways), eosinophils
- Skin testing for specific allergens may be necessary if the client lacks history of allergy

Rx:

- Treatment is usually tailored to individual client's need and focuses on identifying and avoiding predisposing factors. Desensitization of specific antigen may be helpful, but is not effective in persistent asthma.
- Emergency treatment: Oxygen therapy, corticosteroids, and bronchodilators such as subcutaneous epinephrine, IV theophylline, and inhaled agents such as metaproterenol, albuterol, and ipratropium
- Medication:
  - —Bronchodilators
  - —Beta-adrenergic agonists: metered does inhaler—children will need spacers, nebulizer—for infants and toddlers, and rescue drugs for acute attacks.
  - —Corticosteroids: oral for persistent wheezing, inhaled by MDI or nebulizer, IV in the hospital
  - —Nonsteroidal anti-inflamatory agents: nedocromil, cromolyn sodium, and leukotriene inhibitors
  - —Other commonly used medications are as follows:
    - Rapid-acting epinephrine
    - Aminophylline
    - Terbutaline
    - Theophylline
    - Corticosteroids

Step Approach to Asthma Management

Step 1 Long-term control: none

Rescue (Short-term control): short-acting bronchodilator (inhaled beta 2 agonist); if used more than biw; long-term control required.

Step 2 Long-term control: daily anti-inflammatory: low dose inhaled corticosteroid or cromolyn or nedocromil

Rescue: short-acting bronchodilator (inhaled beta 2 agonist); if used daily or with increased frequency, additional long-term therapy is needed.

Step 3 Long-term control: daily anti-inflammatory: medium dose inhaled corticosteroid or low to medium dose inhaled corticosteroid plus long-acting bronchodilator (inhaled or oral).

If needed, medium to high dose inhaled corticosteroid plus long-acting bronchodilator.

Rescue: short-acting bronchodilator (inhaled beta 2 agonist); if used daily or with increased frequency, improved long-term therapy is needed.

—High-dose inhaled corticosteroid plus long-acting inhaled bronchodilator or oral corticosteroid (2 mg/kg/d) and long-acting beta 2 agonist tablets.

—Rescue: inhaled short-acting beta 2 agonist

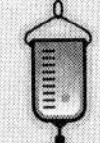

Clinical Alert

Status asthmaticus occurs when there is little or no response to treatment and symptoms persist.

Nursing Process Elements

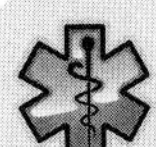

Nursing Intervention Alert

During an acute attack, take appropriate measures to maintain airway and respiratory function, and relieve bronchoconstriction.

- Place the client on semi-Fowler's position
- Administer oxygen
- Encourage diagrammatic breathing
- Administer medication and IV therapy as ordered
- Provide humidification and hydration to loosen secretions
- Monitor for respiratory distress
- Provide chest percussion and postural drainage once symptoms improve
- If the attack was caused by exertion, have the client sit down, rest, and sip warm water if not contraindicated
- For status asthmaticus, humidified oxygen to achieve full saturation; large, frequent doses of inhaled short-acting beta 2 agonists; continuous treatment with bronchodilators until clinical improvement or toxic side effects occur; subcutaneous epinephrine for those refractive to beta 2 agonists

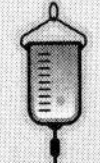

Clinical Alert

Status asthmaticus unrelieved by epinephrine is a medical emergency. Noninvasive positive pressure ventilation is preferable to intubation and mechanical ventilation in its treatment.

Client teaching for self-care

- Prescribed medication
  - —Take missed doses as soon as possible but do not double dose
  - —If using inhaled bronchodilator and corticosteroid, use bronchodilator first and wait for 5 minutes before using the corticosteroid
  - —Rinse mouth with water after inhaling corticosteroid to decrease risk of *Candida*
  - —Contact physician if sore throat or mouth occur

—Don't discontinue cromolyn or nedocromil without consulting physician as exacerbation of symptoms may occur
- Use peak flow monitor to determine respiratory status
- Use of the oral inhaler
  —Remove cap and shake the inhaler
  —Hold the inhaler upside down
  —Breath out as fully as possible
  —Open the mouth and tilt the head slightly back
  —Keep inhaler 2 in. away from the mouth
  —Firmly press the canister down into the mouth piece to release the medication
  —Slowly inhale through mouth
  —Hold breath for 10 seconds
  —Slowly breathe out through the nose
  —Wait for about 5 minutes. Repeat if needed
  —Cap and store the inhaler
  —Rinse mouth
  —Clean mouth piece periodically
- Breathing exercises
- How to control the asthma attack
  —Keep the nebulizer handy at all times
  —Do not take more than two or three inhalations every 4 hours.
  —Call the physician if the symptoms persist after two to three uses of the nebulizer.
- Explain that overuse of the inhaler can weaken response to medication and can also lead to cardiac arrest and death
- Stress the importance of preventing respiratory tract infection.
- Help the client to identify asthma triggers and explain how these triggers cause bronchospasm, airway edema, and mucus production.

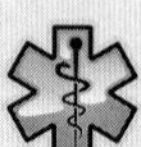

Nursing Intervention Alert

Modification of environment such as providing good ventilation, removing plants and animals is the key to avoiding and reducing exposure to allergens.

- Refer the client to asthma support group as the American Lung Association.

EMPHYSEMA

- Emphysema is a chronic, irreversible, and abnormal enlargement and destruction of alveoli leading to loss of elastic recoil of the lung tissue resulting in the accumulation of sputum and the creation of large air pockets.
- Structural changes result in the accumulation of carbon dioxide, hypoxia, and ultimately respiratory acidosis.

Think Smart/Test Smart

The "arrow method" can be used to interpret arterial blood gas values and determine a client's acid–base balance.

- Place up or down arrows (depending on whether the client's lab values are higher or lower than normal) before the words/phrases pH, $PaCO_2$, and HCO_3^- and follow with an equals sign.
- Look at the direction of the arrows you have made: if the arrow before pH points down, write acidosis after the equals sign. If the arrow before pH points up, write alkalosis.
- Look at the arrow before $PaCO_2$. If it is pointing in the same direction as the pH arrow, write metabolic after the equals sign. If it is pointing in the opposite direction to the pH arrow, write respiratory after the equals sign.
- The two words to the left of the equals sign name the type of acid–base imbalance the client has.
- To determine if the client's body is trying to compensate for the problem, look at the arrows before $PaCO_2$ and HCO_3^-; if they point the same way, compensatory effects are present; if they point in opposite directions, the imbalance is uncompensated.

$\downarrow$pH $\downarrow PaCO_2$ $\downarrow HCO_3^-$ = compensated metabolic acidosis

$\downarrow$pH $\downarrow PaCO_2$ $\uparrow HCO_3^-$ = uncompensated metabolic acidosis

$\uparrow$pH $\uparrow PaCO_2$ $\uparrow HCO_3^-$ = compensated metabolic alkalosis

$\uparrow$pH $\uparrow PaCO_2$ $\downarrow HCO_3^-$ = uncompensated metabolic alkalosis

$\downarrow$pH $\uparrow PaCO_2$ $\uparrow HCO_3^-$ = compensated respiratory acidosis

$\downarrow$pH $\uparrow PaCO_2$ $\downarrow HCO_3^-$ = compensated respiratory acidosis

$\uparrow$pH $\downarrow PaCO_2$ $\downarrow HCO_3^-$ = compensated respiratory alkalosis

$\uparrow$pH $\downarrow PaCO_2$ $\uparrow HCO_3^-$ = compensated respiratory alkalosis

- Most common respiratory cause of death in the United States.

Etiology:
- Congenital deficiency of alpha-antitrypsin
- Cigarette smoking

Precipitating/risk factors:
- Inhaled irritants
- Frequent upper respiratory tract infection
- Allergic factors

S&S:

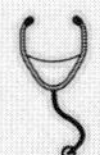

Assessment Alert

Onset is insidious with dyspnea as the predominant symptom

- Long-term respiratory disease symptoms: feeling of breathlessness, cough, sputum production, nasal flaring, use of accessory muscles, and dyspnea.
- Prolonged expiratory period with grunting, pursed lip breathing, and tachypnea
- Barrel chest, resonant to hyperresonant on percussion, and decreased breath sounds with prolonged expiration
- Anorexia and weight loss

Dx:
- Physical exam
- Health History
- Chest X-ray: flattened diaphragm, reduced vascular marking, and large air spaces
- Pulmonary function test
- Arterial blood gases: $PaCO_2$ is elevated and PaO_2 is decreased
- ECG: tall, symmetrical P waves
- CBC: increased RBC

Rx:
- Bronchodilators: aminophylline, albuterol, Isuprel, and theophylline
- Antimicrobials: tetracycline and ampicillin to treat bacterial infection
- Corticosterioids for inflammation

Nursing Process Elements

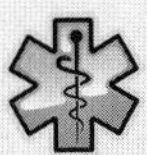

Nursing Intervention Alert

Oxygen to 2 l/min for hypoxia—clients with emphysema depend on hypoxia to drive respiration because they become used to elevated levels of carbon dioxide which is the main drive to breathe in normal individuals. If a client with emphysema receives enough oxygen to eliminate hypoxia entirely, there is a risk of respiratory arrest because there is no impetus to breathe.

- Administer medication as ordered
- Institute measures to improve ventilation such as positioning the client in semi-to high-Fowler's position, and encouraging diagrammatic breathing, productive coughing, and pursed-lip breathing
- Facilitate removal of secretions by increasing fluid intake and providing chest PT as ordered.
- Provide oral hygiene after chest PT

Client teaching for self-care

- Avoid precipitating/risk factors such as inhalation of irritants and exposure to sources of upper respiratory tract infection
- Importance of getting flu and pneumococcal vaccinations
- Use home humidifier at 30–50%
- Develop activity tolerance gradually starting with mild exercise and slowly increasing duration
- Avoid sudden changes of temperature, e.g., cover nose and mouth with scarf while going out
- Prevent frequent respiratory tract infection:
  —Avoid overcrowded areas
  —Report to physician any sign of respiratory tract infection such as change of sputum color.
- Encourage high-protein, high-calorie, increased vitamin diet

BRONCHIECTASIS

- Bronchiectasis is a chronic, irreversible condition marked by abnormal dilatation of bronchi and destruction of bronchial walls.
- It can occur throughout the tracheobronchial tree or can be confined to one segment or lobe but is usually bilateral involving basilar segments of the lower lobes.

Etiology/precipitating/risk factors:
- Immunologic disorders such as gammaglobulinemia
- Recurrent bacterial respiratory tract infections such as tuberculosis.
- Measles, pneumonia, pertussis, or influenza
- Obstruction by foreign body

S&S:

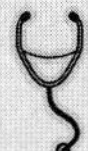

Assessment Alert

Chronic cough that produces copious, foul-smelling, mucopurulent secretion, possibly totaling several cupfuls daily is characteristic.

- Occasional wheezes
- Dyspnea
- Weight loss
- Clubbing
- Recurrent fever, chills, and other signs of infection

Dx:
- Bronchography: most reliable test, reveals the location and extent of the disease
- Chest X-ray: shows peribronchial thickening, areas of atelectasis, and scattered cystic changes
- Bronchoscopy: helps to identify the sources of secretions or the site of bleeding
- Sputum culture to identify infective organisms

Rx:
- IV antibiotics for 7–10 days
- Bronchodilators with postural drainage and chest PT
- Oxygen therapy
- Lobectomy

Nursing Process Elements

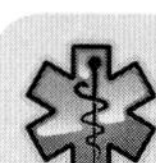

Nursing Intervention Alert

Warm, quiet environment and rest is very important for recovery.

- Administer antibiotics as ordered
- Perform chest PT as ordered, include postural drainage
- High-protein, high-carbohydrate diet
- Mouth care after chest PT

Client teaching for self-care
- Teach family members how to perform PT and postural drainage
- Discuss the importance of mouth care postpostural drainage
- Teach the client deep breathing and coughing exercises to promote good ventilation and removal of secretions
- Encourage the client to stop smoking
- Teach the client to properly dispose of secretions and other infection control measures
- Teach the client the importance of childhood vaccines in decreasing risk of this disease.

ATELECTASIS

- Atelectasis is collapse or airless condition of all or part of lung.
- It may be chronic or acute.

Etiology:
- Bronchial obstruction from intrabronchial or extrabronchial cause that results in incomplete expansion of clusters of alveoli or lung segments

Precipitating/risk factors:
- Mucus plug, a common problem in smokers and clients with COPD, bronchiectasis, or cystic fibrosis
- Foreign body
- Bronchogenic carcinoma
- Inflammatory lung disease
- Oxygen toxicity
- Pulmonary edema
- Any condition that inhibits full lung expansion such as immobility or makes deep breathing painful such as thoracic surgery
- CNS depression from drug overdose

S&S:

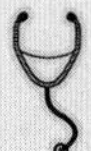

Assessment Alert

Assessment findings may vary depending upon the cause and area involved.

- Dyspnea, possibly mild and subsiding without treatment if atelectasis involves only a small area of the lung; severe if massive collapse occurs.
- Cyanosis
- Decreased breath sounds
- Anxiety, diaphoresis, tachypnea, tachycardia, pain over the affected area, and elevated temperature
- Substernal or intercostal retraction

Dx:
- Chest X-ray shows lobar collapse with dense tissue and decreased size of affected lung. Extensive areas of

microatelectasis may exist without showing abnormalities on the client's chest X-ray.

- Bronchoscopy may or may not reveal obstruction
- PO_2 decreased.

Rx:

- Bronchoscopy
- Chest physiotherapy
- Antibiotics
- Symptomatic treatment
- Drug therapy includes
  - —Bronchodilators such as Proventil
  - —Mucolytic inhalation such as Mucomyst

Nursing Process Elements

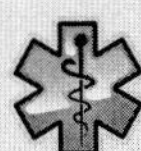

Nursing Intervention Alert

Prevention of atelectasis in hospitalized clients is an important nursing responsibility.

- Prevention of predisposing factors is the key to preventing atelectasis
  - —Turn and reposition the client every 1–2 hours while client is bedridden or immobile.
  - —Use incentive spirometry
  - —Encourage coughing and deep breathing every 1–2 hours as ordered
  - —Provide suctioning as needed
  - —For clients on mechanical ventilation, maintain tidal volume at 10–15 ml/kg of the client's body weight to ensure adequate lung expansion.
  - —Monitor breath sounds and ventilatory status
  - —Promote liquefaction and removal of secretions
  - —Avoid large doses of sedative and opiates that depress the cough reflex
  - —Encourage fluid intake

Client teaching for self-care

- Promote emotional support and reassurance; clients may be frightened by the limited breathing capacity
- Discuss the importance of using incentive spirometer: encourage client to use 10–20 times every hour while awake
- Teach breathing exercises, respiratory care, and postural drainage
- Encourage client to stop smoking

HISTOPLASMOSIS

- Histoplasmosis is a systemic fungal disease.
- Fungus is found in bird manure.
- Histoplasmosis is transmitted by inhalation of *Histoplasma capsulatum* contaminated dust.

Etiology: *Histoplasma capsulatum.*

Precipitating/risk factors:

- Inhalation of dust

S&S:

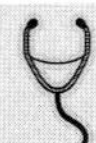

Assessment Alert

Symptoms of histoplasmosis are similar to tuberculosis and pneumonia.

- Cough
- Fever
- Pain in the joints
- Fatigue

Dx:

- Chest X-ray
- Skin test for histoplasmin

Rx:

- Antifungal agent such as amphotericin B
  - —Watch for toxic effects such as anorexia, chills, fever, and renal failure
  - —May give Benadryl before administration to minimize reaction to drug

Nursing Process Elements

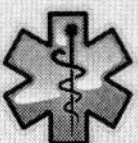

Nursing Intervention Alert

Respiratory precautions similar to client with pneumonia are used.

- Support effective respiratory function
- Monitor renal function before and after medication administration
- Administer medication as ordered

Client teaching for self-care

- Side effects of and toxic reactions to the medication

- Respiratory precautions
- Prevention of recurrence by staying away from dust and birds

PEDS CYSTIC FIBROSIS

- Cystic fibrosis is a chronic multisystem disorder primarily affecting the exocrine (mucus-producing) glands (pancreas, respiratory, gastrointestinal, and reproductive glands).
- It is inherited as an autosomal-recessive defect.
- It is the most common cause of lung disease in children.
- It occurs predominantly in whites as opposed to blacks or Asians

Etiology:

- Genetic predisposition (autosomal-recessive)
- Family history

S&S:

- Respiratory involvement: COPD including wheezing, chronic productive cough, dyspnea, barrel chest, cyanosis, clubbing, chronic infection
- Cardiovascular involvement: right-sided heart enlargement, CHF
- Pancreatic/gastrointestinal involvement: steatorrhea, weight loss, malnutrition, deficiencies of fat-soluble vitamins (A, D, E, K), neonatal history of meconium ileus. Loose, bulky, fatty stool, partial or complete intestinal obstruction known as distal intestinal obstruction syndrome (DIOS)
- Sweat gland involvement: parent reports salt taste when kissing the child, hyponatremia and hypochloremia.

Dx:

- Physical examination
- Sweat test indicates an increase in sodium and chloride in perspiration
- Absence or decrease of trypsin and an increase of fat in stool

Rx:

- Tailored to individual client's need; focuses on facilitating gas exchange and preventing respiratory infection
- Aerosol therapy
- Mist tent
- Breathing exercises
- Medication: bronchodilators, mucolytic agents and expectorants, and antibiotics

Nursing Process Elements

- Check for family history of cystic fibrosis
- Assess for S&S

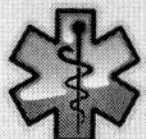

Nursing Intervention Alert

Respiratory assessment for impaired gas exchange; good pulmonary hygiene to promote gas exchange, and prevention of respiratory infection are the priorities of care.

- Provide pulmonary hygiene to clear air passage:
  —Daily postural drainage with percussion and vibration between meals and HS
  —Avoid PD right before and right after meals
  —Follow PD with good oral hygiene and rest
  —Aerosol therapy as ordered
  —Maintain mist tent
- Encourage physical exercise
- Breathing exercises
- Administer bronchodilators, mucolytic agents, and expectorants as ordered
- Prevent respiratory infection; treat vigorously if present
- Maintain adequate nutrition
  —Provide high-calorie, high-protein, normal-fat diet
  —Administer water-soluble preparation for fat-soluble vitamins such as A, D, E, and K
  —Provide salt supplements during hot or febrile periods (soup, and sports drink, salty pretzels)
  —Administer pancreatic enzymes immediately with each meal and each snack. (Mix with cold sauce such as apple or pear sauce)
  —Increase intake of fluids with electrolytes (Gatorade, sports drink)
- Provide emotional support for the child and family
  —Allow verbalization of concerns and feelings
  —Encourage age appropriate independence
  —Suggest genetic counseling
  —Refer family to cystic fibrosis association

Client teaching for self-care

- Discuss the prescribed medication (refer to asthma teaching)
- Explain the importance of good pulmonary hygiene and preventing respiratory tract infection
- Review Dx, disease process, long-term implications, and chronic nature of the condition
- Review dietary instructions

PLEURAL EFFUSION

- Pleural effusion is the collection of excess fluid in the pleural space.

- Normally, pleural space contains a small amount of extracellular fluid that lubricates the pleural surface.
- Inadequate removal or excess production of pleural fluid results in pleural effusion.

Etiology: May result from various conditions.

Precipitating/risk factors:

- Heart disease
- Hepatic disease with ascites
- Kidney disease
- Pneumonia
- Tuberculosis
- Hypoalbuminemia
- Pulmonary edema
- Systemic infection
- Disseminated lupus
- Chest trauma

S&S:

- Dyspnea, dry cough
- Dullness over the affected area upon percussion
- Pleural friction rub
- Pleuritic pain that worsens with cough or deep breathing
- Tachycardia
- Tachypnea
- Decreased breath sounds

Dx:

- Chest X-ray reveals fluid collection in the dependent area
- With emphysema, cell analysis shows leukocytosis
- Fluid collected through thoracentesis may be tested for the following:
  —lupus antinuclear antibodies, analyzed for color, consistency, acid-fast *Bacillus*, fungal or bacterial cultures, triglycerides (to rule out chylothorax)
- Pleural biopsy may be particularly useful for confirming TB or cancer

Rx:

- Treatment of underlying cause is key
- Thoracentesis
- Drug therapy
  —Antibiotic therapy as indicated
  —Trypsin or streptokinase to decrease thickness of pus and dissolve fibrin clots
  —Closed chest drainage or open chest drainage

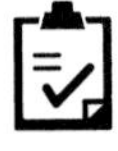

Nursing Process Elements

- Administer oxygen as ordered

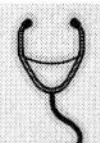

Assessment Alert

Assess client for decreased breath sounds, a sign of plural effusion

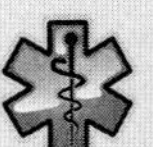

Nursing Intervention Alert

Maintain client in high Fowler's position

- Provide chest tube care
- If the client has open drainage, provide postoperative dressing care
- Administer narcotic and pain reliever as ordered
- Assist with instillation of medication into pleural space

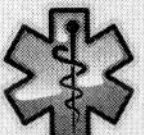

Nursing Intervention Alert

Reposition the client every 15 minutes to distribute drug which has been administered into the pleural space.

Client teaching for self-care

- Discuss and reassure regarding thoracentesis
- Encourage deep breathing and coughing exercise to promote lung expansion

FRACTURED RIBS

- Most commonly fractured ribs are —four to eight, which are protected by the least chest muscle.
- Most common chest injury from a blunt trauma.
- Displaced ribs may cause pleural and lung injury.

Etiology: MVA, accidents, and fight.

Precipitating/risk factors:

- Osteoporosis
- Calcium deficiency

S&S:

- Pain especially on inspiration
- Splitting with shallow respiration

Dx:

- Chest X-ray shows area of fracture
- ABG analysis: elevated $PaCO_2$ and decreased PaO_2

Rx:

- Pain management
  —Drug therapy for pain
  —Intercostal nerve block to relieve pain

Nursing Process Elements

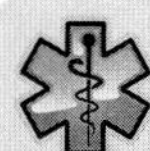

Nursing Intervention Alert

Pain management and preventing complications are goals of care.

- Provide pain relief: administer ordered narcotic and monitor effect
- Position the client semi-Fowler's or Fowler's position
- Monitor client for complications
  —Lung injury
  —Pneumothorax
  —Hemothorax

Client teaching for self-care

- Teach side effects of narcotic analgesics

FAIL CHEST

- Fail chest is fracture of several ribs causing instability of the chest wall.
- Chest wall no longer provides the bony structure to maintain adequate ventilation.
- Flail portion of the chest wall moves in opposition to the rest of the chest wall.

Etiology:

- Trauma, sternal rib fracture with possible costochondral separations

Precipitating/risk factors:

- Long-term calcium deficiency

S&S:

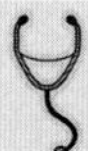

Assessment Alert

Paradoxical chest motion and acute respiratory symptoms are diagnostic signs of flail chest.

- Flail portion of the chest wall is sucked in on inspiration and bulges out on expiration
- Severe dyspnea; rapid, shallow breathing
- Cyanosis, tachycardia, hypotension

Dx:

- Chest X-ray
- ABG analysis:
  —PaO_2 decreased
  —$PaCo_2$ increased
  —pH decreased

Rx:

- Internal stabilization with a volume-cycled ventilator
- Pain reliever

Nursing Process Elements

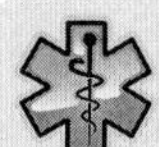

Nursing Intervention Alert

Airway management and monitoring for signs of shock are critical interventions.

- Monitor VS
- Maintain an open airway
- Suction secretions as needed; note color, consistency, and amount
- Provide mechanical ventilator care
- Encourage turning and deep breathing

Client teaching for self-care

- Teach deep breathing technique.
- Importance of turning every 2 hours

PNEUMOTHORAX/HEMOTHORAX

- Pneumothorax
  —Loss of negative intrapleural pressure results in the collapse of the lung.
  —Spontaneous pneumothorax results from the rupture of a bleb.
  —Open pneumothorax occurs when an opening through the chest wall allows air to flow between the pleural space and the outside of the body.
  —Tension pneumothorax results from a buildup of air that can't escape in the pleural space

• Hemothorax
 —Blood accumulates in the pleural space resulting from rupture of pulmonary vessels.
 —Open pneumothorax can lead to hemothorax.

Etiology:
 —Ruptured blebs
 —Insertion of CVP
 —Thoracic surgery
 —Thoracentesis or closed pleural biopsy
 —Penetrating chest injury
 —MVA
 —Transbronchial biopsy
 —Tubercular lesion or malignant lesion that erodes into the pleural space.

S&S:

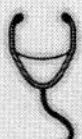

Assessment Alert

Sudden, sharp pain in the chest that increases with respiration and diminished breath sounds unilaterally are diagnostic signs.

- In all types, the surface area for gas exchange is reduced, resulting in hypoxia and hypercapnia
- Dyspnea, tachypnea, subcutaneous emphysema, and cough
- Dullness on chest percussion.
- Weak, rapid pulse; anxiety; diaphoresis

Dx:
- Chest X-ray shows air or fluid collection in the pleural space, tracheal shift, and decreased chest expansion unilaterally.
- $PaCO_2$ elevated
- PaO_2 decreased
- Lung scan revels V\Q ratio mismatch

Rx:
- Bed rest or activity as tolerated
- Chest tube to water seal drainage
- Occlusive dressing for open pneumothorax
- Incentive spirometry
- Oxygen therapy
- Analgesic therapy

Nursing Process Elements
- Monitor VS q 1 hour initially
- Maintain high-Fowler's position
- Maintain proper chest tube function

LARYNGEAL CANCER

- The majority of the laryngeal malignancies are squamous cell carcinomas.
- Types
  —Supraglottic (also called extrinsic laryngeal cancer): involves the epiglottis and false cords and is likely to produce no symptoms until advanced stages.
  —Glottic (also referred to as intrinsic laryngeal cancer): affects the true vocal cord; the most frequently occurring laryngeal cancer.
- Occurs most often in white men in middle or later life.

Etiology: Chronic irritation.

Risk/precipitating factors:
- Caused by cigarette smoking
- Excessive alcohol consumption
- Chronic laryngitis
- Vocal abuse
- Family history

S&S:

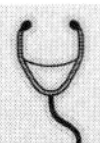

Assessment Alert

Enlarged cervical lymph nodes are common to both types. Symptoms may vary based on the involvement.

Glottic

- Progressive hoarseness that lasts more than 2-weeks duration.

Supraglottic

- Burning while drinking citrus juices or hot liquids
- Localized throat pain
- Lump in the neck region causing dyspnea and dysphagia leading to weight loss
- Cough
- Hemoptysis
- Muffled voice

Dx:
- Laryngoscopy
- Flexible nasopharyngoscope
- CT scan or MRI

Rx:
- Radiation therapy
- Chemotherapy

- Partial laryngectomy: lesion on the true cord on one side removed along with adjoining tissue. Client is able to talk and has a normal airway postoperatively
- Total laryngectomy
- Radical neck dissection

Nursing Process Elements

- See care of the following interventions:
  —Radiation therapy
  —Chemotherapy
  —Laryngectomy
  —Radical neck dissection

LUNG CANCER

- Lung cancer usually develops within the wall or epithelium of the bronchial tree.
- It is the most common cause of cancer responsible for causing death in men and women.
- Prognosis is generally poor, but varies with cell type and extent of spread at the time of diagnosis.
- Types:
  —Squamous cell (epidermoid) carcinoma.
  —Adenocarcinoma, which involves lining of the lung wall.
  —Oat cell (small cell) carcinoma, cancer of the wall of the major bronchus, round or elongated cell.
  —Large cell (anaplastic) carcinoma, a bronchogenic undifferentiated large cell.
- Early metastasis occurs to other thoracic structures such as the hilar lymph nodes and mediastinum. Distant metastasis may involve the brain, liver, bone, and adrenal gland.

Etiology:

- Tobacco smoking: accounts for majority of lung cancers and is closely associated with all histologic types
- Genetic predisposition
- Exposure to carcinogenic industrial or air pollutions such as asbestos, uranium, coal dust, arsenic, and radioactive dust

S&S:

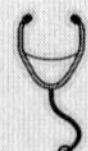

Assessment Alert

Disease is usually well developed by the time clients present with symptoms.

- With large cell cancer and adenocarcinoma, clients present with fever, weakness, weight loss, anorexia, shoulder pain, and other bone and joint pain.
- With small cell (Oat cell) and squamous cell carcinoma, clients present with respiratory symptoms such as smoker's cough, hoarseness, wheezing, dyspnea, hemoptysis, chest pain, flushing, diarrhea, cramps, skin lesions, and palpitations
- S&S of hypercalcemia, and S&S of Cushing's syndrome occur with squamous cell carcinoma
- Gynecomastia with large cell carcinoma

Dx:

- Chest X-ray shows advanced lesions
- Bronchoscopy can locate the tumor site and provide material for cytologic and histologic examination
- Needle biopsy detects peripheral tumors
- Tissue biopsy detects metastasis
- Thoracentesis allows chemical and cytologic examination
- Bone scan, computed tomography scan of the brain, liver function test, gallium scan of the liver, spleen, and bone to locate metastasis

Rx:

- Radiation: radiation therapy is usually recommended for early stage. Preoperative radiation therapy is used to reduce the size of the tumor to allow surgical resection Prophylactic cranial irradiation may be used to prevent brain metastasis
- Chemotherapy:
  —A combination of fluoruracil, vincristine, and mitomycin induces remission of adenocarcinoma
  —For small cell carcinoma, a combination of cyclophosphamide, doxorubicin, and vincristine has proven effective
- Surgical intervention: surgery is the main intervention for squamous, adenocarcinoma, and large cell carcinoma

Nursing Process Elements

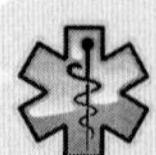

Nursing Intervention Alert

Eventless recovery from treatment and preventing complications are the goals of nursing care.

- Provide psychological support to the client and family
- Provide supportive care to the client

- Take measures to minimize complications and promote recovery from surgery, radiation, or chemotherapy
- Follow strict infection control protocol

Client teaching for self-care

- Behavior/lifestyle modification especially toward smoking/avoidance of cigarette smoke
- Treatment regime, the need for pulmonary hygiene and follow up
- Home oxygen therapy
- Prevention of respiratory infection
- Importance of medical treatment of upper respiratory tract infection

WORKSHEET

FILL IN THE BLANKS

Fill in the blank spaces with the correct word or phrase to complete each statement.

1. Decreased breath sounds accompanied by pleuritic pain that worsens with coughing or deep breathing is consistent with a diagnosis of __________________.
2. The diagnostic test that can identify early *Pneumocystis carinii* pneumonia is a ___.
3. *Legionella* bacteria are found in __________.
4. To minimize a client's reaction to amphotericin B, _______ may be given before the amphotericin B is administered.
5. Barking cough and inspiratory stridor are classic symptoms of _________.
6. A lung scan done on a client with a pneumothorax shows a ____________.
7. A PPD must be read in ______ hours.
8. To decrease the risk of SIDS, infants should sleep in the ______ position.
9. TB is spread by ______________.
10. An elderly confused client with an impaired gag reflex is at high risk for ___________________ pneumonia.
11. Clients with a pleural effusion should be placed in ___ position.
12. When using an inhaler, it should be held ____inches away from the mouth.
13. To remove a foreign body from the lower airway, the ___________ maneuver is performed.
14. The four cardinal S&S of bacterial pneumonia are _____, ______, ______, and _____.

TRUE & FALSE QUESTIONS

Mark each of the following statements True or False. Correct all false statements in the space provided.

1. With squamous cell carcinoma of the lung, the client needs to be monitored for Cushing's syndrome and hypocalcemia. ___ T ___ F
2. A primary therapeutic goal for a child with bronchiolitis is maintaining a patent airway. ___ T ___ F
3. Morphine is the drug of choice for the pleuritic chest pain that accompanies pneumonia. ___ T ___ F
4. Epiglottitis is primarily a problem of expiration. ___ T ___ F
5. The hilar lymph nodes are a site of early metastasis of lung cancer. ___ T ___ F
6. The diet for a client with pneumonia should be high calorie with increased fluids. ___ T ___ F
7. Trypsin is given to a client with a pleural effusion for the purpose of decreasing the viscosity of pus and dissolving fibrin clots. ___ T ___ F
8. Removal of a foreign object from the lower airway is less of an emergency than removing one from the upper airway. ___ T ___ F
9. Inspiratory pain, splinting, and shallow respirations are characteristically seen in client's with fractured ribs. ___ T ___ F
10. Meeting resistance on trying to pass an N/G tube into the stomach is suggestive of a tracheal esophageal defect. ___ T ___ F
11. The nurse should monitor clients with fractured ribs for pneumothorax. ___ T ___ F
12. Paradoxical chest motion is characteristic of hemothorax. ___ T ___ F
13. Excessive alcohol consumption is associated with the occurrence of laryngeal cancer. ___ T ___ F
14. Putting an infant into a steamy bathroom at home can be an effective measure in the management of croup. ___ T ___ F
15. Semi-Fowler's position for an infant with a T/E defect is important because it aids in expectoration of mucus. ___ T ___ F
16. Bronchiolitis is an infection caused by gram-negative bacteria. ___ T ___ F
17. Cough, which is initially non-productive and then produces grayish, blood streaked, nonpurulent sputum is characteristic of aspiration pneumonia. ___ T ___ F
18. Sputum specimens from a client with TB should be labeled AFB precautions. ___ T ___ F
19. Clients with TB should be in a positive pressure room with the door closed at all times. ___ T ___ F
20. Prematurity is a risk factor for apnea of infancy. ___ T ___ F
21. Preventing an infant from overheating during sleep reduces the risk of SIDS. ___ T ___ F

22. Sudden change in temperature can induce an asthma attack in susceptible persons. ___ T ___ F

23. A goal of therapy during an acute asthma attack is the relief of bronchoconstriction. ___ T ___ F

24. Increased RBC count is an expected finding in clients with pneumonia. ___ T ___ F

25. Overuse of nebulized asthma medications increases the need for medication but presents no serious health risks. ___ T ___ F

26. Corticosteroids are prescribed for asthma clients for their bronchodilating effect. ___ T ___ F

27. Dyspnea is a prominent symptom of emphysema. ___ T ___ F

28. Pursed-lip breathing improves ventilation. ___ T ___ F

29. Bronchiectasis is typically unilateral. ___ T ___ F

30. Mucous plugs, which are common in clients with COPD, can cause atelectasis. ___ T ___ F

31. Clients with atelectasis have a decreased $PaCO_2$. ___ T ___ F

32. Clients with atelectasis should be taught to use the incentive spirometer for 10–20 breaths per hour while awake. ___ T ___ F

33. After postural drainage, mouth care is essential. ___ T ___ F

34. Epiglottitis may lead to respiratory arrest. ___ T ___ F

35. A congenital deficiency of alpha-antitrypsin predisposes to emphysema in adulthood. ___ T ___ F

APPLICATION QUESTIONS

1. Following insertion of a CVP line, a client suddenly complains of a sharp pain in the right chest that worsens on inspiration. Which assessment data would support the conclusion that the client had developed a pneumothorax?
   a. Tracheal shift with unilateral decreased chest expansion
   b. Increased $PaCo_2$ and decreased PaO_2
   c. Crackles on affected side
   d. Hyporesonance on affected side

2. What advice should be given to a client's spouse who apologizes for his hoarse voice saying he has had the problem for almost a month and it just seems to get worse not better?
   a. "Gargle with salt and warm water three to four times per day."
   b. "If blood-streaked sputum develops, go to a clinic right away."
   c. "Have it checked without delay."
   d. "Rest your voice and drink a lot of fluid."

3. Which would be the priority expected outcome when caring for an infant with croup?
   a. Infant remains free of infection.
   b. Infant takes clear fluids as prescribed.
   c. Infant's temperature returns to normal within 24 hours of antibiotic therapy.
   d. Infant remains free of laryngospasm.

4. Which client would be most at risk for developing aspiration pneumonia?
   a. An infant with a tracheoesophageal defect repair
   b. An alert 10-year-old with cystic fibrosis

(continued)

c. A 50-year-old with fractured ribs and a fractured leg from a MVA
d. A confused 75-year-old with a CVA

5. When teaching at a health fair, the nurse is asked if there is really a relationship between tobacco smoke and lung cancer. Which information should serve as the basis for the nurse's response?
a. There is a relationship and it is between certain types of lung cancer and both smoking and being exposed to second-hand smoke.
b. Exposure to carcinogens such as asbestos and uranium account for a greater portion of lung cancer than does tobacco use.
c. Radon takes precedence over tobacco smoke as a factor responsible for lung cancer.
d. Tobacco smoking is associated with the majority of lung cancers of all types.

6. Management of an acute attack of asthma might include administration of which medications? Mark all that apply.
a. Subcutaneous epinephrine
b. Inhaled albuterol
c. Oral corticosteroids
d. IV theophylline
e. Inhaled cromolyn sodium

7. When assessing a client with emphysema, which finding would the nurse conclude needed further investigation because it is not an expected characteristic of the disease?
a. Pursed-lip breathing
b. Persistent productive cough
c. Grunting at the end of expiration
d. Prolonged expiration

8. Which laboratory results are consistent with long term COPD? Mark all that apply.
a. Erythrocytosis
b. Hypoxemia
c. Hypercapnia
d. Leukopenia

9. When should a newborn be assessed for a T/E defect?
a. Before the first feeding
b. After the first cry
c. As soon as meconium is passed
d. As soon as body temperature is stable

10. How should the nurse interpret the assessment finding that a client with bronchiectasis expectorated three cupfuls of foul-smelling mucopurulent secretions in the last 24 hours?
a. A secondary infection has developed.
b. The disease process is resolving.
c. Client is exhibiting usual symptoms of the disease.
d. Chest physical therapy needs to be adjusted to client's need.

11. When teaching a client about prevention of Legionnaires' disease, instructions for avoiding contact with the infecting organisms should be based on which fact?
a. *Legionella* is found in soil.
b. *Legionella* is found in water.
c. *Legionella* is found in bird feces.
d. *Legionella* is found in roach debris.

12. How should an infant awaiting repair of a T/E fistula be positioned?
a. Side lying
b. Dorsal recumbent
c. Semi-Fowler's
d. Trendelenburg

13. How should the nurse interpret the finding of a "barrel chest" on examination of a client?
a. Sign of long-term hypoxia
b. Sign of chronic air trapping
c. Sign of excess mucus production
d. Sign of congenital bronchospasm

14. When teaching about the prevention of SIDS, which is an appropriate guideline to be included?
a. Always place a baby on the side during naps and at night.
b. Place babies on a soft sleep surface that is covered with a fitted sheet.
c. Do not smoke during pregnancy or near babies.
d. Do not let a baby get chilled during sleep.

15. Report of which activity would suggest the possibility of histoplasmosis in a client presenting with cough, fever, joint pain, and fatigue?
a. Swallowing water from a hose
b. Eating rare meat
c. Cleaning dirt from a bird roost
d. Handling unwashed fruits

16. Which finding when a PPD is read 2 ½ days after it is planted indicates a positive reaction?
a. Reddened area 10 mm in diameter
b. Indurated area 12 mm in diameter
c. Blistered area 4 mm in diameter
d. Blanched area of at least 8 mm in diameter

17. The nurse should expect to include bed rest, a high-calorie diet, and extra fluids in the care plan for a client with which disorder?
    a. Cystic fibrosis
    b. Emphysema
    c. Pneumonia
    d. Lung cancer

18. An infant with a T/E defect requires careful assessment for abnormalities affecting which other structure(s)?
    a. Brain
    b. Kidneys
    c. Liver
    d. Lungs

19. Which is a characteristic assessment finding in clients with bacterial pneumonia?
    a. Increased PaO_2
    b. Rust-colored sputum
    c. Expiratory wheeze
    d. Nonproductive cough

20. In what way are croup and laryngotracheobronchitis significantly similar?
    a. Client is afebrile with both.
    b. Both are viral in origin.
    c. Age range of susceptibility is the same.
    d. Speed of onset is identical.

21. A client with histoplasmosis is receiving amphotericin B. Which S&S should the nurse interpret as a common toxic reaction to the drug?
    a. Jaundice
    b. Tinnitus
    c. Irritability
    d. Fever

22. When assessing a client with a pleural effusion, which would be an expected finding?
    a. Expiratory wheeze
    b. Productive cough
    c. Decreased breath sounds
    d. Stridor

23. Which would be the position of choice for a client with a pleural effusion?
    a. Side lying with affected side down
    b. Side lying with affected side up
    c. High-Fowler's position
    d. Low-Fowler's position

24. When assessing a client with fractured ribs, which ABG values would be expected?
    a. PaO_2 89 mm Hg, $PaCO_2$ 41 mm Hg
    b. PaO_2 101 mm Hg, $PaCO_2$ 50 mm Hg
    c. PaO_2 94 mm Hg, $PaCO_2$ 35 mm Hg
    d. PaO_2 76 mm Hg, $PaCO_2$ 48 mm Hg

25. On assessing a client brought into emergency following a motor vehicle accident, the nurse notes that an area of the lateral, right chest bulges on expiration and appears to be sucked in on inspiration. Which problem should the nurse suspect?
    a. Flail chest
    b. Atelectasis
    c. Pneumonia
    d. Hemothorax

26. Which assessment data would support the conclusion that the client had likely developed a pneumothorax?
    a. Sudden sharp pain in the chest which increases on inspiration
    b. Production of blood-streaked sputum
    c. Stridor with diaphoresis
    d. Prolonged inspiration with wet rales

ANSWERS & RATIONALES

ANSWERS FOR FILL IN THE BLANKS

Fill in the blanks spaces with the correct word. or phrase to complete each statement.

1. Decreased breath sounds accompanied by pleuritic pain that worsens with coughing or deep breathing is consistent with a diagnosis of pleural effusion.

(continued)

2. The diagnostic test that can identify early *Pneumocystis carinii* pneumonia is a V/Q scan.
3. *Legionella* bacteria are found in water.
4. To minimize a client's reaction to amphotericin B, Benadryl may be given before the amphotericin B is administered.
5. Barking cough and inspiratory stridor are classic symptoms of laryngotracheobronchitis.
6. A lung scan done on a client with a pneumothorax shows a V/Q mismatch.
7. A PPD must be read in 48–72 hours.
8. To decrease the risk of SIDS, infants should sleep in the supine position.
9. TB is spread by droplets.
10. An elderly confused client with an impaired gag reflex is at high risk for aspiration pneumonia.
11. Clients with a pleural effusion should be placed in Fowler's position.
12. It is important to assess for and identify a T/E defect promptly because of the risk of pneumonia developing from fluids and secretions being aspirated into the lungs.
13. When using an inhaler, it should be held 2 in. away from the mouth.
14. To remove a foreign body from the lower airway, the Heimlich maneuver is performed.
15. The four cardinal S&S of bacterial pneumonia are cough, sputum production, pleuritic chest pain, and fever.

TRUE & FALSE ANSWERS

Mark each of the following statements True or False. Correct all false statements in the space provided.

1. With squamous cell carcinoma of the lung, the client needs to be monitored for Cushing's syndrome and hypocalcemia. *False*
   The client needs to be monitored for Cushing's syndrome and hypercalcemia.
2. A primary therapeutic goal for a child with bronchiolitis is maintaining a patent airway. *True*
3. Morphine is the drug of choice for the pleuritic chest pain that accompanies pneumonia. *False*
   Morphine can depress respirations; codeine is the drug of choice.
4. Epiglottitis is primarily a problem of expiration. *False*
   It is an upper airway obstruction and therefore is an inspiratory problem.
5. The hilar lymph nodes are a site of early metastasis of lung cancer. *True*

6. The diet for a client with pneumonia should be high calorie with increased fluids. *True*

7. Trypsin is given to a client with a pleural effusion for the purpose of decreasing the viscosity of pus and dissolving fibrin clots. *True*

8. Removal of a foreign object from the lower airway is less of an emergency than removing one from the upper airway. *False*
The greater emergency is a foreign object in the lower airway because it is blocking the only passage for air to enter the lungs.

9. Inspiratory pain, splinting, and shallow respirations are characteristically seen in client's with fractured ribs. *True*

10. Meeting resistance on trying to pass an N/G tube into the stomach is suggestive of a tracheal esophageal defect. *True*

11. The nurse should monitor clients with fractured ribs for pneumothorax. *True*

12. Paradoxical chest motion is characteristic of hemothorax. *False*
Paradoxical chest movement is characteristic of flail chest.

13. Excessive alcohol consumption is associated with the occurrence of laryngeal cancer. *True*

14. Putting an infant into a steamy bathroom at home can be an effective measure in the management of croup. *True*

15. Semi-Fowler's position for an infant with a T/E defect is important because it aids in expectoration of mucus. *False*
It is important because it eases respiratory effort and prevents reflux of gastric contents into the trachea.

16. Bronchiolitis is an infection caused by gram-negative bacteria. *False*
Bronchiolitis is a viral infection.

17. Cough which is initially nonproductive and then produces grayish, blood-streaked, nonpurulent sputum is characteristic of aspiration pneumonia. *False*
It is characteristic of Legionnaires' disease.

18. Sputum specimens from a client with TB should be labeled AFB precautions. *True*

19. Clients with TB should be in a positive pressure room with the door closed at all times. *False*
The client with TB should be in a negative pressure room.

20. Prematurity is a risk factor for apnea of infancy. *True*

21. Preventing an infant from overheating during sleep reduces the risk of SIDS. *True*

22. Sudden change in temperature can induce an asthma attack in susceptible persons. *True*

23. A goal of therapy during an acute asthma attack is the relief of bronchoconstriction. *True*

24. Increased RBC count is an expected finding in clients with pneumonia. *False*
An increased RBC count is expected in chronic respiratory diseases such as emphysema which are characterized by hypoxia.

25. Over use of nebulized asthma medications increases the need for medication but presents no serious health risks. *False*
Overuse can weaken response to medications but can also lead to cardiac arrest.

(continued)

26. Corticosteroids are prescribed for asthma clients for their bronchodilating effect. *False*
Corticosteroids are given to clients with asthma for their anti-inflammatory effect.

27. Dyspnea is a prominent symptom of emphysema. *True*

28. Pursed-lip breathing improves ventilation. *True*

29. Bronchiectasis is typically unilateral. *False*
Bronchiectasis is typically bilateral affecting the basilar segments of the lower lobes of the lungs.

30. Mucous plugs, which are common in clients with COPD, can cause atelectasis. *True*

31. Clients with atelectasis have a decreased $PaCO_2$. *False*
Clients with atelectasis have a decreased PaO_2 *because of the decrease in aerated lung tissue.*

32. Clients with atelectasis should be taught to use the incentive spirometer for 10–20 breaths per hour while awake. *True*

33. After postural drainage, mouth care is essential. *True*

34. Epiglottitis may lead to respiratory arrest. *True*

35. A congenital deficiency of alpha-antitrypsin predisposes to emphysema in adulthood. *True*

APPLICATION ANSWERS

1. Following insertion of a CVP line, a client suddenly complains of a sharp pain in the right chest that worsens on inspiration. Which assessment data would support the conclusion that the client had developed a pneumothorax?
   a. Tracheal shift with unilateral decreased chest expansion
   b. Increased $PaCO_2$ and decreased PO_2
   c. Crackles on affected side
   d. Hyporesonance on affected side

Rationale

Correct answer: a.

As air or fluid collects in the pleural space, the trachea is forced out of the midline toward the unaffected side. Simultaneous expansion of the lung and chest on the affected side is inhibited causing a unilateral decrease. Hypoxia and hypercapnia occur with pneumothorax so $PaCo_2$ is decreased with pneumothorax and O_2 is increased. No air is entering affected area so no breath sounds are heard. Hyperresonance occurs on affected side.

2. What advice should be given to a client's spouse who apologizes for his hoarse voice saying he has had the problem for almost a month and it just seems to get worse not better?
   a. "Gargle with salt and warm water three to four times per day."
   b. "If blood-streaked sputum develops, go to a clinic right away."
   c. "Have it checked without delay."
   d. "Rest your voice and drink a lot of fluid."

Rationale

Correct answer: c.

Progressive hoarseness of more than 2-weeks duration is a symptom of glottic laryngeal cancer. Therefore, the client should be advised to see a physician right away. Telling the client to gargle or suggesting rest, although soothing, does not address the basic concern.

3. Which would be the priority expected outcome when caring for an infant with croup?
   a. Infant remains free of infection.
   b. Infant takes clear fluids as prescribed.

c. Infant's temperature returns to normal within 24 hours of antibiotic therapy.
d. Infant remains free of laryngospasm.

Rationale

Correct answer: d.

Croup is a condition that results from acute obstruction at or just below the larynx. Laryngospasm, which is the spasmodic closure of the larynx produces the brassy or barking cough, hoarseness, and respiratory distress that are the S&S of croup and therefore must be prevented. Avoiding infection is a desirable goal but it is not the priority for this infant who already has experienced croup. Similarly, clear fluids are prescribed for infants with croup but laryngospasm that can block the airway is a greater priority than fluid intake. Infants with croup are typically afebrile and since croup is viral, not bacterial, in origin antibiotics are not needed.

4. Which client would be most at risk for developing aspiration pneumonia?
   a. An infant with a tracheoesophageal defect repair
   b. An alert 10-year old with cystic fibrosis
   c. A 50-year old with fractured ribs and a fractured leg from a MVA
   d. A confused 75-year old with a CVA

Rationale

Correct answer: d.

Confusion and impaired gag reflex are two of the major risk factors for aspiration pneumonia. Following a repair, an infant is not at particularly high risk for aspiration nor is an alert 10-year old with cystic fibrosis. A 50-year old with fractured ribs and a broken leg has some degree of immobility but no other risk factors.

5. When teaching at a health fair, the nurse is asked if there is really a relationship between tobacco smoke and lung cancer. Which information should serve as the basis for the nurse's response?
   a. There is a relationship and it is between certain types of lung cancer and both smoking and being exposed to second-hand smoke.
   b. Exposure to carcinogens such as asbestos and uranium account for a greater portion of lung cancer than does tobacco use.
   c. Radon takes precedence over tobacco smoke as a factor responsible for lung cancer.
   d. Tobacco smoking is associated with the majority of lung cancers of all types.

Rationale

Correct answer: d.

Tobacco smoking has been shown to be related to the development of all types of lung cancer, not just certain types. Second-hand smoke is also a risk factor as is exposure to chemicals including asbestos, uranium, and radon but they do not account for more cases of lung cancer than tobacco use.

6. Management of an acute attack of asthma might include administration of which medications? Mark all that apply.
   a. Subcutaneous epinephrine
   b. Inhaled albuterol
   c. Oral corticosteroids
   d. IV theophylline
   e. Inhaled cromolyn sodium

Rationale

Correct answers: a, b, and d.

Epinephrine stimulates the beta-2 adrenergic receptors on the respiratory smooth muscle resulting in bronchodilation. Albuterol is a short-acting, beta 2 agonist bronchodilator. Theophylline is a methylxanthine bronchodilator. Subcutaneous administration or inhalation yields a rapid onset of action. Oral corticosteroids are used for persistent wheezing not for emergency management of an acute attack. Cromolyn sodium is not used for acute attacks; it is a mast cell stabilizer whose effectiveness depends on regular use.

7. When assessing a client with emphysema, which finding would the nurse conclude needed further investigation because it is not an expected characteristic of the disease?
   a. Pursed-lip breathing
   b. Persistent productive cough
   c. Grunting at the end of expiration
   d. Prolonged expiration

Rationale

Correct answer: b.

Persistent productive cough is not a symptom of emphysema rather there is minimal cough and sputum production. Clients with emphysema automatically use pursed-lip breathing to facilitate exhalation, which is prolonged due to airway narrowing or collapse on expiration and ends with a grunt.

8. Which laboratory results are consistent with long-term COPD? Mark all that apply.
   a. Erythrocytosis
   b. Hypoxemia
   c. Hypercapnia
   d. Leukopenia

Rationale

Correct answers: a, b, and c.

COPD is characterized by a decrease in oxygen and increase in carbon dioxide so hypoxemia and hypercapnia

(continued)

are expected. Erythrocytosis or an increase in RBCs also occurs as a compensatory effort to maintain tissue oxygenation. It is frequently seen as PaO_2 levels fall below 55 mm Hg.

9. When should a newborn be assessed for a T/E defect?
   a. Before the first feeding
   b. After the first cry
   c. As soon as meconium is passed
   d. As soon as body temperature is stable

Rationale

Correct answer: a.

Assessment for T/E defect should be done immediately after birth and before the first feeding. Usually, sterile water is given first since the infant may swallow normally but suddenly coughs and struggles and fluid is aspirated or returned through the nose and mouth. Presence of frothy saliva in the mouth, difficulty handling secretions, or periods of unexplained cyanosis require that an infant be referred immediately for medical evaluation for T/E defect.

10. How should the nurse interpret the assessment finding that a client with bronchiectasis expectorated three cupfuls of foul-smelling mucopurulent secretions in the last 24 hours?
    a. A secondary infection has developed.
    b. The disease process is resolving.
    c. Client is exhibiting usual symptoms of the disease
    d. Chest physical therapy needs to be adjusted to client's need.

Rationale

Correct answer: c.

Bronchiectasis is characterized by a chronic cough with production of several cupfuls of foul-smelling mucopurulent sputum per day. Production of large amounts of this type of sputum does not indicate suprainfection, disease resolution or that chest physical therapy needs to be changed.

11. When teaching a client about prevention of Legionnaires' disease, instructions for avoiding contact with the infecting organisms should be based on which fact?
    a. *Legionella* is found in soil.
    b. *Legionella* is found in water.
    c. *Legionella* is found in bird feces.
    d. *Legionella* is found in roach debris.

Rationale

Correct answer: b.

Legionella bacillus is found in water; so a person can become infected by aspirating contaminated water or inhaling spray from a shower of contaminated water. Tetanus is found in soil and the organism causing histoplasmosis is found in bird feces.

12. How should an infant awaiting repair of a T/E fistula be positioned?
    a. Side lying
    b. Dorsal recumbent
    c. Semi-Fowler's
    d. Trendelenburg

Rationale

Correct answer: c.

An infant awaiting repair of a T/E fistula should be positioned in semi-Fowler's position to decrease the risk of stomach contents being regurgitated and entering the trachea. Side lying and dorsal recumbent positions do not contribute to the pull of gravity in preventing backflow of stomach contents into the esophagus and Trendelenburg position in which the head is lower than the body actually encourages the backflow.

13. How should the nurse interpret the finding of a "barrel chest" on examination of a client?
    a. Sign of long-term hypoxia
    b. Sign of chronic air trapping
    c. Sign of excess mucus production
    d. Sign of congenital bronchospasm

Rationale

Correct answer: b.

Barrel chest, a condition in which the anterior–posterior diameter of the chest is greater than normal results from hyperinflation due to chronic air trapping.

14. When teaching about the prevention of SIDS, which is an appropriate guideline to be included?
    a. Always place a baby on the side during naps and at night.
    b. Place babies on a soft sleep surface that is covered with a fitted sheet.
    c. Do not smoke during pregnancy or near babies.
    d. Do not let a baby get chilled during sleep.

Rationale

Correct answer: c.

Exposure of a fetus/infant to cigarette smoke is believed to increase the risk of SIDS. a, b, and d are not correct guidelines because babies should be placed on their back not on their sides to sleep; babies should sleep on firm not soft surfaces; and overheating, not chilling, predisposes to SIDS.

15. Report of which activity would suggest the possibility of histoplasmosis in a client presenting with cough, fever, joint pain, and fatigue?
    a. Swallowing water from a hose
    b. Eating rare meat
    c. Cleaning dirt from a bird roost
    d. Handling unwashed fruits

Rationale

Correct answer: c.

The causative organism of histoplasmosis is the fungus *Histoplasma capsulatum,* which is found in bird feces so cleaning a bird roost is a source of exposure. It is not passed person to person. Neither is it contracted by swallowing water, eating rare meat, or handling unwashed fruit.

16. Which finding when a PPD is read 2 ½ days after it is planted indicates a positive reaction?
    a. Reddened area 10 mm in diameter
    b. Indurated area 12 mm in diameter
    c. Blistered area 4 mm in diameter
    d. Blanched area of at least 8 mm in diameter

Rationale

Correct answer: b.

Ten mm or more of induration is highly significant for past or present infection with the tubercle bacillus. Erythema alone does not indicate a positive result. Blistering or blanching do not indicate a positive result.

17. The nurse should expect to include bed rest, a high-calorie diet, and extra fluids in the care plan for a client with which disorder?
    a. Cystic fibrosis
    b. Emphysema
    c. Pneumonia
    d. Lung cancer

Rationale

Correct answer: c.

Bed rest, a high-calorie diet and extra fluids are essential parts of the therapeutic plan for the client with pneumonia. For cystic fibrosis, a high-calorie, high-protein, normal-fat diet is desirable but bed rest is not required; in fact, physical exercise is encouraged. For emphysema, a high-protein, high-calorie, vitamin-rich diet is encouraged; bed rest is not necessary. Clients with lung cancer need adequate nutrition but not bed rest.

18. An infant with a T/E defect requires careful assessment for abnormalities affecting which other structure(s)?
    a. Brain
    b. Kidneys
    c. Liver
    d. Lungs

Rationale

Correct answer: b.

Associated anomalies with T/E defects involve GU, cardiovascular, vertebral, anorectal, and limb structures. Anomalies of the brain, liver, and lungs are not associated.

19. Which is a characteristic assessment finding in clients with bacterial pneumonia?
    a. Increased PaO_2
    b. Rust-colored sputum
    c. Expiratory wheeze
    d. Nonproductive cough

Rationale

Correct answer: b.

Rust-colored sputum, pleuritic pain, cough, and fever are classic signs of bacterial pneumonia. PaO_2 is decreased secondary to consolidation in the lung. An expiratory wheeze is characteristic of asthma not pneumonia.

20. In what way are croup and laryngotracheobronchitis significantly similar?
    a. Client is afebrile with both.
    b. Both are viral in origin.
    c. Age range of susceptibility is the same.
    d. Speed of onset is identical.

Rationale

Correct answer: b.

Both diseases are viral in origin. With croup, children are afebrile; with laryngotracheobronchitis, children have fever. Croup primarily affects children aged 6 months to 3 years and laryngotracheobronchitis affects children under 5 years of age. Onset of croup is sudden and onset of laryngotracheobronchitis is more gradual.

21. A client with histoplasmosis is receiving amphotericin B. Which S&S should the nurse interpret as a common toxic reaction to the drug?
    a. Jaundice
    b. Tinnitus
    c. Irritability
    d. Fever

Rationale

Correct answer: d.

Toxic effects of amphotericin B include anorexia, chills, fever, and renal failure.

22. When assessing a client with a pleural effusion, which would be an expected finding?
    a. Expiratory wheeze
    b. Productive cough
    c. Decreased breath sounds
    d. Stridor

Rationale

Correct answer: c.

Decreased breath sounds are a major finding associated with pleural effusion. Expiratory wheeze does not occur with pleural effusion; it occurs with asthma. Cough

(continued)

associated with pleural effusion is dry, not productive. Laryngotracheobronchitis is the most common cause of stridor in children.

23. Which would be the position of choice for a client with a pleural effusion?
    a. Side lying with affected side down
    b. Side lying with affected side up
    c. High-Fowler's position
    d. Low-Fowler's position

Rationale

Correct answer: c.

High-fowler's position facilitates chest expansion and eases work of respiration.

24. When assessing a client with fractured ribs, which ABG values would be expected?
    a. PaO_2 89 mm Hg, $PaCO_2$ 41 mm Hg
    b. PaO_2 101 mm Hg, $PaCO_2$ 50 mm Hg
    c. PaO_2 94 mm Hg, $PaCO_2$ 35 mm Hg
    d. PaO_2 76 mm Hg, $PaCO_2$ 48 mm Hg

Rationale

Correct answer: d.

Hypoxemia and Hypercapnia are expected. Hypoxemia is reflected in the PaO_2 (partial pressure of oxygen dissolved in the blood), the normal value of which is 80–100 mm Hg. Hypercapnia is reflected in the $PaCO_2$ whose normal range is 35–45 mm Hg.

25. On assessing a client brought into emergency following a motor vehicle accident, the nurse notes that an area of the lateral, right chest bulges on expiration and appears to be sucked in on inspiration. Which problem should the nurse suspect?
    a. Flail chest
    b. Atelectasis
    c. Pneumonia
    d. Hemothorax

Rationale

Correct answer: a.

Flail chest occurs when multiple contiguous ribs are fractured in more than one place resulting in free-floating rib pieces. This free-floating section is pulled in during inspiration and bulges outward during expiration (paradoxical movement) impeding both intake and outflow of air from the lungs. Paradoxical movement does not occur with atelectasis, pneumonia, or hemothorax. With atelectasis, there are decreased breath sounds over the affected area. With a large hemothorax, decreased chest movement on the affected side and decreased or absent breath sounds occur.

26. Which assessment data would support the conclusion that the client had likely developed a pneumothorax?
    a. Sudden, sharp pain in the chest that increases on inspiration
    b. Production of blood-streaked sputum
    c. Stridor with diaphoresis
    d. Prolonged inspiration with wet rales

Rationale

Correct answer: a.

Sudden, sharp chest pain that increases on inspiration and unilaterally diminished breath sounds are classic signs of pneumothorax. Blood-streaked sputum, stridor, diaphoresis, prolonged inspiration, and wet rales are not S&S of pneumothorax.

Test Plan Category:

Physiological Integrity

Sub-category: Physiological Adaptation—Part 1

Topics: Alterations in Body Systems
Illness Management
Section 4: Neurologic Problems

MENINGITIS

- Meningitis is an acute inflammation of the meninges surrounding the brain and spinal cord.

Etiology: It is most often caused by a viral infection, but it can also be caused by a bacterial, amebic, or fungal infection. Bacterial infections are more life threatening.

Risk factors:

- Fall, winter, or early spring months
- Poor hand hygiene, sewage infected water, and individuals in crowded areas or dorms that have not been immunized against meningococcal, pneumococcal, Hib, and TB bacteria
- The disease may follow a viral infection occurring elsewhere in the body

PEDS Bacterial meningitis is common in infancy and young children as the immature immune system is unable to isolate the infection in the body and it will spread to the meninges. With the advent and use of vaccines against *H. influenzae* and pneumococcal, the incidence of bacterial meningitis in children has decreased.

S&S:

- Severe headache
- High fever
- Lethargy, irritability, and muscular weakness
- Nausea, vomiting, stomach cramps, and diarrhea
- Stiff neck and nuchal rigidity
- Photophobia
- Decreased level of consciousness
- Rash
- Bulging fontanel
- High-pitched, moaning cry in infants
- Seizures-in 20% of cases
- Coma—rare, but carries poor prognosis

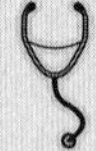

Assessment Alert

Distinction between meningitis and encephalitis needs to be made. Clients with meningitis have no abnormalities in brain function, but changes are common in clients with encephalitis.

PEDS

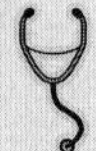

Assessment Alert

Any child who develops a purpuric rash along with symptoms of meningitis may have meningococcemia, a virulent form of meningitis. This child may develop disseminated intravascular coagulation. Meningococcemia has a high mortality rate. Individuals who have been exposed to this child will need to contact their physicians for follow-up care.

Dx: Diagnosis is made from clinical S&S and diagnostic information. Positive Kernig's and Brudzinski signs correlate with meningitis. Most common diagnostic tools are spinal tap, to assess cerebrospinal fluid, and CT scan or MRI to assess for edema, hydrocephalus, or bleeding in the brain. Blood tests are used to assess for an infectious process and determine causative agent; skull X-rays may be done to assess for sinus infection.

Rx: Treatment depends upon type of meningitis. It is aimed at symptomatic relief, rest, and treating disease process. Prevention is the best cure.

- Drug therapy.
  - —Diuretics—mannitol (Osmitrol) or furosemide (Lasix) to decrease cerebral edema.
  - —Antileptics—used to treat or prevent seizures. (See section "Seizures" for description of antileptic medication.)
  - —Antibiotics—cephalosporin (cefotaxime [Claforan], ceftriaxone [Rocephin], cefuroxime [Ceftin], ceftizoxime [Cefizox], ceftazidime [Ceptaz]), ampicillin, or penicillin are used due to their ability to cross the blood–brain barrier and get to the infectious process in bacterial meningitis. Antibiotics are only used for bacterial infections.
- Hypothermia, acetaminophen (Tylenol), or aspirin.
- Codeine to treat severe headache, muscle, and joint pain.
- Sedatives to decrease irritability and restlessness.

Nursing Process Elements

Supportive therapy and prevention of secondary infection are treatment goals.

- Clear liquids and advance as tolerated. Nutritional supplements may be necessary. Monitor intake and output at least every 8 hours.
- Assess neurological status and for S&S of increasing intracranial pressure. Notify physician immediately if the pressure occurs.
- Provide intravenous fluids for administration of medication and fluid support.
- Provide pain medication as needed for headache, muscle, and joint pain.

- Monitor vital signs and give acetaminophen (Tylenol) or aspirin for fever as directed.
- Monitor for seizures and contact physician if occur.
- Keep room quiet and dim lights to allow for frequent rest periods throughout the day.
- Assist to position of comfort with head of bed slightly elevated.
- Increase fluids and offer nutritional supplements throughout the day.

Client teaching for self-care

- Stay away from individuals who are ill.
- Use good hand washing techniques at all times.
- Have your children immunized against Hib and tetanus.
- Drink plenty of liquids daily.
- Maintain high-protein, high-calorie diet to allow for recovery.
- Use range of motion and warm baths to ease stiff, sore muscles.
- Increase activity as tolerated.
- Get at least 8 hours sleep per night and rest during the day.
- Take your medication as directed and do not discontinue abruptly.
- To treat fever and headache, take acetaminophen (Tylenol) or aspirin every 4 hours as directed by your physician.
- Get immunized against meningococcal, TB, Hib, and pneumococcal bacteria particularly if you are planning on living in a crowded area or dorm.
- Follow up with your physician if S&S do not go away or if they increase in severity. Contact immediately for infants with bulging fontanels.

ENCEPHALITIS

- Encephalitis is an acute inflammation of the brain.
- Two forms of the disease occur:
  —Primary encephalitis: Infection begins in the brain and/or spinal cord. This form is more serious, but less common.
  —Secondary encephalitis: Infection begins in one part of the body and then invades the brain and/or spinal cord. This form is more common and usually less severe than primary encephalitis.

Etiology: Most often caused by a viral infection, but it can also be caused by a bacterial or parasitic infection.

Risk factors: Primary encephalitis may occur any time of the year. Secondary encephalitis is more common during the warm summer months. Outdoor activities, weakened immune system, and young or old age increase risk.

Precipitating factors: Persons outside during warm summer months, those that have not been immunized against chicken pox, measles, mumps, or rubella, individuals receiving cancer treatment, and individuals that have had an organ donation are most susceptible.

S&S:

- Headache
- Fever
- Lethargy, irritability, and muscular weakness
- Altered mental status
- Motor or sensory deficits
- Speech abnormalities
- Nausea and vomiting
- Stiff neck
- Ataxic gate
- Tremor or convulsions
- Confusion/sleepiness
- Bulging fontanel
- Milder cases may not have any S&S of the disease

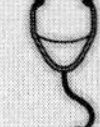

Assessment Alert

Because encephalitis may be secondary, it is important to obtain clients' past medical history and previous illness prior to the new S&S to help determine type of encephalitis and treatment options. Distinction between meningitis and encephalitis needs to be made. Clients with meningitis have no abnormalities in brain function, but these are common in clients with encephalitis.

Dx: Most common diagnostic tools are the spinal tap to assess cerebrospinal fluid, EEG to assess brain wave activity, and CT scan or MRI to assess for edema or bleeding in the brain. A CT scan or MRI may be done before spinal tap to assess for increased intracranial pressure. Blood tests to assess for an infectious process and test for West Nile virus may also be done.

Rx: Treatment depends upon type of encephalitis. Antiviral medication is only given in severe cases of viral encephalitis or for herpes encephalitis. Treatment is aimed at symptomatic relief and treating disease process. Prevention is the best cure.

- Drug therapy
  - —Antiviral—acyclovir (Zovirax), ganciclovir (Cytovene), and vidarabine (Vira-A) to treat infection caused by herpes simplex virus.
  - —Diuretics—mannitol (Osmitrol) to decrease cerebral edema.
  - —Corticosteroids—dexamethasone (Decadron) to decrease edema and inflammation of the brain and spinal cord.
  - —Antileptics used to treat or prevent seizures. (See section "Seizures" for description of antileptic medication.)
  - —Antibiotics may be prescribed for underlying bacterial infection.
  - —Sedatives to decrease irritability and restlessness.

Nursing Process Elements

Supportive therapy and prevention of secondary infection are treatment goals.

- Provide airway management and respiratory support.
- Assess neurological status and for S&S of increasing intracranial pressure. Notify physician immediately if S&S for occur.
- Provide intravenous fluids for administration of medication.
- Provide pain medication as needed for headache.
- Monitor vital signs and give acetaminophen (Tylenol) for fever as directed.
- Assist client with ambulation and activities of daily living as needed.
- Allow client time to answer and ask questions. If client has memory deficits, repeat teaching information as indicated.
- Assess need for physical, occupational, and/or speech therapy and refer as needed.
- Keep room quiet and allow for frequent rest periods throughout the day.
- Increase fluids and offer nutritional supplements throughout the day.
- Teach medication administration techniques for home therapy.

Client teaching for self-care

- If outside during early morning or at dusk, wear long sleeved shirts and long pants and use mosquito repellent with 10–30% DEET.
- Get rid of areas in your home that have standing water such as bird baths, drains, old tires, flower pots, and unused open containers that may hold water.
- Watch for signs of active viral disease—watch for sick or dying birds.
- Stay away from individuals that are ill if you have a weakened immune system.
- Have your children immunized against chicken pox, measles, mumps, and rubella.
- Drink plenty of liquids daily.
- Get at least 8 hours sleep per night and rest during the day.
- Take your medication as directed and do not discontinue abruptly.
- To treat fever and headache, take acetaminophen (Tylenol) every 4 hours as directed by your physician.

PEDS REYE'S SYNDROME

- Reye syndrome is an acute encephalopathy with liver dysfunction
- The five stages of this syndrome are:
  - —vomiting, lethargy, and drowsiness;
  - —confusion, combativeness, and hyperactive reflexes;
  - —decorticate posturing and coma;
  - —decerebrate posturing; and
  - —seizures, respiratory arrest, and death.

Etiology: Unknown

Risk Factors:

- Reye's syndrome usually followed by a viral infection such as varicella.
- It is associated with aspirin use.

S&S:

- Preceding viral infection
- Fever
- Decreasing level of consciousness with combativeness
- Vomiting
- Cerebral edema

Dx:

- Elevated liver enzymes
- Hypoglycemia
- Definitive diagnosis is based on liver biopsy

Rx: Supportive therapy aimed at reducing cerebral edema and maintaining body functions including respirations and coagulation. Outcome varies from full recovery to permanent sequelae or death during the acute disease process. Drug therapy may include:

- corticosteroids and osmotic diuretics to reduce cerebral edema
- anticonvulsants
- vitamin K to aid coagulation

Nursing Process Elements

- Monitor level of consciousness
- Maintain fluid restrictions
- Monitor laboratory values
- Support respiratory function
- Provide physiologic support for the comatose child
- Provide emotional support to the family

Client teaching for self-care

- Teach parents to avoid aspirin in children, especially in relation to a viral infection
- Explain disease and medical treatment to the family
- Explain medical equipment in use with their child
- Rehabilitate on discharge

GUILLAIN–BARRÉ SYNDROME

- Guillain–Barré syndrome is an acute inflammatory polyneuropathy.
- Disease occurs in three stages:
  —1–3 weeks of onset and deterioration of physical status
  —Plateau of a few days to weeks
  —Recovery period of 6 months to more than a year
- Demyelinization occurs between nodes of Ranvier blocks transmission of impulses primarily in motor fibers.
- Recovery occurs in most cases as remyelination takes place; if axons are damaged recovery is slower or disease becomes chronic or recurrent.

Etiology: Autoimmune disease of unknown cause, which often develops few days after a bacterial or viral infection of the respiratory or GI tract.

Risk/precipitating factors: Bacterial or viral infection, surgery, transplant, immunization, other immune disorder such as Hodgkin's disease or AIDS

S&S:

- Varying degrees of symmetrical weakness and flaccid paralysis most often occurring in ascending progression starting with the feet and moving upward to the thorax, upper extremities, and face. Half of affected clients have respiratory insufficiency.
- Sensory involvement manifested as paresthesias (numbness, tingling, and hypersensitivity to touch) and pain are also common.
- Autonomic dysfunction: Labile blood pressure, tachycardia or bradycardia, dysrhythmias, flushing, sweating, urinary retention, and paralytic ileus

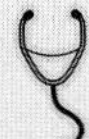

Assessment Alert

Facial nerve (fifth cranial) is often affected. Difficulty in swallowing, speaking, and breathing occur if 7th, 9th, and 10th cranial nerves are affected. There is no effect on the client's alertness or cognitive function.

Dx: History and clinical presentation, elevated CSF protein, and EMG studies

Rx: Supportive and designed to prevent complications

- Respiratory support (ventilator required by up to one third of clients because of respiratory failure)
- Corticosteroids to try and decrease autoimmune inflammation
- Plasmapheresis to remove antibodies, immunoglobulins, and other proteins during first 2 weeks; IVIG is also used
- Nutritional support because complete immobility causes rapid loss of muscle mass: tube feedings or if paralytic ileus is a problem, parenteral nutrition
- May have low dose anticoagulant therapy to prevent venous thrombosis
- Comprehensive plan for rehabilitation

Nursing Process Elements

- Assess for and intervene for sensory deprivation as it is a major potential problem

- Monitor motor, sensory, and cranial nerve status
- Monitor vital capacity, tidal volume, or minute volume: mechanical ventilation is initiated when tidal volume falls below a predetermined level usually 1.0–1.5 l for an average sized adult
- Monitor weight
- Monitor for signs of complications: venous thrombosis, pulmonary embolism, atelectasis, and pneumonia are common
- Maintain range of motion
- Prevent skin breakdown
- Institute bowel program
- Provide care for bladder: indwelling catheter or intermittent catheterization
- Provide meaningful stimulation and regular communication
- Include client in care decisions as cognition is not impaired

MULTIPLE SCLEROSIS

- Multiple sclerosis is a chronic, progressive, and degenerative disorder that affects the central nervous system (CNS).
- It is an autoimmune disorder characterized by exacerbations and remissions causing deterioration of the myelin sheath of the brain and spinal cord with resultant characteristic plaque formation and scarring throughout the CNS.
- Four main patterns:
  —Relapsing remitting—clearly defined relapses followed by periods of remission. Exacerbations appear suddenly, last for weeks or months, and gradually disappear.
  —Primary progressive—disease progression with a gradual decline, with temporary minor improvement.
  —Secondary progressive—continuous deterioration with or without sudden relapses, plateaus, or minor remissions.
  —Progressive relapsing—progressive from onset with sudden episodes of acute relapses with or without full recovery.

Etiology: Unknown.

Risk factors: First, second, and third degree relatives of individuals with multiple sclerosis, people of Northern European descent, and individuals living in temperate climates. Many bacteria and viruses have been thought to be a trigger of the disease.

Precipitating factors: Emotional distress, excessive fatigue, pregnancy, physical injury, and infection.

S&S:

- Unsteady gait or lack of coordination
- Tremor
- Sensation of electric shock radiating down spine with movement of head
- Dizziness
- Paresthesias in one or more limbs on one side of the body or the lower half of the body
- Vertigo, tinnitus, or decreased hearing
- Partial or complete loss of vision, blurred vision, or diplopia
- Fatigue
- Spastic bladder with urinary frequency, urgency, dribbling, and incontinence or hypotonic bladder with urinary retention.
- Erectile dysfunction
- Decreased libido
- Forgetfulness and difficulty concentrating
- Slurred speech
- Paralysis
- Muscle stiffness or spasticity

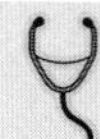

Assessment Alert

S&S such as slurred speech, muscle weakness, paralysis, dizziness, and visual disturbances can mimic persons having a transient ischemic attack (TIA) or cerebrovascular accident (CVA). Careful differentiation between MS, CVA, and TIA is critical.

Dx: No definitive diagnosis, thus based on past medical history, clinical manifestations, and diagnostic studies. MRI to assess for multiple lesions or scarring over time, spinal tap to test CSF for abnormal levels of white blood cells or proteins, evoked responses to check for delayed nerve conduction.

Rx: No cure for MS. Treatment aimed at symptomatic relief and treating disease process.

- Corticosteroids to reduce inflammation and shorten duration of exacerbations

- Muscle relaxants to treat muscle spasticity, stiffness, and spasms
- Bladder control treatments
  —Cholinergics—bethanechol (Urecholine), neostigmine (Prostigmin) to treat urinary retention from a flaccid bladder.
  —Anticholinergics—probanthine (Pro-Banthine), oxybutynin (Ditropan) to treat urinary urgency, frequency from spastic bladder.
- Immunomodulators
  —Beta interferons—Betaseron, Avonex, Rebif to help fight viral infection, regulate the immune system, and decrease exacerbations. Betaseron and Rebif are given subcutaneously. Avonex is given intramuscularly.
  —Glatiramer acetate (Copaxone) subcutaneously once weekly as an alternative to Beta interferons to help block the immune system's attack on the myelin sheath.
- Immunosuppressants given intravenously every 3 months for clients with more severe attacks or rapidly advancing disease not responding to other treatments.

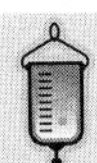

Clinical Caution

Immunosuppressants and immunomodulators may cause serious birth defects or miscarriage. It is, therefore, not used for women who are pregnant or plan to become pregnant. Corticosteroids must not be discontinued abruptly.

- Physical and occupational therapy to increase strength and teach use of assistive devices.
- Plasmapheresis to help restore neurologic function in clients not responding to high-dose corticosteroid therapy.
- Surgery (neurectomy, rhizotomy, cordotomy) to decrease muscle spasticity. Thalamotomy or deep brain stimulation to treat tremors.
- Intrathecal baclofen (Lioresal) pump or electrical stimulation to treat spasticity.
- Counseling—individual or group therapy to help client and family cope with MS and relieve emotional stress.

Nursing Process Elements

- Assess for S&S of acute exacerbation or progression of disease.
- Assess activities of daily living and need for referral for physical and/or occupational therapy.
- Assess need for referral for counseling.
- Teach medication administration techniques for home therapy.
- Assess urinary and bowel patterns. Teach urinary catheter care or self-catheterization techniques (see SCCI) to client and caregiver.

Client teaching for self-care

- Take medication as prescribed.
- Do not discontinue medications abruptly.
- Follow a high-protein, high-fiber diet to help maintain dietary needs and prevent constipation.
- Get adequate rest.
- Avoid extreme heat such as hot tubs and saunas especially if alone.
- Avoid factors that may increase risk for exacerbation such as crowded areas, temperate climates, pregnancy, or infection.
- Seek health care provider if you become ill and before taking any OTC medications.

MYASTHENIA GRAVIS

- Myasthenia gravis is a chronic, autoimmune neuromuscular disorder characterized by fluctuating muscular weakness of voluntary muscle groups.
  —It can occur at any age. Peak age is in the fourth to fifth decade of life for females and sixth to seventh decades in males.
  —It is more common in females with a 3:2 ratio. Ocular myasthenia gravis is higher in males.
- Common voluntary muscle groups affected include facial, chewing, eye, swallowing, and shoulder and hip muscles.
- Acetylcholine receptor antibodies are produced and block the target receptors with a resultant decrease in available acetylcholine receptors available at the postsynaptic membrane.

Etiology: Unknown; however, there is increasing evidence that the thymus might play an important role.

Risk factors: Other autoimmune disorders such as systemic lupus erythematosus (SLE), and rheumatoid arthritis (RA), extrathymic tumors, hyperthermia, hyperthyroidism, and medications such as aminoglycosides, polymyxins and

D-penicillamine, alpha-interferon, and botulinum toxin have been associated with myasthenia gravis.

Precipitating factors: Exposure to bright sunlight, viral illness, surgery, immunization, emotional stress, menstruation, and physical factors might trigger or worsen the exacerbations.

S&S:

- Specific muscle weakness that increases as the day progresses
- Ocular disturbance such as ptosis and diplopia
  —Ptosis may be unilateral or bilateral and may shift from eye to eye
- Difficulty swallowing, chewing, and talking
- Fatigability showing incremental weakness following same motor movements
- Difficulty taking a deep breath
- Weak cough
- Shortness of breath
- Unstable gait
- Impaired speech

Dx: May be delayed for 1–2 years due to commonality of muscular weakness. Laboratory tests include: anti-AChR antibodies assay, thyroid function test, antinuclear antibody test, and rheumatoid factor to test for myasthenia gravis and rule out other disorders; MRI or CT to rule out lesions or thymoma; anticholinesterase test using edrophonium chloride (Tensilon), and electromyography (EMG).

Rx: There is no cure for myasthenia gravis. Common treatments include medication, plasmapheresis, and thymectomy.

- Corticosteroids (Prednisone) to suppress the abnormal action of the immune system.
- Anticholinesterase agents, pyridostigmine bromide (Mestinon), neostigmine bromide (Prostigmin) to allow acetylcholine to remain at the neuromuscular junction longer.
- Immunosuppressants azathioprine (Imuran) and cyclosporine (Gengraf, Neoral, Sandimmune) to depress the immune system. Used when corticosteroids fail. Effect is delayed four to 8 months; symptoms may recur when discontinued.
- Immunoglobulins (IVIG) sometimes used to decrease the production of abnormal antibodies.

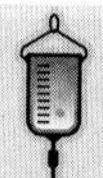

Clinical Caution

Immunosuppressants may cause serious birth defects or miscarriage, therefore, they are not used for women who are pregnant or plan to become pregnant. Corticosteroids must not be discontinued abruptly. Do not mix azathioprine with other drugs.

- Plasmapheresis to remove anti-AChR antibodies from the circulation. It is reserved for myasthenic crisis and refractory cases. Improvement is noted in a couple of days, but does not last for more than 2 months.
- Thymectomy
- Physical and occupational therapy, speech therapy to assist with swallowing, chewing, speech, and assist with ADLs and IADLs.

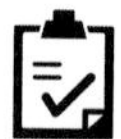

Nursing Process Elements

- Assess for S&S of acute exacerbation or progression of disease.
- Assess airway patency, strength of cough, respiratory rate and effort, mental status, and cardiac status.
- Pace activities throughout the day to allow for rest periods in between. Complete major care activities in the morning when the client is usually stronger.
- Elevate head and shoulders close to 90 degrees for all meals.
- Utilize mechanical soft diet during periods of dysphagia, and thicken clear fluids to avoid aspiration.
- Assess activities of daily living and need for referral for physical, occupational, and/or speech therapy.
- Assess need for referral for counseling.
- Teach medication administration techniques for home therapy.

Client teaching for self-care

- Take medication as prescribed.
- Record the response after each dose of pyridostigmine during the initial period of medication treatment.
- Keep medications with you at all times; keep in carry-on luggage when traveling.
- Avoid the use of D-penicillamine, alpha-interferon, and botulinum toxin.
- Do not discontinue medications abruptly.
- Seek immediate medical attention if difficulty breathing or swallowing occurs.
- Follow a healthful diet utilizing a variety of foods that chew easily. Eat slowly and rest between bites.
- Sit upright in a chair and lean forward when eating.
- Do not complete a large amount of activity prior to meals.
- Get adequate rest, and space activities throughout the day.
- Wear a medical identification bracelet.
- Wear low-heeled shoes that are comfortable and have nonskid soles.
- Use a walker or cane if you have an unsteady gait.
- Sit in a chair that has armrests to assist you when you get up.

PARKINSON'S DISEASE

- Parkinson's disease is a chronic, progressive disease in which nerve cells in the midbrain, called the substantia nigra, die or are impaired.
- A loss of 70–80% of these dopamine-producing neurons occurs before development of symptoms.

Etiology: Causes are not specifically known. Contributing factors include a combination of genetic factors and environmental exposures.

Precipitating factors: Environmental insults such as pesticides or illicit drug use, progression of age. Usually develops in individuals older than 60 years of age.

S&S:

- Resting tremor
- Rigidity or stiffness
- Slowness of movement (bradykinesia), or shuffling gait
- Postural instability
- Muffled speech
- Stiff facial appearance (mask-like appearance)
- Small, cramped handwriting
- Initially, symptoms may be on only one side of the body

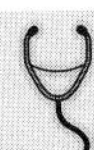

Assessment Alert

Some of the S&S are similar to common manifestations of the aging process, particularly in clients with arthritis. Medication-induced parkinsonism may occur with use of antipsychotics, metoclopramide, reserpine, tetrabenazine, and some calcium-channel blockers. The parkinsonism usually resolves within weeks to months after discontinuation of the medication. Careful differentiation between arthritis, parkinsonism and Parkinson's disease is critical.

Dx: Diagnosis is usually based on clinical presenting symptoms. Presentation of two or more of the above S&S, particularly with a resting tremor, and a unilateral onset are utilized to help distinguish between Parkinson's disease and parkinsonism. An MRI may be useful in distinguishing true Parkinson's disease from other neurodegenerative disorders.

Rx: Currently, there is no cure for Parkinson's disease or treatment that is able to slow or stop the progression of the disease. Treatment is aimed at symptomatic relief and treating disease process.

- Symmetrel (amantadine) to reduce fatigue, tremor, and bradykinesia.
- Eldepryl (selegiline HCL) to inhibit the action of monoamine oxidase B, the enzyme that breaks down dopamine, thereby prolonging the action of dopamine in the brain.
- Anticholinergics—biperiden HCL (Akineton), benztropine mesylate (Cogentin), procyclidine (Kemadrin), trihexyphenidyl (Artane), orphenadrine (Norflex) to help reduce tremor or rigidity.
- Levodopa preparations—to reduce slowness, stiffness, and tremor
  —Standard preparations: levodopa/carbidopa (Sinemet or Atamet)
  —Extended release preparations: levodopa/carbidopa (Sinemet CR), levodopa/benserazide (Madopar HBS)
- Dopamine agonists—bromocriptine (Parlodel), pergolide (Permax), ropinirole (Requip), and pramipexole (Mirapex) to stimulate dopamine receptors.

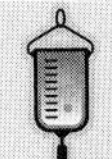

Clinical Caution

Sleepiness, drowsiness, or sedation may be significant in some individuals taking dopamine agonists and may interfere with activities such as driving.

- Physical and occupational therapy to increase strength and teach use of assistive devices.
- Surgery (pallidotomy) to decrease tremor, bradykinesia, rigidity, and dyskinesia.
- Deep brain stimulation procedures—thalamic stimulation, VIM DBS, pallidal stimulation, subthalamic nucleus stimulation to reduce tremor, rigidity, and bradykinesia, gait disorder.

Nursing Process Elements

- Assess for S&S of progression of disease.
- Assess activities of daily living and need for referral for physical and/or occupational therapy.
- Assess need for referral for counseling.
- Teach medication administration techniques for home therapy.

Client teaching for self-care

- Take medication as prescribed.
- Do not discontinue medications abruptly.
- Follow a high-calorie, high-fiber diet and increase fluids to help maintain dietary needs and prevent constipation.
- Teach purposeful movements and concentrating on gait when walking.
- Teach diaphragmatic breathing and taking deep breaths before speaking to facilitate communication.
- Seek health care provider if you become ill and before taking any OTC medications.

AMYOTROPHIC LATERAL SCLEROSIS

- It is also called Lou Gehrig's disease
- Degeneration of upper and lower motor neurons occurs causing weakness and paralysis
- Amyotrophic lateral sclerosis is chronic and rapidly progressive with survival about 5 years from time of diagnosis.

Etiology: Unknown; theories include autoimmune reaction, defect in metabolism of the neurotransmitter glutamate, and cell damage from free radicals. Autosomal dominant gene present in about 1 in 10 cases.

S&S: It typically begins with weakness and atrophy of the skeletal muscles of the upper body due to damage to lower motor neuron manifest as decline in ability to perform fine motor skills and dropping things. Muscle fasciculations and fibrillations, decreased tendon reflex, muscle cramping, and generalized fatigue occur. As upper motor neurons degenerate, hyperactive reflexes, jaw clonus, tongue fasciculations, and a positive Babinski reflex present. With involvement of muscles of neck and throat, difficulty articulating words and difficulty swallowing occur. Ultimately, generalized paralysis including the respiratory muscles occurs and death from pneumonia and respiratory failure results.

Dx: There is no definitive diagnostic test; it is a diagnosis of exclusion. Muscle biopsy documents source of muscle weakness and EMG documents denervation of muscle, fibrillation, and fasciculation.

Rx: There is no cure; symptom relief is goal; tube feedings to maintain nutrition when needed. Riluzole (Rilutek) used for its apparent neuroprotective effect and ability to prolong life by several months.

Nursing Process Elements

- Promote good nutrition.
- Balance activity and rest.
- Promote adequate sleep.
- Prevent complications.
- Support client's functional abilities encouraging use of self-help devices as needed.
- Support families' coping and refer to services such as Hospice and area support groups.

Client teaching for self-care

- Sit up to eat or drink.
- Tuck chin in toward neck when eating to aid swallowing.
- If cough is weak, suction mouth to clear as needed.

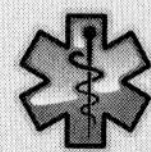

Nursing Intervention Alert

Facilitate client/family decision about the use of ventilator support. This decision should be made before a respiratory crisis occurs.

ALZHEIMER'S DISEASE

- Alzheimer's disease is the amost common cause of severe intellectual deterioration and extreme physical degeneration in the elderly population.
- One in 10 individuals older than age 65 and about half of older adults aged 85 and older have AD.
- *Amyloid plaques* and *neurofibrillary tangles* are found in the brains of AD victims.

Etiology: Unknown

Risk factors: Age, family history

S&S:

- Memory loss (short-term memory first)
- Difficulty performing tasks
- Difficulties with language (forget words, cannot name objects) and communication
- Disorientation to place and time
- Impaired judgment
- Personality changes, delusions, paranoia, and hallucinations

Dx: Based on symptoms and rule out of other causes for dementia with physical and psychiatric examination, laboratory tests, and brain scan

Rx: No cure; drug therapy may improve symptoms and lessen behavioral problems.

Nursing Process Elements

- Provide for safety
- Provide consistency in daily routine
- Provide for socialization
- Use reality orientation
- Maximize independence with ADLs; break down tasks into short simple tasks

Educate the Caregiver on the following points:

- Provide literature, for example, *The 36 Hour Day*
- Teach importance of caregiver support group, and importance of respite for caregiver
- Teach therapeutic modalities including therapeutic touch, validation therapy, and reminiscence

CEREBROVASCULAR ACCIDENT (CVA)

- Cerebrovascular accident is an inadequate blood supply to the brain due to ischemia or hemorrhage with resultant decreased oxygen supply and death of brain cells.
- It may also be classified as a brain attack or stroke.

Etiology: Atherosclerosis, venous thrombosis, embolic and small vessel diseases, hypercoagulopathies, and genetic predisposition.

Precipitating factors: Hypertension, diabetes mellitus, sickle cell disease, obesity, hyperlipidemia, hypercholesterolemia, hypercoagulability, heavy alcohol consumption, smoking, oral contraceptive use, heart disease, physical inactivity, and atrial fibrillation. Nonmodifiable risk factors include African American ethnicity, increasing age, and male gender. Persons with a previous transient ischemic attack (TIA) are at increased risk for developing a CVA.

S&S: Dependent upon which area of the brain affected.

- Right side of brain
  - —Left side of body is affected.
  - —Right side of face is affected.
  - —Vision problem: left homonymous hemianopsia (loss of vision in the left half of the visual field in both eyes)
  - —Memory loss
  - —Problems recognizing faces
  - —Gets lost easily
  - —Short attention span
  - —Concrete thinking
  - —Left hemiplegia
  - —Left hemiparesis
  - —Altered sensation on left side
  - —Impulsive, inquisitive, uninhibited, and socially inappropriate behavior
  - —Verbal outbursts
  - —Left-sided neglect of body
  - —Impaired time and judgment
  - —Overestimation of own abilities with poor judgment regarding safety
- Left side of brain
  - —Right side of body is affected
  - —Left side of face is affected
  - —Right homonymous hemianopsia (loss of vision in the right half of the visual field in both eyes)
  - —Memory impaired for verbal and auditory stimuli
  - —Poor naming ability
  - —Right hemiplegia
  - —Right hemiparesis
  - —Altered sensation on right side
  - —Speech/language impairment (aphasia): auditory speech interpretation, word selection, and motor aspects (articulation) of speech
  - —Reading comprehension impaired
  - —Agraphia (inability to write)
  - —Slow, cautious behavior
  - —Easily frustrated
  - —Disorganized in approach to new problems
  - —Depression and anxiety
  - —Impaired comprehension of language and mathematics concepts, difficulty telling left from right

Dx: Usually based on clinical presenting symptoms, client history, and diagnostic tests. A CT is the primary diagnostic tool used to differentiate type of stroke, indicate size and location of the lesion, and guide treatment modality. MRI—to determine extent of brain injury, angiography for carotid artery imaging, transcranial Doppler (TCD)—to measure velocity of blood flow and assess for vasospasm in cerebral arteries. An EEG may be done to show brain wave activity and differentiate hemorrhagic from ischemic stroke. A lumbar puncture may be done if subarachnoid hemorrhage is suspected and CT is not definitive.

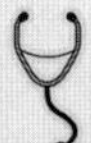

Assessment Alert

Differentiation between ischemic and hemorrhagic stroke is imperative so that emergency treatment can begin immediately. A thorough review of client history to determine exact time of S&S will help facilitate expedient care. Emergency medication "clotbusters" must be given within 3 hours after the symptoms of an ischemic stroke began. The use of clotbusters is contraindicated in a hemorrhagic stroke.

Rx: Determined by type of stroke. Treatment is aimed at restoring blood flow to the brain, preventing further brain damage, and reducing disability.

- Drug therapy
  - —The following are utilized only for ischemic stroke.
    - Recombinant tissue plasminogen activator (tPA), streptokinase, or urokinase to break down clots.
    - Anticoagulant therapy—warfarin (Coumadin), heparin, or low molecular weight heparin to increase time for blood to coagulate.
    - Acetylsalicylic acid (aspirin), ticlopidine (Ticlid), clopidogrel (Plavix), and dipyridamole (Persantine) to inhibit platelet aggregation.
  - —Calcium channel blockers—nimodipine (Nimotop) to decrease and/or prevent vasospasm in hemorrhagic stroke.
  - —Antiseizure medication if seizure has occurred.
  - —Aspirin or acetaminophen (Tylenol) for treatment of hyperthermia.
- Surgical treatment to remove cerebral hematoma due to hemorrhagic stroke. May include clipping, wrapping, or inserting microcoil in a ruptured cerebral aneurysm.

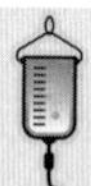

Clinical Caution

The tPA must be given within 3 hours of initial symptoms of ischemic stroke. Candidacy for use of drug therapy must be determined before beginning treatment. Contraindications include uncontrolled blood pressure (>185/110 mm Hg on repeated measurements), a history of brain hemorrhage, abnormal coagulation factors, and a history of major surgery during the previous 14 days.

- Physical and occupational therapy to increase strength, teach use of assistive devices, memory, and cognitive exercises.
- Speech therapy for swallowing and speech difficulties.

Nursing Process Elements

- Assess for S&S of progression of disease.
- Cardiac/respiratory assessment and support during acute phase.
- Oral hygiene, swallowing assessment, and assessment for pocketing of food while client is eating.
- Oral and endotracheal suctioning.
- Monitor for aspiration pneumonia; keep head of bed elevated during and after feedings.
- Prevention of deep vein thrombosis—provide range of motion exercises, utilize compression stockings, and assess lower extremities.
- Assist with activities of daily living, turn client every 2 hours, and assist with ambulation. Keep high-top tennis shoes on client's feet; do not pull on affected limbs.
- Monitor urinary and bowel function.
- Assist family to understand the client's behavior.
- Assess need for referral for counseling.
- Teach medication administration techniques for home therapy.
- Adaptations of care for left hemisphere damage
  - —Speak slowly to allow time for processing
  - —Use simple, short, one- or two-word phrases and commands.
  - —Gesture and demonstrate along with using words to convey meaning.
  - —Repeat often.
  - —Use large print and other visual input.
  - —Use music to provide information.
  - —Help family to understand the communication impairment and how to circumvent it; including fact that comprehension is unimpaired.
- Adaptations of care for right hemisphere damage
  - —Decrease environmental sensory stimuli
  - —Move and speak slowly around client.
  - —Use auditory and visual input together to communicate.
  - —State names of objects as they are touched.
  - —Break tasks into small steps.
  - —Orient the client frequently.
  - —Provide reminders for activities.
  - —Take precautions in regard to client safety.
  - —Prepare family members for behavior changes and for inability to recognize faces.

Client teaching for self-care

- Take medication as prescribed.
- Do not discontinue medications abruptly.
- Follow a high-calorie, high-fiber diet and increase fluids to help maintain dietary needs and prevent constipation. Take stool softeners as prescribed and indicated.
- Teach family members/caregivers to speak slowly and give ample time for client to respond. Use communication board as needed.
- Remove clothes from unaffected side first, followed by affected side. Dress affected side before unaffected side.
- Use assistive devices as taught by therapists.
- Continue with exercises taught by physical, occupational, and speech therapy.
- Follow up with home care and rehabilitation team as ordered.
- Remove unnecessary items from table when eating to avoid spills. Use assistive equipment to assist with eating. Allow client to feed self as much as possible.

CEREBRAL ANEURYSM

- Cerebral aneurysm is an area of a blood vessel in the brain that weakens over time and begins to bulge like a balloon.
- Over time the area can become weaker. Increased pressure exerted in the vessel increases the likelihood that the vessel may rupture.
- The aneurysm may not rupture, but may cause S&S due to the pressure exerted on brain tissue and cranial nerves.

Etiology: Uncontrolled blood pressure, head injury or trauma, and congenital due to weakness in the circle of Willis.

Risk factors: May occur at any age, but more common in adults than children. Occur slightly more often in women than men.

Precipitating factors: High blood pressure, arteriosclerosis/atherosclerosis in the brain, arteriovenous malformation (AVM), injury or trauma to the head, habitual use of cocaine, and genetics.

S&S:

- Sudden, severe headache often classified as "the worst headache ever"
- Nausea and/or vomiting
- Sensitivity to light
- Weakness on one side of the body
- Dizziness or loss of consciousness
- Diplopia
- Neck pain
- Drowsiness or difficulty awakening

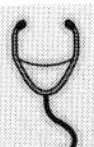

Assessment Alert

Emergency treatment needs to begin as soon as possible. S&S such as severe headache with nausea, vomiting, and sensitivity to light can mimic persons with a migraine headache. S&S such as weakness or paralysis on one side of the body, loss of consciousness, drowsiness, nausea, vomiting, and dizziness can mimic persons having a brain attack (stroke, cerebral vascular accident or CVA). Careful differentiation between aneurysm, migraine, and CVA is critical.

Dx: Based on past medical history, clinical manifestations, and diagnostic studies. CT most common procedure used—to assess for bleeding into brain tissue; lumbar puncture to test for blood and other elements in the cerebrospinal fluid; angiogram to assess for circulation of blood flow in the brain.

Rx: Ruptured cerebral aneurysm treatment aimed at restoring deteriorating vital signs and decreasing intracranial pressure. Surgical intervention to clip the aneurysm and prevent rebleeding is usually required and done within the first 3 days unless the client is unstable. For clients at high risk for surgery or for clients that have an aneurysm that has not ruptured a microcoil thrombosis or balloon embolization may be performed.

- Bed rest
- Hypertensive-hypervolemic therapy to increase pressure on the bleeding vessels in the brain and "thin" the blood to assure adequate blood supply to the brain and decrease vasospasm in cerebral vessels.
  - —Vasoconstricting agents—dopamine (Intropin) and phenylephrine.
  - —Volume expansion using crystalloid or colloid solutions.

- Calcium channel blocker—nimodipine (Nimotop) to prevent and treat vasospasms.
- Stool softeners to keep client from straining with stool.
- Diuretics such as mannitol (Osmitrol) or furosemide (Lasix) to reduce fluid overload and increased ICP.
- Respiratory and cardiac support as indicated.
- Hyperthermia—acetaminophen (Tylenol) and/or use of a cooling blanket.
- Rehabilitation therapy dependent on client's prognosis, overall health, and effects from cerebral bleed.
  - —Physical and occupational therapy to increase strength and teach use of assistive devices.
  - —Speech therapy to improve speech and swallowing.
  - —Counseling—individual or group therapy to help client and family cope with any lasting debilitative effects and relieve emotional stress.

Nursing Process Elements

- Primary assessment: Focus on respiratory, cardiac, and neurologic status.
- Assess respiratory status and need for ventilatory/oxygen support.
- Maintain airway patency and suction as needed.
- Monitor ICP.
- Monitor Glasgow Coma Scale (GCS) and level of consciousness (LOC) and notify primary physician immediately for any decreased LOC or decrease in GCS.
- If client has had surgical intervention, monitor dressing for amount, color, and consistency or drainage. Report any serous drainage with "halo" on gauze and/or positive for glucose immediately to physician.
- Provide oral hygiene every 2 hours for clients on ventilatory support to prevent skin breakdown and keep mucous membranes moist.
- Provide active and passive range of motion to prevent muscle wasting and rigidity.
- Elevate the head of the body and keep head and neck in alignment and avoid hip flexion to prevent increases in ICP.
- Administer nutritional support with use of enteral or parenteral feeding.
- Monitor urine output to assess for possible syndrome of inappropriate antidiuretic hormone (SIADH) and fluid retention.
- Turn client every 2 hours to prevent skin breakdown.
- Assess activities of daily living and need for referral for physical and/or occupational therapy.
- Assess need for referral for counseling.
- Teach medication administration techniques for home therapy.

Client teaching for self-care

- Stop or avoid smoking.
- Control blood pressure and take antihypertensive medication as directed.
- Maintain weight within normal limits for age and height.
- Avoid use of cocaine.
- Follow therapy exercises as prescribed by physical, occupational, and speech therapy.
- Report any sudden, severe headache, diplopia, hemiparesis, or hemiplegia to primary physician immediately.
- Get adequate rest.

HEADACHE

- Primary headaches: These are not symptoms of another known disease, they include: migraine, cluster, tension headaches
- Secondary headaches: These are symptoms of a known disease such as meningitis, brain tumor, and aneurysm.
- Migraine and cluster headaches are also classified as vascular headaches.

MIGRAINE HEADACHE

- Develops in teen to young adult years
- Occurs predominantly in women
- Episodic, lasts hours to days

Etiology: Hereditary pattern evident but precise cause unknown. Believed to be related to vasoconstriction followed by vasodilatation and neurogenic inflammation of cerebral blood vessels causing release of serotonin.

Risk/Precipitating Factors: Stress and hormone changes

S&S: May be an aura 10–30 minutes before acute attack: lights dancing in front of the eyes, photophobia, confusion, or sensorimotor symptoms; pain predominant on one side of the head and increases in severity as attack proceeds; may be accompanied by nausea, vomiting, fatigue, and irritability

Dx: History and clinical presentation

Rx:

Prevention:

- Pharmacological
  - —beta blockers: Inhibit vasodilation of cerebral vessels and the reuptake of serotonin
  - —Tricyclic antidepressants: block uptake of catecholamines and serotonin
  - —Diuretics: prevent fluid retention
- Biofeedback
- Relaxation techniques

Symptom management:

- Triptans—cause vasoconstriction by binding to serotonin receptors on cranial arteries.
- Ergot alkaloids—cause vasoconstriction
- Antiemetics for nausea and vomiting
- Nonopioid analgesics

Nursing Process Elements

- Determine how client manages headaches including use of OTC medications
- Encourage client to keep a headache diary and record occurrence of headaches and surrounding events such as amount of sleep, foods eaten, activities, etc. to help identify triggering factors.

Client teaching for self-care

- Correct use of preventative and symptom relief medications: preventative drugs must be taken on schedule without missed doses to be effective. Take drugs for symptomatic relief as soon as aura or symptom occurs.
- Avoidance of identified triggering factors: common triggers are nitrates, nitrites, alcohol, monosodium glutamate, and high salt intake with fluid retention, nicotine.
- Once headache starts, rest in a quiet, darkened room
- Referrals as appropriate to dietician and/or support groups

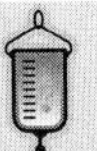

Clinical Alert

Women with migraines should not take oral contraceptives because these have been found to increase migraine occurrence.

CLUSTER HEADACHE

- Occurs in clusters over periods of a week to a year with remissions between clusters.
- Lasts minutes to a few hours
- Severe neurologic pain syndrome

Etiology: Similar to migraine

Risk/precipitating factors: Alcohol and nitrates

S&S: Deep, throbbing, often one-sided pain starting under the orbit of the eye and spreading to head and neck; may be accompanied by tearing, flushing, nasal stuffiness, sweating, swelling of temporal blood vessels; no aura

Rx: Opioid analgesics

Nursing Process Elements

Similar to migraine

TENSION HEADACHE

Etiology: Tension and anxiety

S&S: Dull, constant pain, usually bilateral and involving neck and shoulders; contracted head and neck muscles; no aura; not affected by activity

Rx: Nonopioid analgesics, amitriptyline (Elavil), relaxation exercises

Client teaching for self-care

- Help client identify sources of stress
- Encourage use of stress management and relaxation strategies

SEIZURES

- A seizure is a temporary brain dysfunction caused by aberrant electrical activity in the brain.
- About 30% seizure incidences begin in childhood. Next area of increased incidence occurs in individuals older than 65 years of age.
- One seizure alone does not constitute having a seizure disorder.
- International Classification of Seizure Disorders classifies seizures into the following categories:
  - —Generalized seizures: bilaterally, symmetrically, and without local onset
    - Absence seizures (brief loss of consciousness, staring, unresponsiveness), myoclonic seizures (brief jerking of a muscle group which may cause falling), clonic

seizures (rhythmic jerking of muscles), tonic seizures (rigidity of all muscles) tonic–clonic seizures (rigidity of muscles followed by rhythmic jerking sometimes accompanied by tongue biting and urinary and fecal incontinence), and atonic seizures (brief loss of muscle tone which may cause falling).

—Partial seizures

- Simple partial seizures without impairment of consciousness (focal twitching of an extremity, halt in speech, visual phenomena like seeing lights, feeling of fear or doom)
- Complex partial seizures with impairment of consciousness
  - Simple partial seizures (automatic behavior such as lip smacking, chewing or picking at clothes) with progression to impairment of consciousness
  - Impairment of consciousness at onset

—Unclassified: inadequate or incomplete data

- Status epilepticus: A seizure that does not stop or rapidly occurring seizures without a break in between for recovery. Status epilepticus is a medical emergency requiring immediate treatment to prevent harm and brain damage.

Etiology: Usually not identifiable. The seizure may be caused by underlying physiologic or psychogenic processes.

Precipitating factors: Hypoxia during birth, head injury, Alzheimer's, cerebral bleeding, cerebrovascular accident, hypoparathyroidism, hypocalcemia, hypoglycemia, hypomagnesemia, hypernatremia, hyponatremia, brain malformations, brain tumor, maternal drug use, prescription drugs, alcohol withdrawal, cerebral edema, fever, infection, congenital conditions, cardiac arrhythmia, syncope, and stressful psychological experiences.

S&S: Dependent upon location of abnormal electrical activity in the brain. (See types of seizures above.)

- Convulsions on one side of the body, one area of the body, or entire body
- Loss of consciousness
- Inability to speak or respond
- Staring
- Pleasant or unpleasant sense of smell
- Confusion or altered consciousness
- Loss of bowel or bladder control
- Numbness or tingling in specific body area
- Abnormal movements
- Twitching of eyelids and facial muscles
- Abruptly stopping activity; may fall to the ground

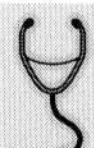

Assessment Alert

In older clients, "Senior moments" characterized by blank stares, temporary confusion or even short gaps in conversation may actually be signs of a seizure disorder.

Dx: Based on client history, eyewitness account of the occurrence, and diagnostic studies. Blood test to determine levels of electrolytes, glucose, white blood cells, and red blood cells; liver and kidney function tests; EEG to assess electrical activity in the brain; CT scan or MRI to assess for cerebral abnormalities, and an EKG to assess cardiac rhythm.

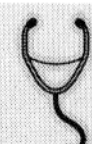

Assessment Alert

Testing is usually done after the client has experienced at least two unprovoked seizures. Many times once the underlying cause of the seizure is corrected, no further seizures will occur. Thus, it is imperative to get an accurate and complete client history to help determine diagnosis and treatment options. If the client experiences a seizure, it is important to note the length of the seizure, symptoms, what the person was doing before the seizure, and whether there were any lasting effects afterward.

Rx: Dependent upon type of seizure and whether there is any underlying physiology or psychogenic processes.

- Anticonvulsant medication dependent upon type of seizure. Lowest possible dose with fewest side effects that stops all seizures is the goal of treatment.
- Medication used for generalized tonic–clonic and partial seizures
  —carbamazepine (Tegretol), divalproex (Depakote), lamotrigine (Lamictal), gabapentin (Neurontin), felbamate (Felbatol), phenytoin (Dilantin), tiagabine (Gabitril), topiramate (Topamax), zonisamide (Zonegran), valproic acid (Depakene) phenobarbital, levetiracetam (Keppra), oxcarbazepine (Trileptal), and primidone (Mysoline).
- Medication used for absence and myoclonic seizures
  —clonazepam (Klonopin), divalproex (Depakote), phenobarbital, valproic acid (Depakene), or ethosuximide (Zarontin).
- Medication used to stop a seizure that has occurred or for status epilepticus
  —fosphenytoin, lorazepam (Ativan), diazepam (Valium) or midazolam (Versed).

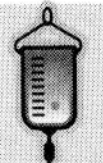

Clinical Caution

Many anticonvulsant medications are harmful to pregnant and lactating women. It is imperative that female clients are made aware of this and pregnancy status determined before beginning treatment therapy to assist in which medication to use. Medication may need to be changed during pregnancy or lactation but only on orders from the physician.

- Surgery—cutting of the nerves in the corpus callosum to decrease seizures that occur in several areas and spread to other parts of the brain.
- Correction of the underlying cause of the seizures—correcting fluid and electrolyte levels, removing tumor, decreasing stress, decreasing cerebral edema, decreasing fever, correcting cardiac arrhythmia, and removing alcohol from client's diet.
- Electrical stimulation of the vagus nerve to reduce number of partial seizures.

Nursing Process Elements

- Protect the client from injury
  —Pad siderails
  —Remove objects close to client
  —Loosen clothing around neck
  —Do not restrain client
  —Do not place anything in the mouth
  —Keep oxygen and suction equipment nearby
  —Do not leave client alone until fully conscious and can move about on own again.
- Keep the room quiet and decrease stimuli.
- Allow for periods of rest, especially after client experiences a seizure.
- Administer anticonvulsant medication as ordered. Do not administer other medications at the same time as anticonvulsant medication unless directed by physician.
- Notify physician when client experiences a seizure.

Client teaching for self-care

- Take medication as directed at the same time every day.
- Do not discontinue medication.
- Do not take your anticonvulsant with any other medication unless directed by your physician.
- Do not drink alcoholic beverages.
- Do not swim alone.
- Do not engage in activities that may result in a loss of consciousness.
- Get plenty of sleep every day.
- Always wear a Medic Alert bracelet.
- Follow up with laboratory work as directed by your physician.
- Exercise or walk as often as possible.
- Decrease stress at work and home as much as possible.
- Do not operate heavy machinery or power tools.
- Do not drive a vehicle until you have been free of seizures for at least 6 months to 1 year. Many states prohibit driving for at least this amount of time.

FEBRILE CONVULSIONS

Etiology: It is one of the most common neurologic problems seen in children. It is usually a symptom of an infectious process. The most common infection associated with febrile convulsions is otitis media.

Risk factors:

- Age between 3 months and 3 years
- Boys more often than girls
- Familial tendency

S&S:

- Rise in temperature, usually above 101.
- Sudden onset of tonic–clonic seizure

Dx: Diagnosis is usually based on the presence of an infectious process and temperature elevation. An EEG may be performed at a later date to rule out underlying neurologic pathology.

Rx: Usually the seizure has ended prior to reaching medical help. Treatment is aimed at the underlying infection and preventing future temperature elevations.

Nursing Process Elements

- Antipyretics such as acetaminophen. Aspirin is not used because of the danger of Reye's syndrome
- Remove excessive clothing
- Maintain cool room temperature
- Tepid bath or sponge: Pat the child dry; do not rub
- Do not cause the child to shiver as that will raise temperature
- Offer cool clear liquids

Client teaching for self-care

- Teach parents how to take the child's temperature
- Explain temperature reducing methods
- Remind parents that children that have had febrile convulsion are at risk of additional febrile convulsions; so temperatures should be treated immediately.
- Explain to parents that there is rarely permanent sequelae from a febrile convulsion

CEREBRAL PALSY

- Nonprogressive brain dysfunction
- Leads to disorders involving movement, muscle tone and coordination
- Classified by clinical characteristics
  —Spastic: Hypertonic muscles, develops contractures, scissoring of legs
  —Athetoid: Also called dyskinetic. Slow, wormlike movements, involuntary movements of extremities
  —Ataxic: Muscles and reflexes hypotonic. Coordination difficulty
  —Mixed: Combination of types of cerebral palsy
- May affect one side of the body (hemiplegia), or all four extremities (quadriplegia).

Etiology: Cerebral injury occurring during the fetal or neonatal period. Asphyxia and intrauterine infections, birth injuries and intracranial hemorrhage. The type of cerebral palsy is dependent upon the area of the brain affected

Risk factors: Prematurity, kernicterus, and low Apgar scores

S&S:

- Failure to meet expected development milestones
- Excessive or diminished muscle tone
- Feeding difficulties
- Seizures may be present
- Mental retardation may accompany CP
- Visual and auditory deficits may be present

Dx: Based on clinical findings with CT and MRI

Rx: Early recognition with interventions designed to promote normal growth and development

- Mobility aids such as bracing, crutches, walkers, and wheelchairs as needed
- Anticonvulsants if needed
- Surgical release of contractures may be necessary
- Intrathecal baclofen infusions may be used to reduce spasticity

Nursing Process Elements

- Multidisciplinary approach individualized to the needs of the child.
- Early intervention such as passive range of motion exercises can reduce the development of contractures and promote muscle development.
- The child will need assistance with daily hygiene and other self-care activities. The skin will be prone to breakdown in the area of bony prominences. Bracing can also contribute to skin breakdown.
- Nutritional support may be necessary if facial involvement makes chewing and swallowing difficult. This support can range from adaptation of feeding methods and the use of high-calorie foods or the insertion of a gastrostomy tube.
- Speech therapy may be necessary to improve communication. Use of computer assisted communication may be necessary for the more severely involved child.
- The child may be at greater risk for aspiration due to involvement of the oral muscles. Whenever possible, the child should be fed in an upright position.
- Emotional support for the child and family throughout the life of the child. Identify and refer to appropriate community resources.

Client teaching for self-care

- Teach the parents means of promoting growth and development by identifying areas of delay and developing a plan that will promote development in that area

- Teach the parents how to apply the braces and means of protecting the underlying skin. Provide information that will assist the parents in early recognition of skin breakdown
- Work with the parents on developing feeding methods that safely promote growth.
- Teach the parents how to administer the medications as well as side effects of the medications their child is receiving.
- The parents may need guidance in adapting safety equipment, toys and other devices for their child.

HYDROCEPHALUS

- Hydrocephalus is an accumulation of cerebral spinal fluid in the ventricles of the brain
- If untreated or treatment is unsuccessful, hydrocephalus will lead to brain damage and could cause eventual herniation of the brain stem through the foramen magnum and death

Etiology:

- May be congenital or acquired.
- May be due to an obstruction of the CSF flow preventing the normal reabsorption of the CSF by the subarachnoid spaces. Termed "noncommunicating hydrocephalus," this form may be caused by tumors, hemorrhage, infection or structural abnormalities.
- Impaired absorption by the subarachnoid spaces, this form is called "communicating hydrocephalus" and is less common than the noncommunicating form
- Accumulation of CSF in the ventricles leads to compression of the surrounding brain tissue and if the sutures are not closed, to an enlarging head circumference.

Risk factors:

- Associated with spina bifida cystica (meningoceles and myelomeningoceles) defects due to structural abnormalities. May be apparent at birth or may not be symptomatic until the sac is closed surgically.
- Intracranial hemorrhage, especially in the premature, meningitis, and brain tumors.

S&S: Symptoms will be dependent upon the age of the child and whether the sutures have closed.

- In the young infant:
  —Increasing head circumference
  —Bulging fontanels
  —Thin scalp with fine appearing hair and obvious scalp veins
  —Setting sun sign, white sclera showing above the iris
  —Shrill, high-pitched cry
- In the older child:
  —Headaches, initially early morning
  —Vomiting without nausea, initially early morning
  —Papilledema
- In all children:
  —Varying degrees of irritability, lethargy progressing to mental slowness

Dx:

- Hydrocephalus may be diagnosed in utero. The earlier the diagnosis and surgical intervention, the greater will be the preservation of brain function.
- CT and MRI

Rx:

Surgery aimed at re-establishing the CSF flow by removing the obstruction (tumor) or by providing an alternate route to CSF reabsorption (shunt)

- Shunts involve a small tube with a one-direction valve taking CSF from the ventricles to a distant site. The CSF fluid is reabsorbed by the body into the blood stream
- Two types of shunts are commonly used
  —Ventriculoatrial shunt: CSF is directed from the ventricle into the atrium of the heart. The advantage to this type of shunt is there is little risk of the distal tip becoming clogged. The disadvantages of this shunt include the need for revisions to allow for the child's growth and the risk that if infection occurs, endocarditis may result.
  —Ventriculoperitoneal shunt: The distal tip of this shunt is in the peritoneal cavity. Extra tubing can be placed in the abdomen to allow for growth and there is no risk of endocarditis with this type of shunt. However, the fatty omentum frequently occludes the distal tip requiring revision.

Nursing Process Elements

Preoperative care

- Measure daily head circumference.
- Promote nutrition. Refeed if the child vomits as vomiting may temporarily relieve the intracranial pressure.
- Elevate the head as it may reduce headaches by reducing the contents of the skull. Medication may be required but care should be taken not to depress the mental status

Postoperative care

- Position the child's head according to medical orders and on nonsurgical side. Elevation of the head may cause the shunt to reduce the intracranial volume too rapidly.
- Monitor for signs of intracranial infection

Client teaching for self-care

- Parents should be aware that the return of symptoms of increased intracranial pressure may indicate that the shunt is not functioning.
- If brain damage has occurred, information should be provided about promoting growth and development as well as community resources available for the child with mental retardation.
- Children who have recurrent neurosurgical procedures have an increased risk of developing latex allergies. Parents should be taught to avoid exposure to latex products including pacifiers and toys.

HEAD INJURY

- Head injury refers to injury to scalp, cranium, and/or brain
- Motor vehicle accidents are the most common cause followed by alcohol and drug ingestion, assaults, and sports related accidents
- Major concern: amount of damage to brain

SKULL FRACTURE

- Break in the bone of the cranium; occurs due to trauma; may be associated cerebral edema and other complications or may result in no further injury
- Linear or simple—crack in bone; may be asymptomatic; no treatment required
- Comminuted—bone is broken or crushed into small pieces
- Depressed—bone fragments are depressed inward into brain tissue
  - —Open if dura is torn
  - —Closed if dura is intact
  - —Requires immediate surgical intervention to prevent brain damage
- Basilar—break at base of skull
  - —May result in CSF drainage from the nose or ear
  - —Treated with antibiotics because of the risk of meningitis

Dx: Skull fracture is visualized by CT or MRI. Basilar is difficult to see if dura is torn and may have CSF leaking from nose (rhinorrhea) or ear (otorrhea), periorbital ecchymoses "Raccoon eyes"; ecchymosis over the mastoid; air in frontal sinuses on CT.

Rx: The treatment varies with type and location

- Linear—no treatment just close monitoring for underlying brain injury
- Depressed—surgery usually within 24 hours to raise bone, remove fragments, close dura if possible. Cranioplasty with insertion of acrylic bone immediately or if cerebral edema or infection is a problem, in 3–6 months. Dexamethasone given for cerebral edema and prophylactic antibiotics for 24–48 hours postoperatively.
- Basilar—if dura is torn and CSF leaking continues for more than 7–10 days the time in which most dural tears close, craniotomy to repair the tear may be necessary. Prophylactic antibiotics are given whenever there is a suspected CSF leak.

Nursing Process Elements

- Assess for signs of a torn dura: CSF leaking from nose or ears. All drainage is tested for glucose; CSF is positive for glucose.
- If dura is known to be torn,
  - —instruct clients to refrain from activities such as coughing, sneezing, nose blowing, and the Valsalva maneuver that increase ICP. Monitor for signs of encephalitis or meningitis.
  - —keep head of bed flat or elevated to no more than 30 degrees as per physician's order.
  - —all procedures involving entry into the ear canal or nasal cavity are avoided.

BRAIN INJURY

- *Concussion*—transient, neurologic dysfunction occurring as a result of head injury
- *Contusion*—area of brain tissue into which bleeding has occurred as a result of trauma that causes the brain to strike the inside of the skull
- *Coup injury*—injury of the brain tissue directly underneath the site of trauma
- *Contra-coup injury*—injury of the brain tissue on the opposite side of the brain from where the injury occurred as a result of trauma causing the brain to move back and forth within the skull.

Etiology: Falls, child abuse, motor vehicle accidents, and other trauma

S&S:

Concussion

- *Mild*: No loss of consciousness, confusion and disorientation may occur but clear in seconds or minutes, dizziness, spots before the eyes, recovery is complete
- *Severe*: Loss of consciousness lasting less than 24 hours, headache, vomiting, irritability; recovery of consciousness usually associated with brief period of confusion/disorientation; amnesia for injury and immediately preceding events, bulging fontanels in infants younger than 18 months, vomiting

Contusion

- More severe S&S than concussion. Loss of consciousness with stupor and confusion and focal neurological deficits including seizures reflecting area of brain that is damaged. Ipsilateral pupil changes, weak pulse, shallow respirations, incontinence, and cerebral edema may also occur.

Dx: History, neurological examination, CT or MRI to rule out underlying injury such as hematoma

Rx: Prevention or management of cerebral edema is of primary importance as well as prevention or reduction of brain compression. Surgical intervention may be required. Contusion: dexamethasone to reduce cerebral edema. Supportive care is based on symptoms.

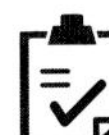

Nursing Process Elements

- Monitor neurologic status. This may include the Glasgow Coma Scale and:
  —vital signs including blood pressure,
  —level of consciousness,
  —strength/ability to move all extremities,
  —pupil reactions, and
  —headache, dizziness, vomiting, confusion, and weakness.
- Limit fluid intake to reduce the development of cerebral edema
- Monitor for drainage that suggests basalar skull fracture
- Monitor pain but analgesics and sedatives are not recommended as their use may mask a decreasing level of consciousness
- Monitor for seizures and be prepared to respond should they occur
- Provide physiologic support for the comatose client
- Instruct the client with a concussion to resume ADLs slowly and progressively

Client teaching for self-care

- All children should wear protective equipment when involved in activities which can cause head injury including bicycle riding and skateboarding
- If the child is to be discharged and monitored at home, teach the parents to awaken the child several times during the night to assess level of consciousness.
- Explain to the parents symptoms they might note that would require immediate notification of the physician.
- Many children will experience a postconcussion syndrome that can include forgetfulness, behavioral changes, and learning difficulties that may last for several months.

EPIDURAL HEMATOMA

- Epidural hematoma is bleeding, usually arterial, into the epidural space, which is between the skull and the dura.
- It creates pressure on the brain and clots rapidly.
- It is a medical emergency.

Etiology: Often associated with fracture of the temporoparietal bones

S&S: Decreasing level of consciousness 1 or even 2 days after initial return to being alert and lucid following injury.

Headache, vomiting, and same side pupil (ipsilateral) dilation. If brain stem herniation occurs due to pressure of the hematoma, contralateral (opposite-side) motor paralysis with increased tendon reflexes, positive Babinski sign, coma, and decerebrate posturing develop.

Dx: Emergency CT to determine location of hematoma and amount of cerebral edema.

Rx: Immediate surgical evacuation; in some cases, craniotomy necessary to top hemorrhaging.

SUBDURAL HEMATOMA

- Subdural hematoma is venous bleeding into the suddural space, which is between the dura and the arachnoid.
- It develops more slowly than arterial hematomas.
- Types:
  —Acute: symptomatic within 48 hours of initial injury
  —Subacute: symptomatic 2 days to 2 weeks after injury
  —Chronic: symptomatic 2 weeks to months after injury

S&S:

- Acute and subacute: Increased intracranial pressure, headache, drowsiness, and confusion that insidiously worsen; ipsilateral pupil dilation.
- Chronic: headache, variable LOC, personality changes, and motor weakness.

Dx: CT scan

Rx: Small hematomas reabsorb; larger clots may require repeated subdural taps to remove the clot or surgical evacuation.

Nursing Process Elements

- Immobilize clients with head trauma until coexistent spinal cord injury has been ruled out.
- Priority assessment is airway: check rate and depth of respirations.
- Assess LOC
- Monitor for VS changes indicative of increasing intracranial pressure: increasing systolic pressure causing widened pulse pressure and decreasing respiratory rate.
- Obtain description of accident.
- Ask about client's use of drugs and alcohol.
- Perform baseline neurological assessment: check PERRLA and lifts and grips.
- Inspect nose and ears for blood or cerebrospinal fluid.
- If alert, ask if client lost consciousness at time of accident
- Monitor neurological status every 2 hours using Glasgow Coma Scale; report change from baseline.
- Monitor VS every 2 hours.
- Administer medications to control cerebral edema.
- Control environmental stimuli to prevent increase in ICP.
- Maintain side lying position to keep airway patent.
- Monitor ABGs because hypoxia and hypercarbia can potentiate an increase in ICP.
- Change position every 2 hours to prevent pooling of secretions and skin breakdown.

BRAIN TUMOR

- Brain tumor is a tumor located anywhere in the brain.
- Primary tumors originate in the brain or spinal cord and rarely spread elsewhere in the body.
- Secondary brain tumors may metastasize to the brain from other tumors in the body.
- Brain tumors can be benign or malignant.

Etiology: Unknown, family history may increase predisposition.

Precipitating factors: Exposure to radiation, formaldehyde, vinyl chloride, or acrylonitrile (textiles and plastics) at work, family history of gliomas, increasing age, and being male. Secondary tumors may arise from a primary lesion elsewhere in the body and spread or metastasize to the brain.

S&S: Dependent upon tumor size, type, and location

- Headache that may awaken the client
- Problems with balance

- Muscle weakness
- Aphasia
- Memory problems
- Nausea or vomiting
- Changes in hearing, vision, or speech
- Paresthesias in arms or legs
- Seizures
- Mood or personality changes

Dx: Usually based on clinical presenting symptoms, client history, complete neurological examination, and diagnostic tests. A CT scan to determine the location of the lesion. MRI and PET to determine location of the lesion; useful in detecting smaller lesions that may not be evident on other studies. Angiography to determine blood flow and localize the tumor. Endocrine studies may be done to detect pituitary adenoma. A biopsy for histology testing is the most accurate way to diagnose a brain tumor.

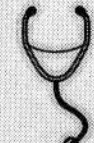

Assessment Alert

Many of the S&S are due to increasing intracranial pressure caused by the growing tumor. An accurate baseline neurological assessment is critical when determining any change in level of consciousness with increasing intracranial pressure. Immediate action should be taken in case of any decreasing level of consciousness.

Rx: A combination of therapies may be used and is determined by tumor type, location, and stage.

- Surgery is preferred treatment for removal of brain tumor.
- Chemotherapy may be given intravenously, orally, intrathecally, or via a wafer implanted during surgery.
  - —Chemotherapeutic agents are limited due to their difficulty in crossing the blood–brain barrier. Many malignant tumors break down the barrier increasing the likelihood that chemotherapeutic agents will cross to the tumor and be more effective.
- Radiation therapy using X-rays, gamma rays or protons, or radiation seeds implanted during surgery. Follows surgery or is used when surgery is not an option.
- Corticosteroids such as dexamethasone (Decadron), prednisone, or methyl-prednisolone (Solu-Medrol) may be administered to decrease cerebral edema and increasing intracranial pressure that may occur after surgery and/or radiation therapy.
- Anticonvulsant medication may be utilized if the client experiences seizures.
- Antiemetics may be given to decrease nausea the client may experience after radiation and chemotherapy treatments.
- Physical therapy may be used to increase strength and balance.
- Occupational therapy may be used to manage activities of daily living and teach use of assistive devices.
- Speech therapy may be used to assist with speaking, swallowing, and cognition.

Nursing Process Elements

- Assess for S&S of infection after surgical interventions.
- Assess for changes in level of consciousness, and complete a thorough neurological assessment.
- Allow for periods of rest. Treatments can be very taxing.
- Administer pain medication as ordered and indicated.
- Assess for nausea and administer antiemetics as needed.
- For radiation treatments, assess areas surrounding treatment for increased redness and skin breakdown.
- Implement seizure precautions for clients experiencing seizures.
- Assess need for referral for social services, physical, occupational, or speech therapy.
- Allow ample time for client to answer questions.

Client teaching for self-care

- Your hair will grow back in a few months. Use a wig, scarf or hat to keep head from becoming sunburned.
- Do not wash off marks made for radiation therapy.
- Do not operate heavy machinery or a vehicle if you have experienced seizures.
- Allow client ample time to answer questions and use communication board if indicated.
- Allow client to perform as much of own care as possible.
- Follow up with therapy as ordered.
- Take oral chemotherapy as directed.
- Take antiemetics half an hour before radiation or chemotherapy treatments.
- Get plenty of rest.
- Drink plenty of fluids and eat high-protein, high-calorie foods.

PEDS NEUROBLASTOMA

- Solid, malignant tumor arising from the neural crest cells or adrenal glands.
- Tumor may originate in the sympathetic nervous system from the base of the neck to the tailbone.

Etiology: Not specifically known. Occasionally found in children with neurofibromatosis.

Precipitating factors: Usually found by the age of two. Boys are at slightly increased risk over girls.

S&S:

- Pain in the abdomen
- Dark circles under the eyes
- Hypertension
- Weakness/paralysis or fatigue
- Lump in abdomen, neck, or chest
- Bone pain
- Bulging eyes
- Breathing difficulties in infants
- Easy bruising
- Uncontrolled eye movements
- Edema of legs, feet, ankles or scrotum
- Petechiae
- Severe diarrhea
- Jerky muscle movements/ataxia
- Fever
- Shortness of breath

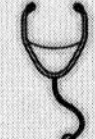

Assessment Alert

Clinical differentiation can be difficult because neuroblastoma can mimic so many other disease processes. By the time the diagnosis is made, many times the disease has already spread. Careful attention to presenting S&S is critical in assisting with diagnosis.

Dx: Usually based on clinical presenting symptoms and diagnostic studies. Twenty-four-hour urine test to check for elevated levels of catecholamines. Blood chemistry to check for elevated levels of dopamine and norepinephrine. CT scan, MRI, or ultrasound to assess for tumor size and location. Neurological examination to assess neurologic function, mental status, and reflexes. Bone marrow aspiration or biopsy to assess for tissue and chromosomal changes, and test for the presence of antigens.

Rx: Prognosis and treatment are dependent on age of the child at diagnosis, stage of the cancer, tumor location, and histology. Treatment is also affected by the rate of tumor cell growth, number of chromosomes in tumor cells, pattern of tumor cells, tumor differentiation, and how many copies have been made.

- Surgery to remove all or most of the tumor cells. A biopsy may be indicated if the entire tumor cannot be removed.
- External radiation therapy to kill cancer cells. Internal radiation using needles seeds, wires, or catheters placed directly into or near the tumor cells to kill the tumor.
- Chemotherapy—daunorubicin, cyclophosphamide, carboplatin, and etoposide to stop the growth of cancer cells.
- Bone marrow transplantation may be used following aggressive chemotherapy.
- Dopamine agonists—bromocriptine (Parlodel), pergolide (Permax), ropinirole (Requip), and pramipexole (Mirapex) to stimulate dopamine receptors.

Nursing Process Elements

- Assess need for referral for counseling.
- Teach medication administration techniques for home therapy.
- Assess need for nutritional support.
- Maintain accurate record of intake and output and weight. Weigh all diapers and assess for increased diarrhea.
- Assess surgical site for S&S of infection.
- Assess vital signs/blood pressure every 4 hours and PRN.
- Assess abdomen for presence of lumps.
- Do not palpate abdomen on clients with adrenal tumors.

Client teaching for self-care

- Take medication as prescribed.
- Do not discontinue medications abruptly.
- Follow a high-calorie, high-protein diet and increase fluids to help maintain dietary needs.
- Seek health care provider if child becomes ill, has difficulty breathing, or if increased nausea and vomiting occur due to treatment.
- Keep a record of how well the child tolerated treatment modalities.
- Maintain record of child's daily weight.
- Do not wash off radiation markers from skin.
- Apply sunscreen if outside and watch for increased redness and dryness at the site of therapy.

PEDS MENTAL RETARDATION

Mental retardation is a cognitive dysfunction that dates from the developmental period (prenatal or postnatal) and results with difficulty in function and adaptability. Mental retardation is measured on the intelligence quotient below 70 or 75 when normal IQ is considered 100. IQ is a measure of mental age divided by chronologic age.

Etiology: Selected chromosomal anomalies such as Down's syndrome, and fragile X syndrome, periods of hypoxia, and infections have all been associated with mental retardation.

Risk factors: Prenatal factors include infection and alcohol and drug abuse. Poor nutrition and hypoxia are risk factors in both the prenatal and postnatal periods.

S&S:

- Diagnosis may be made at birth secondary to select characteristics as in Down's syndrome or microcephaly or after delays occur in development
- Parents are often the first to recognize that the child's development differs from normal
- Development follows the same pattern as the normal child but at a slower pace
- Degree of mental retardation is determined by IQ scores which are used educationally to determine the optimal learning environment
  —Mild MR ranges from 50 to 75 and the child usually reaches the mental age of 8–12 years. This child may be classified as educable and may be main streamed for some classes while receiving additional help for other subjects
  —Moderate MR ranges on the IQ scale from 35 to 50, reaching a mental age of 3–7 years. This child may be classified educationally as trainable and will require supervision throughout life
  —Severe MR has an IQ of 20–35 and the child will attain a mental age of a 2–3-year old. The child will learn to walk and have limited speech requiring lifelong support and supervision
  —Profound MR has an IQ of less than 20. The child will need custodial care and educational goals will be aimed at basic skills of eating and use of extremities

Dx: Chromosomal studies, IQ tests, CT scans and MRIs may be ordered

Rx: Medical care will be directed toward diagnosis and supportive care. Seizures may accompany MR and anticonvulsants may be indicated. Genetic counseling may be included in selected situations.

Nursing Process Elements

- Emotional support to the family during the diagnostic period and throughout the life of the child
- Meeting the needs of the child such as innovative feeding techniques for the child who has a poor suck and swallow

Client teaching for self-care

- Explain about the diagnostic procedures
- Provide information about supporting growth and development
- Instruct parents about anticonvulsant therapy and management during a seizure if needed
- Refer to community resources to provide support to the family

PEDS NEURAL TUBE DEFECTS

Neural tube defects are congenital defects affecting the spinal canal including the vertebrae and spinal cord. The defects can occur anywhere alone the spinal canal but are most frequent in the sacral area

There are several types of neural tube defects with varying degrees of involvement:

- Spina bifida occulta: In this form of neural tube defect, the posterior vertebral bodies fail to completely form. The individual may be symptom free. The defect may be an incidental finding on an X-ray.
- Spina bifida cystica: In addition to the bony vertebral defect, there is a herniation of spinal material through the defect. There are two primary forms of Spina bifida cystica:
  —Meningocele: In the milder form, the meninges protrudes through the bony defect. This form will display a saclike protrusion over the spine, which may be covered by skin or only by the thin meninges. The individual may display weakness below the defect. Without intact skin, meningitis is a risk.

—Myelomeningocele: In this severe form of spina bifida cystica, the protrusion contains not only the meninges and CSF, but also the spinal cord (or more frequently the cauda equina). Blood supply to the nerves will be impaired resulting in permanent nerve damage. The child will be paralyzed from that point down.

Etiology: Unknown

OB **Risk factors:** Folic acid deficiency during early pregnancy has been associated with neural tube defects. It is recommended that all pregnant women and women who want to become pregnant take a folic acid supplement.

S&S:

- Spina bifida occulta may display a tuft of hair or a dimple at the site or be nonapparent.
- Spina bifida cystica is obvious defect present at birth.
  - —Sac-like protrusion over lower spine. The sac may be covered with intact skin or by a thin membrane.
  - —Weakness or paralysis of lower extremities.
  - —Neurogenic bladder and bowel.
  - —Hydrocephalus may be present at birth or develop after closure of the meningocele/myelomeningocele

Dx: An alpha-fetoprotein blood test run on the pregnant woman may yield high levels which may indicate neural tube defects. The finding can be confirmed by ultrasound. Further radiologic studies will differentiate the defects. Testing of neurologic function will determine the level of damage.

Rx: No treatment is required for spina bifida occulta. The child with meningocele/myelomeningocele will have surgery to repair the defect. A shunt device will be placed.

- For meningocele/myelomeningocele, surgical repair will be performed within 48 hours of birth to reduce the risk of infection.
- A shunt device may be needed to control the hydrocephalus.
- Bracing and other mobility assistive devices will be added as the child grows.

Nursing Process Elements

Preoperative care

- Position the child to protect the sac. This usually requires a prone position
- A nonadherent dressing may be applied to protect the sac from contamination.
- Avoid powdering the diaper area as the powder may contaminate the sac.
- Monitor bladder function. The child may dribble continuously placing skin integrity at risk or may not spontaneously void at all. The nurse may need to crede the bladder.
- Monitor bowel function. In the preoperative period, care must be taken that stool does not contaminate the meningocele sac.
- Provide normal infant nutrition. Position the infant during feedings to protect the sac.
- Monitor for infection including signs of meningitis
- Measure head circumference daily
- Provide emotional support to the parents. Infant may be transferred shortly after birth from the birth hospital and separated from mother. Encourage parental visits and include them in the care of their newborn.

Postoperative care

- Sterile dressings over surgical site
- Continue to monitor bladder and bowel function
- Promote nutrition for healing
- Measure head circumference daily
- Monitor for infection including signs of meningitis

Client teaching for self-care

- Prepare the parents for eventual discharge and normal infant care.
- Teach the parents to monitor and manage bladder and bowel function.
- Provide information on skin care focusing on paralysis.
- Provide information on promoting growth and development.
- Teach parents to monitor for signs of infection and hydrocephalus.
- As child grows, provide information to parents on using bracing and other assistive devices.
- Teach parents to avoid exposure to latex products including pacifiers and toys because children who have recurrent neurosurgical procedures have an increased risk of developing latex allergies.

SPINAL CORD INJURY

- Above C3 injuries are generally fatal.
- Above C4 respiratory failure is common.
- *Complete transection of the cord*—complete loss of sensory and motor function below level of injury.
- *Incomplete transection*—some spinal cord tracts are intact so there is some sensory or motor function below the level of injury.

- *Tetraplegia* (formerly quadriplegia)—loss of function in arms, legs, trunk, bowel, and bladder due to a cervical cord injury.
- *Quadriparesis*—weakness of both upper and lower extremities.
- *Paraplegia*—loss of function in legs, bowel, and bladder resulting from a thoracic, lumbar, or sacral cord injury.
- *Paraparesis*—weakness of lower extremities.
- *Level of injury*—lowest neurologic segment with normal sensory and motor function.

Etiology:

- Hyperflexion injury
  —Head and neck are forced into hyperflexion as in a head on motor vehicle accident.
  —Usually affects C5-C6
- Hyperextension injury
  —Head and neck are forced back and downward as in rear end motor vehicle accidents and falls striking the chin
  —Middle to lower cervical spine most often affected
  —Damage is often major
- Compression injury
  —Results from extreme vertical force as in being hit on top of the head or forceful landing on the feet or buttocks
  —Cervical and thoracolumbar spine most often affected
- Rotational injury
  —Extreme lateral flexion or twisting of the head

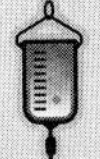

Clinical Alert

Many SCIs involve more than one direction of force so often mixed injuries occur.

- Penetrating injury
  —Direct contact of an object such as a bullet or knife with the spinal cord
  —Low-impact (low-speed) injury results in damage localized at site of impact; high-impact (high-speed) injury as from a gunshot results in widespread damage.
- Primary injury
  Results from initial damage to the cord and is irreversible
  —Types:
  - Cord concussion
    - Occurs due to severe jarring or squeezing as in many sports injuries
    - No structural injury to cord
    - May cause 1–2-day loss of sensory and motor function
    - Function returns spontaneously
  - Cord contusion
    - Bleeding into cord occurs causing swelling and bruising
    - Effect depends on overall perfusion of cord and extent of inflammatory response
    - Often caused by compression
  - Cord laceration
    - Tear in cord causes permanent injury
  - Cord transection
    - May be complete or incomplete
    - Function lost below level of injury
  - Vascular injury
    - Causes decreased perfusion and ischemia
    - If ischemia loses, cell death will occur
- Secondary injury
  —Begins within minutes of the initial injury and results from it.
  —Can destroy full thickness of cord and extend injury both above and below the site of injury.

Risk/precipitating factors: Age: greater frequency among young (16–30 years); sex: males four times as likely to sustain an SCI; alcohol use

S&S: Depend primarily on amount and level of injury to the cord

- *Spinal shock*
  —It is temporary suppression of reflexes below level of injury (spinal reflexes do not require connection to the brain as functions like sensation and voluntary movement do)
  —Spinal shock occurs in all SCI clients
  —Reappearance of spinal reflexes indicates end of period of spinal shock
- *Neurogenic shock*
  —Neurogenic shock is a hemodynamic instability secondary to the loss of neuroconnection between the brain and the sympathetic nervous system
  —It occurs with injuries to cervical or high thoracic spine
  —S&S are hypotension caused by venous pooling in lower extremities and splanchnic circulation
  —Bradycardia occurs due to unopposed parasympathetic stimulation
  —Warm, dry skin occurs due to peripheral vasodilation
  —Neurogenic shock gradually resolves over 10–14 days

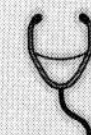

Assessment Alert

When assessing a trauma victim and trying to differentiate between hypovolemic shock and neurogenic shock, consider that bradycardia occurs with neurogenic shock and tachycardia is typical of hypovolemic shock.

Syndromes of incomplete transection

- *Central cord syndrome:* frequently occurs with cervical hyperextension injury
  - —Motor weakness, which is more pronounced in arms than legs
  - —Variable degree of sensory impairment but always more pronounced in arms than legs
  - —Possible effect on bowel and bladder function
  - —Tends to improve over time
- Anterior cord syndrome
  - —Frequently occurs due to damage to the anterior spinal artery or from pressure of a tumor or a herniated disc
  - —Loss of strength, pain perception, and temperature perception below the level of injury
  - —Can sense position, vibration and light touch
- Posterior cord syndrome
  - —Rare
  - —Position and vibration sense lost
  - —Movement, pain, and temperature sense are lost.
- Brown–Séquard syndrome
  - —Occurs with a penetrating injury involving half the cord
  - —Motor ability, touch, vibration, and pressure sense lost on side of injury; loss of pain and temperature sense on side opposite the injury
- Conus medullaris syndrome
  - —Injury at L1–2 level frequently due to vertebral fracture of disc herniation
  - —Urinary retention, loss of anal sphincter tone, constipation, impotence, slight motor weakness, loss of sensation in perineum, parts of thighs, and buttocks
- Cauda equina syndrome
  - —Asymmetrical weakness, numbness, and pain along the nerve roots, sometimes neurogenic bladder and bowel dysfunction

It is rare that any of these syndromes occur just as described; most often injuries result in a combination of syndromes.

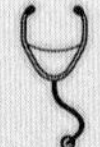

Assessment Alert

There is greater potential for some recovery of function with incomplete transection of the cord but it is not possible to differentiate complete from incomplete until after the period of spinal shock is over.

Respiratory symptoms

- Paralysis of muscles of respiration; if injury above C3, respirations cease.
- C3 to C4 injuries result in decreased inspiratory volumes because the diaphragm and some intercostals muscles are innervated from nerves at this level.
- C5 to T1 injury results in hypoventilation as a result of weak intercostals and accessory muscle strength with reduced vital capacity and inspiratory force. Inability to clear secretions occurs because of inability to take a deep breath and impaired use of abdominal muscles.
- Below T1, buildup of secretions is the major problem.

Bladder, bowel, and sexual symptoms

- Micturition reflex center, the spinal defecation reflex center, and the sexual reflex center (controls erection and labial–clitoral engorgement and vaginal lubrication) are located at S2 and S4 levels
- Injury above these reflex centers results in:
  - —Spastic automatic bladder with voluntary control of urination lost; no perception of bladder fullness or urge to void; incontinence with the bladder often not fully emptying.
  - —Loss of voluntary control over the anal sphincter, which is flaccid during spinal shock and then becomes spastic; no sense of rectal fullness and no urge to defecate; defecation may occur if the reflex arc is stimulated.
  - —Loss of sexual response to psychological stimuli but able to respond reflexively to direct stimulation of the genitals and surrounding areas.
- Injury below these reflex centers results in:
  - —An autonomous, flaccid bladder with urinary retention and overflow common.
  - —Flaccid bowel and anal sphincter with both constipation and incontinence
  - —Loss of reflex erections, engorgement and lubrication but can respond to psychologic stimuli
- Ejaculation is rare with spinal cord injury.

Dx: Neurological examination; X-rays, MRI, CT scan, and myelography

Rx:

- Immediate immobilization with a rigid cervical collar and backboard; cardiorespiratory support.
- Mechanical ventilation required for injury above C3; mechanical ventilation required at least during acute phase for C3 and C4 injury but ultimately may breathe independently for at least short intervals; temporary mechanical ventilation may be required for clients with middle to lower cervical injury who can initiate and maintain breathing but can need assistance in compensating for decreased tidal volume and difficulty maintaining a clear airway.
- IV fluids along with inotropic and chronotropic agents are administered to counteract hypotension of neurogenic shock and maintain systolic BP between 85 and 90 mm Hg to ensure good perfusion of the cord and decrease secondary injury.

- Pharmacological treatment:
  - —Methylprednisolone (Solu-Medrol) in first 8 hours after injury; not given later than 8 hours
  - —Anticoagulant prophylaxis
  - —Muscle relaxants to control spasticity
  - —Histamine 2 receptor antagonist or proton pump inhibitor to protect against gastric ulcers
- Decompression and stabilization
  - —Nonsurgical: immobilization and traction
    - Cervical tongs (Crutchfield) with a prescribed amount of weight to provide pull and realign vertebrae.
    - Halo device for cervical skeletal fixation; may be used similarly to tongs or attached to a body vest which allows the client to be ambulatory and shortens hospitalization.
    - Bedrest may initially stabilize thoracolumbar injuries; injuries at this level cannot be stabilized with traction so braces, corsets or other devices may be used; surgical repair is needed for unstable fractures.
  - —Surgical treatment
    - Remove bony fragments; relieve cord compression, correct alignment by means of screws, plates, rods, or wiring to improve stability, or to treat a penetrating wound.

Surgery is immediate if realignment is not possible in any other way or if there is unrelieved compression.

As soon as client is stable and alignment and cord compression are not problems, mobilization and rehabilitation are begun.

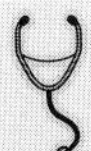

Assessment Alert

Motor and sensory function is assessed before and after the addition of each weight used for traction.

Complications:

- Autonomic hyperreflexia (previously dysreflexia)
  - —Emergency that can result in stroke, blindness, or death
  - —Over response of the sympathetic nervous system because below the injury it is shut off from inhibitory control of centers in the brain
  - —Occurs with injuries at T6 or above after period of spinal shock is over
  - —Stimuli initiating the response include: bladder distention (most common cause), bowel distention, local pressure or irritation in groin, sacral or penile areas, tight clothing, urethral catheterization or digital or other stimulation of anus, abdominal or pelvic stimulation as from sexual activity, menses, UTI, cholecystitis, gastritis, cold, heat, and drafts.
  - —Sympathetic stimulus from below area of injury causes vasoconstriction and paroxysmal hypertension; this in turn leads to bradycardia and vasodilation above level of injury in an unsuccessful attempt to lower BP.
  - —Pounding headache, nausea, nasal stuffiness, and blurred vision often accompany the hypertension.
  - —Below injury, skin is pale or mottled, cool and has goosebumps due to profound vasoconstriction; above injury, skin is flushed and diaphoretic due to the vasodilation.
- Pneumonia
- DVT
- Pain muscular, visceral, or neuropathic
  - —Neuropathic pain is burning, sharp, or shooting above, below, or at level of injury
  - —Often more responsive to treatment with antidepressants or anticonvulsants then to analgesics
- Spasticity
  - —Develops when stage of spinal shock is over
  - —May be sustained (tonic) or intermittent (clonic)
  - —Spasticity may worsen with other stresses such as UTI
  - —Degree of spasticity stabilizes in about 24 months after injury
- Altered thermoregulation
  - —Injury at or above T6 results in an inability to sweat or shiver below injury
- Adynamic ileus
  - —Result of loss of autonomic innervation to gut
  - —NG tube for gastric distention
  - —Resolves in 3 days to a week
- Gastric ulcers
  - —Secondary to stress and steroids
  - —Prophylactic medications to decrease gastric acid
  - —Monitor for bloody or coffee ground vomitus or aspirate; tarry stools
- Orthostatic hypotension
- UTI
- Renal calculi
- Osteoporosis

Nursing Process Elements

Immediate Care

- First priority: immobilize spinal cord: neck securely immobilized and lower spine aligned
- Log roll or lift.
- Ensure a patent airway
- Assess rate and depth of respirations
- Obtain baseline neurological status (see Chapter 9)

Continuing Care

- Maintain effective respiration
  - —Position for ease of respiration—breathing may be easiest in supine position because when sitting, the abdomen protrudes and the flaccid intercostals muscles collapse inward on inspiration decreasing chest capacity; as muscles become spastic over ensuing months, the chest stops collapsing on inspiration. Use of an abdominal binder may facilitate breathing in the sitting position.
  - —Facilitate clearing of secretions: with injuries below T1 this is the major respiratory problem; secretions build up.
    - Guide in use of incentive spirometer every 1–2 hours while awake
    - Thin secretions with humidity and good fluid intake
    - Monitor oxygen saturation and administer supplemental oxygen PRN
    - Turn clients every 2 hours. If spine not yet stable, a specialty bed is used
    - Use assisted cough techniques to promote airway clearance:
      - Manual assist: place hands above umbilicus and below the xiphoid; press strongly inward and upward as the client exhales
      - Mechanical assist—use of a machine, which delivers a deep breath with positive pressure and then applies negative pressure to simulate a cough.

Assessment Alert

A moist, nonproductive cough indicates inadequate airway clearance.

- Chest PT, for example, percussion and postural drainage as ordered.
- Suction clients with tracheostomies PRN

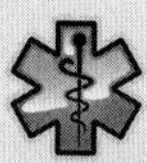

Nursing Intervention Alert

Clients with high cervical injuries can develop bradycardia, which sometimes progresses to asystole when being suctioned or moved. If it occurs during suctioning, manually ventilate and provide supplemental oxygen during the procedure.

- Assess and intervene for autonomic dysreflexia
  - —Close monitoring essential: if hypertension occurs, elevate head of bed to 90 degrees.
  - —If bowel is impacted, manually remove feces.
  - —Respond immediately to autonomic hyperreflexia.
  - —Elevate head of bed to Fowler's position if possible.
  - —Loosen clothing and any constricting equipment, for example, compression stockings or devices.
  - —Monitor BP and pulse every 2–5 minutes.
  - —Check for bladder distention. If catheterized, check for blocks, replace catheter PRN; if not, catheterize stat; instill anesthetic gel before catheterizing as per agency policy.
  - —If condition persists: check for bowel distention. Apply Nupercaine or similar local anesthetic to rectal area; check response; remove stool as needed. If there is no resolution, administer vasodilators such as nifedipine or captopril as per order; assess for sources of irritation; change position; and send a urine specimen for C&S.

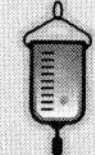

Clinical Alert

Autonomic dysreflexia can result in CVA if untreated.

- DVT prophylaxis for 3 months after injury
  - —Position without pressure behind knee and to prevent edema from gravity to decrease risk of DVT; limit tactile stimulation and change position every 2 hours keeping joints in a functional position to combat spasticity and maintain rehabilitation potential.
  - —Put joints through regular ROM exercise at least four times per day to prevent DVT and prevent contractures from spasticity.
  - —Use compression devices such as stocking or pneumatic sleeves.
  - —Administer anticoagulant prophylaxis as ordered.

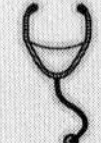

Assessment Alert

Client cannot feel calf pain or tenderness and so warmth, erythema, and edema are the warning signs of DVT. Low-grade fever may also present. Bedside duplex ultrasound can assist in diagnosis.

- Promote effective urinary elimination
  - —Maintain indwelling catheter initially to prevent overdistention of bladder and allow close monitoring of output.
  - —Subsequently implement an individualized bladder management program.
    - Intermittent catheterization (IC)
      - Most common type of management
      - Catheterize every 3–4 hours using aseptic technique (clean technique used when client goes home)
      - Volume of urine at any catheterization should not exceed 400 ml for women or 500 ml for men; if volume is consistently greater then reinsert indwelling

catheter and try IC again later. If it is consistently less than 400–500 ml, gradually lengthen time between IC with goal to stabilize at a 4–6 hour interval. If volume of greater than 400–500 ml occurs at anytime, shorten the length of time between catheterizations.
- Valsalva and Crede (compression of bladder by manually pushing on the lower abdomen) maneuver voiding
  - Initiates voiding when injury is to the UMN but bladder emptying is often incomplete and incontinence results.
- Reflexive voiding
- With lower motor neuron injury, the micturition reflex may be triggered by tapping the suprapubic area, pulling on pubic hair, or stroking the inner thigh. Initially this method is used with IC, when reflexive voiding occurs, residual urine is checked. Once residual drops to less than 100ml then IC may be eliminated.
- Suprapubic catheter if none of the above is effective.

—Monitor for UTI: hematuria, clouding of urine, foul smell, increased sediment, mucus, chills, fever, and autonomic hyperreflexia).

- Institute a bowel program to prevent constipation.

—Determine what client's bowel habits were before injury.

—Set a consistent time for bowel elimination, ideally 30 minutes after a meal to take advantage of the gastrocolic reflex and as close to preinjury pattern as possible.

—Establish a proper balance of fiber and fluids; clients are usually begun with 5–25 g of fiber daily.

—Administer stool softeners or bulk formers as ordered.

—Provide privacy.

—Do a digital rectal examination to check for fecal impaction using anesthetic ointment if injury is at or above T6 to decrease the risk of autonomic hyperreflexia.

—Administer stimulant suppository if ordered; using anesthetic ointment as above.

- Place client in sitting position or, if not possible, left side lying position.
- May apply pressure manually or with a binder to the abdomen to facilitate defecation.
- 20–30 minutes after giving the suppository, may digitally stimulate reflex defecation in clients with UMN injury by moving a gloved, lubricated, finger in circular motion inside the rectum (anesthetic ointment used as above); if LMN injury, no reflex stimulation is possible, so feces is manually removed.

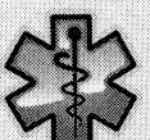

Nursing Intervention Alert

Frequency and consistency of stool is the guide to the development of an effective bowel program.

- Maintain skin integrity

—See pressure ulcers in Chapter 29

—Skin assessment twice daily by self or other

—For clients with SCI, relieve pressure with weight shifts every 15–20 minutes when sitting up.

—Use of a wheel chair pillow.

- Promote effective coping
- Accept and support client through stages of grief.
- Provide information according to what client desires.
- Give client a sense of control by offering choices, involving in care and making as many decisions as possible.
- If client is unable to speak, provide alternate form of communication.
- Set limits as needed.
- Use a nonjudgmental approach.

Client teaching for self-care

- Relationship of injury to sensory motor function
- Expected functional outcomes
- Use/care of stabilization devices
- Respiratory support strategies
- Signs of respiratory infection: fever, cough, sputum change, noisy breathing.
- Bladder care
- Signs of UTI
- ROM
- Moving and positioning techniques
- Skin care regimen
- Sexual function
- Autonomic hyperreflexia
- Coping strategies
- Resources

SPINAL CORD TUMOR

- Spinal cord tumors may be primary or metastatic tumors
- They most commonly occur in the thoracic spine
- Primary tumors are often benign but cause motor or sensory defects because they compress the cord
- Metastatic tumors erode the vertebrae and increase the risk of fracture and spine instability

Etiology: Common sources of metastatic tumors are the lungs, breast, and prostate.

S&S: Mild to severe pain is usually the first symptom; either localized or radicular (along the spinal nerve root path); weakness, sensory and motor loss develop and bladder, bowel, or sexual problems may also occur. The exact symptoms depend on level of lesion.

Dx: MRI

Rx:

- Corticosteroids, usually dexamethasone (Decadron), to decrease edema and, therefore, decrease cord compression; surgical removal of primary tumors; surgery to decompress cord and debulk the tumor for metastatic lesions; radiation for palliation when surgical excision is impossible.
- Immobilization if spine is unstable

Nursing Process Elements

Nursing care varies according to whether tumor is primary or metastatic; the medical treatment plan; and functional deficits.

TRIGEMINAL NEURALGIA

- Trigeminal neuralgia is a disorder affecting one or more branches of the fifth cranial nerve (trigeminal)
- It is chronic with exacerbations and remissions; over time exacerbations become longer and remissions shorter.

Etiology: Unknown but vascular compression of the nerve root, trauma, pressure from a tumor, or dental infection are theorized to contribute.

Risk/precipitating factors: Age and sex—more common in middle aged and older women

S&S: Abrupt onset, unilateral, and paroxysmal pain along the nerve pathway—usually the maxillary and/or mandibular branch of the nerve, lasting from a few seconds to a few minutes. Pain described as intense, piercing, burning; no motor or sensory defects occur. Often a pain trigger can be identified by the client such as a draft of air, brushing teeth, talking, smiling, chewing, or touching the face.

Dx: Based on classic pain pattern and exclusion of other causes

Rx:

- Pharmacological: Anticonvulsant medications such as carbamazepine (Tegretol which inhibits pain impulses)
- Surgery for refractory disease:
  - —Neurodestructive procedures, done through the skin, usually result in almost immediate pain relief but cause partial facial numbness and sometimes loss of innervation to the cornea. Recurrence is common.
  - —Stereotactic radiosurgery (Gamma knife) irradiates trigeminal nerve resulting in pain relief in 4–6 weeks; facial sensation remains intact.
  - —Microvascular decompression involves cutting away the compressing blood vessel by visualizing the nerve by means of a craniotomy

Nursing Process Elements

- Assist client in identifying pain triggers and identifying methods of avoiding or minimizing them
- Assess nutrition because of risk of less than body requirements as a result of pain interfering with eating.

Client teaching for self-care

- Take medications on a strict schedule to maintain optimal blood levels.
- Take analgesics as soon as pain starts to maximize their effectiveness.
- Use relaxation techniques and imagery to aid in pain control.
- Eat small, frequent meals composed of soft, nutritious foods or nutritional supplements chewing on unaffected side to minimize pain and increase caloric intake.
- Monitor weight weekly; report weight loss
- If oral care is painful, use soft swabs, mouthwashes or a water-based system
- Rinse mouth after eating to remove food particles and cleanse breath.
- See dentist every 6 months.

BELLS PALSY

- Bells Palsy is a disorder of cranial nerve VII (facial nerve)
- Most common in men and women aged 20–60
- Recovery is generally complete in a few weeks but may take up to a year

Etiology: Herpes simplex virus

S&S: Rapid weakening of muscles of one side of face sometimes preceded by a feeling of facial stiffness or pain behind the ear, inability to blink or close eyelid, constant tearing, decreased taste, difficulty swallowing. Increased sensitivity to sound on affected side

Dx: History and presentation; a diagnosis of exclusion

Rx: Corticosteroids, antiviral medications

Complications: Corneal abrasions, permanent facial weakness

Nursing Process Elements

- Nursing Intervention Goals: prevent eye injury; prevent aspiration and related respiratory problems
- Ease anxiety by reassuring client that condition is temporary

Client teaching for self-care

- Use artificial tears
- Patch or tape eyelid shut at night and when outdoors.
- Eat and drink only when upright; eat foods with consistency that is easiest to swallow.
- Perform facial exercises as nerve function begins to return to help regain muscle tone.

WORKSHEET

MATCHING QUESTIONS

Match the following:

Column A	Column B
1. ___ concussion	a. tumor of the neural crest cells or adrenal gland
2. ___ cerebrospinal rhinorrhea	b. drug used to decrease cerebral edema
3. ___ beta interferons	c. venous bleeding into space between dura and arachnoid
4. ___ subdural hematoma	d. sign of brain contusion
5. ___ cerebral aneurysm	e. transient, neurologic dysfunction occurring as a result of head injury
6. ___ hemiparesis	f. injury of brain tissue directly underneath the site of trauma
7. ___ tonic seizure	g. drug used for seizures
8. ___ carbamazepine	h. associated with cocaine use
9. ___ coup injury	i. immunomodulators used in treatment of multiple sclerosis

(continued)

10. __ bradykinesia — j. slowness of movement seen in Parkinson's disease

11. __ ipsilateral pupil dilation — k. used in management of Guillain–Barré syndrome

12. __ neuroblastoma — l. surgical procedure used in management of myasthenia gravis

13. __ lorazepam — m. paralysis of half the body

14. __ myoclonic seizure — n. drug used for status epilepticus

15. __ hemiplegia — o. sign of a tear in the dura

16. __ thymectomy — p. weakness on one side of the body

17. __ dexamethasone — q. abnormal sensation

18. __ plasmapheresis — r. brief jerking of a muscle group

19. __ paresthesia — s. impairment of motor or sensory function of lower extremities

20. __ paraplegia — t. rigidity of all muscles

TRUE & FALSE QUESTIONS

Mark each of the following statements True or False. Correct all false statements in the space provided.

1. A major difference between meningitis and encephalitis is that brain function is normal with meningitis and abnormal with encephalitis. ___ T ___ F
2. For clients with meningitis, the room should be kept quiet and lights dimmed to allow for frequent rest periods throughout the day. ___ T ___ F
3. Long term memory loss is an early sign of Alzheimer's disease. ___ T ___ F
4. The priority intervention for a client who has sustained head trauma is immobilization because of the risk that damage to the spinal cord has also occurred. ___ T ___ F
5. One seizure alone does not constitute having a seizure disorder. ___ T ___ F
6. Pallidotomy is performed on selected clients with Parkinson's disease to decrease muscle stiffness and increase mobility. ___ T ___ F
7. A subacute, subdural hematoma becomes symptomatic 24–48 hours after injury. ___ T ___ F
8. Rhinorrhea consisting of clear fluid is suggestive of a tear in the dura in a client with a basilar skull fracture. ___ T ___ F
9. Decadron decreases spinal cord compression by decreasing inflammation and, therefore, decreasing edema. ___ T ___ F

10. It is not possible to differentiate complete from incomplete transection of the spinal cord until the period of spinal shock is over; thus it is impossible to estimate recovery potential until this time. ___ T ___ F

11. Methylprednisolone (Solu-Medrol) when given for SCI cannot be given later than the first 4 hours after injury. ___ T ___ F

12. Clients with SCI must be monitored for tarry stools because of the risk of gastric bleeding. ___ T ___ F

13. Breathing is generally easiest when clients with a recent SCI are in an upright sitting position. ___ T ___ F

14. Bells palsy is a disorder of cranial nerve V. ___ T ___ F

15. A symptom of hydrocephalus in an older child is vomiting without nausea. ___ T ___ F

16. The client with meningitis is best positioned flat with a small pillow. ___ T ___ F

17. A child who has a febrile convulsion is at risk for having a seizure from another type of environmental stimulus at another time. ___ T ___ F

18. Teaching the parents of a child with cerebral palsy how to care for the skin underlying the braces is essential. ___ T ___ F

19. For a client with a fractured skull the bed should be flat or no higher than 30 degrees if ordered. ___ T ___ F

20. Symptoms of postconcussion syndrome include forgetfulness, changes in behavior, and learning problems. ___ T ___ F

FILL IN THE BLANKS

Fill in the blank spaces with the correct word or phrase to complete each statement.

1. The most commonly used test for the diagnosis of meningitis is the ______________.
2. When caring for a client with a subdural hematoma the nurse would monitor neurological status every 2 hours using the ____________.
3. The neurological disorder characterized by progressive ascending sensory and motor defects is ________________.
4. Treatment with tPA must be given within ______ hours of initial symptoms of ischemic stroke.
5. A fracture at the base of the skull is called a ____ fracture.
6. Deep, throbbing, one-sided head pain starting under the orbit of the eye and spreading to the head and neck are symptoms of a ______headache.
7. A decline in fine motor skills is an early symptom of _____.

(continued)

8. In the treatment of a client with myasthenia gravis, the class of drug used when corticosteroids fail is the ______.

9. The tremor characteristic of Parkinson's disease is a ______ tremor.

10. Sleepiness, drowsiness, and sedation are side effects of the _____ used in the treatment of Parkinson's disease.

APPLICATION QUESTIONS

1. A client with Guillain–Barré syndrome has an order for low dose anticoagulation. Which finding best indicates that this treatment is having the desired effect on this client?
   a. Client reports of paresthesias have decreased.
   b. Client's blood pressure is stable.
   c. Client's cerebrospinal fluid is clear.
   d. Client is free of S&S of thromboembolism.

2. Which characteristic must an antibiotic have in order to be used in the treatment of meningitis?
   a. Low protein binding in the bloodstream
   b. Ability to cross the blood–brain barrier
   c. Effectiveness against gram-negative organisms
   d. Resistance to neurotransmitter effects.

3. A client with encephalitis has an order for a diuretic. Which assessment data would provide the best evidence of the drug having its desired effect related to the disease process?
   a. Fever returns to normal.
   b. DTRs are intact.
   c. Seizure activity is absent.
   d. ICP decreases.

4. Which assessment findings would the nurse expect when admitting a client with a diagnosis of bacterial meningitis? Mark all that apply.
   a. High fever
   b. Nausea and vomiting
   c. Stomach cramps
   d. Diarrhea
   e. Nuchal rigidity
   f. Photophobia

5. Which nursing order should be included in the plan of care for a 2-year old with an adrenal neuroblastoma?
   a. Palpate abdomen for increased distention daily.
   b. Weigh all diapers.
   c. Limit fluids to 1000 cc/24 hours.
   d. Provide a high-carbohydrate, low-protein diet.

6. Occurrence of which symptom best differentiates between mild and severe concussion?
   a. Loss of consciousness
   b. Tremor
   c. Unstable gait
   d. Impaired speech

7. A client with a seizure disorder whose disease is well controlled with medication tells the nurse she is trying to get pregnant. Which would be the most appropriate response for the nurse to make?
   a. You should see your neurologist as soon as you get a positive pregnancy test because you may need to discontinue your seizure medications.
   b. Be sure to see your neurologist if you should have a seizure once you are pregnant because you may need increased doses of medication.
   c. You should see your neurologist now because some seizure medications are harmful during pregnancy.
   d. You should see your gynecologist to determine if you can get pregnant because seizure drugs can cause changes in the uterus that prevent pregnancy.

8. A child is admitted to the hospital with symptoms of meningitis and a purpuric rash. Until the diagnosis is confirmed, the child should be:
   a. entertained to prevent boredom.
   b. placed in contact and respiratory isolation
   c. kept in a well-lit room to be observed for cyanosis.
   d. encouraged to drink fluids to counteract dehydration.

9. The nurse in the physician's office completes the nursing history on a 6-month-old infant. Which statement by the mother would make the nurse suspect cerebral palsy?
   a. I've noticed my baby often crosses his eyes.
   b. My baby is on schedule with his development.
   c. My baby often crosses his legs when I pick him up.
   d. When I feed my baby, he often pushes the food back out of his mouth.

10. A newborn has been admitted to the pediatric hospital with a large, high myelomeningocele. The child displays paralysis of the lower extremities. To monitor for a common associated defect, the nurse will
    a. monitor cardiac function.
    b. measure intake and output
    c. do daily head circumferences.
    d. measure abdominal circumferences.

11. When a mother of a child with a viral illness asks the nurse what she should do when her child runs a fever, the nurse would recommend:
    a. placing the child in a bathtub of cold water.
    b. giving the child acetaminophen according to the label directions.
    c. giving the child baby aspirin according to the label directions.
    d. bringing the child to the emergency room if the child's temperature was over 99 °F.

12. When comparing the development of a mentally retarded child to a normal child, the nurse would note
    a. the development patterns will be exactly the same.
    b. the pattern of development for the mentally retarded child is unpredictable.
    c. the development of the mentally retarded child follows the same pattern as the normal child does except at a slower pace.
    d. the normal child develops cephalocaudally, the mentally retarded child develops in the reverse pattern.

13. A child is admitted to the hospital unit after a car accident in which his/her head struck the windshield. The child is alert and oriented. While cleaning up the child's lacerations, the nurse notes serosanguineous drainage from the right ear. The nurse would suspect
    a. ruptured ear drum.
    b. basilar skull fracture.
    c. depressed skull fracture.
    d. linear skull fracture.

14. A newborn is admitted to the pediatric hospital with a meningocele. In which position would the nurse place the infant during the preoperative period?
    a. Prone
    b. Supine
    c. High Fowler's
    d. Semi-Fowler's

15. An infant has had a meningocele repair. After surgery, the mother is at the baby's crib and asks the nurse: "When will my baby start moving his legs?" The nurse's best response would be based on the knowledge that:
    a. damage to the spinal cord is permanent.
    b. no one knows if the baby will regain leg use or not.
    c. it takes several weeks after surgery for the swelling to go down.
    d. the baby will gain movement following the insertion of a shunt for hydrocephalus.

16. Which direction would be included when teaching a client with multiple sclerosis?
    a. Use strict aseptic technique for self-catheterization.
    b. Report slurred speech to the health care provider.
    c. Eat a high-protein, low-fiber diet.
    d. Avoid extremes of heat such as hot tubs or saunas if alone.

17. When caring for a client with an upper motor neuron spinal cord injury, on what basis would the nurse conclude that the period of spinal shock is over?
    a. Client is hemodynamically stable.
    b. Client's spinal reflexes have returned.
    c. Client experiences an episode of autonomic hyperreflexia.
    d. Client sweats above the level of injury.

18. What direction regarding nutrition should the nurse give to a client with trigeminal neuralgia?
    a. Drink large amounts of clear fluids each day.
    b. Eat three meals per day taking an analgesic a half hour before each.
    c. Stick to a full liquid diet until pain is relieved.
    d. Use unaffected side of mouth to manage food and chew.

19. Which assessment findings would be expected in a client with Brown–Séquard syndrome resulting from a stab wound? Mark all that apply.
    a. ipsilateral loss of pain perception
    b. ipsilateral paralysis

(continued)

c. ipsilateral vasomotor loss
d. contralateral loss of position sense
e. contralateral temperature sensation
f. contralateral paralysis

20. Which is a priority concern when planning teaching for a client with Bell's palsy?
a. Exercises to combat facial weakness
b. Precautions to prevent spread to others
c. Eye care to prevent corneal abrasion
d. Nutritional requirements to support healing.

21. For which client would planned reflexive bladder emptying be a possibility?
a. A client with an upper motor neuron injury
b. A client with a lower motor neuron injury
c. A client with Brown–Séquard syndrome
d. A client with anterior cord syndrome

22. What is the first action the nurse should take when a client with a cervical SCI develops hypertension, bradycardia, a throbbing headache, blurred vision and marked diaphoresis above the level of the injury?
a. Notify the physician.
b. Raise the head of the bed to Fowler's position.
c. Check for bladder distention.
d. Remove restrictive clothing.

23. Why is it important to determine the exact time that the S&S developed in a client who presents at the emergency room with a stroke?
a. Diagnostic laboratory values change during the first 8 hours after stroke.
b. The tPA therapy if appropriate, must be given within the first 3 hours after the onset of symptoms.
c. Differentiation between ischemic and hemorrhagic stroke is not possible once 4 hours have elapsed.
d. Size of the lesion cannot be determined for at least 48 hours.

24. Flaccid paralysis would be an expected assessment finding in which client?
a. A client with an upper motor neuron injury
b. A client with a lower motor neuron injury
c. A client with Brown–Séquard syndrome
d. A client with anterior cord syndrome

25. Which nursing order should be part of the plan of care for a client with SCI?
a. Assess skin every morning.
b. Monitor for calf pain.
c. Use a gloved finger to stimulate bowel elimination 30 minutes after arising in the morning.
d. Have client shift weight every 15–20 minutes when sitting up.

ANSWERS & RATIONALES

MATCHING ANSWERS

Column A	Column B
1. _e_ concussion	a. tumor of the neural crest cells or adrenal gland
2. _o_ cerebrospinal rhinorrhea	b. drug used to decrease cerebral edema
3. _i_ Beta interferons	c. venous bleeding into space between dura and arachnoid
4. _c_ subdural hematoma	d. sign of brain contusion
5. _h_ cerebral aneurysm	e. transient, neurologic dysfunction occurring as a result of head injury
6. _p_ hemiparesis	f. injury of brain tissue directly underneath the site of trauma
7. _t_ tonic seizure	g. drug used for seizures
8. _g_ carbamazepine	h. associated with cocaine use

9. __f__ coup injury	i. immunomodulators used in treatment of multiple sclerosis
10. __j__ bradykinesia	j. slowness of movement seen in Parkinson's disease
11. __d__ ipsilateral pupil dilation	k. used in management of guillain–barré syndrome
12. __a__ neuroblastoma	l. surgical procedure used in management of myasthenia gravis
13. __n__ lorazepam	m. paralysis of half the body
14. __r__ myoclonic seizure	n. drug used for status epilepticus
15. __m__ hemiplegia	o. sign of a tear in the dura
16. __l__ thymectomy	p. weakness on one side of the body
17. __b__ Dexamethasone	q. abnormal sensation
18. __k__ plasmapheresis	r. brief jerking of a muscle group
19. __q__ paresthesia	s. impairment of motor or sensory function of lower extremities
20. __s__ paraplegia	t. rigidity of all muscles

TRUE & FALSE ANSWERS

1. A major difference between meningitis and encephalitis is that brain function is normal with meningitis and abnormal with encephalitis. *True*
2. For clients with meningitis, the room should be kept quiet and lights dimmed to allow for frequent rest periods throughout the day. *True*
3. Long term memory loss is an early sign of Alzheimer's disease. *False*
   Short-term memory is an early symptom.
4. The priority intervention for a client who has sustained head trauma is immobilization because of the risk that damage to the spinal cord has also occurred. *True*
5. One seizure alone does not constitute having a seizure disorder. *True*
6. Pallidotomy is performed on selected clients with Parkinson's disease to decrease muscle stiffness and increase mobility. *False.*
   It is performed to decrease tremor.
7. A subacute, subdural hematoma becomes symptomatic 24–48 hours after injury. *False*
   An acute subdural hematoma becomes symptomatic 24–48 hours after injury; a subacute hematoma becomes symptomatic 2 days to 2 weeks after injury.

(continued)

8. Rhinorrhea consisting of clear fluid is suggestive of a tear in the dura in a client with a basilar skull fracture. *True*

9. Decadron decreases spinal cord compression by decreasing inflammation and, therefore, decreasing edema. *True*

10. It is not possible to differentiate complete from incomplete transaction of the spinal cord until the period of spinal shock is over; thus it is impossible to estimate recovery potential until this time. *True*

11. Methylprednisolone (Solu-Medrol) when given for SCI cannot be given later than the first 4 hours after injury. *False*

    It must be given within the first 8 hours after injury.

12. Clients with SCI must be monitored for tarry stools because of the risk of gastric bleeding. *True*

13. Breathing is generally easiest when clients with a recent SCI are in an upright sitting position. *False*

    Breathing is often easiest in the supine position because the flaccid intercostals muscles collapses inward on inspiration thereby decreasing chest capacity.

14. Bell's palsy is a disorder of cranial nerve V. *False.*

    Bell's palsy affects cranial nerve VII, the facial nerve. Trigeminal neuralgia affects cranial nerve V.

15. A symptom of hydrocephalus in an older child is vomiting without nausea. *True*

16. The client with meningitis is best positioned flat with a small pillow. *False*

    The client is best positioned with the head slightly elevated.

17. A child who has a febrile convulsion is at risk for having a seizure from another type of environmental stimulus at another time. *False*

    A child who has a febrile seizure is likely to have another seizure if he/she develops another fever so fevers must be treated promptly. The child is not at greater risk for any other type of seizure.

18. Teaching the parents of a child with cerebral palsy how to care for the skin underlying the braces is essential. *True*

19. For a client with a fractured skull the bed should be flat or no higher than 30 degrees if ordered. *True*

20. Symptoms of postconcussion syndrome include forgetfulness, changes in behavior, and learning problems. *True*

ANSWERS FOR FILL IN THE BLANKS

1. The most commonly used test for the diagnosis of meningitis is the spinal tap.

2. When caring for a client with a subdural hematoma the nurse would monitor neurological status every 2 hours using the Glasgow Coma Scale.

3. The neurological disorder characterized by progressive ascending sensory and motor defects is Guillain–Barré syndrome.

4. Treatment with tPA must be given within 3 hours of initial symptoms of ischemic stroke.

5. A fracture at the base of the skull is called a basilar fracture.

6. Deep, throbbing, one-sided head pain starting under the orbit of the eye and spreading to the head and neck are symptoms of a cluster headache.

7. A decline in fine motor skills is an early symptom of amyotrophic lateral sclerosis.

8. In the treatment of a client with myasthenia gravis, the class of drug used when corticosteroids fail is the immunosuppressants.

9. The tremor characteristic of Parkinson's disease is a resting tremor.

10. Sleepiness, drowsiness, and sedation are side effects of the dopamine agonists used in the treatment of Parkinson's disease.

APPLICATION ANSWERS

1. A client with Guillain–Barré syndrome has an order for low dose anticoagulation. Which finding best indicates that this treatment is having the desired effect on this client?
   a. Client reports of paresthesias have decreased.
   b. Client's blood pressure is stable.
   c. Client's cerebrospinal fluid is clear.
   d. Client is free of S&S of thromboembolism.

Rationale

Correct answer: d.

Clients with Guillain–Barré syndrome receive low dose anticoagulation because of the risk for thromboembolism secondary to immobility. Therefore, the desired effect of the treatment is that the client remains free of thromboembolism. This is indicated by absence of the S&S of the disorder. Anticoagulation is not given for paresthesias or unstable blood pressure, neither does it affect the spinal fluid.

2. Which characteristic must an antibiotic have in order to be used in the treatment of meningitis?
   a. Low protein binding in the bloodstream
   b. Ability to cross the blood–brain barrier
   c. Effectiveness against gram-negative organisms
   d. Resistance to neurotransmitter effects

Rationale

Correct answer: b.

Antibiotics must be able to cross the blood–brain barrier in order to reach the infective organisms. Not all organisms causing meningitis are gram negative and so this is not a characteristic that must apply to all antibiotics used to treat it. Low protein binding in the blood and resistance to neurotransmitter effects are irrelevant to the ability of an antibiotic to combat meningitis.

3. A client with encephalitis has an order for a diuretic. Which assessment data would provide the best evidence of the drug having its desired effect related to the disease process?
   a. Fever returns to normal.
   b. DTRs are intact.
   c. Seizure activity is absent.
   d. ICP decreases.

Rationale

Correct answer: d.

A diuretic such as Osmitrol or Furosemide is prescribed for clients with meningitis to decrease cerebral edema. The best measure of cerebral edema is intracranial pressure (ICP).

4. Which assessment findings would the nurse expect when admitting a client with a diagnosis of bacterial meningitis? Mark all that apply.
   a. High fever
   b. Nausea and vomiting
   c. Stomach cramps
   d. Diarrhea
   e. Nuchal rigidity
   f. Photophobia

Rationale

Correct answer: all.

In addition to the S&S listed, rash, lethargy, irritability, muscular weakness, seizures and decreased level of consciousness, even coma also occurs. In infants a bulging fontanel and high-pitched moaning may also be present.

(continued)

5. Which nursing order should be included in the plan of care for a 2-year old with an adrenal neuroblastoma?
   a. Palpate abdomen for increased distention daily.
   b. Weigh all diapers.
   c. Limit fluids to 1000 cc/24 hours.
   d. Provide a high-carbohydrate, low-protein diet.

Rationale

Correct answer: b.

All diapers should be weighed as part of monitoring output. The abdomen is not palpated when an adrenal tumor is present. Fluids are encouraged not limited. Diet is high calorie and high protein.

6. Occurrence of which symptom best differentiates between mild and severe concussion?
   a. Loss of consciousness
   b. Tremor
   c. Unstable gait
   d. Impaired speech

Rationale

Correct answer: a.

Loss of consciousness does not occur with a mild concussion.

7. A client with a seizure disorder whose disease is well controlled with medication tells the nurse she is trying to get pregnant. Which would be the most appropriate response for the nurse to make?
   a. You should see your neurologist as soon as you get a positive pregnancy test because you may need to discontinue your seizure medications.
   b. Be sure to see your neurologist if you should have a seizure once you are pregnant because you may need increased doses of medication.
   c. You should see your neurologist now because some seizure medications are harmful during pregnancy.
   d. You should see your gynecologist to determine if you can get pregnant because seizure drugs can cause changes in the uterus that prevent pregnancy.

Rationale

Correct answer: c.

Some seizure medications are harmful to the fetus/infant when taken by pregnant or lactating women so the client's neurologist should be consulted prior to her getting pregnant. Pregnancy may require a change in seizure medication but it does not require drug therapy to be discontinued. Seeing a neurologist only if a seizure occurs during pregnancy does not protect the fetus from possible untoward effects of prescribed drugs. Anticonvulsants do not affect the uterus.

8. A child is admitted to the hospital with symptoms of meningitis and a purpuric rash. Until the diagnosis is confirmed, the child should be:
   a. entertained to prevent boredom.
   b. placed in contact and respiratory isolation
   c. kept in a well-lit room to be observed for cyanosis.
   d. encouraged to drink fluids to counteract dehydration.

Rationale

Correct answer: b.

Until meningococcal meningitis has been ruled out, the child should be placed on isolation. Photophobia is a common symptom of meningitis so a well-lit room will add to the discomfort. The child will probably be placed on fluid restrictions to reduce cerebral edema.

9. The nurse in the physician's office completes the nursing history on a 6-month-old infant. Which statement by the mother would make the nurse suspect cerebral palsy?
   a. I've noticed my baby often crosses his eyes.
   b. My baby is on schedule with his development.
   c. My baby often crosses his legs when I pick him up.
   d. When I feed my baby, he often pushes the food back out of his mouth.

Rationale

Correct answer: c.

Children with spastic cerebral palsy often display "scissoring" of the legs. Babies with cerebral palsy are often described as delayed in development. The tongue thrust is a normal feeding mechanism of infancy and pseudostrabismus (cross eyes) is a sign of immaturity.

10. A newborn has been admitted to the pediatric hospital with a large, high myelomeningocele. The child displays paralysis of the lower extremities. To monitor for a common associated defect, the nurse will
    a. monitor cardiac function.
    b. measure intake and output.
    c. do daily head circumferences.
    d. measure abdominal circumferences.

Rationale

Correct answer: c.

A large percentage of infants with myelomeningoceles also develop hydrocephalus. Daily head circumferences may indicate hydrocephalus.

11. When a mother of a child with a viral illness asks the nurse what she should do when her child runs a fever, the nurse would recommend
    a. placing the child in a bathtub of cold water.
    b. giving the child acetaminophen according to the label directions.

c. giving the child baby aspirin according to the label directions.

d. bringing the child to the emergency room if the child's temperature was over 99°F.

Rationale

Correct answer: b.

Never give a child with a viral illness aspirin as it is associated with Reye's syndrome. Cold water would bring the child's temperature down too fast and could cause seizures. A fever of 99°F is not considered serious.

12. When comparing the development of a mentally retarded child to a normal child, the nurse would note:
    a. the development patterns will be exactly the same.
    b. the pattern of development for the mentally retarded child is unpredictable.
    c. the development of the mentally retarded child follows the same pattern as the normal child does except at a slower pace.
    d. the normal child develops cephalocaudally, the mentally retarded child develops in the reverse pattern.

Rationale

Correct answer: c.

The pattern is the same but the mentally retarded child develops at a slower rate.

13. A child is admitted to the hospital unit after a car accident in which his/her head struck the windshield. The child is alert and oriented. While cleaning up the child's lacerations, the nurse notes serosanguineous drainage from the right ear. The nurse would suspect:
    a. ruptured eardrum.
    b. basilar skull fracture.
    c. depressed skull fracture.
    d. linear skull fracture.

Rationale

Correct answer: b.

The bloody drainage could be cerebrospinal fluid, an indication of a basilar skull fracture.

14. A newborn is admitted to the pediatric hospital with a meningocele. In which position would the nurse place the infant during the preoperative period?
    a. Prone
    b. Supine
    c. High Fowler's
    d. Semi-Fowler's

Rationale

Correct answer: a

The child is placed in a position to protect the sac. All other positions would put pressure on the sac.

15. An infant has had a meningocele repair. After surgery, the mother is at the baby's crib and asks the nurse: "When will my baby start moving his legs?" The nurse's best response would be based on the knowledge that:
    a. damage to the spinal cord is permanent.
    b. no one knows if the baby will regain leg use or not.
    c. it takes several weeks after surgery for the swelling to go down.
    d. the baby will gain movement following the insertion of a shunt for hydrocephalus.

Rationale

Correct answer: a.

Damage to the spinal cord that has occurred during the fetal period is permanent. The paralysis will not change because the sac has been removed.

16. Which direction would be included when teaching a client with multiple sclerosis?
    a. Use strict aseptic technique for self-catheterization.
    b. Report slurred speech to the health care provider.
    c. Eat a high-protein, low-fiber diet.
    d. Avoid extremes of heat such as hot tubs or saunas if alone.

Rationale

Correct answer: d.

Client should avoid exposure to extreme heat when alone. Self-catheterization in the home is done using clean, not sterile technique. Slurred speech is a symptom of multiple sclerosis. The diet for a client with MS should be high protein, high fiber. Fiber is needed to facilitate bowel function.

17. When caring for a client with an upper motor neuron spinal cord injury, on what basis would the nurse conclude that the period of spinal shock is over?
    a. Client is hemodynamically stable.
    b. Client's spinal reflexes have returned.
    c. Client experiences an episode of autonomic hyperreflexia.
    d. Client sweats above the level of injury.

Rationale

Correct answer: b.

Resolution of spinal shock is indicated by a return of spinal reflexes. Hemodynamic instability is associated with autonomic hyperreflexia, which is a condition that results from over response of the sympathetic nervous system because below the injury is shut off from inhibitory control of centers in the brain

(continued)

18. What direction regarding nutrition should the nurse give to a client with trigeminal neuralgia?
    a. Drink large amounts of clear fluids each day.
    b. Eat three meals per day taking an analgesic a half hour before each.
    c. Stick to a full liquid diet until pain is relieved.
    d. Use unaffected side of mouth to manage food and chew.

Rationale

Correct answer: d.

The client should be encouraged to eat soft, nutritious foods using the unaffected side of the mouth to hold and move food and chew. Drinking large amounts of clear fluids per day would not be a good suggestion because fluids are hard to manage using only one half of the mouth and clear fluids are not nutrient rich. Since eating can be painful anything the client eats should contribute significantly to meeting nutritional needs. A full liquid diet is not desirable because of the difficulty managing liquids.

19. Which assessment findings would be expected in a client with Brown-Séquard syndrome resulting from a stab wound? Mark all that apply.
    a. ipsilateral loss of pain perception
    b. ipsilateral paralysis
    c. ipsilateral vasomotor loss
    d. contralateral loss of position sense
    e. contralateral temperature sensation
    f. contralateral paralysis

Rationale

Correct answers: b, c, and e.

Paralysis and loss of position sense, and vasomotor control occur on the same side as the lesion (ipsilateral). Loss of pain and temperature sensation is contralateral, that is, it occurs on the side opposite the lesion. This is because the nerve fibers that carry the sensations of pain and temperature immediately cross over and ascend on the other side of the cord.

20. Which is a priority concern when planning teaching for a client with Bell's palsy?
    a. Exercises to combat facial weakness
    b. Precautions to prevent spread to others
    c. Eye care to prevent corneal abrasion
    d. Nutritional requirements to support healing.

Rationale

Correct answer: c.

Inability to blink or close the eye on the affected side creates risk of corneal abrasion. Client is taught to use artificial tears and to wear a patch when outdoors to prevent particles from entering the eye and to prevent drying and exposure to the environment. At night the client is instructed to wear an eye patch or tape the lid shut. Exercises may be done to strengthen facial muscles but preserving eyesight is the priority. Bell's palsy is caused by the Herpes simplex virus, which the majority of people in the population are already exposed to. Nutrition does not play a significant role in treatment of the disease.

21. For which client would planned reflexive bladder emptying be a possibility?
    a. A client with an upper motor neuron injury
    b. A client with a lower motor neuron injury
    c. A client with Brown–Séquard syndrome
    d. A client with anterior cord syndrome

Rationale

Correct answer: a.

Upper motor neuron lesions result in a loss of brain control over the lower motor neurons. Initially an UMN injury causes muscles to be flaccid and hyporeflexic but reflex arcs gradually become reactive resulting in spasticity of the muscles in response to muscle stretch or autonomic or noxious stimuli. With a lower motor neuron injury, impulses from the cord do not reach the peripheral nerves, which innervate muscles. The result is flaccid weakness or paralysis, loss of reflexes, and atrophy of the involved muscle. Brown–Séquard syndrome occurs with a penetrating injury involving half the cord. It involves loss of motor ability, touch, vibration, and pressure sense on side of injury; and loss of pain and temperature sense on the side opposite injury. Anterior cord syndrome is frequently due to damage to the anterior spinal artery or from pressure of a tumor or a herniated disc. It involves loss of strength, pain perception, and temperature perception below the level of injury.

22. What is the first action the nurse should take when a client with a cervical SCI develops hypertension, bradycardia, a throbbing headache, blurred vision and marked diaphoresis above the level of the injury?
    a. Notify the physician.
    b. Raise the head of the bed to Fowler's position.
    c. Check for bladder distention.
    d. Remove restrictive clothing.

Rationale

Correct answer: b.

Hypertension, bradycardia, a throbbing headache, blurred vision, and marked diaphoresis above the level of the injury are S&S of autonomic hyperreflexia, which is a medical emergency. The nurse's first action when autonomic hyperreflexia occurs is to raise the head of the bed to 45 degrees to lower pressure in cranial arteries. The physician is notified because this is a medical emergency. The bladder is checked for distention because this along with bowel distention are the most common causes of autonomic hyperreflexia. Restrictive clothing is removed because autonomic hyperreflexia can be caused by a variety of stimuli which include heat and pain.

23. Why is it important to determine the exact time that the S&S developed in a client who presents at the emergency room with a stroke?
    a. Diagnostic laboratory values change during the first 8 hours after stroke.
    b. The tPA therapy if appropriate, must be given within the first 3 hours after the onset of symptoms.
    c. Differentiation between ischemic and hemorrhagic stroke is not possible once 4 hours have elapsed.
    d. Size of the lesion cannot be determined for at least 48 hours.

Rationale

Correct answer: b.

Ischemic strokes can be treated with "clot buster" drugs such as tPA but treatment must be given within the first 3 hours after symptoms occur. Therefore it is important to determine the exact time of symptoms in order to know if clot buster treatment is possible. CT scans are used to differentiate hemorrhagic from ischemic strokes and to determine the size and location of the lesion.

24. Flaccid paralysis would be an expected assessment finding in which client?
    a. A client with an upper motor neuron injury
    b. A client with a lower motor neuron injury
    c. A client with Brown–Séquard syndrome
    d. A client with anterior cord syndrome

Rationale

Correct answer: b.

With a lower motor neuron injury, impulses from the cord do not reach the peripheral nerves, which innervate muscles. The result is flaccid weakness or paralysis, loss of reflexes, and atrophy of the involved muscle. Upper motor neuron lesions result in a loss of brain control over the lower motor neurons. Initially an UMN injury causes muscles to be flaccid and hyporeflexic but reflex arcs gradually become reactive resulting in spasticity of the muscles in response to muscle stretch or autonomic or noxious stimuli. Brown–Séquard syndrome occurs with a penetrating injury involving half the cord. It involves loss of motor ability, touch, vibration, and pressure sense on side of injury; and loss of pain and temperature sense on the side opposite injury. Anterior cord syndrome is frequently due to damage to the anterior spinal artery or from pressure of a tumor or a herniated disc. It involves loss of strength, pain perception, and temperature perception below the level of injury. Senses of position, vibration, and light touch remain intact. Both of these two syndromes can involve either upper or lower motor neurons and, therefore, can result in either flaccid or spastic paralysis.

25. Which nursing order should be part of the plan of care for a client with SCI?
    a. Assess skin every morning.
    b. Monitor for calf pain.
    c. Use a gloved finger to stimulate bowel elimination 30 minutes after arising in the morning.
    d. Have client shift weight every 15–20 minutes when sitting up.

Rationale

Correct answer: d.

Clients with SCI are at risk for skin breakdown. An important preventative measure is weight shifting every 15–20 minutes when sitting up. Clients' skin should be assessed to ensure early detection and treatment of any skin problems but it must be checked twice a day; once per day is not sufficient. Clients would not be monitored for calf pain because they are unable to feel pain. A gloved finger moved in a circular motion within the rectum may be used to stimulate defecation 20–30 minutes after administration of a suppository to a client with an UMN injury. It is not a routine aspect of care; the finger must be lubricated and an anesthetic ointment applied in accord with agency policy.

Test Plan Category:

Physiological Integrity

Sub-category: Physiological Adaptation—Part 1

Topics: Alterations in Body Systems
Illness Management
Section 5: Eye and Ear Problems

Think Smart/Test Smart

As you review the care of clients with eye and ear disorders, keep in mind that safety is always a particular concern for these clients. Not only does the nurse have to institute safety measures when giving direct care to the client but the nurse also has an important role in teaching about safety measures applicable to daily life. Examples of the latter include teaching clients with loss of peripheral vision to turn the whole head in order to look to the sides and informing clients with a hearing deficit about devices such as fire alarms that use light rather than sound to alert to a problem.

EYE PROBLEMS

CATARACTS

- Cataract is the clouding or opacity of the lens resulting in blurred vision and leading ultimately to the loss of vision.
- It is the leading preventable cause of blindness in United States.

Etiology:

- Senile cataract—associated with aging

- Congenital cataract—present at birth, may be due to maternal exposure to rubella in the first trimester
- Traumatic cataract—resulting from trauma such as a contusion or a penetrating injury
- Secondary cataract—resulting from other eye or systemic diseases such as uveitis, diabetes mellitus, and sarcoidosis
- Also associated with ultraviolet radiation and medications such as phenothiazines, corticosteroids, and certain chemotherapeutic agents

S&S:

- Gradual painless blurring and loss of vision
- Glare at night when driving is often the first symptom
- Improved vision with pupil dilation
- Inability to discriminate hues
- Cloudy white opacity behind pupil

Dx: Direct visualization with an ophthalmoscope

Rx: Monitoring with surgical removal and lens implantation at the point at which cataract interferes with the client's daily activities

Nursing Process Elements

For care of clients having cataract surgery, see Chapter 18. For those not having surgery, recognize that the ability to read, drive, see family members' faces clearly, cook, sew, or to perform any other activities that require clear eyesight may be compromised.

Client teaching for self-care

- Keep eyeglasses or contact lens prescription up-to-date
- Have plenty of lighting in your home—incandescent, not fluorescent—to reduce glare
- Reduce glare by wearing sunglasses outside, having windows with sheer curtains, tinted glass, or adjustable shades
- Explain availability and use of appropriate vision aids such as magnifiers, clear sheets of yellow plastic to reduce glare and make print darker for easier reading, overlays for check writing, large print materials, stove dials with raised markings, telephones that have large buttons with raised numbers, etc. Stress that all aids are not right for everyone

RETINAL DETACHMENT

- Retinal detachment refers to the painless separation of the outer and inner layers of the retina.
- It may be sudden or gradual.

Etiology: Myopic degeneration, trauma, inflammation, and bleeding from a retinal blood vessel.

S&S:

- Floating spots before the eyes
- Flashes of light
- Loss of vision in affected area
- If sudden and extensive, the sensation is of a curtain being lowered over the eye; if the macula involved, blindness results

Dx: Ophthalmoscopic examination shows the tear and its location

Rx:

- If the vision is impaired, surgery is done to reattach retina
- Small areas or holes are sealed with laser or cryopexy (cold)

Nursing Process Elements

See Chapter 18 for perioperative care

After laser therapy

- Ensure that the client has someone to drive him or her home

Client teaching for self-care

- Expect sensitivity to light so wear dark glasses and avoid direct light exposure
- There are no activity restrictions

MACULAR DEGENERATION

Macular degeneration is a chronic, degenerative disease of the aging retina that occurs in neovascular (exudative or wet) and nonneovascular (dry) forms.

- Wet form: In this, a sudden proliferation of new, fragile blood vessels that leak and cause damage occurs in the normally avascular macula; it may result in rapid loss of central vision over days or weeks.
- Dry form: Macular thins or atrophies and functions poorly.

Etiology Unknown:

S&S: Blurred vision, distortion, loss of central vision, and decreased ability to distinguish color

Dx: Missing areas and distorted, wavy lines seen on the Amsler grid; fluorescein angiography confirms neovascularization

Rx:

Dry form: No effective treatment

Wet form: No restoration of vision but additional loss prevented by laser or photodynamic therapy (PDT), which consists of IV verteporfin activated by low-level laser light

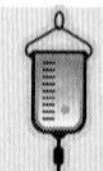

Clinical Alert

Drusen (subretinal hyaline deposits) indicate risk of age-related macular degeneration (AMD); if seen on ophthalmic examination of persons above the age of 55 years. An antioxidant plus zinc supplement is recommended.

Nursing Process Elements

- Assess how change in vision has affected lifestyle
- Explain that vision loss is permanent but total loss is rare
- Refer to state agencies such as Bureau for Vocational Rehabilitation if retraining is needed

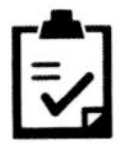

Client teaching for self-care

- Use of Amsler grid to determine progressive visual change: Check each eye daily with glasses on
- Use an object in the living area such as a doorframe or clock to check vision daily
- Report to ophthalmologist if new or enlarged areas of distortion occur
- Maximize vision by using incandescent light, 75–100-watt bulbs with light rays directed at the area to be seen, and other visual aids such as magnifiers, overlays, etc.

GLAUCOMA

- Glaucoma is an eye disorder characterized by an intraocular pressure (IOP) too high for the health of the eye, optic nerve damage, and loss of peripheral vision, which, if untreated, can cause blindness.
- It is controllable but not curable.
- In glaucoma, lost vision cannot be restored.
- There are two major forms of glaucoma: open-angle, which forms 90% of all cases, and angle-closure.

Etiology: Normal IOP which reflects balance between formation and drainage of aqueous humor is 10–21 mm Hg. Cause of elevation to damage-causing levels is most often unknown; can occur as a result of another eye problem and is then called secondary glaucoma.

S&S:

Open-angle

- No early signs and symptoms are seen; slow, progressive peripheral vision loss occurs later
- IOP over 24 mm Hg
- Tunnel vision
- Persistent dull brow pain
- Inability to detect color changes
- Difficulty adjusting to darkness
- Cupping of the optic disc on ophthalmic examination.

Acute angle-closure

- Severe eye pain often with N&V (nausea and vomiting)
- Decreased vision with halos around lights
- Enlarged, fixed pupil
- Erythematous conjunctiva
- IOP severely elevated (may be 50 mm Hg or over)
- Permanent blindness occurs if IOP remains severely elevated for 24–48 hours

Dx: Tonometry to determine IOP, tonography to check resistance in outflow channels, ophthalmoscopy to assess optic disc, perimetry to check visual fields, and gonioscopy to check for abnormalities in the angle (where iris, ciliary body, and cornea meet) of the eye

Rx: The goal is to lower and maintain IOP at a level that does not cause vision loss. First line Rx is with medications to either increase outflow of aqueous humor (prostaglandin agonists) or decrease its production (beta-adrenergic blockers and carbonic anhydrase inhibitors) or both (alpha-adrenergic agonists). If control is not achieved with medications, argon-laser trabeculoplasty or surgical trabeculotomy to create new drainage channels for aqueous humor is done. Medications are usually still needed after surgery to control IOP.

Acute angle-closure is a medical emergency due to potential loss of vision if IOP is not lowered. Management may require IV carbonic anhydrase inhibitors in combination with osmotic agents along with topical beta blockers and miotics. Topical steroids may be given to minimize tissue damage. If due to a nonreversible cause, laser peripheral iridotomy or surgical peripheral iridectomy is done to create a permanent opening between the anterior and posterior chambers of the eye.

Nursing Process Elements

- For care of client having surgery for glaucoma, see Chapter 18
- Assess client's understanding of the disease specifically its chronicity, need for treatment to prevent further loss of vision, and the fact that once vision is lost it cannot be restored

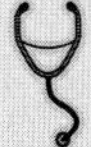

Assessment Alert

If client has been previously diagnosed, determine what medications are used and the frequency of their use; compare with the list of prescribed medications and note differences.

- Approach client from front and not from side
- If approaching from a direction out of line of vision, call out a greeting to avoid startling client

Client teaching for self-care

The client should be taught the following:

- how to administer prescribed eye drops
- importance of adherence to prescribed medication regime for a lifetime if loss of vision is to be avoided
- importance of keeping a reserve bottle of eye drops on hand and of carrying eye drops on one's person when traveling

- need for regular follow-up care to determine effectiveness of treatment
- need to avoid heavy lifting, isometric exercises, straining at stool, and wearing tight collars, all of which can increase IOP
- importance of taking the required safety precautions related to vision changes from medications or the disease: blurring, delayed dark adaptation, and loss of peripheral vision
  —Turn head to look to sides to make up for loss of peripheral vision
  —Remove small objects from frequently traveled paths
  —Have good lighting in all rooms
  —Use night lights
  —Wait for eyes to adjust before walking in dark areas
  —Avoid driving at night

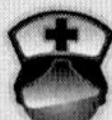

Practice Alert

Persons with a family history of glaucoma should have an eye examination with IOP measurement every 2 years after the age of 40 years.

CONJUNCTIVITIS

Conjunctivitis is the inflammation or infection of the conjunctiva.

Etiology: It may be caused due to allergies, exposure to irritants, bacteria, or viruses.

S&S: Itching, burning, photophobia, foreign-body sensation, tearing or drainage, and hyperemia or redness

Rx: Antibiotic eye drops for bacterial; anti-allergy drops, corticosteroid drops, and vasoconstrictors may be used for allergic; avoidance of irritants and allergens

Nursing Process Elements

- Use cool compresses and refrigerated eye drops to reduce itching and soreness
- Wear sunglasses or a wide-brimmed hat and use window shades to reduce the effects of photophobia
- Do not rub eyes; replace with substitute action such as rubbing chin if necessary
- Avoid perfumed soaps and make up
- Prevent transmission and reoccurence if infective:
  —Avoid touching the infected eye
  —Wash hands before and after doing compresses or instilling medications
  —Use disposable tissues to wipe drainage; dispose of in proper container; wash hands
  —When cleansing face, wash uninfected eye, infected eye; then rinse cloth and continue
  —Keep washcloth and towel separate from those of other people
  —Launder washcloth, towel, and pillowcase separately from others
  —If eye drops are needed in both eyes for another problem, use two bottles—one for each eye, clearly labeled for each

KERATITIS

Keratitis refers to the inflammation or infection of the cornea; it is called corneal ulcer if a microorganism is involved.

Etiology: Exposure or microorganisms (bacteria, viruses, fungi, amoebae); herpes simplex virus 1 is major cause.

S&S:

Exposure keratitis: dry, scratchy, foreign-body sensation; red, swollen conjunctiva; small erosions on lower half of cornea

Microbial keratitis: epiphora, decreased visual acuity, photophobia, iridescent vision, mucopurulent discharge, pain

Rx: Varies with cause.

Exposure keratitis: ocular lubricant, eye patch or soft contact lens if necessary; eyelid sutured shut is final measure

Microbial keratitis: anti-infective drops. Severity of ulcer determines the frequency of administration of ophthalamic drops. Frequency may be as often as every hour. If two drops must be given every hour, one is administered on the hour and the second on the half hour

Nursing Process Elements

- Assess for precipitating events: eye injury, travel, and use of homemade contact lens cleaning solution

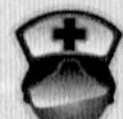

Practice Alert

Prevent exposure keratitis by instilling ocular lubricants at least every 8 hours in susceptible clients; apply eye patch PRN.

- Institute measures to maximize vision, decrease glare, and ease photophobia

EAR PROBLEMS

HEARING LOSS

- Conductive hearing loss: Results from any obstruction to the passage of sound waves through the external ear canal to the bones of the middle ear.
- Sensorineural hearing loss: Sensory hearing loss results from lesions in the cochlea; neural loss results from lesions in the cochlear nerve or higher auditory pathways.

  Symptoms along with deafness can include distortion of sound, unusual difficulty hearing in the presence of background noise, impaired discrimination (can hear people talk but do not know what is being said), difficulty localizing sound, intolerance for even low noises, tinnitus, and vertigo. Sounds of high frequency are affected first.
- Mixed hearing loss: Combination of conductive and sensorineural hearing loss.

Etiology:

Sudden loss (most often from trauma): Risk of sensorineural hearing loss exists with all ear surgeries, head injuries, blast trauma or barotraumas.

Progressive loss: Ototoxic drugs such as aminoglycoside antibiotics, salicylates, quinine, and loop diuretics (e.g., furosemide and ethacrynic acid), exposure to noise, and infections.

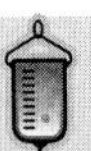

Clinical Alert

All clients with meningitis should have their hearing tested immediately on recovery. Meningitis is one of the most common causes of severe bilateral deafness in infants and children.

Dx:

Tuning fork tests: allow differentiation between conductive and sensorineural hearing loss

- Rinne Test—A sounded tuning fork is held beside the head just in front of the ear and the client is asked to say when the sound is no longer heard. The base of the tuning fork is then placed against the mastoid process. If sound is not heard the client is Rinne-positive, which means that air conduction is better than bone conduction and the client either has normal hearing or a sensorineural hearing loss; if sound is heard, the client is Rinne-negative meaning that bone conduction is better than air conduction and the client has a conductive hearing loss.
- Weber's Test—A sounded tuning fork is placed in the middle of the client's forehead or vertex; the client is asked if the sound is heard, is it louder in one ear, and if so, which one? In case of conductive hearing loss, sound is heard loudest in the ear with the greatest loss while in sensorineural loss, sound is heard loudest in the least affected ear.

Audiometry

- Pure-tone audiometry is an indicator of sensorineural function; it is a part of any hearing assessment particularly if surgery is being considered to improve hearing.
- Speech audiometry is an indicator of the client's ability to discriminate speech; it is important in assessing suitability for surgery and hearing aids.

PROBLEMS OF THE EXTERNAL EAR

Wax Buildup

Etiology: Excessive production or change in consistency.

S&S: Hearing loss which may be sudden is chief; pain and irritation may also occur

Rx: Removal with a curette or by ear irrigation; wax may need to be softened first

Dx: Otoscopic examination

Nursing Process Elements

To irrigate an ear, a stream of fluid is directed up and back along the posterior wall of the external auditory canal so it gets behind the wax or other detriment and washes it back toward the entrance of the canal.

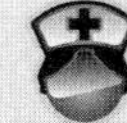

Practice Alert

A stream of water under great pressure aimed directly at the eardrum can perforate it.

Otitis Externa

Otitis externa refers to the inflammation of the skin of the external auditory canal and the surface of the tympanic membrane.

Etiology: Infection either primary or spread form middle ear through a perforated eardrum, eczema, or allergy to eardrops.

Risk factors: Hot, humid climates, moisture in the ear canal, and exposure to irritants which lead to scratching the ear

S&S: Acute: red, swollen meatus weeping freely and very painful; in less acute cases, ear is tender to touch and glands in front of or behind the ear may be enlarged

Rx: Analgesics and local heat application to control pain; steroid drops to control inflammation; antibiotic drops to combat infection; canal may need to cleansed

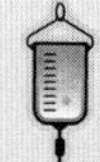

Clinical Alert

Antibiotic drops must be given with great care if a perforation exists because some antibiotics may be ototoxic if they enter the middle ear.

Nursing Process Elements

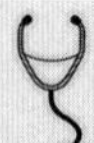

Assessment Alert

Hearing loss is usually not a significant symptom of otitis externa unless it is secondary to middle-ear infection.

Client teaching for self-care

Prevention of external otitis

- Keep ears dry—wear ear plugs when showering, washing hair, or swimming
- Never poke anything in the ears
- Avoid cosmetic products such as hair dyes and sprays, which can cause irritation or itching
- Seek health care at earliest sign of itching or discomfort

Otomycosis

It is a fungal infection of the ear; key characteristic is finding of white to brown or black masses of material like wet paper in the ear. It may occur as a complication of antibiotic treatment of external otitis.

Rx: Cleansing and a local fungicide, e.g., nystatin or clotrimazole for at least 3 weeks

PERFORATED TYMPANIC MEMBRANE

Etiology: Puncture by a foreign object such as a match or a hair pin, blow on the external ear, or compression of air in the external air as from a shotgun blast.

S&S: Pain and discharge. If due to infection, pain is relieved on perforation; if due to trauma, pain occurs at the moment of perforation but does not persist

Rx: "Less is better"—sterile dressing over ear, antibiotic–steroid eardrops if infection likely. Complicated cases may require surgical repair

Nursing Process Elements

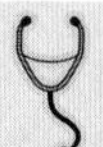

Assessment Alert

Clients with trauma to the ear must be assessed for signs of damage to the facial nerve and for dizziness, nystagmus, and sensorineural hearing loss as any of these indicate the need for surgical exploration of the ear via tympanotomy. If there is recent trauma, consider that clear fluid drainage may be cerebrospinal fluid and be a symptom of a skull fracture.

Client teaching for self-care

- Keep ear canal dry during healing
- Avoid vigorous nose blowing which can disrupt healing
- Contact health care provider if signs of infection such as fever, pain, drainage, or warmth occur

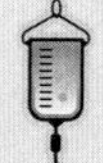

Clinical Alert

Never irrigate an ear when there is the possibility of a perforated tympanic membrane.

PROBLEMS OF THE MIDDLE EAR

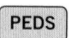

Otitis Media

Acute or chronic infection of the lining of the middle ear, common in children, nearly always preceded by an upper respiratory infection (URI).

Etiology: Infection can spread up into middle ear via the Eustachian tube in which case the tube becomes blocked and air is reabsorbed and replaced with exudates or the infection can spread from the external ear via a perforation of the eardrum. Most commonly due to *Streptococcus pneumoniae* or *H. influenzae*.

S&S:

- Sharp, stabbing pain in ear itself
- Hearing loss with fluid accumulation in the middle ear, discharge and lessening of pain if perforation of the tympanic membrane occurs
- Tinnitus, dizziness, fever, and malaise may also occur
- In infants and young children, discharge from the ear may be the first sign; or fever and acting not well may be present; in all cases, screaming, especially at night, rolling the head on the pillow, or putting the hand up to the ear suggest need for ear examination

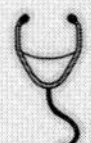

Assessment Alert

Progressive conductive hearing loss is best indicator of progressing otitis media; return of hearing indicates resolving of the infection.

Normal: hear whisper at 8 m

Moderate hearing loss: hear whisper at 2 m

Great hearing loss: whisper can just be heard

Severe hearing loss: conversational voice heard only at 1–2 m

Rx: The goal is return of normal hearing. Analgesics or local heat for pain relief; decongestant nose drops and oral medications, mucolytics, and inhalations to reestablish Eustachian tube function; amoxicillin or other antibiotic if deemed indicated

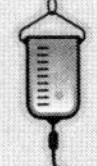

Clinical Alert

Once the middle ear has drained either through perforation or myringotomy, pain should decrease. If pain persists or worsens, it indicates progression of disease and requires intervention.

Chronic Otitis Media

Chronic otitis media can be suppurative or nonsuppurative. Nonsuppurative is known as secretory otitis media, otitis media with effusion or "glue ear"-fluid is in middle ear without acute inflammation—is the most frequent cause of acquired hearing loss in childhood.

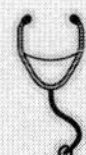

Assessment Alert

Signs of hearing loss vary with child's age: Under the age of 3 years, it may manifest as delayed speech and language development, for example, by 12 months, a child should be able to localize familiar sounds and by the age of 2 years, to understand simple commands and put spoken words together; older children may appear as inattentive and uncooperative.

Rx: Insertion of small plastic tubes through incisions in the eardrums (myringotomy) to ventilate the middle ear and bypass Eustachian tube function; they are not drainage tubes. Tubes are slowly extruded over several months

PROBLEMS OF THE INNER EAR

Otosclerosis

Otosclerosis is the overgrowth of a spongy bone around the oval window and stapes footplate resulting in progressive conductive hearing loss because the resulting fixation prohibits transmission of sound waves to the cochlea. It is often bilateral, is common in young adult females, and shows familial disposition.

S&S: Progressive hearing loss, sometimes tinnitus

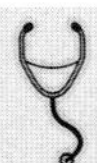

Assessment Alert

Paracusis (ability to hear better in a noisy environment) is characteristic of early otosclerosis. Reason for this is that the client hears background noises less clearly while others hear it well and raise their speaking voices to overcome it. This louder speech without hearing background noise enables the person with otosclerosis to hear better than others.

Rx: Stapedectomy with insertion of a prosthesis to restore mobility of the ossicles (see Chapter 18).

Meniere's Disease

Etiology: Usually idiopathic.

S&S: Recurrent episodes (20 minutes to several hours) of spontaneous rotary vertigo, fluctuating hearing loss, tinnitus, and a feeling of fullness in the ear, often accompanied by nausea, vomiting, and sweating and sometimes loss of consciousness. After acute symptoms subside, balance is poor and client feels unwell for up to 24 hours

Rx: Low-salt diet, betahistine hydrochloride and a mild diuretic given to reduce number and severity of attacks;

vestibular sedative such as prochlorperazine to abort acute attacks. Surgery may be done in refractory cases.

Nursing Process Elements

Help the client identify precipitating events or forewarning of attacks

Client teaching for self-care

- Aim to reduce severity of attacks by taking medication as prescribed when attack starts and lying down on the unaffected side in a quiet, darkened room and avoiding sudden movements and activities including reading
- Try to prevent attacks by avoiding exposure to loud sounds, bright light including sunlight, rapid jerky movements, bending at the waist, or twisting the head, all of which predispose to vertigo
- Encourage avoidance of nicotine, caffeine, and decongestants all of which have a vasoconstrictive effect
- Avoid fatigue and stress
- Use a white-noise machine to mask tinnitus PRN

WORKSHEETS

TRUE & FALSE QUESTIONS

Mark each of the following statements True or False. Correct all false statements in the space provided.

1. The one symptom of a retinal detachment is the sensation of a curtain being pulled down over the eye. ___ T ___ F
2. Tonometry is done to check for abnormalities in the angle of the eye. ___ T ___ F
3. Prostaglandin agonists work to lower IOP by increasing outflow of aqueous humor. ___ T ___ F
4. Following surgery for glaucoma, topical eye medications are no longer required. ___ T ___ F
5. Retinal detachment is a painless event. ___ T ___ F
6. Hearing loss is commonly associated with external-ear infection. ___ T ___ F
7. Progressive hearing loss particularly in young adult females is suggestive of otosclerosis. ___ T ___ F
8. Vertigo due to ear disease is usually accompanied by other signs of ear disease such as hearing loss or tinnitus as opposed to signs of central nervous system dysfunction. ___ T ___ F
9. Signs of hearing loss vary with a child's age. ___ T ___ F
10. Fluid in the middle ear without acute inflammation is the most common cause of acquired hearing loss in childhood. ___ T ___ F

FILL IN THE BLANKS

Fill in the blank spaces with the correct word or phrase to complete each statement.

1. Blindness can result if IOP is elevated to 50 mm Hg or more for ____ to ____ hours.
2. An ear is never irrigated when there is the possibility of __________.
3. Persons with a family history of glaucoma should have IOP measured every 2 years after the age of ____.
4. Antibiotic eardrops must be used carefully and selectively when the eardrum is perforated because some antibiotic drops may be __________ if they enter the middle ear.
5. Wavy lines seen on an Amsler grid are symptomatic of __________.

MATCHING QUESTIONS

Match the following:

1. ____ Acute angle-closure glaucoma	a. Glare at night when driving is often first symptom
2. ____ Meniere's disease	b. Sudden hearing loss
3. ____ Retinal detachment	c. Persistent dull brow pain, slow dark adaptation
4. ____ Otosclerosis	d. Masses of white to brown wet paper-like material in ear
5. ____ Cataracts	e. Sharp, stabbing pain in ear
6. ____ Macular degeneration	f. N&V, enlarged fixed pupil
7. ____ Otitis media	g. Moving spots in front of the eyes
8. ____ Otomycosis	h. Recurrent episodes of vertigo
9. ____ Open-angle glaucoma	i. Paracusis
10. ____ Ear wax buildup	j. Distorted vision with central loss

APPLICATION QUESTIONS

1. Which are the risk factors for infection of the external ear? (Select all that apply.)
   a. Hot, humid environment
   b. Moisture in the ear canal
   c. Upper respiratory infection
   d. Scratching the ear
   e. Change in altitude and air pressure

(continued)

2. How should the nurse interpret persistent pain in a client with a middle-ear infection whose tympanic membrane has ruptured?
   a. Expected since drainage takes 24–48 hours to occur
   b. Expected because of the trauma of the perforation
   c. Disease is progressing since pain should decrease immediately with rupture
   d. Secondary infection has occurred as a result of the break in the membrane

3. Clients with ear trauma must be assessed for which of the following problems? (Select all that apply.)
   a. Facial nerve damage
   b. Sensorineural hearing loss
   c. Dizziness
   d. Nystagmus

4. When assessing the effectiveness of prochlorperazine therapy for a client with Meniere's disease which data is the most important for the nurse to obtain?
   a. the number of attacks per week
   b. the length of time between attacks
   c. the duration of an attack
   d. the perceived severity of an attack

5. Which information would be correct to give to the parents of a child having myringotomy tubes inserted for the treatment of chronic otitis media?
   a. Tubes will come out by themselves in a few months
   b. Small amounts of drainage from the tubes will occur, especially in the morning
   c. Tubes cause periodic discomfort, which is treated with acetaminophen
   d. Prophylactic antibiotics are needed while the tubes are in place

6. Which is the best indicator that an acute middle-ear infection is resolving?
   a. Tinnitus disappears
   b. Drainage thins
   c. Hearing improves
   d. Pain dulls

7. A mother tells the nurse at a Health Fair that her 5-month old has been screaming at night and tossing his head back and forth on the pillow for the last few nights. Which type of examination would the nurse suggest for the infant?
   a. Dental examination
   b. Ear examination
   c. Throat examination
   d. Neurological examination

8. The daughter of an elderly client keeping an appointment for an eye examination asks the nurse how cataracts are diagnosed. Which is an accurate reply?
   a. "Cataracts are seen with an ophthalmoscope."
   b. "Decreased central vision is diagnostic of cataracts."
   c. "Cataracts are visualized using fluorescein dye."
   d. "MRIs of the head are used to make the diagnosis."

9. For which disease would the nurse would plan to evaluate the ability of a client to use an Amsler grid?
   a. Glaucoma
   b. Macular degeneration
   c. Retinal detachment
   d. Uveitis

10. Which finding indicates a risk for AMD?
    a. Decreased visual fields
    b. Sluggish pupillary response to light
    c. Presence of drusen
    d. IOP measurement of 22

11. A client tells the nurse that the eye doctor said the pressure in her right eye was 19 and asks if this is normal. Which is the most appropriate answer?
    a. "19 is within the normal range of 10–21."
    b. "19 is low but not dangerously so."
    c. "19 is borderline high and needs monitoring."
    d. "19 is high and treatment is needed."

12. Which are characteristic assessment findings in a client with acute closed-angle glaucoma? (Select all that apply.)
    a. persistent dull brow pain
    b. inability to detect color changes
    c. severe eye pain
    d. N&V
    e. decreased vision with halos around lights
    f. difficulty adjusting to darkness
    g. enlarged, fixed pupil
    h. erythematous conjunctiva

13. Which is an appropriate answer to a client who asks "When do cataracts get removed"?
    a. "When they reach a diameter of 3 mm or more."
    b. "When they have turned from light gray to milky white in color."
    c. "When they have a distinct capsule around them."
    d. "When they interfere with daily activities."

14. Reports of floating spots before the eyes, flashes of light, and loss of an area of vision as part of the client's description of the reason for seeking health care should be interpreted by the nurse as possible signs of which problem?
    a. acute glaucoma
    b. wet macular degeneration
    c. corneal abrasion
    d. retinal detachment

15. Which statement made by a client with conjunctivitis indicates the need for further teaching?
    a. "I will not touch the affected eye unnecessarily."
    b. "I will instill prescribed eye drops at room temperature."
    c. "I will wash the infected eye after the uninfected eye."
    d. "I will use disposable tissues to wipe drainage from my eye."

16. What advice is appropriate for the nurse to give to a client who complains of problems with tinnitus?
    a. "You can block it with a white noise machine."
    b. "A radio set at low volume will help."
    c. "Wearing ear plugs is a very effective solution."
    d. "Obtaining a hearing aid can help."

17. When caring for a client at risk for exposure keratitis, how often should the nurse plan to instill ophthalmic lubricant drops?
    a. Once a day
    b. Every 12 hours
    c. Every 8 hours
    d. Every 4 hours

18. Which of the following activities should be avoided by a client with Meniere's disease? (Select all that apply.)
    a. Sun bathing
    b. Attending a rock concert
    c. Bending at the knees to pick a spoon off the floor
    d. Turning the body to look to the left
    e. Traveling by plane
    f. Drinking coffee

19. Which measure would the nurse recommend for a client who needs to reduce glare?
    a. Use of fluorescent lighting in the home
    b. Use of 60-watt bulb in a lamp directly aimed at the reading surface
    c. Use of a hand-held magnifier
    d. Use of a yellow plastic overlay for reading

20. After laser therapy for a small retinal tear, the client complains of sensitivity to light. Which is an appropriate response by the nurse?
    a. "This sometimes occurs. If it continues over the next 8 hours you will need to be checked."
    b. "This is normal. Let me review some things you can do to avoid exposure to direct light."
    c. "Apply cool compresses; if you do not have relief in 2 hours, call me back."
    d. "You need to come in right away to check for abnormal swelling in your eye."

ANSWERS & RATIONALES

TRUE & FALSE ANSWERS

Mark each of the following statements True or False. Correct all false statements in the space provided.

1. The one symptom of a retinal detachment is the sensation of a curtain being pulled down over the eye. *False*
   This is the symptom that is experienced if the detachment is sudden and extensive; symptoms of smaller, slower detachments include floating spots before the eyes, flashes of light, and blind spots.

2. Tonometry is done to check for abnormalities in the angle of the eye. *False*
   Tonometry measures intraocular pressure (IOP).

(continued)

3. Prostaglandin agonists work to lower IOP by increasing outflow of aqueous humor. *True*
4. Following surgery for glaucoma, topical eye medications are no longer required. *False*
   In most cases, medication is still needed to keep IOP in a safe range.
5. Retinal detachment is a painless event. *True*
6. Hearing loss is commonly associated with external-ear infection. *False*
   Hearing loss generally occurs with external otitis only if it is secondary to a middle-ear infection.
7. Progressive hearing loss particularly in young adult females is suggestive of otosclerosis. *True*
8. Vertigo due to ear disease is usually accompanied by other signs of ear disease such as hearing loss or tinnitus as opposed to signs of central nervous system dysfunction. *True*
9. Signs of hearing loss vary with a child's age. *True*
10. Fluid in the middle ear without acute inflammation is the most common cause of acquired hearing loss in childhood. *True*

ANSWERS FOR FILL IN THE BLANKS

Fill in the blank spaces with the correct word or phrase to complete each statement.

1. Blindness can result if IOP is elevated to 50 mm Hg or more for 24 to 48 hours.
2. An ear is never irrigated when there is the possibility of tympanic membrane perforation.
3. Persons with a family history of glaucoma should have IOP measured every 2 years after the age of 40.
4. Antibiotic eardrops must be used carefully and selectively when the eardrum is perforated because some antibiotic drops may be ototoxic if they enter the middle ear.
5. Wavy lines seen on an Amsler grid are symptomatic of macular degeneration.

MATCHING ANSWERS

Match the following:

1. f Acute angle-closure glaucoma
2. h Meniere's disease
3. g Retinal detachment
4. i Otosclerosis

a. Glare at night when driving is often first symptom
b. Sudden hearing loss
c. Persistent dull brow pain, slow dark adaptation
d. Masses of white to brown wet paper-like material in ear

5. __a__ Cataracts	e. Sharp, stabbing pain in ear
6. __j__ Macular degeneration	f. N&V, enlarged fixed pupil
7. __e__ Otitis media	g. Moving spots in front of the eyes
8. __d__ Otomycosis	h. Recurrent episodes of vertigo
9. __c__ Open-angle glaucoma	i. Paracusis
10. __b__ Ear wax buildup	j. Distorted vision with central loss

APPLICATION ANSWERS

1. Which are the risk factors for infection of the external ear? (Select all that apply.)
   a. Hot, humid environment
   b. Moisture in the ear canal
   c. Upper respiratory infection
   d. Scratching the ear
   e. Change in altitude and air pressure

Rationale
Correct answers: a, b, and d.
Microorganisms tend to thrive in warm, moist environments and scratching the ear increases the likelihood of breaking the skin and introducing pathogens. URIs and changes in altitude and air pressure affect the middle ear.

2. How should the nurse interpret persistent pain in a client with a middle-ear infection whose tympanic membrane has ruptured?
   a. Expected since drainage takes 24–48 hours to occur
   b. Expected because of the trauma of the perforation
   c. Disease is progressing since pain should decrease immediately with rupture
   d. Secondary infection has occurred as a result of the break in the membrane

Rationale
Correct answer: c.
Rupture should result in immediate relief of pain. Persistent or worsening pain needs to be reported because intervention is required. Drainage can occur as soon as the membrane is perforated. Pain is not experienced from the perforation itself. Secondary infection takes time to develop and therefore persistent pain is not consistent with this occurrence.

3. Clients with ear trauma must be assessed for which of the following problems? (Select all that apply.)
   a. Facial nerve damage
   b. Sensorineural hearing loss
   c. Dizziness
   d. Nystagmus

Rationale
Correct answers: a, b, c, and d.
Because of its location close to the ear, facial nerve damage is a risk when ear trauma occurs. Sensorineural hearing loss can occur due to damage to the cochlear. Dizziness also can result from inner ear damage and nystagmus, which is an involuntary, rapid, rhythmic movement of the eyeball, can result from damage to the labyrinth of inner ear.

4. When assessing the effectiveness of prochlorperazine therapy for a client with Meniere's disease which data is the most important for the nurse to obtain?
   a. the number of attacks per week
   b. the length of time between attacks
   c. the duration of an attack
   d. the perceived severity of an attack

Rationale
Correct answer: c.
Prochlorperazine, a vestibular sedative, is designed to abort acute attacks. It does not reduce the number, frequency, or severity of attacks.

5. Which information would be correct to give to the parents of a child having myringotomy tubes inserted for the treatment of chronic otitis media?
   a. Tubes will remain in place until removed by the physician

(continued)

b. Small amounts of drainage from the tubes will occur, especially in the morning
c. Tubes cause periodic discomfort, which is treated with acetaminophen
d. Prophylactic antibiotics are needed while the tubes are in place

Rationale

Correct answer: a.

Tubes are slowly extruded over a few months. Small amounts of drainage, especially in the morning, are not expected; tubes do not cause discomfort and prophylactic antibiotics are not given.

6. Which is the best indicator that an acute middle-ear infection is resolving?
   a. Tinnitus disappears
   b. Drainage thins
   c. Hearing improves
   d. Pain dulls

Rationale

Correct answer: c.

Progressive hearing loss indicates progressive infection; return of hearing indicates resolution of the infection. Tinnitus may or may not occur with middle-ear infection. Pain is sharp and stabbing—it disappears with perforation of the tympanic membrane or with the resolution of the infection; it does not become dull. Drainage occurs only if the tympanic membrane ruptures.

7. A mother tells the nurse at a Health Fair that her 5-month old has been screaming at night and tossing his head back and forth on the pillow for the last few nights. Which type of examination would the nurse suggest for the infant?
   a. Dental examination
   b. Ear examination
   c. Throat examination
   d. Neurological examination

Rationale

Correct answer: b.

The symptoms described are classic signs of an earache so an ear examination would be the first type of examination suggested.

8. The daughter of an elderly client keeping an appointment for an eye examination asks the nurse how cataracts are diagnosed. Which is an accurate reply?
   a. "Cataracts are seen with an ophthalmoscope."
   b. "Decreased central vision is diagnostic of cataracts."
   c. "Cataracts are visualized using fluorescein dye."
   d. "MRIs of the head are used to make the diagnosis."

Rationale

Correct answer: a.

Cataracts can be directly visualized with an ophthalmoscope. Decreased central vision is the major symptom of macula degeneration. Fluorescein dye is used to detect corneal abrasions when placed on the surface of the eye and when given IV is used to illuminate the blood vessels of the retina.

9. The nurse would plan to evaluate the ability of a client with which disease, to use an Amsler grid?
   a. Glaucoma
   b. Macular degeneration
   c. Retinal detachment
   d. Uveitis

Rationale

Correct answer: b.

The Amsler grid allows areas of blindness and distortion to be identified; it is used by the client with AMD daily to monitor disease progression. The Amsler grid is not used by clients with the other disorders.

10. Which finding indicates a risk for AMD?
   a. Decreased visual fields
   b. Sluggish pupillary response to light
   c. Presence of drusen
   d. IOP measurement of 22

Rationale

Correct answer: c.

Drusen are subretinal hyaline deposits that are risk factors for AMD. Decreased visual fields can occur from a wide variety of problems including visual problems such as retinitis pigmentosa and central nervous system problems such as pituitary adenomas. Sluggish pupillary response to light accompanies a large variety of neuro-ophthalmic disorder and can also be caused by Addison's disease or diabetes mellitus. Increased IOP is associated with glaucoma.

11. A client tells the nurse that the eye doctor said the pressure in her right eye was 19 and asks if this is normal. Which is the most appropriate answer?
   a. "19 is within the normal range of 10–21."
   b. "19 is low but not dangerously so."
   c. "19 is borderline high and needs monitoring."
   d. "19 is high and treatment is needed."

Rationale

Correct answer: a.

IOP normally ranges between 10 and 21.

12. Which are characteristic assessment findings in a client with acute closed-angle glaucoma? (Select all that apply.)
   a. persistent dull brow pain
   b. inability to detect color changes

c. severe eye pain
d. N&V
e. decreased vision with halos around lights
f. difficulty adjusting to darkness
g. enlarged, fixed pupil
h. erythematous conjunctiva

Rationale

Correct answers: c, d, e, g, and h.

Persistent dull brow pain, inability to detect color changes, and difficulty adjusting to darkness are all signs/symptoms of chronic open-angle glaucoma.

13. Which is an appropriate answer to a client who asks "When do cataracts get removed?"
    a. "When they reach a diameter of 3 mm or more."
    b. "When they have turned from light gray to milky white in color."
    c. "When they have a distinct capsule around them."
    d. "When they interfere with daily activities."

Rationale

Correct answer: d.

In the past, it was believed that cataracts had to ripen before they could be removed; current practice is they are removed when the client reports significant interference with daily activities. Size, color, and distinct capsule are all irrelevant.

14. Reports of floating spots before the eyes, flashes of light, and loss of an area of vision as part of the client's description of the reason for seeking health care should be interpreted by the nurse as possible signs of which problem?
    a. acute glaucoma
    b. wet macular degeneration
    c. corneal abrasion
    d. retinal detachment

Rationale

Correct answer: d.

Floating spots before the eyes, flashes of light, and loss of an area of vision are indicative of retinal detachment. With a large detachment, the client may experience a "curtain being pulled" effect on vision. Acute glaucoma is characterized by severe pain and elevated IOP; macular degeneration whether wet or dry is characterized by loss of central vision; corneal abrasion is characterized by tearing, pain, and a foreign-body sensation in the eye.

15. Which statement made by a client with conjunctivitis indicates the need for further teaching?
    a. "I will not touch the affected eye unnecessarily."
    b. "I will instill prescribed eye drops at room temperature."
    c. "I will wash the infected eye after the uninfected eye."
    d. "I will use disposable tissues to wipe drainage from my eye."

Rationale

Correct answer: b.

Eye drops should be cool for comfort. If the client says they will be instilled at room temperature then he or she needs to be instructed to cool them.

16. What advice is appropriate for the nurse to give to a client who complains of problems with tinnitus?
    a. "You can block it with a white noise machine."
    b. "A radio set at low volume will help."
    c. "Wearing ear plugs is a very effective solution."
    d. "Obtaining a hearing aid can help."

Rationale

Correct answer: a.

Tinnitus can be blocked with a white noise machine. A radio or TV will not help; ear plugs will not help since the source of the sound is internal not external; and a hearing aid does not help either.

17. When caring for a client at risk for exposure keratitis, how often should the nurse plan to instill ophthalmic lubricant drops?
    a. Once a day
    b. Every 12 hours
    c. Every 8 hours
    d. Every 4 hours

Rationale

Correct answer: c.

Ophthalmic lubricant drops need to be instilled at least every 8 hours.

18. Which of the following activities should be avoided by a client with Meniere's disease? (Select all that apply.)
    a. Sun bathing
    b. Attending a rock concert
    c. Bending at the knees to pick a spoon off the floor
    d. Turning the body to look to the left
    e. Traveling by plane
    f. Drinking coffee

Rationale

Correct answers: a, b, and f.

Clients with Meniere's disease need to avoid exposure to bright light, loud noise, caffeine, and nicotine. They should also avoid sudden, jerky movements, bending at the waist, and twisty movements of the head.

(continued)

19. Which measure would the nurse recommend for a client who needs to reduce glare?
    a. Use of fluorescent lighting in the home
    b. Use of 60-watt bulb in a lamp directly aimed at the reading surface
    c. Use of a hand-held magnifier
    d. Use of a yellow plastic overlay for reading

Rationale

Correct answer: d.

Fluorescent lights create glare so incandescent are better. Use of a 75–100-watt bulb aimed at what is to be read and/or use of a hand magnifier can facilitate reading but does not affect glare per se.

20. After laser therapy for a small retinal tear, the client complains of sensitivity to light. Which is an appropriate response by the nurse?
    a. "This sometimes occurs. If it continues over the next 8 hours you will need to be checked."
    b. "This is normal. Let me review some things you can do to avoid exposure to direct light."
    c. "Apply cool compresses; if you do not have relief in 2 hours, call me back."
    d. "You need to come in right away to check for abnormal swelling in your eye."

Rationale

Correct answer: b.

There is light sensitivity after laser therapy and sunglasses should be worn and window shades used for comfort.

CHAPTER 24

Test Plan Category:

Physiological Integrity

Sub-category: Physiological Adaptation—Part 1

Topics: Alterations in Body Systems
Illness Management
Section 6: Musculoskeletal Problems

FRACTURES

A fracture is a break in the bone. Types of fractures are:

- Linear—fracture line is parallel to the bone's axis
- Longitudinal—fracture line extends in a longitudinal direction along the bone's axis
- Oblique—fracture line crosses the bone at a 45-degree angle to the bone's axis
- Spiral—fracture line crosses the bone at an oblique angle creating the spiral pattern; typically occurs in long bones

- Transverse—fracture forms a right angle with the bone's axis

Etiology: Trauma; pathological conditions that weaken the bone (osteoporosis, bone tumors, metabolic disease)

S&S:

- Pain and joint tenderness
- Pallor
- Pulse loss distal to fracture
- Deformity
- Swelling
- Discoloration
- Crepitus

Open fractures can present with

- blood loss and
- hypovolemic shock.

Dx: Anteroposterior and lateral X-rays; angiography may be done if vascular compromise is noted.

Rx: Emergent treatment includes splinting above and below the fracture, applying ice or a cold pack, elevating the limb to reduce swelling and pain. Severe fractures may require the application of pressure to stop bleeding and fluid replacement. Following diagnosis, there will be application of a splint, cast, or traction to immobilize the fracture.

Complications:

- Compartment syndrome
- Fat emboli

Nursing Process Elements

- Assess neurovascular status
- Administer analgesics
- Maintain proper body alignment
- Provide pin care, if in skeletal traction
- Reposition frequently if on bed rest due to traction
- Assist with range of motion exercises
- Encourage deep breathing and coughing if on bed rest due to traction
- Monitor for S&S of fat emboli
- Monitor for S&S of compartment syndrome (increased pain in limb, skin color changes, absent pulse, edema distal to injury, pain with passive muscle stretching, sensory changes)
- Encourage fluids to prevent constipation and urinary stasis

Client teaching for self-care

- S&S of impaired circulation to be reported
- Keep cast dry, if appropriate
- Do not insert foreign objects into cast
- Encourage ambulation as permitted

See Chapter 16 for discussion of casts and traction.

Think Smart/Test Smart

Almost all clients with a musculoskeletal problem have some degree of immobility. The immobility may be the result of the disease process itself, a result of the treatment required, or a result of the client's reaction to the symptoms or the treatment i.e., clients limit activity because of discomfort or fear. This means there is a risk of one or more effects of immobility and so preventative measures must be a part of every plan of care. Be sure to recognize that the degree of risk will vary with the client's problem as will the specific risk. For example, a client with rheumatoid arthritis does not have the same risk as a client with paraplegia.

HIP FRACTURE

Fracture of the proximal femur may be intracapsular (within hip joint and capsule), extracapsular, or intertrochanteric (outside the hip joint and capsule to an area approximately 5 cm below the lesser trochanter), and subtrochanteric (below the lesser trochanter).

Etiology: Falls

Risk factors:

- Osteoporosis
- Advanced age
- Female and Caucasian
- Decreased estrogen levels
- Prior hip fractures
- Alzheimer's dementia
- Institutional residence
- Sedentary lifestyle

S&S:

- Severe pain at fracture site
- Inability to move leg
- Shortening and external rotation of leg

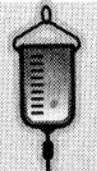

Clinical Alert

Hospital stay of the elderly is often complicated and long with hip fracture being the leading cause of morbidity and mortality.

Dx: X-ray

Rx: Conservative management with traction or surgical repair.

Complications:

- Thromboembolism
- Pneumonia
- Alteration in skin integrity
- Voiding dysfunction

Nursing Process Elements

- Provide pain management
- Perform neurovascular assessment
- Maintain hip precautions (avoid hip flexion beyond 60 degrees, avoid adduction beyond midline, maintain weight bearing status per MD orders)

Client teaching for self-care

- Follow medication regime for pain management, anticoagulants, and/or treatment of osteoporosis
- Practice hip precautions (avoid hip flexion beyond 90 degrees for up to 2 months, avoid adduction past midline for up to 2 months)
- Monitor S&S of complications for thromboembolism, pneumonia, and infection
- Use adaptive or assistive devices
- Restrict weight bearing while ambulating
- Prevent falls
- Have sufficient dietary intake of calcium and vitamin D

SPRAINS

A sprain is a complete or incomplete tear of supporting ligaments surrounding a joint.

Etiology: Sharp twist to the joint

S&S:

- Localized pain
- Swelling
- Ecchymosis
- Decreased use of the joint several hours after injury

Dx: X-rays are performed to rule out fracture

Rx: Immobilize the joint and control pain and swelling

Nursing Process Elements

- Immobilize joint with splint or soft cast
- Administer analgesic or nonsteroidal anti-inflammatory drug
- Apply heat

Client teaching for self-care

- Elevate joint for 48–72 hours
- Apply heat
- Apply ice periodically for the initial 24–48 hours following the injury
- Apply elastic wrapping

DISLOCATION

Dislocation is a displaced joint causing loss of contact of the articulating surfaces.

Etiology: Congenital abnormality, trauma, disease of surrounding joint tissue.

S&S:

- Deformity around joint
- Altered length of the extremity
- Impaired joint mobility
- Point tenderness or extreme pain

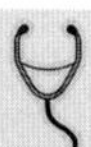

Assessment Alert

Dislocation occurs at the joints of the shoulder, elbow, wrist, digits, hips, knees, ankles, and feet.

Dx: X-ray, client history, and clinical examination

Rx: Reduction of the dislocation should be performed immediately. Closed reduction occurs when manual traction is applied with the client either under local or generalized anesthesia. Open reduction may be required to repair ligaments, use of wire fixation of the joint, or for skeletal traction.

Complications: Tissue damage and vascular impairment if reduction is not done immediately.

Nursing Process Elements

- Apply ice to relieve pain until reduction is attempted
- Splint the extremity as it lies even though angle may be awkward and not normal body alignment
- Keep emergency resuscitation equipment nearby when client receives IV morphine sulfate or diazepam during reduction of dislocation
- Immobilize joint

Client teaching for self-care

S&S of neurovascular compromise (numbness, pain, cyanosis, coldness of extremity)

STRAIN

- A strain is an injury to a muscle or tendon.
- The common sites of strain are the back and hamstring.

Etiology: Twisting or pulling of muscle

S&S:

- Rapid swelling
- Ecchymosis after several days
- Muscle tenderness

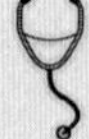

Assessment Alert

A chronic strain will have the client complaining generalized tenderness, stiffness, and soreness of the injured muscle or tendon.

Dx: X-ray to rule out fracture and injury to ligaments.

Rx: Immobilize; control pain and swelling.

Complications: Muscle rupture if strain is severe.

Nursing Process Elements

- Apply ice to relieve pain
- Splint the extremity
- Elevate the limb
- Administer analgesic and/or muscle relaxant as needed

Client teaching for self-care

- Maintain a healthy, well-balanced diet to keep muscles strong.
- Maintain a healthy weight.
- Practice safety measures to help prevent falls (for example, keep stairways, walkways, yards, and driveways free of clutter, and salt or sand icy patches in the winter).
- Do stretching exercises daily.
- Warm up and stretch before participating in any sports or exercise.
- Wear protective equipment when playing.
- Avoid exercising or playing sports when tired or in pain.
- Run on even surfaces.

OSTEOMYELITIS

- Osteomyelitis is an acute or chronic bone infection caused by bacteria
- It can cause tissue necrosis, breakdown of bone structure, and decalcification

Etiology: Combination of trauma and acute infection. Most common organisms are *Staphylococcus aureus* as well as *Streptococcus pyogenes, Pneumococcus, Pseudomonas areuginosa, Escherichia coli,* and *Proteus vulgaris.*

Risk factors:

- Hematoma
- Local site of infection

S&S:

Localized symptoms:

- Sudden pain
- Tenderness
- Heat
- Swelling
- Restricted movement
- Drainage from a sinus tract

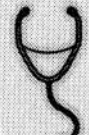

Assessment Alert

PEDS Occurs more commonly in children than adults and most often in boys. In children the most common sites are the upper or lower ends of the tibia, humerus, and radius. In adults the most common locations are the pelvis and vertebrae.

Dx: X-rays, bone scans, CBC, blood cultures, bone lesion aspiration, or biopsy.

Rx: Large dose intravenous penicillinase-resistant penicillin (nafcillin, oxacillin); immobilization of the bone; analgesics; intravenous fluids; local wound care.

Complications:

- Chronic osteomyelitis
- Local spread of infection
- Reduced function of limb or joint
- Amputation

Nursing Process Elements

- Practice strict aseptic technique when doing wound care
- Administer intravenous fluids
- Assess vital signs every 4 hours
- Administer analgesics
- Provide a balanced diet that is high in calcium, vitamin D, and protein
- Provide preventative skin care if client is on bed rest
- Take care of cast and/or traction if the affected bone has been immobilized
- Provide safety measures as needed depending on level of immobility

Client teaching for self-care

- Explain the disease process to both client and family
- Teach medication regime, including side effects and when to contact health care provider
- Educate about management of wound care
- Tell S&S of a recurring infection

OSTEOPOROSIS

Thinning of bone tissue with loss of density over time

Risk factors:

- Insufficient calcium intake or impaired absorption of calcium
- Menopause
- Smoking
- Heavy alcohol consumption
- Amenorrhea
- Use of steroids or anticonvulsants

S&S:

- No symptoms in early stage of disease
- Fractures of vertebrae, wrists, or hips
- Low back pain
- Neck pain
- Bone pain or tenderness
- Loss of height over time
- Stooped posture

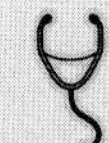

Assessment Alert

Most common in menopausal women

Dx: Bone marrow density testing

Rx: Bisphosphonates, such as alendronate (Fossomax) and risedronate (Actenol); raloxifene (Evista); hormone replacement therapy; calcitonin, such as Miacalcin (nasal spray) and Calcimar (injectable)

Complications:

- Compression fractures of the spine
- Hip and wrist fractures

Nursing Process Elements

- Check skin daily for signs of possible fracture (redness, warmth, and pain)
- Provide a balanced diet high in vitamin D, calcium, and protein
- Administer analgesics as needed
- Apply heat to relieve pain

Client teaching for self-care

- Encourage exercise that includes weight-bearing and resistance
- Diet that includes adequate amounts of calcium (e.g., low-fat milk, yogurt, cheese, tofu, and salmon) and protein
- Supplemental calcium 1200 mg per day
- Supplemental vitamin D 400–800 IU per day
- Smoking cessation

OSTEOARTHRITIS

Degeneration of the joint cartilage and formation of reactive new subchondral bone which causes joint deformity and pain on motion.

Etiology: Cause is unknown

Risk factors:

- Metabolic conditions such as acromegaly
- Injury
- Inflammatory disorders

S&S:

- Gradual and subtle onset of joint pain that is worse after exercise and relieved by rest
- Joint swelling
- Limited movement
- Morning stiffness
- Grating of the joint with motion

Dx: Physical examination, X-ray

Rx: Medications for pain relief and inflammation include aspirin, phenylbutazone, indomethacin, ketorolac, ibuprofen (Motrin, Advil, Nuprin), naproxen (Aleve, Naprosyn, Naprelan, Anaprox) propoxyphene, hydrochloride, rofecoxib, and intra-articular injections of corticosteroids; surgical procedures for clients with disabilities and severe pain include arthroplasty (replacement of a deteriorated joint with a prosthesis), arthrodesis (surgical fusion of bones), and osteotomy (excision of bone to change alignment and relieve stress).

Nursing Process Elements

- Promote adequate rest, particularly following activities
- Encourage client to perform gentle range of motion exercise
- Provide emotional support
- For the hands, apply hot soaks and paraffin dips as ordered
- Check for redness and irritation of the skin, if client is wearing a cervical collar.
- Administer prescribed medications for pain, spasms, and inflammation

Client teaching for self-care

- Maintain proper body alignment to avoid excessive stress on joints
- Install safety devices at home, if appropriate
- Avoid over exertion and plan for adequate rest throughout the day
- Tell about side effects of medications and when to contact health care provider
- Advise weight loss, if appropriate

RHEUMATOID ARTHRITIS

Chronic, systemic disease that causes inflammation of the joints and surrounding tissues

Etiology: Unknown; considered an autoimmune disease

S&S:

- Fatigue
- Morning stiffness lasting more than 1 hour
- Generalized muscle aches
- Loss of appetite
- Weakness
- Joint pain

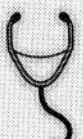

Assessment Alert

Joint destruction starts 1–2 years after the appearance of the disease.

Dx: Joint X-rays; rheumatoid factor test; erythrocyte sedimentation rate; CBC (low hematocrit and platelet count); C-reactive protein; synovial fluid analysis

Rx: Disease-modifying antirheumatic drugs (DMARD): Methotrexate (Rheumatrex), leflunomide (Arava), gold thiomalate (Myochrysine), aurothioglucose (Solganal), auranofin (Ridaura); anti-inflammatory agents: aspirin and nonsteroidal anti-inflammatory agents; COX-2 inhibitors; antimalarial drugs such as hydroxychloroquine (Plaquenil) and sulfasalazine (Azulfidine); tumor necrosis factor (TNF) inhibitors such as etanercept (Enbrel), infliximab (Remicade), and adalimumab (Humira); corticosteroids; immunosuppressive agents such as azathioprine (Imuran), cyclophosphamide (Cytoxan)

Nursing Process Elements

- Administer appropriate medication
- Apply heat to relax muscles and relieve pain
- Apply ice pack during acute episodes
- Provide splints to rest inflamed joints
- Encourage diversionary activities
- Provide range of motion to maintain function of joints

Client teaching for self-care

- Disease process
- Need for 8–10 hours of sleep per night
- Importance of maintaining treatment regime
- Medications, their adverse affects and when to contact health care provider

PEDS JUVENILE RHEUMATOID ARTHRITIS

- Juvenile rheumatoid arthritis (JRA) is a chronic inflammation of the synovium with joint effusion
- JRA is also known as juvenile idiopathic arthritis
- There are three types of JRA
  —Pauciarticular: affects four or fewer joints
  —Polyarticular: affects five or more joints
  —Systemic onset: affects at least one joint but causes inflammation of internal organs as well.

Etiology: Unknown; considered an autoimmune process

S&S:

- Joint pain
- Swollen joint(s)
- Limping
- Stiffness when waking
- Fever
- Rash

Dx: Diagnosis is by exclusion; plain X-rays. Laboratory tests most often performed include complete blood count (CBC), erythrocyte sedimentation, rheumatoid factor, antinuclear antibody (ANA), blood culture, bone marrow examination, and bone scan.

Rx: Nonsteroidal anti-inflammatory drugs (naproxen, ibuprofen, tolmetin), methotrexate, tumor necrosis factor inhibition drugs (etanercept), slow-acting antirheumatic drugs (sulfasalazine, hydroxychloroquine, gold, D-penicillamine); physical therapy

Nursing Process Elements

- Pain management
- Encourage a well-balanced diet
- Promote maintaining a normal life style, such as attending school and getting adequate rest
- Encourage compliance with health care regime (medication, physical therapy, use of assistive devices)

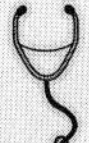

Assessment Alert

Emotional and behavioral function is not linked to the severity of the child's disability but to maternal depression and parental distress over the child's condition.

Client teaching for self-care

- Participate in a support group
- Follow the prescribed therapeutic regime (medication, physical therapy, application of heat)
- Incorporate physical therapy and exercise into favorite play activities

SYSTEMIC LUPUS ERYTHEMATOSUS

- Systemic lupus erythematosus is a chronic, inflammatory autoimmune disorder
- It may affect the skin, joints, and kidneys
- It can be fatal
- Recurring remissions and exacerbations most often occur in Spring and Summer

Etiology: Mechanism is not known; it is speculated that following an infection with an organism that is similar to a particular protein in the body, the protein is at a later date mistaken for the original organism and destroyed by the body's natural defenses.

Risk factors:

- Genetic predisposition
- Stress
- Streptococcal or virus infections
- Exposure to sunlight or ultraviolet light
- Immunizations
- Pregnancy
- Abnormal estrogen metabolism
- Medications, such as procainamide, hydralazine, anticonvulsants, penicillins, sulfa drugs, and oral contraceptives

S&S: The most common are:

- Facial erythema (butterfly rash)
- Nonerosive arthritis
- Photosensitivity

Other symptoms include

- Aching
- Malaise
- Fatigue
- Low-grade or spiking fever
- Chills
- Anorexia
- Weight loss
- Lymph node enlargement
- Abdominal pain
- Nausea and vomiting
- Diarrhea or constipation
- Irregular menstrual periods or amenorrhea
- Discoid rash
- Oral or nasopharyngeal ulcerations
- Pleuritis
- Psychoses
- Patchy alopecia

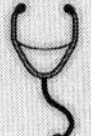

Assessment Alert

Most prevalent among Asians and African-Americans.

Dx: Blood tests for ANA, antideoxyribonucleic and lupus erythematosus cell

Rx: Mild disease requires little to no management. Nonsteroidal anti-inflammatory drugs and aspirin are used to manage arthritis symptoms. Skin lesions are treated topically with corticosteroids as well as with oral antimalarial (hydroxychloroquine) medication. Corticosteroids are the treatment of choice for systemic symptoms.

Complications:

- Infection
- Kidney failure
- Thrombocytopenia
- Hemolytic anemia
- Myocarditis
- Seizures

Nursing Process Elements

- Monitor for bleeding by checking urine, stool, gums, and skin for bruising
- Monitor weight and intake and output
- Monitor vital signs, particularly for hypertension
- Provide a balanced diet
- Apply heat packs to relieve joint pain and stiffness
- Monitor for neurological changes, such as personality change, paranoid or psychotic behavior, ptosis or diplopia

Client teaching for self-care

- Encourage client to get adequate rest
- Perform range of motion and maintain proper body alignment
- Explain the need for prescribed medications and side effects and when to contact health care provider
- For photosensitivity wear protective clothing (long sleeves, hat, slacks, and sunglasses) and sun-screen containing para-aminobenzoic acid

GOUT

Gout is a chronic, systemic, metabolic inflammatory disease.

Etiology:

- Buildup of uric acid in the blood which leads to deposit of urate crystals in joints and soft tissues
- Primary gout due to a genetic error in purine metabolism.

Risk factors:

- Diet high in rich food (e.g., red meat, cream sauces, and red wine)
- Kidneys unable to filter uric acid from blood

S&S: Joint symptoms—base of large toe most often affected

- Swelling
- Pain
- Stiffness
- Redness

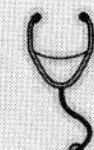

Assessment Alert

Most common in menopausal women

Dx: Synovial fluid contains uric acid crystals, elevated serum uric acid

Rx: NSAID (e.g., naproxen) and indomethacin. Cortisone may be injected into the joint.

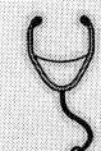

Assessment Alert

There may not be an elevation of uric acid during an acute attack.

Client teaching for self-care

- Dietary restriction for alcohol and foods high in purine (e.g., scallops, sardines, red wine, cream sauces, and sweet breads)
- Increased intake of fluids, such as water
- Pain control
- Rest for affected joints during acute episodes
- Weight control measures if needed

MULTIPLE MYELOMA

- Multiple myeloma is a cancer of the plasma cells in the bone marrow
- It infiltrates the bone to produce osteolytic lesions throughout the skeleton
- The late stages of the disease will have infiltration of internal organs
- Prognosis is poor

Etiology: Cause is unknown

S&S:

- Severe back pain that increases with exercise
- Achiness
- Joint swelling and tenderness
- Fever
- Malaise
- Paresthesia
- Pathologic fractures

Advanced disease symptoms

- Anemia
- Weight loss
- Thoracic deformities
- Height loss

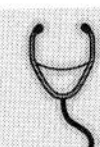

Assessment Alert

Early diagnosis and treatment may prolong life by 3–5 years.

Dx: Bone marrow biopsy, serum protein electrophoresis, bone X-rays, CBC (low hematocrit, RBCs, platelets, and WBCs), serum chemistry profile (high calcium and total protein)

Rx: Goal of treatment is to relieve symptoms, since there is no permanent cure. Chemotherapy and localized radiation therapy. Combinations of chemotherapy include melphalan and prednisone or vincristine, doxorubicin, and dexamethasone. Treatment of hypercalcemia would include hydration, diuretic, corticosteroids, oral phosphate, and IV mithramycin.

Complications:

- Renal failure
- Increased susceptibility to infection
- Paralysis
- Pathological fractures

Nursing Process Elements

- Observe for S&S of infection
- Monitor intake and output (daily output should not be less than 1500 cc)
- Reposition every 2 hours if on bed rest
- Administer analgesics as ordered
- Assist with passive range of motion exercises
- Encourage respiratory hygiene activities, such as deep breathing and coughing
- Provide emotional support for client and family
- Refer to appropriate community resource, such as the Leukemia Society of America

Client teaching for self-care

- Drink 3–4 liters of fluids daily
- Encourage exercise to minimize bone demineralization
- Use of assistive devices when ambulating to prevent falling

OSTEOGENIC SARCOMA

- Osteogenic sarcoma is a malignant bone tumor which occurs during periods of rapid growth in adolescence
- It is also known as osteosarcoma

Etiology: Cause is unknown

Risk factors:

- Family history
- Repeated trauma to an area of long bone
- Exposure to ionizing radiation for the treatment of other cancers
- History of retinoblastoma

S&S:

- Bone pain
- Tenderness, swelling, or redness at site of bone pain
- Pathological fracture
- Limping

Dx: X-ray, CT scan, open biopsy at time of surgery for definitive diagnosis

Rx: Limb-saving surgery, but amputation may be necessary for a permanent cure. Chemotherapy includes high dose methotrexate with leucovorin, doxorubicin (Adriamycin), cisplatin, carboplatin (Paraplatin), cyclophosphamide (Cytoxan), and ifosfamide (Ifex).

Complications:

- Lung metastasis
- Effects of chemotherapy

Nursing Process Elements

- Emotional support
- Referral to a cancer support group
- Administering analgesics
- Postoperative care including monitoring for infection, pain management, neurovascular assessment, monitoring for DVT

Client teaching for self-care

- Use of assistive devices and/or prosthesis
- Compliance with medical regime

EWING'S SARCOMA

- Bone tumor occurring in the marrow of the femur, tibia, ulna, humerus, vertebrae, scapula, ribs, and skull.
- Second most common bone tumor in children and adolescents. Occurs in persons less than 30 years of age.

Etiology:

Primitive neuroectodermal tumor

S&S:

- Pain, initially intermittent and then becomes intense
- Intermittent fever
- Mild anemia
- Leukocytosis
- Increased sedimentation rate

- Increased serum lactic dehydrogenase level
- Weight loss
- Palpable mass that grows rapidly with tense, tender local swelling

Dx: X-ray, CT scan, MRI

Rx: Combination of radiation and combination chemotherapy (vincristine, actinomycin D and cyclophosphamide or ifosfamide, VP-16, and Adriamycin); surgical amputation is only performed when necessary.

Nursing Process Elements

- Skin assessment for signs of reaction to radiation therapy
- Administer chemotherapy agents
- Monitor for S&S of reaction to chemotherapy
- Monitor for S&S of infection
- Encourage food and fluid intake to maintain nutritional health
- Encourage the use of loose clothing during radiation therapy
- Encourage ambulation
- Refer to American Cancer Society for wigs and other devices to maintain a satisfactory body image
- Provide opportunities for child and family to discuss concerns and feelings related to diagnosis and treatment
- Manage pain as appropriate

Client teaching for self-care

- Preparation for diagnostic tests, such as bone marrow aspiration
- Preventative skin care while receiving radiation therapy, such as wearing loose clothing, protecting skin from sunlight, avoiding heating pads or ice packs
- Management of dry and/or moist desquamation of skin from radiation therapy
- Side effects of chemotherapy, such as hair loss, nausea, vomiting, peripheral neuropathy, and cardiotoxicity
- Encouraging a normal lifestyle, including physical activities

INTERVERTEBRAL DISC DISEASE

- Intervertebral disc disease is also known as degenerative disc disease
- It is a degeneration of the spine due to dehydration of the intervertebral disc
- It is a common disorder of the lower spine

Etiology: Aging process results in loss of gelatinous mucoid material of the nucleus pulpous due to loss of water content which is replaced by fibrocartilage.

S&S:

- Low back pain radiating to hips

Dx: Spinal X-ray, myelography, CT scan, and MRI

Rx: Anti-inflammatory medications such as nonsteroidal anti-inflammatory drugs, physical therapy, and spinal injections. Surgery may be beneficial to some clients not receiving adequate pain relief

Complications:

- Bone spurs that can pinch or put pressure on the nearby nerve roots or spinal canal

Nursing Process Elements

- Neurovascular assessment
- Application of corset or back brace

Client teaching for self-care

- Notify health care provider if pain increases or there is loss of sensation to extremities
- Apply corset or back brace
- Reduce weight, if appropriate

HERNIATED NUCLEUS PULPOSUS

- In herniated nucleus pulposus, all or part of the nucleus pulposus leaks out from the intervertebral disc
- It is also known as herniated disc

Etiology: May be the result of trauma, strain, or intervertebral disc degeneration

S&S:

- Severe low back pain radiating to buttocks, legs, and feet
- Increase in pain with Valsalva maneuver, sneezing, coughing, bending

- Possible motor and sensory loss
- Weakness and atrophy of leg muscles

Dx: Straight leg raising test (posterior leg pain without back pain), Lasègue's test (with thigh and knee flexed at a 90-degree angle there is resistance and pain with either absence or decrease of ankle and deep tendon reflexes), CT scan, MRI, and myelography

Rx: Conservative treatment with bed rest, pelvic traction, application of heat; aspirin, corticosteroids, muscle relaxants (diazepam, methocarbamol), and analgesic (hydrocodone with APAP); chemonucleolysis (injection of chymopapain (enzyme) into herniated disc to dissolve nucleus pulposus (an alternative to laminectomy); surgical management such as, microdiskectomy, laminectomy, and/or spinal fusion

Complications:

- Deterioration of neurological status

Nursing Process Elements

- Assess neurological status
- Maintain antiembolism stockings
- Encourage fluids
- Provide skin care
- Administer analgesics and/or muscle relaxants
- Provide emotional support

Client teaching for self-care

- Physical therapy exercises as appropriate
- Proper body mechanics
- Proper weight
- Adverse reactions to medications (analgesics, muscle relaxants)

PEDS SCOLIOSIS

- Scoliosis is a descriptive term referring to the curve of the spine

Risk factors:

Congenital spinal deformities, genetic conditions, neuromuscular disease, cerebral palsy, spina bifida, muscular dystrophy, and tumors.

S&S:

- Shoulders are at different heights
- Head is not centered directly over pelvis
- One hip appears higher than the other
- Sides of rib cage are at different heights
- Uneven waist
- Skin over spine may have dimples, hairy patches, or color changes
- Body leans to one side

Dx: Adam's Forward Test; confirmed by X-ray, CT scan, and MRI

Rx: Nonsurgical treatment includes observation and braces (Boston & Wilmington, Thoracolumbosacral orthosis (TLSO), Milwaukee brace, Charleston nighttime bending brace); surgery

Nursing Process Elements

- Preoperative
  —NPO prior to surgery
  —Instruction on log rolling
- Postoperative
  —Monitor neurovascular status of extremities
  —Pain management
  —Monitor skin integrity
  —Monitor intake and output
  —Perform abdominal assessment

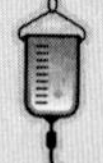

Clinical Alert

Common postoperative complications of spinal fusion include spinal cord injury, hypotension from blood loss, wound infection, and implanted hardware complications.

Client teaching for self-care

- Application of molded plastic brace

PEDS LEGG-CALVÉ-PERTHES DISEASE

Legg-Calvé-Perthes disease is a self-limiting juvenile idiopathic avascular necrosis of the femoral head

Etiology: Lack of blood supply to the bone

Risk factors: Trauma, lupus, kidney and liver disease, sickle cell anemia, and blood clotting disorders

S&S:

- Limping, becomes pronounced with activities
- Pain in hip, the entire thigh, or knee joint
- Limited range of motion

Dx: X-ray, MRI

Rx: Nonsurgical management for up to 4 years using abduction brace, leg cast, leather harness sling, and restricted weight-bearing on affected leg; surgical reconstruction would return the child to normal activities within 4 months

Nursing Process Elements

- Referral for medical evaluation
- Maintaining corrective appliance/device chosen for conservative (nonsurgical) therapy

Client teaching for self-care

- Provide activities to meet creative needs of child while maintaining restrictive activity

PEDS DEVELOPMENTAL DYSPLASIA OF THE HIP

Developmental dysplasia is an abnormal formation of the hip joint resulting in the femoral head not being stable in the acetabulum.

Etiology: Unknown

Risk factors: Familial tendency, crowding of the fetus inside the uterus (large birth weight, oligohydramnios)

S&S: Asymmetrical thigh and buttock skin folds or creases

- Legs may appear a different length
- Hip may have decreased motion
- Toddler or child may walk with a limp or altered gait

Dx: Physical examination, hip ultrasound

Rx: Pavlik harness (soft dynamic brace that maintains the hip in flexion and abduction); Spica cast

Nursing Process Elements

- Teach parents to apply and maintain the reduction device
- Provide cast care, if appropriate
- Monitor skin for alteration in skin integrity

Client teaching for self-care

- Apply reduction device
- Provide activities and/or distraction appropriate to the child's age
- Provide cast care, if appropriate

PEDS SLIPPED FEMORAL CAPITAL EPIPHYSIS (COAX VARA)

- Slipped femoral capital epiphysis is an unusual disorder of the adolescent hip occurring during growth spurts
- The ball of the upper femur slips backward

Etiology: Weakness of the growth plate

Risk factors: Obesity, physical architecture and orientation, pubertal hormone changes, minor fall, or trauma

S&S:

- Hip or knee pain for several weeks
- Intermittent limp
- Unable to bear weight on affected leg, if severe
- Affected leg turned outward
- Affected leg may appear shorter
- Loss of range of motion in affected leg

Dx: X-ray

Rx: Surgical stabilization of femoral head

Nursing Process Elements

- Maintain cast or traction as appropriate
- Provide cast care, if appropriate

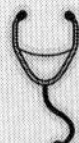

Assessment Alert

Slipped femoral capital epiphysis can be associated with endocrine disorders, renal osteodystrophy, and radiation therapy.

Client teaching for self-care

- Cast care

PEDS OSTEOGENESIS IMPERFECTA

- Osteogenesis imperfecta causes bones to break easily.
- It is the most common osteoporosis syndrome in children.
- There are five types with type I being the least severe.

Etiology: Genetic disorder affecting the body's production of collagen

Risk factors: Hereditary (autosomal dominant)

S&S:

- Bone fragility, deformity, or fracture
- Blue sclera
- Hearing loss
- Dentinogenesis imperfecta (hypoplastic discolored teeth)

Dx: Physical examination, family history, bone density testing, X-ray, skin biopsy for collagen testing

Rx: Supportive therapy to prevent positional contractures/deformities, muscle weakness, osteoporosis, and malalignment of lower extremities.

Nursing Process Elements

- Gently handle the infant with slow movements of the extremities
- Maintain Immobilization of fractures
- Refer to Osteogenesis Imperfecta Foundation

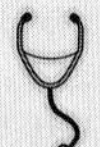

Assessment Alert

Children with new or healing fractures should be screened for osteogenesis imperfecta rather than immediately assuming child abuse.

Client teaching for self-care

- Gentle handling of the infant with slow movements of the extremities, never hold by the ankles when changing diaper
- Recognition of a fracture and how to transport child to emergency room
- Referral for genetic counseling

PEDS TIBIAL TORSION

- It is the twisting of the tibia.
- As the tibia lengthens the unnatural twisting is resolved.

Etiology: In utero development

Risk factors: Genetic

S&S:

- Toes turn inward
- Stumbling or tripping when walking

Dx: Prenatal ultrasonography, assessment at birth

Rx: Surgery will be done if the child is 8–10 years old and has a severe twisting of the tibia causing ambulation problems.

Nursing Process Elements

- Cast care
- Skin assessment

Client teaching for self-care

- Provide cast care
- Encourage normal growth and development activities

PEDS MUSCULAR DYSTROPHY

- Muscular dystrophy (MD) is a group of familial disorders.
- Progressive weakness and degeneration of the skeletal muscles that control movement may lead to disability and deformity.
- This is a general diagnosis for several types of muscle diseases: Duchenne's (most common), Emery–Dreifuss, Becker's, Limb-girdle, Congenital, Facioscapulohumeral, Distal Welander, and Myotonic.
- Children rarely live past 25 years of age.

Etiology: Genetically determined

S&S:

- Progressive muscle wasting, weakness, and eventual loss of function
- Delayed development of basic muscle skills and coordination in children (Duchenne's MD)
- Obesity
- Joint contractures
- Intellectual impairment (occurs in a few of the types of MD)

Dx: Clinical presentation, muscle biopsy, electromyography, and serum muscle enzyme levels

Rx: Treatment varies on the basis of the type of MD

Duchenne's: Physical therapy, orthoses, braces, wheelchair, spinal fusion, release of contractures, and respiratory exercises.

Becker's: Surgical release of contractures, maintain ambulation

Limb-girdle: Physical therapy

Facioscapulohumeral: Physical therapy, orthoses, maintain ambulation and use wheelchair for distances, surgical stabilization of scapula, arthrodesis of scapula to ribs

Myotonic: Aspiration precautions, tube feeding might be needed for decreased esophageal motility, cataract surgery, medication for somnolence

Nursing Process Elements

- Administer steroids and immunosuppressants
- Refer to genetic counseling
- Encourage ambulation
- Provide assistive devices, such as a lift

Client teaching for self-care

- Knowledge of S&S and complications of MD
- Prevention of complications associated with immobility
- Transfer techniques to and from wheel-chair

WORKSHEET

FILL IN THE BLANKS

Fill in the blank space with the correct word or phrase to complete each statement.

1. Describe three hip precautions that should be taught to a client following a total hip replacement.

   A. ______________________________

   B. ______________________________

   C. ______________________________

(continued)

2. List five localized symptoms of osteomyelitis.
   A. ______________________________
   B. ______________________________
   C. ______________________________
   D. ______________________________
   E. ______________________________

3. Identify four risk factors for osteoporosis.
   A. ______________________________
   B. ______________________________
   C. ______________________________
   D. ______________________________

4. Explain the difference between a sprain and a strain of an extremity.
   ____
   ____
   ____

5. Describe limitation of range of motion.
   ____
   ____
   ____

6. Identify three specific diseases or injuries that can result in limitation of range of motion.
   A. ______________________________
   B. ______________________________
   C. ______________________________

7. Describe four nursing interventions to prevent the occurrence of complications related to immobility.
   A. ______________________________
   B. ______________________________
   C. ______________________________
   D. ______________________________

MATCHING QUESTIONS

Match the following.

Problem	**Cause**
1. _____ Sprain	a. Grating joint sounds
2. _____ Dislocation	b. Twisting injury to a muscle
3. _____ Crepitation	c. Tear of a ligament
4. _____ Strain	d. Loss of contact between bony articulating surfaces

Disease Process	Etiology
5. _____ Gout	e. Lack of blood supply to the bones
6. _____ Legg-Calvé-Perthes	f. Develops in utero
7. _____ Lyme Disease	g. Build up of uric acid in the joints
8. _____ Osteogenesis imperfecta	h. *Borrelia burgdorferi* transmitted to humans by ticks
9. _____ Tibial torsion	i. Genetic disorder affecting production of collagen

MATCHING QUESTIONS

Match the following.

Diagnostic Test	Disease Process
1. _____ Elevated serum uric acid	a. Osteosarcoma
2. _____ Adam's forward test	b. Systemic lupus erythematosus
3. _____ Bone marrow biopsy	c. Scoliosis
4. _____ Open biopsy at time of surgery	d. Herniated nucleus pulposus
5. _____ Lasègue's test	e. Gout
6. _____ Antinuclear antibody	f. Multiple myeloma

Match the following.

Type of Fracture	Definition of Fracture
1. _____ Transverse	a. Fracture line crosses bone at a 45-degree angle to bone's axis
2. _____ Longitudinal	b. Fracture forms a right angle with bone's axis
3. _____ Spiral	c. Fracture line is parallel to bone's axis
4. _____ Linear	d. Fracture line crosses bone at an oblique pattern
5. _____ Oblique	e. Fracture line extends along bone's axis

Match the following.

Diagnostic test	Definition
1. _____ Gallium scan	a. Visualization of bone or joint using a radioisotope
2. _____ Arthrogram	b. Removal of fluid from the joint
3. _____ Bone scan	c. Visualization of inflammatory areas using a radioactive medium
4. _____ Arthrocentesis	d. Visualization of the joints using a radiopaque dye

MATCHING QUESTIONS

Match the following.

Immobility Complication	Body System
1. _____ Decreased peristalsis	a. Cardiovascular
2. _____ Decreased hydration of dermis	b. Gastrointestinal
3. _____ Loss of detrusor tone	c. Integument
4. _____ Decreased vital capacity	d. Metabolic
5. _____ Osteoporosis	e. Musculoskeletal
6. _____ Orthostatic hypotension	f. Respiratory
7. _____ Negative nitrogen balance	g. Urinary tract

TRUE & FALSE QUESTIONS

Mark each of the following statements True or False. Correct all False statements in the space provided.

1. Maintaining proper body alignment is an important part of teaching for the client with osteoarthritis because it prevents excessive strain on the joints. ___ T ___ F
2. Ewing's sarcoma is the second most common bone tumor in children. ___ T ___ F
3. A complication of a muscle strain is muscle rupture. ___ T ___ F
4. Joint pain can be the result of injury, arthritis, infection, gout, and medication. ___ T ___ F
5. Trauma and demineralization are the only causes of bone pain. ___ T ___ F
6. Both kidney stones and kidney dysfunction are complications of gout. ___ T ___ F
7. A diagnostic sign of a herniated disc is pain that is relieved by the Valsalva maneuver. ___ T ___ F
8. The importance of 8–10 hours of sleep per night should be stressed to the client with rheumatoid arthritis. ___ T ___ F
9. Aspiration precautions should be included in the plan of care for a child with myotonic muscular dystrophy. ___ T ___ F
10. Care must be taken not to conclude an infant is a victim of child abuse before the possibility of osteogenesis imperfecta has been ruled out. ___ T ___ F
11. Surgery for tibial torsion needs to be scheduled before the infant begins to walk. ___ T ___ F
12. Ewing's sarcoma is a bone cancer of the lower extremities which affects children, teens, and young adults. ___ T ___ F

APPLICATION QUESTIONS

1. Which complaint would be expected when reviewing the health history of a client with rheumatoid arthritis?
   a. Rash over the nose and cheeks
   b. Joint stiffness for 1–2 hours on arising
   c. Reddened edematous joints
   d. Intolerance of vegetable protein

2. Which topic would be included in the teaching plan for a client with gout?
   a. Need to include foods high in purine in the daily diet
   b. Importance of restricting use of alcohol
   c. Necessity of limiting fluid intake
   d. Benefits of decreasing intake of dairy products

3. Which factors are associated with an increased risk of osteoporosis? Mark all that apply.
   a. Menopause
   b. Anticonvulsant medications
   c. Smoking
   d. Obesity
   e. Early menarche
   f. Prolonged use of NSAIDs

4. Which intervention would appropriately be included in the care plan of a client experiencing an acute episode of rheumatoid arthritis?
   a. Guide the client in active exercises for the affected joints twice a day.
   b. Apply ice packs to affected joints.
   c. Maintain affected joints in a hyperextended position.
   d. Assist the client to weight bear on affected joints for at least 15 minutes tid.

5. A complaint of a joint "grating when moved" should be interpreted by the nurse as consistent with which condition?
   a. Rheumatoid arthritis
   b. Osteoarthritis
   c. Osteomyelitis
   d. Osteoporosis

6. Which statement made by a client who has a fractured hip indicates understanding of "hip precautions"?
   a. "I can't fully extend my leg at the hip for 1 month."
   b. "I won't be able to cross my knees for at least 12 weeks."
   c. "I can put weight on the affected leg as long as it doesn't cause pain."
   d. "I can flex my hip but not more than 90 degrees for up to 2 months."

7. Which finding would be expected when assessing a client with a herniated nucleus pulposus?
   a. Anterior leg pain when flexing and extending the knee
   b. Decreased deep tendon reflexes when the leg is rapidly raised and lowered
   c. Relief of low back pain when thigh and knee are flexed at a 90-degree angle
   d. Posterior leg pain without back pain when straight legs are raised

8. Nonsurgical management of Legg-Calvé-Perthes disease involves maintaining the affected leg in which position?
   a. abduction
   b. adduction
   c. flexion
   d. hyperextension

9. Which instructions would the nurse include when teaching self-care to a client with osteoporosis? Mark all that apply.
   a. Stop smoking
   b. Take 1200 mg of supplemental calcium daily
   c. Take 400–800 IU of supplemental vitamin D daily
   d. Do weight bearing and resistance exercises daily
   e. Make certain your diet is not deficient in calcium or protein

10. Which statement made by a client indicates a correct understanding of systemic lupus erythematosus?
    a. Sunlight can help clear skin lesions that develop.
    b. Exacerbations are most likely to occur in the winter and spring.
    c. Pulmonary function tests are needed annually because of frequent lung involvement.
    d. Blood pressure needs monitoring because of the risk of hypertension.

11. Emergent treatment of a simple long bone fracture includes which measure?
    a. Application of heat
    b. Positioning the limb in a dependent position

(continued)

c. Splinting above and below the fracture
d. Application of a pressure bandage

12. A client being treated for intervertebral disc disease calls to report that he has no feeling in his left leg. Which is an appropriate response for the nurse to make?
a. "This is a common symptom of your disease; no treatment is needed."
b. "Most likely it's not a problem but let's schedule an appointment for a checkup when it's convenient for you."
c. "I will tell the doctor and have him call you this afternoon."
d. "You need to be checked; come in right away."

13. Monitoring for signs of a fat embolus is of particular importance when caring for a client with which problem?
a. Degenerative disc disease
b. Systemic lupus erythematosus
c. Osteogenesis imperfecta
d. Femoral fracture

14. Emergent care for a client with a dislocation includes which intervention?
a. Putting the joint through passive range of motion
b. Splinting the joint in the dislocated position
c. Keeping the area warm
d. Providing tactile stimulation distal to the affected joint

15. Which statement made by a client being treated for a badly sprained ankle indicates a need for further explanation of self-care during the first 2 days after injury?
a. "I will keep my foot elevated."
b. "I will apply ice periodically."
c. "I will keep my ankle wrapped in an elastic bandage."
d. "I will bear full weight on my injured leg for no more than 15 minutes at a time."

16. Which goal related to fluid balance for a client with multiple myeloma would be appropriate?
a. Daily output should be at least 1000 ml.
b. Daily output should be at least 1500 ml.
c. Daily intake should not exceed 2000 ml.
d. Daily intake should not exceed 2500 ml.

17. Which client presenting with a limp would be at the greatest risk for osteogenic sarcoma?
a. A 72-year-old man
b. A 46-year-old woman
c. A 16-year-old boy
d. A 7-year-old girl

18. A client presents with a dislocated wrist. The hand on the affected side is cold and blue. How should the nurse interpret these findings?
a. Bleeding into the soft tissues has occurred
b. Neurovascular compromise exists
c. Lymphatic channels are blocked
d. A bone fracture coexists

19. When planning care for a client with a fractured hip, the nurse would plan to monitor for which common complications?
a. Urinary tract infection
b. Pneumonia
c. Candidiasis
d. Herniated nucleus pulposus
e. Thromboembolism

20. Hip precautions would be part of the plan of care for a client with which disorder?
a. Osteogenesis imperfecta
b. Tibial torsion
c. Juvenile rheumatoid arthritis
d. Hip fracture

21. The teaching plan for the parents of an infant with which problem would include the instruction "Never hold by the ankles when changing the diaper"?
a. Muscular dystrophy
b. Osteomyelitis
c. Club foot
d. Osteogenesis imperfecta

22. Which statement made by the relative of a child with muscular dystrophy indicates understanding of at least one aspect of the disease?
a. "I'm relieved that this is a noninherited, developmental defect."
b. "There may be some disability but at least there is a normal life expectancy."
c. "If intellectual impairment was not always a part of the disease, it would be easier to deal with."
d. "It will be very hard watching as the muscle wasting and loss of function occur."

23. Which client has risk factors and/or signs most characteristic of Ewing's sarcoma?
a. A 24-year old with a rapidly growing mass palpable on the tibia
b. A 40-year old with a history of retinoblastoma
c. A 55-year old with severe back pain that increases with exercise
d. A 73-year old with multiple pathological fractures

24. What findings on physical examination of a client brought into Emergency are consistent with a fractured hip?
    a. Lengthening and internal rotation of the affected leg
    b. Lengthening and external rotation of the affected leg
    c. Shortening and internal rotation of the affected leg
    d. Shortening and external rotation of the affected leg
25. When monitoring a client for compartment syndrome, which question should be included in the assessment?
    a. "Does it hurt when you flex the muscle of your arm?"
    b. "Has the pain increased in your arm?"
    c. "Has the swelling increased near your shoulder?"
    d. "Is there a red line going down your arm?"
26. Foods such as scallops, red wine, and gravies should be restricted in the diet of clients with which disease?
    a. Rheumatoid arthritis
    b. Systemic lupus erythematosus
    c. Gout
    d. Muscular dystrophy

ANSWERS & RATIONALES

ANSWERS FOR FILL IN THE BLANKS

1. Describe three hip precautions that should be taught to a client following a total hip replacement.
   A. ____________________
   B. ____________________
   C. ____________________
   Answers may include: Do not cross legs, do not adduct operative leg beyond midline of body, avoid flexing hips more than 90 degrees when rising from chair or bed, avoid turning affected leg inward, use high seated chairs, use raised toilet seat, do not flex hip to put on clothing.
2. List five localized symptoms of osteomyelitis.
   A. ____________________
   B. ____________________
   C. ____________________
   D. ____________________
   E. ____________________
   Answers may include: Sudden pain, tenderness, heat, swelling, restricted movement or drainage from a sinus tract.
3. Identify four risk factors for osteoporosis.
   A. ____________________
   B. ____________________
   C. ____________________
   D. ____________________
   Answers may include: Insufficient calcium intake, menopause, smoking, heavy alcohol consumption, amenorrhea, use of steroids, and use of anticonvulsants.
4. Explain the difference between a sprain and a strain of an extremity.
   ____
   ____
   ____
   Answer: A sprain can be either a complete or incomplete tear of supporting ligaments surrounding a joint. A strain is an injury to a muscle or tendon.

(continued)

5. Describe limitation of range of motion.
____
____
____
Answer: There is a decrease in the normal distance and direction through which a joint can move.

6. Identify three specific diseases or injuries that can result in limitation of range of motion.
A. ______________________________
B. ______________________________
C. ______________________________
Answers may include arthritis, cerebral palsy, dislocation, fracture, or spondylosis.

7. Describe four nursing interventions to prevent the occurrence of complications related to immobility.
A. ______________________________
B. ______________________________
C. ______________________________
D. ______________________________
Answers may include: Range of motion, monitor for dehydration, monitor serum electrolytes (sodium, potassium, chloride, calcium), assess for DVT, apply compressive stockings (TEDS) or device (SCD), encourage deep breathing and use of incentive spirometry, administer calcium and phosphorous supplements, monitor for infection, monitor bowel function, administer stool softener, encourage foods high in fiber, assess vulnerable body surfaces for changes in skin integrity, reposition at least every 2 hours, provide a pressure relief surface that is appropriate for client.

MATCHING ANSWERS

Problem	Cause
1. __c__ Sprain	a. Grating joint sounds
2. __d__ Dislocation	b. Twisting injury to a muscle
3. __a__ Crepitation	c. Tear of a ligament
4. __b__ Strain	d. Loss of contact between bony articulating surfaces
Disease Process	**Etiology**
5. __g__ Gout	e. Lack of blood supply to the bones
6. __e__ Legg-Calvé-Perthes	f. Develops during utero
7. __h__ Lyme Disease	g. Build up of uric acid in the joints
8. __i__ Osteogenesis imperfecta	h. *Borrelia burgdorferi* transmitted to humans by ticks
9. __f__ Tibial torsion	i. Genetic disorder affecting production of collagen

MATCHING ANSWERS

Diagnostic Test	Disease Process
1. _e_ Elevated serum uric acid	a. Osteosarcoma
2. _c_ Adam's Forward Test	b. Systemic lupus erythematosus
3. _f_ Bone marrow biopsy	c. Scoliosis
4. _a_ Open biopsy at time of surgery	d. Herniated nucleus pulposus
5. _d_ LeSegue's Test	e. Gout
6. _b_ Antinuclear antibody	f. Multiple Myeloma

Type of Fracture	Definition of Fracture
1. _b_ Transverse	a. Fracture line crosses bone at a 45-degree angle to bone's axis
2. _e_ Longitudinal	b. Fracture forms a right angle with bone's axis
3. _d_ Spiral	c. Fracture line is parallel to bone's axis
4. _c_ Linear	d. Fracture line crosses bone at an oblique pattern
5. _a_ Oblique	e. Fracture line extends along bone's axis

Diagnostic test	Definition
1. _c_ Gallium scan	a. Visualization of bone or joint using a radioisotope
2. _d_ Arthrogram	b. Removal of fluid from the joint
3. _a_ Bone scan	c. Visualization of inflammatory areas using a radioactive medium
4. _b_ Arthrocentesis	d. Visualization of the joints using a radiopaque dye

MATCHING ANSWERS

Immobility Complication	Body System
1. __b__ Decreased peristalsis	a. Cardiovascular
2. __c__ Decreased hydration of dermis	b. Gastrointestinal
3. __g__ Loss of detrusor tone	c. Integument
4. __f__ Decreased vital capacity	d. Metabolic
5. __e__ Osteoporosis	e. Musculoskeletal
6. __a__ Orthostatic hypotension	f. Respiratory
7. __d__ Negative nitrogen balance	g. Urinary Tract

TRUE & FALSE ANSWERS

1. Maintaining proper body alignment is an important part of teaching for the client with osteoarthritis because it prevents excessive strain on the joints. *True*
2. Ewings sarcoma is the second most common bone tumor in children. *True*
3. A complication of a muscle strain is muscle rupture. *True*
4. Joint pain can be the result of injury, arthritis, infection, gout, and medication. *False*
   Medication is not a cause of to joint pain.
5. Trauma and demineralization are the only causes of bone pain. *False*
   Bone pain has many etiologies, which include trauma, demineralization, overuse, infection, malignancy, disruption of blood supply and leukemia.
6. Both kidney stones and kidney dysfunction are complications of gout. *True*
7. A diagnostic sign of a herniated disc is pain that is relieved by the Valsalva maneuver. *False*
   With a herniated disc, pain increases with the Valsalva maneuver, coughing, sneezing, or bending.
8. The importance of 8-10 hours of sleep per night should be stressed to the client with rheumatoid arthritis. *True*
9. Aspiration precautions should be included in the plan of care for a child with myotonic muscular dystrophy *True*
10. Care must be taken not to conclude an infant is a victim of child abuse before the possibility of osteogenesis imperfecta has been ruled out. *True*
11. Surgery for tibial torsion needs to be scheduled before the infant begins to walk. *False*
    Surgery for tibial torsion is done between 8 and 10 years of age if twisting is severe and creates problems with ambulation.
12. Ewing's sarcoma is a bone cancer of the lower extremities which affects children, teens and young adults. *False*
    Ewing's sarcoma effects persons under age 30 but can occur in the marrow of the femur, tibia, ulna, humerus, vertebrae, scapula, ribs, or skull.

APPLICATION ANSWERS

1. Which complaint would be expected when reviewing the health history of a client with rheumatoid arthritis?
   a. Rash over the nose and cheeks
   b. Joint stiffness for 1–2 hours on arising
   c. Reddened edematous joints
   d. Intolerance of vegetable protein

Rationale
Correct answer: b.
Joint stiffness for more than 1 hour on arising in the morning is characteristic of rheumatoid arthritis. Rash over the nose and cheeks is a symptom of systemic lupus erythematous. Reddened erythematosus joints are signs of gout. Intolerance to vegetable program is unrelated to a musculoskeletal disorder.

2. Which topic would be included in the teaching plan for a client with gout?
   a. Need to include foods high in purine in the daily diet
   b. Importance of restricting use of alcohol
   c. Necessity of limiting fluid intake
   d. Benefits of decreasing intake of dairy products

Rationale
Correct answer: b.
Alcohol restriction is an essential treatment measure for clients with gout. Clients with gout need to limit intake of high purine foods, not to increase it; and increase fluid intake to aid renal filtration of uric acid from the blood. Dairy products do not have to be decreased.

3. Which factors are associated with an increased risk of osteoporosis? Mark all that apply.
   a. Menopause
   b. Anticonvulsant medications
   c. Smoking
   d. Obesity
   e. Early menarche
   f. Prolonged use of NSAIDs

Rationale
Correct answers: a, b, and c.
Menopause, anticonvulsant medications and smoking are all associated with an increased risk for osteoporosis. Obesity, early menarche and prolonged use of NSAIDs are not known to be related to the development of osteoporosis.

4. Which intervention would appropriately be included in the care plan of a client experiencing an acute episode of rheumatoid arthritis?
   a. Guide the client in active exercises for the affected joints twice a day.
   b. Apply ice packs to affected joints.
   c. Maintain affected joints in a hyperextended position.
   d. Assist the client to weight bear on affected joints for at least 15 minutes tid.

Rationale
Correct answer: b.
Ice helps reduce inflammation and relieve pain during acute episodes; heat is used to relax muscles and relieve pain at other times. During acute episodes affected joints are splinted for rest; they are not exercised; used to bear weight; nor placed in a hyperextended position.

5. A complaint of a joint "grating when moved" should be interpreted by the nurse as consistent with which condition?
   a. Rheumatoid arthritis
   b. Osteoarthritis
   c. Osteomyelitis
   d. Osteoporosis

Rationale
Correct answer: b.
A major symptom of osteoarthritis is grating of the affected joint with motion. Joint pain and morning stiffness are characteristic of rheumatoid arthritis. Restricted movement is a sign of osteomyelitis. Bone pain or tenderness are characteristic of osteoporosis.

6. Which statement made by a client who has a fractured hip indicates understanding of "hip precautions"?
   a. "I can't fully extend my leg at the hip for 1 month."
   b. "I won't be able to cross my knees for at least 12 weeks."
   c. "I can put weight on the affected leg as long as it doesn't cause pain."
   d. "I can flex my hip but not more than 90 degrees for up to 2 months."

Rationale
Correct answer: d.
Hip flexion of more than 90 degrees must be avoided for up to 2 months. Adduction past the midline must be avoided for up to 2 months so the knees cannot be crossed for 2 months. Weight bearing is restricted and doctor's orders regarding extent of restriction need to be followed. There is no restriction on extending the leg.

7. Which finding would be expected when assessing a client with a herniated nucleus pulposus?
   a. Anterior leg pain when flexing and extending the knee

(continued)

b. Decreased deep tendon reflexes when the leg is rapidly raised and lowered.
c. Relief of low back pain when thigh and knee are flexed at a 90-degree angle
d. Posterior leg pain without back pain when straight legs are raised

Rationale

Correct answer: d.

A positive straight leg raising test (posterior leg pain without back pain) is diagnostic of herniated nucleus pulposus.

A positive Lasègue's test (with thigh and knee flexed at a 90-degree angle, there is resistance and pain with ankle and DTRs either decreased or absent) is also indicative of herniated nucleus pulposus.

8. Nonsurgical management of Legg-Calvé-Perthes disease involves maintaining the affected leg in which position?
   a. abduction
   b. adduction
   c. flexion
   d. hyperextension

Rationale

Correct answer: a.

An abduction brace or leg cast can be used.

9. Which instructions would the nurse include when teaching self-care to a client with osteoporosis? Mark all that apply.
   a. Stop smoking.
   b. Take 1200 mg of supplemental calcium daily.
   c. Take 400–800 IU of supplemental vitamin D daily
   d. Do weight bearing and resistance exercises daily
   e. Make certain your diet is not deficient in calcium or protein

Rationale

Correct answer: All of the above.

10. Which statement made by a client indicates a correct understanding of systemic lupus erythematosus?
   a. Sunlight can help clear skin lesions that develop.
   b. Exacerbations are most likely to occur in the winter and spring.
   c. Pulmonary function tests are needed annually because of frequent lung involvement.
   d. Blood pressure needs monitoring because of the risk of hypertension.

Rationale

Correct answer: d.

There is a risk of hypertension with lupus erythematosus so blood pressure monitoring is needed. Sunlight can exacerbate the disease not help clear skin lesions. Exacerbations occur most often in the spring or summer.

Pleuritis can be a symptom of the disease but monitoring with annual pulmonary function tests is not part of the medical routine.

11. Emergent treatment of a simple long bone fracture includes which measure?
   a. Application of heat
   b. Positioning the limb in a dependent position.
   c. Splinting above and below the fracture
   d. Application of a pressure bandage

Rationale

Correct answer: c.

Above and below the fracture is stabilized to prevent movement of the bone segments and further damage. Cold not heat is applied immediately and the limb is elevated not lowered. A pressure bandage would not be used for a simple fracture.

12. A client being treated for intervertebral disc disease calls to report that he has no feeling in his left leg. Which is an appropriate response for the nurse to make?
   a. "This is a common symptom of your disease; no treatment is needed."
   b. "Most likely it's not a problem but let's schedule an appointment for a checkup when it's convenient for you."
   c. "I will tell the doctor and have him call you this afternoon."
   d. "You need to be checked; come in right away."

Rationale

Correct answer: d.

Loss of sensation indicates pressure on a nerve and it needs to be treated immediately to prevent permanent damage.

13. Monitoring for signs of a fat embolus is of particular importance when caring for a client with which problem?
   a. Degenerative disc disease
   b. Systemic lupus erythematosus
   c. Osteogenesis imperfecta
   d. Femoral fracture

Rationale

Correct answer: d.

Fat embolism is a risk associated with a break in a long bone. Degenerative disc disease places the client at risk for compression damage to nerves; risks associated with SLE include infection, kidney failure, myocarditis, seizures, hemolytic anemia, and thrombocytopenia.

14. Emergent care for a client with a dislocation includes which intervention?
    a. Putting joint through passive range of motion
    b. Splinting the joint in the dislocated position
    c. Keeping the area warm
    d. Providing tactile stimulation distal to the affected joint

Rationale
Correct answer: b.
The joint would be splinted in the dislocated position until controlled reduction is possible. Cold, not heat, is applied initially to reduce swelling. The joint is immobilized not moved through a ROM. Tactile stimulation distal to the affected joint serves no purpose.

15. Which statement made by a client being treated for a badly sprained ankle indicates a need for further explanation of self-care during the first 2 days after injury?
    a. "I will keep my foot elevated."
    b. "I will apply ice periodically."
    c. "I will keep my ankle wrapped in an elastic bandage."
    d. "I will bear full weight on my injured leg for no more than 15 minutes at a time."

Rationale
Correct answer: d.
Weight bearing is contraindicated or restricted. The foot should be elevated, ice applied periodically for the first 1–2 days and an elastic bandage applied.

16. Which goal related to fluid balance for a client with multiple myeloma would be appropriate?
    a. Daily output should be at least 1000 ml.
    b. Daily output should be at least 1500 ml.
    c. Daily intake should not exceed 2000 ml.
    d. Daily intake should not exceed 2500 ml.

Rationale
Correct answer: b.
Renal failure is a complication of the disease. Intake is not restricted rather 3–4 liters per day is encouraged since hypercalcemia which occurs with this disease is treated with hydration.

17. Which client presenting with a limp would be at the greatest risk for osteogenic sarcoma?
    a. A 72-year-old man
    b. A 46-year-old woman
    c. A 16-year-old boy
    d. A 7-year-old girl

Rationale
Correct answer: c.
Osteogenic sarcoma occurs during periods of rapid growth in adolescents.

18. A client presents with a dislocated wrist. The hand on the affected side is cold and blue. How should the nurse interpret these findings?
    a. Bleeding into the soft tissues has occurred.
    b. Neurovascular compromise exists.
    c. Lymphatic channels are blocked.
    d. A bone fracture coexists.

Rationale
Correct answer: b.
Symptoms of neurovascular damage include numbness, pain, cyanosis, and coldness of an extremity. Bleeding does not typically occur with a dislocation; lymphatic blockage does not cause cyanosis; and coldness and blue color are not specific signs indicative of a fracture.

19. When planning care for a client with a fractured hip, the nurse would plan to monitor for which common complications?
    a. Urinary tract infection
    b. Pneumonia
    c. Candidiasis
    d. Herniated nucleus pulposus
    e. Thromboembolism

Rationale
Correct answers: b and e.
Pneumonia and thromboembolism are complications related to immobility and are significant risks in clients with fractured hips. Urinary tract infection and candidiasis may occur but clients with fractured hips are not at particular risk for them. Herniated nucleus pulposus is a problem of the intervertebral discs that may be the result of degeneration or trauma to the spine.

20. Hip precautions would be part of the plan of care for a client with which disorder?
    a. Osteogenesis imperfecta
    b. Tibial torsion
    c. Juvenile rheumatoid arthritis
    d. Hip fracture

Rationale
Correct answer: d.
Hip precautions—no hip flexion beyond zero degrees, no adduction beyond the midline, and weight bearing restriction as prescribed—are part of the plan of care for the client with a fractured hip. Osteogenesis imperfecta requires

(continued)

careful handling to avoid breaking bones. There are no special positioning precautions for JRA or tibial torsion.

21. The teaching plan for the parents of an infant with which problem would include the instruction "Never hold by the ankles when changing the diaper"?
    a. Muscular dystrophy
    b. Osteomyelitis
    c. Club foot
    d. Osteogenesis imperfecta

Rationale

Correct answer: d.

Holding the infant by the ankles to change the diaper is contraindicated in osteogenesis imperfecta because of the ease with which any stress can cause a bone to break. Holding by the ankles is not contraindicated by any of the other disorders.

22. Which statement made by the relative of a child with muscular dystrophy indicates understanding of at least one aspect of the disease?
    a. "I'm relieved that this is a noninherited, developmental defect."
    b. "There may be some disability but at least there is a normal life expectancy."
    c. "If intellectual impairment was not always a part of the disease, it would be easier to deal with."
    d. "It will be very hard watching as the muscle wasting and loss of function occur."

Rationale

Correct answer: d.

Muscle wasting, weakness, and loss of function are characteristic of muscular dystrophy. Muscular dystrophy is an inherited disorder, with a shortened life expectancy. Intellectual impairment occurs with a few forms of MD but not with all.

23. Which client has risk factors and/or signs most characteristic of Ewing's sarcoma?
    a. A 24-year-old with a rapidly growing mass palpable on the tibia
    b. A 40-year-old with a history of retinoblastoma
    c. A 55-year-old with severe back pain that increases with exercise
    d. A 73-year-old with multiple pathological fractures

Rationale

Correct answer: a.

Ewing's sarcoma is a disease of those under 30 years of age and is characterized by a rapidly growing mass on the affected bone with tense, tender local swelling. History of retinoblastoma is a risk factor for osteogenic sarcoma. Back pain that increases with exercise is characteristic of multiple myeloma. Pathological fractures are associated with multiple myeloma.

24. What findings on physical examination of a client brought into Emergency are consistent with a fractured hip?
    a. Lengthening and internal rotation of the affected leg
    b. Lengthening and external rotation of the affected leg
    c. Shortening and internal rotation of the affected leg
    d. Shortening and external rotation of the affected leg

Rationale

Correct answer: d.

The leg shortens and externally rotates when the hip fracture allows the femur to move up and it is no longer held in position within the acetabulum.

25. When monitoring a client for compartment syndrome, which question should be included in the assessment?
    a. "Does it hurt when you flex the muscle of your arm?"
    b. "Has the pain increased in your arm?"
    c. "Has the swelling increased near your shoulder?"
    d. "Is there a red line going down your arm?"

Rationale

Correct answer: b.

A sign of compartment syndrome is increased pain in the extremity. Other signs are pain on passive muscle stretching of the part and edema distal to the site of injury. A red line down the arm is indicative of infection.

26. Foods such as scallops, red wine, and gravies should be restricted in the diet of clients with which disease?
    a. Rheumatoid arthritis
    b. Systemic lupus erythematosus
    c. Gout
    d. Muscular dystrophy

Rationale

Correct answer: c.

Foods high in purines should be avoided because primary gout is caused by a genetic error in purine metabolism the end result of which is the over production or retention of uric acid. There are no dietary restrictions for any of the other diseases.

Test Plan Category:

Physiological Integrity

Sub-category: **Physiological Adaptation—Part 1**

Topics: **Alterations in Body Systems**
Illness Management
Section 7: Gastrointestinal Problems

FACIAL/ORAL PROBLEMS

PEDS CLEFT LIP/CLEFT PALATE

- Cleft lip and cleft palate refer to facial malformations that evolve during embryonic development, resulting in nonunion of the bones and tissues of the lip and palate.
- Cleft lip and cleft palate may occur independently or together.
- There may be a combination of defects and degrees of involvement.
- Facial defects are noticeable at birth.

Etiology: Cleft lip occurs when the medial nasal and maxillary processes fail to form. Cleft palate occurs when the bone and tissue of the primary palatial shelves or processes fail to fuse, causing a communication between the mouth and nose.

Precipitating factors: Combination of genetic and environmental factors; cleft palate is found mostly in girls and cleft lip alone or together with cleft palate is found mostly in boys; maternal smoking during the first trimester may contribute to the development of these defects.

S&S:

- Incompletely formed lip
- Opening in roof of the mouth can be palpated
- Unilateral or bilateral cleft lip
- With cleft palate, milk or formula escapes through the nose
- Abdominal distention due to swallowing air
- Slow weight gain

Dx: Visual assessment of defects at birth and by palpation; ultrasound to identify cleft lip or cleft palate in utero; MRI to detect the extent of the abnormality; evaluation of the infant's ability to suck, swallow and breathe; a genetic evaluation to determine reoccurrence

Rx: Modification of feeding technique with adaptive devices (nipples) to ensure growth; extra-and intraoral prosthesis used before surgery to aid in feeding and speech and to prevent maxillary collapse; cleft lip is usually corrected before cleft palate; immediate repair focuses on the first few weeks after birth; repair of cleft palate is at about eighteen months. Surgery offers optimal cosmetic and functional results; scheduled when the infant is without any infections (respiratory, oral, or systemic), surgical treatments begin early and continue into adolescence; scheduling depends on the severity of the cleft.

Chiloplasty used for correction of a cleft lip; the involvement of a multidisciplinary team is needed: pediatrician, plastic surgeon, orthodontist, audiologist, speech therapist, prosthodontist, and psychiatrist

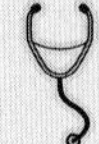

Assessment Alert

When taking temperature, avoid the oral route.

Nursing Process Elements

- Provide emotional support to parents as they experience the emotional reactions to the infant's appearance
- Offer information to provide a better understanding about the infant's deformity, that the infant is normal and that surgery will correct the problem
- If sucking is ineffective use a cross-cut soft nipple or other specially adapted nipples
- When the infant is unable to suck, use a syringe with a rubber tip to place the formula into the mouth
- Hold the infant's head upright when feeding, to prevent aspiration
- Make the infant burp often, this helps prevent regurgitation and aspiration
- Monitor feeding-tube function if the infant cannot feed orally
- Postoperative nursing
  —Assess respiratory status
  —Monitor vital signs
  —Check weight periodically to evaluate adequate nutritional intake
  —Clean suture line to prevent infection
  —Use a gentle restraint to prevent the infant from placing hands on its mouth
  —Position infant so that rubbing of lip is prevented
  —Use wrist restraints after cleft-lip repair and elbow restraints following cleft-palate repair to prevent the child from putting anything into the mouth
  —Use a rubber-tipped asepto syringe to feed after cleft-lip repair
  —Following cleft-palate repair, limit the child to fluids, which the child can drink from a cup
  —Do not use eating utensils or straws to prevent traumatizing the palate repair
  —Avoid any activity that might strain the suture line, including crying, in the postoperative period

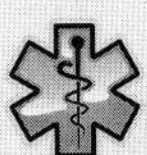

Nursing Intervention Alert

The infant requires stimulation after surgery to provide distraction, to prevent reaching for the mouth and to decrease crying which increases tension on the suture line. Provide age-appropriate toys and music; encourage the parents to hold, cuddle, and comfort the infant.

Client teaching for self-care

- Teach parents that cleft lip or palate interferes with the ability to suck and feeding is difficult
- Encourage family to participate in both physical and emotional care
- Teach feeding methods: to feed small amounts, slowly and for a short time, to hold the infant upright and to burp often
- Review the need to observe for respiratory difficulty and aspiration
- Monitor for weight gain
- Prepare for discharge home by allowing time for parents to practice feeding
- Answer parents' questions about care and initiate referrals to the American Cleft Palate Association

JAW FRACTURE

- Jaw fracture includes broken jaw, trauma to the mandible, and also possible trauma to the maxillary bones, teeth, face, and mouth framework.

Etiology: Caused by a direct blow to the jaw; related to a motor vehicle accident, assault, a sport or recreation injury; a powerful blow may also injure the cervical spine.

Precipitating factors: Males are 3 times more prone to jaw fracture; ages 20–29 years form a common group with this injury.

S&S:

- Difficulty in breathing
- Pain
- Edema
- Bleeding
- Bruising
- Difficulty in opening mouth
- Temporary problem during talking and eating

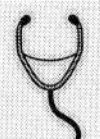

Assessment Alert

Monitor general condition for shock; check neurovascular status.

Dx: Assessment of symptoms; X-rays to determine the type of fracture and position of any bone fragments; MRI

Rx: The goal is to reduce the fracture and restore function—apply ice to reduce edema and pain; use analgesics; wire jaws together to keep bones in place; surgery involves repositioning and reconstruction of the jaw and insertion of a rigid plate fixation with screws into the bone to stabilize fracture

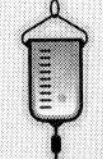

Clinical Alert

The following complications are medical emergencies that may accompany a fractured jaw and need immediate attention: airway obstruction, cervical spine injury, or hemorrhage.

Nursing Process Elements

- Monitor for increased respiratory effort
- Address concerns about body image
- Evaluate neurovascular status
- Treat pain with analgesics
- Help clear secretions from oropharynx
- Keep wire cutter nearby

Client teaching for self-care

- Offer guidelines for mouth care and feeding
- Instruct client with wired jaw or postsurgery to follow a liquid diet, not to chew, and to use protein drinks
- Teach to call physician for: difficult breathing, severe jaw pain not relieved by medication, elevated temperature, and loose wires
- Provide wire cutters for client's use

ORAL CANCER

- The most commonly occurring oral cancers are squamous cell carcinomas.

- Oral cancer may occur anywhere in mouth: lips, palate, floor, etc., but tongue is the most common site.
- Metastasis from the tongue is especially rapid because of lymph and blood supply.

Etiology: Precise cause unknown.

Risk factors: Smoking and alcohol use linked to all but tongue cancers.

Leukoplakia are white lesions appearing on the oral mucosa. More common in men, and those over the age of 60 years, one type linked to heavy smoking, also cheek or lip biting or friction from dentures. Associated with increased cancer risk only if occur on the floor of mouth.

Erythroplakia are red, velvety lesions associated with cancer risk. Biopsy recommended.

S&S: Single asymptomatic lesion like a painless, nonhealing ulcer, often unnoticed by client

Dx: Biopsy is definitive. Ultrasonography or CT scans may be done to evaluate masses

Rx: Depends on size and stage.

- Early: radiation or surgery; highly curable with radiation if confined to mucosa
- More invasive: both surgery and radiation.
- Late: palliative

Surgery often includes neck dissection because of early metastasis to cervical nodes

Nursing Process Elements

Assess and manage side effects of treatment

- Surgery: Airway, chewing, swallowing, or speech problems
- Radiation: stomatitis, xerostomia, dental decay, change/loss of taste

(See section on radiation Rx.)

Client teaching for self-care

Following oral surgery instruct the client to:

- Follow program of mouth care carefully to help prevent infection and tooth decay. Use sterile water, dilute peroxide, and saline and/or bicarbonate solution as prescribed; no commercial mouth washes until healed
- Select foods of a consistency which is easiest to swallow and least uncomfortable
- Avoid damage to healing tissues: Eat slowly, avoid very hot or cold foods; do not use a fork or other potentially traumatic utensil
- Take nutritional supplements as needed to maintain weight and balanced nutrition
- Rinse mouth as directed after eating

GASTROESOPHAGEAL REFLUX DISEASE

- Gastroesophageal reflux disease (GERD) refers to a relapsing, chronic disorder in which gastric and duodenal contents move back into the lower esophagus resulting in a break in the mucosa and inflammation.
- In the long term, this can result in the development of Barrett's epithelium, which is more resistant to acid but has a significant malignant potential.
- Ulceration and hemorrhage as well as fibrosis and esophageal stricture can also occur.

Etiology: Inappropriate relaxation of the lower esophageal sphincter (LES), possibly delayed gastric emptying.

Precipitating factors: Ingestion of foods that lower LES pressure (fatty foods, chocolate, alcohol, caffeine containing cola, coffee, and tea); nicotine; drugs such as calcium channel blockers, theophylline, maybe NSAIDs; elevated estrogen or progesterone levels; conditions such as obesity or pregnancy that elevate intra-abdominal pressure.

S&S:

- Heartburn—substernal or retrosternal burning pain that may radiate to the back or jaw
- Regurgitation, belching, flatulence, and difficult or painful swallowing in severe cases
- Nocturnal cough, wheezing, or hoarseness

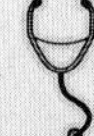

Assessment Alert

The heartburn of reflux can mimic angina. Careful differentiation between reflux and cardiac disease is critical.

Dx: Often based on symptoms. 24-hour pH monitoring is the gold standard, endoscopy to check mucosal damage; biopsy to check for Barrett's epithelium or cancer; manometry to check muscle and sphincter function

Rx: Drug therapy to neutralize acid and/or suppress its secretion

Antacids or alginates (Gaviscon) and histamine 2 (H2) receptor antagonists for mild symptoms; proton pump inhibitors (PPIs) (once a day, 15–20 minutes before breakfast) for severe cases

Surgery (fundoplication) to reinforce the LES may be done in severe, refractive cases

Nursing Process Elements

- Assess for S&S
- Obtain baseline weight to determine need for weight loss
- Support efforts to lose weight and/or stop smoking

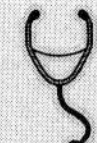

Assessment Alert

Clients generally do not report heartburn unless specifically asked or symptoms are very severe. It is important to ask specifically and explore the use of OTC remedies.

Client teaching for self-care

Teach the client to

- take medication as prescribed
- follow a low-fat, adequate-protein diet; fatty foods delay gastric emptying
- avoid foods that lower LES pressure or that consistently cause heartburn
- eat four to six small meals daily to avoid gastric distention, to eat slowly and chew thoroughly
- sit up for 1–2 hours after meals
- avoid eating or drinking for at least 3 hours before bedtime; evening snacking makes problem worse
- elevate head of bed 6–8 inches with foam wedge to discourage reflux secondary to the recumbent position
- lose weight if needed
- stop smoking
- avoid factors that increase intra-abdominal pressure: constrictive clothing, straining, weight lifting, and working bent over

ESOPHAGEAL CANCER

- Esophageal cancer is a rare but aggressive form of cancer. It is almost never diagnosed early.
- There are two distinct types:
  —Squamous cell esophageal cancer, which occurs predominantly in African-American men and arises in the middle and lower third of the esophagus.
  —Adenocarcinoma esophageal cancer, which primarily affects Caucasian men and arises in the distal third of the esophagus.

Etiology: Unknown.

Risk factors:

- Squamous cell: Tobacco use, heavy alcohol use, dietary nitrates, deficient intake of fresh fruits and vegetables, vitamin deficiency, mucosal irritants, African-American ethnicity, male sex.
- Adenocarcinoma: Barrett's epithelium (age 10–20 years, Caucasian ethnicity, male sex).

S&S: Typically asymptomatic until advanced

- Progressive dysphagia is the most common symptom; client often automatically eliminates difficult-to-swallow foods from the diet and is unaware of the problem until diet is predominantly liquid
- Vague sense of substernal discomfort or feeling of fullness after eating only a small amount may occur
- Halitosis, anorexia, weight loss, and emaciation in later stages of disease
- N&V occurs if esophagus completely obstructed
- Cough if tracheoesophageal fistula or other tracheal involvement occurs
- Steady, boring pain on swallowing and/or hoarseness if mediastinum involved

Dx: X-ray esophagram with barium swallow indicates mass present; esophagoscopy with biopsy determines the specific pathology. Workup for metastasis

Rx: Varies with tumor location, client condition, and stage of disease

- Resection of the esophagus to eliminate obstruction and restore swallowing
- Radiation pre- or postoperatively or for palliation when surgery not feasible
- Endoscopic laser destruction of the tumor, which requires repeated treatments but has no undesirable systemic effects and is unaffected by tumor location in the esophagus
- Prosthetic intubation—pliable tube inserted in esophagus to keep it open and/or bypass a tracheoesophageal (T/E) fistula
- Gastrostomy to maintain nutrition

Nursing Process Elements

- Assess for S&S with particular attention to nutritional status
- Monitor I&O
- Provide care as described under esophageal resection for clients having surgery
- Provide care as described under radiation therapy for clients having radiation
- For clients having laser palliation:
  —Explain that a temporary increase in dysphagia and discomfort is expected

—Begin oral diet a few days after last treatment

—Monitor for complications: aspiration, bleeding, and perforation of esophagus

HIATAL HERNIA

Hiatal hernia refers to the movement of the distal esophagus and a part of the stomach up through the esophageal hiatus (opening) in the diaphragm into the thoracic cavity. It is called

- sliding hernia if the gastroesophageal junction is above the diaphragm and part of the stomach slides up into the thorax when the client lies down and slides back into the abdomen on standing.
- paraesophageal hernia if the junction remains below the diaphragm but a section of the gastric fundus and greater curvature rolls up into the thorax forming a pouch.

Etiology: May be a congenitally enlarged opening.

Risk factors: Weakening of the diaphragmatic muscle, aging, trauma, surgery, prolonged increased intra-abdominal pressure from obesity, tumors, ascites, pregnancy, and strenuous activity.

S&S:

- Most hiatal hernias are asymptomatic
- S&S that occur with sliding hernias, are due to chronic reflux so are the same as in GERD
- With paraesophageal hernias, S&S are due to distention and obstruction so heartburn and chest pain are common. Occult bleeding secondary to rubbing of the mucosal surfaces of the herniated portion of the stomach also occurs

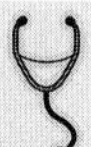

Assessment Alert

Occult bleeding associated with a hiatal hernia can lead to iron-deficiency anemia. Be sure to assess for related S&S.

Complications: Paraesophageal hernia—obstruction, strangulation, acute volvulus, regurgitation with tracheal aspiration

Dx: Visualized on barium swallow; mostly found during workup for GERD

Rx:

- Medical—Treat reflux as described under GERD
- Surgical—Only effective Rx for paraesophageal hernias. Hernia and its sac is reduced and the widened hiatus is partially closed; a fundoplication antireflux procedure may also be done

Nursing Process Elements

Same as for the client with GERD

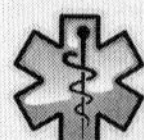

Nursing Intervention Alert

Warn client not to take alcohol for pain relief because it lowers LES pressure and worsens the problem.

GASTRITIS

Gastritis refers to the inflammation of the stomach mucosa.

- It may be acute or chronic, diffuse or localized.
- Acute gastritis is self-limiting and is characterized by superficial ulcerations, which heal with time.
- Hemorrhagic type may be a result of the use of NSAIDS or due to stress.

Acute Gastritis

Etiology: Injury to the gastric mucosa from chemical, thermal, or bacterial factors, which include drugs such NSAIDS, steroids, digitalis; large amounts of irritating foods such as tea, coffee, spices; very hot, rough, or bacterially contaminated foods; alcohol; radiation exposure. Also occurs in association with severe physiologic stress.

S&S:

- Often asymptomatic
- When symptomatic: epigastric pain, abdominal tenderness, N&V, eructation. If hemorrhagic gastritis: hematemesis, melena, decreased HCT, increased BUN

Dx: Endoscopy or biopsy

Rx: Only when symptomatic

- Eliminate precipitating factor
- Treat symptoms: NPO during acute symptoms progressing to bland diet as tolerated, antiemetics, antacids, and H2-antagonist to decrease irritating gastric secretions; fluid and blood replacement, NG lavage PRN for hemorrhagic type

Nursing Process Elements

- Assess for S&S using PQRS format
- Pay particular attention to

—pain
—use of alcohol
—following of prescription
—use of OTC and herbal drugs
—usual diet and any changes in eating habits
—appetite and weight
—signs of dehydration

- Monitor electrolyte values
- Monitor emesis for signs of bleeding
- Discourage cigarette smoking because nicotine increases gastric acidity

Client teaching for self-care

In case of acute gastritis:

- Avoid risk factors: drugs such as NSAIDs, steroids, digitalis; large amounts of irritating foods such as tea, coffee, spices; very hot, rough, or bacterially contaminated foods; alcohol; radiation exposure; nicotine because it increases gastric activity
- Handle, store, and prepare food properly
- Follow directions for taking medications
- Read OTC drug labels or ask pharmacist to check for ASA content in medicines
- Change to nonirritating foods and flavorings in the daily diet and limit alcoholic beverages
- Participate in a stop smoking program

Chronic Gastritis

In case of chronic gastritis, gastric mucosa atrophies, parietal and chief cells disappear, secretions decrease, and digestion becomes impaired.

Etiology:

- Type A: autoimmune associated with pernicious anemia.
- Type B: associated with *Helicobacter pylori* infection.

S&S:

- Mimic peptic ulcer disease or gastric cancer with epigastric fullness, burning or pain, N&V, and flatulence, especially after a large meal
- Anorexia, weight loss, and symptoms of anemia can also develop

Dx: Endoscopy and biopsy

Rx: Only when symptomatic

- Lifestyle changes to eliminate contributing factors
- Antibiotic therapy for *H. pylori* infection
- Bland diet and antacids
- Cobalamin injections for pernicious anemia

Nursing Process Elements

Assess for S&S, also for signs of developing B-12 deficiency associated with pernicious anemia, such as glossitis and stomatitis

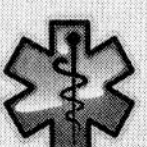

Nursing Intervention Alert

Gastric cancer occurs more commonly in those with chronic gastritis than in the general population. Teaching the client about the importance of regular medical follow-up is important.

PEPTIC ULCER DISEASE

Peptic ulcer disease (PUD) is a break in the mucosa of any area of GI tract exposed to gastric secretions containing acid and pepsin. Thus, peptic ulcers can occur in lower esophagus, stomach, duodenum or any part of GI tract surgically connected to stomach

Duodenal or Gastric Ulcers

Etiology: Most cases are related to mucosal injury secondary to *H. pylori* infection, though only a small percent of people with *H. pylori* infection develop ulcers. Remaining cases are a result of mucosal injury secondary to chronic NSAID use.

Risk factors: Smoking: as amount and duration of smoking increases, so does risk. Alcohol has no proven role nor do diet, stress, or excess acid production.

S&S:

- Pain:
  —Gastric ulcer: Dull epigastric pain near midline, unrelieved by antacids or food
  —Duodenal ulcer Gnawing, burning or aching, midline epigastric pain sometimes with radiation around costal border to back, 1–3 hours after meals and at night (12pm–3am), lasting 30 minutes to 2 hours, often relieved by food or antacid
- Early satiety with gastric ulcer
- Dyspepsia, i.e., fullness, vague nausea, bloating/distention, anorexia, and weight loss

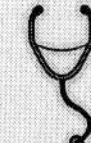

Assessment Alert 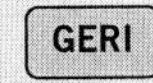

S&S of PUD are often atypical in the elderly. Pain may be absent or poorly localized and similar to that associated with angina, gall bladder disease, or dysphagia.

Dx: Suggested by history, confirmed by endoscopy, presence of *H. pylori* confirmed by biopsy or serology test

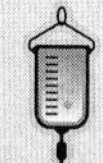

Clinical Alert

Serology test can confirm presence of *H. pylori* but cannot be used to monitor therapeutic results because it remains positive for an indefinite period of time.

Rx:

- Antibiotics to eliminate *H. pylori* infection
- H2 receptor antagonists or proton pump inhibitors to decrease gastric acid production
- Antacids to decrease irritation from gastric acid and permit healing; used predominantly for symptomatic relief; aluminum hydroxide preparations preferred
- Mucosal protective agents
  —sucralfate coats mucous membrane and ulcer crater providing a barrier against gastric acid
  —GERI Misoprostol, synthetic prostaglandin analog, used preventatively in high-risk older clients who need NSAIDS

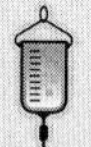

Clinical Alert OB

Misoprostol can cause abortion so it is not used for women of child-bearing age.

- Surgery primarily for complications though selective vagotomy may be done to decrease HCl production
- Diet: Restrict foods that cause distress

Complications:

- Hemorrhage from damage to a large blood vessel
- Peritonitis secondary to perforation and release of contaminated GI contents into peritoneal cavity
- Obstruction (partial or total) as a result of edema in narrow pyloric area
- Gastric cancer

GERI Most complications occur in elderly. Elderly more likely to be colonized with *H. pylori*, more frequently use NSAIDS, often have dyspepsia making diagnosis more difficult, and less often seek treatment.

Nursing Process Elements

- Assess S&S with particular attention to pain, signs of GI bleeding including occult blood in feces, changes in Hgb, HCT, and RBC count, weight gain or loss
- Obtain history of medication use with focus on ulcerogenic drugs especially ASA and NSAIDs, alcohol use, smoking, and dietary habits
- Refer to smoking cessation program if needed

Client teaching for self-care

Provide the following instructions to the client:

- Adhere to prescribed drug regimen. This includes continuing to take all medications even if pain or other S&S are relieved
- Do not take antacids at the same time as other anti-ulcer medications such as H2 blockers because the antacids decrease absorption of the other drugs by a significant amount
- Never abruptly discontinue anti-ulcer medications because of risk of severe acid rebound
- Substitute acetaminophen for ASA or other NSAIDs for routine pain or fever management
- Use good eating habits:
  —Avoid foods that cause discomfort
  —Avoid overeating
  —Eat slowly and chew thoroughly
  —Avoid snacking at bedtime because it increases nighttime acid secretion
- Use alcohol in moderation if at all; do not drink on an empty stomach because of irritating effect on the mucosa
- Obtain adequate rest
- Engage in stress-reducing activities

GASTROENTERITIS

- Gastroenteritis refers to an inflammation of the stomach and small intestine.
- The most common causative agents of gastroenteritis are bacteria and viruses, and then parasites or toxins.
  —Bacteria: *Escherichia coli*, *Salmonella*, *Staphylococcus aureus*, and *Shigella*.
  —Parasites: Ascaris, enterobius, and trichomonas.
  —Viruses: Norwalk, retrovirus, adenoviruses, echoviruses, and coxsackievirus.
  —Toxins: Poisonous plants, lead, mercury, arsenic, and toadstools.

Etiology: Tissue damage and inflammation lead to the release of exotoxins that cause a secretion of electrolytes and water into the intestine; as a result, diarrhea and fluid loss occur.

Precipitating factors: Ingestion of feces-contaminated food and water; food borne viral infections caused by feces-contaminated shellfish; the use of antibiotics which decrease normal intestinal flora that usually protects the bowel from pathogens; travelers to countries with poor sanitation are prone to gastroenteritis or traveler's diarrhea; not washing hands before handling food and after using the bathroom.

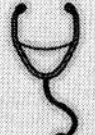

Assessment Alert

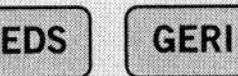

Those at greatest risk are infants, the elderly, and dehabilitated clients, due to immature or impaired immune systems.

S&S:

- Diarrhea, mild to severe
- Anorexia, N&V
- Excessive vomiting may lead to metabolic alkalosis due to loss of hydrochloric acid from the stomach
- Malaise
- Abdominal distention, pain, cramps
- Borborygmi
- Electrolyte imbalances such as hypokalemia, hyponatremia
- Fever
- Headache

Dx: Laboratory tests such as HCT (decreased due to dehydration and hypovolemia), creatinine, and BUN; assessment of electrolyte values and acid–base balance; tests to identify the causative agent such as Gram stain, stool culture, blood culture, and ELISA to specifically identify *Clostridium difficile*; endoscopic examinations show an inflamed, edematous bowel mucosa

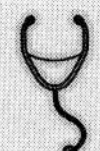

Assessment Alert

Complications include shock, dehydration, and renal failure.

Rx: Acute gastroenteritis resolves quickly; if client is severely ill, medications are prescribed, antibiotics are used if cause is bacterial (obtain a stool culture first), occasionally antidiarrheals used to increase comfort and decrease fluid loss or cathartics may be used to remove toxins from the bowel and antiemetics for severe vomiting; supportive measures as bed rest, nutritional supplements, increasing fluids and a bland diet; electrolytes are replaced; IV fluids are administered if necessary, as glucose in normal saline or lactated ringers solution

Nursing Process Elements

- When client can tolerate fluids, offer ginger ale, lemonade, or broth to replace fluids and electrolytes
- Ask about recent travel and antibiotic therapy
- Wash hands thoroughly after administering care to prevent spread of infection
- Plan care so that the client has uninterrupted periods of rest to improve resistance and conserve strength
- Administer IV fluids as ordered
- If food poisoning is the cause, contact the public health department to find source of the problem

Client teaching for self-care

- Teach to wash hands before handling food and after using the bathroom
- Instruct to clean cooking utensils well
- Teach to identify foods that need immediate refrigeration as dairy products, meats, and fresh fish
- Teach client to avoid raw meat
- Instruct to cook meat well to prevent salmonellosis or staphylococcal food poisoning
- Teach about the cause, symptoms, and treatments of gastroenteritis
- Inform clients who travel to drink only bottled water, not to use ice in their drinks, and to avoid raw fruits and vegetables

PEDS PYLORIC STENOSIS

- Pyloric stenosis is a hypertrophy (thickening) of the circular muscles surrounding the pylorus resulting in stenosis and obstruction.

Etiology: Exact cause unknown; develops during infant's first weeks of life; hypertrophy and hyperplasia cause the circular muscles of the pylorus to enlarge, resulting in narrowing of the pyloric canal between the stomach and duodenum; later, inflammation and edema add to constriction of the lumen and to obstruction.

Precipitating factors: May be familial or acquired; more common in Caucasians; affects males more than females; associated with anorectal abnormalities and intestinal malrotation.

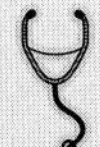

Assessment Alert

Most often seen in full term first-born male infants.

S&S:

- Vomiting (usually stale milk), 30–60 minutes after feeding, becomes forceful and projectile
- Visible peristalsis
- Infant is irritable, hungry, and without weight gain
- Few, small stools
- Distended upper abdomen
- Dehydration—poor skin turgor, sunken fontanels, lethargy
- Palpable olive-shaped mass in the epigastrium
- Development of alkalosis and hyperbilirubinemia

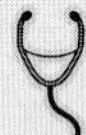

Assessment Alert

Infants are at high risk for dehydration due to fluid deficit and altered nutrition as a result of vomiting.

Dx: Ultrasound to confirm diagnosis, Upper GI to rule out any other cause of vomiting; evaluation of laboratory values to detect anemia and metabolic alkalosis, increased blood urea nitrogen and/or decreased sodium, potassium, and chloride levels

Rx: Correct fluid and electrolyte imbalances; surgery: a pyloromytomy (Fredet-Ramstedt procedure) performed to enlarge the pyloric outlet or opening of the obstruction to allow for passage of fluids and food; may use laparoscopic surgery which involves a shorter surgical time and an earlier feeding and discharge time

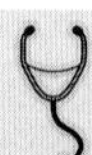

Assessment Alert

Complications that may occur postoperatively: wound dehiscence, continued pyloric obstruction, and gastroesophageal reflux.

Nursing Process Elements

- Monitor vital signs, daily weights, I&O, urine specific gravity
- Assess vomiting episodes and assess for aspiration
- Evaluate for fluid and electrolyte imbalances
- Restoration of hydration
- Evaluate NG tube function, type and amount of drainage
- Assess parent's anxiety and offer reassurance about problem
- Postoperative care:
  —Promote rest and comfort
  —Prevent infection
  —Maintain IV fluids and I&O
  —Encourage parents to remain with infant and to participate with care

Client teaching for self-care

- Encourage parents to hold child and provide pacifier for comfort
- Instruct family to monitor intake of food and fluids and vomiting episodes
- Inform parents about pre- and postoperative interventions
- Offer discharge instructions to parents: check incision for redness and drainage, when temperature is elevated call the physician, give written instructions about feedings, to fold diaper off incision site to prevent infection, give analgesics as acetaminophen as ordered, warn parents that some postsurgery vomiting may occur.
- Provide resources for parents to contact for any questions about infant's needs

PEDS FAILURE TO THRIVE

- Failure to thrive (FTT) refers to growth failure.
- It is the inability to utilize or obtain enough food, resulting in poor growth patterns.
- It represents a continual deceleration on the growth curve.

Etiology: Organic FTT caused by the presence of a major disease, inorganic FTT caused by many psychosocial factors. Mixed FTT may also occur.

Precipitating factors: Presence of a disease such as AIDS, congenital heart defects, metabolic disorders, esophageal reflux, or a neurological abnormality; psychosocial problems as parent's misunderstanding of the infant/child's nutritional requirements, disturbances in the parent–child relationship, poverty, or immature parents.

S&S:

- Weight and/or height falls below the fifth percentile for child's age
- Developmental milestones are not achieved
- Slow social, lingual, and motor development
- Irregular sleep patterns

- Weakness
- Limited smiling
- Absence of appropriate stranger anxiety

Dx: Health and dietary history; physical examination and diagnostic tests to rule out major illnesses; developmental screening; evaluation of growth patterns; family assessment; evidence of growth retardation

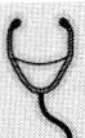

Assessment Alert

It is normal for American-Asian children to be lower than the fifth percentile on growth charts.

Rx: Reversal of malnutrition; adequate nutrition to increase calorie intake; treat psychosocial problems with a multidisciplinary team; multivitamins and minerals

Nursing Process Elements

- Assess parent and child behavior during feeding: how child is held, eye-to-eye contact, sensitivity to child's needs
- Provide feedings by consistent nursing staff, to learn child's feeding behavior
- Take initial height and weight and weigh daily
- Evaluate when hungry and when hunger is met
- Record food intake
- Use a structured feeding schedule
- Provide quiet nonstimulating surroundings
- Offer appropriate developmental stimulation
- Arrange home care visits, contact social agencies for financial assistance to family

Client teaching for self-care

- Give instruction and guidance about meeting child's nutritional needs
- Demonstrate feeding techniques to parent
- Encourage parents to hold, touch, and cuddle when feeding infant
- Teach to maintain scheduled, quiet meal times
- Suggest that parents eat with the child or that the child eat with others can be more enjoyable for the child
- Instruct parent to create eye contact when feeding infant or child
- Teach to offer foods first and liquids later, liquids have fewer calories and create a feeling of fullness
- Instruct to limit junk food in a child's diet

PEDS COLIC

- Colic is a disorder characterized by periods of excessively loud crying associated with proxysmal abdominal cramping and pain.

Etiology: Unknown, possibly swallowing air during feeding; newer theory suggests an association with CNS maturation; there is no apparent medical reason for crying; infant does gain weight and thrives.

Precipitating factors: Feeding too fast; swallowing large amounts of air; generally present in infants under 3 months; may be a symptom of cow's milk allergy or allergy to something in mother's diet.

S&S:

- Continuous loud crying for hours
- Infant may draw up legs to chest
- Clenched hands
- Distended abdomen
- Symptoms may resemble intestinal obstruction
- Refuses breast or bottle
- Usually occurs in late afternoon or early evening
- When crying stops, see exhaustion and/or passage of gas or stool

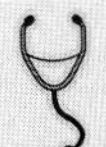

Assessment Alert

Assess for abuse; parents become frustrated when caring for difficult infants.

Dx: Based on symptoms, infant is inconsolable

Rx: No medical treatment; outgrow problem; sometimes use drugs as antispasmodics, sedatives, and antiflatulents may be useful; if breast-feeding mother notes certain foods in her diet cause increased crying, these foods should be eliminated; if cow's milk is a problem, trial use of another formula; burping to relieve air in GI tract

Nursing Process Elements

- Support parent's every effort to comfort infant; listen attentively and offer suggestions
- Observe feeding process, relationship between feeding and crying, diet type, and amount of burping
- Evaluate colic episodes
- Reduce stimuli, provide soothing music, and respond to crying
- Swaddle and hold

- Place infant in crib or bassinet on back if all efforts fail, will eventually fall asleep

Client teaching for self-care

- Explain to parents that although crying is stressful, colic disappears in about 3 months and leaves no long-term effects
- Hold and rock infant, give rhythmic movement using either infant swing or front baby carrier
- Reduce stimuli, no loud noises, provide quiet, soothing environment
- Massage abdomen, try pacifier or warm bath to relieve discomfort
- Feed small amounts and burp often
- Try bottle with collapsible bag to prevent sucking air
- Change formula, or mother's diet if necessary

CELIAC DISEASE

- Celiac disease is a chronic malabsorption syndrome.
- It involves inability to digest gliadin, formed from the breakdown of gluten, a protein found in wheat, rye, oats, and barley.
- It is also called gluten-induced enteropathy or celiac sprue.

Etiology: Malabsorption develops when a child or adult is unable to absorb and digest nutrients; celiac disease, lactose intolerance, and short bowel syndrome are examples of malabsorption. Specific cause is unknown; ingestion of gluten causes an immune response that damages the small intestine villi, resulting in malabsorption; affects fat metabolism.

Precipitating factors: Genetic and environmental influences or immune factors; more common in Caucasians; affects young children and adults; present more often in females; untreated celiac disease can develop into associated lactose intolerance due to intestinal mucosa lesions.

S&S:

- Distended abdomen and wasted extremities
- Steatorrhea, foul-smelling stools
- Irritability
- Anemia
- Extreme malaise
- Anorexia

Dx: Measurement of stool fecal fat; assessment of failure to thrive; jejunal biopsy to evaluate changes in the intestinal mucosa; serologic testing for IgA endomysial antibodies and IgA and IgG antigliadin antibodies for diagnosis and for evaluation of compliance to diet; CBC to evaluate anemia, prothrombin time to check for vitamin K deficiency

Rx: Gluten-free, high-calorie, high-protein diet: the elimination of wheat, rye, oats, and barley from the diet; limited fat in diet; use corn and rice as wheat substitutes; vitamins, minerals, and also iron and folic acid for anemia; vitamin K if prothrombin time is prolonged; corticosteroids if modified diet is not successful, used to reduce the inflammatory response

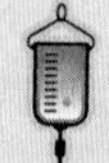

Clinical Alert

Noncompliance with diet results in risk for relapse, retarded growth, anemia, and development of gastrointestinal cancers when an adult.

Nursing Process Elements

- Continuing support to parents, provide information about celiac disease and about dietary restrictions
- Observe for normal growth patterns after treatment
- Evaluate stools: should be soft and formed
- Reinforcement needed for school age children and adolescents to maintain their diet since they are influenced by peers to try other foods
- Arrange for home care

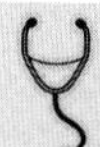

Assessment Alert

Celiac crisis, a sudden buildup of glutamine, which destroys the intestinal mucosa cells and causes severe watery diarrhea and vomiting results in a quick onset of dehydration and metabolic acidosis, which is treated with IV fluids and electrolytes and corticosteroids.

Client teaching for self-care

- Reinforce importance of following the prescribed diet
- Give information about preparing foods with rice and corn products
- Teach to read all food labels
- Schedule regular visits with a dietician
- Instruct to take vitamins, minerals, folic acid, and iron as prescribed
- Refer to resources for assistance as: American Celiac Society, Gluten Intolerance Group

INFLAMMATORY BOWEL DISEASE

Inflammatory bowel disease (IBD) has two major forms: Crohn's disease and ulcerative colitis. The pathology of both the forms is different but they are similar in other aspects; both are chronic and recurrent.

Etiology: Genetic factors: IBD associated with permissive genes on chromosomes 5 and 6 and CARD 15 gene mutations are associated with some forms of Crohn's disease. Positive family history is the most important risk factor but these are permissive; actual triggering factors not known. Smoking is one environmental factor

S&S:

- Ulcerative colitis—Continuous inflammation with edema and shallow ulcers primarily affecting the distal colorectal area (left-sided disease); ultimately the colon wall becomes inelastic and thick like a pipe and can no longer absorb. Pseudopolyps that can become malignant may result. Classic symptoms are bloody diarrhea (3–4 times per day up to hourly, mushy, urgent) and abdominal pain (left-sided, colicky, relieved by defecation); incontinence can occur because the urge to defecate can be lost as bowel thickens
- Crohn's disease—Cobblestone (affected areas separated by normal tissue) inflammation primarily affecting the proximal colon and ileum (right-sided disease); bowel wall thickens, ulcerates, and lumen narrows; fistulas to bladder, vagina, or other areas of bowel may form; scar tissue may obstruct the bowel, absorptive capacity may be lost. Diarrhea and abdominal pain are classic but pattern varies with location and severity of disease. Ileal disease: 3–5 large semisolid stools containing mucus and pus but no blood. Colorectal disease: urgent, small volume diarrhea and tenesmus. Severe, colicky pain after eating may be diffuse or localized in right lower quadrant (RLQ).
- Systemic symptoms of IBD: Anorexia, nausea, weakness, malaise, weight loss, anemia, fever, and leukocytosis. Almost any organ can be affected by a related systemic disorder that are believed to result from some underlying immune phenomenon, for example, arthritis and renal stones

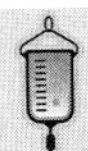

Clinical Alert

Primary complications of IBD are hemorrhage, obstruction, perforation, toxic megacolon, and malignancy developing in area of cellular dysplasia.

Dx: Stool culture and other laboratory work to rule out infectious origin; serologic antibody assay to help distinguish type of IBD; barium enema which can show "string lesions" of ulcerative colitis and cobblestones of Crohn's disease; endoscopy for direct visualization of characteristic changes; ultrasound to identify abscesses and fistulas

Rx:

- Stepped protocol in which drug regimen progressed until a response occurs
  - —Step 1(a): Aminosalicylates
    - 5-ASA preparations such as sulfasalazine, mesalamine, and olsalazine are not absorbed and have an anti-inflammatory effect on the colon inducing and sustaining remission in clients with mild to moderate IBD. Aminosalicylates can be used topically via enema or suppository
  - —Step 1(b): Antibiotics (metronidazole and ciprofloxacin)
  - —Step 2: Corticosteroids (prednisone and budesonide)
    - IV, PO, PR used to treat acute flares; never for maintenance therapy because of severe side effects (fluid and electrolyte abnormalities, osteoporosis, aseptic necrosis, peptic ulcers, cataracts, neurologic and endocrine problems, infection, and psychiatric problems)

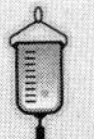

Clinical Alert

When corticosteroids are given, dose is tapered as soon as clinical response occurs, usually in 1–2 days.

  - —Step 3: Immunomodulators (azathioprine, mercaptopurine) or in Crohn's, the monoclonal antibody infliximab
    - Slow onset of action; may take 4 months to have effect

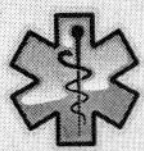

Nursing Intervention Alert

Clients on immune modifiers need CBC with differentials and platelets monthly for at least a year to check for neutropenia or pancytopenia, less frequently thereafter, if stable. LFTs also need monitoring.

  - —Step 4: Agents known to work on selected clients only
- Supportive care for severe episodes: bed rest, NPO, IV rehydration, parenteral nutrition for malnutrition
- Surgery: For ulcerative colitis, total colectomy with ileostomy is curative; in Crohn's disease, surgery avoided when possible because disease tends to recur in remaining bowel

Nursing Process Elements

- Assess S&S with particular attention to pain, bowel elimination pattern, and nutritional status
- Check usual meal pattern and intake, recent weight changes, food intolerances, bowel sounds, condition of perianal skin, skin turgor, condition of mucous membrane, fluid and electrolyte values, and current medication regimen
- Assess impact of illness on daily activities, family, and social relationships
- Encourage client to keep a record of pain and its relationship to eating, drinking, and passing stool or flatus; also of the frequency, severity, and urgency of defecation and whether blood or pus was present
- Monitor daily weight, I&O, signs of dehydration
- Administer anticholinergic or antispasmodic drugs as prescribed to reduce cramping
- Recommend attendance at support group

Client teaching for self-care

Instruct client to

- eat a high-calorie, well-balanced diet of whatever appeals when feeling well; limit raw fruits and vegetables and spicy or fatty foods or other aggravating foods when experiencing pain or diarrhea
- drink 2500–3000 ml of fluid per day to make up for losses with diarrhea
- use salt and drink Gatorade if tolerated during flares to replace electrolytes
- limit activity when diarrhea is severe and to lie down for 20 minutes after meals to limit peristalsis
- keep anal area clean and dry; use sitz baths, medicated wipes, and/ or a protective ointment
- monitor weight during flares
- use bulk-forming hydrophilic laxatives as directed if constipation is a problem
- apply warm heating pad to abdomen for comfort but not during acute exacerbations
- maintain a balanced schedule of rest and activity with regular sleep pattern
- use stress-reduction strategies
- report signs of problems requiring intervention: change in pattern of pain or diarrhea, change in stool characteristics, unusual rectal discharge, fever
- keep appointments for regular follow-up care

PEDS INTUSSUSCEPTION

- Intussusception refers to an intestinal obstruction that occurs when one portion of the bowel slips into an adjacent section.
- It is also called invagination or telescoping.

Etiology: Usually has an unknown cause; the passage of stool is obstructed beyond the defect; most common site is the ileocecal valve; onset can be abrupt, a previously healthy client suddenly develops abdominal pain and vomiting.

Precipitating factors: Present more often in males; most common at about 6 months, majority of cases are under the age of 2 years; associated with cystic fibrosis, celiac disease, Merkel's diverticulum, and Down's syndrome.

S&S:

- History of a piercing cry, severe abdominal pain, and pulling legs up to the trunk
- Currant jelly like stools with mucous and blood
- Failure to grow and weight loss
- Vomiting that is bile stained with a foul odor
- Increasing absence of stools
- A palpable sausage-like mass in the upper right quadrant of the stomach
- Between episodes the child is comfortable

Dx: Based on infant's or child's history; barium enema shows obstruction to the flow of barium; ultrasound of abdomen to identify the location

Rx: To reduce the intussusception, a nonsurgical hydrostatic reduction of the bowel is attempted with a barium enema or use of a water-soluble contrast and air pressure. Surgery is used if treatments are not successful. First, a manual reduction of the telescoping bowel is tried. If this is not effective and if the bowel is gangrenous or strangulated, a resection of the affected bowel is performed

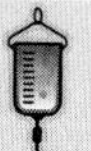

Clinical Alert

Hydrostatic reduction is not recommended when the infant or child shows signs of perforation or shock.

Without treatment, necrosis with hemorrhage, strangulation of the intestine, perforation, gangrene, and peritonitis occur. This is considered a pediatric emergency; these complications may be fatal.

Nursing Process Elements

- Check vital signs frequently, increased pulse and decreased blood pressure may indicate peritonitis

- Monitor I&O
- Check for bleeding
- Evaluate for fluid and electrolyte imbalances
- Offer reassurance and information about treatment to the parents
- Observe for passage of barium or contrast material
- Encourage parents to participate in child's care to help reduce stress
- Postoperative care
  —manage pain
  —assess vital signs
  —maintain NG tube functioning
  —evaluate bowel sounds

Client teaching for self-care

- Encourage parents to monitor stools and note any changes
- Instruct parents to notify physician if symptoms reoccur, appetite is poor, and a fever develops
- Teach parents that reoccurence can occur after nonsurgical treatment
- Provide pre- and postoperative teaching about abdominal surgery

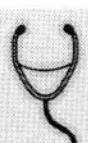

Assessment Alert

Report passage of a normal stool, this indicates that the intussusception has been reduced.

BOWEL OBSTRUCTION

- Bowel obstruction may be mechanical if a result of narrowing of the bowel lumen.
- It may be nonmechanical if a result of impaired peristalsis.
- Either type may be partial or complete.

Etiology:

- Mechanical—adhesions, hernias, volvulus (twisting of intestine on self), tumors, intussusception (leading segment of bowel invaginates into an adjacent segment), strictures from IBD, fecal impaction.
- Nonmechanical—paralytic or adynamic ileus (impaired or absent peristalsis for 72 hours, common after abdominal surgery), failure of nervous innervation as seen in Parkinson's disease, MS, Hirschsprung's disease, metabolic factors as seen with endocrine disorders such as diabetes mellitus, effects of drugs.

When an obstruction causes ischemia of the bowel, the bowel becomes increasingly permeable to bacteria and the risk of peritonitis increases. Paralytic ileus rarely causes ischemia.

S&S:

- Abdominal pain: crampy, poorly localized
- N&V: profuse with small bowel obstruction, may have fecal odor if distal small bowel, occurs late in process if large bowel obstructed
- Frequent high-pitched bowel sounds early; decreased or absent, late in obstruction
- Abdominal distention
- Obstipation
- Signs of dehydration and fluid shifts: dry mucous membrane, decreased skin turgor, decreased urinary output, hemoconcentration, hypokalemia, and hyponatremia

Dx: Based on S&S, abdominal X-ray shows air and fluid trapped in obstructed area; once hypovolemia is severe, Hct and Hgb increase and serum K+ decreases

Rx:

- Correct fluid and electrolyte imbalance
- Decompress the GI tract by means of an NG tube and suction to relieve distention, pain, and vomiting
- Prevent infection by use of antibiotics to combat bacterial overgrowth in the bowel
- Promotility drugs may be used for nonmechanical obstruction
- Usually bowel resection with end-to-end anastomosis though an ostomy is sometimes necessary, for acute, complete obstruction
- Endoscopic balloon dilation or laser removal of tumor segments may be done for mechanical obstruction

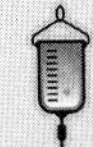

Clinical Alert

Opioids are not given because of their negative effects on peristalsis. Other analgesics are used sparingly because they can conceal the pattern and severity of pain needed for diagnosis.

Nursing Process Elements

- Assess vital signs, urinary output, NG tube output, pain, fluid and electrolyte values, especially serum K+
- Check for edema and measure abdominal girth every 2–4 hours because of third spacing of fluids
- Be alert for signs of shock

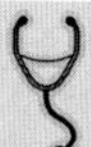

Assessment Alert

Immediately report pain that changes from crampy to constant and/or increases significantly. This can mean perforation or strangulation of the bowel.

- Administer IV fluids and potassium supplement as ordered to make up for loses due to vomiting and fluid shifts
- Elevate the head of the bed to relieve pressure on abdomen; side lying often comfortable
- Assist OOB and ambulate to promote peristalsis as ordered
- Keep NPO with small amounts of ice chips for thirst
- Provide frequent oral and nasal care

PERITONITIS

- Peritonitis refers to a local or generalized inflammation of the peritoneum.
- In response to this acute inflammation, large amounts of fluid shift into the abdominal cavity, blood is shunted to the involved area, and peristalsis slows or stops. Bowel becomes distended with gas and fluid.

Etiology: Most often due to bacteria entering the peritoneal cavity

- through an opening in the intestinal wall due to trauma, surgical injury, ruptured appendix, perforation associated with peptic ulcer, diverticulitis, ulcerative colitis, Crohn's disease, or malignancy.
- by extension of infection through the wall of a hollow organ such as the gall bladder, uterus, or urinary bladder.
- secondary to continuous ambulatory peritoneal dialysis.

Also may occur due to chemical irritation from GI secretions secondary to a leak in a GI suture line or hemorrhagic pancreatitis.

S&S:

- Local or diffuse abdominal pain, rebound tenderness, guarding, and rigidity
- Distention and absence of bowel sounds as inflammation progresses
- Generalized: fever (100–101 F), elevated WBC, N&V
- S&S of early shock (tachycardia, tachypnea, oliguria, restlessness, weakness, pallor, diaphoresis)
- GERI S&S initially significantly less severe in older clients

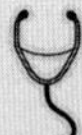

Assessment Alert

Pain may be absent in elderly clients as well as those with severe diabetic neuropathy, those on high doses of corticosteroids or analgesics, or those under the influence of alcohol.

Dx: Based on history, physical findings, abdominal X-ray showing abnormal gas and air patterns

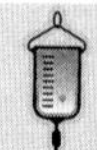

Clinical Alert

WBC counts elevated to 20,000/mm^3 or higher with a shift to the left are the most common indicators of peritonitis in immunocompromised clients.

Rx: Fluid and electrolyte replacement; antibiotics based on culture of blood and peritoneal fluid; NG tube to relieve gastric distention; surgery to correct underlying problem and remove infected material. Parenteral nutrition if sepsis is severe and prolonged recovery is expected

Nursing Process Elements

- Assess S&S, vital signs, and I&O including NG tube drainage. Be particularly alert for signs of shock and for impaired ventilation secondary to pain and abdominal distention
- Monitor electrolyte values for deviations from normal range
- Maintain bed rest in semi-Fowler's position to promote ventilation and comfort
- Encourage deep breathing because of the risk of hypoventilation
- Institute measures to reduce client and family anxiety, which tends to be significant because of the rapid onset of the disease

APPENDICITIS

Etiology: Perhaps obstruction.

S&S:

- Pain is the primary symptom; classical presentation—vague periumbilical or epigastric discomfort, which intensifies, becomes colicky, and localizes in LRQ in about 4 hours.

Variations—diffuse, lower abdominal pain, which may radiate to R thigh or testicle or even localize in LLQ. Sudden relief of pain if rupture occurs, subsequently pain from peritonitis develops. Pain worse on coughing; relieved with flexion of right knee on abdomen

- Tenderness over McBurney's point (midway between umbilicus and right anterior iliac spine)
- Anorexia, nausea with or without vomiting
- Rigidity of rectus muscle and rebound tenderness
- Low grade fever (100.4–101.4°F); higher if appendix ruptured
- Leukocytosis (12,000/mm^3 or more) with increased neutrophils

Dx: Often difficult especially in young children and elderly clients

Rx: NPO, no analgesics which can mask symptoms; no laxatives or enemas which can stimulate peristalsis and cause perforation; IV antibiotics, appendectomy ASAP

Nursing Process Elements

See appendectomy in the section on surgery

DIVERTICULAR DISEASE

- Diverticulum: a small, finger-like, outpouching of the mucosa through the muscle bands of the colon.
- Diverticulosis refers to the presence of diverticula.
- Number of diverticula increases with age. GERI
- Most diverticula are asymptomatic.
- Diverticulitis—acute inflammation of a diverticulum secondary to obstruction with mucus or fecal matter.

Etiology: Increased intraluminal pressure and decreased muscle strength in the colon.

Risk factors: Low-fiber diet and aging.

S&S:

- Crampy LLQ abdominal pain with low-grade fever is classic presentation of diverticulitis
- N&V and bloating also common
- Occasionally abrupt, copious, self-limited rectal bleeding and urinary symptoms occur

Complications: Abscess, (symptoms of local peritonitis), perforation with peritonitis

Dx: CT scan shows diverticula and abscesses; episode of diverticulitis diagnosed based on Hx and physical examination

Rx: NPO or clear fluid diet to rest the bowel, IV fluids, antibiotics, analgesics, anticholinergics to decrease bowel spasms

- Relief in 48–72 hours
- Surgical bowel resection with or without a temporary colostomy may be necessary to treat abscesses or perforation

Nursing Process Elements

- Assess for S&S with special attention to
  - —pain and fluid and electrolyte balance
  - —response to therapy
  - —development of complications such as bleeding, perforation, and peritonitis

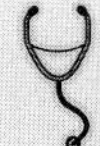

Assessment Alert

Usual symptoms are less pronounced or underreported in older clients. GERI

Client teaching for self-care

- For prevention of episodes of diverticulitis, instruct client to
  - —consume diet to prevent constipation—2500–3000 ml fluids per day, high-fiber, soft foods such as fruits, vegetables, and whole grains with small amounts of bran added to foods or use of bulk forming agents as needed
  - —avoid activities that increase intra-abdominal pressure
  - —lose weight if needed to lower resting intra-abdominal pressure
- Teach client to avoid high-fiber foods during episodes of diverticulitis because of irritating effect

ABDOMINAL HERNIAS

Hernia refers to the protrusion of an organ through an abnormal opening. Abdominal hernias are most common and involve protrusion of intestine out of the abdominal cavity.

Abdominal hernia is classified based on location:

- Inguinal—Occurs in the groin where the spermatic cord in men and the round ligament in women emerge through the abdominal wall.
- Femoral—Occurs at the femoral ring, usually in women.
- Incisional—Occurs at the site of a surgical incision.

Hernias are further classified as the following:

- Reducible—can be manually placed back into abdominal cavity.
- Irreducible or incarcerated—cannot be pushed back into abdominal cavity.

- Strangulated—irreducible with obstruction of both blood flow to the involved intestine and flow of contents through the intestine.

S&S: Visible or palpable protrusion, more obvious on coughing or bearing down, discomfort at site, S&S of intestinal obstruction if strangulated

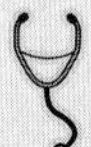

Assessment Alert

Crampy abdominal pain and abdominal distention are symptoms of bowel obstruction due to a strangulated hernia.

Dx: Physical examination

Rx: Manual reduction, use of a truss (pad placed over hernia and held in place with a belt). Herniorrhaphy (hernia repair) with or without hernioplasty (reinforcement of weakened area) if strangulated or as prophylaxis against strangulation

Nursing Process Elements

- Assess for skin irritation in clients who wear a truss
- Teach client about the symptoms of strangulation and the importance of immediate report to a health care provider
- For pre- and postoperative care, see section on herniorrhaphy

COLORECTAL CANCER

- Most colorectal cancers develop from epithelium; they may project into lumen or the encircle bowel and cause stenosis, ulceration, or perforation.
- They spread through the bowel wall into the small intestine or uterus or via lymph and portal vein to liver (most common), lungs, kidneys, or bones.

Etiology: Interaction of genetic and environmental factors.

Risk factors:

- Family history or previous self-history of colorectal cancer; familial polyposis, colorectal polyps, or chronic IBD.
- Diet has not been shown to increase risk; heavy alcohol intake and smoking appear to slightly increase the risk. Long-term use (5 years) of ASA or NSAIDs appears to decrease risk.

S&S: Often asymptomatic early in disease; then vary with tumor location.

- Left colon: constipation or diarrhea along with gradual development of flat, ribbon-like or pencil-shaped stool, crampy gas pains, bright red blood in stool, and abdominal distention
- Right colon: vague, dull abdominal pain worsened with walking, and dark red or mahogany blood in stool
- Rectal cancer: straining at stool, mucous discharge, sense of incomplete rectal emptying, bright red bleeding, and pain in late disease
- Systemic S&S of late disease: weakness, anorexia, weight loss, and anemia

Dx: Biopsy, which can be done via colonoscope, provides the definitive diagnosis. Tumors low in the rectum are often found on digital rectal examination, higher tumors on colonoscopy or suggested by a positive stool for occult blood. Other studies include CT of the abdomen and pelvis to size and localize the tumor and check for local invasion and metastases to the liver or other area. CEA levels are useful in judging response to therapy

Rx:

- Surgery is preferred therapy because it offers potential for cure. Procedure depends on location of tumor:
  —Left hemicolectomy
  —Right hemicolectomy
  —Abdominal—perineal resection
  —Laparoscopic colectomy
- Radiation may be used preoperatively or to shrink tumors and relieve symptoms in advanced disease
- Chemotherapy is used when lymph nodes are positive or metastases are found. Common drugs used are: 5-FU, methotrexate, levamisole, and irinotecan

Nursing Process Elements

See sections on intestinal resection, abdominal–perineal resection, radiation therapy, and chemotherapy. Also see sections on screening and health promotion

HEMORRHOIDS

Hemorrhoids refer to dilated, swollen rectal veins and are of the following types:

- Internal—protrude within the rectal canal.
- External—protrude at the anal opening.

Etiology: Stasis in anal veins.

Risk factors: Straining at stool, prolonged sitting on the toilet, heavy lifting, prolonged standing, pregnancy, infiltrating cancer, portal hypertension secondary to liver disease.

S&S:

- Internal—pain and bleeding on defecation; bleeding is red, often appears as red streaks on stool or toilet tissue

- External—rectal itching, lumps of pink to red tissue at anus (tender, tense, and blue if thrombosed)

Dx:

- External—visual inspection
- Internal—Visualization with an anoscope

Rx:

- Symptomatic treatment:
  - —Sitz baths and topical preparations such as dibucaine ointment to shrink mucous membrane and relieve pain
  - —High-fiber diet, 2000 ml or more fluid per day, stool softeners or mild laxatives to keep stool soft and formed and prevent straining
- Alternative treatment of internal hemorrhoids:
  - —Rubber band ligation
    - Rubber bands placed at bottom of hemorrhoids that bleed or are prolapsed
    - Result is ischemia with necrosis and sloughing in about a week
    - Outpatient procedure not requiring anesthesia
    - Slight postoperative discomfort easily managed with OTC analgesic
  - —Sclerosing Rx: An agent such as 5% phenol in oil is injected subcutaneously between and around hemorrhoids; results in sclerosis and shrinking of tissue; one to four injections 5–7 days apart
- Neither Rx used for external hemorrhoids—too painful due to sensory innervation of area.
- Hemorrhoidectomy—removal of hemorrhoids—done in cases of multiple prolapsed or thrombosed hemorrhoids with severe symptoms (see hemorrhoidectomy under surgery)

Nursing Process Elements

- Assess for S&S with particular attention to frequency and severity of each
- Assess for lifestyle factors such as prolonged standing at work, heavy lifting, bowel and toilet habits that can predispose to hemorrhoids

Client teaching for self-care

Instruct client to

- avoid activities that can contribute to development or worsening of hemorrhoids when possible
- prevent constipation and straining at stool by eating a high-fiber diet with 2000 ml of fluid per day, taking stool softeners or mild laxatives as directed, and exercising regularly
- use sitz baths and topical preparations such as cold witch hazel compresses or dibucaine ointment for relief of symptoms
- report excessive pain, bleeding, or prolapse of hemorrhoids

PEDS HIRSCHSPRUNG'S DISEASE

- Hirschsprung's disease refers to an obstructive disorder of the colon caused by the absence of autonomic parasympathetic ganglion cells resulting in inadequate motility.
- It is also called congenital aganglionic megacolon.

Etiology: The precise etiology is unclear; absence of ganglion cells in the GI tract results in a lack of enervation needed for peristalsis or propulsive movements. This results in accumulation of intestinal contents proximal to the problem; usually includes the rectum and proximal portion of the large intestine; develops during embryonic development.

Precipitating factors: Occurs more often in males in the ratio 4:1; the greatest percentage of cases are detected by the first year while some remain undetected by 3 years of age; may develop along with Down's syndrome, congenital heart defects, and Waardenburg syndrome; disease is related to a genetic component.

S&S: Vary with age

- Newborn and infant:
  - —newborn's failure to pass meconium within approximately 24–48 hours
  - —reluctance to take feedings, failure to suck
  - —abdominal distention
  - —bile stained and fecal vomiting
  - —constipation
  - —dehydration
  - —failure to thrive
- Older child:
  - —without symptoms at birth
  - —progressive abdominal distention
  - —stools are watery, ribbon or pellet-like
  - —vomiting
  - —constipation
  - —failure to gain weight and delayed growth

Dx: Assessment for signs of bowel obstruction; newborn's failure to pass meconium; barium enema reveals structural changes: client may fail to evacuate the barium; rectal biopsy to check for presence or absence of ganglion cells; an anorectal manometry demonstrates failure of the intestinal sphincter to relax in response to distention and palpation reveals a small rectum

Rx: For a mild defect treatment, it is based on relieving constipation; dietary modification; administering stool softeners and using isotonic irrigations to prevent impaction. Surgery is required for most infants and children, removal of the ganglion portion of the intestine relieves obstruction and provides for normal bowel function or a temporary colostomy is formed and repaired when the child is about 20 lbs or 9 kg

Nursing Process Elements

- Obtain a complete history of nutritional intake, weight gain, and bowel habits
- Evaluate bowel sounds and abdominal distention; measure abdominal circumference at the umbilicus
- Maintain fluid and electrolyte balance
- Provide adequate nutrition to promote healing and to prepare for surgery if needed
- Administer daily irrigation with normal saline solution to promote adequate elimination
- Assess family concerns and how they will deal with the problem; support parent and promote infant bonding
- To relieve anxiety for an older child, evaluate his/her feelings about constipation and treatments
- Refer parents to a home care agency for supportive continuing care

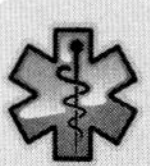

Nursing Intervention Alert

If Hirschsprung's disease does occur in an older child, he or she can be taught to take total care of the colostomy.

Client teaching for self-care

- Instruct parents to notify the physician if no stool is passed
- Teach parents about the infant's or child's health needs such as irrigation, low-residue diet
- Offer pre- and postoperative teaching: place diapers below site to avoid infection
- Instruct parents to participate in colostomy care and child care also. Inform parents that the colostomy is temporary

PEDS IMPERFORATE ANUS

- Imperforate anus refers to the absence of a normal rectal opening.
- It is also called anal atresia.

Etiology: Malformation occurring during fetal development; rectum can end and not connect to the anus or may connect to wrong location as the vagina, urethra, or bladder; anal agenesis in which rectal pouch ends blindly above the perineum, can be an anal fistula formation or anal stenosis; defect is classified as high or low according to the relationship to the levator ani muscles; no prevention is known.

Predisposing factors: Due to an abnormal congenital defect formed during fetal development; associated with other congenital defects as Down's syndrome, cardiac defects, esophageal atresia, or renal anomalies.

S&S:

- Without an anal opening, or misplaced anal opening
- No passage of stool 24–48 hours after birth
- Passage of meconium from vagina or urinary meatus
- Abdominal distention

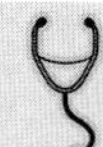

Assessment Alert

Evaluate for complications such as bowel incontinence, intestinal obstruction, constipation, or infection.

Dx: Made by examination of the perineum, abdominal X-ray, ultrasound of rectal and vaginal areas to evaluate for malformations

Rx: Prophylactic antibiotics; excision of membrane; daily anal dilation by nurse and at home by parents; surgical reconstruction, called an anoplasty, to repair malformations; postoperative pain medications; temporary colostomy may be performed if classified as high

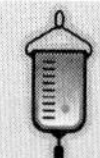

Clinical Alert

Successful treatment depends upon location of the abnormality and age and sex of client.

Nursing Process Elements

- Assess newborn for malformations
- Instruct parents about the problems caused by imperforate anus
- Assess for other congenital problems
- Perform manual dilation, as ordered

- Preoperative care
  - —Administer broad-spectrum antibiotics as ordered
  - —Maintain NG tube, used for decompression
- Postoperative care
  - —Keep perineum very clean
  - —Position client on side for easy access to perineum and to prevent pressure on site
- Monitor vital signs and general condition
- Begin formula when normal peristalsis is present

Client teaching for self-care

- Offer reassurance to parents, especially for a child with a colostomy; inform that colostomy will later be reanastomased
- Teach parents correct technique for manual dilation of anus
- Instruct parents to perform scrupulous care of perineal area
- Review care of colostomy, if needed
- Inform parents not to take a rectal temperature

WORKSHEET

SHORT ANSWER QUESTIONS

1. Why is it important to decrease crying in an infant who has had cleft-palate repair?
2. Which piece of equipment should be available at the bedside of a patient with a fractured jaw that has been wired in place?
3. Why does cancer of the tongue metastasize rapidly?
4. What surgical procedure treats GERD by reinforcing the LES?
5. Which is the most common symptom of esophageal cancer?
6. What are the two major causes of hemorrhagic gastritis?
7. Gnawing epigastric pain occurring 1–3 hours after meals and at night is characteristic of which GI problem?
8. In what position would an infant be placed after surgery for an imperforate anus?
9. When are antibiotics used to treat gastroenteritis?
10. Vomiting a half to one hour after feeding and visible peristalsis in an infant are symptoms of which problem?
11. At what age does colic usually disappear?
12. Results of which laboratory tests must be monitored in patients taking immune modulators?
13. What observation indicates that intussusception has been reduced?
14. Which type of analgesic is contraindicated for pain associated with bowel obstruction?
15. Promotility drugs may be used to treat which type of bowel obstruction?

(continued)

16. What is the most common sign of peritonitis in immunocompromised clients?
17. How should a client with peritonitis be positioned while on bed rest?
18. Which two categories of drugs are contraindicated in a client with possible appendicitis?
19. What type of diet should a client ingest during an episode of diverticulitis?
20. What are the two major symptoms that occur when a strangulated hernia causes a bowel obstruction?
21. Stool containing mahogany-colored blood is indicative of cancer in which part of the colon?
22. What is the goal of radiation therapy when it is used in advanced cases of colorectal cancer?
23. What makes a hemorrhoid tender, tense, and blue?
24. Failure of a neonate to pass meconium within 24–48 hours after birth is indicative of which genetically related disease?
25. What type of diet supports the symptomatic relief of hemorrhoids?
26. Why is alcohol contraindicated for clients experiencing symptoms of GERD?
27. What lifestyle habit puts a client at risk for peptic ulcer disease?
28. Why are infants at particular risk for gastroenteritis?
29. Which anomaly has as a major symptom projectile vomiting of stale milk 30–60 minutes after a feeding?
30. Which substance found in some foods cannot be digested by clients with celiac disease?

APPLICATION QUESTIONS

1. When evaluating the ability of a mother to care for her newborn, who has a cleft palate, which maternal behavior would indicate to the nurse that the mother needs teaching?
   a. Supports infant in a low Fowler's position to feed
   b. Burps the infant frequently during feeding
   c. States that weight gain will have to be carefully monitored
   d. Feeds small amounts slowly
2. What symptom reported in the health history of a 55-year-old woman should be interpreted by the nurse as requiring immediate follow-up evaluation for cancer of the right colon?
   a. Black, tarry stools
   b. Loose, frothy stool
   c. Flat, ribbon-shaped stool
   d. Mahogany-colored, formed stool
3. When planning teaching for a client with chronic gastritis, which information should be included?
   a. "Decrease acid secretion by drinking a glass of milk an hour before bedtime."
   b. "Remain in an upright position for at least 30 minutes after meals."
   c. "Avoid foods that are high in simple carbohydrates and fiber or roughage."
   d. "Report development of a sore tongue or sore gums to the health care provider."

4. When teaching at a health fair about the prevention and treatment of hemorrhoids, which information should the nurse include?
   a. "Avoid use of laxatives."
   b. "Avoid strenuous sports."
   c. "Avoid dietary roughage."
   d. "Avoid extended sitting on the toilet."

5. Which symptoms in a man with a left inguinal hernia are indicative of development of hernia strangulation?
   a. Crampy abdominal pain and abdominal distention
   b. Fever and abdominal rigidity
   c. Absence of bowel sounds and LLQ tenderness
   d. RUQ rebound tenderness and flatulence

6. Which is a priority nursing goal, specific to a neonate who has had a cleft-lip repair?
   a. Decrease crying
   b. Keep nares patent
   c. Protect from exposure to cold
   d. Prevent dehydration

7. Allowing parents to practise feeding their infant is a critical aspect of care when the child has which problem?
   a. Failure to thrive
   b. Hirschsprung's disease
   c. Cleft palate
   d. Pyloric stenosis

8. What should a client with a wired jaw following a traumatic fracture be instructed to do if difficulty in breathing occurs?
   a. Cut the wires
   b. Take prescribed decongestant
   c. Use a humidifier
   d. Call the physician

9. When teaching a local club group about oral cancer, which comment by a participant indicates that the nurse needs to clarify the information presented?
   a. "Most oral cancers occur on the tongue."
   b. "The most rapidly spreading oral cancer is on the floor of the mouth."
   c. "Early oral cancers are generally asymptomatic."
   d. "Smoking is a risk factor for cancer of the lip."

10. A client under treatment for GERD asks why she needs to avoid caffeine. What fact should form the basis of the nurse's response?
   a. Caffeine delays gastric emptying
   b. Caffeine lowers LES pressure
   c. Caffeine increases secretion of gastric acid
   d. Caffeine thins the mucus coating of the esophagus

11. The need to avoid factors that increase intra-abdominal pressure is an important part of client teaching about the management of which problem?
   a. Acute gastritis
   b. Paralytic ileus
   c. Diverticulosis
   d. Irritable bowel disease

12. When a patient's medical history indicates Barrett's epithelium, questions should be asked which would elicit information about symptoms of which disease?
   a. Esophageal cancer
   b. Peptic ulcer disease
   c. Crohn's disease
   d. Ulcerative colitis

13. Which findings would the nurse expect when assessing a client with celiac disease? (Select all that apply.)
   a. Steatorrhea
   b. Respiratory alkalosis
   c. Anemia
   d. Leukocytosis
   e. Melena
   f. Anorexia

14. Which is the primary goal of care for a child with a mild case of Hirschsprung's disease?
   a. Promote parent–child bonding
   b. Teach colostomy care
   c. Avoid exposure to gluten products
   d. Relieve constipation

15. Which interventions are appropriate when caring for an infant with colic? (Select all that apply.)
   a. Provide rhythmic movement
   b. Swaddle
   c. Give a cool bath
   d. Massage abdomen
   e. Increase environmental stimuli

16. When corticosteroids are prescribed for a client with Crohn's disease, which dosage protocol should the nurse expect?
   a. Dose will be calculated daily based on serum levels of drug
   b. Loading doses will be given for the first 5 days of therapy
   c. Daily maintenance doses will be initiated after 2–3 days of therapy
   d. Dose will be tapered as soon as symptoms decrease

(continued)

17. Which is a priority teaching point for the client with inflammatory bowel disease (IBD) who is placed on immunomodulator therapy?
    a. "Take with at least 200 ml of Gatorade."
    b. "Expect initial worsening of symptoms."
    c. "Renal function must be regularly monitored."
    d. "No effect may be seen for up to 4 months."
18. Which is an appropriate nursing goal for the client experiencing a flare of ulcerative colitis?
    a. Encourage rest for half an hour before meals to decrease peristalsis
    b. Maintain NPO status
    c. Decrease dietary sodium
    d. Promote relaxation by application of heat to the abdomen
19. When caring for a child who has had a nonsurgical hydrostatic reduction of an intussusception, which finding indicates that the procedure was successful in reducing the intussusception?
    a. Presence of bowel sounds
    b. Absence of abdominal distention
    c. Passage of normal stool
    d. Cessation of abdominal pain
20. When a bowel obstruction causes ischemia of the bowel, the patient is at significantly increased risk for which complication?
    a. Hemorrhage
    b. Peritonitis
    c. Embolus
    d. Hyponatremia
21. Which client would most likely *not* experience abdominal pain associated with peritonitis?
    a. Client with diabetes
    b. Client with HIV infection
    c. Client on high dose of corticosteroids
    d. Client taking an anticholinergic drug
22. Which dietary instruction should be given to a client when the nurse is teaching him or her about the prevention of episodes of diverticulitis?
    a. "Eat low-fiber foods and avoid seeds."
    b. "Avoid spicy, high-fat foods."
    c. "Eat soft, high-fiber foods with 2500–3000 ml of fluid daily."
    d. "Avoid raw fruits, vegetables, and bran products."
23. Which factors found in a client's health history indicate increased risk for colorectal cancer? (Select all that apply.)
    a. Family history of colon polyps
    b. Chronic inflammatory bowel disease
    c. Long-term use of NSAIDs
    d. Diet high in fat and carbohydrate
    e. Chronic constipation
24. Which assessment finding is suggestive of an imperforate anus in a newborn?
    a. Hyperactive bowel sounds
    b. Passage of meconium from the vagina
    c. Fecal vomiting
    d. Sausage-like mass in lower, left quadrant
25. Which assessment finding suggests that the appendix of a client with appendicitis has ruptured?
    a. WBC of 15,000/mm^3
    b. Temperature of 101 F
    c. Sudden relief of abdominal pain
    d. Onset of rebound tenderness

ANSWERS & RATIONALES

SHORT ANSWER QUESTIONS

1. Why is it important to decrease crying in an infant who has had cleft-palate repair?

Answer
Crying increases stress on the suture line.

2. Which piece of equipment should be available at the bedside of a patient with a fractured jaw that has been wired in place?

Answer

Wire cutter.

3. Why does cancer of the tongue metastasize rapidly?

Answer

The tongue has a rich blood and lymph supply.

4. What surgical procedure treats GERD by reinforcing the LES?

Answer

Fundoplication.

5. Which is the most common symptom of esophageal cancer?

Answer

Progressive dysphagia.

6. What are the two major causes of hemorrhagic gastritis?

Answer

NSAID use and stress.

7. Gnawing epigastric pain occurring 1–3 hours after meals and at night is characteristic of which GI problem?

Answer

Duodenal ulcer.

8. In what position would an infant be placed after surgery for an inperforate anus?

Answer

Side lying.

9. When are antibiotics used to treat gastroenteritis?

Answer

If the gastroenteritis is severe and caused by bacteria.

10. Vomiting a half to one hour after feeding and visible peristalsis in an infant are symptoms of which problem?

Answer

Pyloric stenosis.

11. At what age does colic usually disappear?

Answer

At the age of 3 months.

12. Results of which laboratory tests must be monitored in patients taking immune modulators?

Answer

CBC with differential and platelets and LFTs.

13. What observation indicates that intussusception has been reduced?

Answer

Passage of stool.

14. Which type of analgesic is contraindicated for pain associated with bowel obstruction?

Answer

Opioid.

(continued)

15. Promotility drugs may be used to treat which type of bowel obstruction?

Answer

Nonmechanical obstruction.

16. What is the most common sign of peritonitis in immunocompromised clients?

Answer

White blood cell count of 20,000/mm^3 or higher with a shift to the left.

17. How should a client with peritonitis be positioned while on bed rest?

Answer

In semi-Fowler's position.

18. Which two categories of drugs are contraindicated in a client with possible appendicitis?

Answer

Analgesics and laxatives.

19. What type of diet should a client ingest during an episode of diverticulitis?

Answer

Low-fiber diet.

20. What are the two major symptoms that occur when a strangulated hernia causes a bowel obstruction?

Answer

Crampy abdominal pain and abdominal distention.

21. Stool containing mahogany-colored blood is indicative of cancer in which part of the colon?

Answer

Right colon.

22. What is the goal of radiation therapy when it is used in advanced cases of colorectal cancer?

Answer

Relief of symptoms.

23. What makes a hemorrhoid tender, tense, and blue?

Answer

Thrombosis.

24. Failure of a neonate to pass meconium within 24–48 hours after birth is indicative of which genetically related disease?

Answer

Hirschprung's disease.

25. What type of diet supports the symptomatic relief of hemorrhoids?

Answer

High-fiber diet with at least 2000 ml of fluid per day.

26. Why is alcohol contraindicated for clients experiencing symptoms of GERD?

Answer

Alcohol lowers LES pressure and therefore worsens the problem.

27. What lifestyle habit puts a client at risk for peptic ulcer disease?

Answer

Smoking.

28. Why are infants at particular risk for gastroenteritis?

Answer

Infants are at risk for gastroenteritis because their immune systems are immature.

29. Which anomaly has as a major symptom projectile vomiting of stale milk 30–60 minutes after a feeding?

Answer

Pyloric stenosis.

30. Which substance found in some foods cannot be digested by clients with celiac disease?

Answer

Clients with celiac disease cannot digest gluten.

APPLICATION ANSWERS

1. When evaluating the ability of a mother to care for her newborn, who has a cleft palate, which maternal behavior would indicate to the nurse that the mother needs teaching?
   a. Supports infant in a low Fowler's position to feed
   b. Burps the infant frequently during feeding
   c. States that weight gain will have to be carefully monitored
   d. Feeds small amounts slowly

Rationale

Correct answer: a.

The infant's head should be held upright for feeding therefore option "a" is an incorrect behavior which indicates the mother needs more teaching. Options "b," "c," and "d" are all correct. The infant with a cleft palate should be fed small amounts slowly and for a short time; burped frequently to help prevent regurgitation and aspiration; and weight needs to be monitored to determine if the infant is getting sufficient nourishment.

Think Smart/Test Smart

Note: This question asks what behavior indicates the mother needs more teaching. More teaching is required when something is not known or something is wrong. Therefore, you are looking for a behavior that is incorrect.

2. What symptom reported in the health history of a 55-year-old woman should be interpreted by the nurse as requiring immediate follow-up evaluation for cancer of the right colon?
   a. Black, tarry stools
   b. Loose, frothy stool
   c. Flat, ribbon-shaped stool
   d. Mahogany-colored, formed stool

Rationale

Correct answer: d.

A symptom of right-sided cancer of the colon is mahogany-colored stool due to the presence of blood from the tumor being mixed with the stool and exposed to digestive tract secretions as it progresses through the remaining colon. Black, tarry stools are indicative of blood from the upper GI tract which has been in the GI tract long enough to be completely digested. Loose, frothy stool is indicative of high fat content and is associated with malabsorptive disorders. Flat, ribbon-shaped stool is consistent with a tumor which alters the shape of the left colon and prevents formation and passage of normally formed stool.

3. When planning teaching for a client with chronic gastritis, which information should be included?
   a. "Decrease acid secretion by drinking a glass of milk an hour before bedtime."
   b. "Remain in an upright position for at least 30 minutes after meals."
   c. "Avoid foods that are high in simple carbohydrates and fiber or roughage."
   d. "Report development of a sore tongue or mouth to the health care provider."

Rationale

Correct answer: d.

Clients with chronic gastritis are at risk for developing pernicious anemia because of a deficiency of intrinsic factor produced in the stomach, which is necessary for the

(continued)

absorption of vitamin B 12 in the ileum. Glossitis, sore tongue, and stomatitis (sore oral mucous membranes) are two presenting symptoms of pernicious anemia.

4. When teaching at a health fair about the prevention and treatment of hemorrhoids, which information should the nurse include?
   a. "Avoid use of laxatives."
   b. "Avoid strenuous sports."
   c. "Avoid dietary roughage."
   d. "Avoid extended sitting on the toilet."

Rationale

Correct answer: d.

Extended sitting on the toilet increases stasis of blood and pressure in the anal veins and predisposes to hemorrhoid formation so it should be avoided.

Routine use of laxatives is not a good health practice but laxatives do not directly contribute to hemorrhoid development. Roughage in the diet is essential for good bowel function. Prolonged standing and heavy lifting are contraindicated but strenuous sports as a group are not.

5. Which symptoms in a man with a left inguinal hernia are indicative of development of hernia strangulation?
   a. Crampy abdominal pain and abdominal distention
   b. Fever and abdominal rigidity
   c. Absence of bowel sounds and LLQ tenderness
   d. RUQ rebound tenderness and flatulence

Rationale

Correct answer: a.

Crampy abdominal pain and distention are symptoms of bowel obstruction due to strangulation (irreducible hernia with obstruction of both blood flow and bowel contents). Fever and abdominal rigidity are signs of peritonitis. Absence of bowel sounds occur late in obstruction not when it first develops. Pain is poorly localized and crampy. Flatulence is not associated with hernia strangulation.

6. Which is a priority nursing goal, specific to a neonate who has had a cleft-lip repair?
   a. Decrease crying
   b. Keep nares patent
   c. Protect from exposure to cold
   d. Prevent dehydration

Rationale

Correct answer: a.

Crying increases tension on the suture line and can disrupt it. Keeping nares patent is not specific to an infant with a cleft-palate repair because all neonates are nose breathers so keeping nares patent is important for all. Similarly all neonates need to be protected from cold and from dehydration, not just those with a cleft-lip repair.

7. Allowing parents to practice feeding their infant is a critical aspect of care when the child has which problem?
   a. Failure to thrive
   b. Hirschsprung's disease
   c. Cleft palate
   d. Pyloric stenosis

Rationale

Correct answer: c.

Cleft palate results in feeding difficulties with risk of regurgitation, aspiration, and inadequate nutrition and in addition, requires use of various techniques and adaptive devices depending on the extent of the abnormality. As a result, it is critical that parents have the opportunity to practice feeding the infant.

8. What should a client with a wired jaw following a traumatic fracture be instructed to do if difficulty in breathing occurs?
   a. Cut the wires
   b. Take prescribed decongestant
   c. Use a humidifier
   d. Call the physician.

Rationale

Correct answer: d.

Call the physician for direction appropriate to the problem. Wires would be cut if the patient started to choke or vomit and needed to expel material from the mouth to avoid blocking the respiratory tree.

9. When teaching a local club group about oral cancer, which comment by a participant indicates that the nurse needs to clarify the information presented?
   a. "Most oral cancers occur on the tongue."
   b. "The most rapidly spread oral cancer is on the floor of the mouth."
   c. "Early oral cancers are generally asymptomatic."
   d. "Smoking is a risk factor for cancer of the lip."

Rationale

Correct answer: b.

The most rapidly spread oral cancer is not cancer of the floor of the mouth but the cancer of the tongue because of its rich blood and lymph supply.

Think Smart/Test Smart

The question asks which information must be clarified. That means you must identify which information is wrong or misunderstood. Option "b" contains incorrect information because the most rapidly spread oral cancer is the cancer of the tongue.

10. A client under treatment for GERD asks why she needs to avoid caffeine. What fact should form the basis of the nurse's response?
    a. Caffeine delays gastric emptying
    b. Caffeine lowers LES pressure
    c. Caffeine increases secretion of gastric acid
    d. Caffeine thins the mucus coating of the esophagus

Rationale

Correct answer: b.

Caffeine lowers lower esophageal sphincter pressure and thus increases the likelihood of reflux of gastric contents into the esophagus. Delayed gastric emptying may contribute to GERD but it is not caused by caffeine. Increased gastric acid is unrelated to the development of GERD. The stomach mucosa has a thick mucus coating to aid in protecting against gastric enzymes; the esophagus does not.

11. The need to avoid factors that increase intra-abdominal pressure is an important part of client teaching about the management of which problem?
    a. Acute gastritis
    b. Paralytic ileus
    c. Diverticulosis
    d. Irritable bowel disease

Rationale

Correct answer: c.

Diverticuli are outpouchings of intestinal mucosa through the muscle bands of the colon associated with increased intraluminal pressure and muscle weakness. Increasing intra-abdominal pressure can increase or worsen diverticula. It is unrelated to acute gastritis, paralytic ileus, or irritable bowel disease.

12. When a patient's medical history indicates Barrett's epithelium, questions should be asked which would elicit information about symptoms of which disease?
    a. Esophageal cancer
    b. Peptic ulcer disease
    c. Crohn's disease
    d. Ulcerative colitis

Rationale

Correct answer: a.

Barrett's epithelium, which is abnormal epithelium in the lower esophagus, is a risk factor for adenocarcinoma of the esophagus after 10–20 years. Barrett's epithelium is not a risk factor for PUD, Crohn's disease, or ulcerative colitis.

13. Which findings would the nurse expect when assessing a client with celiac disease? (Select all that apply.)
    a. Steatorrhea
    b. Respiratory alkalosis
    c. Anemia
    d. Leukocytosis
    e. Melena
    f. Anorexia

Rationale

Correct answers: a, c, and f.

Celiac disease is a malabsorption syndrome related to the inability to breakdown gluten, a protein found in wheat, rye, oats, and barley. Steatorrhea results from the inability to absorb fats and anemia from iron and protein deficiency. Anorexia also occurs. Respiratory alkalosis, leukocytosis, and melena are not signs or symptoms of celiac disease.

14. Which is the primary goal of care for a child with a mild case of Hirschsprung's disease?
    a. Promote parent–child bonding
    b. Teach colostomy care
    c. Avoid exposure to gluten products
    d. Relieve constipation

Rationale

Correct answer: d.

Mild defects only require measures to prevent constipation. More severe defects, which are the majority, require surgical removal of the affected area of intestine. Occasionally, a temporary colostomy is created. Parent–child bonding is important for all children and the child with mild Hirschsprung's disease does not present a significant risk for impaired bonding. Avoidance of gluten products is essential for the child with celiac disease, not Hirschsprung's disease.

15. Which interventions are appropriate when caring for an infant with colic? (Select all that apply.)
    a. Provide rhythmic movement
    b. Swaddle
    c. Give a cool bath
    d. Massage abdomen
    e. Increase environmental stimuli

Rationale

Correct answers: a, b, and d.

There is no medical treatment for colic however rhythmic movement, swaddling, and abdominal massage are often effective in soothing the infant. Decreasing environmental stimuli, not increasing stimuli, and warm, not cold, baths may also be helpful.

16. When corticosteroids are prescribed for a client with Crohn's disease, which dosage protocol should the nurse expect?
    a. Dose will be calculated daily based on serum levels of drug
    b. Loading doses will be given for the first 5 days of therapy

(continued)

c. Daily maintenance doses will be initiated after 2–3 days of therapy

d. Dose will be tapered as soon as symptoms decrease

Rationale

Correct answer: d.

Doses are tapered as soon as a clinical response is obtained. Doses are not calculated on serum levels of blood and loading doses and maintenance doses do not apply.

17. Which is a priority teaching point for the client with inflammatory bowel disease (IBD) who is placed on immunomodulator therapy?
   a. "Take with at least 200 ml of Gatorade."
   b. "Expect initial worsening of symptoms."
   c. "Renal function must be regularly monitored."
   d. "No effect may be seen for up to 4 months."

Rationale

Correct answer: d.

The effect of immunomodulator therapy such as mercaptopurine for ulcerative colitis or infliximab for Crohn's Disease may not be seen for 4 months. Symptoms do not worsen with initiation of these drugs and they do not have to be taken with Gatorade. CBCs with platelets and liver function need to be monitored but not renal function

18. Which is an appropriate nursing goal for the client experiencing a flare of ulcerative colitis?
   a. Encourage rest for half an hour before meals to decrease peristalsis
   b. Maintain NPO status
   c. Decrease dietary sodium
   d. Promote relaxation by application of heat to the abdomen

Rationale

Correct answer: b.

For severe episodes, clients are NPO, on bed rest, and receive IV rehydration and parenteral nutrition, if needed, for malnutrition. Rest after meals decreases peristalsis and is helpful in decreasing diarrhea. Dietary salt is needed during flares to make up for loss. A warm heating pad to the abdomen can provide comfort but should not be used during acute flare-ups of the disease.

19. When caring for a child who has had a nonsurgical hydrostatic reduction of an intussusception, which finding indicates that the procedure was successful in reducing the intussusception?
   a. Presence of bowel sounds
   b. Absence of abdominal distention
   c. Passage of normal stool
   d. Cessation of abdominal pain

Rationale

Correct answer: c.

Passage of normal stool beyond the point of intussusception is impossible. Once the intussusception is reduced the bowel is no longer obstructed so normal stool can pass. Bowel sounds, absence of distention, and cessation of abdominal pain are not specific indicators of reduction.

20. When a bowel obstruction causes ischemia of the bowel, the patient is at significantly increased risk for which complication?
   a. Hemorrhage
   b. Peritonitis
   c. Embolus
   d. Hyponatremia

Rationale

Correct answer: b.

When an obstruction causes ischemia of the bowel, the bowel becomes increasingly permeable to bacteria and the risk of peritonitis also increases. Ischemia is not associated with increased risk for hemorrhage, embolism, or hyponatremia.

21. Which client would be most likely *not* experience abdominal pain associated with peritonitis?
   a. Client with diabetes
   b. Client with bone marrow disease
   c. Client on high dose of corticosteroids
   d. Client taking an anticholinergic drug

Rationale

Correct answer: c.

High doses of corticosteroids inhibit the inflammatory reaction of which pain is a classic sign. Diabetic clients if they have severe neuropathy, and clients taking high doses of analgesics or under the influence of alcohol may also not experience pain. Bone marrow diseases as a group and anticholinergic drugs are unrelated to the occurrence of pain with peritonitis.

22. Which dietary instruction should be given to a client when the nurse is teaching him or her about the prevention of episodes of diverticulitis?
   a. "Eat low-fiber foods and avoid seeds."
   b. "Avoid spicy, high-fat foods."
   c. "Eat soft, high-fiber foods with 2500–3000 ml of fluid daily."
   d. "Avoid raw fruits, vegetables, and bran products."

Rationale

Correct answer: c.

To prevent episodes of diverticulitis, constipation must be prevented. Thus, a diet of soft foods that are high in fiber such as fruits, vegetables and whole grains with small amounts of bran and 2500–3000 ml of fluid daily is recommended. NPO or clear fluid diet is used in treatment of acute episodes to rest the bowel.

Think Smart/Test Smart

Note the question asks about preventing episodes of diverticulitis, not treating them.

23. Which factors found in a client's health history indicate increased risk for colorectal cancer? (Select all that apply.)
    a. Family history of colon polyps
    b. Chronic inflammatory bowel disease
    c. Long-term use of NSAIDs
    d. Diet high in fat and carbohydrate
    e. chronic constipation

Rationale

Correct answers: a and b.

Chronic inflammatory bowel disease and self or family history of colon polyps or colorectal cancer are major risk factors. Heavy alcohol use and smoking increase risk slightly. Long-term use of NSAIDs appears to decrease risk. Diet and constipation have not been shown to be risk factors.

24. Which assessment finding is suggestive of an imperforate anus in a newborn?
    a. Hyperactive bowel sounds
    b. Passage of meconium from the vagina
    c. Fecal vomiting
    d. Sausage-like mass in lower, left quadrant

Rationale

Correct answer: b.

Passage of meconium from vagina or urethral meatus suggests an imperforate anus. Hyperactive bowel sounds are characteristic of a variety of intestinal disorders including gastroenteritis and early bowel obstruction. Fecal vomiting can occur with distal small bowel obstruction. A sausage-like mass in the Upper Right Quadrant (URQ), not the LLQ, is symptomatic of intussusception.

25. Which assessment finding suggests that the appendix of a client with appendicitis has ruptured?
    a. WBC of 15,000/mm^3
    b. Temperature of 101 F
    c. Sudden relief of abdominal pain
    d. Onset of rebound tenderness

Rationale

Correct answer: c.

Pain is the primary symptom of appendicitis; sudden relief of the pain is associated with rupture and release of pressure. Subsequently, pain from the resulting peritonitis develops. WBC of 12,000/mm^3 or higher, low-grade fever (100.4–101.4 F), and presence of rebound tenderness are all characteristic of appendicitis prior to rupture.

Test Plan Category:

Physiological Integrity

Sub-category: Physiological Adaptation—Part 1

Topics: Alterations in Body Systems
Illness Management
Section 8: Hepatic and Biliary Tract Problems

HEPATITIS

- Hepatitis is widespread inflammation and necrosis of the liver, which alters structure and function causing impaired metabolism of carbohydrates, fats, proteins, and drugs, impaired detoxification of alcohol and toxins, impaired immune function, and impaired blood clotting.
- It can be acute or chronic with mild to severe symptoms.
- Forms: hepatitis A, HAV; hepatitis B, HBV; hepatitis C, HCV; hepatitis D, HDV; hepatitis E, HEV; and hepatitis G, HGV.
- Hepatitis D occurs only in those infected with hepatitis B.
- Hepatitis E, rare in United States, generally affects young adults.
- Hepatitis B is a main cause of cirrhosis and liver cancer.

Etiology: Viral infection or non-viral inflammation is caused by exposure to drugs, toxins, and chemicals.

Risk factors, mode of transmission, and mean incubation period:

- Hepatitis A: fecal–oral transmission: poor sanitation and overcrowding, ingestion of foods and liquids infected by human waste (shellfish can be a particular risk as can travel to underdeveloped areas), poor hygiene, infected food handlers, and presence of HIV infection. Incubation: 28–30 days
- Hepatitis B: spread by infected blood or body fluids: contact with blood or body fluids including needlesticks, and sexual activity with multiple partners. Incubation: 6–9 weeks
- Hepatitis C: primarily transmitted by contaminated blood and blood products: also suspected from tattooing, body piercing, manicures, and air gun vaccinations
- Hepatitis D: same as hepatitis B

- Hepatitis E: fecal–oral route: fecal contamination of water supplies in developing areas is a high risk. Incubation: 26–42 days

Think Smart/Test Smart

When a risk factor for a disease is contact with blood or body fluids, then groups that are at particular risk include health care workers (MDs, RNs, EMTs, paramedics, phlebotomists, laboratory technicians), recipients of blood transfusions, dialysis clients, transplant recipients, those with multiple sexual partners, IV drug users, etc.

S&S:

- N&V and anorexia
- Dark urine and clay-colored stool
- General aching
- Jaundice
- Pruritus
- Fatigue
- Low-grade fever
- Muscle and joint pain

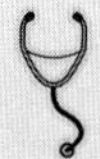

Assessment Alert

Usual course of hepatitis has three stages:

- Preicteric: headache, fatigue, and poor appetite
- Icteric: jaundice, weight loss, and liver tenderness
- Posticteric: energy improved, appetite better, and jaundice decreased.

Dx: Presence of S&S, elevated liver enzymes, serum bilirubin level, ESR, and PT; specific serology tests to identify hepatitis A, B, and C; liver biopsy evaluates chronic hepatitis.

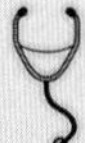

Assessment Alert

In most acute cases, pharmacological treatment is not recommended since most drugs are metabolized in the liver.

Rx: Low-fat, high-carbohydrate diet with increased calories and protein, (not high-protein diet during the acute phase), frequent fluids, small meals as tolerated; IV fluids PRN. Interferon alpha for chronic hepatitis B and C and for acute hepatitis C, this interferes with viral replication, alternative drug for hepatitis B—lamivudine (Epivin HBV), treatment of choice for chronic hepatitis C—interferon alpha plus (Rebetol) ribavirin. Antiemetics for nausea, vitamin K if PT prolonged.

Vaccines:

- Hepatitis A: initial dose then booster in 6–12 months, used if visiting an area with poor sanitation or if IV drug user. For those not vaccinated, immunoglobulin administered IM during incubation period.
- Hepatitis B: three doses, initial dose then second in 1–2 months and a third dose 4–6 months after the first. Third dose results in prolonged immunity. If a dose is not received on schedule, there is no need to start over simply get it as soon as possible. Hepatitis B immunoglobulin provides passive immunity, used for exposure to HBV when not vaccinated.

Nursing Process Elements

- Obtain history of IV drug use, multiple partners, ingestion of contaminated foods or water, and previous history of liver disease
- Monitor VS and I&O
- Assess color of sclera and skin; color of stool and urine; and abdominal contour and tenderness
- Administer IV fluids if unable to tolerate fluids
- Provide periods of rest
- Maintain a quiet, calm environment
- Offer emotional support and diversional activities when recovery is prolonged
- Evaluate PT and administer vitamin K as ordered
- Evaluate for complications such as hypokalemia, dehydration, and fulminant hepatitis

Client teaching for self-care

- Teach client about disease and treatment
- Explain to client and family about prevention of transmission: proper hygiene such as hand washing, food preparation, not sharing eating utensils, use of condoms
- Instruct about prophylactic treatment for those in close contact with infected clients, not necessary if exposed person is vaccinated or known to be immune
- Teach to avoid agents toxic to the liver such as alcohol
- Encourage to drink fluids frequently as tolerated
- Instruct about gradual participation in activities and exercise during convalescence
- Recommend hepatitis A and B vaccine for those in high-risk groups
- Inform adolescents about risks of piercing and tattooing related to transmission of hepatitis C

PEDS BILIARY ATRESIA

- Biliary atresia is the congenital absence of the biliary duct system or acquired fibrosis of the bile duct.
- Accumulation of bile in the liver (cholestasis) takes place.
- Bile fails to reach duodenum
- Untreated biliary atresia leads to cirrhosis of the liver and liver failure in the toddler/preschool period.

Etiology: Unknown. May be the result of an infection or other injury resulting in fibrosis of the bile duct.

Risk factor: More common in girls than boys. Seen more frequently in African-American children than in Caucasians.

S&S:

- Normal appearance at birth
- Symptoms begin to appear at 2–3 months of life
- Accumulation of direct bilirubin leads to jaundice, liver enlargement, and abdominal distention
- Absence of bile in the duodenum leads to clay-colored stools
- Bile salts are excreted in the urine causing tea-colored urine
- Damage to the liver leads to diminished clotting factors with bruising and easy bleeding

Dx: Elevated bilirubin levels; liver tests indicate dysfunction—elevated liver enzymes and prolonged clotting times. Liver biopsy confirms the diagnosis.

Rx: Palliative treatment includes the Kasai surgical procedure (also called a hepatic portoenterostomy), where a portion of the intestine is anastomosed to the hepatic portal extravascular structures to establish bile drainage and reduce liver damage. In a small percentage of children, this may permanently resolve the problem. The majority of children will eventually require a liver transplant. The child will require vitamin K to support clotting, vitamin D to prevent rickets. Antihistamines and cholestyramine may reduce itching from bile excretion through the skin.

Nursing Process Elements

- Emotional support for family during diagnosis and treatment
- Lack of bile salts interferes with absorption of fat-soluble vitamins. Nutritional guidance is given to promote nutrition
- Itching is a major concern that can affect skin integrity and sleep. Tepid baths may promote comfort in addition to medication. Nails should be kept short to prevent skin damage
- Postoperative care is the same as for other abdominal surgeries
- Care after a transplant includes monitoring the child for infection, and liver rejection

Client teaching for self-care

- Teach parents about disease and treatment
- Teach nutritional needs of the child
- Explain to the parents that the child may have bleeding tendencies and teach means of protection for the child as well as bleeding control methods
- Teach the parents measures to reduce itching
- Teach the parents about the surgical procedures
- Explain proper drug administration including the reasons for the medication and side effects of the medications
- Teach the parents of a child with a liver transplant the signs of liver rejection (vomiting, jaundice, and fever)

CIRRHOSIS

- Cirrhosis is a destructive, progressive liver disease resulting in damage to hepatic cells.
- It eventually leads to liver failure.

Etiology:

Two most common causes:

- Alcohol abuse of 10 years or more—can be as little as — two to three drinks per day in women and three to four in men; appears to injure liver by blocking normal metabolism of proteins, fats, and carbohydrates
- Chronic hepatitis C. Infection with this virus causes inflammation of and low-grade damage to the liver that over several decades can lead to cirrhosis

Other causes: Chronic hepatitis B and D, Autoimmune hepatitis, inherited diseases such as alpha-1 antitrypsin deficiency, hemochromatosis, Wilson's disease, galactosemia, and glycogen storage diseases; nonalcoholic steatohepatitis (NASH) that appears to be associated with diabetes, protein malnutrition, obesity, coronary artery disease, and treatment with corticosteroid medications; reactions to drugs, exposure to environmental toxins, infections such as schistosomiasis, and repeated episodes of heart failure (HF). Blocked bile ducts (primary biliary or obstructive cirrhosis): liver damage due to back up of bile. Biliary atresia (bile ducts are absent or injured) is most common cause in infants; in adults, the most common cause is inflammation, blockage, and scarring of the ducts.

Risk factors:

- Alcohol, poor nutrition, bile obstruction, viral hepatitis, drugs, toxins, and chemicals.

S&S:

- Early: anorexia, nausea, vomiting, weight loss, weakness, tender enlarged liver, dull liver pain
- Late: ascites in peritoneal cavity, distended abdomen, peripheral edema, jaundice, and pruritus due to impaired bile excretion and metabolism, brownish urine due to presence of uroblinogen, clay-colored stool due to absence of bilirubin, easy bruising and bleeding due to decreased absorption of vitamin K and low production of prothrombin, splenomegaly, and spider angiomas, gynecomastia, amenorrhea, impotence, infertility due to altered hormone metabolism, hepatic encephalopathy—personality change, mild mental confusion, restlessness, personality change, and possible progression to irreversible coma, changes in handwriting, slurred, slow speech, and unkept appearance
- Complications:
  —Esophogeal Varices—enlarged esophageal veins that rupture and bleed, which develop as a result of elevated pressure in the portal vein (portal hypertension)
  —Insulin resistance and ultimately type 2 diabetes
  —Liver cancer
  —Immune system dysfunction
  —Kidney dysfunction and failure
  —Osteoporosis

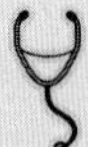

Assessment Alert

Asterixis or liver flap is a symptom defined as jerky movements of the hands and wrists in advanced cirrhosis.

Dx: Elevated alanine aminotransferase, ALT; aspartate aminotransferase, AST; gamma globulin transferase, GTT. Coagulation studies, PT and PTT are prolonged. CT scan shows enlarged liver nodules and vascular changes. Liver scan indicates abnormal thickening of the liver mass. Liver biopsy confirms the diagnosis.

Rx: Directed toward slowing the disease process and treating complications.

- Treat underlying cause, e.g., avoid alcohol, relieve bile obstruction
- Dietary support with vitamins and minerals, reduced protein
- Rest and moderate exercise
- Medications
  —Antiemetics for nausea
  —Diuretics to decrease edema
  —Antihistamines to relieve pruritus
  —Neomycin and lactulose to reduce ammonia-producing bacteria in the GI tract are given for hepatic encephalopathy, which is due in part to the accumulation of ammonia in the blood due to the liver's inability to remove it.
  —Beta-blockers for portal hypertension; for bleeding varices.
- Injection with a clotting agent or a rubber-band ligation.
- Liver transplant for liver failure or uncontrollable complications

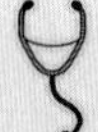

Assessment Alert

Medications cannot reverse the disease process. Hepatotoxic drugs such as opioids, sedatives, INH, acetaminophen, and aspirin are avoided.

Nursing Process Elements

- Assess for fluid retention, check weight, edema, and I&O
- Observe for behavior changes
- Assess skin (prone to breakdown associated with pruritus, decreased mobility, compromised nutrition and edema)
- Maintain bleeding precautions, avoid IM and SC injections.
- Evaluate nutrition
- Promote comfort
- Monitor fluid and electrolyte balance, especially for hypokalemia and sodium retention.
- Long-term, low-protein diet, preferably high in dairy products and vegetables that contain less ammonia than meat.

Client teaching for self-care

- Avoid alcohol
- Follow prescribed diet
- Avoid spicy, hot foods that may irritate esophageal varices
- Avoid exposure to infectious diseases

- Monitor for bleeding tendencies, check for blood in urine or stool, check gums for bleeding
- Use an electric razor and soft tooth brush
- Conserve energy
- Make an appointment for follow-up care with a health professional

LIVER CANCER

- Liver cancer may be primary (hepatocellular cancer) or a result of metastasis from another site.
- Primary liver cancer grows rapidly and metastasizes early most often to the lung, lymph nodes, adrenal glands, the stomach, ovary, and kidney.
- More than half of advanced liver cancers are a result of spread from another source.
- Liver cancer is usually detected at a late stage and the prognosis is poor.

Etiology: Primary liver cancer can be caused by damage to hepatocellular DNA from hepatitis B and C viruses leading to DNA mutations. Metastatic tumors reach the liver through lymphatic channels, the portal system, and by extension of an abdominal tumor to the liver.

Risk factors: Primary cancer: history of HBV, HCV and cirrhosis; smoking; alcohol use; exposure to chemicals and toxins; male sex; and hereditary influences.

S&S:

- Pain, dull or aching
- A palpable mass in the right upper lobe of the liver
- Abdominal distention with ascites
- Fatigue, anorexia, and malaise
- Jaundice if larger bile ducts are occluded
- Symptoms of liver failure which are portal hypertension, splenomegaly, and hepatomegaly.

Dx: Based on history and physical and S&S. AFP, AST, ALD and alkaline phosphatase are elevated, ultrasound, CT scan and MRI to locate tumor and identify site for biopsy which is done to confirm diagnosis and identify tumor type and origin.

Rx: Lobectomy or liver transplant; chemotherapy to slow growth but not cure; radiation for pain relief; percutaneous biliary drainage for comfort and to decrease pruritus and jaundice.

Nursing Process Elements

- Provide emotional support for the client and family
- Offer pre- and postoperative teaching PRN, answer questions about the procedure (see Chapter 19)
- Discuss pain management and response to pain control measures
- Consult with other health team members to manage client problems
- Initiate a referral to Home Care, if the client can live at home. The Home Care RN can treat and evaluate needs such as comfort, nutrition and use of alternative measures of pain relief such as massage or guided imagery.

Client teaching for self-care

- Encourage independence and activity as tolerated
- Assist with referral to support groups, Hospice
- Encourage client and family to discuss and participate in care
- Teach about the complications of chemotherapy, radiation or surgery and the need to report to the nurse or physician if a problem occurs
- Discuss end-of-life issues
- Encourage small meals and supplementary feedings

CHOLELITHIASIS

Cholelithiasis is a disease characterized by stones in the gall bladder, cystic duct, or common bile duct.

Etiology: Unknown.

Risk factors: Five Fs: fair, fat, female, forty, and flatulent. Also, use of oral contraceptives, history of pregnancy, and family history of disease.

Precipitating factors: Bile stasis, imbalances of cholesterol metabolism, and infection

S&S: Asymptomatic and not treated unless cause cholecystitis (see below)

CHOLECYSTITIS

Cholecystitis is inflammation of the gall bladder.

Etiology: Most often associated with cholelithiasis.

S&S:

- Early disease: intolerance of fatty foods, nausea with or without vomiting, flatulence, fever, right upper quadrant discomfort after a heavy meal or at night
- Acute episode: RUQ pain, may radiate to right scapula and shoulder
- Elevated WBC count, alkaline phosphatase, amylase, and lipase
- If bile flow is obstructed, jaundice, clay-colored stool, dark amber-colored urine, and elevated serum bilirubin

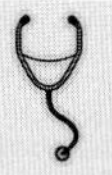

PEDS **Assessment Alert**

Gallstones are rare in children with the exception of children with sickle cell.

Dx: Visualization of gallstones usually with ultrasound imaging or oral cholecystogram.

Rx:

- Acute episode: supportive treatment
  —IV antibiotics for infection
  —Narcotic analgesics (Demerol not morphine) and anti-cholinergics (atropine)for pain
  —NPO, NG tube to suction, antiemetics for N&V
  —F&E replacement
  —Diet as tolerated clear or minimum-fat full liquids progressing to a fat restricted soft diet
- Removal of gallstones:
  —Surgical: open or laparoscopic cholecystectomy is the most common procedure. Choledochostomy—opening of common bile duct with stone removal and T-tube insertion
  —Gallstone dissolution therapy—substances that dissolve stones administered orally or via percutaneous catheter
  —Mechanical litholysis of common bile duct stones—crushing and removal of stones via an endoscope
  —Extracorporeal shock wave lithotripsy—use of high pressure, high-energy sound waves to crush stones

Nursing Process Elements

See cholecystectomy in Chapter 18 for perioperative care.

Client teaching for self-care

To manage symptoms of chronic indigestion related to cholecystitis and lower the risk of gallstone formation:

- Reduce weight to normal range
- Eat a high-fiber, high-calcium diet
- Reduce intake of saturated fatty acids
- Eat at regular intervals
- Exercise regularly

PANCREATITIS

- Pancreatitis is inflammation of pancreas.
  —It may be acute or chronic.
  —It is mild and self-limiting to life-threatening with severe hemorrhagic necrosis.
  —It is most common in middle-aged men.

Etiology: Apparently due to autodigestion secondary to pancreatic cell injury or activation of pancreatic enzymes in pancreas rather than small intestine.

Risk factors: Alcoholism, biliary tract disease, trauma, viral infection, drugs such as steroids, thiazides, oral contraceptives, NSAIDs, sulfonamides, metabolic disorders such as hyperparathyroidism, hyperlipidemia, and renal failure.

S&S: Acute:

- LUQ pain radiating substernally or to the back or flank, worsened by eating and unrelieved by vomiting, abdominal tenderness with guarding; N&V; jaundice; decreased or absent bowel sounds; tachycardia and hypotension; presence of Grey-Turner spots (flank ecchymoses); positive Cullen's sign (periumbilical ecchymoses)

Chronic:

- malabsorption, weight loss, mild jaundice, dark urine, and diabetes mellitus

Dx: Elevated serum amylase, urinary amylase, renal amylase-creatinine clearance, blood glucose, lipids; decreased serum calcium; pancreatic enlargement on CT scan. Secretin stimulation test showing reduced volume of pancreatic secretions is most diagnostic of chronic disease.

Rx:

- Analgesics and smooth muscle relaxants such as papaverine and nitroglycerine for pain.

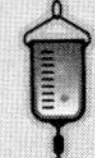

Clinical Alert

Morphine is not given because of its ability to cause spasm in the muscles of the ducts.

- Anticholinergics (atropine, Pro-Banthine) and antacids, NPO, NG suction to prevent acidic gastric contents from entering small intestine; small amounts of bland, high - CHO, high PRO, low-fat foods when oral intake resumed to decrease pancreatic stimulation.
- Fluid and electrolyte replacement
- Pancreatic enzyme replacement for chronic pancreatitis

Complications: Pseudocyst, abscess, pleural effusion, atelectasis, pneumonia, hypocalcemic tetany, fluid and electrolyte imbalance, and hemorrhagic shock

Nursing Process Elements

- Assess S&S, effect of medications; fluid and electrolyte status because risk of imbalance due to vomiting and NG suction. Monitor I&O and for signs of hypocalcemic tetany.

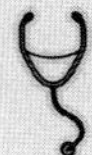

Assessment Alert

First sign of hypocalcemia: numbness and tingling in fingers and around lips.

- Eliminate environmental sources of pancreatic stimulation: sight, smell, and talk of food
- Implement nonpharmacologic measures to manage pain; positioning (fetal); relaxation techniques; calm, quiet environment
- Turn, cough and deep breathe to prevent respiratory infection which is a risk due to pain and elevation of diaphragm secondary to effects of inflammation
- Monitor blood glucose to check for damage to insulin-producing cells

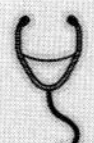

Assessment Alert

Monitor closely for infection because inflamed, necrotic pancreatic tissue is at high risk for bacterial invasion.

Client teaching for self-care

- Avoid alcohol, caffeine, smoking, and stress all of which stimulate the pancreas
- Eat a high-carbohydrate, high-protein, low-fat diet
- Eat small frequent meals
- Maintain a relaxed atmosphere for meals
- Report signs of complications: continued N&V; increasing abdominal distention; continued weight loss; severe epigastric or back pain; frothy, foul-smelling stool; elevated temperature of 48-hours duration; irritability; and confusion

PANCREATIC CANCER

Prognosis is poor, usually well advanced, and metastasized at diagnosis.

Etiology: Unknown but some association with diabetes mellitus and chronic pancreatitis.

Risk factors: Smoking, high-fat diet, diabetes, exposure to chemicals such as benzidine.

S&S:

- Dull, aching upper abdominal pain, which may radiate to the back and occurs after eating or at night
- Anorexia, nausea, rapid weight loss, and jaundice
- Tumors in body or tail of pancreas often asymptomatic until well advanced.

Dx: Difficult; ERCP demonstrates obstructions in ducts. Cytology of pancreatic juice may show malignant cells. CEA is elevated in advanced disease but is nonspecific; CA1-9 is a more specific tumor marker. CT scan shows tumor mass and lymph node spread.

Rx: Surgery: Whipple procedure. Palliative procedures for bile duct obstruction such as a cholecystojejunostomy bypass or placement of a biliary stent. Radiation for pain relief; chemotherapy has a limited effect.

Nursing Process Elements

- Combines care of the client with pancreatitis, general care of the client with cancer, and care of the client at end-of-life
- Assess and manage pain
- Assess for bleeding secondary to impaired vitamin K synthesis
- Control N&V
- Stimulate appetite

WORKSHEET

TRUE & FALSE QUESTIONS

Mark each of the following statements True or False. Correct all false statements in the space provided.

1. A risk factor for hepatitis A is poor hygienic practices. ___ T ___ F
2. Liver tenderness is a sign associated with the preicteric phase of hepatitis. ___ T ___ F
3. Hepatitis A vaccine is given as an initial dose and then a booster in 6–12 months. ___ T ___ F
4. Flapping hand tremors (asterixis) are characteristic of hepatic encephalopathy. ___ T ___ F
5. Clients with cirrhosis must be assessed for thrombus formation due to altered clotting factors. ___ T ___ F
6. Hepatitis B and C viruses can damage DNA of liver cells and result in the development of primary liver cancer. ___ T ___ F
7. Intramuscular and subcutaneous injections should be avoided in the client with cirrhosis. ___ T ___ F
8. Morphine is the analgesic of choice for clients with pancreatitis. ___ T ___ F
   Morphine is not given to clients with pancreatitis because it can cause spasm in the muscles of the pancreatic ducts.
9. To avoid stimulating the pancreas, high-fat foods should be avoided when oral intake is resumed in clients with pancreatitis. ___ T ___ F
10. The surgical procedure of choice for cancer of the pancreas is a Whipple procedure. ___ T ___ F
11. An elevated AFT confirms the diagnosis of primary liver cancer. ___ T ___ F
12. CA1-9 is more reliable than CEA as a marker for pancreatic cancer. ___ T ___ F

13. Part of the nursing care plan for the client with pancreatitis should be avoidance of the sight, smell, or talk of food. ___ T ___ F

14. Pancreatitis places the client at risk for concurrent renal infection. ___ T ___ F

15. Signs of severe hemorrhagic pancreatitis include a positive Cullen's sign and presence of Grey-Turner spots. ___ T ___ F

16. Hepatic damage associated with alcoholic cirrhosis can be reversed by abstaining from alcohol and eating a nutritionally complete diet. ___ T ___ F

MATCHING QUESTIONS

Match the following.

1. ____ Risk factor for cholelithiasis
2. ____ Clay-colored stool
3. ____ Sign associated with cirrhosis
4. ____ Drug to be avoided in cirrhosis
5. ____ Hypocalcemic tetany
6. ____ Secretin stimulation
7. ____ Pancreatic enzyme replacement
8. ____ CT scan
9. ____ Biliary stent
10. ____ Portal hypertension
11. ____ Vasopressin
12. ____ Interferon alpha
13. ____ Anticholinergics
14. ____ Biopsy
15. ____ Neomycin

a. Test for chronic pancreatitis
b. Treatment of chronic pancreatitis
c. Palliative treatment for bile duct obstruction
d. Acetaminophen
e. Necessary for diagnosis of liver cancer
f. Gynecomastia
g. Oral contraceptives
h. Treatment for esophageal varices
i. Complication of cirrhosis
j. Treatment for chronic hepatitis B
k. Treatment of pain of acute cholecystitis
l. Treatment of hepatic encephalopathy
m. Demonstrates vascular changes in the liver associated with cirrhosis
n. Complication of pancreatitis
o. Sign of hepatitis or cholecystitis

APPLICATION QUESTIONS

1. Which forms of hepatitis can be transmitted by contaminated blood and blood products? Mark all that apply.
   a. ___ Hepatitis A
   b. ___ Hepatitis B
   c. ___ Hepatitis C
   d. ___ Hepatitis D
   e. ___ Hepatitis E

2. Which lab values are consistent with a diagnosis of hepatitis? Mark all that apply.
   a. ___ Increased AST
   b. ___ Increased ESR
   c. ___ Increased serum bilirubin
   d. ___ Increased ALT

3. How should the nurse interpret the development of frothy, foul-smelling stool in a client with pancreatitis?
   a. Expected sign of the disease
   b. Reportable sign of a complication
   c. Sign that bilirubin drainage is reestablished
   d. Indication that liver damage has occurred

4. Which assessment data would the nurse gather to monitor for damage to the cells in the Islet of Langerhans in the client with pancreatitis?
   a. Serum bilirubin levels
   b. Urobilinogen levels
   c. Creatinine levels
   d. Blood glucose levels

5. When caring for the client with pancreatitis, which question should be asked to check for the onset of hypocalcemia?
   a. Do you have numbness or tingling in your fingers or around your lips?
   b. Do you have any muscle cramps in your feet or legs?
   c. Do you have any difficulty swallowing?
   d. Do you feel weak or dizzy when you stand up?

6. Vaccines are available against which forms of hepatitis? Mark all that apply.
   a. ___ Hepatitis A
   b. ___ Hepatitis B
   c. ___ Hepatitis C
   d. ___ Hepatitis D
   e. ___ Hepatitis E

7. In what stage(s) of hepatitis would the nurse expect the client to have liver tenderness and weight loss?
   a. preicteric
   b. icteric
   c. posticteric
   d. both icteric and posticteric

8. The mother of an 11-year-old girl with hepatitis asks why her daughter is not receiving any medication for the disease. Which fact should serve as the basis for the nurse's answer?
   a. Most drugs are metabolized in the liver.
   b. There are no drugs for hepatitis, which are safe for children.
   c. Drug therapy is only used when jaundice has resolved.
   d. The risk of kidney damage from drugs when the liver is impaired is high.

9. Which statement about the hepatitis A vaccine made by a client at an immunization clinic indicates understanding about the vaccine?
   a. I have to come back in 6 months to a year for the booster dose.
   b. I won't have lasting protection until after the third dose of the vaccine.
   c. I'll be able to get a tattoo without worry once I get all these injections.
   d. I need to avoid shellfish now that I have had this first injection.

10. Which unvaccinated client would be a candidate for hepatitis A immunoglobulin?
    a. Client planning to visit a developing country in 10-months time
    b. Client who had a tattoo 2 weeks ago
    c. Client with a history of drug abuse
    d. Client with a spouse diagnosed with hepatitis A

11. Which are risk factors for cholelithiasis? Mark all that apply.
    a. ___ Use of oral contraceptives
    b. ___ Female gender
    c. ___ Elevated serum bilirubin
    d. ___ Fair skin
    e. ___ Obesity
    f. ___ Elevated serum calcium
    g. ___ Diet high in legumes

12. Which classes of drugs would the nurse expect to be ordered for the treatment of an acute episode of cholecystitis? Mark all that apply.
    a. ___ Narcotic analgesics
    b. ___ Antiemetics
    c. ___ Anticholinergics
    d. ___ Parasympathomimetics
    e. ___ Antilipemics
    f. ___ Antibiotics

13. A client asks what is the difference between gallstone dissolution therapy and lithotripsy. On which fact should the nurse's response be based?
    a. Lithotripsy involves crushing gallstones through an endoscope; dissolution therapy involves using a chemical.
    b. Dissolution therapy involves inserting a T-tube; lithotripsy involves use of radiation.
    c. Lithotripsy uses sound waves to break up stones; dissolution therapy uses p.o. or IV substances to dissolve them.
    d. Dissolution therapy uses a combination of drugs and radio waves; lithotripsy uses a laser to destroy stones.

14. A client suspected of having cirrhosis asks what test will confirm the diagnosis. What is the nurse's most appropriate reply?
    a. Measures of liver enzymes: ALT and AST
    b. CT scan
    c. Liver biopsy
    d. Prothrombine Time (PT)

15. Impaired bile metabolism and excretion are directly related to which symptom of cirrhosis?
    a. Prolonged PTT
    b. Pruritus
    c. Ascites
    d. Esophageal varices

16. Which direction would not be given to a client with cirrhosis?
    a. Take not more than 1300 mg of acetaminophen per day for pain
    b. Avoid IM or SC injections
    c. Use an electric razor
    d. Avoid exposure to people with colds or other infections

17. When caring for a client with cholecystitis, the nurse would question an order calling for administration of which drug?
    a. Morphine
    b. Demerol
    c. Atropine
    d. Compazine

18. Which are risk factors for primary cancer of the liver?
    a. Hepatitis A and cirrhosis
    b. History of gastric cancer and alcohol abuse
    c. Portal hypertension and exposure to environmental toxins
    d. Smoking and hepatitis C

19. A client says his physician told him he has a liver tumor and before it is treated it has to be determined if it started in the liver or if it came from somewhere else. The client asks what test is used to figure this out. Which test would the nurse say is used to identify the origin of a liver tumor?
    a. CT scan of the liver
    b. MRI of the liver
    c. Liver biopsy
    d. Test for alpha-fetoprotein

20. The nurse would expect a history of left upper quadrant pain worse after eating and not relieved by vomiting when assessing a client with which problem?
    a. Cholecystitis
    b. Splenomegaly
    c. Acute pancreatitis
    d. Liver cancer

21. Which is a major indicator of chronic pancreatitis?
    a. Positive Cullen's sign
    b. Postprandial elevated serum amylase
    c. Decreased pancreatic secretion with secretin stimulation
    d. Midepigastric pain worsened by fasting

22. The spouse of a client with pancreatitis asks what is the reason for the NG tube? Which fact should form the basis of the nurse's reply?
    a. To prevent vomiting
    b. To remove gastric contents so they don't enter the intestine
    c. To allow for monitoring of gastric pH
    d. To protect the gastric lining from pancreatic enzymes

23. For which complication of pancreatitis is the nurse monitoring when the client is asked about the presence of numbness and tingling around the lips?
    a. Hyperkalemia
    b. Hypocalcemic tetany
    c. Hemorrhagic shock
    d. Hyponatremia

(continued)

24. Which assessment finding would indicate that papaverine administered to a client with pancreatitis is exerting the desired effect?
    a. Pancreatic secretions have increased.
    b. Pain has decreased.
    c. Oral fluids are tolerated
    d. Electrolyte values are within normal range.

25. Teaching about the need for a long-term, low-protein diet would be part of the plan of care for a client with which problem?
    a. Chronic pancreatitis
    b. Liver cancer
    c. Pancreatic cancer
    d. Hepatic encephalopathy

ANSWERS & RATIONALES

TRUE & FALSE ANSWERS

Mark each of the following statements True or False. Correct all false statements in the space provided.

1. A risk factor for Hepatitis A is poor hygienic practices. *True*
2. Liver tenderness is a sign associated with the preicteric phase of hepatitis. *False*
   Liver tenderness occurs in the icteric phase; the preicteric phase is characterized by headache, fatigue, and anorexia.
3. Hepatitis A vaccine is given as an initial dose and then a booster in in 6–12 months. *True*
4. Flapping hand tremors (asterixis) are characteristic of hepatic encephalopathy. *True*
5. Clients with cirrhosis must be assessed for thrombus formation due to altered clotting factors. *False*
   With cirrhosis the ability of the liver to produce clotting factors is often decreased therefore the client must be assessed for signs of abnormal bleeding.
6. Hepatitis B and C viruses can damage DNA of liver cells and result in the development of primary liver cancer. *True*
7. Intramuscular and subcutaneous injections should be avoided in the client with cirrhosis. *True*
8. Morphine is the analgesic of choice for clients with pancreatitis. *False*
   Morphine is not given to clients with pancreatitis because it can cause spasm in the muscles of the pancreatic ducts.
9. To avoid stimulating the pancreas, high-fat foods should be avoided when oral intake is resumed in clients with pancreatitis. *True*
10. The surgical procedure of choice for cancer of the pancreas is a Whipple procedure. *True*
11. An elevated AFT confirms the diagnosis of primary liver cancer. *False*
    Diagnosis of any liver cancer, primary or metastatic, can only be confirmed by liver biopsy.
12. CA1-9 is more reliable than CEA as a marker for pancreatic cancer. *True*
13. Part of the nursing care plan for the client with pancreatitis should be avoidance of the sight, smell, or talk of food. *True*

14. Pancreatitis places the client at risk for concurrent renal infection. *False*
Pancreatitis puts the client at risk for respiratory infection because pain and elevation of the diaphragm predispose to shallow breathing and stasis of secretions.

15. Signs of severe hemorrhagic pancreatitis include a positive Cullen's sign and presence of Grey-Turner spots. *True*

16. Hepatic damage associated with alcoholic cirrhosis can be reversed by abstaining from alcohol and eating a nutritionally complete diet. *False*
Cirrhotic damage is irreversible; good nutrition and abstinence from alcohol can prevent further damage.

MATCHING ANSWERS

Match the following:

1. __g__ Risk factor for cholelithiasis
2. __o__ Clay-colored stool
3. __f__ Sign associated with cirrhosis
4. __d__ Drug to be avoided in cirrhosis
5. __n__ Hypocalcemic tetany
6. __a__ Secretin stimulation
7. __b__ Pancreatic enzyme replacement
8. __m__ CT scan
9. __c__ Biliary stent
10. __i__ Portal hypertension
11. __h__ Vasopressin
12. __j__ Interferon alpha
13. __k__ Anticholinergics
14. __e__ Biopsy
15. __l__ Neomycin

a. Test for chronic pancreatitis
b. Treatment of chronic pancreatitis
c. Palliative treatment for bile duct obstruction
d. Acetominophen
e. Necessary for diagnosis of liver cancer
f. Gynecomastia
g. Oral contraceptives
h. Treatment for esophageal varices
i. Complication of cirrhosis
j. Treatment for chronic hepatitis B
k. Treatment of pain of acute cholecystitis
l. Treatment of hepatic encephalopathy
m. Demonstrates vascular changes in the liver associated with cirrhosis
n. Complication of pancreatitis
o. Sign of hepatitis or cholecystitis

APPLICATION ANSWERS

1. Which forms of hepatitis can be transmitted by contaminated blood and blood products? Mark all that apply.
   a. ___ Hepatitis A
   b. ___ Hepatitis B
   c. ___ Hepatitis C
   d. ___ Hepatitis D
   e. ___ Hepatitis E

Rationale

Correct answers: b, c, and d.
Incorrect answers: a and e both of which are transmitted by the fecal–oral route.

2. Which lab values are consistent with a diagnosis of hepatitis? Mark all that apply.
   a. ___ Increased AST
   b. ___ Increased ESR
   c. ___ Increased serum bilirubin
   d. ___ Increased ALT

Rationale

Correct answers: a, b, c, and d.
AST and ALT are liver enzymes, which become elevated with liver damage. ESR is elevated due to the inflammation in the liver. Serum bilirubin is increased as a result of impaired bilirubin metabolism and obstruction of the hepatobiliary duct.

3. How should the nurse interpret the development of frothy, foul-smelling stool in a client with pancreatitis?
   a. Expected sign of early disease
   b. Reportable sign of progressive disease
   c. Sign that bilirubin drainage is reestablished
   d. Indication that liver damage has occurred

Rationale

Correct answer: b.
Frothy, foul-smelling stool is characteristic of steatorrhea, which is indicative of malabsorption. Malabsorption that leads to nutritional deficiencies occurs when the pancreas no longer produces sufficient amounts of enzymes needed for digestion. Bilirubin does not drain; it is the pigment, which gives bile its color. It is a product of RBC breakdown by the spleen and circulates in the blood stream to the liver where it is used in the production of bile. When bile is released into the intestine, bilirubin is metabolized and gives stool its color.

4. Which assessment data would the nurse gather to monitor for damage to the cells in the Islet of Langerhans in the client with pancreatitis?
   a. Serum bilirubin levels
   b. Urobilinogen levels
   c. Creatinine levels
   d. Blood glucose levels

Rationale

Correct answer: d.
Monitoring for elevations in blood glucose checks for damage to insulin producing cells because if insulin production is impaired, blood glucose will rise. Bilirubin is the pigment, which gives bile its characteristic green color; urobilinogen is a breakdown product of bilirubin metabolism in the small intestine that gives stool its color. These are unrelated to the function of the Islet of Langerhans, which produce insulin. Creatinine is a metabolic end product of a substance in skeletal muscle. It is formed and excreted through the glomerulus of the kidney in constant amounts and therefore is used to approximate glomerular filtration rate.

5. When caring for the client with pancreatitis, which question should be asked to check for the onset of hypocalcemia?
   a. Do you have numbness or tingling in your fingers or around your lips?
   b. Do you have any muscle cramps in your feet or legs?
   c. Do you have any difficulty swallowing?
   d. Do you feel weak or dizzy when you stand up?

Rationale

Correct answer: a.
The first sign of onset of hypocalcemic tetany is numbness and tingling in the hands and around the mouth. This progresses to paresthesias in the legs and feet, caropedal spasm and ultimately to laryngeal, glottic and bronchial spasms and respiratory arrest as the calcium level falls below 7 mg/dL.

6. Vaccines are available against which forms of hepatitis? Mark all that apply.
   a. ___ Hepatitis A
   b. ___ Hepatitis B
   c. ___ Hepatitis C
   d. ___ Hepatitis D
   e. ___ Hepatitis E

Rationale

Correct answers: a and b.
Hepatitis A vaccine requires an initial dose and a booster in 6–12 months. Hepatitis B vaccine requires three injections with dose two at least 1 month after dose one and the third dose at least 2 months after the second and 4 months after the first.

7. In what stage(s) of hepatitis would the nurse expect the client to have liver tenderness and weight loss?
   a. Preicteric
   b. Icteric

c. Postičteric
d. Both icteric and posticteric

Rationale

Correct answer: b.

Weight loss, jaundice, and liver tenderness are characteristics of the icteric stage of hepatitis. Headache, fatigue, and anorexia are characteristics of the preicteric stage. Decreased jaundice and improved appetite are characteristics of the posticteric stage.

8. The mother of an 11-year-old girl with hepatitis asks why her daughter is not receiving any medication for the disease. Which fact should serve as the basis for the nurse's answer?
   a. Most drugs are metabolized in the liver.
   b. There are no drugs for hepatitis, which are safe for children.
   c. Drug therapy is only used in acute cases when jaundice is prominent.
   d. The risk of kidney damage from drugs when the liver is impaired is high.

Rationale

Correct answer: a.

Most drugs are metabolized in the liver so pharmacological treatment is not recommended for acute cases of hepatitis to avoid further stress and damage to the liver and to avoid other problems related to impaired drug metabolism. The other options are not valid.

9. Which statement about the hepatitis A vaccine made by a client at an immunization clinic indicates understanding about the vaccine?
   a. I have to come back in 6 months to a year for the booster dose.
   b. I won't have lasting protection until after the third dose of the vaccine.
   c. I'll be able to get a tattoo without worry once I get all these injections.
   d. I need to avoid shellfish now that I have had this first injection.

Rationale

Correct answer: a.

Hepatitis A vaccine requires a booster dose in 6–12 months after the initial dose is given. It does not require a third dose; that is hepatitis B vaccine. Hepatitis A is transmitted by the fecal–oral route—the danger with tattoos is from bloodborne hepatitis viruses so hepatitis A offers no protection. Shellfish contaminated with fecal matter can be a source of hepatitis A virus and hence disease; contaminated shellfish should always be avoided. Receiving a dose of hepatitis A vaccine has no relationship to avoiding shellfish.

10. Which unvaccinated client would be a candidate for Hepatitis A immunoglobulin?
    a. Client planning to visit a developing country in 10-months time
    b. Client who had a tattoo 2 weeks ago
    c. Client with a history of heroin abuse
    d. Client with a spouse diagnosed with hepatitis A

Rationale

Correct answer: d.

Persons exposed to hepatitis A who have not been vaccinated can receive passive immunity through administration of immunoglobulin. A person planning to visit a developing country in 10 months has time to receive the vaccine and develop active immunity which is preferable. Tattoos have a potential risk of hepatitis B not A as does heroin abuse.

11. Which are risk factors for cholelithiasis? Mark all that apply.
    a. ___ Use of oral contraceptives
    b. ___ Female gender
    c. ___ Elevated serum bilirubin
    d. ___ Fair skin
    e. ___ Obesity
    f. ___ Elevated serum calcium
    g. ___ Diet high in legumes

Rationale

Correct answers: a, b, d, and e.

Risk factors for cholecystitis are the five Fs (fair, fat, forty, female, and flatulent) as well as use of oral contraceptives, history of pregnancy, and family history of the disease. Elevated serum bilirubin or serum calcium or a diet high in legumes have no relationship to risk for gall bladder disease.

12. Which classes of drugs would the nurse expect to be ordered for the treatment of an acute episode of cholecystitis? Mark all that apply.
    a. ___ Narcotic analgesics
    b. ___ Antiemetics
    c. ___ Anticholinergics
    d. ___ Parasympathomimetics
    e. ___ Antilipemics
    f. ___ Antibiotics

Rationale

Correct answers: a, b, c, and f.

Narcotic analgesics, but not morphine because of its ability to cause spasm of the ducts, are given for pain. Antiemetics are given for N&V. Anticholinergics are given to ease pain by reducing tone and contraction of smooth muscle. Antibiotics are given for infection. Antilipemics and parasympathomimetics have no role in the treatment of acute cholecystitis.

(continued)

13. A client asks what the difference is between gallstone dissolution therapy and lithotripsy. On which fact should the nurse's response be based?
    a. Lithotripsy involves crushing gallstones through an endoscope; dissolution therapy involves using a chemical.
    b. Dissolution therapy involves inserting a T-tube; lithotripsy involves use of radiation.
    c. Lithotripsy uses sound waves to break up stones; dissolution therapy uses p.o. or IV substances to dissolve them.
    d. Dissolution therapy uses a combination of drugs and radio waves; lithotripsy uses a laser to destroy stones.

Rationale

Correct answer: c.

Lithotripsy uses the pressure of high-energy sound waves to crush stones so they can be passed into the intestine and out of the body. Dissolution therapy involves the administration, either oral or through percutaneous catheter, of substances which dissolve gallstones. Mechanical litholysis (grasping and crushing a stone with an instrument designed for the purpose) is performed through an endoscope; a T-tube is inserted when a choledochostomy (opening of the common bile duct) is done to remove stones. Radiation or lasers are not used for gallstone removal.

14. A client suspected of having cirrhosis asks what test will confirm the diagnosis. What is the nurse's most appropriate reply?
    a. Measures of liver enzymes: ALT and AST
    b. CT scan
    c. Liver biopsy
    d. Prothrombin Time (PT)

Rationale

Correct answer: c.

Liver biopsy allows for microscopic examination of liver tissue in which changes diagnostic of cirrhosis can be identified. Liver enzymes are elevated by many different liver problems; CT scans show structural changes but are also nonspecific. PT is a measure specific to blood clotting and may be lengthened with cirrhosis but it can also be affected by many other disorders.

15. Impaired bile metabolism and excretion are directly related to which symptom of cirrhosis?
    a. Prolonged PTT
    b. Pruritus
    c. Ascites
    d. Esophageal varices

Rationale

Correct answer: b.

Pruritus results from deposition of bile salts in the skin. Prolonged PTT, ascites, and esophageal varices all accompany cirrhosis but are not direct results of impaired bile metabolism and excretion.

16. Which direction would not be given to a client with cirrhosis?
    a. Take not more than 1300 mg of acetaminophen per day for pain
    b. Avoid IM or SC injections
    c. Use an electric razor
    d. Avoid exposure to people with cold or other infections

Rationale

Correct answer: a.

Acetaminophen is hepatotoxic and contraindicated in cirrhosis. Avoiding injections and using an electric razor are appropriate because of the risk of bleeding due to impaired clotting. Avoiding exposure to infection is appropriate because of decreased immune function.

17. When caring for a client with cholecystitis, the nurse would question an order calling for administration of which drug?
    a. Morphine
    b. Pro-Banthine
    c. Atropine
    d. Compazine

Rationale

Correct answer: a.

Morphine is not given because it can cause spasms in the muscles of the ducts. The anticholinergics atropine and Pro-Banthine are used for pain and antiemetics such as Compazine is used for N&V.

18. Which are risk factors for primary cancer of the liver?
    a. Hepatitis A and cirrhosis
    b. History of gastric cancer and alcohol abuse
    c. Portal hypertension and exposure to environmental toxins
    d. Smoking and hepatitis C

Rationale

Correct answer: d.

Smoking and hepatitis C are identified as risk factors for liver cancer. Other risk factors are HBV, cirrhosis, alcohol use, exposure to chemicals and toxins, male sex, and heredity factors.

19. A client says his physician told him he has a liver tumor and before it is treated it has to be determined if it started in the liver or if it came from somewhere else. The client asks what test is used to figure this out. Which test would the nurse say is used to identify the origin of a liver tumor?
    a. CT scan of the liver
    b. MRI of the liver

c. Liver biopsy
d. Test for alpha-fetoprotein

Rationale

Correct answer: c.

A liver biopsy confirms the presence of cancer and shows the tumor type and origin. CT scans and MRIs show liver enlargement and nodules as well as vascular changes and indicate if tumor removal is possible. Alpha-fetoprotein is elevated in liver cancer but it is nonspecific and has no relationship to the origin of a liver cancer.

20. The nurse would expect a history of left upper quadrant pain worse after eating and not relieved by vomiting when assessing a client with which problem?
    a. Cholecystitis
    b. Splenomegaly
    c. Acute pancreatitis
    d. Liver cancer

Rationale

Correct answer: c.

Acute pancreatitis is characterized by left upper quadrant pain, which is worse after eating but unrelieved by vomiting. Cholesystitis causes right upper quadrant pain referred to the back under the shoulder blade. Enlarged spleen can press on the diaphragm and stimulate the phrenic nerve resulting in referred shoulder pain. Liver cancer causes dull, aching pain in the right abdomen.

21. Which is a major indicator of chronic pancreatitis?
    a. Positive Cullen's sign
    b. Postprandial elevated serum amylase
    c. Decreased pancreatic secretion with secretin stimulation
    d. Midepigastric pain worsened by fasting

Rationale

Correct answer: c.

Reduced volume of pancreatic secretions on a secretin stimulation test is the most diagnostic measure of chronic disease. Positive Cullen's sign is symptomatic of acute disease. Elevated serum amylase is found with both acute and chronic disease. LUQ pain radiating to the back, not midepigastric pain, is characteristic of acute disease; pain is not prominent with chronic disease.

22. The spouse of a client with pancreatitis asks what is the reason is for the NG tube? Which fact should form the basis of the nurse's reply?
    a. To prevent backup of secretions to the liver
    b. To remove gastric contents so they don't enter the intestine
    c. To allow for monitoring of gastric pH
    d. To protect the gastric lining from pancreatic enzymes

Rationale

Correct answer: b.

The NG tube serves to remove acidic gastric contents so they don't enter and damage the intestine since alkaline pancreatic secretions are not available to neutralize them. Gastric secretions do not back up to the liver; gastric pH is not measured; and pancreatic enzymes back flowing to the stomach is not a problem.

23. For which complication of pancreatitis is the nurse monitoring when the client is asked about the presence of numbness and tingling around the lips?
    a. Hyperkalemia
    b. Hypocalcemic tetany
    c. Hemorrhagic shock
    d. Hyponatremia

Rationale

Correct answer: b.

The first sign of onset of hypocalcemic tetany is numbness and tingling in the hands and around the mouth. If untreated, carpopedal spasm and tetany ensue. Numbness and tingling are not associated with hyperkalemia, hemorrhagic shock, or hyponatremia.

24. Which assessment finding would indicate that papaverine administered to a client with pancreatitis is exerting the desired effect?
    a. Pancreatic secretions have increased.
    b. Pain has decreased.
    c. Oral fluids are tolerated
    d. Electrolyte values are within normal range.

Rationale

Correct answer: b.

Papaverine is a muscle relaxant used along with analgesics for the control of pain in clients with pancreatitis. It is not used for any effect on pancreatic secretions, ability to tolerate oral intake, or electrolyte values.

25. Teaching about the need for a long-term, low-protein diet would be part of the plan of care for a client with which problem?
    a. Chronic pancreatitis
    b. Liver cancer
    c. Pancreatic cancer
    d. Hepatic encephalopathy

Rationale

Correct answer: d.

Buildup of ammonia in the blood due to the inability of the liver to clear it, is a major factor in hepatic encephalopathy. Ammonia is produced in the body by intestinal bacteria as an end product of protein metabolism. Therefore, decreasing protein in the diet decreases ammonia available to accumulate to toxic levels.

Test Plan Category:

Physiological Integrity

Sub-category: Physiological Adaptation—Part 1

Topics: Alterations in Body Systems
Illness Management
Section 9: Endocrine Problems

Think Smart/Test Smart

As you study the endocrine diseases, remember that there are S&S related to the hypersecretion and hyposecretion of each. Overtreatment of hypersecretion results in the symptoms of hyposecretion. Overtreatment of hyposecretion results in the symptoms of hypersecretion. With undertreatment of either, symptoms may be reduced but will not be different.

GROWTH HORMONE (GH) HYPERSECRETION

- PEDS Called gigantism when it occurs in children before epiphyses close
  —Causes excessive growth of both bones and connective tissue; height of 8 ft may be reached with proportional growth in head and other body parts.
  —Bony changes are permanent but connective tissue changes may regress somewhat when excess GH is removed.

- Called acromegaly when it occurs after epiphyses close; growth is horizontal rather than vertical.
  - —Causes excessive growth of connective tissues in every part/organ of the body.
  - —Signs of acromegaly evolve slowly over a period of years.

Etiology: Hypersecretion of GH (somatotropin) usually as a result of a pituitary tumor; ectopic GH-secreting tumor in the pancreas; GH-releasing, hormone-producing tumors.

S&S:

- PEDS Children: increased weight, height, muscle mass, and size of viscera; with pituitary tumor, headache and other signs of increasing intracranial pressure may be present.
- Adults: thickened facial features, enlarged hands and feet, deep voice from thickened vocal cords, enlarged heart with resultant increased BP and signs of congestive heart failure, pressure on nerves and related symptoms, arthritis, backache, and kyphosis from bony overgrowth, snoring, altered glucose tolerance leading to diabetes mellitus (DM), and lipidemia from changes in fat metabolism. If etiology is a pituitary tumor, headaches and vision changes may occur. Premature death from the cardiovascular effects is typical.

Dx: Clinical presentation and measurement of GH secretion.

Rx: Goal: prevent worsening of disorder.

- Removal of the GH-producing tumor
- Adjunctive pharmacological treatment: Octreotide acetate (Sandostatin LAR) injection given monthly; effectiveness is assessed by serial IGF-1 and GH levels.

Nursing Process Elements

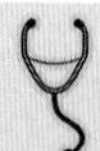

Assessment Alert

Clients with acromegaly are at risk for carbohydrate intolerance or outright DM.

- Promote self-esteem
  - —PEDS Reinforce to tall preadolescent girls that boys will grow taller and many will match or exceed their height
- Support confidence by capitalizing on idol worship in adolescents by noting famous couples in which the woman is taller than the man
- Encourage participation in a support group
- Promote coping

PEDS Growth Hormone (GH) Deficiency

- GH deficiency is defined as the deficient secretion of somatotropin.
- It is idiopathic in more than half the cases with site of dysfunction believed to be the hypothalamus.

Etiology: Known causes include tumors, trauma, vascular abnormalities, and hereditary disorders.

S&S: Short stature: normal at birth but progressively drops behind growth charts.

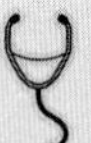

Assessment Alert

Most children presenting with short stature have a constitutional delay not hypopituitarism.

Dx: Radioimmunoassay of plasma GH levels stimulated pharmacologically in two tests below 10 ng/ml.

Rx: Treat underlying cause and/or administration of GH. Before GH is given, an extensive workup is done including family history, imaging to check for brain abnormalities, and evaluation of growth through radiographic study of ossification centers in the hands and wrist.

Nursing Process Elements

- Encourage parents to treat the child in an age-appropriate manner: it is easy to treat the child as younger than he or she is because they look younger
- Encourage parents to work with family members and teachers to treat child in an age-appropriate manner

Client teaching for self-care

- Take injections at bedtime to approximate normal circadian rhythm
- Reinforce realistic expectations of therapy: response to GH varies with young, obese, and severely GH-deficient children responding best; even with good response, adult height is reached more slowly than normal

DIABETES INSIPIDUS (DI)

- DI occurs when there is deficiency in the secretion of antidiuretic hormone (ADH) by the posterior lobe of the pituitary gland or an inability of the kidneys to respond to ADH.
- It causes reduced ability of the renal tubules to reabsorb water and concentrate urine.
- Because the distal tubules remain impermeable to water, large amounts of fluid and electrolytes are excreted in dilute urine.

Etiology:

- Primary DI: tumor of the hypothalamus or posterior pituitary gland
- Secondary DI: head injury or surgical irradiation of the gland

- Transient DI: sequela to transsphenoidal surgery for pituitary adenoma

S&S:

- Polyuria: 4–20 l of dilute urine voided per 24 hours
- Polydipsia (excessive thirst) from dehydration related to excessive water loss in urine
- Decreased urine specific gravity (1.005 or less), hypo-osmolar urine (200 or less), and only slightly increased serum osmolality as long as fluid intake is maintained
- With inadequate water replacement,
  —hypotension, tachycardia, and weight loss develop, without treatment vascular collapse ensues, and the client may develop shock from the fluid loss.
  —hypernatremia coexists as a result of this rapid fluid loss and the concurrent neurological complications of this electrolyte imbalance including irritability, decreased cognition, lethargy, and coma develop.
- Sleep problems due to frequent voiding
- PEDS In children, the first sign may be enuresis
- PEDS In infants, irritability that is relieved by feeding water but not milk is the initial symptom

Dx:

- Water deprivation test to determine ability of renal tubule to concentrate urine
  —Positive for DI if after fluid is restricted, there is no change in urine formation; urine osmolality and specific gravity do not rise

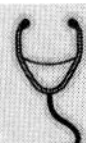

Assessment Alert

Children need close supervision during fluid restriction because they may drink fluid from any available source including toilet bowls and puddles.

- Vasopressin stimulation test to determine if ADH is being secreted from the posterior pituitary gland
  —Positive for DI if after subcutaneous administration of five units of aqueous vasopressin, increased specific gravity and decreased urine output occur
- Serum findings:
  —Decreased levels of ADH
  —Increased osmolality
  —Increased sodium
- Urinary findings:
  —Specific gravity less than 1.005
  —Decreased osmolarity (50–200 mOsm/kg)

Rx:

- Long-term ADH replacement therapy
  —Desmopressin (DDAVP)
    - 0.1–0.4 ml in single or divided doses
    - Nasal spray
    - An upright position promotes better absorption
    - Parenteral administration used for transient DI when use of a nasal spray is impossible due to nasal packing
  —Aqueous vasopressin (Pitressin)
    - 5–20 units in divided doses
    - Subcutaneous, IM, or nasal spray
    - Monitor client weight and I&O

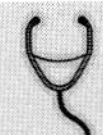

Assessment Alert

Overdosage of ADH replacement therapy is indicated by S&S of water intoxication and SIADH.

  —Chlorpropamide (Diabinese)
    - Thought to stimulate the production of ADH
    - Used for its antidiuretic effects
    - Monitor for signs of hypoglycemia
- Oral and hypotonic IV therapy hydration and replacement:
  —Given if clinical signs of hypernatremia are present
  —Calculated by adding insensible water loss and urinary output to estimated water deficit
  —Administered slowly over 48 hours to avoid cerebral edema and/or seizures
- For nephrogenic DI (caused by lack of responsiveness of the kidney to ADH), low-protein, low-sodium diet and thiazide diuretics.

Nursing Process Elements

- Assess for early signs of dehydration and maintain adequate hydration
  —Ensure IV access site and monitor hourly infusion
- Assess neurologic status
- Measure fluid I&O
  —Urge client to drink fluids in an amount equal to output
- Check urine specific gravity
- Record daily client weight
- Monitor client for education need and ability to participate in health care
- PEDS Counsel parents to speak with school personnel regarding the problems so that the child has unrestricted access to the lavatory

Client teaching for self-care

- Weigh self daily using the same scale at the same time of day

- Notify health care provider if weight loss occurs; notify health care provider if polydipsia and polyuria occur because this signals the need for additional medication doses
- Wear a Medic-Alert bracelet
- Older children and adults should carry the vasopressin nasal spray with them for temporary symptom relief when needed

SYNDROME OF INAPPROPRIATE ANTIDIURETIC HORMONE (SIADH)

- Syndrome of inappropriate antidiuretic hormone (SIADH) occurs when vasopressin (ADH) is secreted even when plasma osmolarity is low or normal.
- The feedback mechanism that regulates ADH does not function properly and ADH continues to be released.
- A nonendocrine source of ADH develops such as when malignant cells synthesize and release ADH.

Etiology:

- Disorders of the CNS, such as head injury, stroke, brain surgery or tumor and infection, which are thought to produce direction stimulation of the pituitary gland
- Medication induced SIADH: vincristine, phenothiazines, tricyclic antidepressants, thiazide diuretics, general anesthetics, opioids, and nicotine have been implicated
- Pulmonary disorders such as tuberculosis, ventilator clients receiving positive pressure, lung abscess
- Malignancies such as small cell lung adenoma, pancreatic and prostate cancer, Hodgkin's and non-Hodgkin's disease, lymphoma, sarcoma, and leukemia that tend to synthesize and release ADH

S&S:

- Early manifestations are related to water retention, the inability to excrete diluted urine, and the resultant hyponatremia: oliguria, anorexia, N&V, muscle weakness, irritability, disorientation, malaise, anxiety, anger, and uncooperativeness
- Because free water (no salt) is retained, weight gain but not edema also occurs
- Neurologic manifestations can progress to lethargy, headache, decreased responsiveness, seizures, and coma with a decrease in deep tendon reflexes
- Decreased plasma sodium and osmolality

Dx:

- Radioimmunoassay of ADH can diagnose SIADH when ADH levels are inappropriately elevated if the plasma osmolarity is normal or decreased
- Serum tests
  - —Plasma osmolarity rises
  - —Serum sodium levels are decreased, often as low as 110/mEq/l
- Urine tests
  - —Urine volume decreases
  - —Urine osmolarity increases
  - —Urine sodium levels rise
  - —Urine specific gravity rises, as a result of the increased urine concentration

Rx:

- Treat cause
- Restricted fluids to 500–600 ml/24hr
- High-sodium diet if client is able to take foods orally
- Use saline to dilute tube feedings, irrigate GI tubes, and mix drugs
- Diuretic therapy, particularly if heart failure is present from fluid overload, but manage concurrent sodium loss
- IV hypertonic saline (3% NaCl), given cautiously to avoid adding to existing fluid overload and a loop diuretic for serum sodium less than 12 mEq/l and CNS symptoms, which requires more rapid replacement. Goal is to raise serum sodium, not to normal but to 125–130 mEq/l or to relieve symptoms or to raise serum sodium by 25 mEq/l
- Demeclocycline (Declomycin) blocks action of ADH on renal tubules

Nursing Process Elements

- Identify clients at risk
- PEDS Institute seizure precautions for children
- Obtain daily serum and urinary sodium and osmolality levels
- Measure I&O
  - —a 1-kg weight increase is equal to a 1000-ml fluid retention
- Record daily client weight
  - —Teach client to use the same scale at the same time
  - —Notify health care provider if weight gain occurs
- Monitor client for education need and ability to participate in health care
- Observe changes in client neurologic status
  - —Assess for muscle twitching
  - —Check orientation to time, place, and person
  - —Reduce environmental noise to prevent overstimulation

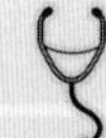

Assessment Alert

Report immediately, if serum sodium is less than 125 mEq/l or any decline in neurological status occurs.

- Give ice chips to combat thirst when fluids are restricted; they must be counted as part of the fluid intake but relieve thirst with less fluid intake than if drinking water.
- Provide mouth care often

HYPOTHYROIDISM (MYXEDEMA)

- Hypothyroidism is the inadequate secretion of thyroid hormones triiodothyronine (T3) and thyroxine (T4), which affects all body functions and can range from mild, subclinical forms to myxedema, an advanced form.
- Sometimes thyroid cells are functional but the person does not ingest enough of the substances needed to make thyroid hormones function properly, especially iodide and tyrosine.
- Failure of the anterior pituitary gland, hypothalamus, or both will cause central hypothyroidism with decreases in TRH and TSH.
- It can occur anytime throughout the life span, more common in older women.

Etiology:

- Most common cause in adults is autoimmune thyroiditis (Hashimoto's disease), in which the immune system attacks the thyroid gland
- Occurs in clients who are being treated for hyperthyroidism with radioiodine, antithyroid medication, or surgical removal of the gland

S&S:

Adults

- Weight gain and constipation
- Thickened skin
- Cold intolerance
- Dull mental processes
- Subnormal temperature and pulse rate
- Development of iodine-deficient goiter
- Other manifestations of decreased metabolism
  —Extreme fatigue
  —Hair loss, brittle nails, and dry skin
  —Menstrual disturbances, and loss of libido
  —Possible atherosclerosis as a result of decreased myocardial metabolism

Children (Juvenile hypothyroidism)

- Decelerated growth
- Dry skin
- Puffiness around the eyes
- Sparse hair
- Sleepiness
- Constipation
- Mental decline

MYXEDEMA COMA

- Myxedema coma is the most extreme stage of hypothyroidism manifestations; precipitated by factors such as cold, surgery, infection, or trauma in any client with severe, prolonged hypothyroidism.
  —Hypothermia and bradycardia
  —Increasing lethargy, stupor, and coma
  —Abnormal sensitivity to opioids, sedatives, and anesthetic agents
  —Depressed respiratory drive, cardiovascular collapse, and shock develop

Dx:

- Decreased levels of serum T3, T4, FT4, and T3 resin uptake
- Delayed TSH response to TRH stimulation test
  —Increased TRH and TSH serum levels if primary hypothyroidism and hypothalamus and pituitary are intact
- Elevated levels of cholesterol due to hypometabolic state
- Decreased results to radioactive iodine uptake test
- Determine whether client has taken medications (contrast agents) or foods (shellfish or cough syrups) containing iodine as these may alter test results

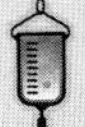

Clinical Alert

Prompt treatment is needed for the infant in order to avoid mental retardation or other neurologic effects because the brain's growth occurs primarily in the first 2–3 years of life.

Rx:

- Primary objective is to restore a normal metabolic state by replacing the missing hormone.
  —Synthetlic levothyroxine (Synthroid or Levothroid)
    - Dosage is based upon the client's TSH serum concentration
- Prevention of cardiac dysfunction
  —Cardiac monitoring
- Prevention of medication interactions
  —Increases in metabolism may affect insulin needs
  —Increases in blood glucose levels, Dilantin levels, digitalis glycoside levels, and anticoagulant levels affected by replacement drugs

Nursing Process Elements

- Alert physician to medications taken that can alter results of diagnostic tests, especially estrogen, salicylates, amphetamines, antibiotics, corticosteroids, and mercurial diuretics
- Modify client activity to accommodate fatigue
  —Promote independence in self-care activities
- Provide extra layers of clothing or extra blanket
  —Monitor body temperature and report decreases from baseline
- Provide foods high in fiber

- Monitor respiratory rate, depth, pattern, pulse oximetry, and arterial blood gas
- Orient client to time, place, and events
- Monitor for increasing severity of S&S of hypothyroidism
  - —Decreased LOC, VS changes, and increasing difficulty in arousal

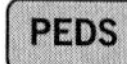

- Position a newborn with a goiter with the neck hyperextended to aid breathing; provide supplemental oxygen; and have a tracheostomy set immediately available in case tracheal compression by the goiter requires emergency ventilation.

Client teaching for self-care

- Take levothyroxine on an empty stomach
- Side effects relate to under or over replacement and therefore are signs of hypo or hyperthyroidism
- Explain rationale for thyroid hormone replacement
  - —Describe desired effects of medication
  - —Explain the necessity for long-term follow-up to client and family

HYPERTHYROIDISM

- Hyperthyroidism is the second most prevalent endocrine disorder, after DM.
- Results from an excessive secretion of thyroid hormones, T3 and T4, which may be temporary or permanent depending upon the cause.
- The normal feedback control over thyroid hormone secretion fails producing a state of hypermetabolism.
- Oversecretion of the releasing and stimulating hormones from the hypothalamus and anterior pituitary gland play a role in the excess of the thyroid hormones.
- Thyrotoxicosis occurs due to toxic effects of excess thyroid hormone.

Etiology:

- The most common cause is a toxic diffuse goiter, autoimmune in nature, which increases the size of the gland and production of its hormones (Graves' disease).
- Thyroid adenoma, a benign thyroid tumor, secretes hormone without stimulus of TSH.

S&S:

- The hallmark of hyperthyroidism is heat intolerance.
  - —Diaphoresis even when the environmental temperatures are comfortable for others
- Visual changes
  - —Blurred or double vision
- Palpitations or chest pain
  - —Changes in breathing patterns due to dyspnea
- Weight loss and diarrhea are often reported.
- Fatigue and weakness are common due to the hypermetabolic demands of the disorder.
- Opthalmopathy
  - —Exopthalmus
    - Bulging eyes, "startled" look
  - —Proptosis
    - Eyelid retraction and eyeball lag
- Thyroid gland enlargement
- Increased systolic BP and tachycardia
- Increased restlessness and irritability

THYROID STORM

- Thyroid storm is a life-threatening event, which consists of rapid onset of exaggerated symptoms of hyperthyroidism.
  - —Abnormally elevated temperature (may be as high as 105–106°F), tachycardia, dysrhythmia, and systolic hypertension
  - —Abdominal pain, N&V, and excessive diarrhea
  - —As the crisis progresses, increased restlessness, confusion, disorientation, psychosis, and seizures ensue

Precipitating factors: Discontinuing needed medications for hyperthyroidism; overreplacement of thyroid hormone; recent treatment with radioactive iodine; surgery, trauma, severe infection, myocardial infarct, or other severe illness in a client with hyperthyroidism.

Dx: Based on clinical presentation and presence of elevated serum levels of T3 and T4.

- Mortality rate is 25% even with treatment

Dx:

- Increased levels of serum T3, T4, FT4, T3 resin uptake
- Thyroid suppression test fails to suppress RAIU or T4 levels
- Elevated titer of antithyroglobulin antibodies
- Elevated thyrotropin receptor antibodies
- Decreased levels of TRH and TSH if primary hyperthyroidism and hypothalamus and pituitary are intact

Rx:

- Nonsurgical management
  - —The most commonly used antithyroid drugs are the thioamides, including propylthiouracil (PTU) and methimazole (Tapazole), which block synthesis of thyroid hormone in the gland.
    - Spreading out dosage helps maintain hormone suppression.

- It takes several weeks before the effect of these drugs is seen because already synthesized hormone must be used up.
- Dose of antithyroid drug is gradually tapered as the client regains euthyroid ststus.
- A side effect of these drugs is agranulocytosis so baseline and periodic WBC count is needed and client must be monitored for signs of infection or jaundice.
- PEDS In children, sore throat and fever can be the first indicators of drug-induced leukopenia so occurrence of these symptoms requires a checkup by the health care provider.

—Iodine preparations that decrease blood flow to the gland thereby reducing the release of the hormones.
- Saturated solution of potassium iodide (SSKI), Lugol's solution, taken after meals to enhance absorption
- Beta-adrenergic blocking agents such as propranolol (Inderal), relieve diaphoresis, anxiety, tachycardia, and palpitations
- Radioactive iodine therapy (I 131) that destroys some of the thyroid cells, which produce the hormone; effects seen in 6 weeks to 6 months; most clients will become hypothyroid after treatment because of the difficulty in titrating the dose of I 131 and will need thyroid hormone replacement

• Surgical management (Also see thyroidectomy in Chapter 18)

—May be needed for clients who have a large goiter causing tracheal or esophageal compression or who do not respond to antithyroid drugs.

—Lifelong thyroid replacement therapy is required after a total thyroidectomy.

—Accidental removal of the parathyroid glands may result in hypocalcemia and tetany, damage to the laryngeal nerves, and thyroid storm.

• Emergency measures include providing a patent airway and adequate ventilation
• Pharmacotherapy

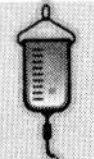

Clinical Alert

Doses of drugs used to treat the client in thyroid storm are higher than for other clients because of the accelerated metabolism of the client in thyroid storm.

—PTU: oral loading dose then 200–300 mg every 6 hours

—Iodide preparations

—Dexamethasone 2 mg IV every 6 hours; helps inhibit release of thyroid hormone

—Beta-adrenergic blockers IV for dysrhythmias as needed

—Nonsalicylate antipyretics

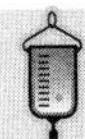

Clinical Alert

Salicylates are contraindicated for clients with thyroid storm because they increase free thyroid hormone levels by interfering with the hormone binding to protein carriers.

• Apply cool blanket or ice packs
• Monitor for cardiac arrhythmias
• Monitor VS
• Identify the cause and stabilize hemodynamic status

Nursing Process Elements

• Monitor VS especially heart rate and rhythm
• Monitor serum albumin, hemoglobin, and lymphocyte levels
• Encourage a diet high in calories, proteins, and carbohydrates to replace energy stores lost due to the hypermetabolic states
• Encourage six meals per day to ensure nutritional needs are consistently and adequately met
• Weigh at least weekly
• Assess for visual changes: photophobia, decreased acuity, or ability to close eyes
• If exophthalmos is present, protect eyes with glasses, wet with artificial tears, elevate head of bed at night; avoid sleeping in a prone position and wear a patch at night if eyelids do not fully close
• Assess level of mentation for impending storm

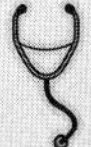

PEDS Assessment Alert

Exophthalmos may be the initial sign. Later "weight loss" despite an excellent appetite, short attention span, and inability to sit still interfering with school performance, unexplained tiredness, and inability to sleep, and impaired fine motor skills may develop.

• PEDS Limit activity of children with symptomatic hyperthyroidism; restrict vigorous exercise until thyroid levels approach normal
• Instruct client how to support neck when coughing or moving after surgery

—Place in semi-Fowler's position that decreases suture line tension to avoid hematoma

—Provide humidified oxygen and ice collar to avoid swelling at the surgical site

- Have tracheostomy available set at bedside in the event of an airway emergency
  —Assess for postoperative hemorrhage, especially at the posterior neck dressing
  —Monitor calcium levels
    - Have client report circumoral tingling or numbness of toes and fingers
- Muscle twitching is a sign of calcium deficiency
    - Have calcium gluconate available at the bedside in the event of hypocalcemic emergency

Client teaching for self-care

- I 131 treatment
- May cause nausea so limit oral intake 2 hours before and after treatment
- Take acetaminophen for sore throat, which may occur a few days after the treatment
- I 131 is eliminated in urine over 4–5 days so drink a lot of fluid, void frequently and flush twice, and thoroughly clean up any spilled urine
- Wash laundry separately if the treated person has sweated heavily, such as after exercise
- Keep an arm's length from anyone who will be in contact with you for more than 2 hours in every 4-hour period; especially if in contact with children and pregnant women. Sleeping together, watching television, going to movies, long car, or plane trips should be avoided for approximately 11 days after treatment
- Small amount found in saliva so avoid kissing and any sharing of food, fluids, or utensils
- After I 131 treatment, women should not get pregnant or breast-feed for 6 months
- Report palpitations, chest pain, or dizziness
- PEDS Counsel parents to establish a regular routine for the child with frequent rest periods

THYROID CANCER

Etiology: Papillary cancer, the most common type of thyroid cancer, is related to prior radiation exposure to the head and neck.

Dx: Fine needle biopsy of the thyroid nodule, which may have been discovered by the client or on physical examination or during diagnostic imaging for other problems.

TSH assay: Suppressed TSH suggests a benign nodule.

RAI uptake: Hot nodules (those that pick up the radioactive iodine are always benign); cold nodules may be benign or malignant.

Rx: Most curative therapy is total thyroidectomy with I 131 ablation of any remaining thyroid tissue followed by levothyroxine replacement beginning the day after surgery.

Neck dissection is also done if metastases in cervical lymph nodes are palpable.

T4 and TSH levels are monitored 6–12 weeks after surgery. Serum thyroglobulin is monitored as a marker for remaining functioning thyroid tissue.

Nursing Process Elements

- Support the client during the diagnostic process
- Provide perioperative care as described under thyroidectomy
- Following I 131 ablation therapy,
  —place client in private room
  —collect all urine and feces in a radiation sewage disposal system
  —ensure disposable dishes and utensils are used for the client
  —allow no visitors
- When I 131 falls to less than 30 mCi as measured by a Geiger counter (usually about 3 days if kidney function is normal), follow radiation safety guidelines as for client having I 131 treatment of hyperthyroidism
- Restrict contact with health care personnel

HYPOPARATHYROIDISM

- Hypoparathyroidism is the disorder of calcium metabolism due to inadequate production of parathyroid hormone.
- Decreased parathormone (PTH) causes decreased resorption of calcium from bone, decreased intestinal absorption, and decreased reabsorption of calcium in the renal tubules with increased retention of phosphate.
- Resultant hypocalcemia increases neuromuscular excitability.

Etiology:

- Most often iatrogenic: result of removal of parathyroid glands or injury from radiation to the neck
- Idiopathic disease may have an autoimmune basis
- Chronic hypomagnesemia inhibits release of parathyroid hormone from normal glands.
- PEDS May occur transiently in infants fed—a milk formula with a high phosphate to calcium ratio.

S&S:

- Early: irritability, apprehension, muscle cramps in abdomen and extremities, photophobia; numbness and tingling around the mouth, nose, ear lobes, hands and feet; and positive Chvostek and Trousseau's signs
- Late: hypocalcemic tetany, respiratory stridor, crowing on inspiration due to laryngospasm, cardiac dysrhythmis, seizures, and respiratory arrest

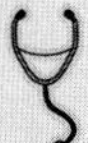

Assessment Alert

Stridor, hoarseness, and a sense of tightness in the throat are signs of laryngospasm.

- PEDS Retarded skeletal growth; dental and enamel hypoplasia; possible mental retardation; thin, brittle nails with transverse grooves; brittle hair; dry, scaly skin with eruptions

Dx: Radioimmunoassay to measure serum level of PTH and concurrent measures of serum calcium and phosphorous. With hypoparathyroidism, serum hormone and calcium is low; phosphorus is high.

Rx: Tetany is an emergency and is treated with IV calcium gluconate or calcium chloride until serum calcium is above 7 mg/dl. When serum calcium above 7 mg/dl, oral vitamin D and calcium is prescribed.

Nursing Process Elements

- Monitor serum calcium
- If client complains of paresthesias suggestive of hypocalcemia check for Chvostek and Trousseau's signs
- Report signs of impending tetany immediately
- Make certain a tracheostomy set and IV calcium gluconate or calcium chloride is immediately available

Client teaching for self-care

- Ingest diet high in calcium, low in phosphorus
- Foods to be limited are high-protein foods (meat, fish, poultry, eggs, legumes, nuts) because they are also high in phosphorus
- Take calcium and vitamin D supplements together preferably with meals
- Regular follow-up is needed to prevent hypercalcemia from the increased calcium and vitamin D
- Report signs of vitamin D toxicity: dry mouth, N&V, metallic taste, or constipation
- Report signs of hypercalcemia: urinary frequency, thirst, slow mentation, fatigue, and muscle weakness
- Report signs of hypocalcemia

HYPERPARATHYROIDISM

- Hyperparathyroidism is a disorder of calcium metabolism due to overproduction of parathyroid hormone.
- It is found most often in clients over age 50.
- It is characterized by increased resorption of calcium from bone and in renal tubules; increased absorption from the intestine; increased urinary excretion of phosphorus.
- Resultant hypercalcemia decreases neuromuscular excitability and calcium is deposited in tissues throughout the body.

Etiology:

- Primary disease: enlargement and increased secretion of one or more glands due to adenoma or other cause
- Secondary disease: compensatory response of normal glands to mild long-term hypocalcemia from problems such as vitamin D or calcium deficiency, elevated serum phosphate, malabsorption, chronic renal failure, or pregnancy

S&S: Fatigue, malaise, lethargy, muscle weakness, memory lapses, poor concentration, depression from slowed nerve impulse transmission; abdominal pain, N&V, constipation from decreased peristalsis; renal calculi from precipitation of calcium; metabolic acidosis, bradycardia, hypertension, osteoporosis, and renal calculi.

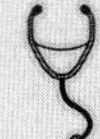

Assessment Alert

The client in acute hypercalcemic crisis can progress from the symptoms above to severe dehydration, coma, cardiac dysrhythmia, and cardiac arrest.

Dx: Elevated serum PTH and serum calcium; decreased serum phosphorus.

Rx: Subtotal parathyroidectomy.

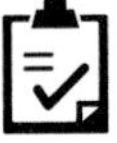

Nursing Process Elements

- See parathyroidectomy in Chapter 18
- Hypercalcemic crisis:
  - —Monitor VS, CVP, and output hourly while administering high-volume IV normal saline (NS)
  - —Administer medications to lower serum calcium
  - —Assess for early signs of hypocalcemia, which are indicative of overtreatment

ADRENAL GLAND HYPOFUNCTION (ADDISON'S DISEASE)

- Production of adrenocortical steroids may decrease as a result of inadequate secretion of adrenocorticotropic hormone (ACTH).
- This decrease may also result from a dysfunction of the hypothalamic–pituitary control mechanism.

- Insufficient secretion of ACTH causes decreases in aldosterone and cortisol secretion from the adrenal gland.
- Manifestations may develop gradually or quickly with stress and life-threatening manifestations may appear without warning.

Etiology:

- Adrenal cortex function is inadequate to meet the physiological need for cortical hormones.
- Can be the result of malfunction anywhere along the hypothalamic–pituitary adrenal axis.
- Called primary when problem is with the adrenal glands themselves.
- Autoimmune or idiopathic atrophy of the adrenal glands is responsible for 80% of the cases.
- Infection or surgical removal of the glands.
    - —Tuberculosis and histoplasmosis are the most common infections
- Hemorrhage into the gland from trauma or a prolonged, difficult delivery.
- Therapeutic use of corticosteroids or abrupt cessation of exogenous adrenocortical hormone therapy results in temporary or permanent adrenal insufficiency.

S&S:

- Muscle weakness, fatigue, and dark skin pigmentation, especially of the knuckles, knees, and elbows
- Hypoglycemia, hyponatremia, and hyperkalemia
    - —Sweating, tachycardia, and tremors
    - —Postural hypotension, and dysrhythmias
- Depression and apathy from glucocorticoid deficiency are frequent
- In severe cases, the disturbance of sodium and potassium metabolism may be marked by depletion of water and severe dehydration: decreased weight, increased BUN, increased Hct, decreased skin turgor, and hypovolemic shock

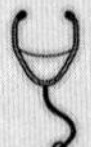

Assessment Alert

With primary disease, ACTH level is high in an effort to compensate for the insufficient amount of hormones in the body and this results in a concomitant increase of melanin-stimulating hormone and the marked bronzy discoloration of the skin.

Clients with primary disease are mineralcorticoid deficient; those with secondary disease are not.

Deficiency of aldosterone, the major mineralcorticoid, causes major loss of sodium and water and retention of potassium. Deficiency of glucocorticoids causes a milder effect.

Addisonian Crisis

- Addisonian crisis is the most severe form of the disorder as the disease progresses, commonly as a result of a stressful event (surgery, trauma, or severe infection).
    - —Cyanosis and the classic signs of circulatory shock
        - Pallor, apprehension, rapid and weak pulse, rapid respirations, low BP, confusion, and restlessness
- If left untreated, may eventually lead to death
- PEDS In the neonate: hyperpyrexia, tachypnea, cyanosis, seizures and if due to hemorrhage into the gland, palpable retroperitoneal mass

Dx:

- Low levels of serum cortisol
- Low- fasting serum glucose and serum sodium
- Elevated serum potassium and ACTH
- ACTH stimulation test is the most definitive test for primary disease: plasma cortisol levels do not rise after administration of ACTH
- Head CT and MRI may help to determine if a pituitary problem is responsible for the adrenal insufficiency, or if atrophy of the adrenal gland is present

Rx:

- Immediate treatment is directed toward combating circulatory shock.
    - —Restoring blood circulation, administering fluids and corticosteroids, and monitoring VS
        - Hydrocortisone (Solu-Cortef) IV followed with 5% dextrose in NS
        - Vasopressor amines if hypotension persists
        - Antibiotics if infection is the precipitator
- Lifelong replacement of corticosteroids (Hycort); for primary disease, replacement of mineralocorticoids (Florinef) is also needed to prevent reoccurrence
- Different schedules of daily dosing are used and there is no agreement on which is best; often two-thirds of the dose is given in the morning and one-third at night; alternatively three doses per day may be given to more closely mimic the normal diurnal rhythm
- Additional supplementary therapy with glucocorticoids during stressful events: for minor stress, the glucocorticoid dose is generally doubled; for major stress 200 mg/d is given in divided doses and then tapered as recovery occurs

Nursing Process Elements

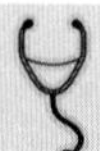

Assessment Alert

With adrenal crisis, assessing for changes in mental status due to hyponatremia and respiratory depression is critical. EKG monitoring with hyperkalemia.

- Interventions to promote fluid balance and monitor for fluid deficit
  - —Weigh daily, record I&O
- Assess VS every 1–4 hours
  - —Depending upon client status and presence of dysrhythmias or postural hypotension
    - Kayexalate may be needed if severe hyperkalemia is present
- Monitor blood glucose levels every 4 hours for hypoglycemia.
- Monitor effects of replacement medication effects
  - —Generally divided doses are given, with two-thirds in the morning and one-third in the late afternoon
- Manage activity intolerance with gradual increases in self-care activities
- Alert client to strategies to minimize anxiety and stress

Client teaching for self-care

- Wear Medic-Alert with the name of disease, medications, doses, and physician
- Always carry medication with you when traveling and be sure to bring extra doses in case of unexpected need
- Never skip a dose of medication: take parenteral form of medication if unable to take oral
- Increase dose of glucocorticoid as directed when minor stresses occur such as personal or family issues, accidents, dental work, or infection
- Report signs of inadequate dosing immediately: anorexia, N&V, weakness, depression, dizziness, polyuria, or weight loss. Report signs of overmedication immediately: rapid weight gain, round face, edema, or hypertension
- Maintain a regular schedule of eating, sleeping, and exercising
- Maintain a fluid intake of at least 2 l/d unless contraindicated
- Eat a diet with normal amounts of sodium; increase sodium, if diaphoresis is expected

EXCESS ADRENAL CORTICAL HORMONES

- Cushing's syndrome results from excess circulating glucocorticoids.
- Hyperaldosteronism results from excess circulating mineralcorticoids.

Cushing's Syndrome

Etiology:

- Use of corticosteroid medications is a common cause.

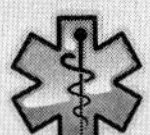

Nursing Intervention Alert

When symptoms are due to steroid therapy, administering the drug early in the day or on alternate days can decrease symptoms.

- Excessive corticosteroid production by the adrenal cortex (less frequently cause)
- A tumor of the pituitary gland that produces ACTH and stimulates the adrenal cortex.
- Regardless of the cause, the normal feedback mechanisms that control the function of the adrenal cortex become ineffective and the pattern of cortisol control is lost.
- Manifestations are usually a result of oversecretion of glucocorticoids and androgens (sex hormones), although mineralcorticoid secretion also may be affected.
- Women 20–40 years are five times more likely to develop Cushing's syndrome.

S&S:

- Changes in physical appearance are the classic signs
  - —"Moon face," central obesity, "buffalo hump" in the neck, heavy trunk, and thin extremities
- Thin, fragile skin with development of ecchymoses, petechiae, red cheeks, and striae
- Excessive protein catabolism produces muscle wasting and osteoporosis, which leads to vertebral compression fractures, kyphosis, backache, and retarded linear growth in children
- Retention of sodium and water occurs producing hypertension and heart failure
- Increased susceptibility to infection, hyperglycemia, and poor wound healing
- Decreased inflammatory response
- Renal calculi
- Peptic ulcer
- If Cushing's syndrome is from a pituitary tumor, visual disturbances may occur because of pressure on the optic chiasm
- Virilization: hirsutism, acne, deepening of the voice, clitoral enlargement, and tendency to a male body shape in females
- Amenorrhea
- Impotence
- Psychological effects: irritability, insomnia, euphoria, depression, and psychosis

Dx:

- Indicators of Cushing's syndrome include an increase in serum sodium and blood glucose levels and a decrease in serum concentration of potassium, eosinophils, and lymphoid tissue.

- Elevated serum cortisol levels are present in clients with hypercortisolism.
- An overnight dexamethasone suppression test is the most widely used screening test.
  —Dexamethasone: 1 mg is administered orally at 11 p.m. and a plasma cortisol level is obtained at 8 a.m. the next morning
  —Suppression of cortisol to less than 5 mg/dl indicates that the hypothalamic–pituitary axis is functioning properly.
- 24-hour urinary free cortisol level is elevated.
- CT, MRI, and angiography may identify lesions of the adrenal or pituitary glands.

Rx:

- Goals of treatment are the reduction of plasma cortisol levels, removal of tumors, prevention of complications, and restoration of normal or acceptable body appearance.
  —Nonsurgical management
  - Radiation therapy if hypercortisolism is caused by a pituitary adenoma
  - Drugs that interfere with adrenocorticotropic hormone production: mitotane (Lysodren), Aminoglutethimide (Cytradren)

  —Surgical management
  - Hypophysectomy (removal of the pituitary gland) if caused due to pituitary adenoma

  —Transsphenoidal approach is usually used
  - Adrenalectomy (removal of the adrenal gland) if cause is an adrenal tumor

Nursing Process Elements

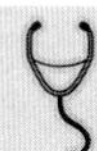

Assessment Alert

Clients with Cushing's syndrome are at risk for carbohydrate intolerance or frank DM.

- Monitor for electrolyte imbalances, hyperglycemia, and opportunistic infections
  - Common signs of infection may be masked by the anti-inflammatory effects of corticosteroid production.
- Provide a diet low in sodium, high in potassium, limited in calories and with increased amounts of calcium and vitamin D
- Provide measures to prevent skin breakdown
  - Use lift sheet to avoid skin tears and shearing
- Assist the client in avoiding pathologic fractures
  - Use of assistive devices if needed
- Monitor and manage potential for Addisonian crisis, which can result from withdrawal of exogenous corticosteroids, adrenalectomy, or by removing a pituitary tumor

Client teaching for self-care

- Advise the client to avoid caffeine and alcohol, which increase risk of GI ulcers and bone density loss
- Lifelong ACTH replacements are needed if adrenal or pituitary gland is removed
- Need to consult with health care provider to adjust doses of replacement hormones when periods of marked physical or emotional stress occur
- Importance of wearing a Medic-Alert

PHEOCHROMOCYTOMA

- Catecholamine-producing tumor of the adrenal medulla and sympathetic ganglia
- Main catecholamine produced is norepinephrine.
- Most are within the adrenal gland but can be extra-adrenal as well.
- Most are benign but if untreated can be fatal.

S&S: Labile hypertension, which may be resistent to control with unusual treatment; palpitations; pallor; profuse generalized perspiration; paroxysmal pulsing headaches, chest and abdomen pain, orthostatic hypotension, hypoglycemia, and hypercalcemia. Episodes of symptomatology may be spontaneous or associated with activities that increase intra-abdominal pressure or by diagnostic tests or anesthesia. Arrhythmias and stroke are risks.

Dx: Screening test: 24-hour urine total metanephrines.

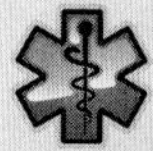

Nursing Intervention Alert

Urine collection for 24 hour; urine total metanephrines should start at the beginning of a hypertensive episode.

MRI or CT imaging of adrenals and abdomen

Rx: Laparoscopic surgical removal of the tumor. Catecholamine blockade with the alpha-adrenergic blocker phenoxybenzamine started 2 weeks prior to surgery followed by beta-blockers. Metyrosine (Demser) also may be given to decrease catecholamine content of the tumor and thereby decrease blood loss and the amount of vasoactive medication needed to control BP during surgery.

Catecholamine levels return to normal in 6 weeks in most clients and normal life activities are resumed.

Nursing Process Elements

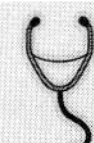

Assessment Alert

Abdominal palpation can precipitate a hypertensive episode.

- During hypertensive crisis, client should be in ICU to allow for needed cardiac, BP, and neurological monitoring
- Manage postoperative pain because untreated it can cause hypertension
- Avoid activities that increase intra-abdominal pressure

Client teaching for self-care

- Self BP measurement
- Avoidance of precipitating factors: straining at stool, bending , lifting, etc.
- Importance of a Medic-Alert bracelet

DIABETES MELLITUS (DM)

- DM is a metabolic disorder characterized by elevated levels of glucose in the blood as a result of a defect in insulin secretion, insulin action, or both.
- Type 1 diabetes
  - —Formerly referred to as insulin-dependent diabetes or juvenile diabetes.
  - —Insulin-producing pancreatic beta cells are destroyed by an autoimmune process.
    - The beta cells produce little or no insulin. People with type 1 diabetes, therefore, require an exogenous form of insulin (injections or inhaled form) in addition to diet and exercise to control blood glucose levels.
- Type 2 diabetes
  - —Formerly referred to as non-insulindependent DM or maturity onset diabetes.
  - —Results from decreased sensitivity to insulin (called insulin resistance) and impaired beta cell functioning results in decreased insulin production.
    - Standard, cornerstone treatment is diet and exercise.
    - May be supplemented with an oral hypoglycemic agent.
    - Insulin injections may be required during periods of acute stress (physiological or psychological), which can markedly increase blood sugar levels and compromise control of the diabetes.
    - Insulin is usually used to control type 2 diabetes during periods of hospitalization for either uncontrolled diabetes or concomitant illness.

Incidence/Prevalence

- Affects 20 million people, 5.9 million (approximately 1/3) of whom are undiagnosed.
- Type 2 diabetes is especially prevalent in the elderly, with up to 50% of people older than 65 years of age suffering some form of glucose intolerance.
  - —Type 2 diabetes occurs more frequently among people who are older than 40 years of age and obese.
  - —Recently, there has been an increased incidence of type 2 diabetes in children and adolescents, as a result of the high incidence of obesity in this population.
- Minority groups share a disproportionate burden of diabetes compared to nonminority groups.
- Non-Hispanic black women have the highest incidence of diabetes.
- Hispanic people also have very high incidence.
- Native American population has very high incidence as well.

Etiology:

Genetic predisposition for both type 1 and type 2

- Type 1 diabetes is thought to be the result of an autoimmune response following viral infection.
- Type 2 diabetes occurs as a result of a variety of risk factors including obesity, sedentary life style, increasing age, past history of gestational diabetes, past history of glucose intolerance, and ethnicity.

Pathophysiology

- Type 1
  - —Genetic, immunologic, and possibly environmental factors contribute to beta cell destruction in the pancreas.
  - —Results in decreased insulin production, unchecked glucose production by the liver, which in turn results in a fasting hyperglycemia.
  - —Glucose derived from food cannot be utilized for energy and metabolic processes without insulin, causing it to remain in the bloodstream and contribute to postprandial (after meals) hyperglycemia.
  - —Increased levels of sugar in the blood cause fluids to be pulled from the intracellular and interstitial spaces into the bloodstream or vascular space (osmosis). Once this extra fluid circulating in the bloodstream reaches the kidneys, diuresis occurs as the kidneys try to maintain normal fluid volume; hence the term "osmotic diuresis." The urine takes with it some of the excess sugar (glucosuria) as well as electrolytes. This can result in profound dehydration and electrolyte imbalance.
  - —Insulin normally inhibits glycogenolysis (breakdown of stored glucose) and gluconeogensis (production of new glucose from amino acids). With defective insulin

production or action, both occur in an unrestrained fashion and further contribute to hyperglycemia

- —Since the body is unable to utilize carbohydrates or sugar for energy, it resorts to breaking down fats, proteins, and body fat for energy; the by-product of which is ketones. This accounts for the ketoacidosis associated most commonly with type 1 diabetes.

- TYPE 2
  - —The main problems associated with type 2 diabetes are insulin resistance and impaired insulin secretion.
  - —The body attempts to counteract the effects of insulin resistance by secreting increased amounts of insulin in an effort to keep blood sugar levels near normal.
    - When the beta cells can not keep up with this increased demand for insulin, clinical symptoms of type 2 diabetes occur.
  - —There is usually enough insulin present to prevent the breakdown of fats and proteins. As a result unless the client is experiencing some type of physiological or severe psychosocial stress that demands increased amounts of energy, ketoacidosis does not occur.
  - —Ketoacidosis may occur when infection, dental problems, or other medical conditions that require increased energy production are present. If quantity or effectiveness of insulin is insufficient to meet these energy demands through metabolism of carbohydrates, proteins and fats are used for energy.

S&S:

- Onset of S&S
  - —Abrupt in type 1 diabetes since there is very little insulin present
  - —Insidious in type 2, a contributing factor to the high number of undiagnosed people living with type 2 diabetes
- Development of the 3 Ps
  - —Polyuria (increased urination): This is the result of osmotic diuresis.
  - —Polydipsia (increased thirst): This is the result of the dehydration that occurs as a result of diuresis.
  - —Polyphagia (increased appetite): Result of decreased satiety (inability to metabolize carbohydrates for energy).
- Other symptoms: fatigue, weakness, vision changes, tingling in hands or feet, dry skin, and wounds that are slow to heal

Dx:

- Symptoms of diabetes

OR

- Fasting plasma glucose levels of 126 mg/dl or more and random plasma glucose levels exceeding 200 mg/dl

OR

- 2-hour postload glucose equal to or greater than 200 mg/dl on a Glucose Tolerance Test (GTT) using 75 g of anhydrous glucose dissolved in water
  - —2-hour GTT is not routinely performed if a fasting plasma glucose of 126 mg/dl or more or random sugar of greater than 200 mg/dl is established because these are diagnostic.

Rx:

Treatment goals:

- Normalize insulin activity and blood glucose levels to reduce the development of vascular and neuropathic complications
  - —Achieve normal glucose levels without hypoglycemia and without disrupting the client's normal lifestyle
  - —Research indicates that maintaining glycemic control can reduce the incidence of complications as much as 50%
- Minimize likelihood of complications that include
  - —Retinopathy: vascular changes in the retina which if untreated may lead to blindness
  - —Neuropathy
    - Peripheral neuropathy that results in loss of sensation, pain, burning in extremities beginning with toes/fingers, and working its way up
    - Autonomic neuropathy that results in loss of nervous innervation to vital organs such as the cardiovascular system and gastrointestinal tract
  - —Renal failure from changes in microvasculature of kidneys, which results in need for dialysis or transplant
  - —Amputation can be required as a result of vascular changes and decreased blood flow to the lower extremities, or sores and infections that do not respond to therapies
  - —Cardiovascular disease: higher incidence of stroke and heart disease in people with diabetes
- Client education in diabetes self-management: Diabetes is a condition that requires that the clients take an active role in managing their disease. Clients make day-to-day choices regarding behaviors that influence their blood sugars or glycemic control. As such, clients must be knowledgeable about their condition, the factors that influence changes in blood sugar, and be able to make informed decisions regarding their illness. The role of the nurse is to facilitate education and promote autonomy in clients with diabetes. The American Diabetes Association standards for education include teaching the client about:
  - —Diet/nutrition
  - —Exercise
  - —Complications: acute and long-term
    - Acute-hypo/hyperglycemia
    - Long-term heart disease, stroke, renal failure, or blindness
  - —Blood glucose monitoring
  - —Stress management/social support
  - —Pharmacological therapies

—Care during periods of illness
—Traveling with diabetes
—Follow-up resources

- Nutrition
  —Primary goal of nutrition therapy is to control blood sugar.
  —Secondary goal may include weight loss and maintenance (particularly in type 2).
  —Higher distribution of calories in carbohydrates than fats and proteins (consistent with food pyramid).
  - 50–60% carbohydrates
  - 20–30% fats
  - 10–20% proteins

  —Exchange lists provide information on serving size and categories of foods so that patients may enjoy a variety of foods by "exchanging" those within each food group.
  - For example, one slice of bread is equal to one serving or 15 gm of carbohydrates or one serving of carbohydrates; three squares of graham crackers are also equal to 15 gm or one serving of carbohydrate, so that patients may "exchange" i.e. choose either a slice of bread; or three squares of graham crackers as one of their carbohydrate servings based on personal preference.
  - The same holds true for proteins, fats, fruits, milk, and vegetables.
  - The number of servings of each group that a patient is allowed is based on the recommendations set forth by the US government food pyramid as well as the total number of calories the patient is prescribed daily.
  - So, while a patient on a 2500-calorie diet is permitted 11 servings of starch and 8 servings of meat daily, a patient on a 1200-calorie diet would be allowed only 5 servings of starch and 4 servings of meat.
  - The primary goal in diet therapy is to attain glycemic control, secondary goals may be related to body weight.

  —Carbohydrate counting; measuring the total grams of carbohydrate contained in a food; 15 grams of carbohydrate is equal to 1 starch (carb) exchange. This provides increased freedom of choices. Also, clients using insulin therapy may be taught to calculate insulin dose based on the number of carbohydrates to be consumed. Commonly, 1 unit of regular or short-acting insulin will cover 1 carbohydrate (15 grams). This is modified based on individual client response.
  —Clients are encouraged to choose foods with lower glycemic index (foods that take longer to break down to sugar in the body), e.g., select whole grains over products containing white flour.
- Exercise
  —Lowers the blood glucose level by increasing the uptake of glucose by body muscles and improving insulin utilization.
  - Clients should not begin exercising if glucose is above 250mg/dl and ketones are present in the urine.
  - Clients are encouraged to exercise daily at the same time, using the same type of activity if exercise is used to control blood sugar.

  —Exercise also may be used as a method to control weight.
  —Because there is a strong relationship between diabetes and heart disease, clients must be cautioned to consult their primary care providers before beginning an exercise program.
  —Clients should be encouraged to monitor blood sugar before, during, and after exercise particularly if there is a potential for hypoglycemia (particularly so for clients using insulin therapy and sulfonylurea treatment).
  —Clients should be encouraged to exercise with a "buddy" who knows about their diabetes and is aware of methods to treat hypoglycemia.
- Monitoring glucose levels
  —Self-monitoring of blood glucose
  - Two to four times daily if insulin is required.
  - Three times daily if insulin is required before all meals.
  - Two to three times per week if insulin is not required, including one test that is done after meals (2 hours is suggested time).
  - Whenever hypoglycemia or hyperglycemia is suspected.
  - Increase frequency of testing with changes in medications, activity, or diet and with stress or illness.

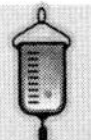

Clinical Alert

Ketone bodies in the urine indicate that control of type 1 diabetes is deteriorating and the risk of diabetic ketoacidosis (DKA) is high.

  —Glycosylated hemoglobin (HgbA1c)
  - HgbA1c contains glucose molecules, which attach to red blood cells; RBCs live in body for 2–3 months; therefore, the HgbA1c reflects the average blood glucose level over 2–3 months.
  - Normal ranges are usually 4–6% and indicate an almost normal blood glucose control.
  - Levels over seven would indicate less than optimal control, putting the client at risk for complications.

  —Research indicates that every decline of one in HgbA1c produces up to a 40% risk reduction; for example decrease in level from 8 to 7.
  —Clients are encouraged to know their values and plan care with the goal of achieving an HgbA1c as close to normal as possible.

- Pharmacological therapy
  - —Rapid-acting insulin: for rapid reduction of glucose before a meal; in some cases taken after meals, e.g., clients with a history of N&V may wait to see if meal is retained
    - Humalog/Novolog
      - Onset; 10–15 minutes
      - Peak; 1 hour
      - Duration; 3 hours
  - —Short-acting insulin: taken 20–30 minutes before a meal
    - Humalog R/Novolog R
      - Onset; 1 hour
      - Peak; 2–3 hours
      - Duration; 4–6 hours
  - —Intermediate-acting insulin: taken after food
    - NPH/Humulin N/Lente/Novolin L
      - Onset; 2–4 hours
      - Peak; 6–12 hours
      - Duration; 16–20 hours
  - —Long-acting insulin: controls fasting glucose level
    - Ultralente
      - Onset; 6–8 hours
      - Peak; 12–16 hours
      - Duration; 20–30 hours
  - —Very long-acting insulin: used for basal dose
    - Lantus
      - Onset; 1 hour
      - Peak; continuous, very little peak
      - Duration; 24 hours
      - Note: Lantus may not be mixed in same syringe with any other insulin
  - —Inhaled insulin: short-acting form, does not come in long-acting form
  - —Exubera
    - Used only in absence of lung disease.
    - No history of smoking for at least 6 months prior to beginning therapy.
    - Pulmonary function tests must be monitored.
  - —Insulin therapy complications
    - Systemic allergic reactions
    - Insulin lipodystrophy; loss of subcutaneous adipose tissue or development of fibrotic tissue in areas of injection—seen less frequently in younger patients since use of human insulin minimizes development, also minimized by site rotation
    - Insulin resistance
    - Morning hyperglycemia
  - —Insulin waning
    - Increase evening dose of intermediate or long-acting insulin
    - Dawn phenomenon—result of normal nighttime release of hormones, which are counterregulatory to insulin and cause an increase in blood sugar level
      - Change time of injection of evening intermediate-acting insulin from dinnertime to bedtime
    - Somogyi effect—result of medications acting at the wrong time, blood sugar drops during night, liver attempts to correct hypoglycemia and client arises with high blood sugar levels
      - Decrease evening dose of intermediate-acting insulin
      - Snack before bedtime
- Oral antidiabetic agents, used in addition to other treatment modalities in type 2 diabetes.
  - —Sulfonylureas
    - Glucotrol
    - Diabeta
    - Amaryl
      - Increase insulin secretion
      - As a result, side effects include weight gain and hypoglycemia
  - —Biguanides
    - Glucophage; Metformin
      - Insulin sensitizer does not cause hypoglycemia
      - Some clients lose weight
      - GI side effects are usually self-limiting to 2 weeks
      - Lactic acidosis rare but requires client teaching
  - —Alpha glucosidase inhibitors
    - Acarbose and glycet
    - Inhibit glucose absorption
    - Major deterrent severe flatulence
  - —Thiazolidinediones
    - Avandia: recent research indicates high incidence of MI in clients using this drug
    - Actos
    - Insulin sensitizers
    - Liver enzymes must be monitored
    - Delayed onset of action: 2 weeks
  - —Meglitinides
    - Prandin
    - Starlix
    - Insulin secretagogues
    - Used to control postprandial rises in blood sugar
    - Taken with first bite of food at each meal
  - —Alternate insulin delivery methods
    - Insulin pens, injectors, and pumps
    - Insulin pumps can
      - deliver a premeal dose of insulin before each meal;
      - deliver a varying hourly basal rate of insulin;

- deliver a dose of insulin based on a pre-programmed insulin to carbohydrate ratio; and
- monitor blood sugar levels at preset intervals
- Implantable and inhalant insulin delivery

Nursing Process Elements

- Education is the ongoing focus of care to aid clients in mastering the concepts and skills necessary for long-term management of diabetes and its potential complications.
- Recognize that NPO status requires adjustments in usual insulin regimens:
  —Eliminating insulin for type 1 diabetes may lead to DKA; eliminating insulin for type 2 is safer
  —Question regarding continuing administration of oral hypoglycemic agents even when NPO
- Monitor for and manage episodes of hypoglycemia:
  —Symptoms are shakiness, sweating, hunger, and weakness, which are caused by too much insulin, exercise, or not enough food.
  —Treat with 15 g concentrated carbohydrate such as two to three glucose tablets , half cup juice, 8-oz skim milk
  —Follow with snack such as cheese or milk and crackers.
  —Clients at risk for hypoglycemia should be instructed to always carry some form of simple carbohydrate with them such as glucose tabs, lifesavers or other candies, crackers, or juice.
  —Significant others of those clients receiving insulin therapy must be instructed on the administration of glucagon in the event of severe hypoglycemia where the patient is unable to ingest oral forms of glucose.
- Monitor for and manage DKA, which is a consequence of severe insulin deficiency in the adipose tissue, liver, and skeletal muscle.
  —Symptoms are hyperglycemia (300–800 mg/dl), signs of dehydration, electrolyte loss, and ultimately acidosis: N&V, abdominal pain, acetone breath (fruity odor), hyperventilation (Kussmaul respirations), and mental status changes caused by absence or markedly inadequate amount of insulin.
  —Treat with IV regular insulin, rehydration with NS at 500 ml/hr for 1 hour and then 250 ml/hr, electrolyte restoration (IV K^+ if serum level is less than 3.5 mEq/l once renal output is established) and acidosis reversal to arterial pH of 7.0 or greater.
- Monitor for and manage hyperglycemic hyperosmolar nonketotic coma which is an acute complication of type 2 DM
- Symptoms are similar to those of DKA except dehydration is profound; serum glucose ranges from 600 to 2000 mg/dl; serum osmolarity is 350 mOsm/l or higher; ketosis is absent because some insulin is available; thirst perception is usually impaired by some problem; and another illness generally exists; polyuria disappears early; and lethargy and somnolence may be present.
- Treat with hypotonic (0.45% NS) IV and correct precipitating disease; insulin usually not required.

Client teaching for self-care

- Reinforce information and instructions related to daily schedule, diet, exercise, blood glucose monitoring, stress management, and lifestyle changes
- Self-administration of insulin
  —Use correct type and amount of insulin
  —Rotate sites
  —Roll bottle to mix before drawing up
  —Use opened bottles within 30 days
  —Keep refrigerated or at room temperature
  —Rapid-or short-acting forms of insulin can be given simultaneously with longer-acting insulins; mix together in the same syringe, drawing the regular insulin first
- Foot and leg care
  —Thoroughly dry and lubricate feet, no water or lotion between toes
  —Never go barefoot
  —Wear closed-toe shoes, with extra cushioning for bony prominences
  —Trim toenails straight across
  —Avoid walking barefooted, using heating pads on feet or shaving-toe calluses
  —Inspect feet daily for open areas and sores
  —Ask physician or nurse practitioner to examine feet at each office visit
  —Yearly examination by podiatrist
  —Goal: early detection of neuropathy and lesions
- Prevention/early detection of renal disease
  —Screen urine for microalbuminuria, which is an early sign of kidney disease that occurs when small particles of protein are leaking into urine.
  —Clients should be instructed to question provider if microalbuminuria is present.
  —Importance of taking angiotensin-converting enzyme (ACE) inhibitors as prescribed because of their protective effect on the kidneys, which can reverse and/or slow progression of kidney disease.
- Prevention/early detection of eye disease
  —Obtain a dilated eye exam at least annually to detect early signs of retinopathy; eye exam also allows detection of cataracts and macular degeneration for which diabetic clients are at high risk.

- Dental care
  —See dentist at least twice annually because diabetes increases risk of dental problems and conditions such as an abscess can cause blood sugar to rise.

Client teaching for self-care

- Diagnostic criteria:
  Fasting Blood Sugar (FBS): 100–126 mg/dl or
  Oral Glucose Tolerance Test (OGTT): 140–200 mg/dl
- Early detection and treatment may prevent or delay onset of type 2 diabetes in more than 50% of clients
- Treatment consists of lifestyle changes including incorporation of diet and exercise
- Diabetic emergencies
  —DKA
  - Life-threatening condition that occurs as a result of severe insulin deficiency
  - Occurs primarily in type 1 diabetes
  - Clinical manifestations
    - Elevation in blood glucose levels typically between 300–800 mg/dl
    - Decreased pH of blood
    - Ketonuria
    - Electrolyte imbalance
    - Dehydration
- Treatment
  —Rehydration: Restore circulating fluid volume initiated with NS until blood sugar levels reach 250–300 mg/dl at which point the client is typically switched to a solution containing dextrose such D5W or D5NS.
  —Insulin: Regular insulin is administered IV to treat hyperglycemia
  —IV insulin administration will continue until the client is stabilized and subcutaneous administration can be resumed
  —Blood sugar levels are monitored closely sometimes at least hourly until stabilized
  —Potassium levels may be compromised due to dehydration so should be monitored frequently to assess for the need for replacement.
- Hyperglycemic hyperosmolar nonketotic syndrome (HHNS)
  —Extreme hyperglycemia occurring without ketosis
  —Occurs most frequently in clients with type 2 diabetes
  —May occur rapidly or slowly over period of days
  —May occur in individuals with subclinical type 2 diabetes, undiagnosed who are further compromised by the onset of a concurrent illness or condition
  —Clinical manifestations
  —Hyperglycemia manifested in blood glucose levels of 600–1200 mg/dl.
  —Dehydration: often profound resulting in hypotension and compensatory tachycardia
  —Change in mental status
  —Neurological manifestations, coma, and death if not corrected
- Treatment
  —Fluid replacement with NS; and then dextrose solution levels once reach 250–300 mg/dl
  —IV insulin to treat hyperglycemia
  —Monitor electrolyte status/replacement as indicated
  —Monitor mental/neurologic status
  —Monitor VS
  —Rehydration is key in both ketoacidosis and HHNS

WORKSHEET

MATCHING QUESTIONS

Match the following:

Column A	Column B
1. ____ Addison's disease	a. Insulin resistance
2. ____ Myxedema coma	b. Graves' disease
3. ____ Thyroid cancer	c. Extreme stage of hypothyroidism

4. ____ GH deficiency	d. Characterized by elevated serum calcium and decreased serum phosphorus
5. ____ Pheochromocytoma	e. May be precipitated by hypomagnesemia
6. ____ Hyperthyroidism	f. Classic presenting sign is labile hypertension
7. ____ Type 1 DM	g. Only occurs prior to closure of epiphyses
8. ____ Acromegaly	h. Growth deceleration is characteristic of the juvenile form
9. ____ DI	i. Characterized by horizontal growth
10. ____ Hypoparathyroidism	j. May be iatrogenic secondary to use of Prednisone
11. ____ Hypoglycemia	k. Lack of insulin due to beta cell destruction
12. ____ DKA	l. Manifests in the neonate with hyperpyrexia, tachypnea, and seizures
13. ____ SIADH	m. Signs include acetone breath and Kussmaul's respirations
14. ____ Cushing's syndrome	n. Cold nodule
15. ____ Hypothyroidism	o. Short stature is the usual presenting complaint
16. ____ Gigantism	p. Signs predominantly the result of excessive glucocortecoids and androgens
17. ____ Thyroid storm	q. Can be a transient event after transsphenoidal pituitary surgery
18. ____ Type 2 DM	r. Associated with malignancies such as opioids and small cell cancer of the lung
19. ____ Hyperparathyroidism	s. Temperature may reach 105–106°F.
20. ____ Addisonian crisis	t. Precipitated by inadequate food intake

MATCHING QUESTIONS

Match the following:

Column A: Drugs	Column B: Diseases
1. ____ Tapazole	a. Acromegaly
2. ____ Exubera	b. DI
3. ____ Avandia	c. DM
4. ____ SSKI	d. Somatotropin defeiciency
5. ____ Glucophage	e. Nephrogenic DI

(continued)

6. ____ Declomycin	f. Hyperthyroidism
7. ____ Novolog	g. Hypothyroidism
8. ____ Acarbose	h. Hyperparathyroidism
9. ____ Levothyroxine	i. Hypoparathyroidism
10 ____ Metyrosine	j. Addison's disease
11. ____ Humalin	k. Cushing's disease
12. ____ DDAVP	l. Pheochromocytoma
13. ____ Vitamin D	m. SIADH
14. ____ Sulfonylureas	
15. ____ Thiazide diuretics	
16. ____ Solu-Cortef	
17. ____ Octreotide acetate	
18. ____ Calcium gluconate	
19. ____ GH	
20. ____ Mitotane	
21. ____ Aminoglutethimide	
22. ____ Propylthiouracil	
23. ____ Metformin	
24. ____ Prandin	
25. ____ Actos	

FILL IN THE BLANK

Fill in the blank space with the correct word or phrase to complete each statement

1. The client is performing a return demonstration on preparing insulin. The morning dose of insulin is 10 units of regular and 22 units of NPH. The nurse determines that the client has prepared the correct dose when the syringe reads ____ units.

TRUE & FALSE QUESTIONS

Mark each of the following statements True or False. Correct all false statements in the space provided.

1. The alpha-adrenergic blocker phenoxybenzamine is started 2 weeks prior to surgery for a pheochromocytoma. ___ T ___ F

2. Abdominal palpation should be avoided in clients with a pheochromocytoma because it can precipitate a hypotensive episode. ___ T ___ F

3. Peripheral neuropathy is a potential complication of diabetes that places the client at risk for injury such as burns and falls. ___ T ___ F

4. Dental problems in the diabetic client have the potential to trigger ketoacidosis. ___ T ___ F

5. Tube feedings for a client with SIADH should be diluted with saline rather than water. ___ T ___ F

APPLICATION QUESTIONS

1. When assessing a client with a PTH deficiency, the nurse would expect abnormal serum levels of which substances?
   a. Sodium and chloride
   b. Potassium and glucose
   c. Urea and uric acid
   d. Calcium and phosphorous

2. When answering a client's question about the use of a RAIU test, on which fact should the nurse's answer be based?
   a. RAIU increases in hyperthyroidism and decreases in hypothyroidism.
   b. RAIU decreases in hyperthyroidism and increases in hypothyroidism.
   c. RAIU increases in both secretion disorders of the thyroid gland.
   d. RAIU decreases in both secretion disorders of the thyroid gland.

3. When assessing a client diagnosed with Graves' disease, which finding would the nurse consider to be a hallmark of the disease?
   a. Low specific gravity of urine
   b. Heat intolerance
   c. Hirsutism
   d. Dulled mentation

4. A client with a history of mitral valve replacement using long-term warfarin (Coumadin), is diagnosed with myxedema. When levothyroxine is prescribed, which other type of order should the nurse expect the physician to write?
   a. Decrease in warfarin dosage
   b. Protamine sulfate PRN
   c. 2-weeks follow-up with radioactive iodine
   d. Weekly APTT measures

5. A client with thyroid cancer undergoes a thyroidectomy. After surgery, the client develops peripheral numbness, tingling, and muscle twitching. Which type of medication should the nurse be prepared to administer?
   a. Thyroid supplement
   b. Antispasmodic
   c. Barbiturate
   d. Calcium replacement

6. A client with asthma develops Cushing's syndrome and tells the nurse she doesn't understand what could have caused the problem. The nurse's response would be based in part on the understanding that

(continued)

Cushing's syndrome can develop as a complication from the chronic use of which medication?
a. Theophylline
b. Prednisone
c. Alupent
d. Intal

7. Which action helps to combat the Dawn phenomenon in a client with DM?
a. Eat a snack at bedtime
b. Inject evening intermediate-acting insulin at bedtime rather than dinnertime
c. Decrease evening dose of intermediate-acting insulin
d. Increase evening dose of long-acting insulin

8. A client recently diagnosed with type 1 diabetes is learning foot care. Which of the following responses by the client would indicate additional teaching is needed?
(Select all that apply.)
a. "I will never go barefoot outside; only in my house is it permissible."
b. "My toenails need to be trimmed straight across."
c. "I will always wear socks and closed-toe shoes."
d. "I will inspect my feet every week for any sores or open areas."

9. When assessing a client during an acute episode of DI, on which problem would the nurse focus?
a. Imbalanced nutrition
b. Deficient fluid volume
c. Ineffective coping
d. Risk for impaired skin integrity

10. When teaching a diabetic client about his insulin protocol, the nurse explains that intermediate-acting insulin should reach its "peak" in how many hours?
a. 16–20 hours
b. 3–4 hours
c. 6–12 hours
d. 1–2 hours

11. When answering a client's question about insulin pumps and how they work, which information could appropriately be included in the nurse's response? Mark all that apply.
Insulin pumps can
a. deliver a pre-meal dose of insulin before each meal.
b. deliver a varying hourly basal rate of insulin.
c. deliver a dose of insulin based on a preprogrammed insulin to carbohydrate ratio.
d. monitor blood sugar levels at preset intervals.

12. A diabetic client taking an oral antidiabetic agent asks if he will also need parenteral insulin therapy at times. The nurse's response would be based on the knowledge that parenteral insulin therapy will be temporarily substituted for oral antidiabetic agents if the diabetic
a. develops an infection with fever.
b. suffers trauma.
c. undergoes major surgery.
d. all of the above.

13. In evaluating laboratory results, the nurse interprets which findings as indicative of DKA? Mark all that apply.
a. ___ Increased blood pH
b. ___ Decreased total body potassium
c. ___ Elevated blood glucose
d. ___ Decreased serum bicarbonate level

14. A client with DM receives a prescription for an ACE inhibitor and asks what this drug will do for him. The nurse responds that the drug reduces changes in the blood vessels and may help delay the onset of which problem?
a. Chronic obstructive pulmonary disease
b. Pancreatic cancer
c. Renal failure
d. Cerebral vascular accident

15. When teaching a diabetic client, which symptom should the nurse identify as most commonly indicative of hypoglycemia?
a. Nervousness
b. Anorexia
c. Kussmaul's respirations
d. Bradycardia

16. A female client with type 1 DM is experiencing a minor flu-like illness with nausea, muscle aches, and low-grade fever. Which instruction should the nurse give her?
a. Increase the frequency of glucose self-monitoring
b. Try to reduce food intake to diminish nausea
c. Do not take any insulin if she cannot eat
d. Take half of the normal dose of insulin

17. Which of the following is a priority nursing diagnosis for the diabetic client who is taking insulin and has N&V from a viral illness or influenza?
a. Imbalanced nutrition; less than body requirements
b. Impaired health maintenance related to ineffective coping skills
c. Risk for acute pain
d. Activity intolerance

18. During a home visit, a diabetic client begins to cry and say, "I just cannot stand the thought of having to give myself a shot every day." Which would be the best response by the nurse?
    a. "If you do not give yourself your insulin shots, you will die."
    b. "We can teach your daughter to give the shots so you will not have to do it."
    c. "I can arrange to have a home care nurse give you the shots every day."
    d. "What is it about giving yourself the insulin shots that bothers you?"
19. A client presents in the emergency room with DKA. Which nursing diagnosis would be the priority problem?
    a. Disturbed sleep pattern
    b. Impaired health maintenance
    c. Imbalanced nutrition; less than body requirements
    d. Deficient fluid volume
20. Which of the following would the nurse include when developing a teaching plan for a newly diagnosed client with type 2 DM. (Select all that apply.)
    a. A major risk factor for complications is cigarette smoking.
    b. Insulin is mandatory for controlling the disease.
    c. Exercise increases insulin resistance.
    d. The primary nutritional source requiring monitoring in the diet is carbohydrates.
    e. Annual eye and foot examinations are recommended by the American Diabetes Association.
21. Which of the following would the nurse report for a client with unstable type 2 DM? (Select all that apply.)
    a. Systolic BP of 145 mmHg
    b. Diastolic BP of 87 mmHg
    c. HDL of 30 mg/dl
    d. HgbA1c of 10.2%
    e. Triglycerides of 425 mg/dl
    f. Urinary ketones negative
22. When should the diabetic client who is taking insulin (Humalog) injections be advised to eat?
    a. Within 20 minutes after the injection
    b. 1 hour after the injection
    c. At any time, because timing of meals with Humalog is unnecessary
    d. 2 hours before the injection
23. Teaching for a client beginning therapy with methimazole (Tapazole) would appropriately include which information? Mark all that apply.
    a. The effect of the treatment will be noticeable in 7–10 days.
    b. Periodic RBC counts will be needed during therapy.
    c. Any signs of infection need to be reported to the health care provider.
    d. Dose of Tapazole will be tapered as normal thyroid status is attained.
24. A client is being treated for hypercalcemic crisis. Which assessment findings would the nurse interpret as indicating overtreatment of the problem? Mark all that apply.
    a. _____ Decreased bowel sounds
    b. _____ Photophobia
    c. _____ Leg cramps
    d. _____ Positive Chvostek sign
    e. _____ Vomiting
    f. _____ Perioral numbness and tingling
    g. _____ Bradycardia

ANSWERS & RATIONALES

MATCHING ANSWERS

Match the following:

Column A	Column B
1. __j__ Addison's disease	a. Insulin resistance
2. __c__ Myxedema coma	b. Graves' disease

(continued)

3. __n__ Thyroid cancer	c. Extreme stage of hypothyroidism
4. __o__ GH deficiency	d. Characterized by elevated serum calcium and decreased serum phosphorus
5. __f__ Pheochromocytoma	e. May be precipitated by hypomagnesemia
6. __b__ Hyperthyroidism	f. Classic presenting sign is labile hypertension
7. __k__ Type 1 DM	g. Only occurs prior to closure of epiphyses
8. __i__ Acromegaly	h. Growth deceleration is characteristic of the juvenile form
9. __q__ DI	i. Characterized by horizontal growth
10. __e__ Hypoparathyroidism	j. May be iatrogenic secondary to use of Prednisone
11. __t__ Hypoglycemia	l. Manifests in the neonate with hyperpyrexia, tachypnea, and seizures
12. __m__ DKA	k. Lack of insulin due to beta cell destruction
13. __r__ SIADH	m. Signs include acetone breath and Kussmaul's respirations
14. __p__ Cushing's syndrome	n. Cold nodule
15. __h__ Hypothyroidism	o. Short stature is the usual presenting complaint
16. __g__ Gigantism	p. Signs predominantly the result of excessive glucocortecoids and androgens
17. __s__ Thyroid storm	q. Can be a transient event after transsphenoidal pituitary surgery
18. __a__ Type 2 DM	r. Associated with malignancies such as opioids and small cell cancer of the lung
19. __d__ Hyperparathyroidism	s. Temperature may reach 105–106 degrees F.
20. __l__ Addisonian crisis	t. Precipitated by inadequate food intake

MATCHING ANSWERS

Match the following:

Column A: Drugs	Column B: Diseases
1. __f__ Tapazole	a. Acromegaly
2. __c__ Exubera	b. DI
3. __c__ Avandia	c. DM
4. __f__ SSKI	d. Somatotropin defeiciency
5. __c__ Glucophage	e. Nephrogenic DI

6. _m_ Declomycin
7. _c_ Novolog
8. _c_ Acarbose
9. _g_ Levothyroxine
10. _l_ Metyrosine
11. _c_ Humalin
12. _b_ DDAVP
13. _i_ Vitamin D
14. _c_ Sulfonylureas
15. _e_ Thiazide diuretics
16. _j_ Solu-Cortef
17. _a_ Octreotide acetate
18. _i_ Calcium gluconate
19. _d_ GH
20. _k_ Mitotane
21. _k_ Aminoglutethimide
22. _f_ Propylthiouracil
23. _c_ Metformin
24. _c_ Prandin
25. _c_ Actos

f. Hyperthyroidism
g. Hypothyroidism
h. Hyperparathyroidism
i. Hypoparathyroidism
j. Addison's disease
k. Cushing's disease
l. Pheochromocytoma
m. SIADH

ANSWER FOR FILL IN THE BLANK

Fill in the blank space with the correct word or phrase to complete the statement.

1. The client is performing a return demonstration on preparing insulin. The morning dose of insulin is 10 units of regular and 22 units of NPH. The nurse determines that the client has prepared the correct dose when the syringe reads _32_ units.

TRUE & FALSE ANSWERS

Mark each of the following statements True or False. Correct all false statements in the space provided.

1. The alpha-adrenergic blocker phenoxybenzamine is started 2 weeks prior to surgery for a pheochromocytoma. *True*
2. Abdominal palpation should be avoided in clients with a pheochromocytoma because it can precipitate a hypotensive episode. *False*

   Abdominal palpation should be avoided in clients with a pheochromocytoma because it can precipitate a hypertensive episode.
3. Peripheral neuropathy is a potential complication of diabetes, which places the client at risk for injury such as burns and falls. *True*
4. Dental problems in the diabetic client have the potential to trigger ketoacidosis. *True*
5. Tube feedings for a client with SIADH should be diluted with saline rather than water. *True*

APPLICATION ANSWERS

1. When assessing a client with a PTH deficiency, the nurse would expect abnormal serum levels of which substances?
   a. Sodium and chloride
   b. Potassium and glucose
   c. Urea and uric acid.
   d. Calcium and phosphorous

Rationale

Correct answer: d.

Decreased PTH reduces resorption of calcium from bone, reduces intestinal absorption of calcium, and reduces reabsorption of calcium in the renal tubules. At the same time, it increases retention of phosphate in the renal tubules. The net effect of these actions is that serum calcium is low and serum phosphate is high. Changes in serum sodium, chloride, potassium, glucose, urea, or uric acid are not direct effects of PTH deficiency.

2. When answering a client's question about the use of a RAIU test, on which fact should the nurse's answer be based?
   a. RAIU increases in hyperthyroidism and decreases in hypothyroidism.
   b. RAIU decreases in hyperthyroidism and increases in hypothyroidism.
   c. RAIU increases in both secretion disorders of the thyroid gland.
   d. RAIU decreases in both secretion disorders of the thyroid gland.

Rationale

Correct answer: a.

The more active the thyroid gland is, the more iodide it concentrates. Thus in hyperthyroidism with its increase in thyroid activity, radioactive iodine is concentrated in the thyroid in above normal amounts. In hypothyroidism, with its decrease in thyroid activity, lower than normal amounts of radioactive iodine are picked up by the thyroid gland.

3. When assessing a client diagnosed with Graves' disease, which finding would the nurse consider to be a hallmark of the disease?
   a. Low specific gravity of urine
   b. Heat intolerance
   c. Hirsutism
   d. Dulled mentation

Rationale

Correct answer: b.

Heat intolerance with diaphoresis when environmental temperature is comfortable to others is a classic sign of hyperthyroidism or Graves' disease. Low specific gravity of urine is a classic sign of DI. Hirsutism accompanies hypersecretion of glucocorticoids from the adrenal glands. Dulled mentation is a sign of hypothyroidism.

4. A client with a history of mitral valve replacement using long-term warfarin (Coumadin), is diagnosed with myxedema. When levothyroxine is prescribed which other type of order should the nurse expect the physician to write?
   a. Decrease in warfarin dosage
   b. Protamine sulfate PRN
   c. 2-week follow-up with radioactive iodine
   d. Weekly APTT measures

Rationale

Correct answer: a.

Levothyroxine interacts with anticoagulants including warfarin increasing available levels of active anticoagulant. As a result, dosage needs to be decreased to avoid bleeding problems. Protamine sulfate is an antidote for heparin. Follow-up with radioactive iodine is not done. APTT guides the dosage of heparin; INR guides the dosage of warfarin.

5. A client with thyroid cancer undergoes a thyroidectomy. After surgery, the client develops peripheral numbness, tingling, and muscle twitching. Which type of medication should the nurse be prepared to administer?
   a. Thyroid supplement
   b. Antispasmodic
   c. Barbiturate
   d. Calcium replacement

Rationale

Correct answer: d.

The parathyroid glands can be unintentionally removed along with the thyroid gland. If this occurs, hypocalcemic tetany is a risk, the first signs of which include numbness and tingling in the extremities and muscle twitching. The treatment of hypocalcemic tetany is IV calcium gluconate or calcium carbonate, which should be readily available at the bedside.

6. A client with asthma develops Cushing's syndrome and tells the nurse she doesn't understand what could have caused the problem. The nurse's response would be based in part on the understanding that Cushing's syndrome can develop as a complication from the chronic use of which medication?
   a. Theophylline
   b. Prednisone
   c. Alupent
   d. Intal

Rationale

Correct answer: b.

Prednisone is a corticosteroid and long-term use of corticosteroids is a common cause of Cushing's syndrome.

7. Which action helps to combat the Dawn phenomenon in a client with DM?
   a. Eat a snack at bedtime
   b. Inject evening intermediate-acting insulin at bedtime rather than dinner time
   c. Decrease evening dose of intermediate-acting insulin
   d. Increase evening dose of long-acting insulin

Rationale

Correct answer: b.

Inject evening intermediate-acting insulin at bedtime rather than dinnertime. Eating a snack at bedtime and decreasing the evening dose of intermediate-acting insulin combat the Somogyi effect. Increasing the evening dose of long-acting insulin helps combat insulin waning.

8. A client recently diagnosed with type 1 diabetes is learning foot care. Which of the following responses by the client would indicate additional teaching is needed?
   (Select all that apply.)
   a. "I will never go barefoot outside; only in my house is it permissible."
   b. "My toenails need to be trimmed straight across."
   c. "I will always wear socks and closed-toe shoes."
   d. "I will inspect my feet every week for any sores or open areas."

Think Smart/Test Smart

This is a negative question. It asks which statements indicate a need for more teaching. More teaching is needed if the client has not learned needed information correctly. Therefore, you are looking for what the client says that is wrong.

Rationale

Correct answers: a and d.

Option a is an incorrect statement because the diabetic client should never go barefoot. Option d also is incorrect because feet need to be inspected daily not weekly. Therefore, both of these statements indicate a need for further teaching. Options b and c are true statements: toenails need to be trimmed straight across and socks and closed-toed shoes should always be worn.

(continued)

9. When assessing a client during an acute episode of DI, on which problem would the nurse focus?
   a. Imbalanced nutrition
   b. Deficient fluid volume
   c. Ineffective coping
   d. Risk for impaired skin integrity

Rationale

Correct answer: b.

During an acute episode of DI between 4 and 20 l of dilute urine is voided per 24 hours. With inadequate fluid replacement, hypotension, tachycardia, and weight loss develop and ultimately shock from fluid loss can occur. Thus, deficient fluid volume should be the focus of assessment. Imbalanced nutrition, ineffective coping, and risk for impaired skin integrity may be problems but they are not the priority.

10. When teaching a diabetic client about his insulin protocol, the nurse explains that intermediate-acting insulin should reach its "peak" in how many hours?
    a. 16–20 hours
    b. 3–4 hours
    c. 6–12 hours
    d. 1–2 hours

Rationale

Correct answer: c.

Intermediate-acting insulin (NPH/Humulin N/Lente/ Novolin L) has its onset in 2–4 hours, peaks at 6–12 hours, and has a duration of 1–20 hours.

11. When answering a client's question about insulin pumps and how they work, which information could appropriately be included in the nurse's response? (Mark all that apply.) Insulin pumps can
    a. deliver a premeal dose of insulin before each meal.
    b. deliver a varying hourly basal rate of insulin.
    c. deliver a dose of insulin based on a preprogrammed insulin to carbohydrate ratio.
    d. monitor blood sugar levels at preset intervals.

Rationale

Correct answers: a, b, and c.

Insulin pumps can deliver a bolus of insulin before a meal or a continuous basal rate, which can be programmed to vary hourly to best match normal diurnal rhythm. Smart pumps also can be preprogrammed with an insulin to carbohydrate ratio so at mealtime or snack time , the client programs in the number of grams of carbohydrate that he or she plans to eat and the pump calculates the insulin dose accordingly. The pump does not test blood sugar levels but an algorithm allows additional insulin to be administered based on a blood sugar value entered by the client following a fingerstick.

12. A diabetic client taking an oral antidiabetic agent asks if he will also need parenteral insulin therapy at times. The nurse's response would be based on the knowledge that parenteral insulin therapy will be temporarily substituted for oral antidiabetic agents if the diabetic
    a. develops an infection with fever.
    b. suffers trauma.
    c. undergoes major surgery.
    d. all of the above.

Rationale

Correct answer: d.

Any major physical stress such as infection, trauma, or surgery requires the temporary use of insulin rather than an oral antidiabetic agent.

13. In evaluating laboratory results, the nurse interprets which findings as indicative of DKA? (Mark all that apply.)
    a. ___ Increased blood pH
    b. ___ Decreased total body potassium
    c. ___ Elevated blood glucose
    d. ___ Decreased serum bicarbonate level

Rationale

Correct answers: b, c, and d.

In DKA, blood glucose is elevated as a result of glycogen breakdown into glucose and accelerated gluconeogenesis. As the liver produces ketone bodies in excess of the number that can be cleared by the kidney, ketones in the plasma rise. Serum bicarbonate decreases as the acidic ketones are buffered by the bicarbonate. Total body potassium is decreased even though serum potassium is increased, because acidosis is associated with a shift of potassium out of the cells into the serum from which it is lost through the kidney. Blood pH decreases, not increases, as acidosis occurs.

14. A client with DM receives a prescription for an ACE inhibitor and asks what this drug will do for him. The nurse responds that the drug reduces changes in the blood vessels and may help delay the onset of which problem?
    a. Chronic obstructive pulmonary disease
    b. Pancreatic cancer
    c. Renal failure
    d. Cerebral vascular accident

Rationale

Correct answer: c.

ACE inhibitors are renal protective and may reverse or delay the onset of renal disease.

15. When teaching a diabetic client, which symptom should the nurse identify as most commonly indicative of hypoglycemia?
    a. Nervousness
    b. Anorexia
    c. Kussmaul's respirations
    d. Bradycardia

Rationale

Correct answer: a.

Nervousness along with shakiness, weakness, trembling, pallor, diaphoresis, tachycardia, irritability, and palpitations are all adrenergic symptoms associated with hypoglycemia. Headache, mental confusion, circumoral paresthesia, fatigue double vision, incoherent speech, seizures, and coma are neuroglycopenic symptoms. Kussmaul's respirations are a symptom of hyperglycemia.

16. A female client with type 1 DM is experiencing a minor flu-like illness with nausea, muscle aches and low grade fever. Which instruction should the nurse give her?
    a. Increase the frequency of glucose self-monitoring
    b. Try to reduce food intake to diminish nausea
    c. Do not take any insulin if she cannot eat
    d. Take half of the normal dose of insulin

Rationale

Correct answer: a.

The client should be instructed to increase the frequency of glucose self-monitoring in order to determine if insulin dosage needs to be adjusted.

17. Which of the following is a priority nursing diagnosis for the diabetic client who is taking insulin and has N&V from a viral illness or influenza?
    a. Imbalanced nutrition; less than body requirements
    b. Impaired health maintenance related to ineffective coping skills
    c. Risk for acute pain
    d. Activity intolerance

Rationale

Correct answer: a.

Imbalanced nutrition: less than body requirements. Insulin and dietary intake must be in balance for hypoglycemia or hyperglycemia to be avoided. With decreased intake from N&V, the need for insulin will be decreased placing the client at risk for hypoglycemia. Ineffective coping skills and activity intolerance may be problems but are not life-threatening at the moment so are not the priority. Acute pain is not an expected symptom.

18. During a home visit, a diabetic client begins to cry and say, "I just cannot stand the thought of having to give myself a shot every day." Which would be the best response by the nurse?
    a. "If you do not give yourself your insulin shots, you will die."
    b. "We can teach your daughter to give the shots so you will not have to do it."
    c. "I can arrange to have a home care nurse give you the shots every day."
    d. "What is it about giving yourself the insulin shots that bothers you?"

Rationale

Correct answer: d.

Asking "What is it about giving yourself the insulin shots that bothers you?" acknowledges the existence of a problem and gives it validity. It also facilitates identifying the exact nature of the problem so it can be addressed. Threatening the client as in option a does not address the problem or give confidence in one's ability to manage self-care. Having another person—family member or nurse, is not the best approach because not only doesn't it determine what the problem is but puts potentially unnecessary constraints on the client.

19. A client presents in the emergency room with DKA. Which nursing diagnosis would be the priority problem?
    a. Disturbed sleep pattern
    b. Impaired health maintenance
    c. Imbalanced nutrition; less than body requirements
    d. Deficient fluid volume

Rationale

Correct answer: d.

Deficient fluid volume occurs because insulin deficiency results in hyperglycemia as a result of the breakdown of glycogen into glucose and accelerated gluconeogenesis. The progressive hyperglycemia results in glycosuria, which acts as an osmotic diuretic and causes dehydration. Initially, thirst increases fluid intake and dehydration is minimized but with progressive ketosis, N&V ensue and dehydration becomes severe. Thus, deficient fluid volume that can lead to circulatory collapse and shock is the priority diagnosis because it is immediately life-threatening; the other diagnoses are not.

20. Which of the following would the nurse include when developing a teaching plan for a newly diagnosed client with type 2 DM. (Select all that apply.)
    a. A major risk factor for complications is cigarette smoking.
    b. Insulin is mandatory for controlling the disease.
    c. Exercise increases insulin resistance.
    d. The primary nutritional source requiring monitoring in the diet is carbohydrates.
    e. Annual eye and foot examinations are recommended by the American Diabetes Association.

(continued)

Rationale

Correct answers: a and e.

Cigarette smoking is a major risk factor for every known complication of DM. Annual eye and foot examinations are recommended by the American Diabetes Association. Insulin is not always necessary for the control of DM. Type 2 DM is characterized by insufficient insulin or impaired action of insulin, not absence of insulin. Thus diet, exercise, and/or oral antidiabetic medications may control the problem. Exercise lowers blood sugar by increasing uptake of glucose by muscles and improving insulin utilization. Intake of carbohydrates, fats, and proteins must be monitored and should be consistent with the food pyramid with most calories derived from carbohydrates.

21. Which of the following would the nurse report for a client with unstable type 2 DM? (Select all that apply.)
    a. Systolic BP of 145 mm Hg
    b. Diastolic BP of 87 mm Hg
    c. HDL of 30 mg/dl
    d. HgbA1c of 10.2%
    e. Triglycerides of 425 mg/dl
    f. Urinary ketones negative

Rationale

Correct answers: a, b, c, d, and e.

Hypertension in the diabetic exacerbates retinopathy, renal changes, and cardiovascular disease. Therefore, it must be aggressively monitored and treated. For the diabetic person, a BP of 130/85 or higher either systolically or diastolically requires intervention and therefore should be reported. HDL of 30 mg/dl is consistent with dyslipidemia as is the elevated triglyceride level. HgbA1c reflects the average blood glucose of over 2–3 months. Normal range is 4–6%. Over 7% indicates less than optimal control of blood sugar and risk for complications.

22. When should the diabetic client who is taking insulin (Humalog) injections be advised to eat?
    a. Within 20 minutes after the injection
    b. 1 hour after the injection
    c. At any time, because timing of meals with Humalog is unnecessary
    d. 2 hours before the injection

Rationale

Correct answer: a.

The onset of Humalog is in 10–15 minutes with a peak in 1 hour and a duration of 3 hours. It is typically taken before meals to ensure a rapid reduction in glucose. In a few cases, it is taken after a meal as when a client with N&V waits to make certain that the ingested food is going to stay down.

23. Teaching for a client beginning therapy with methimazole (Tapazole) would appropriately include which information? (Mark all that apply.)
    a. The effect of the treatment will be noticeable in 7–10 days.
    b. Periodic RBC counts will be needed during therapy.
    c. Any signs of infection need to be reported to the health care provider.
    d. Dose of Tapazole will be tapered as normal thyroid status is attained.

Rationale

Correct answers: c and d.

Infection may be the first sign of agranulocytosis, which is a side effect of the thiomides which include Tapazole and PTU. The dose of antithyroid drug is gradually tapered as the client regains a euthyroid state. The effect of treatment is not seen for several weeks because hormone which is already synthesized must be used up. Periodic WBC counts are required during therapy.

24. A client is being treated for hypercalcemic crisis. Which assessment findings would the nurse interpret as indicating overtreatment of the problem? (Mark all that apply.)
    a. ___ Decreased bowel sounds
    b. ___ Photophobia
    c ___ Leg cramps
    d. ___ Positive Chvostek sign
    e. ___ Vomiting
    f. ___ Perioral numbness and tingling
    g. ___ Bradycardia

Rationale

Correct answers: b, c, d, and f.

Overtreatment of hypercalcemia results in hypocalcemia. Signs of hypocalcemia include photophobia, cramps in the extremities, positive Chvostek and Trousseau's signs, and numbness and tingling around the mouth and in the hands and feet. Decreased bowel sounds that occur with decreased peristalsis, vomiting and bradycardia are signs of hypercalcemia so they would be associated with undertreatment not overtreatment.

CHAPTER 28

Test Plan Category:

Physiological Integrity

Sub-category: Physiological Adaptation—Part 1

Topics: Alterations in Body Systems
Illness Management
Section 10: Urinary Problems

URINARY TRACT INFECTION (UTI)

- UTI is acute or chronic bacterial infection of the normally sterile lower urinary tract including the urethra (urethritis) and bladder (cystitis).
- Sepsis may result, particularly in the elderly and the immunocompromised.

Etiology: Bacteria (most commonly *E. coli*) enters the urinary tract through the urethra and begins to multiply and produce symptoms of infection.

Risk factors: Incomplete emptying of the bladder; urethral stricture; inadequate fluid intake; bowel incontinence; decreased mobility; improper cleaning of perineal area; urinary catheterization; clothing or personal care products that encourage irritation and inflammation of the perineal area; females and the elderly are at highest risk.

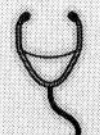

Assessment Alert

UTIs are frequently seen in late pregnancy due to the pressure of the uterus on the urinary structures. UTIs are also frequent in the postpartal period secondary to bladder trauma during the birth process.

S&S:

- Dysuria
- Urinary frequency and urgency
- Suprapubic pain
- Nocturia
- Cloudy, foul-smelling urine

- Hematuria
- N&V
- Fever and chills
- Fatigue

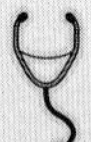

Assessment Alert 

Atypical presentations of infection are common in the elderly. Mental changes or confusion may be the only signs of possible UTI.

Dx: Urinalysis indicates leukocyturia, hematuria, albuminuria; urine C&S identifies causative organism; abdominal ultrasound or X-ray (KUB) may be needed to evaluate the status of the renal system.

Rx: Antibiotic therapy, commonly co-trimoxazole (Bactrim, Septra), nitrofurantoin (Macrodantin), or amoxicillin (Amoxil) to reduce pathogen count; prophylactic antibiotic therapy commonly ordered for recurrent UTIs; phenazopyridine (Pyridium) for its analgesic effects to relieve dysuria; increased fluid intake encourages passage of bacteria out of the body; drinking two to three glasses of cranberry juice a day increases acidity of the urine, which discourages bacteria from attaching to the wall of the bladder.

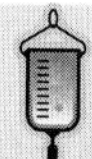

Clinical Alert

Chronic or recurrent episodes must be treated thoroughly to reduce the risk of progression to pyelonephritis and possible permanent kidney damage.

Nursing Process Elements

- Assess for S&S
- Recognize high-risk populations
- Support efforts to prevent recurrence
- Maintain asepsis with urinary catheter insertion and follow standards for routine catheter care

Client teaching for self-care

- Take all medications as prescribed, even if symptoms of infection subside
- Anticipate that urine will be red–orange with Pyridium use
- Void at regular and frequent intervals; void after intercourse
- Increase fluid intake to at least 8 oz/d
- Wear cotton underwear; avoid tight-fitting pants, and nylon pantyhose
- Shower, rather than tub bathe
- Avoid douching, bubble bath, powder, sprays, or harsh soaps
- Keep the genital area clean and wipe from front to back
- Notify physician if symptoms persist or recur

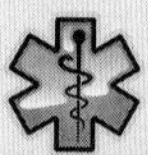

Nursing Intervention Alert OB

Pregnant women with UTIs are at risk for preterm labor. The pregnant client should be monitored closely for S&S of the onset of labor. A preterm infant faces many additional challenges, which can lead to physical and/or mental deficits.

Pyelonephritis

- Pyelonephritis is acute or chronic bacterial infection of the upper urinary tract including the kidneys and ureters.
- It can result in renal failure secondary to damage and atrophy of the nephrons.
- Sepsis may result particularly in the elderly and immunosuppressed.

Etiology: Bacterial pathogens cause inflammation of the renal parenchyma and collecting system; the inflammatory process may result in formation of scar tissue over time; most often occurs as a result of UTI, particularly in the presence of backflow of urine from the bladder into the ureters or kidney pelvis (vesicoureteric reflux).

Risk factors: History of chronic or recurrent UTI, renal papillary necrosis, kidney stones, vesicoureteric reflux, and obstructive uropathy.

S&S:

- UTI symptoms (dysuria, frequency & urgency, pyuria, hematuria, nocturia)
- Fever
- Chills
- Malaise
- Fatigue
- Flank pain
- Costovertebral angle tenderness
- N&V

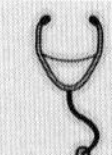

Assessment Alert 

Atypical presentations of infection are common in the elderly. Mental changes or confusion may be the only indication of an acute infection.

Dx: Urinalysis indicates leukocyturia, hematuria, albuminuria; urine C&S identifies causative organism; intravenous pyelogram (IVP) or CT scan of the abdomen may reveal enlarged kidneys with poor flow of dye through the kidneys; blood culture is positive in the presence of sepsis.

Rx: Antibiotic therapy (intravenous or oral depending on severity), commonly cephalosporins, levoflaxin, ciproflaxin, amoxicillin. Prophylactic antibiotics may be prescribed for chronic pyelonephritis; increased fluid intake (up to 3 l/d) encouraged; analgesics to relieve pelvic or flank pain; hospitalization may be required.

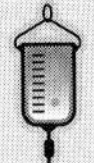

Clinical Alert 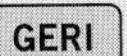

Prompt treatment is critical for the elderly due to the high mortality rate and risk of permanent damage.

Nursing Process Elements

- Assess for S&S
- Recognize high-risk populations
- Administer medications and IV fluids as ordered
- Monitor for complications, including sepsis and acute renal failure, and report immediately if any develop
- Support prompt and complete treatment of UTIs
- Educate the client about ways to prevent UTIs (See client teaching under UTI.)

Glomerulonephritis

- Glomerulonephritis is acute or chronic inflammation of the glomeruli.
- It is among the leading causes of chronic renal failure and end-stage renal disease (ESRD).

Etiology: Infection, injury, or autoantibodies stimulate an immune response within the body and the glomeruli become inflamed, scar tissue forms, and tubular atrophy and loss of renal function ultimately occurs.

Precipitating factors: Acute glomerunephritis can occur 2–3 weeks following streptococcal infection.

Risk factors: Vasculitis, polyarteritis, abscess of any internal organ, collagen vascular diseases, history of malignant tumors, or blood or lymphatic system disorders.

S&S:

- Dark, smoke-colored, or foamy urine
- Edema
- Oliguria or anuria
- Hematuria
- Nocturia
- Resistant hypertension
- Shortness of breath
- Cough
- Fever
- Malaise
- Arthralgia
- Myalgia
- Abdominal pain
- Anorexia and unintentional weight loss
- N&V
- Decreased alertness
- Seizure
- Polyneuropathy

Dx: Urinalysis indicates hematuria, leukocyturia, proteinuria; BUN, creatinine, and potassium levels are elevated; creatinine clearance is decreased; ultrasound, CT, or IVP may reveal altered kidney size; chest X-ray may reveal pulmonary congestion; kidney biopsy indicates inflammation and may identify crescent-shaped abnormalities.

Rx: Hospitalization; bed rest; restriction of fluids, sodium, potassium, and dietary protein; corticosteroids (Prednisone) to suppress inflammatory response; antibiotics to treat infection; ACE inhibitors to reduce proteinuria and control hypertension; diuretics for moderate edema; dialysis or kidney transplant if progresses to ESRD.

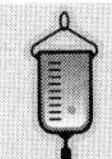

Clinical Alert 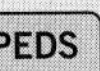

Outcome varies with disease process responsible for the glomerulonephritis. Children tend to recover more quickly and completely.

Nursing Process Elements

- Emphasize importance of early detection and treatment of streptococcal infections
- Monitor for complications, including renal failure, pulmonary edema, and heart failure and notify physician immediately if any S&S develop
- Administer medications as prescribed
- Educate client about the importance of strict compliance with medication and diet regime

Client teaching for self-care

- Take medication as prescribed, even if symptoms subside
- Follow dietary restrictions on salt, fluid, and protein

- Seek treatment for possible streptococcal infections, vascular diseases, hypertension, or fluid retention
- Report development of new symptoms particularly shortness of breath, decreased urine output, or changes in level of alertness

NEPHROSIS (NEPHROTIC SYNDROME)

- A group of symptoms including protein in the urine (exceeding 3.5 g/d), low serum protein, high serum cholesterol, and generalized edema associated with functional damage to glomeruli.
- Outcome varies; may be acute and short-term or chronic and unresponsive to treatment, leading to ESRD.

Etiology: Infection, drug exposure, malignancy, immune disorders, or disease damage the basement membrane of the glomeruli, disrupting the filtering and excretion of protein, lipids, and blood. As vital protein is lost from the intravascular space, extravascular fluid accumulates.

Risk factors: Can affect all age groups; occurs slightly more often in males than females; can accompany kidney disease including glomerulonephritis.

S&S:

- Edema
- Ascites
- Foamy urine
- Unintentional weight gain (edema-related)
- Anorexia
- Hypertension
- Atherosclerosis

Dx: Urinalysis reveals large amounts of protein; urine may also contain fat, which is visible under the microscope; serum protein and cholesterol levels elevated.

Rx: Moderate protein, sodium-restricted diet; corticosteroids (Prednisone) to diminish inflammatory response; ACE inhibitors to reduce proteinuria and control hypertension; cholesterol-reducing medications; antithrombolytics may be ordered to prevent clot formation. Immunosuppressant drugs such as Cytoxan may be added to reduce the risk of relapse. Note: the edema of nephritic syndrome does not usually respond to diuretic agents.

Nursing Process Elements

- Encourage compliance with diet and medication therapy
- Educate client to recognize serious symptoms and seek medical attention
- Monitor blood pressure and cholesterol levels routinely and encourage vigorous treatment
- Monitor for development of complications including atherosclerotic disease, renal vein thrombosis, pulmonary edema, congestive heart failure, and renal failure

Client teaching for self-care

- Take medications as prescribed even if symptoms subside
- Follow dietary restrictions
- Monitor blood pressure, cholesterol levels, and weight changes
- Report if symptoms persist or new symptoms develop, particularly severe headache, fever, sores on the skin, cough, discomfort with urination, or decreased urine output

ACUTE RENAL FAILURE

- Acute renal failure is a sudden loss of the kidney's ability to excrete wastes, concentrate urine, and conserve electrolytes.
- Outcomes are affected by the underlying cause, severity of condition, and timing of treatment initiation.
- It may progress to uremic syndrome, ESRD, or death.

Etiology: Both kidneys rapidly become unable to excrete the daily accumulation of metabolic wastes; toxins build up and damage tissues and impair organ functioning. Acute renal failure is classified as prerenal, intrarenal, or postrenal based on the location of its cause.

Prerenal failure is characterized by diminished renal perfusion resulting from a decrease in blood supplying the kidneys.

Intrarenal failure (also called intrinsic) results from an abrupt decrease in glomerular filtration rate (GFR) due to tubular cell damage because of renal ischemia or nephrotoxic injury.

Postrenal failure is associated with conditions causing an obstruction of urinary flow.

Risk factors: Cardiovascular disorders, hemolytic disorders, autoimmune disorders, sepsis, shock, hypovolemia, exposure to nephrotoxic agents (contrast dyes, aminoglycosides, etc.), surgery, trauma, neurogenic bladder, renal calculi, renal tubular necrosis, and obstruction of the bladder, ureters, or urethra. The elderly and immunosuppressed are at highest risk.

S&S:

- Oliguria (usually the earliest sign)
- Anorexia
- Fatigue
- N&V
- Diarrhea or constipation
- Pruritus
- Edema
- Dyspnea

- Mental status changes
- Dry mucous membranes
- Bleeding and bruising
- Tinnitus
- Uremic breath and metallic taste
- Hypertension and tachycardia
- Hypotension (if renal hypoperfusion)
- Pleuritic chest pain
- Seizures

Dx: Blood tests reveal elevated BUN, creatinine, and potassium levels and decreased pH, bicarbonate levels, and hematocrit/hemoglobin. Urine specimens indicate decreased specific gravity, proteinuria, and urine osmolality close to serum osmolality. Urine sodium is usually <20 mEq/l when the failure is related to hypoperfusion and >40 mEq/l when the cause is intrinsic. Creatinine clearance (measures GFR) is used to estimate the number of remaining functioning nephrons. Kidney ultrasound, CT scan, retrograde pyelography, MRI, and KUB may be needed to evaluate the status of the renal system.

Rx: Goal is to identify and treat any reversible causes and reestablish renal functioning. Hospitalization is usually required. Supportive measures include a high-calorie, vitamin-supplemented diet with restricted fluid, sodium, protein, and potassium. Offending drugs are discontinued; life-threatening hyperkalemia is treated with hypertonic glucose and insulin infusions, oral or rectal Kayexalate, or dialysis; antibiotics are given to treat or prevent infection; ACE inhibitors to control blood pressure; digoxin to improve cardiac function; diuretics to eliminate excess fluid retention; renal replacement therapy (peritoneal dialysis or hemodialysis) to remove the accumulation of nitrogenous waste products.

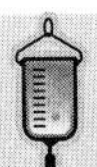

Clinical Alert

Monitor and report elevated serum creatinine levels. Renal dosing should be considered when prescribing medications that are excreted by the kidneys to a client with a serum creatinine level >2.0.

Nursing Process Elements

- Accurately record I&O, vital signs, and daily weight
- Administer medications as ordered
- Support nutrition and hydration status
- Monitor for complications including metabolic acidosis, fluid volume overload, hyperkalemia, and seizures. Report immediately if any develop

Client teaching for self-care

- Take all medications as prescribed
- Follow high-calorie, low-protein, low-sodium, low-potassium diet with vitamin supplements
- Follow fluid restrictions
- Report decreased urine output, weight gain, edema, changes in respiratory and neurological status, or irregular heartbeats

CHRONIC RENAL FAILURE

- Chronic renal failure is a gradual, progressive, irreversible syndrome of impaired renal function resulting from a decreased number of functioning nephrons.
- It occurs in three stages reflecting progressive loss of nephron systems.
  —Stage I (Diminished renal reserve)—50% functional loss, serum creatinine in high normal range (2 mg/dl), and asymptomatic
  —Stage II (Renal insufficiency)—75–80% functional loss, serum creatinine around 4 mg/dL, BUN/creatinine elevated, and anemia present
  —Stage III (ESRD)—90% functional loss, serum creatinine ~8 mg/dl, GFR critically low (≤10), homeostasis cannot be maintained and all body systems are affected

Etiology: Chronic inflammation, renal ischemia, or obstruction leads to progressive nephron and glomerular damage. Remaining healthy nephrons are able to compensate by enlarging and increasing clearance until 75% or more of the nephrons become nonfunctioning. At that point, the kidney's ability to excrete wastes, concentrate urine, and conserve electrolytes is lost and uremic toxins accumulate and produce life-threatening changes in all major organ systems.

Risk factors: Chronic infections, glomerulonephritis, vascular disease, hypertension, diabetes, long-term use of nephrotoxic agents, renal calculi, obstructive uropathy, and acute renal failure that fails to respond to treatment.

S&S (early):

- Fatigue
- Malaise
- Anorexia
- N&V
- Unintentional weight loss
- Nocturia

S&S (late):

- Edema
- Dyspnea

- Severe anemia
- Oliguria or anuria
- Pruritus
- Easy bruising/bleeding
- Mental status changes
- Peripheral neuropathy
- Muscle and bone pain
- Hypertension
- Cardiac arrhythmias
- Uremic breath
- Sexual dysfunction
- Skeletal demineralization

Dx: Progressively increasing BUN and creatinine levels; decreased 24-hour urine creatinine clearance; elevated potassium level; ABGs and blood chemistry may indicate metabolic acidosis; CT, MRI, X-ray, or ultrasound may reveal decreased kidney size.

Rx:

- Diphenhydramine to relieve itching
- Calcium carbonate to lower serum phosphate levels
- Vitamin B & D supplementation to treat deficiencies
- Loop diuretic (Lasix) to reduce fluid retention
- Digoxin to improve cardiac functioning
- ACE inhibitors to control blood pressure
- Antiemetics to relieve nausea
- Famotidine to decrease gastric irritation
- Ducosate sodium to prevent constipation
- Epoetin alfa to increase RBC production
- Blood transfusions to treat severe anemia
- Kayexalate to treat hyperkalemia

Think Smart/Test Smart

Remember that diuretics move fluid out of the body by means of the kidney. In order for a diuretic to work, there must be functioning kidney cells. Diuretics do not cure sick kidneys. Therefore, once ESRD sets in, diuretics are of almost no value and in fact can cause harmful effects.

- Supportive treatment includes a diet restricted in fluid, protein, sodium, potassium, and phosphate and promotion of rest and conservation of energy. Renal replacement therapy (peritoneal dialysis, hemodialysis, or kidney transplant) is necessary when the GFR falls to between 5 and 10

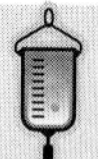

Clinical Alert

Frequent transfusions to treat anemia increase the risk of hepatitis for clients with chronic renal failure.

Nursing Process Elements

- Monitor lab values including BUN/Creatinine, H&H, and potassium levels
- Monitor vital sign changes, daily weight, and strict I&O
- Observe for signs of bleeding
- Educate about dietary restrictions, compliance with medication and treatment plan, importance of maintaining normal glucose levels and blood pressure
- Educate about dialysis treatment and monitor response to therapy (see Chapter 16)
- Provide opportunity for client to vent feelings about imposed diet and activity limitations
- Refer client and family for appropriate counseling and support
- Monitor for complications including infection at dialysis access site, hyperkalemia, and impaired organ functioning

Client teaching for self-care

- Regularly monitor blood glucose levels and blood pressure; report abnormal results
- Avoid foods high in sodium, potassium, and phosphate
- Comply with protein and fluid restrictions
- Take medications as prescribed
- Report decreased urine output, persistent nausea, unexplained weight loss, presence of swelling, shortness of breath, changes in mental status, elevated blood pressure.

URINARY CALCULI (NEPHROLITHIASIS)

- Urinary calculi are stones of varying size which result from the accumulation and precipitation of deposits of mineral crystals.
- Calculi may remain in the renal pelvis or enter the ureters.
- Obstruction of urine flow, infection, and bleeding may result.

Etiology: Inadequate water or excessive mineral levels lead to an accumulation, then precipitation, of substances normally dissolved in the urine. The most common types are calcium oxalate calculi, uric acid calculi, cystine calculi, and struvite calculi.

Risk factors: Dehydration; infection; urinary obstruction; urinary stasis; excessive intake of calcium, vitamin C & D, and protein; immobility; gout; arthritis; hyperparathyroidism; genetically defective metabolism of cystine; consistent urine acidity or alkalinity.

S&S:

- Pain (flank, back, testicle, or groin)
- N&V
- Fever and chills
- Hematuria
- Pyuria
- Anuria (rare)
- Abdominal distention

Dx: Stones or obstruction may be seen on ultrasound, X-rays, IVP, MRI, or CT; urine culture may indicate UTI; urinalysis may be normal or may indicate elevated specific gravity, altered pH, hematuria, and pyuria; 24-hour urine collection may be elevated for calcium oxalate, phosphorus, and uric acid excretion levels; serum uric acid levels may indicate gout as the cause.

Rx: Vigorous hydration and ambulation to encourage natural passage; analgesics (opioid and adjuvant) for pain; antibiotic therapy if infection present; low-purine, low-protein, low-calcium diet; allopurinol to reduce uric acid levels; bicarbonate or potassium citrate to alkalinize urine; ascorbic acid to acidify urine; thiazide diuretics to decrease calcium excretion; parathyroidectomy to treat hyperparathyroidism; ureteroscopy, lithotripsy, or percutaneous nephrolithotomy to surgically remove large stones (>7 mm). Ninety percent of stones are smaller than 5 mm in diameter.

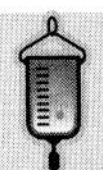

Clinical Alert

Approximately 90% of renal calculi are smaller than 5 mm in diameter; stones larger than 7 mm usually require some form of surgical intervention.

Nursing Process Elements

- Assess and treat pain
- Force fluids
- Encourage ambulation
- Strain urine; save solid material for analysis
- If surgery necessary, explain preoperative and postoperative care
- Monitor for complications including urine flow obstruction, hydronephrosis, infection, or bleeding

Client teaching for self-care

- Take all medications as prescribed
- Increase fluid intake (up to 3–4 l/d)
- Report symptoms of infection, pain, bleeding, and inability to void
- Save urine for straining

Vesicoureteral Reflux

- Vesicoureteral reflux is characterized by the reflux of urine from the bladder back into the ureter and kidney.
- It may lead to pyelonephritis, scarring, nephrotic syndrome, and ESRD.

Etiology: One-way ureteral valve fails, allowing urine to back flow.

Risk factors: Previous or family history; renal calculi; bladder outlet obstruction; congenital abnormalities of the urinary tract; neurogenic bladder; ureteral edema or trauma.

S&S:

- Flank, back, or abdominal pain
- Fever and chills
- Dysuria
- Nocturia
- Hematuria
- Recurrent UTIs
- Hydronephrosis
- Hypertension
- May be asymptomatic if only one kidney involved

Dx: BUN, creatinine, and urine protein levels may be elevated; urine culture may be positive; cystogram, IVP, or abdominal CT may reveal reflux, hydronephrosis, scarring, or small kidney; voiding cystourethrogram (VCUG) confirms diagnosis.

Rx: Antibiotics if infection present; annual ultrasounds to monitor development; ureteral reconstruction or reimplantation if condition is severe.

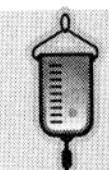

Clinical Alert

Close monitoring is warranted. It may resolve without intervention; however, damage to kidney is irreversible.

Nursing Process Elements

- Educate client about the S&S of reflux; emphasize importance of follow-up
- Monitor for complications including hypertension, pyelonephritis, nephrotic syndrome, and renal failure

Client teaching for self-care

- Keep appointments for monitoring progression
- Report new or persistent symptoms, including pain, fever, bleeding, diminished output, generalized swelling, or high blood pressure

Hydronephrosis

- Hydronephrosis is unilateral or bilateral dilation of renal calyces and pelvis proximal to an obstruction of urine flow.
- Symptoms, treatment, and outcomes are related to the cause of the obstruction.
- The unaffected kidney, in unilateral cases, hypertrophies and may function up to 80% as effectively as both kidneys did before the obstruction.
- Bilateral obstruction leads to renal failure.

Etiology: Obstruction of any part of the urinary system generating backflow of urine, increased pressure, and distention. The urine backup eventually reaches the kidney pelvis and results in increased tubular pressure and damage.

Risk factors: Vesicoureteral reflux, renal calculi, prostate enlargement, advanced pregnancy, uterine cancer, bladder outlet obstruction, neurogenic bladder, acute or chronic obstructive uropathy.

S&S:

- Flank pain
- Abdominal mass
- N&V
- Fever
- Dysuria
- Urinary frequency, urgency, and retention
- Recurrent UTIs
- Sometimes unilateral hydronephrosis does not have symptoms

Dx: Diagnostic studies vary depending on whether the obstruction is in the upper or lower urinary tract; generally an IVP, ultrasound, CT scan, or MRI confirms disorder; urinalysis may suggest etiology; serum BUN, creatinine levels may help to determine degree of renal impairment.

Rx: Surgical management includes balloon dilation, nephrostomy tube placement, or stenting; IV fluids and electrolyte replacements as indicated for postobstructive diuresis; opioid analgesics and antispasmodics for pain management; antibiotics if infection present; prophylactic antibiotics if condition is chronic.

Nursing Process Elements

- Assess and treat pain
- Report fluid and electrolyte imbalances
- If surgery necessary, explain preoperative and postoperative care
- Educate client about S&S of infection and recurrent obstruction
- Monitor for complications including renal failure

Client teaching for self-care

- Reduce occurrence/recurrence of conditions that increase risk (renal calculi, frequent UTIs, vesicoureteral reflux, etc.)
- If postsurgical, follow instructions for incision and drain care
- Take medications as prescribed
- Keep appointments for follow-up
- Report S&S of infection and recurrent obstruction, including pain, fever, diminished urine output, and swelling

Bladder Cancer

- Most common is transitional cell (cells lining the bladder); other types include squamous cell and adenocarcinoma.
- Graded and staged (TNM staging system) based on aggressiveness and degree of mutation; treatment and prognosis varies according to staging category.

Etiology: Unknown, though several factors may contribute to development.

Risk factors: Cigarette smoking; exposure to certain industrial chemicals, chemotherapeutic agents, or pelvic irradiation; chronic infections; three times more common in men.

S&S:

- Painless hematuria
- Urinary urgency
- Dysuria
- Bladder outlet or ureter obstruction
- Cystitis
- Pelvic or abdominal pain and distention
- Anemia
- Weight loss
- Fatigue and lethargy

Dx: Physical exam may reveal rectal or pelvic mass; urinalysis may be positive for blood: urine cytology may identify malignant cells; cystoscopy allows visualization and biopsy; IVP enables evaluation of upper urinary tract for tumors or blockage; chest X-ray, bone scan, CT, and MRI studies rule out metastases

Rx: Intravesical chemotherapy; radiotherapy; surgical options include transurethral resection of tumor; partial cystectomy, or radical cystectomy with urinary diversion (see Chapter 18)

Nursing Process Elements

- Assess presence and severity of unpleasant symptoms; take measures to alleviate
- Explain chemotherapy and radiotherapy procedures
- Teach about preoperative and postoperative care and long-term management
- Assess and treat postoperative pain
- Provide opportunity for venting feelings about diagnosis and change in body appearance; make referrals as appropriate.
- Monitor for complications including anemia, stomal problems, and infection
- Support efforts to reduce occupational exposure to carcinogens and smoking cessation

Client teaching for self-care

- Take medications as directed
- Keep appointments for treatment and follow-up
- Participate in education for urinary diversion care prior to performing independently
- Report complications of disease or treatment including obstructed urine flow, bleeding, fever, pain, malaise, and peristomal skin problems

Renal Cancer

- May be unilateral or bilateral cancer of the kidney.
- Most common is renal cell carcinoma involving the cells of tubule lining.
- Graded and staged based on aggressiveness and degree of mutation; prognosis is based on progression at the time of diagnosis.
- About one-third of clients have metastasis at the time of diagnosis; most common sites of metastasis are the lungs, lymph nodes, liver, and bone.

Etiology: Unknown, though several factors may contribute to development.

Risk factors: Cigarette smoking; positive family history; obesity; occupational exposure to certain industrial chemicals; occurs twice as often in men; usually occurs between the ages of 40–70.

S&S:

- Painless hematuria
- Flank, back, or abdominal pain
- Unexplained weight loss
- Testicular or abdominal distention
- Fever
- Hypertension
- Polycythemia
- Constipation
- Elevated alkaline phosphatase and serum calcium levels

Dx: Kidney X-ray or abdominal CT confirms diagnosis; chest X-ray, bone scan, and MRI may reveal metastasis.

Rx: Chemotherapy, radiotherapy, surgical removal of all or part of the kidney (nephrectomy), or a combination of these treatments.

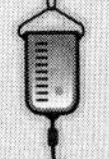

Clinical Alert

Early detection and aggressive treatment improves clinical outcomes.

Five-year survival rate for early stages without metastasis is 60–75%

Five-year survival after lymph node metastasis is 5–15%

Five-year survival after other organ metastasis is less than 5%

Nursing Process Elements

- Educate about preoperative and postoperative care and long-term management
- Explain chemotherapy and radiotherapy procedures
- Assess and treat pain
- Provide opportunity for venting feelings and make referrals as appropriate
- Monitor for complications including hypertension and metastasis
- Support efforts to reduce occupational exposure to carcinogens and smoking cessation

Client teaching for self-care

- Immediately report presence of blood in urine
- Stop smoking
- Take medications as directed
- Keep appointments for treatment and follow-up

PEDS Wilm's Tumor

- Wilm's tumor is the most common renal cancer in children.
- Rapidly developing kidney tumor may become quite large, but usually remains encapsulated.
- Complications include hypertension, impaired renal functioning, possible metastasis to lungs, liver, bone, or brain, or death
- Early detection and aggressive treatment improves clinical outcomes

Etiology: Unknown.

Risk factors: Early childhood (3–8 years); positive history in twin or sibling; presence of certain birth defects including urinary tract abnormalities, absence of an iris, or hemihypertrophy (enlargement of one side of the body).

S&S:

- Abdominal pain and swelling
- Hematuria
- Anorexia
- N&V
- Generalized malaise
- Hypertension
- Constipation

Dx: CBC may reveal anemia; BUN and creatinine elevated; abdominal U/S, X-ray, or CT scan confirm a mass; CXR, bone scan, and MRI studies rule out metastasis.

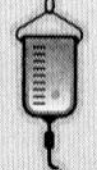

Clinical Alert

Children with a known risk for Wilm's tumor should be routinely screened with kidney ultrasounds.

Rx: Surgery, radiotherapy, chemotherapy, or a combination of these.

Nursing Process Elements

- Report hypertension in children
- Explain chemotherapy and radiotherapy procedures
- Teach about preoperative and postoperative care
- Assess and treat postoperative pain
- Support child and family; make referrals as appropriate
- Monitor for complications including renal failure and metastasis

Client teaching for self-care

- If postsurgical, follow instructions for incision and drain care
- Take medications as prescribed
- Keep appointments for follow-up
- Report development of new or worsening symptoms including pain, fever, bleeding, cough, chest pains, or weight loss.

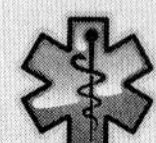

Nursing Intervention Alert

Care should be taken to avoid palpating the abdomen prior to surgical removal of the tumor to reduce the risk of seeding the tumor.

PEDS Extrophy of the Bladder

- Extrophy of the Bladder is an infrequent congenital defect in which the abdominal wall and anterior bladder wall fail to fuse in utero resulting in the posterior wall of the bladder protruding through the abdominal wall
- Accompanied by congenital pelvic bone separation and epispadias (abnormal location of urethral opening)
- Complications include chronic UTIs, incontinence, or erectile/sexual dysfunction

Etiology: Unknown.

Risk factors: Occurs more often in males.

S&S:

- Red, angry-looking mass on abdominal surface, continuous leakage of urine onto surface
- Widened pubic bones
- Outwardly rotated legs and feet
- Short, small penis with urethral opening along top of penis in the male.
- Narrow vaginal opening, wide labia, and short urethra in the female.

Dx: Usually diagnosed by fetal ultrasound before birth and physical examination after birth.

Rx: Surgical repair to internalize the bladder and attach the pelvic bones within the first 48 hours after birth. Epispadias repair may be completed at the same time or repair may be delayed.

Nursing Process Elements

- Sterile, nonadherent dressing covers bladder in preoperative period

- Educate about preoperative and postoperative care and long-term management
- Explain that the child may be in a lower body cast or sling postoperatively
- Assess and treat postoperative pain
- Assess family's coping style and support systems; make referrals as appropriate
- Monitor for complications including skin impairment from urinary incontinence, infection, or sexual dysfunction

Client teaching for self-care

- If postsurgical, follow instructions for incision and drain care
- Take medications as prescribed
- Keep appointments for follow-up
- Anticipate stages of surgical correction
- Report development of new or worsening symptoms including pain, fever, cloudy, foul-smelling urine, or skin impairment

PEDS Cryptorchidism

- Cryptorchidism is a developmental defect in which one or both testicles fail to descend into the scrotum prior to birth.
- About 65% will typically descend without intervention by 9 months of age.
- Infertility, testicular torsion, and an increased risk for testicular cancer may develop if the testicle fails to descend by age 1.

Etiology: Unknown.

Risk factors: Premature birth.

S&S:

- Visual and palpable variance in scrotal assessment

Dx: Examination confirms that one or both testicles are not present in the scrotum.

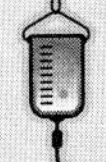

Clinical Alert

The risk for testicular cancer is 40% greater in men with a history of cryptorchidism.

Rx: Testicle most often descends without intervention within the first year of life; hormonal injections (B-HCG or testosterone) may be given to stimulate testicular movement; surgical correction (orchiopexy) is definitive therapy (in rare cases, no testicle may be found upon surgical exploration).

Nursing Process Elements

- Perform scrotal assessments on all male infants; assess for natural testicular descent within first year of life
- Administer medication as ordered and monitor response
- If surgery necessary, educate about preoperative and postoperative care
- Educate about increased risk for infertility and testicular cancer
- Teach males over the age of 15 to perform testicular self-examinations to screen for testicular cancer (see Chapter 8)

Client teaching for self-care

- If postsurgical, follow instructions for incision and drain care
- Take medications as prescribed
- Keep appointments for follow-up
- Perform monthly testicular self-examinations after age 15 because the risk of testicular cancer is 40% greater in men with a history of cryptorchidism

PEDS Hypospadias

- Hypospadias is a congenital condition in which the male urethral opening is located on the ventral surface of the penis and the foreskin is incompletely formed.
- It is associated with chordee (a downward curvature of the penis).
- If left untreated, it may lead to difficulty with toilet training, sexual dysfunction, urethral strictures, and fistulas

Etiology: Unknown.

S&S:

- Urethra is displaced to the underside, midshaft, or base of the penis
- Downward curvature of penis

Dx: Physical examination reveals disorder; radiologic studies rule out other congenital anomalies.

Rx: Surgical revision of the urethral tract and meatus; may require temporary urinary diversions; repair may need to be performed in stages, requiring multiple surgeries. Results typically good, both cosmetically and functionally, approximately 10–20% require revision for fistulas and chordee recurrence.

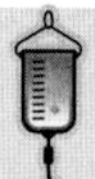

Clinical Alert

Infants with hypospadias should not be circumcised. The foreskin should be preserved for use in later surgical repair.

Nursing Process Elements

- Assess presence of disorder
- Educate about preoperative and postoperative care
- Monitor for complications including strictures or fistulas

Client teaching for self-care

- Anticipate stages of surgical correction
- Do not have child circumcised if hypospadias is suspected
- If postsurgical, follow instructions for incision and drain care
- Keep appointments for follow-up
- Report new or recurring symptoms including urinary straining or an abnormal location of urine passage

WORKSHEET

TRUE & FALSE QUESTIONS

Mark each of the following statements True or False. Correct all false statements in the space provided.

1. Confusion may be the only clinical sign of a UTI in the older adult. ___ T ___ F
2. Recurrent episodes of UTIs could progress to permanent kidney damage. ___ T ___ F
3. Placement of an indwelling catheter to treat urinary incontinence decreases the risk for a UTI. ___ T ___ F
4. A client with nocturia should be instructed to schedule the majority of fluid intake prior to 4 p.m. ___ T ___ F
5. Symptoms of renal failure occur when 40% of nephrons become nonfunctioning. ___ T ___ F
6. Renal calculi larger than 7 mm usually require some form of surgical intervention. ___ T ___ F
7. Surgical correction of cryptorchidism is usually performed prior to the age of 6 months. ___ T ___ F
8. Infants with hypospadias should not be circumcised. ___ T ___ F
9. Dehydration is a risk factor for urinary calculi. ___ T ___ F
10. Flank pain is a prominent symptom of hydronephrosis. ___ T ___ F

FILL IN THE BLANKS

Fill in the blank spaces with the correct word or phrase to complete each statement.

1. What lifestyle habit puts a client at risk for prostatitis? ____________________
2. What is the term for the amount a client should weigh after urinating if renal functioning is not impaired? ____________________
3. What type of screening is needed by a child with a known risk of Wilm's tumor?____________________
4. What volume per hour of urine is considered significantly low and warrants notifying the physician? ____________________
5. What percentage of cardiac output circulates each minute through the kidneys? ____________________
6. Polyuria is described as a daily urine output exceeding ____________________

MATCHING QUESTIONS

Match the following:

Column A	Column B
1. _____ Hematuria	a. Inability to filter and excrete proteins
2. _____ Glomerulonephritis	b. Glomerulonephritis is among the leading cause
3. _____ Nephrotic syndrome	c. Symptom of pyelonephritis
4. _____ Dysuria	d. Urine output between 100–400 cc in 24 hours
5. _____ Renal insufficiency	e. Urinary analgesic that discolors urine
6. _____ Costovertebral angle tenderness	f. Can follow untreated streptococcal infections
7. _____ Pyridium	g. May obstruct urine flow
8. _____ ESRD	h. Connects artery and vein
9. _____ Oliguria	i. Urethra on ventral surface of penis
10. _____ Kayexalate	j. Surgical removal of the kidney
11. _____ Calcium carbonate	k. Surgical removal of the bladder
12. _____ Anuria	l. Lowers serum potassium levels

(continued)

13. _____ Renal calculi	m. Lowers serum phosphate levels
14. _____ AVF	n. 75–80% loss of nephron functioning
15. _____ Hydronephrosis	o. Urine output <100 cc in 24 hours
16. _____ Hypospadias	p. Helps keep urine acidic
17. _____ Nephrectomy	q. Bladder must be full at onset of procedure
18. _____ Cystectomy	r. Applying pressure over symphysis pubis to expel urine
19. _____ Ureterosigmoidostomy	s. Percutaneously introduced urinary catheter
20. _____ Vitamin C	t. Measures bladder pressure and volume during filling and storage
21. _____ Cystoscopy	u. Urinary diversion that mixes urine and stool
22. _____ Urinary flow rate	v. Endoscopic visualization of the bladder and urethra
23. _____ Cystometrogram	w. Bloody urine
24. _____ Suprapubic catheter	x. Painful urination
25. _____ Credé maneuver	y. Stretching of the renal pelvis as a result of obstruction

APPLICATION QUESTIONS

1. A client develops renal failure from a massive hemorrhage following a motor vehicle accident. This client's renal failure would be classified as
   a. Prerenal
   b. Intrarenal
   c. Postrenal
   d. Chronic

2. The nurse has completed client education on a renal diet. The nurse will recognize that the client understands the teaching when the client states that he will restrict (Mark all that apply)
   a. calories
   b. proteins
   c. fluids
   d. potassium

3. The client is diagnosed as being in acute renal failure. The nurse would expect the lab results to show
   a. metabolic acidosis
   b. metabolic alkalosis
   c. respiratory acidosis
   d. respiratory alkalosis

4. The nurse is teaching a group of women about UTIs. The nurse would identify risk factors for developing UTIs as including (Mark all that apply)
   a. decreased mobility
   b. wearing cotton underwear
   c. bowel incontinence
   d. consumption of cranberry juice

5. A client is being treated for renal failure. Which assessment data would indicate a progression of the disease?
   a. Lowering GFR
   b. Rising hematocrit and hemoglobin
   c. Decreased blood glucose levels
   d. Elevated urine bicarbonate

6. The client has a history of painless hematuria. The client asks the nurse what to do if it occurs again. The nurse would respond by
   a. reassuring the client that bleeding is only significant if it is accompanied by pain.
   b. instructing the client to seek treatment if it persists past 3 days.
   c. encouraging prompt reporting of any visible bleeding.
   d. informing the client that painless hematuria is diagnostic of bladder cancer.

7. When asked about organisms causing UTIs, which bacteria would the nurse identify as the most common cause?
   a. Streptococcus
   b. *E. coli*
   c. Staphylococcus
   d. Bacillus anthracis

8. A client has a surgical procedure on the urinary system. Which are potential postoperative problems for which the nurse must monitor? (Mark all that apply)
   a. surgery on any part of the urinary tract may result in bleeding.
   b. surgical blood loss could decrease renal perfusion.
   c. anesthetics may decrease the perception of the need to void.
   d. urethra may swell following cystoscopy or catheterization.

9. A pregnant woman seeks help for a UTI. The physician places the client on antibiotics. Which of the following nursing actions is appropriate for this client?
   a. Stop medication as soon as symptoms subside
   b. Stop medications if symptoms do not improve the 3rd day of administration
   c. Obtain specimen for culture and sensitivity immediately after initiating
   d. Administer around the clock at timed intervals

10. The nurse working on a urology hospital unit monitors clients for urosepsis. The nurse would recognize that the population most at risk for the development of urosepsis is
    a. females
    b. males
    c. elderly
    d. athletes

11. The nurse is evaluating a client for a UTI. To correctly assess for costovertebral angle tenderness, the nurse would
    a. use fist percussion performed bilaterally on the posterior chest below the rib cage.
    b. have the client contract pelvic floor muscles for 10 seconds, then relax them for 10 seconds.
    c. apply pressure over symphysis pubis.
    d. have the client contract abdominal muscles and hold his or her breath while straining.

12. A woman is 28-weeks pregnant and develops a UTI. The maternity nurse will monitor the client for
    a. uterine contractions
    b. hypertension
    c. a white, cheesy vaginal discharge
    d. varicose veins

13. A nurse inserts a urinary catheter into the bladder immediately after the child has voided. The child's mother asks why the nurse does this since the child has voided. The nurse explains that this procedure checks for retained urine referred to as
    a. Insensible
    b. Residual
    c. Incidental
    d. Tubular

14. A client has returned from surgery for a radical prostatectomy. The nurse would adjust the flow of sterile normal saline in a three-way bladder irrigation to keep the urine
    a. bright red
    b. pale yellow
    c. pink-tinged
    d. dark amber

15. The urology clinic nurse conducts a class on urinary health for a group of clients. After teaching, the nurse asks the clients "What volume of daily fluid intake is recommended for a healthy adult?" The client that best understands the concept is the client who answers
    a. 750 ml/d
    b. 1000 ml/d
    c. 2000 ml/d
    d. 3000 ml/d

(continued)

16. A client is being admitted for urinary retention and bladder distention. On completing the admission history, the nurse would expect the client to describe which urinary symptom as preceding the development of urinary retention and bladder distention?
    a. Nocturnal enuresis
    b. Hesitancy
    c. Dysuria
    d. Hematuria

17. The mother of a child diagnosed with glomerulonephritis asks about the normal function of the kidney. Which functions would be correct for the nurse to identify?
    a. Excretion of waste products
    b. Control of blood pressure
    c. Manufacture of electrolytes
    d. Regulation of red blood cell production

18. The nurse hears a group of mothers discussing their children, all of whom have nocturnal enuresis. The mothers ask the nurse if it is normal that their children are bed-wetting. The nurse would explain that nocturnal enuresis is considered abnormal after
    a. age 2
    b. age 4
    c. age 6
    d. the onset of puberty

19. The client has a history of nephrolithiasis. The nurse has completed the appropriate client teaching. Which statement by the client demonstrates an understanding of the teaching?
    a. "I will decrease fluid intake to 1000 ml/d."
    b. "I will strain urine and save solid material for analysis."
    c. "I will avoid calcium-rich foods or calcium supplements."
    d. "I will maintain bed rest with bathroom privileges."

20. A nurse assesses four pediatric clients and finds each client has one of the following symptoms. The nurse would suspect a Wilm's tumor in the child with
    a. hypertension
    b. nocturnal enuresis
    c. oliguria
    d. painful hematuria

21. The nurse reviews the medical orders for a client with acute prostatitis. The nurse would question the order for which intervention?
    a. NSAIDS
    b. Broad-spectrum antibiotics
    c. Massage prostate
    d. Sitz baths

22. After being diagnosed with pyelonephritis, the client asks the nurse what causes this disorder. The nurse's response would be based on the knowledge that the most common cause of pyelonephritis is/are
    a. urethritis and cystitis
    b. potassium imbalances
    c. sodium imbalances
    d. uremic syndrome

23. A client is being treated for nephrolithiasis. The nurse should monitor the client for the common complication of
    a. hydronephrosis
    b. gout
    c. immobility
    d. defective cystine metabolism

24. The nurse observes that the client's urine is dark yellow and appears very concentrated. The lab test that would correlate with this data would be
    a. high urine specific gravity.
    b. low hemoglobin and hematocrit.
    c. elevated WBC count.
    d. proteinuria.

25. A child has been diagnosed with nephritic syndrome. The nurse tells the mother that the child needs to be protected from infection. The mother asks why. The nurse explains the child is susceptible to infection because (Select all that apply)
    a. edema fluid is a good medium for bacterial growth.
    b. decreased blood proteins reduce the production of gamma globulin.
    c. the child is on a low-sodium diet.
    d. the child is lethargic.

ANSWERS & RATIONALES

TRUE & FALSE ANSWERS

Mark each of the following statements True or False. Correct all false statements in the space provided.

1. Confusion may be the only clinical sign of a UTI in the older adult. *True*
2. Recurrent episodes of UTIs could progress to permanent kidney damage. *True*
3. Placement of an indwelling catheter to treat urinary incontinence decreases the risk for a UTI. *False*
   Regardless of the reason for placement, indwelling catheters increase the risk for infection by providing a portal of entry for bacteria.
4. A client with nocturia should be instructed to schedule the majority of fluid intake prior to 4 p.m. *True*
5. Symptoms of renal failure occur when 40% of nephrons become nonfunctioning. *False*
   Healthy nephrons enlarge and compensate until 75% or more of the nephrons become nonfunctioning.
6. Renal calculi larger than 7 mm usually require some form of surgical intervention. *True*
7. Surgical correction of cryptorchidism is usually performed prior to the age of 6 months. *False*
   Testicles often descend without intervention in the first year of life.
8. Infants with hypospadias should not be circumcised. *True*
9. Dehydration is a risk factor for urinary calculi. *True*
10. Flank pain is a prominent symptom of hydronephrosis. *True*

ANSWERS FOR FILL IN THE BLANKS

Fill in the blank spaces with the correct word or phrase to complete each statement.

1. What lifestyle habit puts a client at risk for prostatitis? Multiple sexual partners.
2. What is the amount a client should weigh after urinating if renal functioning was not impaired? Dry weight.
3. What type of screening is needed by a child with a known risk of Wilm's tumor? Kidney ultrasound.
4. What volume per hour of urine is considered significantly low and warrants notifying the physician? 30 ml.
5. What percentage of cardiac output circulates each minute through the kidneys? approximately 25%.
6. Polyuria is described as a daily urine output exceeding 2500 ml.

MATCHING ANSWERS

Match the following:

1. __w__ Hematuria
2. __f__ Glomerulonephritis
3. __a__ Nephrotic syndrome
4. __x__ Dysuria
5. __n__ Renal insufficiency
6. __c__ Costovertebral angle tenderness
7. __e__ Pyridium
8. __b__ ESRD
9. __d__ Oliguria
10. __l__ Kayexalate
11. __m__ Calcium Carbonate
12. __o__ Anuria
13. __g__ Renal calculi
14. __h__ AVF
15. __y__ Hydronephrosis
16. __i__ Hypospadias
17. __j__ Nephrectomy
18. __k__ Cystectomy
19. __u__ Ureterosigmoidostomy
20. __p__ Vitamin C
21. __v__ Cystoscopy
22. __q__ Urinary flow rate
23. __t__ Cystometrogram
24. __s__ Suprapubic catheter
25. __r__ Credé maneuver

a. Inability to filter and excrete proteins
b. Glomerulonephritis is among the leading cause
c. Symptom of pyelonephritis
d. Urine output between 100–400 cc in 24 hours
e. Urinary analgesic that discolors urine
f. Can follow untreated streptococcal infections
g. May obstruct urine flow
h. Connects artery and vein
i. Urethra on ventral surface of penis
j. Surgical removal of the kidney
k. Surgical removal of the bladder
l. Lowers serum potassium levels
m. Lowers serum phosphate levels
n. 75–80% loss of nephron functioning
o. Urine output <100 cc in 24 hours
p. Helps keep urine acidic
q. Bladder must be full at onset of procedure
r. Applying pressure over symphysis pubis to expel urine
s. Percutaneously introduced urinary catheter
t. Measures bladder pressure and volume during filling and storage
u. Urinary diversion that mixes urine and stool
v. Endoscopic visualization of the bladder and urethra
w. Bloody urine
x. Painful urination
y. Stretching of the renal pelvis as a result of obstruction

APPLICATION ANSWERS

1. A client develops renal failure from a massive hemorrhage following a motor vehicle accident. This client's renal failure would be classified as
   a. Prerenal
   b. Intrarenal
   c. Postrenal
   d. Chronic

Rationale

Correct answer: a.

Prerenal failure results from a decrease in blood supplying the kidneys.

Incorrect answers: b, c, and d.

Intrarenal failure results from renal tubular cell damage; postrenal failure results form obstructed urinary flow; chronic renal failure is a progressive, irreversible loss of renal function not based on the location of its cause.

2. The nurse has completed client education on a renal diet. The nurse will recognize that the client understands the teaching when the client states that he will restrict (Mark all that apply.)
   a. calories
   b. proteins
   c. fluids
   d. potassium

Rationale

Correct answers: b, c, and d.

Incorrect answer: a.

Renal diets are high in calories.

3. The client is diagnosed as being in acute renal failure. The nurse would expect the lab results to show
   a. metabolic acidosis
   b. metabolic alkalosis
   c. respiratory acidosis
   d. respiratory alkalosis

Correct answer: a.

Clients with acute oliguria cannot eliminate the daily metabolic load of acid-type substances produced by metabolic processes and normal buffering mechanisms fail.

Incorrect answers: b, c, and d.

Metabolic alkalosis occurs with losses of H^+ and chloride acid, most commonly with vomiting, gastric suctioning, or hyperkalemia. Respiratory acidosis and alkalosis are rooted in ventilation problems.

4. The nurse is teaching a group of women about UTIs. The nurse would identify risk factors for developing UTIs as including (Mark all that apply.)
   a. decreased mobility
   b. wearing cotton underwear
   c. bowel incontinence
   d. consumption of cranberry juice

Rationale

Correct answers: a and c.

Incorrect answers: b and d.

Wearing cotton underwear discourages irritation and inflammation and cranberry juice discourages bacterial growth by increasing urine acidity, so both decrease the risk for UTI.

5. A client is being treated for renal failure. Which assessment data would indicate a progression of the disease?
   a. Lowering GFR
   b. Rising hematocrit and hemoglobin
   c. Decreased blood glucose levels
   d. Elevated urine bicarbonate

Rationale

Correct answer: a.

As renal functioning declines, the GFR decreases.

Incorrect answers: b, c, and d.

H&H would decrease as the body retains fluid and production of RBCs is impaired; low blood glucose is not linked with renal impairment; kidneys would not increase bicarbonate excretion in response to the metabolic acidosis associated with renal failure because it would worsen the acidosis.

6. The client has a history of painless hematuria. The client asks the nurse what to do if it occurs again. The nurse would respond by
   a. reassuring the client that bleeding is only significant if it is accompanied by pain.
   b. instructing the client to seek treatment if it persists past 3 days.
   c. encouraging prompt reporting of any visible bleeding.
   d. informing the client that painless hematuria is diagnostic of bladder cancer.

Rationale

Correct answer: c.

Incorrect answers: a, b, and d.

Significant bleeding is often painless and should be investigated promptly; may be associated with genitourinary problems, cancer, or a bleeding disorder.

(continued)

7. When asked about organisms causing UTIs, which bacteria would the nurse identify as the most common cause?
   a. Streptococcus
   b. Escherichia coli (*E.coli*)
   c. Staphylococcus
   d. Bacillus anthracis

Rationale

Correct answer: b.

E. coli is responsible for 80% of UTIs.

Incorrect answers: a, c, and d.

8. A client has a surgical procedure on the urinary system. Which are potential postoperative problems for which the nurse must monitor? (Mark all that apply.)
   a. surgery on any part of the urinary tract may result in bleeding.
   b. surgical blood loss could decrease renal perfusion.
   c. anesthetics may decrease the perception of the need to void.
   d. urethra may swell following cystoscopy or catheterization.

Rationale

Correct answers: a, b, c, and d.

Bleeding, decreased renal perfusion, decreased perception of need to void, and edema are all risks associated with urological surgery.

9. A pregnant woman seeks help for a UTI. The physician places the client on antibiotics. Which of the following nursing actions is appropriate for this client?
   a. Stop medication as soon as symptoms subside
   b. Stop medications if symptoms do not improve the third day of administration
   c. Obtain specimen for culture and sensitivity immediately after initiating
   d. Administer around the clock at timed intervals

Rationale

Correct answer: d.

Incorrect answers: a, b, and c.

Client should take the complete course of medication, even if symptoms of infection subside. Specimens for C&S are collected prior to the administration of antibiotics.

10. The nurse working on a urology hospital unit monitors clients for urosepsis. The nurse would recognize that the population most at risk for the development of urosepsis is
    a. females
    b. males
    c. elderly
    d. athletes

Rationale

Correct answer: c.

The elderly and immunosuppressed are at higher risk and should be closely monitored for S&S of sepsis.

Incorrect answers: a, b, and d.

Gender and athletic activity do not play a role in increasing risks.

11. The nurse is evaluating a client for a UTI. To correctly assess for costovertebral angle tenderness, the nurse would
    a. use fist percussion performed bilaterally on the posterior chest below rib cage.
    b. have the client contract pelvic floor muscles for 10 seconds, then relax them for 10 seconds.
    c. apply pressure over symphysis pubis.
    d. have the client contract abdominal muscles and hold his or her breath while straining.

Rationale

Correct answer: a.

Incorrect answers: b, c, and d.

Pelvic floor muscle contractions are Kegel exercises; pressure over symphysis pubis is Credé maneuver; abdominal muscle contraction while bearing down is Valsalva maneuver.

12. A woman is 28-weeks pregnant and develops a UTI. The maternity nurse will monitor the client for
    a. uterine contractions
    b. hypertension
    c. a white, cheesy vaginal discharge
    d. varicose veins

Rationale

Correct answer: a.

Incorrect answers: b, c, and d.

UTIs during pregnancy are associated with preterm labor. The nurse should monitor for uterine contractions. The other complications occur in pregnancy but not in relation to a UTI.

13. A nurse inserts a urinary catheter into the bladder immediately after the child has voided. The child's mother asks why the nurse does this since the child has voided. The nurse explains that this procedure checks for retained urine referred to as
    a. Insensible
    b. Residual
    c. Incidental
    d. Tubular

Rationale

Correct answer: b.

Incorrect answers: a, c, and d.
Residual urine.

14. A client has returned from surgery for a radical prostatectomy. The nurse would adjust the flow of sterile normal saline in a three-way bladder irrigation to keep the urine
    a. bright red
    b. pale yellow
    c. pink-tinged
    d. dark amber

Rationale

Correct answer: c.

Incorrect answers: a, b, and d.

15. The urology clinic nurse conducts a class on urinary health for a group of clients. After teaching, the nurse asks the clients "What volume of daily fluid intake is recommended for a healthy adult?" The client that best understands the concept is the client who answers
    a. 750 ml/d
    b. 1000 ml/d
    c. 2000 ml/d
    d. 3000 ml/d

Rationale

Correct answer: c.
A healthy adult consumes up to 2000 ml of fluid per day and normally all but 4000–500 ml of this is excreted as urine. The remainder is lost from the skin, lungs, and GI tract.

Incorrect answers: a, b, and d.

16. A client is being admitted for urinary retention and bladder distention. In completing the admission history, the nurse would expect the client to describe which urinary symptom as preceding the development of urinary retention and bladder distention?
    a. Nocturnal enuresis
    b. Hesitancy
    c. Dysuria
    d. Hematuria

Rationale

Correct answer: b.
Hesitancy may impair complete emptying

Incorrect answers: a, c, and d.
Nocturnal enuresis is incontinence while sleeping, dysuria is painful urination, and hematuria is bleeding into the urine.

17. The mother of a child diagnosed with glomerulonephritis asks about the normal function of the kidney. Which functions would be correct for the nurse to identify?
    a. Excretion of waste products
    b. Control of blood pressure
    c. Manufacture of electrolytes
    d. Regulation of red blood cell production

Rationale

Correct answers: a, b, and d.

Incorrect answer: c.
The kidney plays an important role in regulating electrolytes through excretion or retention, but does not actually manufacture them.

18. The nurse hears a group of mothers discussing their children, all of whom have nocturnal enuresis. The mothers ask the nurse if it is normal that their children are bed-wetting. The nurse would explain that nocturnal enuresis is considered abnormal after
    a. age 2
    b. age 4
    c. age 6
    d. the onset of puberty

Rationale

Correct answer: c.
There is a developmental aspect to nocturnal enuresis and it is not considered a problem until age 6.

Incorrect answers: a, b, and d.

19. The client has a history of nephrolithiasis. The nurse has completed the appropriate client teaching. Which statement by the client demonstrates an understanding of the teaching?
    a. "I will decrease fluid intake to 1000 ml/d"
    b. "I will strain urine and save solid material for analysis."
    c. "I will avoid calcium-rich foods or calcium supplements"
    d. "I will maintain bed rest with bathroom privileges."

Rationale

Correct answer: b.
All urine should be strained through gauze

Incorrect answers: a, c, and d.
Fluid intake should be increased to 3000–4000 ml/d; low-calcium intake is generally not recommended and can lead to osteoporosis; ambulation would encourage natural passage.

20. A nurse assesses four pediatric clients and finds each client has one of the following symptoms. The nurse would suspect a Wilm's tumor in the child with
    a. hypertension
    b. nocturnal enuresis
    c. oliguria
    d. painful hematuria

(continued)

Rationale

Correct answer: a.

Wilm's tumor is the most common renal cancer in children and complications include hypertension.

Incorrect answers: b, c, and d.

None are associated with Wilm's tumor.

21. The nurse reviews the medical orders for a client with acute prostatitis. The nurse would question the order for which intervention?
    a. NSAIDS
    b. Broad-spectrum antibiotics
    c. Massage prostate
    d. Sitz baths

Rationale

Correct answer: c.

Massaging an obviously swollen and tender prostate may potentially spread infection and increase the risk for sepsis.

Incorrect answers: a, b, and d.

All are therapeutic for acute prostatitis—NSAIDS relieve inflammation, broad-spectrum antibiotics treat infection, and Sitz baths provide comfort.

22. After being diagnosed with pyelonephritis, the client asks the nurse what causes this disorder. The nurse's response would be based on the knowledge that the most common cause of pyelonephritis is/are
    a. urethritis and cystitis
    b. potassium imbalances
    c. sodium imbalances
    d. uremic syndrome

Rationale

Correct answer: a.

Pyelonephritis most often occurs as the result of chronic or recurring UTIs.

Incorrect answers: b, c, and d.

Electrolyte imbalances and metabolic waste accumulation are the result of renal failure.

23. A client is being treated for nephrolithiasis. The nurse should monitor the client for the common complication of
    a. hydronephrosis
    b. gout
    c. immobility
    d. defective cystine metabolism

Rationale

Correct answer: a.

Dilation of the renal calyces is a potential complication of kidney stones.

Incorrect answers: b, c, and d.

All of these are risk factors for the development of nephrolithiasis.

24. The nurse observes that the client's urine is dark yellow and appears very concentrated. The lab test that would correlate with this data would be:
    a. high urine specific gravity
    b. low hemoglobin and hematocrit
    c. elevated WBC count
    d. proteinuria

Rationale

Correct answer: a.

Concentrated urine is measured by specific gravity of the urine.

Incorrect answers: b, c, and d.

These findings are not specific to concentrated urine.

25. A child has been diagnosed with nephritic syndrome. The nurse tells the mother that the child needs to be protected from infection. The mother asks why. The nurse explains the child is susceptible to infection because (Select all that apply.)
    a. edema fluid is a good medium for bacterial growth.
    b. decreased blood proteins reduce the production of gamma globulin.
    c. the child is on a low-sodium diet.
    d. the child is lethargic.

Rationale

Correct answers: a and b.

Incorrect answers: c and d.

These responses are related to nephritic syndrome but do not relate to fighting infection.

Test Plan Category:

Physiological Integrity

Sub-category: Physiological Adaptation—Part 1

Topics: Alterations in Body Systems
Illness Management
Section 11: Skin Problems

SKIN PROBLEMS

Think Smart/Test Smart

As you review problems of the skin, remember that the skin plays a critical role in how the world views the client and in turn, how the client views himself or herself. As a result, there is significant psychological overlay to almost every skin problem. Further, many skin problems are difficult to treat and treatment regimes must be followed carefully for an extended length of time before any improvement is seen. Many problems are often recurrent. Thus being supportive and sensitive to the client's feelings and aware of the potential impact of the disease on the client's self concept and social interactions are essential components of care.

ACNE VULGARIS

Etiology: Multifactorial: free fatty acids, hormones, stress, heredity, infection all seem to play a role. Diet not a causative factor.

S&S: Hair follicles plugged with sebum and other cellular debris to form open (at the skin surface) or closed (under the surface) comedos (blackheads, color due to melanin not dirt, or whiteheads), inflammation occurs when sebum escapes into dermis; occurs mostly on face and neck, upper chest, and back. Healing occurs in 5–10 days without scarring; large, deep lesions last for weeks and typically cause ice-pick-type scars.

Dx: Clinical presentation

Rx:

- Topical—benzoyl peroxides, retinoids, retinoid-like drugs, for example, tretinoin, and antibiotics, for example, sulfa, erythromycin, etc.
- Systemic—antibiotics, for example, tetracylines and erythromycin for inflammatory lesions, low-progestin oral contraceptives help some; isotretinoin (accutane) also an option

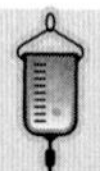

Clinical Alert

Isotretinoin causes birth defects and cannot be used if pregnant or likely to become pregnant so the client must be on birth control.

- Intralesional—corticosteroids for severe lesions
- Surgical—dermabrasion and laser resurfacing for scars
- Chemical peels may be used in addition to topical or systemic drug therapy

Nursing Process Elements

Client teaching for self-care

Teach client to

- keep hands and hair away from face
- avoid use of oily products
- shampoo daily
- use a gentle, nongreasy cleanser on skin; do not overwash
- use only water-based cosmetics and never leave on overnight
- avoid vigorous rubbing
- exercise care if using medication
  —avoid sun exposure if using tretinoin, tetracycline, or sulfa
  —recognize that it takes up to 8 weeks for improvement with therapy

ACNE ROSACEA

Acne rosacea is a follicular eruption of the skin with acne and a vascular component. It affects 30–50-year olds; more women are affected than men.

Etiology: Unknown.

Risk factors: Fair complexion, genetic predisposition, and easy flushing and blushing.

S&S: Erythema, papules, pustules, and enlarged superficial blood vessels of central face, cheeks and nose; ultimately, skin of nose can become thickened, and reddish purple in color (rhinophyma)

Dx: Clinical presentation

Rx: Topical antibiotics such as Metrogel; responds slowly with frequent relapses

Nursing Process Elements

Client teaching for self-care

Teach client to

- avoid triggers, i.e., anything that induces flushing such as heat, cold, sunlight, alcohol, and spicy foods
- use sun protection daily
- use mild cleansers and avoid alcohol-based products

ECZEMA

- Eczema refers to the superficial inflammation of the skin; it is also called dermatitis.
- It occurs in many different forms each of which is triggered by specific flare factors such as dryness, change in environment or temperature, stress, etc.
- The lesions that develop are similar regardless of type. It results in erythema and local edema followed by vesicle formation with oozing and then crusting and scaling.
- The commonly identified forms include
  —contact dermatitis. Which may be allergic or irritant, lesions appear on exposed areas; patch testing may be done to determine responsible agent; Domeboro soaks are used for weeping vesicular lesions; crusts and scales are allowed to drop off naturally; topical steroids may be used along with oral antihistamines, topical antipruritics or colloidal oatmeal baths for itch.
  —atopic dermatitis. Which is a genetically based disorder occurring most commonly in children; it appears first as rough, dry skin at an age as early as 1 month; major symptom is intense pruritus; skin thickening and pigment change can occur due to scratching; hydrating the skin is the most important therapy; topical corticosteroids and immunomodulators as well as oral antihistamines are also used.
  —seborrheic dermatitis. Which occurs on the hairy areas of the body; it often worsens in winter; the cause is unknown but overgrowth of yeast is suspected; scalp sites are treated with tar, selenium, zinc, or ketoconazole preparations; facial sites are treated with topical low-potency steroids or antifungal agents.

Nursing Process Elements

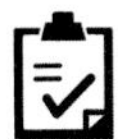

Client teaching for self-care

- For contact dermatitis: teach client about the recognition and prevention of causative agent(s)
- For atopic dermatitis: teach client
  —about the proper application of topical medications (apply a thin layer, rub in well)
  —about the methods of hydrating the skin such as a 15–20 minute a warm bath with immediate application of moisturizer after patting away excess water or use of wet wraps
  —to avoid overheating, which can cause sweating and itching; to wear loose, cool clothing; to use air conditioning
  —to avoid excessive cold, which is drying
  —to avoid sunburn and other irritants such as wool, fur, rough fabrics; to wash new garments before wearing to avoid exposure to potentially irritating chemicals

PSORIASIS

Etiology: T-cell–mediated disease; specific precipitating factors typically unknown though stress, climate change, drugs, trauma, or infection seem to play a role in causing psoriasis in some people.

S&S:

- Scaling, pruritus, and erythema are classic
- Papules and plaques are raised, red, sharply circumscribed, and with a silvery scale; most common on scalp, elbows, knees, and sacrolumbar area
- Removal of scale yields pinpoint bleeding called Auspitz sign
- Characterized by remissions and exacerbations

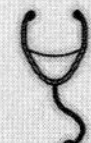

Assessment Alert

Plaques may appear purple in dark-skinned individuals.

Dx: Clinical presentation

Rx:

- Localized disease: topical corticosteroids for a defined time; coal tar remedies for pruritus and epidermal cell turnover
- Diffuse disease: phototherapy (PUVA) therapy in which psoralens are taken 1–2 hours before exposure to UV light
- Advanced disease: methotrexate, acitretin, and the immunosuppressive, cyclosporine

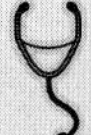

Assessment Alert

Methotrexate, acitretin, and cyclosporine require monitoring of CBC, lipid, and liver function tests (LFTs).

Nursing Process Elements

Assess for effect on self-concept

Client teaching for self-care

Teach client to

- avoid possible precipitating factors: skin trauma including sunburn, extremes of temperature and stress, etc.
- shampoo frequently; use a tar, zinc, or selenium shampoo. If scalp has scales presoften plaques with mineral overnight PRN and use a fine-toothed comb to remove scales.
- apply topical medications in a thin layer as directed
- avoid self-medication

HERPES ZOSTER (SHINGLES)

Etiology: Herpes zoster (chicken pox) virus.

S&S: Clusters of vesicles in a line along the course of peripheral sensory nerves—lesions never cross the midline and typically occur unilaterally. Itching and/or intermittent or constant light burning to deep pain; persists 2–3 weeks or longer.

Complication: Postherpetic neuralgia pain syndrome that may last a year or more.

Dx: Clinical presentation

Rx: Antiviral therapy for high-risk individuals or when diagnosis is made in first 48–72 hours to decrease pain and incidence of postherpetic neuralgia; analgesics for pain; topical antipruritic agents

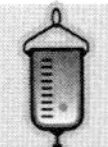

Clinical Alert

NSAIDs are not usually effective for pain.

Client teaching for self-care

Instruct client to

- wear loose clothing
- avoid contact with those who have not had chickenpox or who are immunosuppressed

CANDIDIASIS

- Candidiasis refers to an inflammation caused by an overgrowth of the fungus *Candida albicans* on the skin or the mucous membrane.
- It is normally found in mouth and GI tract and in the vagina.
- Overgrowth on mucous membrane of mouth or GI tract is called thrush or oral candidiasis or oral moniliasis.

Etiology: Overgrowth of Candida albicans; can be transmitted to the neonate from the mother's vagina during delivery, or by contaminated hands, bottles, or nipples. Person-to-person transmission is also possible.

Risk factors: Pregnancy, oral contraceptives, inhaled corticosteroids, poor nutrition, antibiotic therapy, diabetes mellitus, and other endocrine problems, and immunocompromise.

S&S:

- Skin infection: Moist, macerated, itchy/burning patches with vesicles and pustules most often found in warm, moist skin fold areas such as under the breasts, groin, and intergluteal region. Satellite lesions at the periphery of the inflamed area is a classic sign
- Vaginal infection: Thick, white "cottage cheese" like vaginal discharge, itching and burning
- Thrush: White, milk curd-like plaques on buccal mucosa; may extend into esophagus; causes painful burning and dysphagia

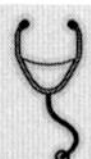

PEDS

Assessment Alert

Plaques of oral thrush look like coagulated milk. To tell the difference, attempt to remove with a tongue blade—thrush plaques do not come off.

Dx: History, clinical presentation, microscopic examination

Rx:

- Antifungal agents such as nystatin (Mycostatin), clotrimazole (Lotrimin), ketoconazole (Nizoral), fluconazole (Diflucan)
  —Topical nystatin (1 ml over oral mucous membrane every 6 hours) effectively treats thrush in most infants
- Long-term antifungal therapy may be prescribed for immunocompromised individuals
- Elimination of predisposing factors

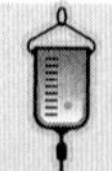

Clinical Alert

Good hand washing is essential in preventing the transmission of candidiasis.

Nursing Process Elements

Client teaching for self-care

Teach client

- to eliminate warm, moist environments that support growth of the fungus by
  —thoroughly drying skin after bathing
  —wearing loose, absorbent clothing
- to use powder to keep skin folds from rubbing against each other
- about the early detection and treatment
- about the antifungal medications, their correct use, side effects, and importance of compliance

IMPETIGO

Etiology: Contagious, superficial skin infection caused by beta hemolytic *Streptococcus* or *Staphylococcus aureus*.

Risk factors: Childhood, *Streptococcus* in nares, spring or fall, tropical climate, poor nutrition or health, and poor hygiene.

S&S: Vesicles that rupture and leave weeping denuded area. With *Streptococcus*, honey-colored crusts form lesions on the face, arms, and legs

Dx: Clinical appearance and culture

Rx:

- Crusts removed and area washed gently bid or tid.
- Topical antibiotics bid × 10 days
- Antimicrobial soaps/washes to decrease bacteria on skin

Nursing Process Elements

Client teaching for self-care

- Teach client about the contagious nature of the disease
- Instruct about good hand washing of client and family members
- Instruct about keeping linens and clothing separate and washing after contact with an infected area

SCABIES

Etiology: Infestation by scabies mite; incubation period: 4–6 weeks.

Risk factors: Crowded living environments, close skin-to-skin contact.

S&S:

- Intense itching, especially at night
- Thread-like linear or serpentine gray-brown burrows visible under skin followed by papules and nodules especially in webs of fingers, on wrists, in axillae, breasts, waist, thighs, lower buttocks, and genitalia

Complication: Infection with excoriation and pustules from scratching.

Dx: Mite removed from burrow and identified under microscope

Rx:

- Permethrin applied topically from head to toe and under nails at bedtime, shower in 8 hours; repeat in 2 weeks if symptoms persist
- Gamma benzene hexachloride applied at bedtime from neck down, washed off in 8–12 hours; repeated in a week if live mites found. Low-dose topical corticosteroids bid for 1–2 weeks for posttreatment itching

Nursing Process Elements

Client Teaching for Selfcare

Instruct client to

- washing underwear, bed linens and towels in hot water and drying in dryer or iron on day of treatment
- putting nonwashable items in a tightly closed, plastic bags for several weeks

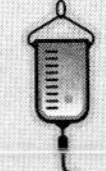

Clinical Alert

Close contacts of client must be treated even if asymptomatic because the mite is so easily transmitted.

SKIN CANCER

- The major types of skin cancer are malignant melanoma (tumor of the melanocytes), squamous cell carcinoma, and basal cell carcinoma.
- Incidence and deaths from melanoma, which metastasizes readily to regional lymph nodes and then to lungs, liver, brain and other areas, and has the worst prognosis of the three types, are increasing.
- Squamous cell carcinoma, arising on hair-bearing skin, rarely metastasizes; lesions on lip or ear may metastasize to regional nodes.
- Basal cell carcinoma rarely metastasizes but can cause extensive local tissue destruction.

Melanoma

Etiology: Often develops from a mole but may arise from healthy skin.

Risk factors:

- Genetic predisposition
- Light complexion especially with light hair and eyes
- History of blistering sunburns as a child
- Presence of multiple atypical nevi (moles)

S&S: Most lesions occur on head, neck, and the lower extremities and vary greatly. Lesions that are suspect are those that are new, have undergone change, or have grown; have deep, variegated (yellow, blue, black, gray), or no pigmentation, irregular borders, surrounding erythema or halo. Late changes are bleeding and ulceration

Dx: Excisional biopsy with sufficient margins to allow depth of invasion to be determined. Other types of biopsy contraindicated

Rx: Wide surgical excision to decrease chance of local recurrence. If invasion is more than 1-mm deep, sentinel lymph node dissection may be done followed by a complete lymphadenectomy, if the sentinel node is positive. Latter is also done when there are enlarged regional nodes found at time of diagnosis. Metastatic melanoma is resistant to chemotherapy

Squamous Cell Carcinoma

Etiology: Unknown.

Risk factors: Long-term sun damage, possibly genetic predisposition, fair skin, light hair, blue-, gray-, or green-eyed individuals, immunocompromised, previous skin cancer.

S&S: If develops from a preexisting lesion, appears indurated and surrounded by an inflammatory base. If new lesion, appears as a firm keratotic nodule with indurated base. Occurs most often on areas of the body exposed to sun with rim of the ear and the lower lip especially vulnerable.

Also can occur in areas of skin damage such as scars, burns, chronic inflammation, and areas exposed to radiation or chemicals

Dx: Biopsy

Rx: Removal by surgical excision, Mohs micrographic surgery, curettage with electrodesiccation, irradiation, or chemosurgery. Area may be treated with methotrexate following excision to destroy any remaining tumor cells and prevent local recurrence

Basal Cell Carcinoma

Etiology: Chronic overexposure to the sun.

Risk factors: Outdoor work, fair skin that sunburns easily, living in an area with long hours of sun.

S&S: Flesh color to pale pink lesion with a translucent pearly appearance with a few telangiectic blood vessels across its surface. Can cause severe tissue destruction, infection, and hemorrhage. Occurs most often on face, ears, scalp, neck, back, and shoulders

Dx: Biopsy

Rx: Same as for squamous cell

Nursing Process Elements

Client teaching for self-care

Teach client about

- how to take care of the wound if surgically treated
- the need for follow-up care to check for recurrence, metastasis, or new lesions
- the methods of reducing skin cancer risk See Chapter •••)
- periodic skin self-examination, which is best done monthly
- the importance of seeking care if any suspicious changes are noted
- washing underwear, bed linens and towels in hot water and drying in dryer or iron on day of treatment
- putting nonwashable items in a tightly closed, plastic bags for several weeks

PRESSURE ULCERS

A pressure ulcer refers to any lesion caused by unrelieved pressure.

Etiology:

- Decreased bloodflow to an area of tissue as a result of compression and damage to blood vessels. This decreases the amount of oxygen and nutrients delivered to the cells and allows waste products to accumulate; ultimately, cells die.
- Friction—can remove superficial skin layers.
- Shearing force—combination of friction and pressure which damages blood vessels and tissues in area where deep and superficial tissues meet—occurs when deeper tissues move and surface tissues stay in place for example, when clients are pulled up in bed and the skin of the lower back and buttocks is in contact with the sheets and drags behind the deeper tissues as the client is moved.

Risk factors: Immobility, inactivity, inadequate nutrition, fecal and urinary incontinence, decreased mental status, diminished sensation, excessive body heat, advanced age, chronic medical conditions such as diabetes and cardiovascular disease that impair delivery of oxygenated blood to the tissues, and care-related factors such as poor positioning, incorrect use of pressure-relieving devices, and inappropriate lifting techniques.

S&S: Decreased blood flow causes pallor; when pressure is relieved reactive hyperemia (bright red flush due to vasodilation) occurs to compensate for the period of ischemia

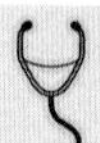

Assessment Alert

The period of reactive hyperemia lasts for a period half to three-fourths as long as the period of ischemia if no permanent tissue damage has occurred. If the red flush lasts longer than this amount of time, tissue has been damaged.

S&S during the four stages of pressure ulcers:

Stage I—Nonblanchable erythema

Stage II—Partial-thickness skin loss as seen with an abrasion or blister, may involve epidermis only or epidermis and some dermis

Stage III—Full-thickness skin loss with damage to subcutaneous tissue that may go as deep as the fascia but not through it—ulcer looks like a deep crater. Undermining of adjacent tissue may or may not be present

Stage IV—Full-thickness skin loss with tissue necrosis or damage to muscle, bone, or supporting structures. Tissue undermining and sinus tracts may also be present

Dx: Clinical appearance

Rx:

- Prevention is the best treatment
- Clean and dress according to the stage of ulcer and agency protocol

—Stage I: Keep ulcer moist by use of a transparent barrier or occlusive hydrocolloid dressing

—Stage II: Keep ulcer moist by use of an occlusive hydrocolloid dressing or a hydrogel dressing

—Stage III: Use dry gauze or wet to dry gauze to wick drainage away from ulcer surface or use hydrocolloid or hydrogel to keep ulcer moist or alginate to both keep moist and absorb exudate

—Stage IV: Use dry or wet to dry gauze, hydrogel, or alginate

- Surgical treatment: Myocutaneous flaps and skin grafts in selected cases
- Diet: Increased protein (1.5–2 g/kg body weight/day) and increased calories

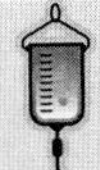

Clinical Alert

Ulcer will not heal unless pressure is relieved.

Complications: Most complications result from infection

- Septicemia
- Osteomyelitis

Nursing Process Elements

- Use risk assessment tools, for example, Braden scale or the Norton scale to identify clients at high risk; use on admission and then at regular intervals
- Assess essential areas such as immobility, incontinence, nutrition, and level of consciousness as part of risk
- Assess common pressure sites (bony prominences) such as sacrum, heels, elbows, shoulder blades, back of head, hip, knee, medial and lateral malleoli, shoulder, side of head, ear, vertebrae for pale or reddened areas; abrasions which occur due to friction, and excoriations which can result from exposure to body secretions/excretions particularly in skin folds
- Palpate skin over pressure areas for increased warmth and for a spongy feel characteristic of edema, both of which can be the result of inflammation
- Assess and document pertinent information about pressure ulcer: Location, size (length, width, and depth measured by inserting a sterile gloved finger or sterile applicator into the deepest part of the wound and then measuring it against a measuring guide) in centimeters, presence of tissue undermining or sinus tracts, stage of the ulcer, color of the ulcer bed and location of necrotic tissue or eschar, appearance of the wound margins and the surrounding skin, presence or absence of signs of infection (redness, warmth, edema, pain, odor, color, and amount of exudates)
- Nursing diagnosis:
  —risk for impaired skin integrity
  —impaired skin integrity (stage I or II pressure ulcers)
  —impaired tissue integrity (stage III or IV pressure ulcers)
- Prevention:
  —Keep skin dry and free of irritating substances such as soap, alcohol, sweat, urine, and feces. Use liquid, spray or moist wipe skin barrier/prep to keep irritants off skin
  —Avoid rubbing and excessive friction during bathing and other activities
  —Use small amounts of mild, nonirritating, nondrying cleansers; avoid harsh soaps; rinse thoroughly
  —Use tepid not hot water
  —Apply moisturizer to dry skin while still moist after bathing.
- Avoid trauma to the skin:
  —Keep the surface smooth and wrinkle free
  —Use layer of cornstarch on sheet or protective film on client to protect from friction
  —Elevate the head of the bed to no more than 30 degrees to protect against shearing
  —Use a trapeze or lift to move client without dragging skin against bed surface
- Use pressure-reducing devices such as foam or gel cushions, sheepskins, wedges, or pillows to keep heels off the bed, heel protectors, egg crate, foam or alternating pressure pads or mattresses, air fluidized (AF), or static low air loss (LAL) bed
- Avoid use of doughnut-type devices, which actually decrease blood flow to central area and can damage tissue in contact with the device

Nursing Process Elements

Client teaching for self-care

- Shift position, even if slightly, every 15–30 minutes
- Report areas of persistent erythema

WORKSHEET

MATCHING QUESTIONS

Match the following:

1. ____ Metrogel	a. Requires monitoring of LFTs
2. ____ Squamous cell carcinoma	b. Infection characterized by honey-colored crusts
3. ____ T-cell-mediated disease	c. Nonblanchable erythema
4. ____ Thrush	d. Absorbs exudates
5. ____ PUVA	e. Itch
6. ____ *Iso*tretinoin	f. Used in treatment of candidiasis
7. ____ Methotrexate	g. Used in treatment of melanoma
8. ____ Stage-I pressure ulcer	h. Used for acne rosacea
9. ____ Melanoma	i. Form of light therapy
10. ____ Intralesional corticosteroids	j. Most likely to metastasize skin cancer
11. ____ Permethrin	k. Protection against effects of ischemia
12. ____ Mohs surgery	l. Oral moniliasis
13. ____ Rhinophyma	m. Long-term effect of acne rosacea
14. ____ Alginate dressing	n. Acne treatment
15. ____ Diflucan	o. Characterized by an indurated base
16. ____ Basal cell carcinoma	p. Lesion with a translucent, pearly appearance
17. ____ Impetigo	q. Occlusive dressing
18. ____ Pruritus	r. Psoriasis
19. ____ Reactive hyperemia	s. Acne therapy causing birth defects
20. ____ Hydrocolloid dressing	t. Kills the scabies mite

FILL IN THE BLANKS

Fill in the blank spaces with the correct word or phrase to complete each statement.

1. Persons using tretinoin, tetracycline, or sulfa for the treatment of acne need to avoid ________.
2. Oral contraceptives are required for women who could become pregnant, if ________ is prescribed for acne.
3. Raised, thread-like lesions located in the webs of the fingers are characteristic of ________.
4. Fair skin and easy flushing are risk factors for ________.
5. The rim of the ear and the lower lip are sites where ________ is particularly likely to occur.
6. Candidiasis of the skin most often occurs in the ________ areas of the body.
7. A long-term complication of herpes zoster infection is ________.
8. Pruritus is the major symptom of ________ dermatitis.
9. The type of dermatitis found primarily in young children is ________.
10. The two types of skin change found as a result of repeated scratching in clients with dermatitis are ________ and ________.

TRUE & FALSE ANSWERS

Mark each of the following statements True or False. Correct all false statements in the space provided.

1. Need to avoid triggers such as hot, spicy foods and alcohol is an important part of the teaching for clients with psoriasis. ___ T ___ F
2. Domeboro soaks are used for the weeping vesicular lesions of contact dermatitis. ___ T ___ F
3. Removal of the scale of psoriasis yields pinpoint bleeding called the Auspitz sign. ___ T ___ F
4. Lesions of herpes zoster never cross the midline. ___ T ___ F
5. NSAIDs are not usually effective for the pain of shingles. ___ T ___ F
6. Inhaled corticosteroids place the client at risk for oral candidiasis. ___ T ___ F
7. Full-thickness skin loss with damage to subcutaneous tissue that may go as deep as the fascia is a stage-IV pressure ulcer. ___ T ___ F
8. Metastatic melanoma is resistant to chemotherapy. ___ T ___ F
9. Intense itching especially in the morning is characteristic of scabies. ___ T ___ F
10. White, milk curd-like plaques on buccal mucosa are characteristic of *Candida albicans* overgrowth. ___ T ___ F

APPLICATION QUESTIONS

1. Which direction must be given to an adolescent being treated with tetracycline for acne?
   a. Eliminate fatty foods from the daily diet
   b. Wash affected areas thoroughly at least every 4 hours during the day
   c. Keep out of direct sunlight
   d. Use only oil-based skin care products
2. Which information should the nurse include in the teaching plan for a woman being treated for acne rosacea?
   a. Alcohol-based products help reduce erythema
   b. Rhinophyma only occurs in men
   c. Metrogel rapidly eliminates large pustules and papules
   d. Sun block needs to be used daily
3. When assessing a dark-skinned client with psoriasis, which finding would be consistent with the S&S of the disorder?
   a. Raised, sharply-demarcated plaques that appear purple in color
   b. Silvery scales on an indurated, erythematous base
   c. Translucent, pearly appearing pink to red papules
   d. Honey-colored crusts on shallow ulcers
4. Which information would the nurse include when developing a teaching plan for a client receiving methotrexate for psoriasis?
   a. Creatinine clearance and other tests of renal function are required weekly for the first month of therapy
   b. Periodic EKGs will be done from the start of therapy until 6 months after its completion
   c. Pulmonary function tests and arterial blood gases need to be checked before the start of therapy
   d. Liver function tests, lipid levels, and blood counts need to be monitored during therapy
5. Which order would the nurse expect to be included in the plan of care for a client with herpes zoster?
   a. Administer ibuprofen 800 mg q 4 hours for pain
   b. Prevent contact with persons who have never had chickenpox
   c. Keep affected area tightly covered with a moisture-preserving dressing
   d. Monitor for change in respiratory status every 4 hours
6. The mother of an infant diagnosed with "diaper" candidiasis (candidiasis affecting the area of the body covered by a diaper) asks what caused this problem. Which information should serve as the basis of the nurse's response?
   a. It is caused by a type of bacteria that is normal on the skin of older children and adults
   b. It is an inflammatory response due to irritation from urine and fecal matter
   c. It is caused by a fungus which normally is found in areas of the body such as the mouth and vagina
   d. Its cause is unknown but likely involves an allergy to some substance that the infant has encountered
7. Escape of sebum into the dermis is the cause of inflammation in which disorder?
   a. Moniliasis
   b. Impetigo
   c. Acne vulgaris
   d. Psoriasis
8. Which direction would be appropriate to give to the mother of an 8-year-old child diagnosed with impetigo?
   a. Allow crusts to drop off the affected area naturally
   b. Keep the child's linens and clothing separate from others
   c. Cover the affected area at night with a dry, sterile dressing
   d. Keep the child away from anyone who has not had chicken pox
9. Which characteristics of a skin lesion make it a suspect for being melanoma? (Select all that apply.)
   a. Congenital
   b. Variegated in color
   c. Irregular border
   d. Ulcerated
   e. Bleeding
   f. Sharply demarcated
10. When gamma benzene hexachloride is prescribed for the management of scabies, which directions should the nurse give the client regarding its use?
    a. Apply from head to toe; wait 4 hours; wash off; repeat in 2 weeks
    b. Apply to intertriginous areas; rub in well; repeat daily until itch disappears

c. Apply from neck down at bedtime; wash off in 8–12 hours; repeat in 1 week if live mites seen

d. Apply to hairy areas of the body; do not rub in; wait 8 hours and rinse off thoroughly

11. When an adolescent who is beginning acne treatment asks if his skin will be clear in time for the junior prom, on which fact should the nurse's reply be based?
   a. The response to therapy is completely unpredictable
   b. Lesions should begin to clear in about 2 weeks
   c. It can take up to 8 weeks for a response to therapy to be noticeable
   d. It will depend on how well the client complies with the prescribed diet

12. Which client would the nurse expect to have an order for antiviral therapy?
   a. 3-month-old boy with diaper candidiasis
   b. 10-year-old girl with eczema affecting the face and neck
   c. 45-year-old woman with impetigo of 10 days duration
   d. 75-year-old man who broke out with herpes zoster 12 hours ago

13. What is the major symptom of atrophic dermatitis in children?
   a. Marked erythema
   b. Intense itching
   c. Pinpoint ecchymoses
   d. Peeling epidermis

14. For which type of skin lesion would Domeboro's solution most likely be used?
   a. Weeping vesicular
   b. Pustular
   c. Dry, scaly
   d. Seborrheic papule

15. A coal tar based topical preparation is prescribed for a client with psoriasis. The client asks what this preparation is expected to do. The nurse's response should be based on which fact?
   a. Coal tar preparations protect against excessive loss of skin oils
   b. Coal tar preparations have an anti-infective effect
   c. Coal tar preparations decrease epidermal cell turnover and pruritus
   d. Coal tar preparations counteract the allergic component of the disease

16. A client with psoriasis who is to begin PUVA therapy calls to verify when the ordered psoralen is to be taken. Which is the appropriate answer to be given?
   a. At bedtime, the night before treatment
   b. With breakfast, on the day of treatment
   c. One and a half to two hours before treatment
   d. Immediately following treatment

17. Which assessment finding best supports the conclusion that the care given to a client with a stage-II pressure ulcer has been effective?
   a. The client changes position every hour
   b. The dressing over the ulcer is intact
   c. Diameter of the ulcer has decreased by 50%
   d. The ulcerated area is free of drainage

18. Which is an appropriate expected outcome for a client with postherpetic neuralgia?
   a. Client states pain is 2 or less on a scale from 1 to 10
   b. Skin lesions have disappeared
   c. Antibody titers are positive for varicella
   d. Affected area is limited to one dermatone.

19. An elderly client at risk for impaired skin integrity is to have moisturizer applied to her skin. When delegating this task to a nursing assistant, which direction should be given?
   a. Dry skin thoroughly and then apply generous amounts of moisturizer
   b. Do not rub in moisturizer that is applied to skin fold areas
   c. Apply moisturizer only to areas of the skin that appear chapped or flaky
   d. Apply moisturizer while skin is still moist from bathing

20. Which measure is effective in preventing shearing forces from causing tissue damage over the lumbosacral area?
   a. Adjusting sheets so they are wrinkle free
   b. Changing client's position every 2 hours
   c. Maintaining head of bed at an elevation of 0–30 degrees
   d. Keeping client's skin clean and dry

21. Assessment of a newly admitted client shows a full-thickness skin loss with an ulcer that looks like a deep crater and clear undermining of adjacent tissue. This finding would be documented as which stage of pressure ulcer?
   a. I
   b. II
   c. III
   d. IV

(continued)

22. An alginate dressing is ordered for a client with a stage-IV pressure ulcer. The client's daughter asks what this type of dressing does. On which fact should the nurse's answer be based?
    a. Alginate dressings are impregnated antibiotics
    b. Alginate dressings keep the wound moist and absorb exudates
    c. Alginate dressings keep the wound dry and encourage granulation
    d. Alginate dressings have an antibacterial effect
23. When planning care of the client with a stage-III pressure ulcer, the nurse must be cognizant of the fact that most complications of pressure ulcers relate to which type of event?
    a. Infection
    b. Immune reaction
    c. Fluid imbalance
    d. Malabsorption
24. Which measure might the nurse use to assess a client's risk for developing a pressure ulcer?
    a. Barthel Index
    b. Glasgow Coma Scale
    c. Katz Index
    d. Braden Scale
25. When assessing the daily diet of a client with a pressure ulcer, how much protein should the nurse consider to be an adequate intake?
    a. 0.5–1 g/kg body weight/day
    b. 1–2 g/kg body weight/day
    c. 1.5–2 g/kg body weight/day
    d. 2–2.5 g/kg body weight/day

ANSWERS & RATIONALES

MATCHING ANSWERS

Match the following:

1. h Metrogel
2. o Squamous cell carcinoma
3. r T-cell-mediated disease
4. l Thrush
5. i PUVA
6. s Isotretinoin
7. a Methotrexate
8. c Stage I pressure ulcer
9. j Melanoma
10. n Intralesional corticosteroids
11. t Permethrin

a. Requires monitoring of LFTs
b. Infection characterized by honey-colored crusts
c. Nonblanchable erythema
d. Absorbs exudates
e. Itch
f. Used in treatment of candidiasis
g. Used in treatment of melanoma
h. Used for acne rosacea
i. Form of light therapy
j. Most likely to metastasize skin cancer
k. Protection against effects of ischemia

12. _g_ Mohs surgery	l. Oral moniliasis
13. _m_ Rhinophyma	m. Long-term effect of acne rosacea
14. _d_ Alginate dressing	n. Acne treatment
15. _f_ Diflucan	o. Characterized by an indurated base
16. _p_ Basal cell carcinoma	p. Lesion with a translucent, pearly appearance
17. _b_ Impetigo	q. Occlusive dressing
18. _e_ Pruritus	r. Psoriasis
19. _k_ Reactive hyperemia	s. Acne therapy causing birth defects
20. _q_ Hydrocolloid dressing	t. Kills the scabies mite

ANSWERS FOR FILL IN THE BLANKS

1. Persons using tretinoin, tetracycline, or sulfa for the treatment of acne need to avoid sun exposure.
2. Oral contraceptives are required for women who could become pregnant, if isotretinoin is prescribed for acne.
3. Raised, thread-like lesions located in the webs of the fingers are characteristic of scabies.
4. Fair skin and easy flushing are risk factors for acne rosacea.
5. The rim of the ear and the lower lip are sites where squamous cell carcinoma is particularly likely to occur.
6. Candidiasis of the skin most often occurs in the skin fold or intertriginous areas of the body.
7. A long-term complication of herpes zoster infection is postherpetic neuralgia.
8. Pruritus is the major symptom of atopic dermatitis.
9. The type of dermatitis found primarily in young children is atopic.
10. The two types of skin change found as a result of repeated scratching in clients with dermatitis are thickening and pigment change.

TRUE & FALSE ANSWERS

Mark each of the following statements True or False. Correct all false statements in the space provided.

1. Need to avoid triggers such as hot, spicy foods and alcohol is an important part of the teaching for clients with psoriasis. *False*
   It is important for clients with acne rosacea, not psoriasis.
2. Domeboro soaks are used for the weeping vesicular lesions of contact dermatitis. *True*
3. Removal of the scale of psoriasis yields pinpoint bleeding called the Auspitz sign. *True*
4. Lesions of herpes zoster never cross the midline. *True*
5. NSAIDs are not usually effective for the pain of shingles. *True*
6. Inhaled corticosteroids place the client at risk for oral candidiasis. *True*
7. Full-thickness skin loss with damage to subcutaneous tissue that may go as deep as the fascia is a stage-IV pressure ulcer. *False.*
   It is a stage-III ulcer; stage-IV ulcer goes through the fascia into the underlying structures.
8. Metastatic melanoma is resistant to chemotherapy. *True*
9. Intense itching especially in the morning is characteristic of scabies. *False*
   Intense itch occurs at night.
10. White, milk curd-like plaques on buccal mucosa are characteristic of *Candida albicans* overgrowth. *True*

APPLICATION ANSWERS

1. Which direction must be given to an adolescent being treated with tetracycline for acne?
   a. Eliminate fatty foods from the daily diet
   b. Wash affected areas thoroughly at least every 4 hours during the day
   c. Keep out of direct sunlight
   d. Use only oil-based skin care products

Rationale

Correct answer: c.

Clients on tetracycline, sulfa, or tretinoin need to avoid exposure to sunlight so this is correct advice. The other options are incorrect because there is no documented relationship between diet and acne; overwashing should be avoided; and only water-based cosmetic and skin products should be used.

2. Which information should the nurse include in the teaching plan for a woman being treated for acne rosacea?
   a. Alcohol-based products help reduce erythema
   b. Rhinophyma only occurs in men
   c. Metrogel rapidly eliminates large pustules and papules
   d. Sun block needs to be used daily

Rationale

Correct answer: d.

Daily sun protectant is needed. Alcohol-based products should be avoided; rhinophyma occurs in both males and females; and acne rosacea responds slowly, not rapidly, to Metrogel.

3. When assessing a dark-skinned client with psoriasis, which finding would be consistent with the S&S of the disorder?
   a. Raised, sharply-demarcated plaques that appear purple in color
   b. Silvery scales on an indurated, erythematous base
   c. Translucent, pearly appearing pink to red papules
   d. Honey-colored crusts on shallow ulcers

Rationale

Correct answer: a.

In dark-skinned persons, the raised, sharply demarcated plaques of psoriasis may appear purple. Silvery scales do occur with psoriasis but the lesions do not have an indurated, erythematous base. Translucent pink to red papules that have a pearly appearance are characteristic of basal cell carcinoma while honey-colored crusts are characteristic of impetigo.

4. Which information would the nurse include when developing a teaching plan for a client receiving methotrexate for psoriasis?
   a. Creatinine clearance and other tests of renal function are required weekly for the first month of therapy
   b. Periodic EKGs will be done from the start of therapy until 6 months after its completion
   c. Pulmonary function tests and arterial blood gases need to be checked before the start of therapy
   d. Liver function tests, lipid levels, and blood counts need to be monitored during therapy

Rationale

Correct answer: d.

Liver function, lipid levels and blood counts need to be monitored during therapy with methotrexate because of its side effects. Routine monitoring of respiratory, cardiac, and renal function is not necessary.

5. Which order would the nurse expect to be included in the plan of care for a client with herpes zoster?
   a. Administer ibuprofen 800 mg q 4 hours for pain
   b. Prevent contact with persons who have never had chickenpox
   c. Keep affected area tightly covered with a moisture-preserving dressing
   d. Monitor for change in respiratory status every 4 hours

Rationale

Correct answer: b.

Herpes zoster is caused by the varicella (chickenpox) virus. Therefore, clients with herpes zoster can pass the viruses to others and if they are not immune to chickenpox, they can develop the disease. Ibuprofen is an NSAID and NSAIDs are generally not effective in treating pain associated with herpes zoster so this order would not be expected. Lesions are left open to the air so an order for a dressing would not be expected; nor would an order for monitoring respiratory status be expected, as this is not altered by herpes zoster infection.

6. The mother of an infant diagnosed with "diaper" candidiasis (candidiasis affecting the area of the body covered by a diaper) asks what caused this problem. Which information should serve as the basis of the nurse's response?
   a. It is caused by a type of bacteria that is normal on the skin of older children and adults.
   b. It is an inflammatory response due to irritation from urine and fecal matter
   c. It is caused by a fungus which normally is found in areas of the body such as the mouth and vagina
   d. Its cause is unknown but likely involves an allergy to some substance that the infant has encountered

Rationale

Correct answer: c.

Candidiasis is caused by a fungus not by bacteria. Irritation may be a risk factor. Allergy is not the cause.

7. Escape of sebum into the dermis is the cause of inflammation in which disorder?
   a. Moniliasis
   b. Impetigo
   c. Acne vulgaris
   d. Psoriasis

Rationale

Correct answer: c.

The inflammation of acne vulgaris is caused by escape of sebum into the dermis. Moniliasis is caused by a fungus, which is the source of irritation, and impetigo is caused by infection with bacteria such as *Staphylococcus aureus* or beta hemolytic *Streptococcus*. Psoriasis is a T-cell-mediated disease.

8. Which direction would be appropriate to give to the mother of an 8-year-old child diagnosed with impetigo?
   a. Allow crusts to drop off the affected area naturally
   b. Keep the child's linens and clothing separate from others
   c. Cover the affected area at night with a dry, sterile dressing
   d. Keep the child away from anyone who has not had chicken pox

Rationale

Correct answer: b.

Impetigo is contagious and therefore keeping potentially contaminated clothing and linens away from those

(continued)

if others is essential. Careful hand washing and laundering of linens and clothing that have come in contact with the affected area is also critical. Crusts should be removed and the area washed two to three times per day; lesions are not routinely covered. Impetigo is typically caused by either beta hemolytic *Streptococcus* or *Staphylococcus aureus* so the varicella virus that causes chicken pox is unrelated. Clients with herpes zoster need to be kept away from persons who have not had chicken pox.

9. Which characteristics of a skin lesion make it suspect for being melanoma? (Select all that apply.)
   a. Congenital
   b. Variegated in color
   c. Irregular border
   d. Ulcerated
   e. Bleeding
   f. Sharply demarcated

Rationale

Correct answers: b, c, d, and e.

Melanoma lesions are typically variegated in color. Lesions occur that are yellow, blue, black, gray, and even colorless. They also typically have an irregular border and may ulcerate and bleed. Melanomas usually occur as new lesions although some develop in preexisting lesions so the fact that a lesion is congenital does not increase the likelihood that it is a melanoma. Melanomas are not sharply demarcated from surrounding tissue.

10. When gamma benzene hexachloride is prescribed for the management of scabies, which directions should the nurse give the client regarding its use?
   a. Apply from head to toe; wait 4 hours; wash off; repeat in 2 weeks
   b. Apply to intertriginous areas; rub in well; repeat daily until itch disappears
   c. Apply from neck down at bedtime; wash off in 8–12 hours; repeat in 1 week if live mites seen
   d. Apply to hairy areas of the body; do not rub in; wait 8 hours and rinse off thoroughly

Rationale

Correct answer: c.

Directions for the application of gamma benzene hexachloride are to apply it from the neck down at bedtime; wash it off in 8–12 hours; and repeat in a week if more live mites are seen.

11. When an adolescent who is beginning acne treatment asks if his skin will be clear in time for the junior prom, on which fact should the nurse's reply be based?
   a. The response to therapy is completely unpredictable
   b. Lesions should begin to clear in about 2 weeks
   c. It can take up to 8 weeks for a response to therapy to be noticeable
   d. It will depend on how well the client complies with the prescribed diet

Rationale

Correct answer: c.

It takes up to 8 weeks for improvement to be seen; this is one reason why compliance with the therapeutic regiment is often a problem—it takes so long for results to be noticeable. Diet restriction is not a part of the treatment plan for acne vulgaris.

12. Which client would the nurse expect to have an order for antiviral therapy?
   a. 3-month-old boy with diaper candidiasis
   b. 10-year-old girl with eczema affecting the face and neck
   c. 45-year-old woman with impetigo of 10 days duration
   d. 75-year-old man who broke out with herpes zoster 12 hours ago

Rationale

Correct answer: d.

Herpes zoster is a viral infection and can be treated with an antiviral medication when it is diagnosed in the first 48–72 hours in an effort to shorten the course of the disease and to prevent complications. Candidiasis is a fungal infection and impetigo is a bacterial infection so antiviral therapy is not used. The cause of eczema is unknown but there appears to be an allergic component; no viral role has been identified.

13. What is the major symptom of atrophic dermatitis in children?
   a. Marked erythema
   b. Intense itching
   c. Pinpoint ecchymoses
   d. Peeling epidermis

Rationale

Correct answer: b.

Intense pruritus is the major symptom of atrophic dermatitis in children.

14. For which type of skin lesion would Domeboro's solution most likely be used?
   a. Weeping vesicular
   b. Pustular
   c. Dry, scaly
   d. Seborrheic papule

Rationale

Correct answer: a.

Domeboro's (Burow's) solution (aluminum acetate solution) exerts an astringent effect and is used on vesicular lesions. It also has antiseptic and antipruritic effects.

15. A coal tar based topical preparation is prescribed for a client with psoriasis. The client asks what this preparation is expected to do. The nurse's response should be based on which fact?
    a. Coal tar preparations protect against excessive loss of skin oils
    b. Coal tar preparations have an anti-infective effect
    c. Coal tar preparations decrease epidermal cell turnover and pruritus
    d. Coal tar preparations counteract the allergic component of the disease

Rationale

Correct answer: c.

Coal tar is an antiproliferative agent that acts by suppressing DNA synthesis in the epidermis. It also has antipruritic, astringent, vasoconstrictive and is infectant effects. Anthralin is a synthetic coal tar used to treat psariatic plaques.

16. A client with psoriasis who is to begin PUVA therapy calls to verify when the ordered psoralen is to be taken. Which is the appropriate answer to be given?
    a. At bedtime, the night before treatment
    b. With breakfast, on the day of treatment
    c. One and a half to two hours before treatment
    d. Immediately following treatment

Rationale

Correct answer: b.

Psoralen is a photosensitizer and is used to potentiate the effects of ultraviolet radiation used in the treatment of psoriasis. It is taken one and a half to two hours before treatment so it is in the system when the therapy is given.

17. Which assessment finding best supports the conclusion that the care given to a client with a stage-II pressure ulcer has been effective?
    a. The client changes position every hour
    b. The dressing over the ulcer is intact
    c. Diameter of the ulcer has decreased by 50%
    d. The ulcerated area is free of drainage

Rationale

Correct answer: c.

Decrease in size of the pressure ulcer is the only definite sign of healing and therefore it supports a conclusion that therapy is working. Changing position every hour can effectively support healing as can an intact dressing but neither indicates healing is occurring. Absence of drainage is not necessarily a sign of healing of a pressure ulcer.

18. Which is an appropriate expected outcome for a client with postherpetic neuralgia?
    a. Client states pain is 2 or less on a scale from 1 to 10
    b. Skin lesions have disappeared
    c. Antibody titers are positive for varicella
    d. Affected area is limited to one dermatone

Rationale

Correct answer: a.

Postherpetic neuralgia is a pain syndrome that can occur as a complication of herpes zoster infection. Therefore, control of pain is the goal of therapy and so relief of pain is an expected client outcome. Skin lesions disappear as part of the course of the disease itself; they are not a postherpetic phenomenon. Antibody titers are irrelevant and the affected area refers to the original outbreak of disease.

19. An elderly client at risk for impaired skin integrity is to have moisturizer applied to her skin. When delegating this task to a nursing assistant, which direction should be given?
    a. Dry skin thoroughly and then apply generous amounts of moisturizer
    b. Do not rub in moisturizer that is applied to skin fold areas
    c. Apply moisturizer only to areas of the skin that appear chapped or flaky
    d. Apply moisturizer while skin is still moist from bathing

Rationale

Correct answer: d.

Applying moisturizer while skin is still moist from bathing better hydrates the skin. Skin should not be thoroughly dried before applying moisturizer as this decreases effectiveness. Moisturizer is not left on the skin surface in areas of skin folds; this would only increase the medium for growth of microorganisms. Particularly dry areas of skin may appear chapped and flaky but dry skin occurs with age so all areas of an elderly person at risk for skin breakdown need to be moisturized.

20. Which measure is effective in preventing shearing forces from causing tissue damage over the lumbosacral area?
    a. Adjusting sheets so they are wrinkle free
    b. Changing client's position every 2 hours
    c. Maintaining head of bed at an elevation of 0–30 degrees
    d. Keeping client's skin clean and dry

(continued)

Rationale

Correct answer: c.

Shearing forces, a combination of friction and pressure which damages blood vessels and tissues in area where deep and superficial tissues meet, occur when deeper tissues move and surface tissues stay in place. When the head of the bed is elevated more than 30 degrees, clients tend to slip down in bed and a shearing force results. Keeping sheets wrinkle free prevents areas of increased pressure as would occur on skin that was on top of wrinkles. Changing position at least every 2 hours prevents prolonged pressure on a single area and permits each area that was subjected to increased pressure to regain normal circulation and tissue oxygenation.

21. Assessment of a newly admitted client shows a full-thickness skin loss with an ulcer that looks like a deep crater and clear undermining of adjacent tissue. This finding would be documented as which stage of pressure ulcer?
    a. I
    b. II
    c. III
    d. IV

Rationale

Correct answer: c.

A stage-III pressure ulcer is characterized by a full-thickness skin loss with damage to subcutaneous tissue that may go as deep as the fascia but not through it and an ulcer that looks like a deep crater. Undermining of adjacent tissue may or may not be present. A stage-I ulcer is characterized by nonblanchable erythema; a stage-II ulcer by partial-thickness skin loss which may involve epidermis only or epidermis and some dermis; and a stage-IV ulcer is characterized by full thickness skin loss with tissue necrosis or damage to muscle, bone, or supporting structures. Tissue undermining and sinus tracts may also be present.

22. An alginate dressing is ordered for a client with a stage-IV pressure ulcer. The client's daughter asks what this type of dressing does. On which fact should the nurse's answer be based?
    a. Alginate dressings are impregnated antibiotics
    b. Alginate dressings keep the wound moist and absorb exudates
    c. Alginate dressings keep the wound dry and encourage granulation
    d. Alginate dressings have an antibacterial effect

Rationale

Correct answer: b.

Alginate dressings both keep the wound moist and absorb exudates. They do not contain antibiotics or have an antibacterial effect.

23. When planning care of the client with a stage-III pressure ulcer, the nurse must be cognizant of the fact that most complications of pressure ulcers relate to which type of event?
    a. Infection
    b. Immune reaction
    c. Fluid imbalance
    d. Malabsorption

Rationale

Correct answer: a.

Most complications of a pressure ulcer result from infection with septicemia and osteomyelitis being two major ones. Immune reactions generally do not play a role. Fluid imbalance and malabsorption can increase risk of pressure ulcers and impair healing but complications per se are not directly related to either.

24. Which measure might the nurse use to assess a client's risk for developing a pressure ulcer?
    a. Barthel Index
    b. Glasgow Coma Scale
    c. Katz Index
    d. Braden Scale

Rationale

Correct answer: d.

The Braden scale is used to predict pressure ulcer risk. It consists of 6 subscales: sensory perception, moisture, activity, mobility, nutrition, and friction and shear. Highest possible score is 23; a score of 18 or lower equals risk with the lower the score, the greater the risk. The Barthel Index and the Katz Index are measures of functional assessment; the Glasgow Coma Scale is a measure of level of consciousness.

25. When assessing the daily diet of a client with a pressure ulcer, how much protein should the nurse consider to be an adequate intake?
    a. 0.5–1 g/kg body weight/day
    b. 1–2 g/kg body weight/day
    c. 1.5–2 g/kg body weight/day
    d. 2–2.5 g/kg body weight/day

Rationale

Correct answer: c.

The client with a pressure ulcer to be healed needs increased protein, 1.5–2 g/kg body weight/day. This client also needs increased calories.

Test Plan Category:

Physiological Integrity

Sub-category: Physiological Adaptation—Part 1

Topics: Alterations in Body Systems
Illness Management
Section 12: Male and Female Reproductive System Problems

REPRODUCTIVE SYSTEM PROBLEMS

FIBROCYSTIC BREAST DISEASE

- Fibrocystic breast disease is the most widely accepted term for benign changes in breast tissue.
- It refers to the most common benign breast disorder.
- It affects an estimated 10% of women of 21 years and younger, 25% of women of 25 years and older, and 50% of postmenopausal women.

- Fibrocystic breast changes include three types:
  —Cystic
    - It involves formation of fluid-filled sacs, which are the most common feature; these changes are easily treated.
  —Fibrous
    - Fibrous tissue increases progressively until menopause and then regresses.
  —Epithelial proliferation
    - It includes structurally diverse lesions, such as sclerosing adenosis and the lobular and ductal hyperplasias.

Etiology: Exact cause unknown; causal theories are

- estrogen excess and progesterone deficiency during the luteal phase of the menstrual cycle and
- environmental toxins that inhibit cyclic guanosine monophosphate enzymes: methylxanthines (caffeine, tea, and chocolate), tyramine (cheese, wine, and nuts), and tobacco.

Predisposing factors: Age, parity, genetic background, history of lactation, caffeine, and use of exogenous hormones.

S&S:

- Breast pain due to inflammation and nerve root stimulation (most common symptom), beginning 4–7 days into the luteal phase of the menstrual cycle and continuing until the onset of menstruation
- Pain in the upper outer quadrant of breasts (usually bilaterally)
- Palpable lumps that increase in size premenstrually and are freely movable
- Granular feeling of breasts on palpation
- Occasional nipple discharge (greenish-brown to black) that contains fat, proteins, ductal cells, and erythrocytes (ductal hyperplasia)

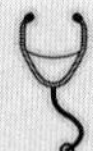

Assessment Alert

If breast pain is not relieved after menses begins, the client should see her primary health care provider.

Dx:

- Ultrasonography distinguishes cystic (fluid-filled) sacs from solid masses
- Tissue biopsy distinguishes benign from malignant changes
- Cytologic analysis of bloody aspirate rules out malignancy

Rx:

- Symptomatic to relieve pain: p.o. anti-inflammatory agent (ibuprofen), supportive bra, diet low in fat, salt, and caffeine
- Draining of painful cysts under local anesthesia
- Synthetic androgen (Danazol) for severe pain
- Oral contraceptives

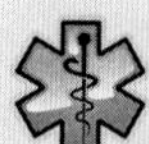

Nursing Intervention Alert

If diuretic agents or oral contraceptives are prescribed, the client needs to know that symptoms usually recur after these medications are discontinued.

Nursing Process Elements

- Identify client's concerns, anxieties, and fears
- Provide psychosocial support
- Reassure client that breast pain is rarely indicative of cancer in its early stages
- Encourage use of oral anti-inflammatory agent as prescribed
- Prior to a breast biopsy procedure, instruct client to avoid use of agents that can interfere with blood clotting and increase the risk of bleeding; NPO after midnight
- Postbiopsy, monitor for effects of anesthesia
- Inspect dressing for bleeding and/or drainage
- Monitor vital signs
- Provide pain relief as prescribed
- Prior to discharge, the nurse must insure that client is tolerating fluids, can ambulate, and is able to void

Client teaching for self-care

- Teach client about taking care of the biopsy site, pain management, and activity restrictions
- Ensure that the client knows how and when biopsy report will be obtained
- Teach client about the need for follow-up with surgeon for discussion of the final pathology report and assessment of the healing of the biopsy site

BREAST CANCER

- Breast cancer arises from the ductal epithelium.
- It is the most common cancer in women with one in every eight women in the United States expected to develop breast cancer in her lifetime.
- It may develop any time after puberty, but is most common after the age of 50 years (80% with 20% in women under the age of 30 years).

- The 5-year survival rate for localized breast cancer has improved from 72% in the 1940s to 97% in 2006.

Etiology: No single, specific cause rather a combination of hormonal, genetic, and possibly environmental events

High risk factors:

- Family history of breast cancer, particularly in first-degree maternal relatives (mother, sister, and/or maternal aunt)
- Positive tests for genetic mutations (*BRCA 1* and *BRCA 2*)
- Long menstrual cycles
- Early menarche, late menopause
- Nulliparous or first pregnancy after age of 30 years
- History of unilateral breast cancer or ovarian cancer
- Exposure to radiation between puberty and age of 30 years

Low risk factors:

- Pregnancy before age of 20 years, history of multiple pregnancies
- Native American or Asian ancestry
- Obesity
- Alcohol intake of one or more drinks daily

S&S:

- Painless lump or mass in the breast
- Breast pain
- Change in symmetry or size of the breast
- Changes in the skin—thickening, scaling skin around the nipple, dimpling, edema, and ulceration
- Change in the skin temperature (warm, hot, or pink area)
- Drainage or discharge
- Changes in nipple—itching, burning, and retraction
- Edema of the arm
- Axillary node enlargement
- Dilated blood vessels visible through the skin of the breast
- Bone pain
- Pathologic bone fractures, hypercalcemia

Dx:

- Mammography reveals tumors that are too small to palpate
- Ultrasonography distinguishes between a fluid-filled cyst and a solid mass
- Alkaline phosphatase levels and liver function tests uncover distant metastases
- Hormonal receptor assay determines whether the tumor is estrogen- or progesterone-dependent
- Fine-needle aspiration and excisional biopsy provide cells for histologic examination to confirm the diagnosis
- Chest X-rays pinpoint metastases in the chest
- Scans of the bone, brain, liver, and other organs detect distant metastases

Rx:

- Surgical:
  —lumpectomy
    - often radiation therapy is combined with this surgery
  —lumpectomy and dissection of axillary lymph nodes
  —quadrant excision
  —simple mastectomy
    - removes breast but not lymph nodes or pectoral muscles
  —modified radical mastectomy
    - removes breast and axillary lymph nodes
  —radical mastectomy (now rarely done)
    - removes breast, axillary lymph nodes, and pectoralis major and minor muscle
- Other treatments:
  —reconstructive surgery if no advanced disease
  —chemotherapy, adjuvant or primary therapy
  —tamoxifen (estrogen antagonist)
    - adjuvant treatment of choice for postmenopausal clients with positive estrogen-receptor status; has also been found to reduce risk of breast cancer in women of high risk
  —peripheral stem cell therapy for advanced disease
  —primary radiation therapy before or after tumor removal
    - effective for small tumors in early stages
    - helps make inflammatory breast tumors more surgically manageable
    - used to prevent or treat local recurrence
  —estrogen, progesterone, androgen, or antiandrogen aminoglutethimide therapy

Nursing Process Elements

- Assess client's understanding of breast cancer and treatment options
- Reduce fear and anxiety and improve coping ability
- Promote decision-making ability
- Maintain skin integrity
- Promote positive body image
- Promote positive adjustment and coping
- Promote participation in care
- Promote sexual functioning
- Encourage participation of partner in care

Client teaching for self-care

Instruct client to

- exhibit knowledge abut diagnosis and treatment options
- demonstrate ability to make decisions regarding treatment options in a timely fashion

- verbalize ability to deal with anxiety and fears related to the diagnosis and the effects of surgery on self-image and sexual functioning

VAGINITIS

- Vaginitis refers to the inflammation of the vagina and vulva; because of their proximity, inflammation of one may cause inflammation of the other.
- It may occur at any age.
- It is common in women who use estrogen-containing birth control pills and among pregnant women due to increased estrogen.

Etiology: Bacterial vaginitis occurs from a disturbance of the normal vaginal flora and an overgrowth of anaerobic bacteria *Trichomonas vaginalis* usually transmitted through sexual intercourse, *Gardnerella vaginalis*, *Candida albicans*, parasitic infection, trauma (skin breakdown may lead to secondary infection), poor personal hygiene, chemical irritants or allergic reactions to hygiene sprays, douches, detergents, clothing, or toilet paper, vulvar atrophy in menopausal women due to decreasing estrogen levels, and retention of a foreign body (tampon, diaphragm).

S&S:

- *Trichomonas vaginalis*: thin, bubbly, green-tinged, malodorous discharge, irritation, itching; urinary symptoms such as burning and/or frequency
- *Candida albicans*: thick, white, cottage cheese-like discharge, red, edematous membranes, intense itching
- Bacterial vaginitis: gray, foul, "fish-smelling" discharge

Dx:

- Wet prep saline examination
- Pap smear
- Urinalysis

Rx:

- Trichomonal vaginitis: oral metronidazole (Flagyl)
- Candida albicans: topical miconazole or clotrimazole; single dose of oral fluconazole
- Gardnerella vaginitis: oral or vaginal metronidazole
- Acute vulvitis: cold compresses or cool sitz baths for pruritus; warm compresses for severe inflammation; and topical corticosteroids to reduce inflammation
- Chronic vulvitis: topical hydrocortisone or antipruritics; good hygiene, especially in elderly or incontinent clients
- Atrophic vulvovaginitis: topical estrogen ointment

Nursing Process Elements

- Adopt the following goals of care:
  - —relieve discomfort
  - —reduce anxiety
  - —prevent reinfection or spread of infection

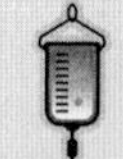

Clinical Alert OB

Avoid using Flagyl during first trimester of pregnancy

Client teaching for self-care

Teach client about

- cause of symptoms to reduce anxiety related to fear of a more serious illness
- importance of treating partner, if indicated, to decrease likelihood of reinfection
- role of abstinence in preventing spread of infection
- the need to avoid tight clothing and to wear cotton underwear
- good hygienic practices including daily bathing
- proper hand washing before and after administration of medication
- need to avoid douching unless therapeutically prescribed
- need to avoid alcohol during treatment with Flagyl

PELVIC INFLAMMATORY DISEASE

- Pelvic inflammatory disease (PID) is an inflammatory condition of the pelvic cavity that may involve the uterus, fallopian tubes, ovaries, pelvic peritoneum, or pelvic vascular system.
- Untreated PID may cause infertility and may lead to potentially fatal septicemia and shock.
- Approximately one million women are treated for PID in the United States each year; most of them are younger than 25 years of age, and one-fourth of them have serious sequelae (chronic pelvic pain, ectopic pregnancy, and infertility).

Etiology: Usually caused by bacterial infection but may be viral, fungal, or parasitic; presumption is that organisms enter the body through the vagina, pass through the cervical canal, colonize the endocervix, and move upward into the uterus. Under various conditions, the organisms may proceed to one or both of the fallopian tubes and ovaries and into the pelvis. In infections that occur after childbirth or abortion, pathogens are disseminated directly through the tissues that support the uterus by way of the lymphatic vessels and blood vessels

Risk/Precipitating factors: Conization or cauterization of the cervix, insertion of an intrauterine device, abortion, pelvic surgery, infections during or after pregnancy, early age of first intercourse, multiple sexual partners, frequent intercourse, intercourse without condoms, sex with a partner with an STI, history of previous STI or previous pelvic infection, use of a biopsy curette or an irrigation catheter, tubal insufflation.

S&S:

- Profuse, purulent vaginal discharge
- Low-grade fever
- Dyspareunia
- Malaise
- Anorexia
- Vomiting
- Lower-abdominal pain
- Headache
- Chills
- Vaginal bleeding
- Severe pain on movement of the cervix or palpation of adnexa

Dx:

- Culture and sensitivity and Gram stain testing of endocervix or cul-de-sac secretions show the causative agent
- Urethral and rectal secretions reveal the causative agent
- Blood test reveals elevated C-reactive protein level
- Transvaginal ultrasonography shows the presence of thickened, fluid-filled Fallopian tubes
- CT scan shows complex tubo-ovarian abscesses
- Culdocentesis obtains peritoneal fluid or pus for C&S testing
- Diagnostic laparoscopy identifies cul-de-sac fluid, tubal distension, and masses

Rx:

- Intensive therapy including bed rest
- Antibiotic therapy beginning immediately after culture specimens are obtained and reevaluated as soon as laboratory results are available
- Analgesics
- IV fluids
- Adequate drainage if pelvic abscess forms
- Ruptured abscess (life-threatening complication): total abdominal hysterectomy with bilateral salpingo-oophorectomy
- Abdominal distension or ileus: nasogastric intubation and suction
- Treat sexual partners to prevent reinfection

Nursing Process Elements

- Relieve anxiety related to treatment/diagnosis
- Maintain on bed rest in semi-Fowler's position to facilitate dependent drainage
- Maintain accurate vital sign recordings
- Maintain accurate recordings of characteristics and amounts of vaginal discharge
- Administer analgesics as prescribed for pain relief
- Apply heat safely to abdomen to promote pain relief and comfort

Client teaching for self-care

Teach client about

- the importance of immediate evaluation of any pelvic pain and/or abnormal discharge, especially after sexual exposure, childbirth, or pelvic surgery
- proper perineal care procedures (wiping from front to back after defecation or urination)
- the fact that douching reduces the natural flora that combat infecting organisms and may introduce bacteria upward
- the importance of consulting a health care professional if unusual vaginal discharge or odor is noted
- the importance of safe sexual practices (i.e., using condoms, avoiding multiple sexual partners, etc.)
- the importance of use of condoms consistently before intercourse or any penile–vaginal contact if there is any chance of transmitting the infection
- the need for gynecologic examination at least once a year

TOXIC SHOCK SYNDROME

Etiology: Toxins produced by *Staphylococcus aureus*.

Risk/Precipitating factors: Menstruation and tampon use, postoperative infection, use of a diaphragm, cervical cap, or vaginal contraceptive sponge, focal infection, and postpartum and nonmenstrual vaginal conditions.

S&S: Flu-like symptoms for 24 hours, rapid onset of high fever, headache, sore throat, vomiting, diarrhea, generalized rash that initially looks like sunburn and subsequently like a drug rash followed in 1–2 weeks by peeling of the skin particularly on the palms and soles, and hypotension. Respiratory, renal, liver, cardiovascular, and central nervous system impairments can also occur

Dx: Presence of symptoms which meet CDC criteria

Rx: Antibiotics, drugs for hypotension, IV fluid and electrolyte replacement, corticosteroids for rash

Nursing Process Elements

- Provide supportive care related to treatment of shock and fluid and electrolyte imbalance.

Client teaching for self care

For prevention of recurrence, instruct client to

- avoid use of tampons
- avoid use of a diaphragm during menses
- wash hands thoroughly before inserting a diaphragm or contraceptive sponge
- avoid the use of sponge if dirty; wet with clean water; and do not leave in place for more than 30 hours at a time
- remove diaphragm within 24 hours; wash thoroughly; dry and store in a clean place

UTERINE PROLAPSE

- Uterine prolapse refers to the descent of the cervix or the entire uterus into the vaginal canal.
- In severe cases, the uterus falls completely through the vagina and protrudes outside of the body.
- As the uterus descends, it may pull the vaginal walls and even the bladder and rectum with it.
- Uterine prolapse is more prevalent in whites than in blacks, and rare in Canadian Indians.

Etiology: Progressive relaxation of the support structures of the pelvis.

Predisposing factors: Trauma to perineum (childbirth, pelvic surgery), occupational activities that require heavy lifting, chronic medical conditions such as lung disease and chronic constipation and straining, neural abnormalities that interfere with the innervation of the levator ani muscles, obesity, and strong familial tendency.

S&S:

- Pelvic pressure
- Urinary problems (retention or incontinence)
- Pain
- Collapse through the vagina
- Pain during sexual intercourse

Dx:

- Physical examination
- Ultrasound, fluoroscope, or magnetic resonance
- Urinary, sexual, anorectal review of systems for pelvic floor disorders provides comprehensive historical data

Rx:

- First-degree uterine prolapse is not treated unless it causes discomfort
- In second- and third-degree prolapse, or in elderly women who may not be candidates for surgery, a pessary (removable mechanical device that holds the uterus in position) may be placed
- The pelvic fascia may be strengthened by Kegel exercises or by a course of estrogen therapy in postmenopausal women; hysterectomy may be done in this age group
- Surgical repair is the last treatment of choice; in this procedure, the uterus is sutured back into place and repaired to strengthen and tighten the muscle bands

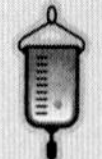

Clinical Alert

Rubber pessaries need to be avoided in women with latex allergies.

Nursing Process Elements

- Relieve anxiety related to treatment

CYSTOCELE

- Cystocele refers to the descent of a portion of the posterior bladder wall into the vaginal canal.
- In severe cases, the bladder and anterior vaginal wall bulge outside the introitus.

Etiology: Usually trauma of childbirth.

Predisposing factors: Pregnancy, obesity, constipation, pelvic tumors, bronchitis, heavy manual labor; hormone deficiency may also play a role

S&S:

- Usually symptoms are insignificant
- Pelvic pressure
- Fatigue
- Pelvic and/or back pain
- Urinary problems such as frequency, incontinence, and urgency

Dx:

- Physical examination
- Detailed genitourinary history

Rx:

- Depends on the age of the woman and severity of the condition; may include isometric exercise (Kegel exercises) to strengthen the pubococcygeal muscle, estrogen to improve tone and vascularity of fascial support, and pessary placement (mechanical device used to hold bladder in place)
- Surgical correction for severe anatomic injury unresponsive to medical treatment

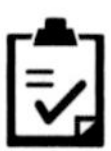

Nursing Process Elements

- Reassure client to help relieve anxiety

Client teaching for self-care

Teach the client about

- importance of eliminating or decreasing or preventing stressors such as obesity, constipation, and heavy manual labor
- method of performing Kegel exercises
- importance of follow-up appointment with health care provider

RECTOCELE

- Rectocele refers to the bulging of the rectum and posterior vaginal wall into the vaginal canal
- Usually the symptoms of rectocele do not occur until several years after menopause.

Etiology: Usually results from injury and strain during childbirth.

Predisposing factors: Childbirth, chronic constipation and straining, and familial and genetic predisposition.

S&S:

- Most rectoceles are asymptomatic
- Vaginal pressure and/or pain
- Rectal fullness
- Incomplete bowel evacuation
- Back pain
- Uncontrollable gas
- Incontinence
- Bleeding
- Ulcerations

Dx:

- Physical examination
- Urinary, sexual, anorectal review of systems for pelvic floor disorders provides comprehensive historical data

Rx:

- Prevention and treatment of constipation
- Pessary insertion
- Rectocele alone (without associated enterocele, uterine prolapse, and cystocele) seldom requires surgery

Nursing Process Elements

- Provide reassurance to the client to relieve anxiety

Client teaching for self-care

Teach client about

- proper technique of performing isometric pelvic exercises (Kegel exercises)
- the need to do Kegel exercises regularly
- measures to prevent constipation (i.e., increase fluids, fruit, fiber, vegetables, etc.)
- the importance of keeping follow-up appointments with health care provider

LEIOMYOMAS (FIBROIDS)

- Leiomyomas refer to the benign, slow-growing, solid tumors of the uterine wall.
- Estrogen appears to stimulate the growth of these tumors.
- These often enlarge with pregnancy and regress after menopause.

Etiology: Unknown, possibly stress on an area of myometrium.

S&S: Often asymptomatic

- Abnormal bleeding is predominant symptom:
  —Menorrhagia refers to increased menstrual bleeding
  —Metrorrhagia refers to bleeding between menstrual periods
- Pelvic pressure
- Constipation
- Urinary frequency or retention

Dx:

- Pelvic examination
- Ultrasound
- Pregnancy test to rule out pregnancy as cause of uterine enlargement
- Endometrial biopsy to rule out malignancy
- CBC to check for anemia secondary to bleeding

Rx: Observation if close to menopause since tumors may shrink; observation or myomectomy (removal of tumors with preservation of uterus) if child bearing is desired; otherwise hysterectomy

Nursing Process Elements

- Reassure the client that tumors are not malignant
- If menopausal, explain that tumors may continue to grow if estrogen replacement therapy is used.
- Perioperative care (see Chapter 18)

CERVICAL CANCER

- Carcinoma of the cervix is predominantly squamous cell cancer.
- It is the third most common cancer of the female reproductive system.
- It is classified as either microinvasive or invasive.
- Preinvasive disease ranges from mild cervical dysplasia in which the lower-third of epithelium contains abnormal

cells, to carcinoma in situ, in which full thickness of epithelium contains abnormally proliferating cells.

- In invasive carcinoma, cancer cells penetrate the basement membrane and can spread directly to contiguous pelvic structures or disseminate to distant sites by lymphatic routes.

Etiology: Major cause is now known to be HPV.

Predisposing factors: Multiple sex partners, early age at first coitus, short interval between menarche and first coitus, sexual contact with men whose partners have had cervical cancer, exposure to the human papilloma virus (HPV), chronic cervical infections, nutritional deficiencies, and smoking.

S&S:

- *Preinvasive disease*
  —often produces no symptoms
- *Early invasive cervical cancer:*
  —abnormal vaginal bleeding
  —persistent vaginal bleeding
  —postcoital pain and bleeding
- *Advanced disease:*
  —pelvic pain
  —vaginal leakage of urine and stool from a fistula
  —anorexia, weight loss, and anemia

Dx:

- Papanicolaou (Pap) test screens for abnormal cells
- Colposcopy shows the source of the abnormal cells seen on the Pap test
- Cone biopsy is performed if endocervical curettage is positive
- Vira-pap test permits examination of the specimen's DNA structure to detect HPV
- Lymphangiography and cystography detect metastasis
- Organ and bone scans show metastases

Rx:

- *Preinvasive lesions:*
  —Loop electrosurgical excision procedure
  —Cryosurgery
  —Laser destruction
  —Conization (with frequent Pap smear follow-up)
  —Hysterectomy
- *Invasive carcinoma:*
  —Radical hysterectomy
  —Radiation therapy (internal, external, or both)
  —Chemotherapy
  —Combination of the above procedures

Nursing Process Elements

- Relieve anxiety related to surgical procedures
- Relieve pain
- Improve skin integrity
- Monitor for and manage potential complications: infection, deep vein thrombosis, and hemorrhage
- Support positive sexuality and sexual function

Client teaching for self-care

Teach client about

- the need for regular pelvic examinations and Pap tests
- reproductive health and safer sex
- smoking cessation program and provide referral

ENDOMETRIAL CANCER

- Endometrial cancer is also known as uterine cancer or cancer of the lining of the uterus.
- It is the most common gynecological cancer.
- It can also lead to adenocarcinoma that metastasizes late, usually from the endometrium to the cervix, fallopian tubes, and other peritoneal structures.

Etiology: Unknown.

Predisposing factors: Anovulation, abnormal uterine bleeding, history of atypical endometrial hyperplasia, unopposed estrogen stimulation, nulliparity, polycystic ovarian syndrome, familial tendency, obesity, hypertension, and diabetes.

S&S:

- Uterine enlargement
- Persistent and unusual premenopausal bleeding
- Any postmenopausal bleeding
- Late signs and symptoms, such as pain and weight loss (do not appear until the cancer is well advanced)

Dx:

- Endometrial, cervical, or endocervical biopsy confirms the presence of cancer cells
- Fractional dilatation and curettage identifies cancer when biopsy is negative
- Cervical biopsies and endocervical curettage pinpoint cervical involvement

Rx:

- Surgery
- Radiation therapy
- Hormonal therapy
- Chemotherapy

Nursing Process Elements

- Relieve anxiety related to surgical procedures
- Relieve pain

- Improve skin integrity
- Monitor and manage for complications: infection, deep vein thrombosis, and hemorrhage
- Support positive sexuality and sexual function

Client teaching for self-care

Teach client

- about stress reducing activities
- to care for incision and surgical site as directed; to observe for healing of surgical site without excoriated skin or purulent discharge
- to properly clean the surgical site after voiding and defecating
- to maintain a low-residue diet to prevent straining on defecation and wound contamination
- to avoid crossing legs or sitting with pressure against knees; to exercise ankles and legs to decrease the risk of venous thrombosis
- to discuss with primary care physician concerns and anxieties about sexual functioning; to discuss options and alternative approaches to sexual intercourse

OVARIAN CANCER

- There are two major types of ovarian cancer: epithelial neoplasms and germ cell neoplasms.
- Ovarian cancer causes more deaths than any other cancer of the reproductive system.
- It spreads rapidly intraperitoneally by local extension or surface seeding, and occasionally, through the lymphatic vessels and the bloodstream.
- Generally, extraperitoneal spread travels through the diaphragm into the chest cavity, where the tumor may cause pleural effusions.
- About 75% of cases are detected at a late stage.

Etiology: Unknown; may be linked to mutations in the *BRCA 1* or *BCRA 2* gene.

Associated factors: Infertility, nulliparity, familial tendency, ovarian dysfunction, irregular menses, exposure to asbestos, talc, industrial pollutants, fertility drugs, diet high in saturated fat, hormone replacement therapy.

S&S:

- May grow to considerable size before overt symptoms begin to appear
- *Occasionally, in the early stages:*
  —vague abdominal discomfort, and distension
  —mild GI discomfort (nausea, vomiting, and bloating)
  —urinary frequency and pelvic discomfort
  —constipation
  —vaginal bleeding
  —weight loss
- *Later stages:*
  —tumor rupture, torsion, or infection
- *Advanced ovarian cancer:*
  —ascites
  —postmenopausal bleeding and pain
  —symptoms of metastatic tumors, commonly pleural effusion

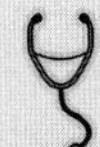

Assessment Alert

Pain associated with ovarian cancer in young clients may mimic appendicitis.

Dx:

- Exploratory laparotomy, including lymph node evaluation and tumor resection, is required for accurate diagnosis and staging
- Laboratory tumor-marker studies (such as ovarian carcinoma antigen, carcinoembryonic antigen, and human choriogonadotropin) show abnormalities that may indicate complications
- Abdominal ultrasonography, CT scan, or X-rays delineate tumor size
- Aspiration of ascitic fluid reveals atypical cell

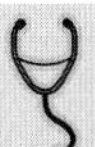

Assessment Alert

A palpable ovary in a woman who has gone through menopause should be investigated because ovaries normally become smaller and less palpable after menopause.

Rx:

- Varying combinations of surgery, chemotherapy, and radiation
- *Conservative treatment for a unilateral, encapsulated tumor in a young girl or a young woman:*
  —Resection of the involved ovary
  —Careful follow-up, including periodic chest X-rays to rule out lung metastasis
- *More aggressive treatment:*
  —Total abdominal hysterectomy and bilateral salpingo-oophorectomy with tumor resection, omentectomy, possible appendectomy, lymphadenectomy, tissue biopsies, and peritoneal washings

- *If tumor has matted around other organs or involves organs that cannot be resected:*
  - —Surgical debulking of tumor implants to less than 2 cm (or smaller) in greatest diameter
- *Chemotherapy:*
  - —may be curative; extends survival time in most clients; largely palliative in advanced disease
  - —standard is combination paclitaxel and platinum-based chemotherapy

Nursing Process Elements

- Provide measures related to the client's treatment plan, be it surgery, chemotherapy, or palliation
- Provide emotional support to client and her family
- Provide comfort measures
- Clients with advanced ovarian cancer may develop ascites and pleural effusion, thus
  - —administer intravenous therapy to alleviate fluid and electrolyte imbalances
  - —initiate parenteral nutrition to provide adequate nutrition
  - —provide postoperative care after intestinal bypass to alleviate an obstruction
  - —provide pain relief and manage drainage tubes
- Provide comfort measures for women with ascites by providing small frequent meals, decreasing fluid intake, administering diuretic agents, and providing rest

Client teaching for self-care

Teach client

- about the need for regular pelvic examinations including Pap test for all women
- about reproductive health
- to eat small, frequent meals
- to take medications as prescribed
- to take frequent rest periods

CANCER OF THE VULVA

- Vulvar neoplasms may develop from various cell origins.
- Because much of the vulva is made of skin, any type of skin cancer can develop on the vulva.
- The majority of vulvar cancers arise from squamous epithelial cells.

Etiology: Primary cause unknown.

Predisposing factors: Leukoplakia in approximately 25% of clients, chronic vulvar granulomatous disease, chronic pruritus of the vulva with friction, swelling, and dryness, pigmented moles that are constantly irritated by clothing or perineal pads, irradiation of the skin such as infection with HPV, obesity, hypertension, and diabetes.

S&S:

- *In 50% of clients:*
  - —vulvar pruritus, bleeding
  - —small vulvar mass
    - may begin as a small ulcer on the surface, which usually becomes infected and painful
- *Less common:*
  - —mass in the groin
  - —abnormal urination and/or defecation

Dx:

- Colposcopy and toluidine-blue staining identify biopsy sites
- Histologic examination of biopsy samples confirm diagnosis and identify the type of cancer

Rx:

- *Small, confined lesions with no lymph node involvement:*
  - —Simple vulvectomy or hemivulvectomy (without pelvic node dissection)
  - —Requires careful postoperative follow-up because it leaves the client at risk for developing a new lesion

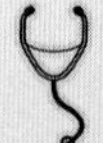

Assessment Alert

Personal considerations such as young age of client and active sexual life may mandate conservative management.

- *For widespread tumor:*
  - —Radical vulvectomy
  - —Radical wide local excision
    - can be as effective as more radical resection, but with much less morbidity
  - —Depending on degree of metastasis, resection may include the urethra, vagina, and bowel, leaving an open perineal wound until healing, that is, for about 2–3 months
  - —Plastic surgery, including mucocutaneous graph to reconstruct pelvic structures
  - —Radiation therapy
- *Extensive metastasis, advanced age, or fragile health:*
  - —Rules out surgery
  - —Palliative treatment with irradiation of the primary lesion or chemotherapy

Nursing Process Elements

- Relieve anxiety—a major goal for the client may include acceptance of and preparation for surgical intervention

- Relieve pain related to the surgical incision and subsequent wound care
- Improve skin integrity
- Support positive sexuality and sexual function
- Monitor and manage potential complications post-surgery: infection, deep vein thrombosis, and hemorrhage

Client teaching for self-care

Teach client

- about stress-reducing activities
- to care for incision and/or surgical site as directed, observe for excoriated skin or purulent drainage
- to take pain medication as ordered
- to prevent deep vein thrombosis, to avoid crossing legs or sitting with pressure against knees, and to exercise ankles and legs
- about the need to discuss with health care provider concerns and anxieties about altered body image and sexual functioning; to discuss options and alternative approaches to sexual intercourse
- to maintain a low-residue diet to prevent straining on defecation

PROSTATITIS

- Prostatitis refers to the sudden (acute) or gradual (chronic) inflammation of the prostate gland.
- It is generally classified as bacterial or nonbacterial.
- The complications include possible infertility and increased risk of prostate cancer.

Etiology: Urethral trauma or bacteria (*E. coli* is the most often identified organism) from the bladder or urethra cause inflammation, congestion, and obstructed urinary flow. Scarring of the prostate and urethra may result in permanent narrowing of the urethra. In nonbacterial prostatitis, the cause is unknown.

Risk factors: Frequent urinary tract infections (UTIs), urethritis, epididymitis, STIs, excessive alcohol intake, perineal injury, multiple sex partners, and advancing age.

S&S:

- Pain (low back, perineal, and testicular) associated with urination, ejaculation, or having a Bowel Movement (BM)
- Fever and chills
- Decrease in force and volume of urinary stream
- Urinary retention
- Hematuria
- Pyuria
- Urethral discharge

Dx: Culture of prostatic fluid, divided urine specimen for segmented urine culture and urinalysis. Physical examination reveals enlarged, tender prostate; groin lymph nodes may be palpable; Prostatic specific antigen (PSA) may be elevated; WBCs elevated and bacteria may be present on urine and semen analysis; blood culture positive if infection is systemic

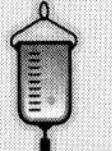

Clinical Alert

Massaging an obviously swollen and tender prostate may potentially spread the infection and increase the risk for sepsis.

Rx: Broad spectrum antibiotics (ciprofloxacin, tetracycline, penicillin, or trimethoprim-sulfamethoxazole) for 10–14 days; hospitalization and IV antibiotic therapy required in severe cases; continuous low-dose antibiotic therapy PRN to suppress infection; NSAIDs to relieve inflammation; stool softeners to relieve discomfort associated with bowel movements; antispasmodics, bladder sedatives, and sitz baths for comfort. Regular ejaculation by sexual intercourse or masturbation to reduce the retention of prostatic fluid. Transurethral resection of the prostate (TURP) may be done if medical therapy is unsuccessful

Nursing Process Elements

- Promote early detection and aggressive treatment of UTIs
- Encourage healthy lifestyle changes
- Provide teaching on effects and side effects of prescribed medications
- Avoid massaging inflamed prostate

Client teaching for self-care

Teach client

- to take medication as prescribed
- to avoid sitting for long periods of time
- to restrict intake of alcohol
- to increase fluid intake (64–128 oz of water per day)
- to avoid foods such as alcohol, coffee, tea, chocolate, cola, and spices that have diuretic action or that increase prostatic secretions
- to avoid sexual arousal and intercourse during periods of acute inflammation
- to limit number of sexual partners and use condoms
- to keep appointments for follow-up
- to report new or recurring symptoms including pain, difficulty with urination, fever, and chills
- about the need for evaluation/treatment of sexual partners to decrease risk of cross-infection

EPIDIDYMITIS

- Epididymitis refers to an infection of the epididymis.

Etiology: Usually descends from an infected prostate or urinary tract; may be a complication of gonorrhea.

Predisposing factors: Chlamydial infection in men under 35 years of age.

S&S:

- Unilateral pain and soreness in the inguinal canal
- Swelling and pain in the scrotum
- Elevated temperature
- Urine may contain pus
- Chills

Dx:

- Swelling in the scrotum and groin
- Urine C&S
- Culture for STIs (chlamydial infection)

Rx:

- Within 24 hours of onset, spermatic cord can be infiltrated with a local anesthetic agent to relieve pain
- Antibiotics for client and partner if from chlamydial infection
- Epididymectomy for recurrent, incapacitating episodes or for chronic, painful disease

Nursing Process Elements

- Assess for signs and symptoms
- Assess for risk factors for STIs

Client teaching for self care

Teach client

- about the need for bed rest with scrotum elevated
- to take antibiotics as ordered
- to use intermittent cold compresses to scrotum to relieve pain
- to apply local heat or take warm sitz baths later to relieve inflammation
- to take analgesics as prescribed and needed
- to expect it to take up to 4 weeks or longer for condition to subside

BENIGN PROSTATIC HYPERPLASIA

- Benign prostatic hyperplasia (BPH) is the enlargement of the prostate gland with extension upward to the bladder resulting in obstruction of the flow of urine.
- It is the most common condition of older men and the second most common cause of surgical intervention in men older than 60 years of age.

Etiology: Uncertain; some evidence that hormones initiate hyperplasia of the supporting stromal tissue and the glandular elements in the prostate.

Risk Factors: Age over 50 years.

S&S:

- Frequency of urination
- Nocturia
- Hesitancy in starting urination
- Abdominal straining with urination
- A decrease in the volume and force of the urinary stream
- Dribbling
- A sensation that bladder has not been completely emptied
- Acute urinary retention
- Recurrent UTIs
- Fatigue
- Anorexia
- Nausea
- Vomiting
- Epigastric discomfort

Dx:

- Physical examination
- Urinalysis and urodynamic studies to assess urine flow
- Renal function tests including serum creatinine levels
- Complete blood studies
- Clients with BPH often have cardiac or respiratory complications because of age so cardiac and respiratory assessments are also done

Rx:

- Treatment depends on cause of BPH, severity of obstruction, and overall condition of the client
- "Watchful waiting" is an appropriate treatment for many because the likelihood of progression is unknown; clients are monitored periodically for severity of symptoms, physical findings, and changes in laboratory and diagnostic urologic tests
- Transurethral resection of the prostate (TURP)
- Balloon dilation
- Alpha-blockers (e.g., terazosin) to constrict prostate reducing pressure on urethral and facilitating urine flow
- 5-alpha-reductase inhibitors (e.g., finasteride) to shrink the prostate by lowering level of dihydrotestosterone, which causes prostatic growth; can take 6 months to have an effect
- Transurethral laser resection
- Transurethral needle ablation
- Microwave therapy

Nursing Process Elements

- Provide information regarding diagnostic tests and procedures
- Encourage client to keep appointments with health care provider to monitor physical findings, laboratory work, and diagnostic tests
- Provide perioperative care if surgery is done (see Chapter 18)

Client teaching for self-care

Teach client to

- prevent overdistention of the bladder:
  - —avoid drinking large amounts at one time
  - —avoid diuretics, caffeine, and alcohol
  - —void when first feel the urge; do not wait
- avoid medications such as anticholinergics, antihistamines, and decongestants that can cause urinary retention

IMPOTENCE (ERECTILE DYSFUNCTION)

- Impotence or erectile dysfunction (ED) refers to a male's inability to attain or maintain penile erection sufficient to complete intercourse.
- Primary impotence—erection sufficient for intercourse has never been achieved.
- Secondary impotence—intercourse has been successful in the past.
- It affects men of all age groups but increases in frequency with age.
- Transient periods of impotence are not considered ED; they probably occur in half of adult males.
- The prognosis depends on the severity and duration of impotence and the underlying causes.

Etiology: Personal and sexual anxieties, disturbed sexual relationships, situational impotence, chronic diseases that cause neurologic and vascular impairment, cirrhosis, spinal cord trauma, complications of surgery, particularly prostatectomy, drug or alcohol-induced ED, genital anomalies, or central nervous system defects.

S&S:

- Anxiety
- Palpitations
- Inability to achieve or sustain a full erection
- Loss of interest in sexual activity
- Depression

Dx:

- Detailed sexual history helps differentiate between organic or psychogenic factors and primary and secondary impotence
- Meeting the diagnostic criteria, either
  - —persistent or recurrent, partial or complete failure to attain or maintain erection until completion of sexual activity or
  - —experience of marked distress or interpersonal difficulty as a result of ED

Rx:

- *Organic impotence:*
  - —Reversing the cause if possible
  - —Psychological counseling to help couple deal realistically with their situation and explore alternatives for sexual expression if reversing the cause is not possible
  - —Sildenafil, tadalafil, or vardenafil to cause vasodilation within the penis
  - —Adrenergic antagonist, yohimbine, to enhance parasympathetic neurotransmission
  - —Testosterone supplementation for hypogonadal men (not for men with prostate cancer)
  - —Prostaglandin E injected directly into the corpus cavernosum (may induce an erection for 30–60 minutes in some men)
  - —Surgically inserted inflatable or noninflatable penile implants
- *Psychogenic impotence:*
  - —Sex therapy including both partners
  - —Improve verbal communication skills, eliminate unreasonable guilt, and/or reevaluate attitudes toward sex and sexual roles

Nursing Process Elements

- Provide support
- Provide information about ED support groups for men and their partners (Impotence Anonymous and I-Anon)

PREMATURE EJACULATION

- Premature ejaculation refers to the inability to voluntarily control the ejaculatory reflex; once aroused, reaches orgasm before or shortly after intromission.
- It is the most common dysfunction in men.

Etiology: Trauma, chronic illness, and physical disability.

S&S:

- Ejaculation, once aroused, without control

Rx:

- Depends on the nature and severity of the problem
- Behavioral therapies often involving the man and his sexual partner

Nursing Process elements

- Provide support
- Reinforce therapeutic plan

RETROGRADE EJACULATION

- Retrograde ejaculation is the involuntary inhibition of the ejaculatory reflex.

Etiology: Disability and medications are the most common causes.

S&S:

- Inability to ejaculate

Rx:

- Usually multidisciplinary in approach; addresses both physical and psychological factors
- Chemical, vibratory, and electrical stimulation have been used with some success
- Urine may be collected after ejaculation and sperm collected from the urine for use in artificial insemination
- In men with spinal cord injury, electroejaculation may be used to produce sperm for artificial insemination

Nursing Process Elements

- Provide support
- Reinforce therapeutic plan

PROSTATE CANCER

- Prostate cancer is the most common cancer in men.
- It is a slow growing cancer.
- It has a predictable pattern of spread: lymph nodes, bone marrow, bones of pelvis, sacrum, and lumbar spine.
- In the later stages, it spreads to lungs, liver, adrenals, and/or kidneys.

Etiology: Androgen-dependent carcinoma.

Predisposing factors: Increasing age, high-fat diet, African-American descent.

S&S:

- Rare in early stages
- Late symptoms include
  - —urinary obstruction: frequency, difficulty in urinating, urinary retention, and decreased size and force of the urinary stream
  - —backache and hip pain from metastases to bone
  - —perineal and rectal discomfort
  - —anorexia, weight loss, weakness, and nausea
  - —oliguria
  - —hematuria

Dx:

- Elevated PSA level: concentration of PSA in the blood is proportional to the total prostatic mass so PSA is elevated with other conditions such as BPH; also elevated in older men
- Digital rectal examination
- Diagnosis confirmed by histologic examination of tissue removed surgically by transurethral resection, open prostatectomy, or transurethral needle biopsy

Rx:

- Based on the stage of the disease, symptoms, and the client's age
- Radical prostatectomy is standard for early-stage, potentially curable disease when life expectancy is at least 10 years
- Curative radiation therapy—for early disease (teletherapy with a linear accelerator or interstitial "seeds" irradiation)
- Androgen deprivation hormonal therapy, controls rather than cures; used for extensive or metastatic disease
  - —Bilateral orchiectomy
  - —Gonadotropin-releasing hormone agonist analogs (GnRH), for example, leuprolide (Lupron), suppress pituitary release of LH and reduces serum testosterone levels
  - —Oral androgen blocking agent, for example, flutamide (Eulexin) blocks uptake of testicular and adrenal androgens by tumor
  - —Estrogens, for example, DES inhibit LH release
- Cryosurgery—to ablate the cancer in clients unable to physically tolerate surgery or with a recurrence

Nursing Process Elements

- Help client identify measures to relieve anxiety
- Provide information about institutional and community resources for coping with prostate cancer: social services, support groups, and community agencies
- Determine effect of disease on sexual functioning; facilitate with partner identification of alternative and satisfying modes of relationship with each other
- Administer analgesics as ordered for pain
- Provide postoperative care, where indicated

Client teaching for self-care

Teach client about

- the medication regimen
- methods of attaining/maintaining bladder control
- prevention of urinary retention

- maintenance of optimal nutritional status
- prevention of infection
- determination of what effect the client's medical condition is having on his sexual functioning; include partner in developing understanding and discovering alternative, satisfying close relations with each other
- the need to avoid activities that aggravate or worsen pain

TESTICULAR CANCER

- Testicular cancer is the most common type of cancer in men aged 15–35 years.
- Ninety-five percent of the cases arise from the germinal cells of the testes.
- The remaining 5% cases are nongerminal tumors arising from epithelium (Leydig cell and Sertoli cell tumors)

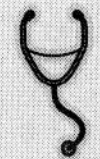

Assessment Alert

Risk of testicular cancer is higher in males with undescended testes.

Etiology: Cause unknown but infections, cryptorchidism, genetic, and endocrine factors appear to be involved.

S&S:

- Mass or lump on the testicle
- Painless enlargement of the testis (significant diagnostic finding)
- "Heaviness" of the scrotum, inguinal area, or lower abdomen
- Backache
- Lower abdominal pain
- Loss of weight
- General weakness

Dx:

- Painless enlargement of the testis
- Mass or lump on the testicle
- Tumor marker levels in the blood (alphafetoprotein [AFP] and the beta subunit of human chorionic gonadotropin [HCG])
- Intravenous urography
- Lymphangiography
- CAT scan of the chest, abdomen, and pelvis

Rx:

- Based on the cell type and the anatomic extent of the disease
- Orchiectomy
- Retroperitoneal lymph node dissection (RPLND)
- Postoperative irradiation of lymph nodes from the diaphragm to the iliac region
- Chemotherapy

Nursing Process Elements

- Encourage verbalization and fears/concerns related to body image and sexuality
- Provide postoperative care (see Chapter 18)

Client teaching for self-care

Teach client

- about sexuality and fertility pretreatment: normal function; potential effects of cancer and therapy; reproductive options including sperm banking:
  —low sperm count may be found at time of diagnosis and eliminate option of sperm banking
- that radiation therapy will not necessarily prevent having children
- that unilateral excision of a tumor does not necessarily decrease virility

WORKSHEET

MATCHING QUESTIONS

Match the following:

1. ______ Prostatitis   a. Result of injury and strain during childbirth

2. ______ Uterine prolapse   b. Removable mechanical device that holds the uterus in position

(continued)

3. ______	Rectocele	c. Isometric exercises that strengthen the pubococcygeal muscle
4. ______	Fibrocystic disease	d. Inability to voluntarily control the ejaculatory reflex once aroused
5. ______	Breast cancer	e. Blood test to detect prostate cancer and monitor effectiveness of therapy
6. ______	Testicular cancer	f. Most widely accepted term for benign changes in breast tissue
7. ______	Pessary	g. Descent of a portion of the posterior bladder wall into the vaginal canal
8. ______	Kegel	h. Most common cancer affecting women
9. ______	Cystocele	i. Descent of the cervix or entire uterus into the vaginal canal
10. ______	Premature ejaculation	j. Involuntary inhibition of the ejaculatory reflex
11. ______	Symptom of PID	k. Laboratory test elevated in a variety of liver and bone disorders
12. ______	Retrograde ejaculation	l. Inability to attain or maintain an erection
13. ______	PSA	m. Undescended testicles are a risk factor
14. ______	Impotence	n. STIs and excessive alcohol intake are risk factors
15. ______	Alkaline phosphatase	o. Pain on manipulation of the cervix

FILL IN THE BLANKS

Fill in the blank spaces with the correct word or phrase to complete each statement.

1. The most common type of gynecological cancer found in women is ____________ cancer.
2. ____________ cancer causes more deaths than any other cancer of the reproductive system.
3. A predisposing factor for epididymitis in males under 35 years of age is ____________ infection.
4. Intermittent cold packs and then later heat application to the scrotum may help relieve the pain of ____________.
5. Nursing care of the client with testicular cancer includes encouraging client to verbalize fears/concerns related to body image and ____________.
6. Noncancerous enlargement of the prostate gland is called ____________.
7. The most common causative organism of prostatitis is ____________.
8. The most common type of cancer found in males 15–35-years old is ____________.
9. Tumor specific antigens found in testicular cancer are ____________ and ____________.

TRUE & FALSE QUESTIONS

Mark each of the following statements True or False. Correct all false statements in the space provided.

1. Acute bacterial prostatitis may produce sudden fever, chills, and perineal, rectal, or low back pain. ____ T ____ F
2. Prostate cancer is the most commonly found cancer in men. ____ T ____ F
3. In prostate cancer, the PSA level in the blood is proportionately related to the total prostatic mass. ____ T ____ F
4. Bilateral upper, outer quadrant breast pain is symptomatic of fibrocystic breast disease. ____ T ____ F
5. All males with testicular cancer can bank sperm prior to treatment and thus preserve reproductive capacity. ____ T ____ F
6. Radiation therapy for testicular cancer results in infertility. ____ T ____ F
7. Unilateral orchiectomy does not necessarily decrease virility. ____ T ____ F
8. Prostate cancer, in the early stages of the disease, produces urinary symptoms such as frequency, urinary retention, and decreased size of the stream. ____ T ____ F
9. Breast lumps associated with fibrocystic disease feel fixed to the chest wall when palpated and regress in size after menses. ____ T ____ F
10. The synthetic androgen (Danazol) is used for severe pain associated with fibrocystic disease. ____ T ____ F
11. Kegel exercises strengthen the muscles of the pelvic floor. ____ T ____ F
12. A course of estrogen therapy may be prescribed for a postmenopausal woman with a uterine prolapse. ____ T ____ F
13. Surgery is the treatment of choice for symptomatic cystocele. ____ T ____ F
14. Ovarian cancer may be linked to mutations in the *BRCA 1* or *BCRA 2* gene. ____ T ____ F
15. "Heaviness" of the scrotum, inguinal area, or lower abdomen is a symptom of testicular cancer. ____ T ____ F
16. Prostaglandin E injected directly into the corpus cavernosum is used to treat impotence and can induce an erection for 30–60 minutes in some men. ____ T ____ F
17. Preventing overdistention of the bladder can be an important part of the management of symptoms related to benign prostatic hypertrophy. ____ T ____ F
18. Prostate cancer metastasizes to the bones of the pelvis before visceral organs such as the lungs. ____ T ____ F
19. Low-grade fever and scant purulent vaginal drainage are symptoms of PID. ____ T ____ F
20. Chlamydial infection predisposes to epididymitis. ____ T ____ F

APPLICATION QUESTIONS

1. The nurse is taking a history of a client who has had benign prostatic hyperplasia (BPH) in the past. To determine whether the client currently is experiencing difficulty, which symptom would the nurse ask the client about?
   a. Hematuria
   b. Urinary incontinence
   c. Urinary retention
   d. Decreased force in the stream of urine

2. A client with prostatitis following a kidney infection has received instructions on management of the condition at home and prevention of recurrence. Which statement by the client indicates that the instructions have been understood?
   a. "I need to keep fluid intake to a minimum to decrease the need to urinate."
   b. "I should exercise as much as possible to stimulate circulation."
   c. "I will take warm sitz baths and analgesics for comfort."
   d. "I can stop taking antibiotics when the pain subsides."

3. The nurse is assessing a client with epididymitis. The nurse anticipates which findings on physical examination?
   a. Fever, diarrhea, groin pain, and ecchymosis
   b. Fever, nausea, vomiting, and painful scrotal edema
   c. Nausea, vomiting, and scrotal edema with ecchymosis
   d. Diarrhea, groin pain, and scrotal edema

4. A client complains of fever, perineal pain, and urinary frequency, urgency, and dysuria. To assess whether the client's problem is related to bacterial prostatitis, the nurse would look at the results of the prostate examination, which should reveal that the prostate gland is
   a. tender and edematous with ecchymosis
   b. reddened, swollen, and boggy
   c. soft and swollen
   d. tender, indurated, and warm to the touch

5. Which information about pelvic inflammatory disease (PID) would the nurse appropriately include when teaching sexually active young adults?
   a. The single most obvious symptom of PID is severe pelvic pain.
   b. PID is an infection of the uterus and Fallopian tubes.
   c. Vaginal discharge is scant but with a foul odor.
   d. PID can result in infertility due to inflammation and scarring.

6. Which treatments are used in the management of PID? (Select all that apply.)
   a. Antibiotics
   b. Analgesics
   c. Bed rest
   d. IV fluids
   e. Douches
   f. Sitz baths
   g. Nasogastric intubation and suction

7. Which classes of drugs are used in the management of fibrocystic breast disease? (Select all that apply.)
   a. Anti-inflammatory agents
   b. Corticosteroids
   c. Synthetic androgens
   d. Oral contraceptives
   e. Vasoconstrictors

8. Which is the most appropriate advice for the nurse to give to help a client with vulvitis cope with severe itch?
   a. Soak in a warm tub
   b. Take cool sitz baths
   c. Wear cotton underwear
   d. Pour water over the perineum after urinating

9. Which information should be included in a teaching plan for a client with prostatitis?
   a. Massage prostate gland daily
   b. Limit alcohol intake
   c. Expect difficulty in initiating urination
   d. Restrict fluid intake to 1500 ml daily

10. Which symptom should the nurse interpret as requiring a check for endometrial cancer?
    a. Postmenopausal bleeding
    b. Persistent leukorrhea
    c. Painful sexual intercourse
    d. Intermittent amenorrhea

11. How should the nurse interpret the leakage of fecal matter from the vagina of a client with advanced cancer?
    a. Anal sphincter has been impaired
    b. Cancer has metastasized to the GI tract

c. Rectovaginal fistula has developed
d. Rectum is being compressed by the tumor mass

12. A woman attending a health fair tells the nurse that her breasts have always gotten very tender during the week before her period but that one breast has stayed sore for the last 2 months. Which is the most appropriate advice for the nurse to give?
 a. "Wear a good support bra to bed for a few nights and see if the pain is relieved."
 b. "Decrease the salt in your diet, the pain probably is due to fluid retention."
 c. "Try taking an OTC anti-inflammatory like ibuprofen for the pain."
 d. "You should see your health care provider and have the breast checked."

13. When teaching about cancer detection, which factors should the nurse identify as predisposing a woman to breast cancer? (Select all that apply.)
 a. Family history of breast cancer, particularly in first-degree maternal relatives (mother, sister, and/or maternal aunt)
 b. Positive tests for genetic mutations (*BRCA 1* and *BRCA* 2)
 c. Long menstrual cycles
 d. Early menarche, late menopause
 e. Dysmenorrheas
 f. Nulliparous or first pregnancy after the age of 30 years
 g. Multiple sexual partners
 h. Extended breast-feeding

14. Which assessment finding is characteristic of advanced ovarian cancer?
 a. Ascites
 b. Purpura
 c. Splenomegaly
 d. Hypoactive DTRs

15. Which are risk factors for endometrial cancer? (Select all that apply.)
 a. Anovulation
 b. Abnormal uterine bleeding
 c. History of atypical endometrial hyperplasia
 d. Multiparity
 e. Polycystic ovarian syndrome
 f. Obesity
 g. Diabetes

16. Which client with breast cancer is a candidate for treatment with Tamoxifen?
 a. A 32-year-old client with a lumpectomy for a small tumor and no sign of spread
 b. A 58-year-old client with negative estrogen receptor (ER) status
 c. A 41-year-old client with metastatic disease
 d. A 66-year-old client with estrogen sensitive disease

17. Following teaching about PID, which statement by a client indicates that clarification is needed?
 a. "Infertility and ectopic pregnancy are complications of PID."
 b. "A risk factor for PID is insertion of an intrauterine device (IUD)."
 c. "Untreated PID can lead to septicemia."
 d. "PID is most often due to fungal overgrowth."

18. When caring for a client with a uterine prolapse who is to have a pessary inserted, which information should the nurse make certain has been checked?
 a. Number of pregnancies
 b. Time since menopause
 c. Allergy to latex
 d. Use of douches

19. Which factors predispose to uterine prolapse or the development of a cystocele? (Select all that apply.)
 a. Child bearing
 b. Obesity
 c. Heavy occupational work
 d. Large pelvic cavity
 e. Bronchitis

20. Which instruction should the nurse include when instructing a client on the use of Flagyl?
 a. "Do not drink alcohol while taking medication."
 b. "Douche daily while taking the medication."
 c. "Discontinue other medications until course of Flagyl is complete."
 d. "Do not use a spermicide while on the medication."

21. Which is a sign of a trichomonas vaginal infection?
 a. Thick, white, cheesy discharge
 b. Relapsing, low-grade fever
 c. Vomiting without nausea
 d. Thin, bubbly, green-tinged malodorous discharge

(continued)

22. Which test confirms the diagnosis of prostate cancer?
    a. PSA
    b. Alkaline phosphatase
    c. Ultrasound of the prostate
    d. Prostate biopsy
23. Lupron is prescribed for a client with prostate cancer. Which assessment data best indicates that the medication is having the desired effect?
    a. Client reports pain is controlled
    b. Vomiting has stopped
    c. Urine is free of blood
    d. PSA level has dropped
24. Which condition can pain in young women with ovarian cancer mimic?
    a. Appendicitis
    b. Constipation
    c. PMS
    d. Urinary tract infection
25. Which finding on the physical examination of a 68-year-old, postmenopausal woman would cause suspicion of disease?
    a. Amenorrhea
    b. Sparse pubic hair
    c. Dry vaginal mucous membrane
    d. Palpable ovary

ANSWERS & RATIONALES

MATCHING ANSWERS

Match the following:

1. __n__ Prostatitis
2. __i__ Uterine prolapse
3. __a__ Rectocele
4. __f__ Fibrocystic disease
5. __h__ Breast cancer
6. __m__ Testicular cancer
7. __b__ Pessary
8. __c__ Kegel
9. __g__ Cystocele
10. __d__ Premature ejaculation
11. __o__ Symptom of PID
12. __j__ Retrograde ejaculation

a. Result of injury and strain during childbirth
b. Removable mechanical device that holds the uterus in position
c. Isometric exercises that strengthen the pubococcygeal muscle
d. Inability to voluntarily control the ejaculatory reflex once aroused
e. Blood test to detect prostate cancer and monitor effectiveness of therapy
f. Most widely accepted term for benign changes in breast tissue
g. Descent of a portion of the posterior bladder wall into the vaginal canal
h. Most common cancer affecting women
i. Descent of the cervix or entire uterus into the vaginal canal
j. Involuntary inhibition of the ejaculatory reflex
k. Laboratory test elevated in a variety of liver and bone disorders
l. Inability to attain or maintain an erection

13. __e__ PSA	m. Undescended testicles are a risk factor
14. __l__ Impotence	n. STIs and excessive alcohol intake are risk factors
15. __k__ Alkaline phosphatase	o. Pain on manipulation of the cervix

ANSWERS FOR FILL IN THE BLANKS

Fill in the blank spaces with the correct word or phrase to complete each statement.

1. The most common type of gynecological cancer found in women is endometrial cancer.
2. Ovarian cancer causes more deaths than any other cancer of the reproductive system.
3. A predisposing factor for epididymitis in males under 35 years of age is chlamydia infection.
4. Intermittent cold packs and then later heat application to the scrotum may help relieve the pain of epididymitis.
5. Nursing care of the client with testicular cancer includes encouraging client to verbalize fears/concerns related to body image and sexuality.
6. Noncancerous enlargement of the prostate gland is called benign prostsatic hypertrophy.
7. The most common causative organism of prostatitis is *E coli*.
8. The most common type of cancer found in males 15–35-years old is testicular.
9. Tumor specific antigens found in testicular cancer are alphafetoprotein (AFP) and beta subunit of human chorionic gonadotropin (HCG).

TRUE & FLASE ANSWERS

Mark each of the following statements True or False. Correct all false statements in the space provided.

1. Acute bacterial prostatitis may produce sudden fever, chills, and perineal, rectal, or low back pain. *True*
2. Prostate cancer is the most commonly found cancer in men. *True*
3. In prostate cancer, the PSA level in the blood is proportionately related to the total prostatic mass. *True*
4. Bilateral upper, outer quadrant breast pain is symptomatic of fibrocystic breast disease. *True*
5. All males with testicular cancer can bank sperm prior to treatment and thus preserve reproductive capacity. *False. Some men are not producing sperm or have low sperm counts at time of diagnosis and so are not candidates for sperm banking.*

(continued)

6. Radiation therapy for testicular cancer results in infertility. *False.*
   Infertility is not always a consequence of radiation therapy for testicular cancer.
7. Unilateral orchiectomy does not necessarily decrease virility. *True*
8. Prostate cancer, in the early stages of the disease, produces urinary symptoms such as frequency, urinary retention, and decreased size of the stream. *True*
9. Breast lumps associated with fibrocystic disease feel fixed to the chest wall when palpated and regress in size after menses. *False*
   Breast lumps associated with fibrocystic disease are freely movable and regress after menses.
10. The synthetic androgen (Danazol) is used for severe pain associated with fibrocystic disease. *True*
11. Kegel exercises strengthen the muscles of the pelvic floor. *True*
12. A course of estrogen therapy may be prescribed for a postmenopausal woman with a uterine prolapse. *True.*
13. Surgery is the treatment of choice for symptomatic cystocele. *False*
    Surgical repair (anterior repair) is done when other treatments have failed.
14. Ovarian cancer may be linked to mutations in the *BRCA 1* or *BCRA 2* gene. *True*
15. "Heaviness" of the scrotum, inguinal area, or lower abdomen is a symptom of testicular cancer. *False*
16. Prostaglandin E injected directly into the corpus cavernosum is used to treat impotence and can induce an erection for 30–60 minutes in some men *True*
17. Preventing overdistention of the bladder can be an important part of the management of symptoms related to benign prostatic hypertrophy. *True*
18. Prostate cancer metastasizes to the bones of the pelvis before visceral organs such as the lungs. *True*
19. Low-grade fever and scant purulent vaginal drainage are symptoms of PID. *False*
    Profuse, purulent vaginal drainage and low-grade fever are two of the many symptoms of PID.
20. Chlamydial infection predisposes to epididymitis. *True*

APPLICATION ANSWERS

1. The nurse is taking a history of a client who has had benign prostatic hyperplasia (BPH) in the past. To determine whether the client currently is experiencing difficulty, which symptom would the nurse ask the client about?
   a. Hematuria
   b. Urinary incontinence
   c. Urinary retention
   d. Decreased force in the stream of urine

Rationale

Correct answer: a.

Decreased force of the stream of urine is an early sign of BPH. The stream later becomes weak and dribbling. Hematuria is a common presenting sign of cancer of the prostate. Urinary incontinence is not generally a problem with BPH. Retention occurs later in the disease.

2. A client with prostatitis following a kidney infection has received instructions on management of the con-

dition at home and prevention of recurrence. Which statement by the client indicates that the instructions have been understood?

a. "I need to keep fluid intake to a minimum to decrease the need to urinate."
b. "I should exercise as much as possible to stimulate circulation."
c. "I will take warm sitz baths and analgesics for comfort."
d. "I can stop taking antibiotics when the pain subsides."

Rationale

Correct answer: c.

Treatment of prostatitis includes medication with antibiotics, analgesics, and stool softeners. The nurse also teaches the client to rest, increase fluid intake, and use sitz baths for comfort. Antibiotic therapy is always continued until the prescription is finished although symptoms may have resolved.

3. The nurse is assessing a client with epididymitis. The nurse anticipates which findings on physical examination?
   a. Fever, diarrhea, groin pain, and ecchymosis
   b. Fever, nausea, vomiting, and painful scrotal edema
   c. Nausea, vomiting, and scrotal edema with ecchymosis
   d. Diarrhea, groin pain, and scrotal edema

Rationale

Correct answer: b.

Typical signs and symptoms of epididymitis include scrotal pain and edema, which often are accompanied by fever, nausea, vomiting, and chills.

4. A client complains of fever, perineal pain, and urinary frequency, urgency, and dysuria. To assess whether the client's problem is related to bacterial prostatitis, the nurse would look at the results of the prostate examination, which should reveal that the prostate gland is
   a. tender and edematous with ecchymosis
   b. reddened, swollen, and boggy
   c. soft and swollen
   d. tender, indurated, and warm to the touch

Rationale

Correct answer: d.

The client with prostatitis has a prostate gland that is swollen and tender but that is also warm to the touch, firm, and indurated. Systemic symptoms include fever with chills, perineal and low back pain, and signs of UTI.

5. Which information about pelvic inflammatory disease (PID) would the nurse appropriately include when teaching sexually active young adults?
   a. The single most obvious symptom of PID is severe pelvic pain.
   b. PID is an infection of the uterus and Fallopian tubes.
   c. Vaginal discharge is scant but with a foul odor.
   d. PID can result in infertility due to inflammation and scarring.

Rationale

Correct answer: d.

PID can result in infertility due to inflammation and scarring. Severe pain is characteristic of PID but it is not the only obvious symptom—profuse vaginal drainage also occurs. PID affects the uterus and Fallopian tubes but can also involve the pelvic vasculature and peritoneum as well as the ovaries.

6. Which treatments are used in the management of PID? (Select all that apply.)
   a. Antibiotics
   b. Analgesics
   c. Bed rest
   d. IV fluids
   e. Douches
   f. Sitz baths
   g. Nasogastric intubation and suction

Rationale

Correct answers: a, b, c, d, and g.

Treatment of PID is intensive and involves all of these modalities. Douches, which can force bacteria and drainage upward, are not given. Sitz baths are used to ease external discomfort from conditions such as vulvitis, episiotomy, and hemorrhoids.

7. Which classes of drugs are used in the management of fibrocystic breast disease? (Select all that apply.)
   a. Anti-inflammatory agents
   b. Corticosteroids
   c. Synthetic androgens
   d. Oral contraceptives
   e. Vasoconstrictors

Rationale

Correct answers: a, c, and d.

Anti-inflammatory agents such as ibuprofen are used for pain. Synthetic androgens can be used to suppress ovarian function and estrogen stimulation of the breast tissue but because of undesirable side effects, use is reserved to unusually severe disease. Oral contraceptives are used to suppress oversecretion of estrogen. Vasoconstrictors and corticosteroids do not have a role in the management of fibrocystic breast disease.

(continued)

8. Which is the most appropriate advice for the nurse to give to help a client with vulvitis cope with severe itch?
   a. Soak in a warm tub
   b. Take cool sitz baths
   c. Wear cotton underwear
   d. Pour water over the perineum after urinating

Rationale

Correct answer: b.

Cooling helps relieve itch. Soaking in a warm tub can soothe inflammation. Wearing cotton underwear helps to prevent vaginitis. Pouring cold water over the perineum after urinating effectively removes irritating urine from the genital area but is not as effective at relieving vulva itch as sitting in cold water.

9. Which information should be included in a teaching plan for a client with prostatitis?
   a. Massage prostate gland daily
   b. Limit alcohol intake
   c. Expect difficulty in initiating urination
   d. Restrict fluid intake to 1500 ml daily

Rationale

Correct answer: b.

Alcohol intake should be limited because of its diuretic effect. An inflamed prostate should not be massaged. Difficulty in initiating urination is a symptom of BPH, not prostatitis. Fluids are not restricted. The man with prostatitis should drink at least 64–128 ounces of fluid per day.

10. Which symptom should the nurse interpret as requiring a check for endometrial cancer?
    a. Postmenopausal bleeding
    b. Persistent leukorrhea
    c. Painful sexual intercourse
    d. Intermittent amenorrhea

Rationale

Correct answer: a.

Postmenopausal bleeding is the primary symptom of endometrial cancer. Persistent leukorrhea occurs with a variety of vaginal and cervical infections. Painful intercourse (dyspareunia) occurs with uterine prolapse. Amenorrhea has a variety of causes. The most frequent is pregnancy but endocrine disturbances, poor diet, excessive exercise, emotional shock, change in climate, etc., are other causes.

11. How should the nurse interpret the leakage of fecal matter from the vagina of a client with advanced cancer?
    a. Anal sphincter has been impaired
    b. Cancer has metastasized to the GI tract
    c. Rectovaginal fistula has developed
    d. Rectum is being compressed by the tumor mass

Rationale

Correct answer: c.

Leakage of fecal matter from the vagina is a sign of rectovaginal fistula. It is not a sign of any of the conditions listed as other options.

12. A woman attending a health fair tells the nurse that her breasts have always gotten very tender during the week before her period but that one breast has stayed sore for the last two months. Which is the most appropriate advice for the nurse to give?
    a. "Wear a good support bra to bed for a few nights and see if the pain is relieved."
    b. "Decrease the salt in your diet, the pain probably is due to fluid retention."
    c. "Try taking an OTC anti-inflammatory like ibuprofen for the pain."
    d. "You should see your health care provider and have the breast checked."

Rationale

Correct answer: d.

Soreness of a breast from fibrocystic disease disappears after menstruation. When soreness persists after menses, assessment by a health care provider is needed to determine the cause. Breast soreness associated with fibrocystic disease can be treated with measures to decrease fluid retention and/or taking an OTC anti-inflammatory. A good support bra can also help but it does not need to be worn at night.

13. When teaching about cancer detection, which factors should the nurse identify as predisposing a woman to breast cancer? (Select all that apply.)
    a. Family history of breast cancer, particularly in first-degree maternal relatives (mother, sister, and/or maternal aunt)
    b. Positive tests for genetic mutations (*BRCA 1* and *BRCA 2*)
    c. Long menstrual cycles
    d. Early menarche, late menopause
    e. Dysmenorrheas
    f. Nulliparous or first pregnancy after the age of 30 years
    g. Multiple sexual partners
    h. Extended breast-feeding

Rationale

Correct answers: a, b, c, d, and f.

Family history of breast cancer, particularly in first-degree maternal relatives (mother, sister, and/or maternal aunt), positive test for mutated *BRCA 1* or *BRCA 2*, long menstrual cycles, early menarche, late menopause, and nulliparity or first pregnancy after the age of 30 years are all risk factors for breast cancer. Multiple sexual partners predisposes to cervical cancer. Breast-feeding appears to exert a protective influence against breast cancer if done for a sufficient length of time.

14. Which assessment finding is characteristic of advanced ovarian cancer?
    a. Ascites
    b. Purpura
    c. Splenomegaly
    d. Hypoactive DTRs

Rationale
Correct answer: a.
Ascites develops late in the course of ovarian cancer. Another sign of advanced ovarian cancer is pleural effusion, which is common with metastases to the lung. Purpura, splenomegaly, and hypoactive DTRs are not related symptoms.

15. Which are risk factors for endometrial cancer? (Select all that apply.)
    a. Anovulation
    b. Abnormal uterine bleeding
    c. History of atypical endometrial hyperplasia
    d. Multiparity
    e. Polycystic ovarian syndrome
    f. Obesity
    g. Diabetes

Rationale
Correct answers: a, b, c, e, f, and g.
Anovulation, abnormal uterine bleeding, a history of atypical endometrial hyperplasia, polycystic ovarian syndrome, obesity, and diabetes are all risk factors for endometrial cancer. Additional risk factors are nulliparity not multiparity, hypertension, and familial history of endometrial cancer.

16. Which client with breast cancer is a candidate for treatment with Tamoxifen?
    a. A 32-year-old client with a lumpectomy for a small tumor and no sign of spread
    b. A 58-year-old client with negative estrogen receptor (ER) status
    c. A 41-year-old client with metastatic disease
    d. A 66-year-old client with estrogen sensitive disease

Rationale
Correct answer: d.
Tamoxifen is adjuvant therapy for early stage ER—positive breast cancer. Tamoxifen is an estrogen antagonist that blocks the ER sites on the tumor cells thus blocking tumor growth. It decreases the risk of metastasis or prolongs survival once metastasis occurs.

17. Following teaching about PID, which statement by a client indicates that clarification is needed?
    a. "Infertility and ectopic pregnancy are complications of PID."
    b. "A risk factor for PID is insertion of an intrauterine device (IUD)."
    c. "Untreated PID can lead to septicemia."
    d. "PID is most often due to fungal overgrowth"

Rationale
Correct answer: d.
PID is most often bacterial in origin; it is not most often the result of fungal infection. Untreated PID can lead to septicemia. Infertility and ectopic pregnancy are complications of PID. Insertion of an IUD is a risk factor for PID. Other risk factors include abortion, pelvic surgery, infections during or after pregnancy, early age of first intercourse, multiple sexual partners, frequent intercourse, intercourse without condoms, sex with a partner with an STI, history of previous STI or previous pelvic infection, use of a biopsy curette or an irrigation catheter, and tubal insufflation.

18. When caring for a client with a uterine prolapse who is to have a pessary inserted, which information should the nurse make certain has been checked?
    a. Number of pregnancies
    b. Time since menopause
    c. Allergy to latex
    d. Use of douches

Rationale
Correct answer: c.
If the client is allergic to latex, a rubber pessary cannot be used. Number of pregnancies, time since menopause, and use of douches are not relevant to the insertion of a pessary.

19. Which factors predispose to uterine prolapse or the development of a cystocele? (Select all that apply.)
    a. Child bearing
    b. Obesity
    c. Heavy occupational work
    d. Large pelvic cavity
    e. Bronchitis

Rationale
Correct answers: a, b, c, and e.
Problems with pelvic support such as uterine prolapse and cystocele can be the result of a congenital defect, prolonged increased intra-abdominal pressure, or traumatic injury to supporting structures. Thus pregnancy and vaginal delivery, obesity, job requiring heavy labor, and chronic cough all predispose to weakened pelvic supports and the development of uterine prolapse and cystocele.

(continued)

20. Which instruction should the nurse include when instructing a client on the use of Flagyl?
    a. "Do not drink alcohol while taking medication."
    b. "Douche daily while taking the medication."
    c "Discontinue other medications until course of Flagyl is complete."
    d. "Do not use a spermicide while on the medication."

Rationale

Correct answer: a.

Alcohol should be avoided because metronidazole (Flagyl) and alcohol together can cause severe nausea, vomiting, cramps, flushing, and headache. Metronidazole also can increase the blood thinning effects of warfarin (Coumadin) and increase the risk of bleeding. All other options are unrelated to the use of Flagyl.

21. Which is a sign of a trichomonas vaginal infection?
    a. Thick, white, cheesy discharge
    b. Relapsing, low-grade fever
    c. Vomiting without nausea
    d. Thin, bubbly, green-tinged malodorous discharge

Rationale

Correct answer: d.

Trichomonas infection causes a thin, bubbly, green-tinged, malodorous vaginal discharge, irritation, itching, and urinary symptoms such as burning and/or frequency. Candida albicans infection causes a thick, white, cheesy discharge. Low-grade fever is a systemic manifestation of infection and is not seen with trichomonas vaginitis. Vomiting without nausea is seen in head injury.

22. Which test confirms the diagnosis of prostate cancer?
    a. PSA
    b. Alkaline phosphatase
    c. Ultrasound of the prostate
    d. Prostate biopsy

Rationale

Correct answer: d.

Diagnosis of cancer can only be confirmed by microscopic examination of tissue. PSA is used for screening for prostate cancer but elevated levels (over 4 ng/ml) can be due to a variety of factors including benign prostatic hypertrophy and prostatitis; they are not specific to prostate cancer. Ultrasound of the prostate is used for follow-up when PSA levels are suspicious but its effectiveness is controversial. Alkaline phosphatase is an enzyme whose serum levels are elevated in hepatobiliary and bone disease.

23. Lupron is prescribed for a client with prostate cancer. Which assessment data best indicates that the medication is having the desired effect?
    a. Client reports pain is controlled
    b. Vomiting has stopped
    c. Urine is free of blood
    d. PSA level has dropped

Rationale

Correct answer: d.

Lupron is a gonadotropin-releasing hormone agonist analog (GnRH), which suppresses pituitary release of LH and reduces serum testosterone levels. Since prostatic cancers require testosterone, reducing testosterone levels causes tumors to regress. Because the concentration of PSA in the blood is proportional to the total prostatic mass as the tumor regresses, PSA level drops. If a client has pain from metastases and these shrink in response to Lupron, pain can be relieved. However, this is not the best measure of Lupron's effectiveness since not all tumors are necessarily causing pain. Vomiting is not common with prostate cancer and hematuria is a late sign. Concentration of PSA in the blood is proportional to the total prostatic mass.

24. Which condition can pain in young women with ovarian cancer mimic?
    a. Appendicitis
    b. Constipation
    c. PMS
    d. Urinary tract infection

Rationale

Correct answer: a.

Ovarian cancer can present in young women with pain similar to that of appendicitis. If pain accompanies constipation it is usually crampy pain or a sense of rectal discomfort. Urinary tract infection causes burning on urination or suprapubic discomfort from the bladder.

25. Which finding on the physical examination of a 68-year-old, postmenopausal woman would cause suspicion of disease?
    a. Amenorrhea
    b. Sparse pubic hair
    c. Dry vaginal mucous membrane
    d. Palpable ovary

Rationale

Correct answer: d.

A palpable ovary in a postmenopausal woman raises suspicion of ovarian cancer. Normally ovaries are not palpable on pelvic examination after menopause. Amenorrhea is absence of menses so is normal postmenopause. Sparse pubic hair and dryness of the vaginal membranes are normal changes with advancing age.

Test Plan Category:

Physiological Integrity

Sub-category: Physiological Adaptation—Part 2

Topics: Fluid and Electrolyte Imbalances
Medical Emergencies

FLUID AND ELECTROLYTE IMBALANCES

BASIC CONCEPTS

Electrolytes are electrically charged ions.

- Cations are positively charged ions, e.g., sodium (Na^+), potassium (K^+), calcium (Ca^{2+}), and magnesium (Mg^{2+}).
- Anions are negatively charged ions, e.g., chloride (Cl^-), bicarbonate (HCO_3^-), phosphate (HPO_4^{2-}), and sulfate (SO_4^{2-}).

Fluid compartments

- Intracellular fluid is the fluid within the cells. The main electrolytes are potassium, magnesium, phosphate$^-$, and sulfate.

- Extracellular fluid is the fluid outside the cells. The main electrolytes in the ECF are sodium, chloride, and bicarbonate.
  —Intravascular fluid (plasma) is the fluid within the blood vessels. Protein-rich albumin is the main protein and is primarily responsible for creating the osmotic pull that holds fluid in the intravascular space.
  —Interstitial fluid contains no protein.
  —Lymph.
  —Transcellular fluid, e.g., synovial, cerebrospinal, intraocular, pericardial, pancreatic, biliary, peritoneal, and pleural.

Fluid balance—I&O:

- Fluid requirement per day for an average adult is 2500-ml intake.
- Average fluid loss per day is 2500 ml.
- Sources of fluid:
  —oral intake is 1200–1500 ml on average;
  —water in foods is 1000 ml;
  —by-product of metabolism water is 200 ml.
- Sources of fluid loss:
  —water loss through urine is 1400–1500 ml;
  —insensible water loss through skin and lungs (vapor in exhaled air) is 350–400 ml and 350–400 ml, respectively;
  —water loss through perspiration is 100 ml;
  —water loss through feces is 100–200 ml.

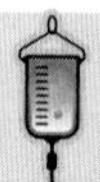

Clinical Alert

Obligatory water losses are essential to maintaining body function. For an adult, the obligatory water loss per day is 1300 ml which includes 500 ml of urine plus the insensible water loss plus water loss in feces).

FLUID IMBALANCES

- Isotonic imbalances occur when water and electrolytes are gained or lost in equal proportions and the osmolarity (concentration of solutes) remains the same.
- Osmolar imbalances occur when only water is gained or lost and the concentration of solutes is changed.

Isotonic Fluid Volume Deficit

- Equal proportions of water and electrolytes are lost from ECF.
- It is also called hypovolemia (decreased blood volume because loss first affects intravascular space).

Etiology: Abnormal loss through skin (fever, diaphoresis, or wound drainage), kidneys, or GI tract (diarrhea, vomiting, gastric suction), bleeding, insufficient intake (anorexia, nausea, dysphagia, inability to access from confusion or immobility), third-spacing shift of fluid into an area where it is sequestered (essentially unavailable), e.g., edema or fluid in bowel.

S&S: Thirst, weakness, weight loss, decreased skin turgor, dry mucous membranes, sunken eyeballs, dry eyes, low-grade fever, weak rapid pulse, drop in blood pressure, orthostatic hypotension, flat neck veins, decreased capillary refill, decreased central venous pressure, decreased urine volume (<30 ml/hr), increased urine specific gravity (>1.030), increased hematocrit, and BUN.

Rx: Isotonic fluid replacement such as lactated Ringer's solution.

Nursing Process Elements

- Monitor VS
- Monitor weight
- Monitor skin turgor
- I&O
- Administer oral and IV fluids as ordered
- Provide mouth care
- Prevent skin breakdown
- Monitor lab values

Isotonic Fluid Volume Excess

- Equal proportions of water and sodium are retained by the body.
- It is also called hypervolemia (increased blood volume).

Etiology: Excessive oral intake of sodium chloride (overuse of sodium-based antacids such as soda bicarbonate or Alka-Seltzer or overuse of hypertonic enemas such as Fleet), too rapid administration of sodium-containing infusions, CHF, renal failure, cirrhosis, and Cushing's syndrome.

S&S: Edema, weight gain, full bounding pulse, tachycardia, increased blood and central venous pressures, distended neck and peripheral veins, slow vein emptying, moist crackles in lungs, dyspnea, and mental confusion.

Rx: Diuretics.

Nursing Process Elements

- Monitor vital signs
- Take daily weight
- Assess for edema
- Measure I&O
- Monitor lab results
- Maintain Fowler's position
- Restrict fluid intake as ordered
- Restrict sodium intake

Dehydration

Hyperosmolar imbalance develops when water is lost from the body and an excess of sodium results.

Etiology: Decreased sensation of thirst, enteral feedings with insufficient water intake, hyperventilation, prolonged fever, diabetes insipidus, di betic ketoacidosis, and osmotic diuresis.

S&S: Dry sticky mucous membranes, flushed dry skin, thirst, fever, irritability, convulsions, and coma.

Rx: Hypotonic IV fluids such as 0.95 sodium chloride.

Nursing Process Elements

- Obtain daily weight
- Monitor I&O
- Monitor serum values
- Administer fluids as ordered

Overhydration

Hypo-osmolar imbalance develops due to the presence of excess water in the body, and low serum osmolality and low serum sodium result.

Etiology: Replacement of only water when loss of both water and electrolytes has occurred as with diaphoresis, SIADH, AIDS, and head injury.

S&S: Impaired neurological function as a result of cerebral edema—confusion, convulsions, and coma.

Rx: Restrict fluid to less than 1000 ml/d.

Nursing Process Elements

- Obtain daily weight
- Monitor I&O
- Monitor serum values
- Restrict fluids as ordered

ELECTROLYTE IMBALANCES

Sodium

- Sodium is the most abundant electrolyte found in ECF.
- Sodium controls water distribution and is the chief regulator of ECF volume; loss or gain of sodium means a loss or gain of water.
- Sodium maintains acid–base balance, transmission of nerve impulses, and osmotic pressure. Balance between dietary intake and renal secretion of sodium determines the sodium content of blood.
- Normal serum sodium is 135–145 mEq/l.

Hyponatremia (serum $Na^+ < 135$ mEq/l)

- Hyponatremia develops due to the presence of excess water in relationship to sodium. It develops when
  - —either there is too much water relative to the amount of sodium (too much water taken into body or not enough water excreted) or
  - —too little sodium relative to the amount of water (too much sodium lost from the body or not enough taken in).

Etiology:

- Loss of fluids high in chloride as in vomiting and diarrhea and gastric suctioning
- Use of medications such as diuretics, lithium, cisplatin, heparin, and NSAIDs
- Decreased aldosterone as in adrenal insufficiency (Addison's disease)
- Water intoxication as from administration of excess volume of D5W
- CHF with decreased cardiac output that leads to fluid retention
- Chronic renal failure

S&S: Lethargy, anorexia, N&V, and muscle cramps. Confusion, muscle twitching, convulsions, and coma occur with serum sodium less than 120 mEq/l.

Dx: Measurement of serum sodium.

Rx:

- Varies with degree of hyponatremia
- Replace sodium orally or intravenously
- Treat underlying cause

Nursing Process Elements

- Monitor I&O and VS
- Obtain daily weight
- Monitor for CNS changes indicative of acute hyponatremia
- Encourage foods high in sodium content
- Administer sodium as ordered
- Restrict fluids as ordered
- Monitor for CHF: crackles, edema, and neck vein distention

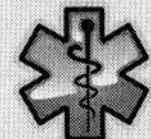

Nursing Intervention Alert

Administer IV hypertonic solutions such as 3% and 5% NaCl carefully; inappropriate administration can cause death.

Client teaching for self-care

- Identification of sources of sodium
- Increase intake of salty foods and fluids
- Hold medications that induce hyponatremia when blood is to be drawn for electrolytes

Hypernatremia (serum $Na^+ > 145$ mEq/l)

- Hypernatremia develops due to the presence of excess sodium in relationship to water. It develops when
  - —either there is too much sodium in relationship to water (too much sodium taken in or too little lost "sodium retention") or
  - —too little water in relationship to sodium (too little water taken in or too much lost—decreased total body water in relationship to sodium).
  - —Hypernatremia results in increased ECF volume.

Etiology:

- Insufficient fluid intake as a result of lack of awareness of thirst as in confusion or altered level of consciousness or inability to access fluids due to immobility.
- Dehydration
- Diabetes insipidus with its excessive water loss
- Lack of antidiuretic hormone
- Cushing's disease
- Potassium depletion
- Hypovolemia
- High-sodium diet
- Excessive administration of IV sodium solution
- Ingestion of large amounts of salt as in salt water drowning
- Use of medications such as methyldopa, oral contraceptives, corticosteroids, and hydrolazine

S&S: Thirst, low-grade fever, sticky mucous membranes, dry swollen tongue, tachycardia, and altered mental status.

Dx: Measurement of serum sodium.

Rx:

- Varies with degree of hypernatremia, hypotonic fluid, sodium restriction, and diuretic
- Treat underlying cause

Nursing Process Elements

- Monitor I&O and VS
- Obtain daily weight
- Assess intake of sodium: dietary (water from a water softener, frozen foods, canned soups, etc.) and in home/OTC remedies such as Alka-Seltzer and baking soda and water
- Assess for excessive thirst, changes in mucous membrane, and fever
- Monitor for changes in behavior
- Restrict sodium
- Administer hypotonic solutions such as D5W as ordered

Client teaching for self-care

- Identification of sources of sodium
- Need to avoid salty foods and fluids
- Hold medications that induce hypernatremia when blood for electrolytes is to be drawn

Chloride

- Chloride is the major extracellular anion found mostly in combination with sodium or hydrogen as NaCl and HCl. Along with sodium, chloride maintains osmolarity of body fluids and acid–base balance.
- Absorption of chloride is controlled indirectly by aldosterone.
- Normal serum chloride is 90–110 mEq/l.
- Hyperchloremia or hypochloremia usually occurs along with shifts in Na^+ or HCO_3^- levels.
- Hyperchloremia is seen with hyperkalemia and hypernatremia, stomach cancer, kidney dysfunction, Cushing's syndrome; medications as KCl, methyldopa, and cortisone preparations are used.
- Hypochloremia is seen with hypokalemia, hyponatremia, gastric suction, prolonged diarrhea, low-sodium diet, diabetic ketoacidosis, Addison's disease; medications as bicarbonate, aldosterone, and thiazide diuretics are used.

Potassium

- Potassium is the most abundant intracellular cation.
- Potassium affects acid–base balance and osmotic pressure.
- Potassium is responsible for electrical conduction in muscle cells.
- Concentration of potassium is dependent on sodium reabsorption, aldosterone (increases loss of) level, and acid–base balance.
- Source of potassium is dietary intake; potassium is excreted or retained by kidneys depending on cellular needs.
- Normal serum potassium is 3.5–5.0 mEq/l.
- Potassium concentration has a narrow range; minor changes in levels have significant effects.
- Serum potassium levels are monitored with health problems such as cardiac dysrhythmias, renal disease, and use of medications such as thiazide diuretics.

Hypokalemia (serum $K^+ < 3.5$ mEq/l)

Hypokalemia develops when there is too little potassium in the body.

- Body does not conserve potassium so intake needs to compensate for loss.

- Intake of potassium can be insufficient and/or loss can be excessive.
- Potassium is secreted by the distal tubule—if secretion is increased, loss can be excessive.
- Loss of potassium can also occur through other routes in the presence of disease, e.g., GI tract with diarrhea.
- Serum K^+ levels can be low due to shift of K^+ to the intracellular space.

Etiology:

- Loss from GI tract: diarrhea, persistent vomiting, ileostomy drainage, GI suction, and overuse of laxatives
- Liver disease
- Diabetic acidosis
- Increased adrenal corticosteroid secretion (Cushing's syndrome)
- Use of medications as thiazide diuretics, aspirin, prednisone, laxatives, and cisplatin
- Anorexia and malnutrition
- Alcoholism
- Dehydration
- Alkalosis

S&S: Muscle weakness, cramps, anorexia, N&V, cardiac dysrhythmias, increased sensitivity to digoxin, lethargy, confusion, and decreased DTRs.

Dx: Measurement of serum potassium.

Rx:

- Administer potassium: dose 40–60 mEq/d
- Treat underlying cause

Nursing Process Elements

- Encourage increase in dietary potassium
- Administer potassium supplements as ordered
- Always dilute potassium when administered intravenously to prevent tissue damage

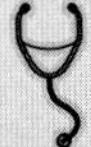

Assessment Alert

Hypokalemia can precipitate toxicity to digoxin. K^+ level should be greater than 3.5 mEq/l when taking digoxin.

Client teaching for self-care

- Eat foods rich in potassium when taking medications that are potassium depleting.

Hyperkalemia (serum $K^+ > 5.5$ mEq/l)

Hyperkalemia develops when there is too much potassium in the body due to inadequate excretion by the kidney or malfunctioning of the distal tubule or decreased renal blood flow with insufficient sodium to be exchanged for potassium or excessive intake or movement of potassium out of cells into ECF.

Etiology:

- Renal failure
- Medications such as tetracycline, antineoplastics, heparin, isoniazid, lithium, and potassium-conserving diuretics
- Acidosis
- Insulin deficiency
- Adrenal insufficiency (Addison's disease)
- High oral or IV intake
- Cell destruction: burns, trauma, and malnutrition

S&S: Weakness, paresthesias of face, tongue, feet and hands; flaccid muscle paralysis, hyperactive DTRs, nausea, confusion, ECG changes: tall, peaked t waves, wide QRS intervals, prolonged PR intervals, bradycardia, cardiac dysrhythmias, heart block, and cardiac arrest with K^+ greater than 7.0.

Dx: Measurement of serum K^+.

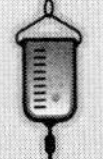

Clinical Alert

Incorrect handling of blood samples can result in hemolysis of blood cells with release of intracellular potassium thereby giving a false, high serum K^+ measurement.

Rx:

- Varies with degree of hyperkalemia
- Restrict K^+—no supplements, no transfusions of whole blood products
- IV sodium bicarbonate to alkalinate plasma causing a shift of K^+ into the cells
- Keyexalate (oral or rectal) to remove K^+
- Dialysis to remove K^+
- Treat underlying cause

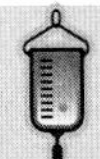

Clinical Alert

Emergency management of hypokalemic cardiac effects: IV calcium gluconate antagonizes effect of K^+ on the heart.

Nursing Process Elements

- Stop any infusions containing potassium and withhold potassium supplements
- Monitor for neuromuscular S&S
- Monitor cardiac function
- Restrict potassium intake: avoid administering potassium supplements, potassium-sparing diuretics, high-potassium foods, and use of salt substitutes all of which are high in potassium

Client teaching for self-care

- Identification of sources of potassium
- Need to restrict intake if level is more then 6 mEq/l

Calcium

- Calcium is the cation primarily concentrated in the skeletal system.
- Concentration of calcium in the body is indirectly controlled by parathormone from the parathyroid gland.
- Calcium is excreted in urine, feces, and sweat.
- Normal serum calcium is 8.5–10 mg/dl.
- Controls transmission of nerve impulses and contraction of all types of muscle; maintains cellular permeability, and is essential for blood coagulation and formulation of teeth and bones.

Hypocalcemia (serum $Ca^{2+} < 8.5$ mg/dl)

Hypocalcemia develops when there is too little calcium in the body. It develops due to inadequate intake or inhibition of absorption from GI tract or excessive loss through GI tract or increased renal excretion.

Etiology:

- Lactose intolerance
- Malabsorption syndrome
- Vitamin D deficiency
- Acute pancreatitis
- Diarrhea
- Ileostomy drainage
- Intestinal suction
- Renal failure
- Removal or destruction of the parathyroid glands
- Medications such as corticosteroids, cisplatin, caffeine, and loop diuretics

S&S:

- Numbness and tingling of fingers and toes
- Hyperactive DTRs
- Positive Trousseau sign—BP cuff inflated on upper arm above systolic pressure for 2 minutes; if carpal spasm occurs, sign is positive.
- Positive Chvostek sign—facial nerve is tapped about 3 cm in front of ear lobe; if unilateral contraction of facial and eyelid muscles occurs, sign is positive.
- Carpo-pedal spasm
- Confusion
- Tetany

Dx: Measurement of serum calcium.

Rx: Medical IV calcium gluconate or calcium chloride for acute symptomatic hypocalcemic emergency.

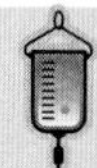

Clinical Alert

Too rapid infusion of IV calcium gluconate or calcium chloride can cause digitalis toxicity and cardiac arrest.

Nursing Process Elements

- Seizure precautions for severe hypocalcemia
- Safety precautions if confused
- Monitor airway because laryngeal stridor can occur

Client teaching for self-care

- Need for high-calcium diet—1000–1500 mg/d
- Dietary sources of calcium: milk and milk products, grains, cereals, fruits, nuts, and greens
- Calcium supplements
- Avoid cigarette smoking since even moderate smoking can increase urinary excretion of Ca^{2+}

Hypercalcemia (serum $Ca^{2+} > 10$ mg/dl; severe >1 mg/dl)

Hypercalcemia develops when there is too much calcium in the body. It occurs due to increased mobilization from bone or increased intake or increased intestinal reabsorption related to excess vitamin D or decreased renal excretion.

Etiology:

- Hyperparathyroidism
- Bone metastases from solid cancers (breast, prostate, lung, head, neck, melanoma), lymphoma, leukemia, and myeloma
- Prolonged immobilization
- Excessive oral intake of calcium supplements
- Excessive intake of vitamin D supplements
- Renal failure
- Use of thiazide diuretics

S&S:

- Muscular weakness
- Tiredness

- Anorexia
- N&V
- Constipation
- Decreased memory span and confusion
- Polyuria
- Polydipsia
- Renal calculi (stones)
- ECG change: shortened QT interval
- Cardiac arrest at >18 mg/dl

Dx: Measurement of serum calcium

Rx:

- Lasix to increase calcium excretion
- IV fluid of 0.45% NS or 0.9% NaCl to dilute serum calcium and promote renal excretion
- Oral, NGT, or IV inorganic phosphate salts: phosphosoda or neutrophos
- Calcitonin for clients with heart or renal damage who cannot manage a large sodium load
- Treat underlying cause

Nursing Process Elements

- Monitor cardiac function
- Assess for signs of toxicity if client is on digoxin
- Administer medications and fluids as ordered and assess for effect on symptoms
- Increase mobilization if possible
- Maintain good fluid intake to decrease risk of renal calculi
- Discourage ingestion of dairy products and other foods high in calcium
- Withhold calcium supplements

Phosphorous

- Phosphorus is essential for function of muscles, nerves, RBCs, and the metabolism of carbohydrates, proteins, and fats.
- Normal serum phosphorus is 2.5–4.5 mg/dl.

Hypophosphatemia (serum level <2.5 mg/dl)

Hypophosphatemia occurs as a result of increased cellular uptake with hyperventilation or poor absorption from the GI tract or excess renal loss.

Etiology:

- Malnutrition or starvation
- Alcohol withdrawal
- Diabetic ketoacidosis
- Recovery phase of severe burns
- Overuse of laxatives
- Hyperalimentation

S&S:

- Memory loss
- Muscle weakness
- Muscle pain and tenderness
- Confusion
- Apprehension
- CHF

Dx: Measurement of serum phosphorus.

Rx: IV phosphorous for serum levels <1 mg/dl; oral otherwise.

Nursing Process Elements

- Monitor for infection because of effect on WBCs
- Begin hyperalimentation slowly in malnourished clients to decrease the risk of a rapid shift of phosphate into the cells
- Encourage intake of phosphorous rich foods: beef, pork, beans, and other legumes
- Stop antacids and calcium supplements

Hyperphosphatemia (serum level >4.5 mg/dl)

Hyperphosphatemia develops when there is too much phosphorous in the body. It occurs due to impaired renal excretion or decreased glomerular filtration rate.

Etiology:

- Renal failure
- Chemotherapy
- Large intake of milk
- Overuse of phosphate-containing cathartics
- Large vitamin D intake
- Overuse of Fleet enemas

S&S:

Same as for hypocalcemia because the problems result from the hypocalcemia associated with hyperphosphatemia.

Dx: Measurement of serum phosphorus.

Rx:

- Treatment of the underlying hypocalcemia
- Low-phosphate diet
- Phosphate-binding gels and dialysis for renal failure

Nursing Process Elements

- Same as for hypocalcemia

Client teaching for self-care

- Low-phosphate diet

Magnesium (normal serum magnesium is 1.6–2.5 mEq/l)

- Magnesium is essential to neuromuscular function.
- Concentration of magnesium in the body is regulated by parathormone which increases or decreases reabsorption of magnesium from the renal tubules.
- Magnesium is absorbed from GI tract.
- If Mg^{2+} level is low, the kidney excretes more K^+.

Hypomagnesemia (serum level <1.6 mEq/l)

Hypomagnesemia develops when there is too little magnesium in the body. It occurs as a result of decreased reabsorption from the GI tract or increased excretion from the kidneys.

Etiology:

- Malnutrition or starvation
- Prolonged gastric suction
- Diarrhea
- Alcoholism
- Alcohol withdrawal
- Drugs such as diuretics, aminoglycosides, cisplatin, excessive doses of vitamin D, and calcium
- Pancreatitis
- Hyperparathyroidism

S&S:

- Neuromuscular irritability: difficulty swallowing, tremors, seizures, positive Chvostek, and Trousseau signs
- CNS changes: mood change and disorientation
- Tachycardia

Dx: Measurement of serum magnesium.

Rx: IV magnesium sulfate or oral magnesium.

Nursing Process Elements

- Assess for symptoms
- Aspiration precautions if difficulty swallowing
- Monitor clients on digoxin for signs of toxicity

Client teaching for self-care

- Dietary sources of magnesium: green vegetables, nuts, legumes, bananas, and oranges

Hypermagnesemia (serum level >2.5 mEq/l)

Hypermagnesemia develops when there is too much magnesium in the body. It occurs due to decreased excretion or excessive intake of magnesium.

Etiology:

- Renal failure
- Excessive use of antacids with a high concentration of magnesium
- Untreated diabetic ketoacidosis

S&S:

- Flushing and sense of skin warmth
- Hypotension
- ECG changes: prolonged PR interval and widened QRS
- Bradycardia
- Altered consciousness: drowsiness and lethargy progressing to coma
- Diminished or absent DTRs
- Depressed respirations

Dx: Measurement of serum magnesium

Rx:

- Hemodialysis with Mg^{2+} free dialysate results in safe serum levels in hours
- IV administration of calcium
- Magnesium-free IV fluids with a diuretic
- Ventilatory support for respiratory depression

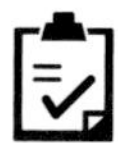

Nursing Process Elements

- Monitor VS for drop in blood pressure, bradycardia, and slow, shallow respirations
- Monitor change in consciousness

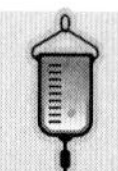

Clinical Alert

Tumor lysis syndrome is an oncologic emergency characterized by hyperphosphatemia, hyperkalemia, hyperuricemia, and hypocalcemia. It is seen with some rapidly growing cancers such as leukemias and lymphomas and following chemotherapy-induced rapid tumor cell destruction. Symptoms include oliguria, azotemia, lethargy, N&V with the release of intracellular contents.

ACID–BASE IMBALANCE

Basic Concepts

- The most important acids and bases in body are
  - —acids such as carbonic acid (H_2CO_3) which dissolves in plasma into carbon dioxide (pCO_2) and water and
  - —bases such as bicarbonate (HCO_3^-).
- Normal acid–base balance is 1 part acid to 20 parts base.
- pH is the concentration of hydrogen ions—a measure of the acidity or alkalinity of a fluid.
  - —Range of pH: The lower the pH, the greater the number of hydrogen ions and the more acidic the fluid; the higher the pH, the fewer the number of hydrogen ions and the more alkaline the fluid.

- Acidosis is a condition in which pH < 7.40.
  - —Respiratory acidosis develops when retention of the volatile gas CO_2 takes place due to inability to blow it off through the lungs.
  - —Metabolic acidosis develops when retention of nonvolatile acids or loss of base takes place.
- Alkalosis is a condition in which pH > 7.40.
  - —Respiratory alkalosis develops when there is an excessive loss of CO_2.
  - —Metabolic alkalosis-develops when retention of nonvolatile bases or loss of nonvolatile acids takes place.
- Regulation of acid–base balance takes place through
  - —chemical buffers: these instantaneously combine with acids or bases in cells and ECF to maintain pH at 7.40. The most important buffer is bicarbonate that accepts a hydrogen ion forming carbonic acid which then becomes CO_2 and H_2O with the CO_2 able to be blown off through the lungs.
  - —respiratory system: it regulates CO_2 in the ECF by changing rate and depth of respiration and therefore the amount of CO_2 blown off. This takes minutes to hours to have effect.
  - —kidneys: these control amount of sodium bicarbonate in the ECF by combining bicarbonate or hydrogen with other substances and excreting them in the urine. This takes hours to days to have effect.
- Measures of acid–base balance: arterial blood gases (see Chapters 16 and 21), serum electrolytes.

Respiratory acidosis

Respiratory acidosis develops due to decreased alveolar ventilation with resulting carbon dioxide retention. Compensatory effects: Kidney retains HCO_3^-, increases elimination of acid, and increased production of ammonia.

Etiology:

- Pulmonary disease: ARDS, pneumonia, flail chest, pneumothorax, smoke inhalation, massive pulmonary embolism, pulmonary edema, COPD, cystic fibrosis, and kyphoscoliosis
- Neuromuscular problems: drugs, toxins, Guillain-Barre syndrome, high spinal cord injury
- Airway obstruction: aspiration, laryngospasm
- CNS depression: sedative overdose, anesthesia, cerebral trauma, brain tumor, polio, multiple sclerosis, ALS, and muscular dystrophy
- Other: cardiac arrest, inadequate tidal volume, or respiratory rate on ventilator

S&S: Dyspnea, tachypnea, restlessness, confusion, diaphoresis, anxiety, headache, tachycardia progressing to lethargy, ventricular dysrhythmia, dilated facial and conjunctival blood vessels, cyanosis, and coma.

Rx: Suction and chest PT to clear airway; intubation and mechanical ventilation for $PaCO_2$ >50–60 mm Hg; low-flow oxygen.

Nursing Process Elements

- Monitor respiratory status: rate, depth, rhythm, and effort
- Encourage coughing or suction to clear airway
- Maintain semi-Fowler's position to promote chest expansion unless contraindicated; sidelying position for mechanically ventilated clients

Respiratory alkalosis

Carbon dioxide is lost as a result of increased alveolar ventilation.

Etiology:

- Stimulation of the respiratory center: anxiety, fever, pain, salicylates, hyperventilation, intracerebral trauma, gram-negative sepsis, pregnancy, and hepatic insufficiency
- Hypoxemia: high altitude, hypotension, severe anemia, and CHF
- Pulmonary disease: pneumonia, pulmonary emboli, inhalation of irritants, and interstitial fibrosis
- Excessive TV or respiratory rate on a ventilator

S&S: Increased rate and depth of respiration, anxiety, lightheadedness, paresthesias, circumoral numbness progressing to confusion, cardiac dysrhythmias, tetany, syncope, and seizures.

Rx: Treat underlying cause.

Nursing Process Elements

- Institute measures to relieve pain or anxiety
- Encourage normal breathing by coaching
- Have client breathe into a paper bag
- Monitor for cardiac dysrhythmias

Metabolic acidosis

Etiology:

- Loss of bicarbonate: diarrhea, ileostomy drainage, biliary and pancreatic drainage, renal tubular disease, and acetazolamide
- Excess production of acid: ketoacidosis, diabetes, alcohol-induced starvation, lactic acidosis, and rhabdomyolysis
- Excess acid ingestion: salicylates, cocaine, ecstasy, and methamphetamine
- Renal inability to excrete hydrogen ions: renal failure, renal tubular type 1 acidosis, hyperaldosteronism, and potassium-sparing diuretics

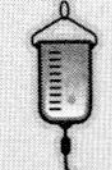

Clinical Alert

Chronic renal failure is the most common cause of chronic metabolic acidosis.

S&S: Increased rate and depth of respiration, fatigue/lethargy, hypotension, tachypnea, cold clammy skin, N&V, diarrhea, confusion, fruity breath odor progressing to Kussmaul's respirations, dry warm flushed skin, dysrhythmias, stupor, and coma.

Rx:

- Treat underlying disorder and correct fluid and electrolyte imbalances; dialysis when renal failure is the cause
- For severe acidosis, IV sodium bicarbonate may be cautiously given especially to clients with CHF or pulmonary edema

Nursing Process Elements

- Monitor for cardiac dysrhythmias
- Check for pulse deficit that indicates weak contractions or cardiac failure
- Monitor ABGs and electrolytes to evaluate treatment

Metabolic alkalosis

Etiology:

- Loss of hydrogen ions: vomiting, nasogastric suctioning, thiazide diuretics, excess mineralocorticoid, hypercalcemia, and hypoparathyroidism
- Hydrogen ion intracellular shift: hypokalemia, refeeding after starvation
- Bicarbonate retention: bicarbonate ingestion or infusion and massive blood transfusion

S&S: Decreased rate and depth of respirations, irritability, restlessness, muscle weakness, hyporeflexia, polyuria/polydipsia, dysrhythmias progressing to tetany, apathy, confusion, convulsions, and stupor.

Rx:

- Correct underlying disease.
- Hypokalemia is usual and is corrected with oral or IV potassium, isotonic saline IV to correct volume deficiencies when cause is diuretics or loss of gastric secretions

Nursing Process Elements

- Monitor for dysrhythmias
- Check for pulse deficits
- Monitor lab data especially pH, serum bicarbonate, and serum potassium
- Weigh daily
- Record I&O including stomach contents removed by suction
- Use isotonic saline to irrigate nasogastric tubes to prevent removal of electrolytes
- Notify physician if serum potassium drops to <3.5 mEq/l

MEDICAL EMERGENCIES

GENERAL PRINCIPLES OF EMERGENCY CARE—REFERS TO CARE GIVEN TO CLIENTS WITH URGENT AND CRITICAL NEEDS

Goal: Preserve life and prevent deterioration before more definitive treatment can be given.

Principles of Assessment and Emergency Management

- Treat the potentially life-threatening problems
- Stabilize the pulmonary cardiovascular and central nervous systems
- Maintain a patent airway and provide adequate ventilation, employing resuscitation measures when necessary
- Assess for chest injuries with subsequent airway obstruction
- Control hemorrhage and its consequences
- Evaluate and restore cardiac output
- Prevent and treat shock; maintain or restore effective circulation
- Perform a rapid initial physical assessment and reassess frequently
- Perform a Glasgow Coma Scale; evaluate best motor, verbal, and pupil response
- Monitor with ECG if appropriate
- Splint suspected fractures; and stabilize c-spine
- Protect wounds with sterile dressings
- Check to see if client has medic-alert identification
- Assess VS frequently
- Provide IV access with large-bore needles

Obtaining Assessment Data

- Obtain a brief history of the accident/illness from the client or accompanying person; include the following questions:
  —What were the circumstances, precipitating events, location, and time of injury/illness?
  —When did symptoms appear?
  — Was the client unconscious after the injury?

— How did the client get to the hospital?
—What was the health status before the client reached the hospital?
— Is there a past history of illness or past admissions?
— Is the client currently taking medications?
— Are there any drug or food allergies?
— Does the client have bleeding tendencies?
—Is the client under a physician's care
—Name of the physician.
— What time was the last meal eaten?
— What is the date of the last tetanus immunization?

Recording of Data

Consent to examine and treat the client is part of the emergency department record. The client must consent to invasive procedures. If the client is unconscious and brought to the emergency department without family or friends, this fact should be documented. Monitoring of the client's conditions and all instituted treatment modalities must be documented. After treatment, a notation is made on the record about the client's condition on discharge or transfer and instructions given to the patient and family for follow-up care.

Psychological Management of Clients and Families in Emergencies

- Understand and accept anxieties
- Keep family members informed
- Provide honest and realistic outcomes
- Help family members cope with impending death or death
- Offer spiritual counseling
- Provide privacy
- Allow immediate family to visit per hospital protocol

CARDIAC ARREST

- Heart ceases to produce an effective pulse and blood circulation.
- Cardiac arrest may follow respiratory arrest.

Etiology:

- Cardiac electrical event: heart rate too fast (especially ventricular tachycardia or ventricular fibrillation), too slow (bradycardia or AV block), or absent (asystole)
- Ventricular fibrillation is the major cause with precipitating factors such as
  —myocardial infarction (MI),
  —congenital heart disease,
  —heart failure,
  —anesthetics and antiarrhythmic drug overdose,
  —electrical shock,
  —electrolyte imbalances,
  —near drowning,
  —hypothermia,
  —ventricular irritation due to cardiac pacing during cardiac catheterization or angiography,
  —acute hemorrhage,
  —hypoxia or acidosis, and
  —myocarditis.
- Precipitating causes of asystole are
  —drug overdose,
  —hemorrhage,
  —anaphylaxis,
  —respiratory acidosis or hypercapnia,
  —left ventricular heart failure, and
  —electromechanical dissociation associated with severe MI, heart wall rupture, and cardiac tamponade.

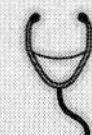

Assessment Alert

Emergency treatment such as CPR must restore circulation within approximately 4 minutes after the onset of cardiac arrest to prevent irreversible brain damage.

S&S:

- Clinical manifestations of cardiac arrest include
  —immediate loss of consciousness,
  —absence of pulses,
  —apnea or gasping respirations, and
  —Ashen-gray skin.

Dx:

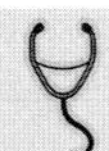

Assessment Alert

Absence of carotid pulses is the most reliable sign.

Nursing Process Elements

- Assess ABCs (airway, breathing, circulation)
- Begin resuscitation measures immediately to prevent irreversible brain damage
- Call for assistance
- Establish a patent airway
- Provide artificial ventilation by mouth-to-mouth resuscitation or with an Ambu bag
- Give oxygen as soon as possible

- Provide artificial circulation through external cardiac compression
- Defibrillate using direct-current countershock for ventricular fibrillation or tachycardia
- Establish a patent IV line if not already in place
- Administer emergency drugs as ordered
- Provide emotional support to family members or significant others

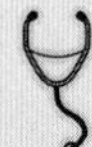

Assessment Alert

Cardiac arrest may occur when electrical activity is present but there is an ineffective cardiac contraction or circulating volume (pulseless electrical activity [PEA]).

Client teaching for self-care

- Teach family members or significant others
  —Steps of CPR
  —Basic pathophysiology of the underlying disease process

RESPIRATORY ARREST

Etiology:

- Airway obstruction, decreased respiratory drive, or respiratory muscle weakness
- Upper airway obstruction: posterior tongue displacement into the oropharynx secondary to a loss of muscular tone in unconscious clients (most common), blood, mucus, vomitus, or foreign body, spasm or edema of the vocal cords, pharyngolaryngeal inflammation, neoplasm, or trauma
- Lower airway obstruction: aspiration of gastric contents, widespread severe bronchospasm, extensive airspace-filling processes (e.g., pneumonia, pulmonary edema, pulmonary hemorrhage)
- Airway obstruction may be partial or complete.

S&S:

- Absence of spontaneous ventilation, cyanosis; if respiratory arrest is prolonged, cardiac arrest quickly ensues as a result of the effect of hypoxemia on cardiac function.
- Impending respiratory arrest: depressed sensorium and feeble, gasping, or irregular respirations, often with tachycardia, diaphoresis, and relative hypertension due to agitation and CO_2 accumulation

Rx:

- Establish patent airway
- Give two rescue breaths (insufflations—mechanical forcing of air into the respiratory system).
- Give artificial respiration if spontaneous respiration is not resumed after rescue breaths.
  —Do only when heart is still beathing
  —Do only for respiratory arrest; not if client is weakly breathing
  —Use a barrier device (even a cotton handkerchief) to protect against exposure to bodily fluids such as blood or vomit.
  —Start by giving two insufflations. These can help a nearly breathing client recover spontaneous respiration.
  —Tilt back the head of the client to extend his airways; the head will remain in this position on itself, you do not have to maintain it so.
  —Open the jaw of the client by pulling on his chin. In some cases (like some cases of epilepsy), the muscles of the clients are so contracted that it is impossible to open the mouth. Contrary to urban legend, the client will not "swallow" tongue. In this situation, it may not be possible to blow into the mouth. Instead, seal the lips together and breathe into the nose while keeping the head tilted back.
  —Close the nose of the client with your free hand.
  —Take a deep breath, put your mouth on the mouth of the client in an airtight manner, and blow into the mouth of the client. These breaths should be gentle and last no longer than 2 seconds to prevent air from entering the stomach.
  —When you have given two insufflations, check the carotid pulse of the client, while keeping an eye on his respiration. Chances are that
  —the client might have recovered spontaneous respiration thanks to "your insufflations" or
  —the client might be in a state of cardio-respiratory arrest.

If the client has recovered spontaneous respiration, put him in *recovery position*, cover him, and monitor his respiration on a regular basis until a mobile medical unit arrives.

If the client is in a state of cardio-respiratory arrest, you will have to perform cardiopulmonary resuscitation (CPR).

- Use a 100% mask (airtight mask) and an air balloon. Ventilate the client with pure oxygen. A client whose lungs are full of pure oxygen can stay in *apnea* for nearly 30 minutes (half an hour).
- Intubate
- ABGs

Nursing Process Elements

- Verify tube placement
- Assess respiratory status
- Monitor cardiac status

SHOCK

- A life-threatening condition which is characterized by inadequate blood flow to the tissues and cells of the body to meet metabolic needs.
- A cellular hypofunction state exists when the body consumes its oxygen more rapidly, and compensatory mechanisms are initiated to meet the increased demands of the body and restore oxygen and perfusion to cells.
- Compensatory mechanisms are the same regardless of the type of shock.
- Shock affects all body systems.
- Cellular hypoperfusion states include hypovolemia, cardiogenic shock, anaphylaxis, neurogenic shock, and septic shock.

Hypovolemic Shock

Etiology: Decreased intravascular volume.

Predisposing factors:

Absolute hypovolemia

- Loss of whole blood (e.g., hemorrhage from trauma, surgery, GI bleeding.)
- Loss of plasma (e.g., burn injuries)
- Loss of body fluids (e.g., vomiting, diarrhea, excessive diuresis, diaphoresis, diabetes insipidus, diabetes mellitus)

Relative hypovolemia

- Pooling of blood or fluids (e.g., ascites, peritonitis, bowel obstruction)
- Internal bleeding (e.g., fracture of long bones, ruptured spleen, hemothorax, severe pancreatitis)
- Massive vasodilation (e.g., sepsis)

S&S:

- Vary with the amount and rate of loss and effectiveness of compensatory mechanisms
- Altered mentation, ranging from lethargy to unresponsiveness
- Rapid, deep respirations that gradually become labored and shallower as the client's condition deteriorates.
- Cool, clammy skin
- Weak and thready pulses
- Tachycardia due to activation of the sympathetic nervous system
- Decreased urine output; urine is dark and concentrated because kidneys are conserving fluid.

Dx:

- Determination of serum lactate
- Arterial pH
- Base deficit to assess the presence of anaerobic metabolism
- Hemoglobin and hematocrit
- Serum potassium

Rx:

- Optimize oxygenation
- Correct the underlying cause of fluid loss as quickly as possible (e.g., bleeding, GI loss)
- Restore intravascular volume to reverse the sequence of events leading to inadequate tissue perfusion
- Administer warmed fluids, blood/blood products, crystalloids, colloids rapidly using two large-bore (14–16 gauge) peripheral IVs
- Goals of resuscitation:
  —CVP 15 mm Hg
  —PAWP 10–12 mm Hg
  —Cl >3 L/min/m^2
  —Blood lactate <4 mmol/l
  —Base deficit −3 to +3 mmol/l

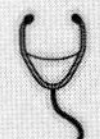

Clinical Alert

Military antishock trousers (MAST) are a garment designed to correct internal bleeding and hypovolemia by the application of counterpressure around the legs and abdomen creating artificial peripheral resistance and helping sustain coronary perfusion.

Nursing Process Elements

- Administer ordered fluids
- Maintain adequate IV access with large-bore needle/catheter
- Assess pulmonary and renal status
- Observe for fluid overload
- Monitor I&O
- Weigh daily

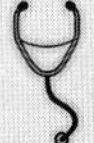

Assessment Alert

Position the client who shows signs of shock with the lower extremities elevated approximately 20 degrees; knees straight, trunk horizontal, and head slightly elevated.

Cardiogenic Shock

Etiology: Loss of ventricular contractile force, which results in decreased stroke volume and decreased cardiac output.

Precipitating factors:

- Systolic dysfunction: inability of the heart to pump blood forward (e.g., MI, cardiomyopathy).

- Diastolic dysfunction: inability of the heart to fill during diastole (e.g., cardiac tamponade).
- Arrhythmias (e.g., bradycardia, tachycardia).
- Structural factors: valvular abnormality (e.g., stenosis or regurgitation), papillary muscle dysfunction, and acute ventricular septal defect.

S&S: Change in mental status, weak, thready pulse of >100 bpm, diminished S1 and S2 heart sounds, pale cool skin, concentrated urine progressively decreasing in amount until <30 ml/hr, tachypnea with auscultory crackles and wheezes, elevated BUN, and serum creatinine.

Hemodynamic Findings

- Systolic blood pressure <90 mm Hg with increased diastolic pressure resulting in a narrowed pulse pressure
- Mean arterial pressure <70 mm Hg
- Cardiac index <2.2 $l/min/m^2$
- Pulmonary artery wedge pressure >18 mm Hg

Noninvasive Findings

- Thready, rapid pulse
- Narrow pulse pressure
- Distended neck veins
- Arrhythmias
- Chest Pain (recurrent chest pain suggests extension of infarct)
- Cool, pale, moist skin
- Oliguria
- Decreased mentation

Pulmonary Findings

- Dyspnea
- Increased respiratory rate
- Inspiratory crackles, possible wheezing
- Arterial blood gases show decrease in PaO_2

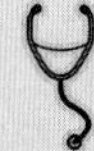

Assessment Alert

The cumulative amount of infarcted muscle is directly related to the risk of developing shock.

Dx:

- Left ventricular damage
- Decreased cardiac output
- Dysrhythmias
- Increased left ventricular end-diastolic pressure (LVEDP)
- Decreased arterial blood pressure

Rx:

- Improve O_2 status by decreasing demand
- Reestablish blood flow with thrombolytics, angioplasty, and emergency revascularization to reestablish blood flow
- Increase O_2 supply by providing supplemental O_2
- Vasoactive drug therapy to increase cardiac output
  - —Dilate coronary arteries (e.g., nitrates)
  - —Improve contractility (e.g., inotropes)
  - —Reduce preload (e.g., nitrates, morphine, diuretics, ACE inhibitors)
  - —Reduce afterload (e.g., ACE inhibitors, phosphodiesterase inhibitors, B-adrenergic agonists, vasodilators)
  - —Reduce heart rate (e.g., B-adrenergic blockers, calcium channel blockers)
  - —Reduce contractility (e.g., B-adrenergic blockers [Contraindicated with decreased ejection fraction])
- Correct arrhythmias
- Circulatory assist devices: IABP, VAD

Nursing Process Elements

- Prevention
- Intra-aortic balloon counter-pulsation (IBAC)
- Hemodynamic monitoring
- Fluid administration
- Safety and comfort

Circulatory Shock or Distributive Shock (Neurogenic, Septic, and Anaphylactic Shock)

Neurogenic shock

Etiology: Massive vasodilation resulting from loss of sympathetic vasoconstrictor tone.

Precipitating factors:

- Hemodynamic consequences of injury and/or disease to the spinal cord at or above T5
- Spinal anesthesia
- Vasomotor center depression (e.g., severe pain, drugs, hypoglycemia, injury)

S&S:

- Dry, warm skin
- Syncope
- Bradycardia
- Hypotension
- Loss of the ability to sweat below the level of the injury

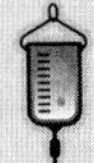

Clinical Alert

An unconscious client is treated as though a spinal cord injury has occurred until proven otherwise.

Dx:

- Radiographs of the spine, chest, and other structures
- CT scan
- MRI
- Somatosensory-evoked potentials
- CBC, electrolytes, glucose, BUN, creatinine, blood type, and crossmatch
- ABGs
- Coagulation studies

Rx:

- Treat underlying cause
- Minimize spinal cord trauma with stabilization
- Careful administration of fluids
- Drug therapy
  —Dopamine for hypotension and bradycardia
  —Phenylephrine or norepinephrine to increase SVR
  —Epinephrine for vasoconstrictive action
- Heparin or low-molecular-weight heparin (Lovenox)

Nursing Process Elements

- Elevate and maintain the head of the bed at least 30 degrees for clients receiving spinal or epidural anesthesia
- Immobilize the client to prevent further damage to the spinal cord
- Apply elastic compression stockings or pneumatic compression hose
- Elevate the foot of bed to minimize pooling of blood
- Check skin for redness, tenderness, and warmth of the calves
- Assess Homans' sign
- Perform passive range of motion
- Monitor for hypothermia and internal bleeding

Septic shock

- Complex and generalized process that involves all organ systems

Etiology: Initiated by infection—most often gram-negative bacterial infection, but can also result from gram-positive bacterial, viral, fungal, or parasitic infection.

Risk Factors:

- Invasive procedure
- Indwelling lines and catheters
- Old age
- Presence of chronic disease (e.g., diabetes mellitus, chronic renal failure, congestive heart failure)
- Immunosuppression
- Malnourishment
- Debilitation
- Malnutrition

S&S:

- Increased cardiac output progressing to low cardiac output
- Decreased urinary output
- Hyperthermia
- Warm flushed skin initially, progressing to cool and pale
- Bounding pulse
- Nausea, vomiting, diarrhea, or decreased bowel sounds
- Confusion or agitation
- Increased heart and respiratory rate

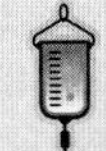

Clinical Alert

Fluid replacement must be instituted to correct the hypovolemia that results from the incompetent vasculature and inflammatory response.

Dx:

- Presence of bacteria in the blood
- Urine, blood, and sputum culture
- WBC with differential leukocyte count
- Hgb and Hct
- Activated protein C
- Changes in plasma D-dimer

Rx:

- Optimize oxygen delivery by increasing supply/decreasing demand
- Fluid resuscitation
- Optimize cardiac output
  —Volume
  —Positive inotropes (e.g., dobutamine)
- Vasopressors (increase blood pressure) (e.g., norepinephrine, phenylephrine)
- Correct acidosis
- Obtain culture before beginning antibiotics
- Antibiotics as ordered
- Debride wounds to remove necrotic tissue
- Institute infection control practices

Nursing Process Elements

- Ensure patent airway
- Start or maintain an established IV catheter
- Administer oxygen
- Administer antibiotics
- Obtain specimens of blood, urine, wound drainage, and sputum for culture
- Observe for overt bleeding
- Administer medications as prescribed

Client teaching for self-care

- Avoid crowds and large gatherings of people
- Do not share eating utensils or personal toilet articles
- Report S&S of infection
- Practise good bodily hygiene
- Do not change pet litter boxes
- Refrigerate and prepare food appropriately
- Take medications as prescribed

Anaphylactic shock

Anaphylactic shock is an immediate, systemic, normovolemic vasogenic reaction that occurs when an antigen interacts with the preformed antibody found on the surface of mast cells and basophils.

Etiology: Result of a systemic antigen–antibody reaction in a client who has preexisting antibodies to an offending antigen.

Precipitating factors:

- Contrast media
- Blood/blood products—transfusion reaction
- Drugs—penicillin sensitivity
- Insect bites—bee stings
- Anesthetic agents
- Food/food additives
- Vaccines
- Environmental agents
- Latex

S&S:

- Uneasiness
- Apprehension
- Weakness
- Impending doom
- Anxious
- Frightened
- Itching and urticaria
- Angioedema
- Crackles, wheezing, and reduced breath sounds
- Congestion, rhinorrhea, dyspnea, and respiratory distress
- Respiratory failure and cardiac dysrhythmias

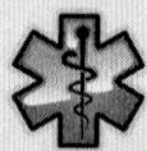

Nursing Intervention Alert

An emergency anaphylaxis kit or and epinephrine injector such as the EpiPen automatic injector should be readily available at all times.

Dx:

- History of severe allergic reaction/anaphylaxis
- Severe bronchospasms
- ABGs
- Angioedema
- Intense itchy skin

Rx:

- Premedication when a history of prior sensitivity (e.g., contrast media) exists
- Identify and remove offending cause if possible, e.g., latex tube
- Maintain patent airway
- Intubation/mechanical ventilation
- Drug therapy
  —Epinephrine: subcutaneous, IV, nebulized
  —Bronchodilators: nebulized, IV
  —Antihistamines
  —Corticosteroids (if hypotension persists)
- Fluid Resuscitation

Nursing Process Elements

- Assess history of allergens
- Institute emergency management of airway
- Start IV access
- Medications as prescribed
- Respiratory support with mechanical ventilation and oxygenation as needed

Client teaching for self-care

- Wear identification that identifies sensitivities
- Prevent further exposure to antigens
- Instructions concerning emergency use of medications to treat anaphylaxis
- Teach S&S of anaphylaxis

DISSEMINATED INTRAVASCULAR COAGULATION (DIC)

Etiology: Inappropriate stimulation of clotting.

Precipitating factors:

- Intrinsic pathway—injury to or alteration of vascular endothelium
- Extrinsic pathway—entry into circulation of procoagulant released from damaged tissue
- Common pathway—platelet adherence to abnormal vascular endothelium or aggregates of platelets or WBCs, which stimulate fibrinogen or prothrombin

S&S:

- CNS changes—restlessness, malaise, confusion, disorientation, and altered level of consciousness
- Cardiovascular—tachycardia, hypotension, nonspecific ST changes on ECG, and increased pulmonary artery pressure
- Pulmonary—hemoptysis, ARDS, tachypnea, orthopnea, dyspnea, hemorrhage, and cyanosis
- Renal—decrased urine output, oliguria, hematuria, urethral bleeding, severe back pain, ↑ BUN and creatinine
- Skin—petechiae, purpura, ecchymosis, oozing from venipuncture sites, bruising under site of BP cuff, hemorrhagic bullae, wound hematomas, cold mottled fingers and toes, and gangrene
- Gastrointestinal—N&V, abdominal pain, hematemesis, or NG drainage with blood, rectal bleeding and hematochezia, GI hemorrhage, and melena
- Musculoskeletal—severe muscle pain
- Legs—severe mottling of skin on lower legs, absent popliteal, posterior tibial, or pedal pulses, calf swelling, pain in foot with dorsiflexion, blood pooling, and cyanosis
- Toes—cool, mottled skin, and gangrenous changes in tips of toes
- Eyes—conjunctival or retinal hemorrhage and blurred vision
- Nasopharyngeal—gingival bleeding, epistaxis, bleeding from NG or endotracheal tube insertion site

Dx:

- Prothrombin time (PT)—prolonged
- Activated partial thromboplastin time (APTT or PT)—prolonged
- Thrombin time—excessively sensitive—20–40 seconds
- Fibrinogen levels—decreased
- Fibrin degradation product—elevated
- d-dimer—specific for fibrin monomer in DIC
- Antithrombin III—decreased
- Ethanol test—positive 1+ and 3+
- Platelets—decreased
- RBC—decreased
- Reticulocytes >4%
- Hgb &Hct—decreased

Rx:

- Correct the primary or underlying disorder if possible (i.e., prompt delivery of dead fetus and placenta or administration of IV antibiotics for sepsis).
- Control the major symptoms, either bleeding or thrombosis
  - —stop hemorrhage
  - —terminate the accelerated coagulation process
  - —minimize development of microthrombi
  - —resolve established thrombi
- Provide prophylaxis to prevent recurrence: heparin accelerates the rate at which antithrombin 3 neutralizes thrombin and activated factor X. This action blocks the coagulation cascade at the common pathway and ultimately prevents conversion of fibrinogen to fibrin.

Nursing Process Elements

- Assess for bloody drainage
- Observe for signs of thrombosis
- Check for petechiae, ecchymosis, or cyanosis
- Provide meticulous care to avoid infection
- Assess for fluid volume
- Assess for respiratory and cardiovascular problems
- Provide gentle care to avoid trauma
- Attend to IV therapy line and heparin infusion
- Provide psychosocial support

CARDIAC TAMPONADE

- Medical emergency
- Rising intracardiac pressure, decreased diastolic filling time, and decreased cardiac output

Etiology: Accumulation of excess pericardial fluid compresses the heart resulting in diminished cardiac filling and deceased cardiac output.

Precipitating factors: Chest trauma (blunt or penetrating) or chest tumor (cancer of esophagus or lung).

S&S:

- Dyspnea
- Chest pain or pressure
- Falling blood pressure
- Rapid, weak pulse
- Increased JVD and CVP
- Distant heart sounds
- Pericardial friction rub

- Diminishing pulse pressure (difference between systolic and diastolic BP)
- Ankle and sacral edema
- Ascites
- Lethargy
- Pulsus paradoxous (lose systolic blood pressure during inspiration)

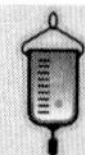

Clinical Alert

Cardiac Tamponade is a life-threatening condition that requires immediate intervention. Pericardial sac normally contains about 50 cc of fluid so even a small increase in fluid causes compression of the heart within the pericardial sac.

Dx: Echocardiogram, chest X-ray (cardiac enlargement), and ECG (nonspecific abnormalities).

Rx: Treat cause; administer oxygen (mechanical ventilation may be needed), drain fluid via pericardiocentesis, if tumor related. Chemotherapy or radiation may be used to decrease tumor size; vasopressors to increase blood pressure and cardiac output.

Nursing Process Elements

- Administer oxygen and position to facilitate breathing
- Treat for signs of shock but avoid fluid overload as cardiac output is already compromised
- Assist with pericardiocentesis
- Check for murmurs
- Assess for signs of fluid reaccumulation after pericardiocentesis

Client teaching for self-care

- Teach client signs of reoccurrence if related to malignancy.

PULMONARY EDEMA

- Acute heart failure
- Usually the result of left heart failure
- Causes severe tissue hypoxia leading to organ system failure and death
- Volume overload increases left atrial, pulmonary vein and capillary pressures; this high pressure forces fluid from the blood into pulmonary interstitial spaces and ultimately into the alveoli.

Etiology: Inadequate left ventricular function with cardiac disease can also result from hypervolemia, pulmonary disorders, and certain cancer-related conditions.

S&S:

- Profound dyspnea, tachypnea, cyanosis, wheezing, production of pink (blood tinged) frothy secretions, and orthopnea
- Wheezing, rales, and crackles
- Severe anxiety and sense of impending doom, restlessness, and confusion
- Tachycardia and hypotension
- Pallor, decrease in oxygen saturation levels, and abnormal ABGs.
- Elevated JVD and CVP

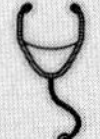

Assessment Alert

Severe life-threatening complication. Client presents in acute respiratory distress and sense of suffocation or "drowning" in secretions. Crackles are heard in the lung bases due to movement of air through the alveolar fluid.

Dx: Clinical manifestations and chest X-ray demonstrate pulmonary. congestion

Rx: Reduce excess fluid and improve gas exchange by means of MOIST.

- M—morphine to reduce anxiety and pain, and to reduce peripheral resistance and venous return
- O—oxygen to respond to hypoxemia; intubation may be needed
- I—IV medications to improve ventricular function including inotropes (dopamine or dobutamine), diuretics (furosemide), aminophylline to relieve bronchospasms, vasodilators (nitroglycerine) to dilate vessels thereby decreasing afterload and preload
- S—suction as needed
- T—treat underlying cause

Nursing care

- Position the client for comfort and support of ventilation and circulation: semi to high Fowler's with legs dangling and arms supported and away from the chest as in leaning on an over-the-bed table
- Maintain airway patency
- Administer oxygen at high concentrations
- Monitor VS, pulse oximetry, ABGs, and hemodynamic status
- Provide emotional support—assume a calm, reassuring manner
- Monitor effects of medications—especially for changes in electrolyte levels

- Accurate I&O
- Prepare for emergency treatments (rotating tourniquets, intubation, phlebotomy)

Client teaching for self-care

- Treatment for underlying cause
- Promote activity without adding to fatigue, so pace and prioritize daily activities
- Avoid extremes in temperature that tax cardiac function
- Stop activity if experiencing light-headedness or shortness of breath
- Plan for periods of rest alternating with periods of activity
- Maintain low-sodium diet
- Potassium replacement if taking a potassium-depleting diuretic and/or include foods high in potassium in the diet. This includes orange and tomato juice, bananas, raisins, figs, prunes, apricots, spinach, cauliflower, and potatoes
- Take diuretics at times that allow for uninterrupted sleep
- Importance of adherence to medical regime
- Weigh self daily and report to physician a greater than 3-lbs weight gain (1 liter = 2.2 lbs; "a pint is a pound the world around")
- How to take pulse and report to physician if pulse is <60 bpm or >120 bpm
- S&S of complications or onset of condition to be reported

ACUTE RESPIRATORY DISTRESS SYNDROME

- Acute respiratory failure
- Clinical syndrome of noncardiogenic pulmonary edema and progressive decrease in arterial oxygen content

Etiology: Always occurs after serious illness or injury either directly to the lungs or after indirect insult to the body.

Precipitating factors:

- Aspiration
- Drug overdose
- Prolonged inhalation of high concentrations of oxygen, smoke, or corrosive substances
- Shock
- Trauma such as pulmonary contusion, multiple fractures, and head injury
- Systemic infection

S&S: Clinical S&S usually 12–48 hours after a serious injury or illness include

- anxiety,
- decreased level of consciousness,
- dyspnea,
- tachypnea,
- auscultated crackles,
- decreased functional residual capacity,
- hypocapnia,
- severe hypoxia, or
- marked buccal peripheral cyanosis.

Dx: Clinical presentation.

- Low partial pressure of arterial oxygen (PaO_2)
- Chest X-ray showing dense pulmonary infiltrates with a white out or ground glass appearance to the lung
- Decreased pulmonary compliance

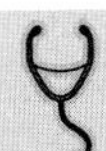

Assessment Alert

ABG analysis: decreased PaO_2 (below 60 mm Hg despite administration of oxygen at a high flow rate (10 l/min)

Rx:

- Oxygen
- Mechanical ventilation
- Extracorporeal lung-assist technology
- Partial liquid ventilation
- Positioning
- Pharmacological therapy
- Nutritional support

Nursing Process Elements

- Assist with endotracheal intubation and mechanical ventilation; as prescribed, institute positive end-expiratory pressure (PEEP) to keep alveoli distended, stretch stiff lungs, and increase oxygen–carbon dioxide diffusion
- Administer corticosteroids as prescribed, to decrease inflammation surrounding the alveoli and to stabilize the capillary membrane
- Encourage semi-Fowler's or high Fowler's position
- Assess for S&S of fluid volume overload including peripheral edema and jugular vein distention (JVD)
- Provide adequate nutritional support that is not high in carbohydrates, which metabolize to form excess CO_2. The diet should include 35–45 kcal/kg a day to meet normal requirements, with enteral or parental feeding support if necessary
- Reassure client, explain all procedures, and remain calm to reduce client's anxiety and thereby decrease oxygen need
- Monitor ABG levels

- Maintain effective tracheobronchial hygiene
- Monitor hemodynamic status

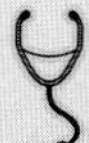

Assessment Alert

Identify clients at high risk for pulmonary hypertension such as COPD, pulmonary emboli, congenital heart disease, and mitral valve disease.

CHOKING

To assist a client who is choking on a foreign object, perform the abdominal thrust maneuver (sometimes called the Heimlich maneuver).

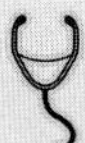

Assessment Alert

Hands crossed at the neck are the universal sign for choking.

- Stand behind the person who is choking
- Place both arms around the person's waist
- Make a fist with one hand with the thumb outside the fist
- Place thumb side of fist against the person's abdomen above the navel and below the xiphoid process
- Grasp fist with other hand
- Quickly and forcefully exert pressure against the person's diaphragm, pressing upward with quick, firm thrusts.
- Apply thrusts 6–10 times until the obstruction is cleared.
- The pressure from the thrusts should lift the diaphragm, force air into the lungs, and create an artificial cough powerful enough to expel the aspirated object.

POISONING

- Exposure to poisons can occur by ingestion, inhalation, or skin or mucous membrane contact.
- Typically occurs in children younger than age 6 years, with a peak incidence between 12 and 24 months.

Etiology:

- Improper or dangerous storage of potentially toxic substances
- Poor lighting resulting in errors in reading
- Human factors are
  —failure to read label properly;
  —failure to return poisons to their proper place;
  —failure to recognize the material as poisonous;
  —lack of supervision of a child.

S&S:

- Vary with poison
- Toxin may have a limited local effect or continue to a stage of absorption and interference with metabolic processes and organ function.
- Acute poisoning may result in arrhythmias or permanent multiorgan damage due to initial loss of airway, breathing, circulation, and specific organ toxicity.

Rx: Emergency management

- Establish and maintain airway, ventilation, and oxygenation. In the absence of cerebral or renal damage, prognosis depends largely on successful management of respiratory and circulatory systems.
- Blood gas analysis or spirometry is used to determine adequacy of ventilation.
- Assess pulse, blood pressure, central venous pressure, and temperature (core and peripheral).
- Mechanical ventilation if respirations are depressed. Positive expiratory pressure applied to the airway (bag mask) may help keep the alveoli inflated.
- Oxygen for respiratory depression, unconsciousness, cyanosis, and shock
- Prevent aspiration of gastric contents by positioning client on side with head down, using an oropharyngeal airway, and suctioning
- Stabilize cardiovascular function and monitor ECG
- Indwelling urinary catheter to monitor renal function
- Obtain blood specimen to test for concentration of drug or poison
- Monitor neurologic status (including cognitive function) and VS for change and direction of change over time
- Determine what product was taken, the amount, time since ingestion, symptoms, age and weight of the client, and pertinent health history.
- Contact poison control center in the area if an unknown toxic agent has been taken or if it is necessary to identify an antidote for a known toxic agent.
- Treatment of shock based on cause: cardiodepressant action of a drug ingested, venous pooling in lower extremities, or reduction in circulating blood volume as a result of increased capillary permeability.
- Remove the toxin or decrease its absorption by emptying the stomach
  —Syrup of ipecac to induce vomiting in the alert client (do not induce vomiting after ingestion of caustic substances or petroleum distillates)
  —Gastric lavage. Save gastric aspirate for toxicology screens.
  —Activated charcoal administration if poison is one that is absorbed by charcoal
  —Cathartic, when appropriate

Table 31–1 Acetaminophen, Salicylate, and Lead Poisoning

Substance	Mechanism of Action	Treatment
Acetaminophen	Can cause fetal hepatonecrosis Toxic dose: 140 mg/kg	O_2, IV, monitor, emesis/lavage, charcoal, cathartic, *N*-acetylcysteine (oral dose: 140 mg/kg, then 70 mg/kg every 4 hours for 17 doses, dilute to 5% solution and add to juice)
Salicylate poisoning aspirin (present in compound analgesic tablets)	Uncouples oxidative phosphorylation; inhibits Krebs cycle • Restlessness, tinnitus, deafness, blurring of vision • Hyperpnea, hyperpyrexia, sweating • Epigastric pain, vomiting, dehydration • Respiratory and metabolic acidosis • Disorientation, coma, cardiovascular collapse	O_2, IV, monitor, emesis/lavage, charcoal, cathartic, alkalinization of urine, replace potassium, dialysis • Treat respiratory distress • Induce gastric emptying emesis or lavage • Give activated charcoal to absorb aspirin: a cathartic may be administered with charcoal to help assure intestine cleaning.
	Phase I (first 24 hours after ingestion) • May be asymptomatic • Anorexia • N&V • Diaphoresis • Malaise • Pallor	• Support client with intravenous infusions as prescribed to establish hydration and correct electrolyte imbalances
	Phase II (24–48 hours after ingestion) • Symptoms of phase I diminish or disappear • Right upper quadrant pain due to liver damage • Liver enlargement with elevated bilirubin and hepatic enzymes and prolonged prothrombin time • Oliguria	• Enhance elimination of salicylates as directed by forced diuresis, alkalinization of urine, peritoneal dialysis, or hemodialysis, according to severity of intoxication. • Monitor serum salicylate level for efficacy of treatment
	Phase III (days 3 to 5 after ingestion) • Signs of hepatic failure such as jaundice, hypoglycemia, coagulopathy, encephalopathy • Peak liver function abnormalities • Anorexia, nausea, vomiting, malaise may reappear • Renal failure and cardiomyopathy may occur	• Administer specific prescribed pharmacologic agent for bleeding and other adverse effects
	Phase IV • Associated with recovery or progression to completed liver failure and death —Pain, vomiting, dehydration —Respiratory and metabolic acidosis —Disorientation, coma, cardiovascular collapse	
Lead Poisoning	• Toxic to CNS, bone marrow, kidneys • Lead attaches to RBCs • Stores in bone and soft tissue • Twice as long to excrete than absorb • Kidneys injured	• Remove lead from environment • Remove child from environment during lead abatement process

- Administer any specific chemical antagonist or physiologic antagonist as early as possible to reverse or diminish effects of the toxin
- Support the client having seizures: poisons may excite the CNS or the client may have seizures from oxygen deprivation.
- Procedures to promote the removal of the ingested substance if the above are not effective:
  —Diuresis for agents excreted by the renal route
  —Dialysis
  —Hemoperfusion (process of passing blood through an extracorporeal circuit and a cartridge containing an adsorbent [such as charcoal or resins], after which the detoxified blood is returned to the client).
  —Multiple doses of charcoal

See Table 31-1 for specific information related to acetaminophen, salicylate, and lead poisoning.

Nursing Process Elements

- Monitor central venous pressure as indicated
- Monitor fluid and electrolyte imbalance
- Reduce elevated temperature
- Cautiously give analgesics as prescribed for pain; severe pain causes vasomotor collapse and reflex inhibition of normal physiologic functions
- Assist in obtaining specimens of blood, urine, stomach contents, and vomitus
- Provide constant nursing surveillance and attention to the client in a coma; coma from poisoning results from interference with brain cell function or metabolism
- Monitor and treat for complications such as hypotension, cardiac dysrhythmias, and seizures
- If the client is discharged, give written material indicating S&S of potential problems and procedures for call-back or return
- Request a psychiatric consultation if poisoning was a suicide attempt
- In cases of accidental poison ingestion, provide poison prevention and home poison-proofing instructions to the client or family

EYE INJURY

Etiology: Trauma to the eye may be caused by blunt or sharp injury, chemical, or thermal burns. The eyelids, protective layers, surrounding soft tissue, or the globe itself may be injured. Vision may be impaired by direct injury or latent scarring. See Table 31-2 for information on specific types of eye injuries and their treatment.

Nursing Process Elements

- Medicate for pain as directed
- Provide ice and cool compresses to relieve swelling and pain
- Provide additional comfort measures such as positioning, dimmed lights, and quiet environment
- Irrigate and patch eye as directed
- Monitor VS and neurological status as indicated
- Watch for and report signs of infection such as fever, drainage, increased pain, warmth, and redness

Client teaching for self-care

- Teach client how to administer medications such as topical antibiotics
- Instruct on use of patch or shield
- Advise client to report increase in pain, decrease in vision, redness, and fever
- Teach safety measures with decreased visual acuity
- Advise use of corrective lenses as prescribed
- Stress follow-up care
- Attempt to prevent future trauma with protective eyewear

WOUND DEHISCENCE AND EVISCERATION

Wound dehiscence—disruption of surgical incision or wound
Evisceration—protrusion of wound contents after dehiscence. These are serious surgical complications.

Etiology: Sutures give way as a result of increased stress related to marked distention or strenuous coughing, infection, or failure of the wound closure technique, e.g., broken sutures, slipped knot, or inadequate muscle bites.

Predisposing factors: Increasing age, poor nutritional status, weak or pendulous abdominal walls, and pulmonary or cardiovascular disease in clients undergoing abdominal surgery.

S&S:

- Gush of bloody peritoneal fluid from the wound
- Something gave way as reported by client
- Pain
- Vomiting
- Protrusion of intestines from an abdominal wound
- Warning signs of dehiscence related to infection: redness or swelling of, or around, incision line, excessive pain and tenderness on palpation, purulent, or odorous drainage

Dx: Clinical presentation.

Rx:

- Opiate for pain
- Sterile dressing to wound
- Fluid resuscitation
- Return to or for resuturing under general anesthesia

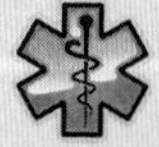

Nursing Intervention Alert

When disruption of a wound occurs, the client is placed in low Fowler's position and instructed to lie quietly. These actions minimize protrusion of body tissues. Protruding coils of intestine are covered with a sterile dressing moistened with sterile saline solution, and the surgeon is notified at once.

Table 31–2 Eye Trauma

Condition	Signs and Symptoms	Treatment
Blunt Contusion—bruising of periorbital soft tissue	• Swelling and discoloration of the tissue • Bleeding into the tissue and structures of the eye • Pain • Increased intraocular pressure	• Treatment to reduce swelling • Pain management dependent on structures involved
Hyphema—presence of blood in the anterior chamber	• Pain • Blood in anterior chamber • Increased intraocular pressure	• Usually spontaneous recovery • If severe, bed rest or chair rest with bathroom privileges, eye shield, interior chamber paracentesis, topical steroids, cycloplegics
Orbital fracture—fracture and dislocation of walls of the orbit, orbital margins, or both	• May be accompanied by other signs of head injury • Rhinorrhea • Contusion • Diplopia • Diagnosis: X-ray, computed tomography (CT)	• May heal on own if no displacement or infringement on other structures • Surgery (repair the orbital floor with plate freeing entrapped orbital tissue)
Foreign body—on cornea (25% all ocular injuries), conjunctiva Intraocular particles penetrate sclera, cornea, globe	• Severe pain • Lacrimation • Foreign body sensation • Photophobia • Redness • Swelling	• Medical emergency • Removal of foreign body through irrigation, cotton-tipped applicator, or magnet • Treatment of intraocular foreign body depends on size, magnetic properties, tissue reaction, location • Surgical removal
Laceration/Perforation cutting or penetration of soft tissue of globe	• Pain • Bleeding • Lacrimation • Photophobia	• Medical emergency • Surgical repair—method depends on severity of injury • Antibiotics—topically and systemically
Ruptured globe concussive injury to globe with tears in the ocular coats, usually the sclera	• Pain • Altered intraocular pressure • Limitation of gaze in field of rupture • Hyphema • Hemorrhage • Diagnosis: CT, ultrasound	• Medical emergency • Surgical repair • Vitrectomy • Scleral buckle • Antibiotics • Steroids • Enucleation
Burns Chemical—caused by alkali or acid agent	• Pain • Burning • Lacrimation • Photophobia	• Medical emergency • Copious irrigation until pH 7.0 • Severe scarring may require keratoplasty • Antibiotics
Thermal—usually burn to eyelids may be first, second, or third degree	• Pain • Burned skin • Blisters	• First aid—apply sterile dressings • Pain control • Fluid blebs left intact • Eyelids sutured together to protect eye if perforation a possibility • Skin grafting with severe second-, and third-degree burns
Ultraviolet—excessive exposure to sunlight, sunlamp, snow blindness, welding	• Pain—delayed several hours after exposure • Foreign body sensation • Lacrimation • Photophobia	• Pain relief • Condition self-limiting • Bilateral patching with antibiotic ointment and cycloplegics

BURNS

Etiology:

- Burns are caused by a transfer of energy from a heat source to the body.
- Types of burns:
  - —Thermal
    - Dry heat—flame, flash
    - Contact—tar, metals, grease
    - Moist heat—steam, scald
  - —Chemical
    - Acids
    - Alkalis
  - —Inhalation
    - Smoke
    - Hot air
    - Chemicals
  - —Electrical
    - Lightning
    - Electric current
  - —Radiation
    - Sunburn
    - Radiation therapy
    - Accidental exposure

Risk factors/groups: Children particularly boys; disabled; older adults with impaired mobility, coordination, judgment; substance abusers, smokers.

S&S:

- Tissue destruction results from coagulation, protein denaturation, or ionization of cellular contents.
- Amount of tissue damage is determined by type, temperature, and amount of causative agent such as flame or scalding liquid, duration of contact, and thickness of the skin.
- Classification of burns:
  - —First-, second-, or third-degree based on depth of the injury. See Table 31-3.
  - —Severity of burn injury: minor, moderate uncomplicated, or major burn injuries (classified according to the American Burn Association criteria). See Table 31-4.
  - —Thermal, chemical, radiation burns.
- Localized effects:
  - —Area of coagulation surrounded by an area of damaged blood vessels and decreased perfusion surrounded by an area of hyperemia
  - —Area of damaged blood vessels is at great risk for necrosis in days following injury
- Systemic effects of major burns—"burn shock"
- Hypovolemia—result of fluid lost from wound and release of vasoactive substances, which cause a massive fluid shift from the intravascular to interstitial space.
- Edema: peaks in 12–24 hours after injury and resolves by 72 hours.
- Results from fluid shift in response to release of vasoactive mediators as above

Table 31–3 Depth of Burn Injury

Depth of Burn and Causes	Skin Involvement	Symptoms	Wound Appearance	Recuperative Course
First degree Superficial Partial-thickness Sunburn Low-intensity flash	Epidermis; possibly a portion of the dermis	Tingling Hyperesthesia (supersensitivity) Pain soothed by cooling	Reddened; blanches with pressure; dry Minimal or no edema Possible blisters	Complete recovery within a week; no scarring. Peeling.
Second degree Deep partial-thickness Scalds Flash flames	Epidermis, upper dermis, portion of deeper dermis	Pain Hyperesthesia Sensitive to cold air	Pale, mottled, pearly white, mostly dry, often insensate; difficult to differentiate from full-thickness injury	Recovery in 2–4 weeks. Some scarring and depigmentation contractures. Infection may convert it to full thickness.
Third degree Full-thickness Flame Prolonged exposure to hot liquids Electric current Chemical	Epidermis, entire dermis, and sometimes subcutaneous tissue; may involve connective tissue, muscle, and bone	Pain free Shock Hematuria (blood in the urine) and possibly hemolysis (blood cell destruction) Possible entrance and exit wounds (electrical burn)	Dry, pale white, leathery, or charred broken skin with fat exposed Edema	Eschar sloughs Grafting necessary Scarring and loss of contour and function; contractures Loss of digits or extremity possible

Table 31–4 Classification of Burns According to the American Burn Association

Minor Burn	Moderate Uncomplicated Burn	Major Burn
• Second-degree burns of <15% TBSA in adults or <10% TBSA in children	• Second-degree burns of 15–25% TBSA in adults or 10–20% TBSA in children	• Second-degree burns of >25% TBSA in adults or >20% TBSA in children
• Third-degree burns of <2% TBSA not involving special care areas (eyes, ears, face, hands, feet, perineum)	• Third-degree burns of <10% TBSA not involving special care areas	• All third-degree burns of 10% TBSA or greater

TBSA, total body surface area

- Other systemic effects—hypermetabolism, myocardial depression, damage to the renal tubules, pulmonary hypertension, pulmonary edema,, suppression of cellular immunity, catabolism of fat and muscle, clotting abnormalities, anemia from early destruction of RBCs, decreased hepatic, and intestinal perfusion
- Decreased cardiac output secondary to vasoconstriction
- Inhalation burns—soot around the mouth, singed eye lashes, brows, nasal hair; respiratory distress
- Electrical burns—cardiac and respiratory arrest due to disruption of electrical conduction throughout body

Rx: Emergent Phase

- First priority: Stop the burning process.
  - —For dry powder burns, brush the powder off first.
  - —For scald, rinse affected area with a large amount of clean water. Never use cold water on extensive burns because of the potential effect on body temperature.
  - —For flash or flame burns, use water or wrap client in a blanket, coat, or other material; then roll on the ground to smother flames; move client to a safe area; cool burn with water; remove clothing and jewelry that is not adherent to the body.
  - —For chemical burns, irrigate with large amounts of water or saline (water for eyes).

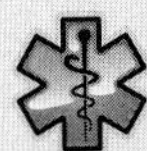

Nursing Intervention Alert

Use litmus paper to test water that has been used to irrigate an eye for acidity or alkalinity; if the injurious chemical has been completely washed out, the pH will be neutral.

- Assess airway, breathing, and circulation. If the client was involved in a fire, assume inhalation injury until proven otherwise, and manage accordingly. Oxygen, suctioning, postural drainage, or endotracheal intubation may be needed.

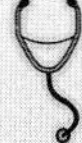

Assessment Alert

Carbon monoxide is probably the most common cause of inhalation injury because it is a by-product of the combustion of organic materials and is therefore present in smoke. Carbon monoxide combines with hemoglobin to form carboxyhemoglobin, which competes with oxygen for available hemoglobin binding sites. The affinity of hemoglobin for carbon monoxide is 200 times greater than for oxygen.

- Perform a quick assessment of neurological status; check for spinal cord injury.
- Remove jewelry and clothing not stuck to burned areas.
- Cover wounds loosely with sterile (if available) or clean dressings dampened with normal saline or water to ease pain and prevent evaporation of body fluids.
- If hands or feet are burned, separate fingers or toes with sterile gauze pads moistened with sterile water. Keep hand in a position of function.
- Do not open eyelids if they are burned; apply moist gauze pads to both eyes. Be certain burn is thermal and not chemical.
- Do not open blisters.
- Do not apply any salves or ointments.
- Wrap entire body in something dry to prevent heat loss.
- Begin volume resuscitation with large bore needle (16–18 gauge) and lactated Ringer's solution or normal saline. If burn is large, keep client NPO to avoid the risk of vomiting and aspiration.
  - —Fluid requirement for 24 hours is based on a formula such as the Parkland or the Brooke; both use isotonic or hypertonic IV solutions and calculate amount to be infused for 24 hours with one-half infused in the first 8 hours and one-fourth infused in each of the next 8-hour blocks.

—Using the Parkland formula, the amount of lactated Ringer's solution (volume expander) to deliver in the first 24 hours after time of injury is calculated as follows:

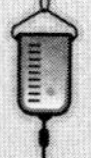

Clinical Alert

Fluid requirements are calculated from the time the burn injury occurred, not from the time fluid resuscitation is being started.

Fluid × 4 cc × %TBSA × weight in kg
%TBSA excludes any first-degree burn

Example: 70-kg client with 50% second-degree burn
4 ml × 70 kg × 50% = 14,000 ml of IV fluid/24 hr.
7000 ml of IV fluid/8 hr

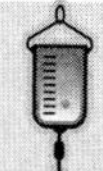

Clinical Alert

The formula is a guide only and infusions must be tailored to urinary output and central venous pressure; if not adjusted to the individual client, under- or over-hydration can result.

Half of this fluid is given in the first 8 hours post injury and the rest in the subsequent 16 hours.

TBSA in the formula is the percentage of body surface area affected by partial thickness or full-thickness burns (superficial thickness burns are not counted). TBSA can be estimated quickly by using the rule of nines (see Table 3-5)

—For smaller or irregular burns, size is estimated by using the surface of the client's hand as about 1% of the TBSA.

- Tetanus toxoid given when immunization status is in doubt.
- Acute phase: focus is treatment of burn wound and prevention of complications
- Medications: analgesics (morphine sulfate, fentanyl, codeine), ranitidine, sucralfate, or other agent to prevent stress ulcers, topical antimicrobial (silver sulfadiazine or mafenide acetate for deep burns; bacitracin or the like for superficial burns) to prevent infection of the burn wound
- Wound care: hydrotherapy to cleanse wound; debridement (surgical or enzymatic) and dressing (closed method) or no dressing (open method)
- Skin grafts
  —Used for full-thickness burns
  —Types of grafts are as follows:
    - autografts: from client's own body
    - allograft: from a live or deceased donor; may be fresh or frozen
    - heterograft: from another species
    - synthetic substitutes
    - biosynthetic dressings
  —Autografts are permanent; all others temporary and are rejected with healing but reduce water, protein and electrolyte loss; decrease pain; and allow mobility.
  —Split thickness grafts: epidermis and part of dermis; allows regeneration of skin at donor site
  —Full-thickness grafts: better cosmetic result so used for face, hands, and neck
- Nutrition: metabolism after a burn injury can be two to three times normal so burn clients are in catabolic state until caloric intake exceeds metabolic demand.
  —Baseline nutritional assessment with anthropometric measurements followed by urea nitrogen and prealbumin measures two to three times weekly
  —Protein requirements increased from 0.8 gm/kg to 1.5–3.0 gm/kg body weight to replace nitrogen lost through wound and urine and to allow healing
  —Caloric need can range from 3500–5000 cal/d and is given as 20% protein, 50% carbohydrate, and 30% fat.
  —Most burn clients require enteral feedings and they are begun as early as possible after burn.

Table 31–5 Rule of Nines

Head	9%
Anterior torso	18%
Posterior	18%
Each leg	18%
Each arm	9%
Genitalia/Perineum	1%

Nursing Process Elements

- Assess severity of injury
  —Depth of burn
  —Extent of burn
  —Age of the client
  —Pulmonary injury
  —Associated trauma
  —Special considerations – electrical, chemical
  —Preexisting illness
- Assess VS frequently
- Assess clients with inhalation burns or burns of the face or neck for signs of laryngeal edema and airway obstruction: severe, brassy cough; stridor, hoarseness, anxiety, confusion, coma and give 100% oxygen by mask

- Protect from hypothermia: keep covered to prevent heat loss from exposure to air; keep room warm; avoid drafts; use warming devices such as heat lamps or warming blankets
- Assess for adequate fluid resuscitation: urinary output of 30–50 ml/hr or 1–2 ml/kg of body weight/hr in children; normal LOC; systolic BP >100 mm Hg with pulse of <100 bpm; pH of 7.35–7.45 and base excess of 6 or greater

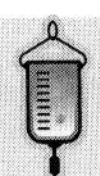

Clinical Alert

Urinary output is used as a guide to fluid resuscitation until edema begins to resolve in 48–72 hours, then serum and urinary electrolyte levels are used to guide fluid administration.

- Maintain cardiac monitoring of clients with electrical burns for 2 hours after dysrhythmias cease
- Maintain indwelling catheter drainage to obtain hourly output, which is used to guide fluid resuscitation
- Monitor urinary output and color or urine

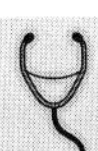

Assessment Alert

Burgundy-colored urine suggests the presence of hemochromogen and myoglobin resulting form muscle damage.

- Weigh daily: gain occurs because of fluid retention; loss occurs as fluid is lost.
- Monitor for glucosuria
- Maintain nasogastric suction if client is nauseated and in absence of peristalsis
- Protect from infection: cleanse dirt from wound; use protective precautions; hair shaved or clipped around area of burn; culture wound after cleaning for baseline and then once or twice per week; encourage as much mobility as possible and deep breathing to prevent pneumonia
- Assess for impaired peripheral tissue perfusion: decreased or absent distal pulses, pallor, coldness, paresthesias, lack of feeling, slow capillary refill. Impaired perfusion can result from edema occurring under areas of eschar because eschar is inelastic
- Assess for respiratory distress resulting from constriction of chest wall by eschar in clients with chest burns
- Control pain: skin anesthetics for first-degree burns, gentle handling, keeping wounds covered to prevent contact with air, and administration of opioids such as morphine sulfate IV in small doses every 5–10 minutes for 24–48 hours

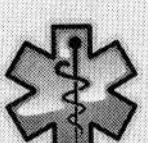

Nursing Intervention Alert

Subcutaneous and intramuscular pain medications are avoided for burn clients because of problems related to absorption from the administration site due to edema and vasoconstriction.

- Administer tetanus toxoid if there is any question about the client's immunization status
- Monitor wound and donor site if applicable, for signs of infection

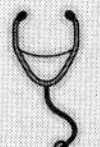

Assessment Alert

Sepsis can occur with serious even deadly consequences. Signs of sepsis are change in mental status, fever, tachypnea, tachycardia, paralytic ileus, abdominal distention, and oliguria.

- Provide wound care:
  —Medicate for pain and time wound care when medication is most effective
  —Provide hydrotherapy (tub immersion, spray table, or shower) to remove topical medications and wound debris:
    - tub immersion: not more than 30 minutes to prevent excess heat loss; promotes range of motion
- Provide graft care:
  —Prevent movement of the graft: maintain immobilizing devices such as bulky dressings or splints for 48–72 hours
  —Remove graft dressings slowly and gently so as not to disturb graft
  —Check full thickness and graft sheets every 24 hours for areas of fluid collection beneath them: collected fluid can be removed by rolling with a q-tip or by making slits in the graft
- Maintain nutrition
- Coordinate with physical and occupational therapists
- Maintain range of motion
- Promote coping
- Support hope
- Provide information for realistic planning for future
- Support client's and family's coping style
- Recognize that anxiety, irritability, sleep, and body image disturbances are common emotional reactions

Client teaching for self-care

- Report: opening of a healed area, blister formation, signs of infection (fever >100.4°F, increased or foul drainage, redness, pain, swelling, hardness or warmth of an area), problems with pressure garment or elastic bandages used to prevent thick, rigid scarring, which is disfiguring and leads to contractures
- Healed burned areas may be hypersensitive to fabric softeners, dyes, detergents: wash new clothing before wearing, use mild soap and no fabric softeners, rinse twice; wash clothes separately if open wound areas exist

PULMONARY EMBOLISM

- Pulmonary embolism is an obstruction of the pulmonary arterial bed. The embolus travels from the venous circulation to the right side of the heart and to the pulmonary artery. Obstruction of blood flow leads to pulmonary hypertension and infarction.
- Can manifest itself as one large clot, several tiny clots, or a shower of clots in the lungs.

Etiology:

- Nondissolved substance such as air, fat, or thrombus in the pulmonary vessels.
  —Most often: dislodged thrombus from leg veins
  —Thrombi may also originate in the pelvic vein, hepatic vein, right side of the heart, or arm vein.

Precipitating/risk factors:

- DVT following orthopedic or abdominal surgery, use of oral contraceptives, pregnancy, prolonged immobility, any conditions characterized by venous stasis, hypercoagulability, and vein wall damage (Virchow's triad)
- Trauma especially with long bone fracture
- Clot dissolution
- Sudden muscle spasm
- Intravascular pressure changes
- IV therapy

S&S:

Symptoms vary depending on the size and location of the emboli.

- Sudden onset of dyspnea, tachypnea, localized, sharp pleuritic chest pain, apprehension, cyanosis, and crackles
- Restlessness
- Cough and hemoptysis
- Splinting of the chest
- Tachycardia
- If DVT is present there will be calf swelling, warmth at site, mild fever
- Signs of shock such as hypotension and cardiac arrhythmia

Dx:

- Chest X-ray shows wedge-shaped infiltrate.
- Lung scan shows V/Q mismatch perfusion defects in areas beyond occluded vessels.
- Pulmonary angiography is the most definitive test (check for dye allergy).
- ECG helps rule out MI versus pulmonary emboli.
- ABGs show alkalosis and hypoxemia.

Rx:

- Oxygen therapy
- Drug therapy: for acute episode IV heparin and thrombolytic agents (urokinase, streptokinase) to inhibit coagulation and prevent further clots; proactive treatment of clients at risk for DVT with low dose SQ heparin and then oral anticoagulants
- If heparin contraindicated may insert inferior vena cava filter, very rarely pulmonary embolectomy
- Pain medication such as morphine (monitor respiratory status before administering)

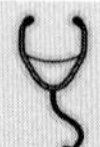

Assessment Alert

PE is difficult to diagnosis therefore the nurse needs to monitor any client at risk for S&S.

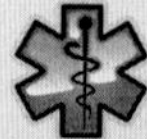

Nursing Intervention Alert

Primary nursing goals are to maintain adequate cardiovascular and pulmonary function as the obstruction resolves and to prevent reoccurrence. Most emboli resolve in about 10 days, therefore care should be given to dissolve the existing emboli and to prevent further formation.

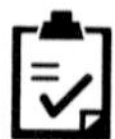

Nursing Process Elements

- Monitor cardiopulmonary status
- Monitor ABGs
- Maintain bed rest in acute stage
- Administer oxygen via nasal cannula
- Place client in high Fowlers position
- Monitor V/S, LOC, and respiratory status
- Auscultate heart and lung sounds

- Controlled breathing technique
- Prepare for endotracheal intubation if need arises
- Administer pain medication as needed
- Monitor coagulation lab results, adjust therapy, give prn medication
- Monitor CVP
- Once client is stable, encourage frequent movement and assist with isometric and ROM exercise
- Reduce anxiety
- No massaging of legs
- Maintain hydration
- Apply elastic stockings (antiembolic) and pneumatic compression devices

Client teaching for self-care

- Deep breathing and coughing exercises using incentive spirometry
- Avoid crossing legs because this can impede circulation and promote thrombus formation
- Anticoagulant therapy regimen if prescribed long-term
- Precautions related to bleeding as a side effect of anticoagulant therapy
- Advise the client to stay away from OTC medication or check with his/her physician before taking OTC medications
- Importance of follow-up care and lab test monitoring for anticoagulant therapy

WORKSHEET

TRUE & FALSE QUESTIONS

Mark each of the following statements True or False. Correct all false statements in the space provided.

1. PEEP is used for clients with ARDS to keep alveoli distended, stretch stiff lungs, and increase oxygen–carbon dioxide diffusion. ___ T ___ F
2. The burned client needs 2 or 4 ml of lactated Ringer's solution/normal saline per kg of body weight per percent of body surface burn in the first 24 hours to maintain blood volume and urinary output. ___ T ___ F
3. When the rule of nines is used to calculate area of a burn, all body areas that have been burned are calculated into the formula. ___ T ___ F
4. When performing the Hiemlich maneuver, the thumb side of fist is placed against the person's abdomen above the navel and below the xiphoid process. ___ T ___ F
5. The fluid that lubricates the pleural space is intracellular fluid. ___ T ___ F
6. An electrolyte imbalane associated with decreased aldosterone is hyponatremia. ___ T ___ F
7. Administration of hypotonic IV solutions would be an expected part of therapy for a client with hypernatremia. ___ T ___ F
8. The most common cause of septic shock is infection with gram-positive bacteria. ___ T ___ F
9. Heparin is used prophylactically in the management of DIC because it blocks the coagulation cascade at the common pathway and ultimately prevents conversion of fibrinogen to fibrin. ___ T ___ F
10. The first priority of the emergent phase of burn care is checking the airway. ___ T ___ F

MATCHING QUESTIONS

Match the value in column B that is realistically consistent with the abnormality named in column A:

Column A	Column B
1. ____ Hyponatremia	a. 1.2 mEq/l
2. ____ Hypokalemia	b. 2.2 mEq/l
3. ____ Hypomagnesemia	c. 3.2 mEq/l
4. ____ Hypochloremia	d. 3.4 mEq/l
5. ____ Hypocalcemia	e. 4.1 mEq/l
6. ____ Hypernatremia	f. 5.4 mEq/l
7. ____ Hyperkalemia	g. 8.2 mEq/l
8. ____ Hypermagnesemia	h. 9.7 mEq/l
9. ____ Hyperchloremia	i. 10.2 mEq/l
10. ____ Hypercalcemia	j. 87 mEq/l
	k. 102 mEq/l
	l. 114 mEq/l
	m. 126 mEq/l
	n. 142 mEq/l
	o. 160 mEq/l

MATCHING QUESTIONS

Match the following:

Column A	Column B
1. ____ sedative overdose	a. Respiratory acidosis
2. ____ hyperventilation	b. Metabolic acidosis
3. ____ diabetes mellitus	c. Respiratory alkalosis
4. ____ gastric suctioning	d. Metabolic alkalosis
5. ____ renal failure	

6. ____ pain

7. ____ vomiting

8. ____ emphysema

9. ____ flail chest

10. ____ diarrhea

MATCHING QUESTIONS

Match the following:

Column A	Column B
1. ____ sweet(acetone) odor to breath	a. Respiratory acidosis
2. ____ decreased rate and depth of respirations	b. Metabolic acidosis
3. ____ tetany	c. Respiratory alkalosis
4. ____ light-headedness	d. Metabolic alkalosis
5. ____ warm, flushed skin	
6. ____ increased respiratory rate and depth	
7. ____ headache	
8. ____ lethargy	
9. ____ tingling in the extremities	
10. ____ hyporeflexia	

FILL IN THE BLANKS

Fill in the blank spaces with the correct word or phrase to complete each statement.

1. The two general types of fluid imbalance are _______ and _______.
2. Cardiac tamponade is best diagnosed based on the results of a(n) _______.
3. PaO_2 below 60 mm Hg despite administration of oxygen at 10 l per minute would be expected in a client with _______.
4. Venous stasis, hypercoagulability, and venous endothelial disease are risk factors for _______.
5. When doing a gastric lavage on a client with an accidental poisoning, the gastric aspirate is saved to allow for a _______.

(continued)

6. The substance that plays the greatest role in holding fluid in the intravascular space is _______.

7. _____ is the predominant cation in the extracellular space.

8. A urine volume of <30 ml/hr and a urine specific gravity of >1.030 are suggestive of isotonic fluid volume _______.

9. Kayexalate is used in the treatment of _______.

10. Morphine is used in the treatment of cardiogenic shock for its effect in reducing _______.

APPLICATION QUESTIONS

1. Which is the most reliable indicator of cardiac arrest?
   a. Loss of consciousness
   b. Apnea of 4-minutes duration
   c. Inaudible blood pressure
   d. Absence of a palpable carotid pulse

2. Which intervention would be expected in the plan of care for a client with hypercalcemia?
   a. Fluid restriction
   b. Low-phosphate diet
   c. Lasix injection
   d. IV calcium gluconate

3. When teaching a client with hypokalemia secondary to decreased intake, which foods would be included in the dietary recommendations?
   a. Cashews and walnuts
   b. Spinach and broccoli
   c. Bananas and apricots
   d. Milk and yogurt

4. A client with which S&S is a candidate for artificial respiration?
   a. No heartbeat or measurable respiration
   b. Barely discernible respirations and a weak carotid pulse
   c. Absence of spontaneous ventilation and tachycardia
   d. Shallow gasping and apical heart rate of 48

5. In which situation would the nurse check Chvostek and Trousseau signs?
   a. Client complains of calf pain
   b. Client complains of headache and photophobia
   c. Client complains of weakness and dysphagia
   d. Client complains of tingling in the feet

6. Which type of treatment would be appropriate for a client with a serum potassium level of 3.3 mEq/l?
   a. Kayexalate
   b. IV sodium bicarbonate
   c. KCl
   d. Dialysis

7. A client has a temperature of 99.4 °F and a urine specific gravity of 1.035. Further assessment discloses poor skin turgor and flat neck veins. Which problem should the nurse suspect?
   a. Isotonic fluid volume deficit
   b. Hypo-osmolar overhydration
   c. Hyponatremia
   d. Hypokalemia

8. A client's laboratory reports show a serum potassium of 3.2 mEq/l. For which symptoms would the nurse assess the client?
   a. Hyperactive DTRs
   b. Flaccid paralysis
   c. Cardiac dysrhythmia
   d. Paresthesias in the extremities

9. A client presents expectorating pink-tinged, frothy respiratory secretions. The nurse would immediately gather additional assessment data related to the possibility of which disorder?
   a. Cardiac tamponade
   b. Pulmonary tuberculosis
   c. Pulmonary edema
   d. Bacterial pneumonia

10. Asking a client about amount and frequency of Alka-Seltzer use would be included in the assessment of a client with which problem?
   a. Hypermagnesemia
   b. Hypernatremia

c. Hypovolemia
d. Hypophosphatemia

11. It is calculated that a burn client needs 1800 ml of fluid in the first 24 hours in order to maintain blood volume and urinary output. How many ml would the nurse plan to infuse in the first 8 hours based on the Parkland formula?
a. 450
b. 600
c. 900
d. 1200

12. What does right upper quadrant pain that develops 48 hours after an overdose of aspirin indicate?
a. Diaphragmatic irritation
b. Lower esophageal ulceration
c. Biliary colic
d. Liver damage

13. When speaking to a group of junior high school students about first aid, the nurse explains there is a universal sign indicating choking and asks if any of the students knows what it is. Which student's response is correct?
a. Mouth open, index finger pointing in
b. Hand on neck over throat area
c. Hands crossed at the neck
d. Mouth open, index fingers pointing at each side of neck.

14. A client, 36 hours after an intestinal resection moves into a sitting position in bed and immediately tells the nurse "Something just 'gave way' under my dressing." On examination, the nurse discovers that the incision has dehisced and a loop of intestine is protruding. Which is the first action the nurse should take?
a. Notify the surgeon
b. Cover the protruding intestine with a sterile dressing wet with normal saline.
c. Assist the client to low Fowler's position.
d. Obtain a wound culture

15. How should the finding of mahogany-colored urine in a burned client be interpreted?
a. Muscle damage has occurred
b. Kidney failure is developing
c. Hemoglobin is being released from the spleen
d. Bladder mucosa has ulcerated

16. A client is admitted with a serum sodium of 128 mEq/l. Which order would the nurse question if it was written on the order sheet for this client?
a. High-protein, low-sodium diet.
b. Restrict fluids to 1500 ml/d
c. IV infusion of 5% NaCl
d. Daily electrolytes

17. Which S&S occurring in a client with burns are indicative of developing sepsis? Mark all that apply.
a. ___ Change in mental status
b. ___ Fever
c. ___ Tachypnea
d. ___ Bradycardia
e. ___ Hepatomegaly
f. ___ Abdominal distention
g. ___ Oliguria

18. Which is a priority goal of nursing care for a client with a burn during the first 48–72 hours after skin grafting?
a. Maintain range of motion
b. Ensure adequate caloric intake
c. Prevent displacement of the graft
d. Suppress an immune reaction

19. What is used as a guide to fluid resuscitation in a client with burns after the edema has resolved?
a. hourly urinary output
b. serum albumin and prealbumin
c. daily weight
d. serum and urinary electrolytes

20. Which client is at risk for metabolic acidosis?
a. A 17-year old with cystic fibrosis
b. A 35-year old pregnant woman
c. A 48-year old with hypoparathyroidism
d. A 65-year old with an ileostomy

21. A client with COPD complains of headache and a "racing" heart; he is also restless and somewhat confused. Which problem would the nurse suspect?
a. Respiratory acidosis
b. Respiratory alkalosis
c. Metabolic acidosis
d. Metabolic alkalosis

22. A 61-year-old client with a history of chronic renal failure is admitted with a possible appendicitis. Based on this history, which acid–base imbalance is most likely to be found when laboratory test results are assessed?
a. Respiratory acidosis
b. Respiratory alkalosis
c. Metabolic acidosis
d. Metabolic alkalosis

23. The plan of care for which client would involve monitoring for respiratory acidosis?
a. A 24-year old with Guillain-Barre syndrome
b. A 37-year old with pancreatic drainage

(continued)

c. A 50-year old who required a massive blood transfusion following a motor vehicle accident
d. A 70-year old with chronic congestive heart failure

24. Which intervention would the nurse expect to be ordered for a client with dehydration?
a. Isotonic IV fluid infusion
b. Hypotonic IV fluid infusion
c. Sodium restriction
d. Diuretic therapy

25. When evaluating fluid resuscitation for a 12-year-old child with a burn injury, which outcome would be one indicator that the client was receiving adequate fluid?
a. Urinary output of 3–5 ml/kg of body weight/hr
b. Normal mentation
c. pH of 7.25–7.35 and base excess of 8 or greater
d. Respiratory rate of 14–20

ANSWERS & RATIONALES

TRUE AND FALSE ANSWERS

Mark each of the following statements True or False. Correct all false statements in the space provided.

1. PEEP is used for clients with ARDS to keep alveoli distended, stretch stiff lungs, and increase oxygen-carbon dioxide diffusion. *True*

2. The burn client needs 2 or 4 ml of lactated Ringer's solution/normal saline per kg of body weight per percent of body surface burn in the first 24 hours to maintain blood volume and urinary output. *True*

3. When the rule of nines is used to calculate area of a burn, all body areas, which have been burned, are calculated into the formula. *False*
Only body surface areas that have partial or full-thickness burns are included; those with superficial thickness burns are not counted.

4. When performing the Hiemlich maneuver, the thumb side of fist is placed against the person's abdomen above the navel and below the xiphoid process. *True*

5. The fluid that lubricates the pleural space is intracellular fluid. *False*
It is transcellular fluid that is part of the extracellular fluid. Other examples of transcellular fluid are synovial, cerebrospinal, intraocular, pericardial, pancreatic, biliary, and peritoneal fluid.

6. An electrolyte imbalance associated with decreased aldosterone is hyponatremia. *True*

7. Administration of hypotonic IV solutions would be an expected part of therapy for a client with hypernatremia. *True*

8. The most common cause of septic shock is infection with gram-positive bacteria. *False*
The most common cause of septic shock is infection with gram-negative bacteria although it can be due to gram-positive as well as to viral, fungal, or parasitic infection.

9. Heparin is used prophylactically in the management of DIC because it blocks the coagulation cascade at the common pathway and ultimately prevents conversion of fibrinogen to fibrin. *True*

10. The first priority of the emergent phase of burn care is checking the airway. *False*
The first priority is to stop the burning; the next concern is airway followed by breathing and circulation.

MATCHING ANSWERS

Match the value in column B that is realistically consistent with the abnormality named in column A:

Column A	Column B
1. _m_ Hyponatremia	a. 1.2 mEq/l
2. _d_ Hypokalemia	b. 2.2 mEq/l
3. _a_ Hypomagnesemia	c. 3.2 mEq/l
4. _j_ Hypochloremia	d. 3.4 mEq/l
5. _g_ Hypocalcemia	e. 4.1 mEq/l
6. _o_ Hypernatremia	f. 5.4 mEq/l
7. _f_ Hyperkalemia	g. 8.2 mEq/l
8. _c_ Hypermagnesemia	h. 9.7 mEq/l
9. _l_ Hyperchloremia	i. 10.2 mEq/l
10. _i_ Hypercalcemia	j. 87 mEq/l
	k. 102 mEq/l
	l. 114 mEq/l
	m. 126 mEq/l
	n. 142 mEq/l
	o. 160 mEq/l

MATCHING ANSWERS

Match the following:

Column A	Column B
1. _a_ sedative overdose	a. Respiratory acidosis
2. _c_ hyperventilation	b. Metabolic acidosis
3. _b_ diabetes mellitus	c. Respiratory alkalosis

(continued)

4. __d__ gastric suctioning — d. Metabolic alkalosis

5. __b__ renal failure

6. __c__ pain

7. __d__ vomiting

8. __a__ emphysema

9. __a__ flail chest

10. __b__ diarrhea

MATCHING ANSWERS

Match the following:

Column A	Column B
2. __b__ sweet(acetone) odor to breath	a. Respiratory acidosis
2. __d__ decreased rate and depth of respirations	b. Metabolic acidosis
3. __c,d__ tetany	c. Respiratory alkalosis
4. __c__ light-headedness	d. Metabolic alkalosis
5. __b__ warm, flushed skin	
6. __b,c__ increased respiratory rate and depth	
7. __a__ headache	
8. __e,f__ lethargy	
9. __g__ tingling in the extremities	
10. __h__ hyporeflexia	

ANSWERS FOR FILL IN THE BLANKS

Fill in the blank spaces with the correct word or phrase to complete each statement.

1. The two general types of fluid imbalance are isotonic and osmolar.
2. Cardiac tamponade is best diagnosed based on the results of a(n) echocardiogram.

3. PaO_2 below 60 mm Hg despite administration of oxygen at 10 l per minute would be expected in a client with acute respiratory distress syndrome.

4. Venous stasis, hypercoagulability, and venous endothelial disease are risk factors for pulmonary embolism.

5. When doing a gastric lavage on a client with an accidental poisoning, the gastric aspirate is saved to allow for a toxicity screen.

6. The substance that plays the greatest role in holding fluid in the intravascular space is albumin.

7. Potassium is the predominant cation in the extracellular space.

8. A urine volume of <30 ml/hr and a urine specific gravity of >1.030 are suggestive of isotonic fluid volume excess.

9. KayExalate is used in the treatment of Hyperkalemia.

10. Morphine is used in the treatment of cardiogenic shock for its effect in reducing pre-load.

APPLICATION ANSWERS

1. Which is the most reliable indicator of cardiac arrest?
   a. Loss of consciousness
   b. Apnea of 4-minutes duration
   c. Inaudible blood pressure
   d. Absence of a palpable carotid pulse

Rationale

Correct answer: d.

Absence of a carotid pulse is a good indicator of cardiac arrest because it is the closest palpable artery to the heart so even a very weak pump can be felt. Loss of consciousness occurs for a variety of reasons—one of the most basic being lack of oxygen to the brain. Lack of oxygen to the brain does result from cardiac arrest but it also occurs from other factors including orthostatic hypotension and blockage or disruption of blood flow through the cerebral arteries. Apnea is not necessarily indicative of cardiac arrest. Cardiac arrest results in apnea or cessation of breathing and apnea, which causes a lack of oxygen, ultimately causes cardiac arrest. Inability to hear blood pressure is not a reliable indicator of cardiac arrest because when the heart pumps very weakly, blood pressure can become inaudible (may still be palpable).

2. Which intervention would be expected in the plan of care for a client with hypercalcemia?
   a. Fluid restriction
   b. Low-phosphate diet
   c. Lasix injection
   d. IV calcium gluconate

Rationale

Correct answer: c.

Lasix is a diuretic that increases calcium excretion. Fluid restriction is inappropriate. Low-phosphate diet is used for hypophosphatemia. IV calcium gluconate is given for the emergency management of hypocalcemia.

3. When teaching a client with hypokalemia secondary to decreased intake, which foods would be included in the dietary recommendations?
   a. Cashews and walnuts
   b. Spinach and broccoli
   c. Bananas and apricots
   d. Milk and yogurt

Rationale

Correct answer: c.

Bananas and apricots are good sources of potassium and therefore are recommended for clients who need to increase intake of potassium.

4. A client with which S&S is a candidate for artificial respiration?
   a. No heartbeat or measurable respiration
   b. Barely discernible respirations and a weak carotid pulse
   c. Absence of spontaneous ventilation and tachycardia
   d. Shallow gasping and apical heart rate of 48.

(continued)

Rationale

Correct answer: c.

Artificial respiration is used for clients who have no spontaneous respiration but whose hearts are still beating. Cardiopulmonary resuscitation is required for clients with neither heartbeat nor spontaneous ventilation. Artificial respiration is not done for clients who have spontaneous breathing. Neither is it done if there is no heartbeat.

5. In which situation would the nurse check Chvostek and Trousseau signs?
   a. Client complains of calf pain
   b. Client complains of headache and photophobia
   c. Client complains of weakness and dysphagia
   d. Client complains of tingling in the feet

Rationale

Correct answer: d.

Positive Chvostek and Trousseau signs are indicative of hypocalcemia that can lead to tetany. Tingling in the hands and feet is an early sign of hypocalcemia but can also have other causes. Chvostek and Trousseau are unrelated to complaints of calf pain, headache, photophobia, weakness, and dysphagia.

6. Which type of treatment would be appropriate for a client with a serum potassium level of 3.3 mEq/l?
   a. Kayexalate
   b. IV sodium bicarbonate
   c. KCl
   d. Dialysis

Rationale

Correct answer: c.

Normal serum potassium is 3.5 to 5.0 mEq/l so a client with a serum potassium of 3.3mEq/l is hypokalemic and needs potassium. Therefore, administration of KCl would be appropriate. Kayexalate and dialysis are used to remove potassium and IV sodium bicarbonate is given to alkalinize the plasma and cause a shift of potassium into the cells.

7. A client has a temperature of 99.4 °F and a urine specific gravity of 1.035. Further assessment discloses poor skin turgor and flat neck veins. Which problem should the nurse suspect?
   a. Isotonic fluid volume deficit
   b. Hypo-osmolar overhydration
   c. Hyponatremia
   d. Hypokalemia

Rationale

Correct answer: a.

Symptoms of isotonic fluid deficit are thirst, weakness, weight loss, decreased skin turgor, dry mucous membranes, sunken eyeballs, dry eyes, low-grade fever, weak rapid pulse, drop in blood pressure, orthostatic hypotension, flat neck veins, decreased capillary refill, decreased central venous pressure, decreased urine volume (<30 ml/hr), increased urine specific gravity (>1.030), increased hematocrit, and BUN. Hypo-osmolar overhydration causes impaired neurological function as a result of cerebral edema: confusion, convulsions, and coma. Symptoms of hyponatremia are lethargy, anorexia, N&V, and muscle cramps. Confusion, muscle twitching, convulsions, and coma occur with serum sodium of less than 120 mEq/l. Hypokalemia causes muscle weakness, cramps, anorexia, N&V, cardiac dysrhythmias, increased sensitivity to digoxin, lethargy, confusion, and decreased DTRs.

8. A client's laboratory reports show serum potassium of 3.2 mEq/l. For which symptoms would the nurse assess the client?
   a. Hyperactive DTRs
   b. Flaccid paralysis
   c. Cardiac dysrhythmia
   d. Paresthesias in the extremities

Rationale

Correct answer: c.

The range of normal for serum potassium is 3.5–5.0 mEq/l so 3.2 mEq/l is indicative of hypokalemia. Cardiac dysrhythmias occur with both hypokalemia and hyperkalemia. DTRs are hypoactive with hypokalemia not hyperactive. Muscle weakness occurs with hypokalemia but paralysis occurs with hyperkalemia. Paresthesias are a symptom of hyperkalemia.

9. A client presents expectorating pink-tinged, frothy respiratory secretions. The nurse would immediately gather additional assessment data related to the possibility of which disorder?
   a. Cardiac tamponade
   b. Pulmonary tuberculosis
   c. Pulmonary edema
   d. Bacterial pneumonia

Rationale

Correct answer: c.

A sign of pulmonary edema is the production of pink-tinged, frothy sputum. Cardiac tamponade is not characterized by any type of expectoration. Clients with tuberculosis first develop a slight cough productive of scant mucoid sputum. If cavitation develops, sputum becomes purulent and blood tinged. Bacterial pneumonia is characterized by the production of rust-colored sputum.

10. Asking a client about amount and frequency of Alka-Seltzer use would be included in the assessment of a client with which problem?
    a. Hypermagnesemia
    b. Hypernatremia
    c. Hypovolemia
    d. Hypophosphatemia

Rationale

Correct answer: b.

Alka-Seltzer is high in sodium and can be a source of high oral intake leading to hypernatremia.

11. It is calculeted that a burn client needs 1800 ml of fluid in the first 24 hours in order to maintain blood volume and urinary output. How many ml would the nurse plan to infuse in the first 8 hours based on the Parkland formula?
    a. 450
    b. 600
    c. 900
    d. 1200

Rationale

Correct answer: c.

One-half of the total fluid required in the first 24 hours is infused in the first 8 hours. One half of the total 1800 ml is 900 ml. The remaining half of the total is infused over the remaining 16 hours.

12. What does right upper quadrant pain that develops 48 hours after an overdose of aspirin indicate?
    a. Diaphragmatic irritation
    b. Lower esophageal ulceration
    c. Biliary colic
    d. Liver damage

Rationale

Correct answer: d.

Right upper quadrant pain due to liver damage is characteristic of the second phase of salicylate poisoning that occurs 24–48 hours after ingestion. Other symptoms of this phase are hepatomegaly, elevated bilirubin and hepatic enzymes, prolonged prothrombin time, and oliguria.

13. When speaking to a group of junior high school students about first aid, the nurse explains there is a universal sign indicating choking and asks if any of the students knows what it is. Which student's response is correct?
    a. Mouth open, index finger pointing in
    b. Hand on neck over throat area
    c. Hands crossed at the neck
    d. Mouth open, index fingers pointing at each side of neck

Rationale

Correct answer: c.

The universal sign indicating choking is hands crossed at the neck.

14. A client, 36 hours after an intestinal resection moves into a sitting position in bed and immediately tells the nurse "Something just 'gave way' under my dressing". On examination, the nurse discovers that the incision has dehisced and a loop of intestine is protruding. Which is the first action the nurse should take?
    a. Notify the surgeon
    b. Cover the protruding intestine with a sterile dressing wet with normal saline
    c. Assist the client to low Fowler's position
    d. Obtain a wound culture

Rationale

Correct answer: c.

A low Fowler's position takes stress off the suture line and prevents further disruption. The intestine is then protected with a sterile, wet with N/S dressing, and the surgeon notified.

15. How should the finding of mahogany-colored urine in a burned client be interpreted?
    a. Muscle damage has occurred
    b. Kidney failure is developing
    c. Hemoglobin is being released from the spleen
    d. Bladder mucosa has ulcerated

Rationale

Correct answer: a.

Muscle damage releases component chemicals that are excreted by the kidneys and turn the urine mahogany in color.

16. A client is admitted with serum sodium of 128 mEq/l. Which order would the nurse question if it was written on the order sheet for this client?
    a. High-protein, low-sodium diet
    b. Restrict fluids to 1500 ml/d
    c. IV infusion of 5% NaCl
    d. Daily electrolytes

Rationale

Correct answer: b.

The normal serum sodium range is 135–145 mEq/l so 128 mEq/l is low so it would not be appropriate to order a low-sodium diet because the client needs sodium. Restricting fluids would help equalize the proportions of sodium and water so the relative amount of sodium in the serum would increase. Infusing a hypertonic solution of 5% NaCl would increase sodium. Daily electrolytes would allow monitoring of electrolyte status.

(continued)

17. Which S&S occurring in a client with burns are indicative of developing sepsis? Mark all that apply.
    a. ___ Change in mental status
    b. ___ Fever
    c. ___ Tachypnea
    d. ___ Bradycardia
    e. ___ Hepatomegaly
    f. ___ Abdominal distention
    g. ___ Oliguria

Rationale

Correct answers: a, b, c, f, and g.
Tachycardia not bradycardia is a sign of developing sepsis. Hepatomegaly is unrelated to sepsis.

18. Which is a priority goal of nursing care for a client with a burn during the first 48–72 hours after skin grafting?
    a. Maintain range of motion.
    b. Ensure adequate caloric intake
    c. Prevent displacement of the graft
    d. Suppress an immune reaction

Rationale

Correct answer: c.
The graft must stay firmly in contact with the graft bed for the first 48–72 hours so immobilization devices such as bulky dressings or splints are left intact for that period of time and when dressings are removed, they are removed slowly and gently.

19. What is used as a guide to fluid resuscitation in a client with burns after the edema has resolved?
    a. Hourly urinary output
    b. Serum albumin and prealbumin
    c. Daily weight
    d. Serum and urinary electrolytes

Rationale

Correct answer: d.
Serum and urinary electrolyte levels are used to guide fluid administration after edema begins to resolve 48–72 hours after the burn injury occurs. Until that time, urinary output is used as a guide to fluid resuscitation. Serum albumin and prealbumin are measures of nutritional status. Daily weight is a measure of fluid retention or loss.

20. Which client is at risk for metabolic acidosis?
    a. A 17-year old with cystic fibrosis
    b. A 35-year old pregnant woman
    c. A 48-year old with hypoparathyroidism
    d. A 65-year old with an ileostomy

Rationale

Correct answer: d.
Ileostomy drainage places a client at risk for metabolic acidosis. Risk associated with cystic fibrosis is for respiratory acidosis. Risk associated with pregnancy is for respiratory alkalosis. Hypoparathyroidism is a risk factor for metabolic alkalosis.

21. A client with COPD complains of headache and a "racing" heart; he is also restless and somewhat confused. Which problem would the nurse suspect?
    a. Respiratory acidosis
    b. Respiratory alkalosis
    c. Metabolic acidosis
    d. Metabolic alkalosis

Rationale

Correct answer: a.
Headache, tachycardia, restlessness, and confusion are S&S of respiratory acidosis for which a client with COPD is at risk. Other S&S include dyspnea, tachypnea, diaphoresis, and anxiety progressing to lethargy, ventricular dysrhythmia, dilated facial and conjunctival blood vessels, cyanosis, and coma.

22. A 61-year-old client with a history of chronic renal failure is admitted with a possible appendicitis. Based on this history which acid–base imbalance is most likely to be found when laboratory test results are assessed?
    a. Respiratory acidosis
    b. Respiratory alkalosis
    c. Metabolic acidosis
    d. Metabolic alkalosis

Rationale

Correct answer: c.
Chronic renal failure is the most common cause of chronic metabolic acidosis.

23. The plan of care for which client would involve monitoring for respiratory acidosis?
    a. A 24-year old with Guillain-Barre syndrome
    b. A 37-year old with pancreatic drainage
    c. A 50-year old who required a massive blood transfusion following a motor vehicle accident
    d. A 70-year old with chronic congestive heart failure

Rationale

Correct answer: a.
Guillain-Barre syndrome because it can affect the muscles of respiration decreasing alveolar ventilation, results in the retention of carbon dioxide, which leads to respiratory acidosis. Pancreatic drainage places the client at risk for metabolic acidosis because of the loss of base. Massive blood transfusion is a risk factor for metabolic alkalosis and CHF is a risk factor for respiratory alkalosis.

24. Which intervention would the nurse expect to be ordered for a client with dehydration?
    a. Isotonic IV fluid infusion
    b. Hypotonic IV fluid infusion

c. Sodium restriction
d. Diuretic therapy

Rationale

Correct answer: b.

A hypotonic solution such as 0.95 sodium chloride solution would be given as dehydration is a hyperosmolar imbalance in which water is lost in excess of sodium. Isotonic IV infusions are used in the treatment of hypovolemia.

25. When evaluating fluid resuscitation for a 12-year-old child with a burn injury, which outcome would be one indicator that the client was receiving adequate fluid?
    a. Urinary output of 3–5 ml/kg of body weight/hr
    b. Normal mentation
    c. pH of 7.25–7.35 and base excess of 8 or greater
    d. Respiratory rate of 14–20

Rationale

Correct answer: b.

One indicator of adequate fluid resuscitation is normal mentation. Other indicators of adequate fluid include urinary output of 30–50 ml/hr or 1–2 ml/kg of body weight/hr in children; and a pH of 7.35–7.45 and base excess of 6 or greater.

Test Plan Category:

Physiological Integrity

Sub-category: Physiological Adaptation—Part 2

Topic: Infectious Diseases

INFECTIOUS DISEASES

GONORRHEA

- Sexually transmitted infection with *Neisseria gonorrhoeae*, a gram-negative *Diplococcus*
- One of the most common STIs
- Over 1 million cases are reported in the United States each year
- Major cause of PID, tubal infertility, ectopic pregnancy, and chronic pelvic pain

- If untreated, it may cause severe disseminated infection: arthritis, dermatitis, pericarditis, endocarditis, and meningitis
- If a pregnant woman is affected, stillbirth, neonatal death, and premature labor can occur
- Infants born to infected mothers may experience prematurity, conjunctivitis, and pneumonia

Etiology: Localized, sexually transmitted infection affecting urethra, endocervix, and/or rectum.

Risk factors: Young, sexually active, multiple sexual partners.

S&S:

- Asymptomatic to mildly symptomatic (50% of women with gonorrhea have no symptoms)
- Dysuria
- Urinary frequency
- Cervical discharge
- Conjunctivitis

Dx:

- Endocervical, oral, or rectal cultures
- Gram stain

Rx:

- Ceftriaxone 125 mg, IM and Cefixime 400 mg p.o.
- Partners must also be treated

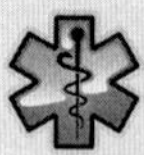

Clinical Alert

Clients who present having been sexually assaulted should be treated prophylactically; repeat cultures should be done in 2 weeks.

Nursing Process Elements

- Assist client in assessing risk for STIs
- Discuss safer sexual practices
- Help clients develop communication skills to initiate discussions with their partners

Client teaching for self-care

- Encourage client to initiate discussions about sex with their partners
- Reinforce the need for client to abstain from sexual intercourse until after all sexual partners are treated
- Reinforce the need for annual screening for STIs

CHLAMYDIA

- Sexually transmitted infection with *Chlamydia trachomatis*
- Most common STI
- An estimated 3–4 million cases occur annually in the United States
- Most commonly found in young, sexually active people with more than one partner
- Up to 40% of untreated women develop PID

OB Increases risk for ectopic pregnancy and infertility

- Chlamydia and gonorrhea often coexist

OB An estimated 30% of pregnant women are affected

Etiology: Sexually transmitted infection.

Predisposing factors: Young, sexually active people with multiple sexual partners; nonbarrier contraceptive methods

S&S:

- Chlamydial infections of the cervix often produce no symptoms
- Cervical discharge
- Dyspareunia
- Dysuria
- Bleeding (friable cervix)
- Conjunctivitis
- Perihepatitis
- Postpartum endometritis

OB If a pregnant woman is affected, stillbirth, neonatal death, or premature birth may occur

- Infants born to infected mothers may experience prematurity, conjunctivitis, and pneumonia

Dx:

- Tissue culture
- Endocervical and urethral culture

Rx:

- Erythromycin or amoxicillin (when pregnant)
- Doxycycline (postpartum)
- Tetracycline (nonpregnant)
- Erythromycin ophthalmic ointment for newborn
- Partners must also be treated

Nursing Process Elements

- Assist client in assessing risk of STIs
- Discuss safer sexual practices
- Help client develop communication skills to initiate discussion with her partners

Client teaching for self-care

- Repeat testing needs to be done 2 weeks posttreatment (test of cure)
- Importance of abstaining from sexual intercourse until all sexual partners have been treated
- Importance of using condoms with all new or noninfected partners
- Annual routine gynecological care, including a PAP test and testing for STIs

SYPHILIS

- Complex, curable sexually transmitted bacterial infection caused by the spirochete *Treponema pallidum*
- Leads to disability and death if left untreated

OB Fetal/neonatal effects: stillbirth, developmental delay, seizures, or neonatal death, symptoms of infection may not be present at birth but develop in a few weeks.

Etiology: Sexually transmitted infection.

Predisposing factors: Young adults, multiple sex partners, inadequate knowledge of transmission and prevention, and unprotected sex.

S&S:

- Divided into primary, secondary, and tertiary stages of infection
  - —Primary: the first sign of primary syphilis is a painless chancre that develops on the genitalia, anus, lips, or in the oral cavity; if untreated, the chancre heals within 6 weeks; the disease is highly infectious during the primary phase.
  - —Secondary: although the chancre disappears, the spirochete lives and is carried by the blood to all parts of the body; about 2 months after the initial infection, symptoms of secondary syphilis appear, which include enlargement of the liver and spleen, headache, anorexia, and a generalized maculopapular skin rash; if left untreated, the disease enters a latent phase that may last several years.
  - —Tertiary: may have heart, blood vessel, and nervous system involvement; general paralysis and psychosis may result.

Dx:

- Primary stage: dark-field microscopy from sample scraped from the base of the chancre; serologic tests are usually negative at this time
- Secondary stage: serologic (VDRL) tests are positive at this time; the rapid plasma regain (RPR) and fluorescent treponemal antibody absorption (FTA-ABS) tests are more specific and are often done to confirm a positive test of VDRL

Rx:

- Best treatment for all stages is with penicillin; doxycycline can be used if client is allergic to penicillin
- Reevaluation should be done at 6 and at 12-month posttreatment

Nursing Process Elements

- Assist client in identifying STI preventive measures that are compatible with age, language, male–female relationships within the client's culture
- Teach the S&S that require medical care
- Refer to support groups

Client teaching for self-care

- Importance of abstaining from sexual intercourse during the prodromal period when lesions are present
- Use of condoms with all new or noninfected partners
- All partners must be treated in order to prevent reinfection
- Comfort measures such as wearing nonconstricting clothing, wearing cotton underwear, taking Sitz baths, and air-drying lesions
- Need for strict hand washing with soap and water
- Importance of returning for follow-up care

HERPES

- Herpes simplex virus (HSV) is an enveloped, double-stranded DNA virus that occurs in two forms: herpes simplex type 1 and type 2
- HSV-1 is transmitted via oral and respiratory secretions; HSV-2 is transmitted via sexual contact
- Transmission is more likely to occur from men to women

Etiology: Herpes simplex virus.

Risk factors: Female sex. African-American ethnic background, Mexican-American ethnic background, older age, poverty, low educational level, cocaine use, multiple sexual partners, unprotected sex, and having a sexual partner with genital herpes.

S&S:

- Painful genital vesicular lesions
- Vesicles can be on cervix, vagina, or external genitalia
- Primary infection is commonly associated with fever, malaise, myalgia; numbness, tingling, burning, itching, redness, swelling, and pain with lesions; urinary retention; lymphadenopathy

Dx:

- Tissue culture (swab specimen from vesicles)
- Immunofluorescent staining of the cell can differentiate HSV-1 from HSV-2

Rx:

- Currently no cure for HSV-2 infection
- Treatment aimed at relieving symptoms
- Acyclovir (Zovirax), valacyclovir (Valtrex), and famciclovir (Famvir)—antiviral agents used to suppress symptoms and shorten the course of infection

OB In pregnant women, acyclovir has been used near date of expected delivery to suppress outbreak

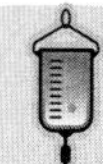

Clinical Alert

OB If a pregnant woman presents to deliver and has active lesions, delivery by cesarean section is the current standard of care because herpes can cause potentially fatal infection in newborns.

Nursing Process Elements

- Listen to client's concerns to reduce anxiety
- Client may need assistance and support in discussing the infection and its implications with partner(s)
- Provide information and instruction
- Encourage use of analgesics as ordered
- Encourage proper hygiene practices (especially hand washing with soap and water)
- Encourage use of Sitz baths for comfort
- Encourage use of clean, soft, loose fitting, and absorbent clothing
- Discourage use of powders, lotions, and occlusive ointments because they prevent lesions from drying
- Encourage client to avoid stress, sunburn, and other stress-producing situations, which can precipitate an outbreak
- Discomfort with urination can be reduced by pouring water over the vulva during voiding
- When oral antiviral agents are taken, client needs to know when to take medication and to alert provider to side effects such as headache and/or rash

Client teaching for self-care

- Disease process:
  —Herpes is transmitted by direct sexual contact
  —Abstinence from sex is required for a brief period during treatment
  —Intercourse during a herpes outbreak not only increases the risk of transmission but also increases the likelihood of contracting HIV and other STIs; makes HIV more infective
  —Transmission is possible even in the absence of lesions
  —Condoms may provide some protection against viral transmission
  —Control of the condition may require a change in sexual behavior and medication use
- Appropriate hygiene practices
- Practices to avoid self-infection
- Health promotion activities such as eating a well-balanced diet, avoiding stress, and getting enough rest
- Importance of taking medications as prescribed, keeping follow-up appointments, and informing health care provider when outbreaks occur
- Support groups and the possible benefits of joining a group where experiences and solutions can be shared

HIV/AIDS

- Human immunodeficiency virus (HIV-1) is a retrovirus transmitted by contact with infected blood or body fluids
- HIV infection may cause acquired immunodeficiency syndrome (AIDS)
- AIDS is the fifth leading cause of death in American women aged 25–44 years; black and Hispanic women make up three-fourth of that statistic
- Women and men are much more likely to get HIV from men than from women
- Heterosexual transmission accounts for the majority of all new cases of HIV in women

OB Seropositive women can transmit HIV to their fetuses across the placenta, at birth when the infant is exposed to maternal blood and vaginal secretions and after birth by breast milk.

Etiology:

- Infection by the HIV retrovirus that affects helper T cells bearing the $CD4^+$ antigen.
- Through the action of reverse transcriptase, HIV produces DNA from its viral RNA. The viral DNA enters the nuclei of affected cells and is incorporated into their DNA, where it's transcribed into more viral RNA. If the host (affected) cells reproduce, the HIV DNA is duplicated along with their own DNA and it is passed on to the daughter cells.
- When activated, host cells replicate the virus. The virus buds out of the cell membrane and emerges from the host cell free to infect other cells.
- HIV replication may lead to cell death or the virus may become latent.
- HIV infection causes pathological effects in two ways: directly through destruction of $CD4^+$ cells, other immune

cells, and/or neuroglial cells, or indirectly through the effects of $CD4^+$ T-cell dysfunction and resulting immunosuppression

Risk factors/at-risk populations: Homosexual or bisexual men, IV drug users, women who exchange sex for drugs, recipients of contaminated blood or blood products, heterosexual partners of those in high-risk groups, neonates of infected women, females in age group 25–44 years old, women who have anal intercourse, unprotected sex, and intercourse during menses

S&S:

- Latency phase: mononucleosis-like syndrome, which may be attributed to flu or another virus; followed by an asymptomatic period which may last for years.
- Symptomatic phase: persistent generalized lymphadenopathy; nonspecific symptoms including weight loss, fatigue, night sweats; fevers related to altered function of $CD4^+$ cells, immunodeficiency, and infection of other $CD4^+$ antigen-bearing cells; neurologic symptoms; opportunistic infections (see Table 32–1); cancer

PEDS

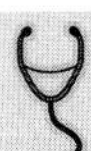

Assessment Alert

HIV/AIDS in children are often manifested by failure to thrive and developmental delays. The child may have recurrent oral candidiasis and chronic diarrhea.

Dx:

- Laboratory studies reveal $CD4^+$ T cell count less than 200 cells per μl and the presence of HIV antibodies
- T cell subsets CD4 and CD8 counts and ratios stage the infection and establish a prognosis.
- Antibody assay tests (ELISA, Western blot, rapid tests including oral fluid HIV-1 antibody test that can be done on plasma or oral fluid obtained by swabbing around gums) take 3 weeks to 3–6 months to be positive after exposure because the body has to have time to produce antibodies to the virus. "Window period": time between exposure and the presence of detectable antibodies.

OB At birth, the infant may have a positive antibody titer as maternal antibodies readily cross the placenta. This does not indicate HIV infection.

PEDS The ELISA and Western blot immunoassay are used to determine HIV infection in children. Infants born to HIV-positive mothers will have positive results due to the presence of maternal antibodies that have crossed the placenta. These antibodies may persist until the child is 18-months old so antibody testing is unreliable until after this age. HIV polymerase chain reaction (PCR) can detect the infection allowing diagnosis by the time the infant is 1-month old.

Rx:

- Protease inhibitors, nucleoside reverse transcriptase inhibitors, and nonnucleoside reverse transcriptase inhibitors
- Highly active antiretroviral therapy (HAART) "cocktail"—combination of a protease inhibitor and two reverse transcriptase inhibitors, which interrupt HIV replication at different places in the cycle, e.g., Laminvudine, Zidovudine, and Nelfinavir
- Additional treatments may include immunomodulatory agents; human granulocyte colony-stimulating growth factor; anti-infective and antineoplastic agents; nutritional support; fluid and electrolyte replacement therapy; treatment of opportunistic infections (See Table 32-1)

OB All pregnant women should be given ZDV orally starting at 14-weeks gestation and continued through pregnancy, intravenously during labor, and to the newborn for the first 6 weeks of life (reduces the risk of maternal–newborn transmission by 66%)

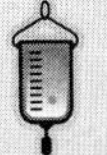

Clinical Alert

Viral load—amount of virus in the serum; measured by Plasma HIV RNA. Used to monitor disease progression and response to antiretroviral therapy.

OB The risk of teratogenic effects of the HIV medications are not known at this time. Some HIV-positive pregnant women choose to suspend therapy during the first 3 months of pregnancy.

OB Although this is a high-risk pregnancy, invasive procedures such as amniocentesis are avoided if possible to reduce the risk of contamination of the fetus. Noninvasive procedures such as nonstress testing and serial ultrasounds are performed at a more frequent rate.

PEDS The child with HIV/AIDS should receive the normal immunizations recommended for all children. Attenuated live virus can be administered when there is no evidence of severe immunocompromise. Children receiving active intravenous gamma globulins (IVIG) may not develop full immunity due to the presence of passive antibodies.

Table 32–1 Common Opportunistic Infections Associated with AIDS

Type of Infection	S&S	Treatment	Comments
M. avian complex (MAC) (bacterial infection)	High fever, night sweats, fatigue, anorexia, weight loss, abdominal pain, diarrhea, enlarged lymph nodes, liver, and spleen.	Prophylaxis: Azithromycin or clarithromycin Rx: Antimycobacterial agents	Most common opportunistic infection in AIDS clients.
Mycobacterium tuberculosis	See TB in Chapter 21	See TB in Chapter 21	Annual PPD needed if HIV positive.
Candidiasis—oral, rectal, vaginal (fungal disease)	White, curd-like patches on erythematous mucous membrane, itching and irritation. White, cheesy vaginal drainage.	Fluconazole, ketoconazole	No prophylaxis given—if client has chronic esophageal infection may be on long-term suppressive therapy.
Disseminated candidiasis	High fever, chills, and hypotension..	Amphotericin B may be needed.	
Cryptococcosis (fungal disease)	Most effects on lungs and CNS: dyspnea, cough, chest discomfort, fever, headache, blurred vision, dizziness, loss of memory,, irritability, fatigue, N&V, and convulsions.	Amphotericin B—primary prophylaxis and long-term suppressive therapy with Fluconazole if CD4 cell counts are less than 50 cells/mm^3.	Dx: fungus in CSF or blood. Source of fungus: pigeon droppings.
Histoplasmosis (fungal infection)	Acute pulmonary symptoms or disseminated disease that is fatal if not treated effectively.	Amphotricin B or fluconazole	Prophylaxis with Itraconazole if CD4 cell count less than 100 cells/mm^3.
Cryptosporidium (protozoan infection)	GI infection: fever, N&V, abdominal pain, cramps, severe watery diarrhea, fluid and electrolyte imbalances, and malnutrition.	No effective cure. Reduce stool volume, decrease peristalsis, and relieve pain.	
Pneumocystis carinii (protozoan infection)	Primarily causes pneumonia: dyspnea on exertion, nonproductive cough, productive cough. Arterial O_2 tension less than 70 mmHg, low respiratory diffusing capacity, or increased alveolar—arterial oxygen tension gradient; no evidence of bacterial pneumonia.	IV pentamidine isethionate or IV or PO or PO trimethoprim-sulfamethoxazole.	Without treatment leads to respiratory insufficiency and death.
Toxoplasma gondii	Encephalitis in AIDS clients: headache, confusion, fever, vomiting, hemiparesis, loss of vision, and seizures.	trimethoprim-sulfamethoxazole (TMP-SMX).	
CMV	Retinitis common in AIDS clients.	Ganciclovir	See individual sections on CMV and Herpes in this chapter
Herpes simplex type 1 and 2	Disseminated effects brain, liver, and lungs.	Acyclovir	

Nursing Process Elements

- Assess for risk factors and S&S of HIV disease
- Assess nutritional status that ranges from normal early in disease to extreme cachexia: weight, appetite, stomatitis, dysphagia, and food tolerance
- Assess fatigue level and ability to perform ADLs

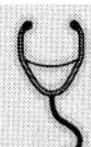

Assessment Alert

Assess carefully persons already infected with HIV for signs of opportunistic infection since opportunistic infections are the major complications of HIV disease.

- Protect clients with AIDS from exposure to other infection
- Promote recognition and discussion of feelings; recognize that clients often are angry or guilty about the diagnosis
- Provide access to counseling for client and partner
- Provide appropriate information to enable informed decisions about care and lifestyle
- For nausea, suggest dry crackers and a beverage half hour before meals; antiemetics if needed.
- Provide high-calorie, high-protein diet divided into six small meals if anorexic or difficulty eating.
- See nutrition section in Chapter 13—for other interventions to support nutrition
- Encourage 8 hours of sleep a night; rest periods as needed during the day; and provide assistance as needed
- Recommend use of appropriate assistive devices

Client teaching for self-care

- For the uninfected, focus on prevention of contracting the virus; for the infected, focus on ways of preventing transmission of the virus
- Provide factual information and correct misconceptions related to diagnosis
- Importance of routine screening
- Safe sexual practices including consistent use of condoms
- Importance of regular follow-up care
- Importance of taking medications as prescribed

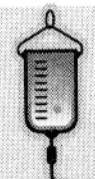

Clinical Alert

Health care workers are at increased risk of exposure to HIV. It is critical that health care workers adhere to protective guidelines meticulously and follow through with postexposure procedures. Basic postexposure procedures are as follows:

- Wash wounds thoroughly with soap and water and irrigate with disinfectant solution; irrigate eyes with water or sterile saline; rinse mucous membranes with water.
- Obtain baseline laboratory tests including serologies.
- Have follow-up testing every 3 months for a year.

PEDS ROSEOLA (EXANTHEM SUBITUM)

Etiology: Human herpes virus type 6 infection.

- At-risk population: children 6 months to 3 years of age
- Incubation period: 5–15 days

S&S: Persistent high fever in apparently well child for 2–3 days; when fever drops nonpruritic, rosy macular rash that fades with pressure appears on trunk and spreads to neck, face, and extremities, and lasts 2–3 days; enlarged cervical and postauricular lymph nodes, cough, pharyngitis, and coryza.

Complications: Febrile seizures.

Rx: Antipyretics for fever.

Nursing Process Elements

- No isolation

Client teaching for self-care

- Measures to control fever
- Febrile seizure precautions if child is at risk

FIFTH DISEASE (ERYTHEMA INFECTIOSUM)

Etiology: Human parvovirus B19 infection from infected person.

- Incubation period: 4–21 days

S&S: Rash occurring in three distinct phases: erythema on cheeks giving an appearance of a "slapped face" lasting 1–4 days; followed in 24 hours by a maculopapular, symmetrical rash, which develops proximally to distally on upper and lower extremities and lasts a week or more. The rash then subsides but reappears if skin is exposed to sun, heat, cold, friction, or other irritant.

Complications: Self-limited arthritis and arthralgia, aplastic crisis in immunosuppressed clients or those with hemolytic disease.

Rx: Antipyretics, analgesics, and anti-inflammatories.

Nursing Process Elements

- Respiratory isolation for hospitalized immunosuppressed child or child with aplastic crisis; otherwise isolation not needed

CHICKEN POX (VARICELLA)

Etiology: Varicella zoster virus infection from direct contact with respiratory secretions or skin lesions of infected persons, from droplet spread or contaminated objects. Communicable 24 hours before rash appears to days after; incubation period: 2–3 weeks.

S&S: Low-grade fever, malaise, and anorexia for 24 hours followed by a severely itchy rash that goes through stages of macule, papule, vesicle, and crust, and begins on the trunk and spreads to face and extremities, enlarged lymph nodes.

Complications: Bacterial infection in skin, pneumonia, and encephalitis.

Rx: Acyclovir (Zovirax); varicella zoster immunoglobulin after exposure for high-risk cliemts; antihistamines or diphenhydramine hydrochloride for itch.

Nursing Process Elements

- Isolation of hospitalized children; isolate at home until vesicles have dried; isolate high-risk children from infected children
- Prevent scratching and risk of secondary infection
  —Give soothing baths
  —Apply calamine lotion
  —Keep child's fingernails short and smooth
  —Put mittens on child
  —Keep child cool
  —Keep child occupied
  —Remove loose crusts
  —Teach child to put pressure on itchy areas rather than scratching
- Do not give aspirin because of risk of Reye's syndrome

MEASLES (RUBEOLA)

Etiology: Viral infection from direct contact with droplets of respiratory secretions, blood or urine of infected person

- Communicable mainly during prodromal period but also 5 days after rash appears; incubation period: 10–20 days

S&S: Fever, malaise, cough, coryza, conjunctivitis, Koplik spots (small, irregular, red spots with a pinpoint blue—white center on oral mucosa opposite molars), red maculopapular rash that starts on face and spreads down over body appearing confluent on upper body and more discrete on lower; turns brownish in 3–4 days and is followed by fine desquamation, anorexia, and generalized lymphadenopathy.

Complications: Otitis media, pneumonia, bronchiolitis, obstructive laryngitis, and encephalitis.

Rx: Supportive care; antipyretics for fever; antibiotics for those at high risk of secondary infection.

Nursing Process Elements

- Respiratory isolation if hospitalized
- Isolation until fifth day of rash at home
- Bed rest while febrile
- Dim lights if photophobia is a problem
- Keep child from rubbing eyes
- Monitor for signs of corneal ulceration
- Use cool mist vaporizer
- Lubricate skin around nares

GERMAN MEASLES (RUBELLA)

Etiology: Rubella virus infection contracted through direct contact with nose or throat secretions of symptomatic or nonsymptomatic infected person, droplet airborne transmission, or indirect contact with articles freshly soiled with secretions from the nose or throat and is communicable for about a week before and 5 days after appearance of rash. Incubation period: 14–21 days.

S&S: Low-grade fever, headache, malaise, anorexia, mild conjunctivitis, coryza, sore throat, cough, lymphadenopathy followed in 1–5 days by discrete, rosy, maculopapular rash which starts on the face and spreads rapidly down over body. Rash disappears in same order it developed and is usually gone in 3 days.

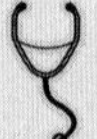

Assessment Alert

PEDS Children exhibit no symptoms before onset of rash.

Complications: Rare.

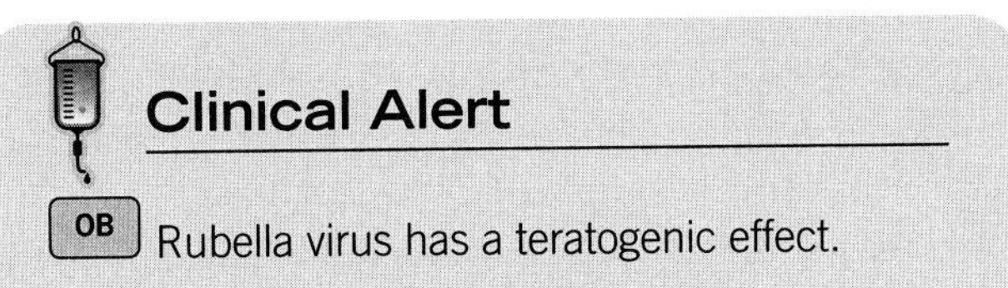

Clinical Alert
OB Rubella virus has a teratogenic effect.

Rx: No specific treatment; antipyretics for fever; and analgesics for discomfort.

Nursing Process Elements

- Provide comfort measures
- Assess knowledge of the disease and immunization

Client teaching for self-care

OB Isolate from pregnant women because of teratogenic effect

MUMPS

Etiology: Paramyxovirus from saliva of infected persons transmitted by direct contact or droplet spread. Communicable from just before to just after swelling begins. Incubation period: 14–21 days.

S&S: Malaise, headache, fever followed in 24 hours by an earache aggravated by chewing; swelling and tenderness of one or both parotid glands by the end of 72 hours.

Complications: Sensorineural deafness, encephalitis, myocarditis, arthritis, hepatitis, epididymo-orchitis with or without sterility, and meningitis.

Rx: Analgesics and antipyretics.

Nursing Process Elements

- Isolation and respiratory precautions if hospitalized
- Isolate at home during communicable stage
- Bed rest until swelling subsides
- Provide soft, bland foods
- Encourage fluids
- Apply hot or cold compresses to swollen parotids for comfort

POLIOMYELITIS

- Poliomyelitis occurs as following three distinct disease forms:
  —Abortive or inapparent
  —Nonparalytic
  —Paralytic

Etiology: Enterovirus type 1 (most often causes paralysis), 2, or 3 (least often causes paralysis) infection contracted by direct contact with oropharyngeal secretions or feces of symptomatic or nonsymptomatic infected persons. Incubation period: 5–35 days.

S&S:

- Abortive disease: fever, sore throat, headache, anorexia, vomiting, abdominal pain for a few hours or days
- Nonparalytic disease: pain and stiffness in neck, back, and legs along with above symptoms in more severe form.
- Paralytic: symptoms of nonparalytic, recovery, then onset of CNS paralysis

Complications: Respiratory arrest, hypertension, and renal calculi from immobilization.

Rx: No specific treatment. Supportive care including mechanical ventilation and physical care, sedatives, and analgesics according to individual needs.

Nursing Process Elements

- Maintain complete bed rest during acute phase
- Monitor for signs of respiratory paralysis: difficulty talking, ineffective cough, inability to hold breath, shallow, and rapid respirations
- Keep tracheostomy tray at the bedside
- Maintain good body alignment
- ROM and footboard to prevent contractures

SEVERE ACUTE RESPIRATORY SYNDROME (SARS)

Etiology: Infection with SARS-associated coronavirus (SARS-CoV), which is spread by respiratory droplets or by touching contaminated objects and then touching own eyes, nose, or mouth.

S&S: Onset: high fever (temperature greater than 100.4°F [>38.0°C]), headache, overall discomfort and aching, occasional mild respiratory symptoms, diarrhea; dry cough after 2–7 days progressing to pneumonia in most clients.

Rx: No effective drug therapy available; symptomatic, supportive treatment may include antiviral medications (such as ribavirin), antibiotics, steroids, IV fluids, and ventilatory assistance.

Nursing Process Elements

- Maintain contact and airborne isolation precautions for persons with SARS or a high suspicion thereof

- Promote respiratory hygiene and coughing/sneezing etiquette among all clients
  - —Provide tissues and hands-free container for disposal of used tissues
  - —Provide accessible alcohol-based hand cleanser
  - —Provide soap and disposable towels for hand washing where sinks are available
- Provide mask for clients with symptoms of a respiratory infection and make them sit apart from other clients in waiting areas
- Use droplet precautions in addition to standard precautions when examining clients with symptoms of respiratory infection

Client teaching for self-care

- Cover mouth when coughing or sneezing
- Use tissues and dispose of in nearest disposal container
- Wash hands after touching respiratory secretions or objects contaminated with them

EASTERN EQUINE ENCEPHALITIS (EEE)

Etiology: Mosquito-borne viral disease

- Occurs in eastern half of the United States
- Incubation period: 3–10 days
- Over age 50 and younger than 15 at greatest risk
- Working or playing outdoors in endemic areas places people at risk

S&S: Many persons who are infected with the virus develop no apparent illness. In those who do develop illness, symptoms range from mild and flu-like to full-blown encephalitis, coma, and death in about one-third of those affected. (See Chapter 22 for S&S of encephalitis.)

Complications: Mild to severe permanent neurologic damage in about 50% of survivors.

Rx: No specific treatment; hospitalization and supportive care, e.g., respiratory support, prevention of secondary bacterial infections, and physical therapy, depending on individual need.

Nursing Process Elements

- Assess for signs and symptoms of complications

Client teaching for self-care

Avoid mosquito bites

- Use an EPA-registered repellent according to manufacturers' instructions
- Wear protective clothing
- Avoid outdoor activity during peak mosquito-biting hours (dusk to dawn) if possible; if not, use double protection: wear long sleeves, and spray repellent directly onto clothes
- Do not apply repellents containing permethrin directly to skin
- Do not spray repellent on the skin under clothing
- Remove standing water that can provide mosquito breeding sites
  - —At least once or twice a week, empty water from flowerpots, pet food, and water dishes, birdbaths, swimming pool covers, buckets, barrels, and cans
  - —Check for clogged rain gutters and clean them out
  - —Remove discarded tires and other items that could collect water
  - —Be sure to check for containers or trash in places that may be hard to see such as under bushes or under your home

WEST NILE VIRUS

Etiology: Infection with West Nile virus from bite of an infected mosquito.

S&S:

- Many infected persons develop no symptoms; about 20% develop mild symptoms and less than 1% develop severe symptoms
- Mild: fever, headache, and body aches, nausea, vomiting, occasional swollen lymph glands or rash on chest, stomach, and back
- Severe: high fever, headache, neck stiffness, stupor, disorientation, coma, tremors, convulsions, muscle weakness, vision loss, numbness, and paralysis
- May last days to several weeks

Complications: Neurological effects may be permanent

Rx: No specific treatment; hospitalization with supportive treatment with IV fluids and ventilatory assistance for severe symptoms.

Nursing Process Elements

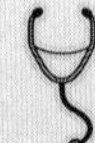

Assessment Alert

People over the age of 50 are more likely to develop serious symptoms.

Client teaching for self-care

- Prevention of mosquito bites (See section EEE.)

RABIES

- Rabies occurs primarily in wild animals like raccoons, skunks, bats, and foxes.
- It can affect domestic animals such as cats, cattle, and dogs.
- It infects the CNS causing encephalopathy and death

S&S: Fever, headache, and general malaise followed by neurological symptoms such as insomnia, anxiety, confusion, slight or partial paralysis, excitation, hallucinations, agitation, hypersalivation, difficulty swallowing, and hydrophobia (fear of water); death usually occurring in few days.

Dx: No single diagnostic test; saliva is tested for virus; serum and spinal fluid are tested for antibodies to the rabies virus; and skin biopsies of hair follicles at the nape of the neck are tested for rabies antigen.

Rx:

- No treatment after symptoms appear
- Rabies vaccine regimen provides immunity when administered after an animal bite or mucous membrane contamination with infectious material such as saliva (postexposure prophylaxis [PEP]) or for protection (preexposure prophylaxis)
- Preexposure prophylaxis: three doses of vaccine given on days 0, 7, and 21 or 28
- PEP begins as soon as possible after exposure: one dose of immunoglobulin and five doses of rabies vaccine over a 28-day period (days 3, 7, 14, and 28 after the first vaccination)

CYTOMEGALOVIRUS (CMV) INCLUSION DISEASE

Etiology: CMV infection from direct contact with saliva, urine, blood, tears, semen, or breast milk of an infected person; virus is absorbed through the mucous membranes of the nose or mouth.

- Fifty to eighty percent of adults in the United States are infected by age 40

OB High-risk groups are

—fetuses of infected mothers, especially mothers first infected while pregnant; fetal effects include lung infection, excessive bleeding, anemia, liver damage, vision impairment, or neurological conditions that include seizures, hearing loss, varying degrees of mental impairment, or problems with physical coordination;

—immunocompromised clients.

S&S: Most infected individuals have no or very mild symptoms and no health consequences. Others have prolonged fever, fatigue, mild hepatitis, and tender lymph nodes. Severe forms of infection, which include CMV retinitis and encephalitis, occur in transplant recipients. Neuromuscular impairments in the form of leg weakness and bladder or bowel dysfunction may occur in end-stage AIDS clients. Symptoms reappear at intervals for life as the virus becomes active after a period of dormancy.

Rx: No cure. Antivirals such as ganciclovir and acyclovir to prevent infection or reduce "viral load" in the immunocompromised. High-titer immunoglobulin (IVIG, CytoGam) for acutely infected individuals with some impaired immunity.

Nursing Process Elements

- Assess client's understanding of the disease course
- Monitor for complications

Client teaching for self-care

- Good hygiene especially hand washing to avoid contracting or spread
- Avoid sharing drinking glasses and utensils
- Carefully dispose of diapers, tissues, and other items contaminated with body fluids

INFECTIOUS MONONUCLEOSIS

Etiology: Infection with Epstein—Barr virus (EBV), a member of the herpes virus family, during adolescence or young adulthood from contact with the saliva of an infected person. EBV infection in children is asymptomatic or not distinguishable from other mild childhood illness.

Following symptomatic infection, EBV remains dormant in some cells of the immune system, throat, and blood, and periodically reactivates asymptomatically and appears in the saliva.

S&S: Fever, sore throat, swollen lymph glands, occasional splenomegaly or liver involvement. No known effect of active EBV infection on pregnancy. Symptoms resolve in 1 or 2 months.

Complications: Burkitt's lymphoma and nasopharyngeal carcinoma occur as a late development in a few carriers of EBV.

Dx: Clinical presentation of fever, sore throat, swollen lymph glands, and client's age, elevated WBC count, greater than 10% atypical lymphocytes, and a positive reaction to a "mono spot" test; positive Paul–Bunnell heterophile antibody test.

Rx: No antiviral drugs, vaccines, or other specific treatment; symptomatic treatment only. Five-day course of steroids to control swelling of the throat and tonsils is sometimes prescribed.

Nursing Process Elements

No special precautions or isolation is needed because transmission only occurs through saliva and most individuals exposed to clients with infectious mononucleosis have previously been infected with EBV and are not at risk for infectious mononucleosis.

TOXOPLASMOSIS

Etiology: Infection with protozoan intracellular parasite, *Toxoplasma gondii* as a result of ingestion of contaminated soil, careless handling of cat litter, ingestion of raw or undercooked meat (lamb, pork, and beef), transmission from a mother to a fetus through the placenta (congenital infection), or by blood transfusion or solid organ transplantation.

S&S:

- Asymptomatic in most people otherwise mild sore throat, headache, muscle pain, lymphadenopathy, and fever
- Immunosuppressed clients: fever, headache, confusion, seizures, and abnormal neurological findings from brain lesions and blurred vision from retinal inflammation

OB Congenital infection: CNS impairments, hepatic and splenic enlargement, rash, fever, jaundice, anemia, blindness from inflammation of the retina, and mental retardation; may be present at birth or develop over the first few months of life

Dx: Serologic titers for toxoplasmosis, MRI of the head, cranial CT scan, brain biopsy, slit lamp examination for retinal lesions.

Rx: Anti-infectives for symptomatic cases: pyrimethamine, sulfonamide drugs, folinic acid, clindamycin, and trimethoprim-sulfamethoxazole. Asymptomatic children are treated to prevent retinal inflammation. Pregnant women are treated despite toxicity of medications. AIDS clients are treated until the CD4 count is over 100 to prevent reactivation of disease.

Nursing Process Elements

- Provide supportive care as necessary

Client teaching for self-care

Prevention:

- Avoid undercooked meats, or freeze meat to −20°C for 2 days.
- Protect children's play areas from cat and dog feces.
- Keep children away from cat litter boxes.
- Wash the hands thoroughly after contact with soil that may be contaminated with animal feces; after cleaning a litter box, and after handling raw meat.

SCARLET FEVER

Etiology: Group A beta-hemolytic streptococci from nose and throat secretions of infected persons or carriers contracted through direct contact, droplets, or contaminated articles or foods. Communicable both during incubation period of 1–7 days and during clinical illness phase. Carriers are communicable for 2 weeks to months.

S&S: Abrupt high fever with disproportionate tachycardia, vomiting, headache, chills, malaise, abdominal pain. Red, swollen tonsils with patchy exudates, beefy-red throat, swollen, white strawberry tongue (white coated with prominent red papillae) followed by red strawberry tongue (white coating sloughs off), red punctuate lesions on palate; red punctate rash most marked in intertriginous areas and absent on face; marked circumoral pallor; subsequent fine skin desuamation sheets on trunk, palms and soles.

Complications: Otitis media, peritonsillar abscess, sinusitis, glomerulonephritis, carditis, and polyarthritis.

Rx: Penicillin; erythromycin if allergic to penicillin; analgesics for sore throat.

Nursing Process Elements

- Respiratory precautions for first 24 hours of antibiotics
- Bed rest while febrile
- Provide quiet activities
- Provide nonirritating liquids and soft foods
- Institute measures to relieve sore throat: gargles, throat spray, cool mist vaporizer, and analgesics
- Client teaching for self-care
- Correct administration of antibiotic and importance of compliance
- Notify health care provider if fever persists with antibiotic therapy

LYME DISEASE

Etiology: *Borrelia burgdorferi* (spirochete) transmitted to humans by ticks.

S&S:

- Headache
- Stiff neck
- Fever
- Muscle aches
- Fatigue
- Rash (may appear up to 1 month after bite)
- Regional lymphadenopathy

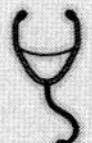

Assessment Alert

- Rash looks like a bull's eye and is called erythema migrans.

Dx: Appearance of erythema migrans, laboratory testing, and at least one of the following: arthritis, facial palsy, meningitis, and carditis.

Rx: Doxycycline (Vibramycin), ceftriaxone (Rocephin), and azithromycin for 3–4 weeks.

Complications:

- Arthritis
- Permanent joint damage
- Meningitis
- Bell's palsy
- Encephalopathy
- Encephalomyelitis
- Severe and/or persistent fatigue
- Hepatitis
- Heart abnormalities
- Eye inflammations
- Muscle aches
- Memory and concentration problems

OB Difficulties with pregnancy including prenatal infection, miscarriage, and still birth

Nursing Process Elements

- Monitor for complications

Client teaching for self-care

- Continue medication to resolve infection

ROCKY MOUNTAIN SPOTTED FEVER

Etiology: *Rickettsia rickettsii* infection transmitted to humans by bite of or exposure to crushed tissues or feces of infected ticks who acquire the infective organism from eating off of rabbits, field mice, and dogs. Occurs spring and summer primarily in the Rocky Mountain and Mid-Atlantic states.

S&S: Sudden onset of fever that typically lasts 14 days, headache, conjunctival infection followed 3 days later by a maculopapular rash, which appears first on the extremities and rapidly spreads to the rest of the body including the palms and soles and subsequently becomes petechial.

Dx: History and clinical presentation.

Rx: Antibiotics, such as tetracycline or chloramphenicol until two or three days after temperature returns to normal for a full 24-hour period. Late or no treatment can result in death.

Nursing Process Elements

- No isolation needed
- Supportive care

Client teaching for self-care

- Avoid known tick-infested areas when possible
- Protect hands when removing ticks from persons or animals
- Remove ticks without crushing them

TETANUS (LOCKJAW)

Etiology: Infection with *Clostridium tetani.*

- Spore-forming organism found in soil, dust, and animal feces
- In puncture or other deep—flesh wounds, spores produce a powerful neurotoxin and tetanospasmin
- Incubation period: 3–21 days with an average of 8

S&S:

- Stiffness of jaw, neck, and other muscles
- Muscular irritability
- Spasms of jaw (lockjaw), neck, throat, chest, and other muscles that cause symptoms such as difficulty swallowing and breathing
- Fever

Complications: Death from constriction of airways, pneumonia, or instability in the autonomic nervous system; permanent brain damage from hypoxemia if muscle spasms have closed the airway.

Rx: Supportive care may include mechanical ventilation, sedation, and pharmacologically maintained muscle paralysis; tetanus antitoxin, such as tetanus immune globulin (TIG) which neutralizes toxin, but only that which hasn't yet combined with nerve tissue; antibiotics; tetanus vaccine to prevent future tetanus infection.

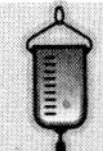

Clinical Alert

- Tetanus infection dose not confer immunity; tetanus vaccination/boosters still are needed throughout life

Nursing Process Elements

- Monitor signs and symptoms with special attention to respiratory status
- Provide supportive care in accord with treatments ordered

Client teaching for self-care

Preventing Tetanus

- Get tetanus toxoid boosters
- Take proper care of wounds
  —Clean wound with soap and a washcloth; rinse thoroughly with water
  —Apply thin layer of a multi-ingredient antibiotic such as Neosporin or Polysporin
  —Cover the wound to keep clean; change dressing daily or when wet or dirty
  —See health care provider for deep, dirty wounds or animal bites especially if immunization not up to date

E. COLI FOODBORNE ILLNESS

Etiology: Infection with *E. coli* O157:H7 from intestines of healthy cattle, deer, goats, and sheep through ingestion of undercooked, contaminated ground beef (most common cause); bean sprouts; fresh, leafy vegetables or raw milk; person-to-person contact; swimming in or drinking sewage-contaminated water.

S&S: Severe, bloody diarrhea; abdominal cramping; little or no fever.

Complications: Hemolytic uremic syndrome (HUS)

- Red blood cells are destroyed and kidneys fail
- Most often occurs in children under age 5 and the elderly
- Principal cause of acute kidney failure in children

Dx: Stool culture.

Rx:

- Most people recover without specific treatment
- Antibiotics are avoided as no benefit is documented and risk of renal disease
- Antidiarrheals such as loperamide are avoided

Nursing Process Elements

- Assess signs and symptoms
- Monitor for fluid and electrolyte imbalance

Client teaching for self-care

- Prevent infection
  —Thoroughly cook ground beef—contaminated meat looks and smells normal
  —Avoid unpasteurized milk
  —Wash hands carefully before preparing or eating food
- Wash well all utensils and counters that have been in contact with raw meat or other food sources of the bacteria
- Keep raw meat and other potential food source separate from other foods
- Wash fruits and vegetables well
- Remove outer leaves from vegetable such as lettuce or cabbage
- Avoid foods as advised by public health officials during outbreaks
- If one has a diarrheal illness,
  —wash hands thoroughly after using the toilet or changing a diaper of an infected child;
  —avoid swimming in public pools or lakes;
  —avoid sharing baths with others;
  —avoid preparing food for others.

WORKSHEET

TRUE & FALSE QUESTIONS

Mark each of the following statements True or False. Correct all false statements in the space provided.

1. Pregnant women do not have to be treated for STIs. ___ T ___ F

2. Douching is necessary for the prevention of STIs and other bacterial infections. ___ T ___ F

3. Client should be aware that any pelvic pain and/or abnormal discharge, especially after sexual exposure, childbirth, or pelvic surgery, should be evaluated as soon as possible. ___ T ___ F

4. Clients who have been sexually assaulted should be treated prophylactically with repeat cultures done in 2 weeks. ___ T ___ F

5. Chlamydia is the most commonly found STI in the United States. ___ T ___ F

6. Pelvic inflammatory disease (PID), if untreated, can cause infertility. ___ T ___ F

7. Syphilis is a serious systemic disease that can lead to disability and death. ___ T ___ F

8. The best treatment for all stages of syphilis is doxycycline. ___ T ___ F

9. Acyclovir is the only known cure for herpes. ___ T ___ F

10. Clients infected with HIV may remain asymptomatic for years. ___ T ___ F

11. The HIV organism can be spread by casual contact. ___ T ___ F

12. The placenta provides protection for the fetus in the HIV-positive pregnant woman. ___ T ___ F

13. A person cannot get the AIDs virus from anal sex. ___ T ___ F

14. HIV is considered a bloodborne pathogen. ___ T ___ F

15. Clients with the HIV infection should be counseled to avoid all sexual contact. ___ T ___ F

16. HIV is a retrovirus. ___ T ___ F

17. Many tests for HIV are looking for antibodies produced by the host against the virus. ___ T ___ F

18. Individuals who become infected with the HIV organism will be seropositive within days of infection. ___ T ___ F

19. AIDS-defining conditions are opportunist infections not normally seen in healthy individuals. ___ T ___ F

20. Antibiotics will not work on an individual with HIV. ___ T ___ F

21. Amniocentesis may be performed on the pregnant HIV-positive woman at 32 weeks to determine if the fetus is infected. ___ T ___ F

22. Only IV drug users are at risk for HIV. ___ T ___ F

23. Gonorrhea is a localized infection of the reproductive organs and pelvic cavity. ___ T ___ F

24. Cervical discharge, which is mucoid and often blood tinged, is the classic sign of chlamydial infection ___ T ___ F

25. The best treatment for all stages of syphilis is penicillin. ___ T ___ F

26. The VDRL test can be used as a screening test for clients with first-stage syphilis. ___ T ___ F

(continued)

27. A nonpruritic rash that appears first on the trunk and faced with pressure is characteristic of roseola. ___ T ___ F

28. An immunosuppressed child diagnosed with Fifth disease must be monitored for aplastic crisis. ___ T ___ F

29. The age group most likely to develop the severe form of West Nile virus are those over age 50. ___ T ___ F

30. The risk of tetanus infection is greatest when a wound is deep. ___ T ___ F

MATCHING QUESTIONS

Matching the following:

Column A	Column B
1. ___ Rabies	a. Undercooked pork
2. ___ EEE	b. Cat feces
3. ___ SARS	c. Contact with respiratory secretions
4. ___ Varicella	d. Infected animal bite
5. ___ Scarlet fever	e. Blood transfusion
6. ___ Chlamydia	f. Contaminated vegetables
7. ___ Rocky Mountain spotted fever	g. Sex with an infected partner
8. ___ Toxoplasmosis	h. Mosquito bite
9. ___ *E.-coli*	i. Contact with skin lesions
10. ___ West Nile virus	j. Tick bite

FILL IN THE BLANKS

Fill in the blank spaces with the correct word or phrase to complete each statement.

1. The disease that Koplik spots are a sign of is ________.

2. An antibiotic used in the treatment of a pregnant woman with chlamydia is ________.

3. Neuromuscular impairments in the form of leg weakness and bladder or bowel dysfunction caused by CMV infection may occur in clients with ________.

4. A child with scarlet fever needs to be on respiratory precautions for ________ hours after antibiotic therapy is started.

5. List four risk factors associated with the development of HIV infections: ________.

6. Name two nonspecific symptoms that are associated with HIV infections in children: ________.

APPLICATION QUESTIONS

1. Which advice would be appropriate for the nurse to give a client who is concerned about preventing EEE?
   a. Avoid swimming in fresh water
   b. Remove ticks from the skin without crushing them
   c. Apply a permethrin-based insect repellant to the skin
   d. Drain standing water from around home

2. Which instruction should the nurse give to a client who is treated for chlamydia?
   a. Use birth control for 30 days after treatment
   b. Do not use tampons for at least months
   c. Return for repeat testing in 2 weeks
   d. Take showers not tub baths

3. Which STIs present a risk to the health of fetuses or neonates? Mark all that apply.
   a. Chlamydia
   b. Syphilis
   c. Gonorrhea
   d. Herpes

4. A client states he was told that one should take care to protect the hands when removing ticks from a dog or cat and asks why this is important. On which fact should the nurse's response be based?
   a. Contact with ticks can cause a desquamation reaction of the skin.
   b. Contact with crushed tick tissues or feces presents a risk of contracting Rocky Mountain spotted fever.
   c. Contact with tick antigens can result in an anaphylactic reaction.
   d. Contact with blood from an engorged tick can transmit the West Nile virus

5. The parents of a child just diagnosed with scarlet fever asks "When we know if our other child is going to get this as well?" Which information should serve as the basis for the nurse's response? Mark all that apply.
   a. The incubation period of scarlet fever is up to a week.
   b. Scarlet fever is communicable both during the incubation and clinical illness phase.
   c. Carriers can be communicable for months.
   d. Transmission is via the fecal–oral route.
   e. Infection is transmitted by tick bites.

6. The nurse is talking to a group of teenagers about the risks involved with drug use. One teenager asks about the relationship between drug abuse and HIV. The student states: "As long as I don't inject the drugs, I won't be at risk of developing HIV." The nurse's best response would include
   a. true, but drugs are not good for you in other ways.
   b. sniffing cocaine can also place you at risk for HIV.
   c. you are right, IV drug use is the only way you can acquire HIV.
   d. it is possible that the drug you are using has been handled by someone with HIV and you could get it from him or her.

7. A pregnant woman who is seropositive for HIV is planning on breast-feeding her infant. As the prenatal nurse, you would explain that
   a. it is a good idea as the baby will receive the HIV antibodies that are in her body.
   b. The HIV virus could be in the breast milk and the mother could give her baby her disease.
   c. The mother should stop taking her HIV drugs if she is going to breast-feed as it could be hazardous to the infant.

(continued)

d. As long as the mother continues to take her HIV drugs, it is OK as the baby will get the drugs at the same time as he/she gets the virus.

8. As a nurse, you should wear gloves for the following activities: (Select all that apply.)
   a. Starting an IV
   b. Hanging a unit of blood
   c. Changing a newborn's diaper
   d. Giving the newborn a first bath
   e. Shaking hands with a new client.

9. While teaching a newly diagnosed HIV client about safe practices, the nurse would teach the client to
   a. avoid kissing his children on the cheek.
   b. use a separate set of dishes for himself.
   c. avoid sharing toothbrushes and razor blades.
   d. wash his clothes separately from the rest of the family.

10. A client says to the nurse: "I sometimes wonder if I should be tested for HIV. What do you think?" The nurse's best response would be
   a. "You wonder if you should be tested?"
   b. "If you are worrying about having HIV, then of course you should be tested."
   c. "The testing for HIV doesn't hurt, so you should go ahead with it."
   d. "Are you worried the information will get out if you are tested?"

11. A woman seropositive for HIV delivers a term infant. While in the newborn nursery, the infant is tested and is found to have HIV antibodies. The mother asks the nurse what this means. The nurse's best response would be based on the knowledge that the antibodies
   a. mean that the baby will develop HIV.
   b. mean that the baby will not develop HIV.
   c. indicate that the baby is infected with HIV.
   d. are maternal antibodies that crossed the placenta.

12. A man is seen in the clinic and asks to be tested for AIDS (HIV). The testing determines that the man's HIV status is negative. The nurse would
   a. congratulate the man on his negative status.
   b. report the man to his employer as a high-risk employee.
   c. explain that the HIV-negative status only provides immunity for 6 months.
   d. provide information about lifestyle changes that may be needed to protect against infection.

13. A 3-month-old infant is showing symptoms of failure to thrive. Because the mother has tested positive for HIV, the physician is planning to test the infant for infection. The nurse would expect the physician to order which HIV test?
   a. PCR
   b. ELISA
   c. Western blot
   d. WBC differential

14. A child is HIV-positive and his immune system is severely compromised. Which vaccination type should be avoided in this child?
   a. Killed vaccine
   b. Toxoid vaccine
   c. Attenuated vaccine
   d. Passive immunization

15. A woman in early pregnancy, asks the nurse whether the HIV drugs she is taking will harm the baby. The nurse's response would be based on the knowledge that
   a. these drugs will harm the baby but without them the mother might die.
   b. nurses should not provide the client with drug-related information.
   c. these drugs do not harm the fetus and may be health promoting for the fetus.
   d. it is not known whether these drugs place the fetus at risk and mothers need to make an informed decision about taking them.

16. Which direction should be given to a client for whom Flagyl is prescribed?
   a. Do not drink alcohol while taking Flagyl
   b. Douche daily while taking Flagyl
   c. Discontinue all other medications while taking Flagyl
   d. Expect gray–green vaginal drainage while taking Flagyl

17. Which is a clinical manifestation of a vaginal trichomonas infection?
   a. thick, white, cheesy discharge
   b. high fever
   c. vomiting
   d. thin, bubbly, green-tinged malodorous discharge

18. Which is an important aspect of care for any client with an STI?
   a. Maintenance of HIPAA standards
   b. Ensuring that both client and partner(s) receive treatment.

c. Reporting the disease to the Department of Health
d. Provision of information on birth control

19. When caring for a client with herpes, which information should be included in the plan for teaching self-care?
    a. The risk of contracting HIV is increased during a herpes outbreak.
    b. Antibacterial powder or lotion can be used to relieve soreness or itch.
    c. Sitz baths should be avoided until lesions heal.
    d. Clean, snug, absorbent underwear should be worn.

20. Which intervention would the nurse expect to be ordered for a woman in labor who has active herpes lesions?
    a. Delivery by cesarean section
    b. IV antibiotics
    c. Stat non-stress test
    d. Buccal pitocin

21. Which STI is the major cause of PID, infertility, ectopic pregnancy, and chronic pelvic pain?
    a. Herpes
    b. Chlamydia
    c. Gonorrhea
    d. Monilia

22. When explaining the importance of treatment, the nurse tells the client that arthritis, dermatitis , pericarditis, endocarditis, or meningitis can result from which STI if it is not treated?
    a. Chlamydia
    b. Herpes
    c. Gonorrhea
    d. PID

23. A client for whom a FTA-ABS test is ordered asks the purpose of the test. The nurse's response should be based on the fact that this test is used to confirm the diagnosis of which STI?
    a. Gonorrhea
    b. Syphilis
    c. Chlamydia
    d. Herpes

24. Which statement made by a client in a clinic waiting room requires correction? Mark all that apply.
    a. You only have to worry about tetanus if you injure yourself on a rusty nail.
    b. Even if you have tetanus, you still need immunizations for the rest of your life.
    c. Tetanus occurs today only in underdeveloped countries.
    d. TIG reverses or prevents the S&S of tetanus.

25. Which instructions should be given to clients when prevention of infection with *E. coli* O157:H7 is the goal? Mark all that apply.
    a. Cook all hamburger to medium or well done
    b. Wash green, leafy vegetables carefully
    c. Stay away from persons with the disease
    d. Avoid contact with sick farm animals
    e. Do not swim where sewage may have escaped into the water
    f. Drink pasteurized, not raw, milk
    g. Wear gloves when changing cat litter boxes

ANSWERS & RATIONALES

TRUE & FALSE ANSWERS

Mark each of the following statements True or False. Correct all false statements in the space provided.

1. Pregnant women do not have to be treated for STIs. *False*
   All women, pregnant or not, need to be treated for STIs.

2. Douching is necessary for the prevention of STIs and other bacterial infections. *False*
   Douching destroys the natural flora that combats infecting organisms and may introduce bacteria upward.

(continued)

3. Clients should be aware that any pelvic pain and/or abnormal discharge, especially after sexual exposure, childbirth, or pelvic surgery, should be evaluated as soon as possible. *True*

4. Clients who have been sexually assaulted should be treated prophylactically with repeat cultures done in 2 weeks. *True*

5. Chlamydia is the most commonly found STI in the United States. *True*

6. PID, if untreated, can cause infertility. *True*

7. Syphilis is a serious systemic disease that can lead to disability and death. *True*

8. The best treatment for all stages of syphilis is doxycycline. *False*
   The best treatment for all stages of syphilis is penicillin; doxycycline can be used if client is allergic to penicillin.

9. Acyclovir is the only known cure for herpes. *False*
   There is no cure for herpes, which is a virus; acyclovir, an antiviral agent, can suppress the symptoms and shorten the course of the infection.

10. Clients infected with HIV may remain asymptomatic for years. *True*

11. The HIV organism can be spread by casual contact. *False*
    The HIV virus cannot be spread by casual contact.

12. The placenta provides protection for the fetus in the HIV-positive pregnant woman. *False*
    The placenta does not prevent the transmission of the HIV virus to the fetus.

13. A person cannot get the AIDS virus from anal sex. *False*
    The AIDS virus can be transmitted from anal sex.

14. HIV is considered a bloodborne pathogen. *True*

15. Clients with the HIV infection should be counseled to avoid all sexual contact. *False*
    Clients with the HIV infection do not need to avoid all sexual contact; they need to be counseled regarding safer sexual practices.

16. HIV is a retrovirus. *True*

17. Many tests for HIV are looking for antibodies produced by the host against the virus. *True*

18. Individuals who become infected with the HIV organism will be seropositive within days of infection. *False*
    Individuals who become infected with the HIV organism are not seropositive within days of infection; it takes 3 weeks to 3–6 months for the client to become seropositive.

19. AIDS-defining conditions are opportunist infections not normally seen in healthy individuals. *True*

20. Antibiotics will not work on an individual with HIV. *False*
    Antibiotics are effective for individuals with HIV provided the organism causing the infection being treated is sensitive to the antibiotic used.

21. Amniocentesis may be performed on the pregnant, HIV-positive woman at 32 weeks to determine if the fetus is infected. *False*
    Amniocentesis does not determine if a fetus is infected with HIV.

22. Only IV drug users are at risk for HIV. *False*
IV drug users are at risk for HIV if dirty needles are used but since HIV can be transmitted by infected blood or blood products or other infected body fluids, anyone including health care workers who has contact with these substances is at risk.

23. Gonorrhea is a localized infection of the reproductive organs and pelvic cavity. *False*
Gonorrhea can cause severe disseminated infection: arthritis, dermatitis, pericarditis, endocarditis, and meningitis.

24. Cervical discharge which is mucoid and often blood-tinged is the classic sign of chlamydial infection. *False*
Chlamydial infection is often asymptomatic. When symptoms do occur discharge or bleeding from the cervix can be among them.

25. The best treatment for all stages of syphilis is penicillin. *True*

26. The VDRL test can be used as a screening test for clients with first-stage syphilis. *False*
The VDRL does not become positive until the second stage of the disease.

27. A nonpruritic rash that appears first on the trunk and faces with pressure is characteristic of roseola. *True*

28. An immunosuppressed child diagnosed with Fifth disease must be monitored for aplastic crisis. *True*

29. The age group most likely to develop the severe form of West Nile virus are those over age 50. *True*

30. The risk of tetanus infection is greatest when a wound is deep. *True*

MATCHING ANSWERS

Matching the following:

Column A	Column B
1. __d__ Rabies	a. Deep flesh wound
2. __h__ EEE	b. Cat feces
3. __c__ SARS	c. Contact with respiratory secretions
4. __i__ Varicella	d. Infected animal bite
5. __a__ Tetanus	e. Blood transfusion
6. __g__ Chlamydia	f. Contaminated vegetables
7. __j__ Rocky Mountain spotted fever	g. Sex with an infected partner
8. __b__ Toxoplasmosis	h. Mosquito bite
9. __f__ *E. coli*	i. Contact with skin lesions
10. __h__ West Nile virus	j. Tick bite

ANSWERS FOR FILL IN THE BLANKS

Fill in the blank spaces with the correct word or phrase to complete each statement.

1. The disease that Koplik spots are a sign of is measles.
2. An antibiotic used in the treatment of a pregnant woman with chlamydia is erythromycin or amoxicillin.
3. Neuromuscular impairments in the form of leg weakness and bladder or bowel dysfunction caused by CMV infection may occur in clients with end-stage AIDS.
4. A child with scarlet fever needs to be on respiratory precautions for 24 hours after antibiotic therapy is started.
5. List four risk factors associated with the development of HIV infections: sexual contact with an infected person, contaminated blood or blood products, drug abuse, particularly IV drug use, and infants born to infected mothers.
6. Name two nonspecific symptoms that are associated with HIV infections in children: failure to thrive and developmental delays.

APPLICATION ANSWERS

1. Which advice would be appropriate for the nurse to give a client who is concerned about preventing EEE?
   a. Avoid swimming in fresh water
   b. Remove ticks from the skin without crushing them
   c. Apply a permethrin-based insect repellant to the skin
   d. Drain standing water from around home

Rationale
Correct answer: d.
EEE is a mosquito-borne disease. Mosquitos breed in still water so draining plant pots and other containers of standing water decreases the number of mosquitos and helps prevent exposure to the EEE virus. Ticks cause Rocky Mountain spotted fever. Swimming in fresh water does not affect exposure to EEE but can be the source of other disease such as infections of the outer ear. Repellants with permethrin are effective in keeping mosquitos away but cannot be applied directly to the skin.

2. Which instruction should the nurse give to a client who is treated for chlamydia?
   a. Use birth control for 30 days after treatment
   b. Do not use tampons for at least months
   c. Return for repeat testing in 2 weeks
   d. Take showers not tub baths

Rationale
Correct answer: c.
Test of cure needs to be done 2 weeks after treatment. Birth control is not needed but sexual activity should be avoided until all sexual partners have been treated. Use of tampons and showers are unrelated.

3. Which STIs present a risk to the health of fetuses or neonates? Mark all that apply.
   a. Chlamydia
   b. Syphilis
   c. Gonorrhea
   d. Herpes

Rationale
Correct answers: a, b, c, and d.
Chlamydia and gonorrhea are associated with neonatal conjunctivitis and pneumonia as well as premature labor, stillbirth, and neonatal death. Syphilis can cause still birth, developmental delay, seizures, or neonatal death.

4. A client states he was told that one should take care to protect the hands when removing ticks from a dog or cat and asks why this is important. On which fact should the nurse's response be based?
   a. Contact with ticks can cause a desquamation reaction of the skin.

b. Contact with crushed tick tissues or feces presents a risk of contracting Rocky Mountain spotted fever.
c. Contact with tick antigens can result in an anaphylactic reaction.
d. Contact with blood from an engorged tick can transmit the West Nile virus.

Rationale

Correct answer: b.

Ticks are the vectors responsible for the transmission of Rock Mountain spotted fever. Desquamation of the skin is seen in Toxic shock syndrome, measles, radiation therapy, and in many other situations; however, it is not characteristic of contact with ticks. Anaphylactic shock from contact with a tick is not documented in the literature. West Nile virus is a mosquito-borne illness.

5. The parents of a child just diagnosed with scarlet fever asks "When we know if our other child is going to get this as well?" Which information should serve as the basis for the nurse's response? Mark all that apply.
   a. The incubation period of scarlet fever is up to a week.
   b. Scarlet fever is communicable both during the incubation and clinical illness phase.
   c. Carriers can be communicable for months.
   d. Transmission is via the fecal—oral route.
   e. Infection is transmitted by tick bites.

Rationale

Correct answers: a, b, and c.

Scarlet fever is communicable both during the incubation phase of 1–7 days and the clinical illness phase. Carriers are communicable from weeks to months. Transmission is by direct contact with nasopharyngeal secretions of infected persons, contact with contaminated items, or by droplet spread. Scarlet fever is not transmitted by ticks, Rocky Mountain spotted fever is.

6. The nurse is talking to a group of teenagers about the risks involved with drug use. One teenager asks about the relationship between drug abuse and HIV. The student states: "As long as I don't inject the drugs, I won't be at risk of developing HIV." The nurse's best response would include
   a. true, but drugs are not good for you in other ways.
   b. sniffing cocaine can also place you at risk for HIV.
   c. you are right, IV drug use is the only way you can acquire HIV.
   d. it is possible that the drug you are using has been handled by someone with HIV and you could get it from him or her.

Rationale

Correct answer: b.

Drug abusers use a straw to sniff the cocaine from the counter into their nares. The nares becomes fragile and bleeds readily. If blood gets on the straw and then the straw is shared with another drug user, that individual may acquire HIV from the straw.

7. A pregnant woman who is seropositive for HIV is planning on breast-feeding her infant. As the prenatal nurse, you would explain that
   a. it is a good idea as the baby will receive the HIV antibodies that are in her body.
   b. the HIV virus could be in the breast milk and the mother could give her baby her disease.
   c. the mother should stop taking her HIV drugs if she is going to breast-feed as it could be hazardous to the infant.
   d. as long as the mother continues to take her HIV drugs, it is OK as the baby will get the drugs at the same time as he gets the virus.

Rationale

Correct answer: b.

HIV is a found in all blood and body fluids. It is recommended that HIV-positive women should not breast-feed.

8. As a nurse, you should wear gloves for the following activities: (Select all that apply.)
   a. Starting an IV
   b. Hanging a unit of blood
   c. Changing a newborn's diaper
   d. Giving the newborn a first bath
   e. Shaking hands with a new client

Rationale

Correct answers: a, b, c, and d.

Any time there could be exposure to blood or body fluid, gloves should be worn. Casual contact does not spread the HIV virus.

9. While teaching a newly diagnosed HIV client about safe practices, the nurse would teach the client to
   a. avoid kissing his children on the cheek.
   b. use a separate set of dishes for himself.
   c. avoid sharing toothbrushes and razor blades.
   d. wash his clothes separately from the rest of the family.

Rationale

Correct answer: c.

Shared toothbrushes and razor blades will lead to exposure to blood and body fluids and should be avoided. All other interventions are not necessary.

10. A client says to the nurse: "I sometimes wonder if I should be tested for HIV. What do you think?" The nurse's best response would be
   a. "You wonder if you should be tested?"
   b. "If you are worrying about having HIV, then of course you should be tested."

(continued)

c. "The testing for HIV doesn't hurt, so you should go ahead with it."

d. "Are you worried the information will get out if you are tested?"

Rationale

Correct answer: a.

This is an open-ended question that encourages the client to respond with more information. More information about the client's concerns are needed before intervening.

11. A woman seropositive for HIV delivers a term infant. While in the newborn nursery, the infant is tested and is found to have HIV antibodies. The mother asks the nurse what this means. The nurse's best response would be based on the knowledge that the antibodies
    a. mean that the baby will develop HIV.
    b. mean that the baby will not develop HIV.
    c. indicate that the baby is infected with HIV.
    d. are maternal antibodies that crossed the placenta.

Rationale

Correct answer: c.

This is passive immunity that crossed the placenta from the mother and provides no indication of the infant's future HIV status.

12. A man is seen in the clinic and asks to be tested for AIDS (HIV). The testing determines the man's HIV status is negative. The nurse would
    a. congratulate the man on his negative status.
    b. report the man to his employer as a high-risk employee.
    c. explain that the HIV-negative status only provides immunity for 6 months.
    d. provide information about lifestyle changes that may be needed to protect against infection.

Rationale

Correct answer: d.

The fact that the man seeks HIV testing indicates he feels he may have been exposed. In addition to providing information about his current status, it is imperative that information about lifestyle changes be included. It is illegal to provide information about HIV status to outside entities.

13. A 3-month-old infant is showing symptoms of failure to thrive. Because the mother has been tested positive for HIV, the physician is planning to test the infant for infection. The nurse would expect the physician to order which HIV test?
    a. PCR
    b. ELISA
    c. Western blot
    d. WBC differential

Rationale

Correct answer: a.

PCR test can be used as early as 1 month of age. The ELISA and Western blot results would be confused by the maternal antibodies in the baby's blood. The WBC differential would not be helpful.

14. A child is HIV-positive and his immune system is severely compromised. Which vaccination type should be avoided in this child?
    a. Killed vaccine
    b. Toxoid vaccine
    c. Attenuated vaccine
    d. Passive immunization

Rationale

Correct answer: c.

Attenuated vaccine contains live but weakened organisms. Because the child's immune system is compromised, these live vaccines may cause illness.

15. A woman in early pregnancy, asks the nurse whether the HIV drugs she is taking will harm the baby. The nurse's response would be based on the knowledge that:
    a. These drugs will harm the baby but without them the mother might die.
    b. Nurses should not provide the client with drug-related information.
    c. These drugs do not harm the fetus and may be health promoting for the fetus.
    d. It is not known whether these drugs place the fetus at risk and mothers need to make an informed decision about taking them.

Rationale

Correct answer: d.

The teratogenic properties of these drugs are not fully known. The clients should be involved in making informed decisions about the health of themselves and their fetus.

16. Which direction should be given to a client for whom Flagyl is prescribed?
    a. Do not drink alcohol while taking Flagyl
    b. Douche daily while taking Flagyl
    c. Discontinue all other medications while taking Flagyl
    d. Expect gray–green vaginal drainage while taking Flagyl

Rationale

Correct answer: a.

Alcoholic beverages should be avoided while taking Flagyl and for 3 days after the last dose. Mixing alcohol with Flagyl can result in abdominal cramps, nausea, vomiting, headaches, and flushing. Caution must be used to avoid accidental ingestion of alcohol from sources such as over the counter cough suppressants or cold products. Douching is unrelated to taking Flagyl. It is not necessary to discontinue all medications and Flagyl does not cause gray–green vaginal drainage.

17. Which is a clinical manifestation of a vaginal trichomonas infection?
    a. thick, white, cheesy discharge
    b. high fever
    c. vomiting
    d. thin, bubbly, green-tinged malodorous discharge

Rationale
Correct answer: d.
A thin, bubbly, green-tinged, foul-smelling vaginal discharge is characteristic of trichomonas infection. A thick, white, cottage cheese like discharge is characteristic of monilia (*Candida albicans*) infection. High fever and vomiting may accompany infections which involve other organisms and more generalized infections such as PID.

18. Which is an important aspect of care for any client with an STI?
    a. Maintenance of HIPAA standards
    b. Ensuring that both client and partner(s) receive treatment
    c. Reporting the disease to the Department of Health
    d. Provision of information on birth control

Rationale
Correct answer: a.
Maintaining client's privacy as regulated by HIPAA is a critical aspect of care of all clients including those with any type of STI. Not all STIs require both the client and partner to be treated and not all are reportable diseases. Information on birth control may be desirable but it is not an essential aspect of care for all clients with STIs as the possibility of pregnancy does not apply to all clients and it is not essential to the cure or prevention of STIs.

19. When caring for a client with herpes, which information should be included in the plan for teaching self-care?
    a. The risk of contracting HIV is increased during a herpes outbreak.
    b. Antibacterial powder or lotion can be used to relieve soreness or itch.
    c. Sitz baths should be avoided until lesions heal.
    d. Clean, snug, absorbent underwear should be worn.

Rationale
Correct answer: a.
The risk of contracting HIV and other STIs is increased during an outbreak of herpes lesions. Use of powders, lotions, or ointments should be avoided; analgesics can be taken as ordered for pain and discomfort on urination can be eased by pouring plain water over the perineum. Sitz bath should be encouraged as they also provide comfort; they do not need to be avoided until the lesions heal. Under clothing covering involved areas should be clean, absorbent, and loose fitting, not snug.

20. Which intervention would the nurse expect to be ordered for a woman in labor who has active herpes lesions?
    a. Delivery by cesarean section
    b. IV antibiotics
    c. Stat nonstress test
    d. Buccal pitocin

Rationale
Correct answer: a.
A woman with active herpes lesions is delivered by caesarean section to avoid exposing the fetus to the herpes virus during passage through the birth canal. Acyclovir is sometimes ordered as the EDC approaches in an attempt to prevent an outbreak at the time of labor so that a C-section is not necessary. IV antibiotics are not administered because herpes is caused by a virus and there is no cure. An immediate non-stress test is ordered to determine fetal well-being and so is not required by the presence of a maternal herpes outbreak. Pitocin is used to induce labor or strengthen contractions and so would be considered for use only with a vaginal delivery.

21. Which STI is the major cause of PID, infertility, ectopic pregnancy, and chronic pelvic pain?
    a. Herpes
    b. Chlamydia
    c. Gonorrhea
    d. *Monilial vaginitis*

Rationale
Correct answer: c.
Gonorrhea is the major cause of PID, infertility, ectopic pregnancy, and chronic pelvic pain. Chlamydia also increases the risk of infertility and ectopic pregnancy but not with the aggressiveness of gonorrhea. *Monilial vaginitis* is a relatively harmless overgrowth of normal vaginal flora brought about by factors such as antibiotic use, changes in hormone levels as in pregnancy, and stress. Herpes is a lifelong problem because there is no cure but it is not a major cause of PID, infertility, ectopic pregnancy, or chronic pelvic pain.

22. When explaining the importance of treatment, the nurse tells the client that arthritis, dermatitis, pericarditis,

(continued)

endocarditis, or meningitis can result from which STI if it is not treated?

a. Chlamydia

b. Herpes

c. Gonorrhea

d. PID

Rationale

Correct answer: c.

Gonorrhea, if not effectively treated, can cause severe disseminated infection causing problems such as arthritis, dermatitis, pericarditis, endocarditis, or meningitis. Chlamydia is the most common STI and it increases the risk of ectopic pregnancy and infertility. Herpes is not curable; antiviral medications are used to suppress outbreaks of the disease and to shorten their duration. PID can be caused by gonorrhea and hence lead to the infections noted but it is not necessarily the cause of PID. Therefore, it cannot be said that untreated PID can lead to these complications.

23. A client for whom a FTA-ABS test is ordered asks the purpose of the test. The nurse's response should be based on the fact that this test is used to confirm the diagnosis of which STI?

a. Gonorrhea

b. Syphilis

c. Chlamydia

d. Herpes

Rationale

Correct answer: b.

VDRL is a basic serologic screening test for syphilis. Because the VDRL can be positive for reasons other than syphilitic infection, a more specific serologic test such as a FTA-ABS or a rapid plasma regain (RPR) test is done to confirm the diagnosis. Gonorrhea, chlamydia, and herpes are all diagnosed based on culture.

24. Which statement made by a client in a clinic waiting room requires correction? Mark all that apply.

a. You only have to worry about tetanus if you injure yourself on a rusty nail.

b. Even if you have tetanus you still need immunizations for the rest of your life.

c. Tetanus occurs today only in underdeveloped countries.

d. TIG reverses or prevents the S&S of tetanus.

Rationale

Correct answers: a, c, and d.

Clostridium tetani, the organism that causes tetanus, is found in soil and dust. Getting a puncture wound from a rusty nail does put one at risk for tetanus, particularly if the nail was in the soil, because the resulting wound is a deep flesh wound and the organism is an anaerobe and therefore more likely to infect a deep wound. Tetanus occurs everywhere in the world even developed countries because the organism forms spores, which can lie dormant for long lengths of time and people do not all receive the required immunizations to protect against the disease. TIG neutralizes the neurotoxin, which causes the S&S of tetanus but only the toxin that has not already attached to nerve cells. Therefore, it does not prevent all S&S or reverse existing S&S.

25. Which instructions should be given to clients when prevention of Infection with *E. coli* O157:H7 is the goal? Mark all that apply.

a. Cook all hamburgers to medium or well done.

b. Wash green, leafy vegetables carefully.

c. Stay away from persons with the disease.

d. Avoid contact with sick farm animals.

e. Do not swim where sewage may have escaped into the water

f. Drink pasteurized, not raw, milk.

g. Wear gloves when changing cat litter boxes.

Rationale

Correct answers: a, b, c, e, and f.

E. coli O157:H7 can be transmitted by ingestion of undercooked contaminated hamburger, contaminated green, leafy vegetables, direct contact with infected persons, by swimming in or drinking sewage contaminated water, or by drinking contaminated raw milk. The organism is found in the GI tracts of healthy cattle, goats, and deer so avoiding contact with sick farm animals does not prevent transmission. The organism is not found in cat urine or feces so precautions in handling soiled litter do not prevent transmission.

Test Plan Category:

Physiological Integrity

Sub-category: Physiological Adaptation—Part 3

Topics: Pathophysiology
Hemodynamics
Radiation Therapy
Unexpected Response to Therapies

CELL INJURY

The three most basic causes of cell injury are

- deficiency—lack of a substance essential to the cell,
- intoxication or poisoning—presence of a substance (toxin) which impairs cell function; toxins may be endogenous (made within the body) or exogenous (from outside the body), and
- trauma or physical injury—damage to the cell's structure.

These in turn may be the result of factors such as hypoxia, chemicals, physical agents such as heat, cold, radiation, electric current, and mechanical force, infectious agents, immune injury, genetic defects, nutritional imbalances, and aging.

EFFECTS OF CELL INJURY

Reversible Effects

- Water accumulation in the cell.
- Fat accumulation in the cell and enlargement of the organ—commonly seen in liver, heart, and kidney.
- Residual body accumulation in the cell—remains of phagosomes (that ingest invading microorganisms and damaged cell organelles, number increases with age).
- Hyaline change in cell—presence of hyaline in or between cells—commonly seen in damaged arterioles, renal tubule cells, liver, and nerves.

- Use of an alternate metabolic pathway: when glucose is lacking; cells burn protein for energy.
- Change in cell size or number
  - —Hypertrophy: Enlargement of cells and organs as a result of increased demand, for example, cardiac hypertrophy and muscle hypertrophy.
  - —Hyperplasia: Increase in the number of cells through cell division, in response to demand.
  - —Atrophy: Shrinking of cells and organs as a result of decreased demand. Types of atrophy are
    - disuse atrophy (due to reduced workload, neurological or hormonal stimuli) and
    - pressure atrophy (decrease in size due to long-term pressure).
  - —Apoptosis: Decrease in the number of cells as a result of self-destruction.
  - —Organelle changes: Increase in the number of specific organelles to meet a functional demand; this occurs over the long term.

Irreversible Effects

Damage to the cell membrane or the membranes of the organelles is a primary cause of irreversible cell injury.

Irreversible cell injury can result in either the cell continuing to function at less than a normal level or in necrosis (cell death).

Types of necrosis

- Coagulation necrosis: This is characterized by initial appearance of a firm area with the structure of normal tissue even though cells are dead; subsequently the area is broken down and cleared by phagocytes. It is common when cells die due to anoxia or toxic injury except in the brain. Examples: gangrene, caseous necrosis seen in TB.
- Liquefaction necrosis: This is characterized by an initial liquid area of dead cells. It is seen in the death of nervous system cells due to anoxia and in death of cells associated with bacterial infections.

Calcification

- Calcification refers to the deposition of calcium in cells.
- It occurs at the sites of necrosis regardless of type; can cause tissue to be brittle and rigid; can interfere with function, for example, calcification of heart valves can prevent proper opening and closing and in arteries can result in loss of elasticity.
- It may occur in normal tissues such as lung, kidney, gastric mucous membranes, and arteries due to hypercalcemia. No effects are seen unless the deposits are very large.

Variation in tissue susceptibility to damage

- Ischemia (decreased blood flow)—CNS 5–10 minutes, Liver and kidney 60 minutes.
- Ionizing radiation—actively dividing cells' DNA in most susceptible.
- Viruses only affect certain types of cells.

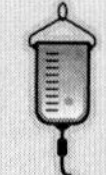

Clinical Alert

The time for which a tissue can withstand ischemia without damage determines the window within which a problem with blood flow needs to be identified and corrected and in which transplants must be done.

INDICATORS OF CELLULAR INJURY

- Decreased function: e.g. change in urine specific gravity when kidneys cannot concentrate urine.
- Release of cell constituents such as potassium and intracellular enzymes such as CPK, GGT.
- Change in electrical activity as on an ECG, EEG, and EMG.
- Direct examination of tissues/cells.

INFLAMMATION

Acute Inflammation

- An acute inflammation is a nonspecific response, i.e., a variety of different initiators (triggering events) produce same vascular and cellular responses.
- Initiators include substances released from injured cells, direct stimulation of mast cells such as from cold or trauma, microbial products, complement activation, exposure of basement membrane or connective-tissue components, deposition of antigen—antibody complexes, and disruption of vascular integrity.
- Initiators activate a variety of chemical mediators, which in turn elicit the vascular and cellular events that comprise the inflammatory response.
- Chemical mediators can be either cell-derived or plasma-derived:
  - —Cell-derived chemical mediators include histamine, which is released from mast cells and promotes vasodilation and increased vascular permeability, and also leukotrienes and prostaglandins, which are released from phagocytes and mast cells in the damaged area.
  - —Plasma-derived mediators are mostly formed from inactive proteins circulating in the plasma as a result of a cascade (sequence of activation events). The one cascade involved solely with inflammation is the kinin cascade. Bradykinin, one of its components, contributes to pain.

- Acute inflammation is a local response with five classic signs: redness, heat, swelling, pain, and loss of function.
- Components of the inflammatory response
  —Vascular component: increased blood flow to damaged tissue and an increase in capillary and venule permeability.
  —Cellular component—movement of leukocytes, which can inactivate bacteria and remove debris, into the tissue spaces of damaged area.

These two components result in exudate formation, which is the movement of fluid with suspended substances and cells into the tissue spaces of the damaged area.

Process of exudate formation

- Hyperemia—increased blood flow occurs as a result of dilation of arterioles and precapillary sphincters, which reduces vascular resistance. Hyperemia causes the area to become red and hot.
- Tissue fluid formation (movement of fluid out of the vascular system into the tissues) increases along the capillary because of the increase in pressure from the increased blood flow. Two other factors that further contribute to formation of tissue fluid are:
  —stasis of blood flow in the capillaries as a result of increased viscosity of blood secondary to fluid being lost into tissue and
  —increased vascular permeability as a result of contraction of the endothelial cells of the venules, which results in spaces between them through which fluid can pass out of the venule.
- Formation of tissue fluid causes swelling and pain.

Benefits of exudate formation

The formation of exudate

- dilutes toxins,
- increases pain as a result of swelling thereby limiting use and preventing further damage,
- allows antibodies to enter the tissues from the blood stream, and
- brings proteins to the damaged tissues, which facilitate phagocytosis.

Types of exudates

Exudates range from thin, and consisting mostly of water, to thick, and consisting of large amounts of fluid, proteins, cellular debris, and blood. The type of exudate formed depends on the nature of the inflammation. Some inflammations and the type of exudates formed in them are:

- Serous—inflammation in response to mild injury; exudate is watery because the vascular permeability is not increased enough to permit the escape of protein from the capillaries. Example, fluid in blisters of a mild sunburn
- Purulent or suppurative—inflammation associated with more severe injury, exudate is thick, white or greenish pus; when localized called an abscess and when diffused called cellulitis.
- Hemorrhagic—inflammation seen in severe injury; capillary damage allows RBCs to escape into tissue spaces.

Leukocytes and the acute inflammatory response

- Initially large numbers of neutrophils arrive at the site of injury; peak at 6–12 hours; then the number declines over the next 12–24 hours.
- Meanwhile mononuclear cells (monocytes) or macrophages begin to increase until they peak at about 5 days.
- In viral rickettsial infections and acute dermatitis—lymphocytes predominate
- Allergies and some parasites—eosinophils predominate

Phagocytosis

- Kills microorganisms.
- Destroys or inactivates toxic agents.
- Degrades macromolecules.

Opsonization enhances phagocytosis—opsonins coat particles to be phagocytized and ease binding to the phagocyte.

Systemic effects of inflammation

S&S: Fever, anorexia, increase in deep sleep, rapid weight loss, residual weakness. Leukocytosis is caused by two- to threefold rapid increase in WBCs on differential with bacterial infection; ischemial damage causes neutrophilia, viral infections cause lymphocytosis, and allergic reactions cause eosinophilia.

Although the inflammatory response is protective, it can also cause tissue damage as in glomerulonephritis in which immune complexes are deposited in the renal basement membrane and cause an inflammatory response. Since the immune complexes cannot be phagocytized because of their attachment to the basement membrane, the result is release of substances from the phagocyte that can damage the membrane and can lead to renal failure. Thus, the challenge is to limit the response sufficiently to prevent tissue damage while maintaining its protective function.

Chronic Inflammation

- Chronic inflammation differs from acute in terms of time and nature of response
  —subacute lasts for more than 1 week while
  —chronic lasts for more than 6 weeks.
- It begins with an acute inflammatory response but the injurious agent is not destroyed. Its long-term presence appears to stimulate the immune response.
- Types of chronic inflammation are
  —nonspecific: diffuse accumulation of macrophages and lymphocytes at site of injury and
  —granulomatous: granulomas form (round masses of transformed macrophages surrounded by lymphocytes and fibroblasts; may be central mass of necrotic tissue

containing the injurious agent (foreign body or bacterium); seen in TB. Cellular response dominates; not the fluid exudative response. There is massive buildup of cells, usually macrophages and lymphocytes. Injurious agent may be minimally invasive bacteria, fungi, parasites, or foreign bodies insoluble in body fluids such as talc.
- Chronic inflammation causes progressive tissue destruction, loss of function, and scarring.

HEALING

Four components of the healing process:
- Regeneration—replacement of parenchyma (functional cells of an organ)
- Repair—replacement of damaged tissue with fibrous scar tissue
- Revascularization—development of vessels to provide bloodflow to new tissue
- Reepithelialization—growth of protective epithelium over damaged surfaces

Regeneration

- Regeneration occurs by mitosis.
- The ability to regenerate varies according to the tissue type.
  —Labile tissues: Cells are continually dividing to replace those lost through normal processes, for example, epithelia of skin and mucous membranes, red bone marrow, and lymphoid tissues; regeneration is easy and rapid.
  —Stable tissues: Cells divide slowly after growth is complete but can increase the rate of mitosis if damage occurs, for example, liver, and fibroblasts and osteoclasts of connective tissue. Regeneration leads to return of function if there is undamaged stroma (supportive connective tissue and blood vessels). If stroma is damaged, regeneration may be disorganized resulting in some functional loss.
  —Permanent tissues: No cell division after growth is complete. Examples nervous, cardiac, and skeletal muscle tissue; lost cells are replaced with scar tissue leaving functional impairment.

Repair

- Repair refers to the formation of scar tissue by fibrosis.
- The main event is the production of collagen fibers by fibroblasts. Collagen formation occurs in the exudates of the acute inflammatory response changing it into ground substance or matrix, which is the intercellular material of the scar. Clots must be removed by phagocytosis before healing can be completed. Organization refers to both phagocytosis of the clot and its replacement with scar tissue.
- Collagen is weak until about 5 days postinjury, then rapidly and steadily increases in strength by means of cross-links between fibers. By 3 months its maximum strength is achieved which is 70–80% of normal.

Revascularization

Revascularization is also called angioneogenesis. As new blood vessels develop, the exudate in which they form appears pink and granular and is called granulation tissue; it is essential to scar formation. New vessels develop from intact vessels adjacent to the damaged site. They begin as endothelial buds which gradually grow into channels through which blood can flow; finally, they differentiate into arterioles, venules, or true capillaries. Lymphatic drainage is also reestablished although later and more slowly than blood supply. Finally, the number of blood vessels in the damaged area is reduced as the metabolic demands associated with healing end. Thus, the scar appears pink and then gradually fades as the blood flow diminishes.

Reepithelialization

A zone of active mitosis develops just at the back of the wound edge and newly formed cells and older cells in front of them slide over the wound surface. When cells from the sides of the wound meet, the newly divided cells begin to move upward and then differentiate into specialized cell types that were lost.

Types of Wound Healing in the Skin

- Primary healing or healing by first intention—Occurs in incision-type wounds with minimal damage and closely approximated edges. Melanocytes are not replaced, so area over scar is pale and does not tan.
- Secondary healing or healing by second intention—Occurs in wounds whose edges are not closely approximated, for example, an ulcer. Secondary healing is similar to primary but it takes longer; much more granulation tissue is needed to fill the wound; and wound contraction occurs. Wound contraction is the drawing in of the wound edges toward the center after granulation tissue forms. This process starts 2–3 days postinjury and can continue for weeks reducing the size of the wound up to 80%.

Table 33–1 discusses the healing characteristics of the tissues in the body.

Conditions Essential for Good Healing

- Site of injury must be free of debris.
- Wound edges need to be immobilized to allow tissues to join across area of injury.
- Adequate blood supply to site of healing.
- Adequate protein, zinc, and vitamin C.

Complications of Healing

- Contracture

  Exaggerated contraction of maturing collagen, mostly affecting large wounds which results in distortion and limited mobility. Example: contracture following burns of the

Table 33–1 Tissue and Healing Characteristics

Tissue	Healing Characteristics
Epithelial	Readily regenerates except for respiratory epithelium in which scar tissue forms if the damage is more than superficial
Connective tissue	Healing is slow because of limited blood supply
• *Bone*	There are 3 stages: Stage 1—Phagocytes clear debris; granulation tissue forms; osteoblasts (bone formers) migrate to site. Takes 4—5 d Stage 2—Osteoblasts form collagen and cartilage (soft callus) in the break and then ossify it into hard callus, which is structurally weak. Takes 3 wks Stage 3—Osteoblasts and osteoclasts (bone dissolvers) work together to model the large mass of hard callus into normal shape. May take many months/years; bone has normal strength during remodeling
• *Tendons and ligaments*	Requires close approximation of wound edges; if not held tightly together or edges are irregular scar tissue forms resulting in a weak area with reduced function
• *Cartilage*	Heals by fibrous repair and the result is some degree of reduced function
• *Adipose tissue*	Fat cells do not divide but precursor cells differentiate to form replacement tissue
Glandular tissue	Most regenerate well although with extensive injury, new tissue may be disorganized with some impairment of function. Parathyroids have limited ability to regenerate; cells of the glomerulus, Bowman's capsule, adrenal medulla, and posterior pituitary do not regenerate
Nervous tissue	No replacement of neurons occurs; injured cells are replaced with nonfunctional neuroglia. If part of a myelinated neuron is lost in the peripheral nervous system, regeneration occurs slowly over weeks if supporting tissue and Schwann cells remain intact but no sensory receptors are replaced so motor function may be restored but there is sensory loss
Muscular tissue	Cardiac and skeletal muscle cells do not divide and produce new cells; healing is by fibrous repair resulting in loss of contraction strength but this is compensated for by hypertrophy of remaining cells. If only a portion of a muscle fiber is injured some regeneration may occur

skin of the ankle can result in reduced motion of these parts.

Contracture causes stricture or narrowing in tubular organs, for example, healing following gonorrheal infection in the oviducts can cause narrowing which prohibits an ovum from reaching the uterus.

- Adhesions

  Joining of serous membranes, which normally move freely against each other, due to organization of inflammatory exudates. Risk is greatest with trauma to abdominal organs, heart, and lungs.

- Dehiscence

  Breaking open of a healing wound usually as a result of pressure on the wound.

  Abdomen is the most common site of dehiscence with paroxysms of coughing, vomiting, or diarrhea increasing risk.

- Keloids

  Irregular masses of scar tissue protruding from the skin that result from overproduction of collagen.

  Most common among young female blacks from Africa or the Caribbean and occur most frequently on the upper body.

INFECTION

Infection is the invasion and proliferation of microorganisms (bacteria, fungi, viruses, and parasites) in body tissues. All infections cause inflammation but not all inflammations are due to infections.

Terminology Related to Infection

- *Virulence*—ability of a microorganism to produce infection.
- *Pathogen*—microorganism that causes infection in a healthy person.
- *Opportunistic pathogen*—microorganism that causes infection only in a susceptible person.
- *Resident flora*—microorganisms that normally live in a specific area of the body, for example, *Escherichia coli* are normal in the gut; *Candida albicans* are normal in the vagina; *Staphylococcus aureus* are normal in the nasal passages and on the skin. Resident flora cause infection when they move to other parts of the body.
- *Transient flora*—microorganisms that attach loosely to the skin and can be removed by washing.

- *Colonization*—process by which strains of microorganisms become resident flora in an area of the body.
- *Local infection*—infection limited to a specific area of the body.
- *Systemic infection*—microorganisms spread and damage a variety of body areas.
- *Bacteremia*—microorganisms found in the blood when it is cultured.
- *Septicemia*—bacteremia with a systemic infection.
- *Nosocomial infection*—infection associated with health care provided in a health care facility; endogenous if the infection spreads from one area of a client to another; exogenous if the source of the infection is the health care environment or personnel.
- *Iatrogenic infection*—type of nosocomial infection that is the direct result of a diagnostic or therapeutic procedure.

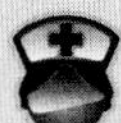

Practice Alert

Most common sites of nosocomial infection: urinary tract, respiratory tract; bloodstream; and wounds.

Most common infecting organisms: *Escherichia coli*, *Staphylococcus aureus*, and *Enterococci*.

Most common type of source: exogenous.

Proper hand washing by heath care providers is essential to prevent exogenous infection; proper washing of client's hands is essential to the prevention of endogenous infection.

Chain of Infection

- *Etiologic agent* (causative microorganism).
- *Reservoir* (source of microorganism; carrier is a human or animal source that does not have signs of disease).
- *Portal of exit from the reservoir* (respiratory tract via coughing, sneezing, breathing, and talking; GI tract via saliva, vomit, and feces; urinary tract via urine; reproductive tract via vaginal or penile discharge and semen; blood via open wounds, needle puncture sites; tissue via drainage from a cut or wound).
- *Modes of transmission*

There are three methods of transmission:

—Direct transfer of microorganisms from person to person through body contact or direct droplet spray.

—Indirect by vehicle (any substance that serves as an intermediate means to transport and introduce a microorganism into a susceptible host; examples include water, blood, serum and fomites (inanimate objects such as tissues, toys, and hospital equipment) or by vector (animal or insect that transports infectious agent).

—Airborne by droplets or dust, which travel on air currents to susceptible host.

- *Portal of entry*—breaks in the skin as well as the usual routes of exit.
- *Susceptible host*—one at risk for infection; compromised host is one at increased risk. Risk results from very young or very old age, chronic illness, suppressed immunity due immunosuppressant drugs, radiation, immunodeficiency diseases; stress with prolonged blood cortisone levels, which suppress inflammatory response and deplete energy, and inadequate nutrition.

Factors Determining the Likelihood of Getting an Infection

- Number of microorganisms—the greater the number, the more likely it is that infection will occur.
- Virulence of the microorganism—the greater the virulence, the more likely the occurrence of infection.
- Ability of the microorganism to enter the body—the greater the ability, the more likely the occurrence of infection.
- Susceptibility of the host—the more susceptible, the greater the likelihood of infection.
- Ability of the microorganism to live in the host's body.

Defenses Against Infection

- Nonspecific defenses
  - —Intact skin and mucous membranes: first line of defense
  - —Cilia and moist membranes that trap microorganisms and other foreign particles
  - —Body fluids such as saliva, highly acidic gastric secretions, acidic vaginal secretions after puberty, and tears
  - —Inflammatory response
- Specific defenses
  - —Antibody-mediated defenses (humoral immunity based on B lymphocytes and mediated by antibodies [immunoglobulins] produced by B cells).
  - —Cell-mediated defenses (cellular immunity based on the T-cells [helper T cells (help immune system), cytotoxic T cells (kill microorganisms), suppressor T cells (suppress function of helper and cytotoxic)] released by lymphoid tissues on exposure to an antigen).

Specific defenses are based in the immune system.

Protection from immunoglobulins from mother protects infants for only 2–3 months.

Signs of Local Infection

- Swelling
- Redness
- Pain or tenderness on touch or movement
- Heat

- Loss of function depending on site and extent

  (Note: These are the five classic signs of inflammation because inflammation always accompanies infection but infection is not always present with inflammation.)

Signs of Systemic Infection

- Fever
- Increased pulse and respiratory rates if fever is high
- Malaise
- Anorexia and sometimes nausea and vomiting
- Enlarged, tender lymph nodes that drain infected area
- Elevated WBC count (>11,000/ml)
- Increase in specific WBCs on differential depending on type of infection
- Elevated ESR
- Positive cultures

NEOPLASIA

CELL CYCLE

- The cell cycle describes the life of a cell.
- It starts at the midpoint of mitosis when a given new cell is being formed and ends at the point when two daughter cells are being formed from that cell.
- The five phases of the cell cycle are
  —G1: postmitotic period of cell growth characterized by development of RNA and protein.
  —G0: resting stage.
  —S: period of DNA synthesis resulting in two sets of chromosomes in the nucleus.
  —G2: premitotic time of RNA and protein synthesis.
  —M: cell splits into two daughter cells.
- From G1 phase, the cell may enter either G0 phase or S phase.
- Length of cycle varies with type of tissue, from 1 hour to 400 hours (liver)—difference results from time spent in G1 and G0.
- Permanent cells such as neurons never enter the cell cycle because they do not replicate.
- Chemotherapeutic drugs act at different stages of the cell cycle.

NORMAL AND ABNORMAL GROWTH

- Aplasia (aplastic growth)—Lack of organ development.
- Hypoplasia (hypoplastic growth)—Inadequate development resulting in immature structure and deficient function.
- Atrophy—Reduction in cell size due to decreased use or demand.
- Hypertrophy—Enlargement of cells that cannot divide in response to use or demand.
- Regeneration—Production of new cells to replace those lost to injury.
- Hyperplasia—Production of new cells by mitosis in response to increased demand, for example, after a nephrectomy, some cells of remaining kidney become hypertrophied and others become hyperplastic and with infection, lymph nodes become hyperplastic and hence lymphadenopathy occurs.
- Metaplasia and dysplasia—Structurally or functionally abnormal tissue due to altered tissue growth in response to intense or prolonged demand, most often affect epithelial tissues.
  —Metaplasia: Conversion of one cell type to another, for example, respiratory epithelium of smokers changes from ciliated pseudostratified to a thicker, well-organized stratification free of cilia and goblet cells that produce mucus so it is more resistant to chronic irritation but does not clear the respiratory tract of inhaled particles and microorganisms as well.
  —Dysplasia: Occurs with more severe and prolonged irritation; dysplastic tissue is disordered and cells vary in size and shape; often precedes neoplasia; some forms of dysplasia are known as precancerous lesions.
- Neoplasia—Overgrowth of tissue resulting in a neoplasm, which is a group of cells with an irreversible abnormal growth pattern. May be benign or malignant.

CHARACTERISTICS OF A BENIGN NEOPLASM

- Benign neoplasm is composed of cells resembling the tissue of origin.
- It grows slowly by expansion.
- It does not recur or metastasize.
- It does not destroy tissue unless it compromises blood supply by pressure.
- It does not cause systemic symptoms or death unless its location interferes with the function of a vital organ such as the brain or the heart.

CHARACTERISTICS OF MALIGNANT NEOPLASMS (CANCER)

- Malignant neoplasms are composed of primitive, undifferentiated cells with limited resemblance to the tissue of origin (anaplastic cells).
- They grow rapidly expanding at periphery and invading and destroying surrounding tissues.
- They tend to recur.
- They metastasize (spread by blood and lymph to distant sites) to create secondary tumors, which in some cases may result in the first signs/symptoms of disease.
- They cause systemic symptoms such as altered taste, anorexia, weight loss, weakness, and ultimately death.

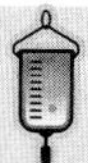

Clinical Alert

Cancers vary in their degree of anaplasia. Generally, the greater the anaplasia, i.e., the more primitive and undifferentiated the cells are, the more malignant the tumor is.

Cancers are not necessarily invasive and metastatic to the same degree—a tumor may be highly metastatic but minimally invasive, minimally metastatic but highly invasive, highly invasive and highly metastatic, or minimally invasive and minimally metastatic.

CLASSIFICATION OF NEOPLASIA

- *Carcinoma*—malignant tumor arising in tissues derived from the ectoderm or endoderm, for example, cancers of the skin, epithelial lining of the respiratory tract or GI tract, or breast.
- *Sarcoma*—malignant tumor arising in tissues derived from the mesoderm, for example, cancers of muscle, bones, or connective tissue.

Specific terminology indicating additional information about the tumor:

- Basal cell carcinoma—cancer of the deepest layer of the skin.
- Squamous cell carcinoma—cancer of skin cells nearer to the surface.
- Adenocarcinoma—cancer of gland cells.
- Leukemia—cancer of the blood.
- Myelomas—cancer of the bone marrow.
- Lymphomas—cancer of the lymphatic system.
- Chondrosarcoma—cancer of cartilage.

CHARACTERISTICS OF MALIGNANT CELLS

- Cell membrane lacks contact inhibition (continues to grow even when touches another cell).
- It does not form intercellular connections.
- Number of free ribosomes is increased.
- Proteins normally synthesized during fetal development are synthesized.
- Fewer enzymes are produced.
- Simpler metabolic pathways are utilized.
- Nucleus is enlarged with abnormal chromosomes and increased amounts of DNA.
- Cells are anaplastic, i.e., primitive and undifferentiated.
- They replicate more quickly than normal—often do not enter the G0 phase of the cell cycle—just keep dividing until blood or nutrient supply runs out.
- They cannot perform functions of the tissue of origin.
- They do not "age" or "die" on time.

CARCINOGENESIS (ONCOGENESIS)

Carcinogenesis refers to the change of normal cells into malignant cells.

Two distinct processes are involved in carcinogenesis:

- *Initiation*—Occurrence of a reversible basic change in the cell, probably in DNA, that creates the potential for tumor development.
- *Promotion*—Exposure to factors which greatly favor tumor growth when initiation has occurred; promoters do not result in tumors in the absence of initiation.

INITIATORS AND PROMOTERS

- Genetic factors
- Environmental chemical and toxic substances
  —nitrosamines in food preservatives
  —benzopyrene in cigarette smoke
  —methylaminobenzene in fabric dyes and food coloring
  —aflatoxin from fungi on improperly stored peanuts and corn
  —asbestos, cobalt, lead, and cadmium
- Tobacco
- Alcohol
- Diet
- Radiation
  —solar radiation (sun)
  —ionizing radiation (radioactive materials, X-ray)

- Viruses
  - —Hepatitis B and C viruses are associated with liver cancer
  - —Human papilloma virus (HPV) causes cervical cancer
  - —Epstein-Barr virus is associated with nasopharyngeal cancer and AIDS-related Burkitt's lymphoma
  - —Human T-cell leukemia virus is associated with some leukemias
  - —Cytomegalovirus is associated with Kaposi's sarcoma
- Immunologic defects
- Psychosocial factors

Most tumors occur in tissues with a high rate of cell reproduction such as epithelia and bone marrow. Permanent tissues such as skeletal muscle and neurons almost never develop tumors.

TUMOR-SPECIFIC ANTIGENS

Tumor-specific antigens (TSAs) form a unique set of antigens found on a tumor's cells. Presence of TSAs suggests "immune surveillance," i.e., that the immune system is capable of recognizing and destroying tumor cells.

TUMOR STAGING

- Tumor staging is the categorization of a cancer based on its potential for invasion and metastasis.
- It is used to describe solid tumors.
- It aids in assessing prognosis and selecting treatment.
- There are many staging systems; in all of them, stage I means growth restricted to primary site and stage IV indicates extensive invasion and metastasis.
- TNM is an international staging system in which T (tumor size), N (regional lymph node involvement), and M (presence of metastasis) are described by subscript numbers from 0 to 3 with 0 meaning none and 1, 2, and 3 meaning increasing disease. Example: for a client with a T1N0M0 breast cancer, there is a single small primary tumor with no involvement of lymph nodes and no metastasis; a T3N2M1 tumor is a large primary tumor with multiple lymph nodes involved and one area of metastasis such as to the bone.

TUMOR GRADING

- Tumor grading is the categorization of a tumor based on histological characteristics of the tumor identified after biopsy.
- Grade 1 has highly differentiated cells with few mitoses and a good prognosis, grades 2, 3, and 4 are progressively less differentiated with more mitoses and a poorer prognosis.

TUMOR EFFECTS

- Tissue destruction secondary to pressure on adjacent cells or blood vessels, release of destructive enzymes, or invasion of adjacent structures, for example, cervical cancer causing kidney failure.
- Obstruction from growth of tumor within a lumen as in esophageal mucosal cancer or from external pressure as in ureteral obstruction from prostate, rectal, or cervical tumors.
- Infection secondary to general suppression of immune system with some cancers; bone marrow suppression that decreases neutrophils and monocytes; disruption of skin or mucous membrane by the tumor; blockage of ureters, GI tract, or respiratory passages causing stagnation which favors bacterial growth.
- Anemia secondary to chronic bleeding from the tumor; bone marrow suppression which also causes clotting deficits due to decreased platelets; autoimmune destruction of circulating RBCs with some tumors and particularly in the elderly; decreased availability of vitamin B12 with GI tumors; or decreased stimulation of RBC production due to decreased erythropoietin with renal tumors.
- Pain, intermittent or constant, due to invasion and destruction of tissue especially bone with fractures, stretching of hollow organs by obstruction, or compression of tissue.
- Cachexia—Syndrome of generalized weakness, fever, wasting, anorexia, and pallor seen in advanced malignancy.
- Hormonal effect

  Hypersecretion of affected glands occurs with benign tumors and with well-differentiated malignant tumors; hyposecretion with anaplastic tumors.

  Ectopic secretion may occur, i.e., tumors of nonendocrine tissue can develop ability to secrete functional hormone.

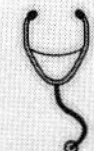

Assessment Alert

Symptoms of hormone excess will present in clients with ectopic secretion of hormones.

Lung cancers may secrete insulin, parathormone, ADH, and ACTH.

Breast, ovarian, and renal cancers may secrete parathormone.

Parathyroid and renal cancers may secrete ACTH.

- Paraneoplastic syndromes—Tumor-related effects that are not well understood, for example, the occurrence of leg vein thrombosis with pancreatic or lung tumors; muscle and peripheral nerve problems with particular lung or breast tumors; increased intracranial pressure from cancers not within the skull.

TUMOR TREATMENT

- Surgery—most successful when tumor is encapsulated and can be removed with minimal disruption of normal tissue; tumors with irregular edges require more removal of normal tissue. If there is node involvement, lymph channels and nodes that drain the tumor site are removed progressively away from the site until no further tumor is detected. Surgical removal of detectable tumor does not guarantee that no microscopic amounts of tumor remain; surgical manipulation may result in embolization of tumor cells.
- Radiation therapy—uses destructive doses of ionizing radiation from radioactive isotopes such as cobalt-60 and devices that produce X-rays to irradiate and destroy tumor cells; also destroys normal cells especially those that are rapidly dividing; produces heat in skin as it passes through and can cause burns (see section "radiation therapy").
- Chemotherapy—toxic chemical substances or hormones, which interfere with the cell's metabolism or division are used to destroy the tumor. Tumors can manifest tolerance to chemotherapy, i.e., antitumor effects are good initially and then diminish (see section "chemotherapy").
- Immunotherapy—uses the immune system to destroy the tumor.
- Combination therapy—uses two or more of the above types of treatment to maximize tumor kill and ideally minimize side effects by limiting the amount of each.

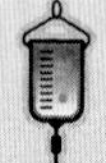

Clinical Alert

Each tumor type differs in its susceptibility to the different types of therapies; therapies used depend on the tumor's susceptibility.

PATHOPHYSIOLOGY OF IMMUNITY

Types of hypersensitivity reactions

- Type I: immediate or anaphylactic hypersensitivity
- Type II: antibody-dependent hypersensitivity
- Type III: immune-complex-mediated hypersensitivity
- Type IV: cell-mediated, delayed-type hypersensitivity

IMMEDIATE OR ANAPHYLACTIC HYPERSENSITIVITY

The first exposure to the antigen, which is usually through skin or mucous membrane, causes no symptomatic reaction but the antigen has been recognized and IgE antibodies specific to it have been produced and have bound to mast cells throughout the body. This is called sensitization and can last for months. When the sensitized system next encounters the antigen, allergen binds to the antibodies causing release of chemical mediators from the mast cells. The result is a two-phase reaction: immediate and late.

- *Immediate phase*
  —Primarily due to histamine.
  —Occurs in 5–30 minutes and can be over in an hour.
  —Effects: increased vascular permeability; constriction of bronchial muscles and narrowed airways; increased secretion from nasal, bronchial, and gastric glands; hives, conjunctivitis, and rhinitis.
  —Antihistamines can lessen early-phase effects by blocking the effects of histamine; epinephrine can block the actual response of mast cells.
- *Late phase*
  —Involves mediators that attract eosinophils and neutrophils, leukotrienes, prostaglandins, platelet-activating factor, and protein-digesting enzymes resulting in cellular infiltration and tissue damage.
  —Occurs in 2–8 hours and may last 2–3 days.
  —Corticoid steroids and NSAIDs block the late phase while leaving the early phase unaffected.

Localized Anaphylaxis

- Forms of localized anaphylaxis include allergic asthma, hay fever, eczema, and urticaria (hives).
- It develops after repeated exposure to low-dose antigen at a mucosal barrier.
- It is controlled by avoiding allergen or desensitization (injections of low but increasing doses of allergen, which increase IgG that removes antigen from the body fluids before it can interact with the mast cells.

Systemic Anaphylaxis

- Within minutes, widespread mast cell release of histamine causes pruritus, urticaria, wheezing, dyspnea, which can progress to laryngospasm and suffocation. Circulatory shock from loss of fluid from the vascular tree also occurs.

- Triggers include drugs, especially antibiotics such as penicillin, insect venoms such as from bee or wasp stings, foods such as shellfish or peanuts, and desensitization injections of allergens.
- Rx: Parenteral histamine competitors such as epinephrine or isoproterenol.

ANTIBODY-DEPENDENT HYPERSENSITIVITY

Antibodies attach to the surface of cells such as RBCs or the glomerular basement membrane of the kidney and initiate a series of cytotoxic mechanisms involving K cells, the complement cascade, and antibody Fc components which destroy the cells.

This reaction in which antibodies are turned against self-cells is the mechanism underlying autoimmune diseases such as myasthenia gravis.

IMMUNE-COMPLEX-MEDIATED HYPERSENSITIVITY

Immune complexes are aggregations of antigens and their antibodies. Large immune complexes, which are removed from the bloodstream by the liver and the spleen, are formed when there are equal amounts of antigen and antibody. When the amounts are unequal, smaller complexes are formed which are deposited in the vascular walls resulting in microthrombi formation and endothelial damage as well as an inflammatory response with basement membrane damage. If the problem is excessive amounts of antibody specific to a tissue, the immune complexes tend to be deposited in that tissue as seen in rheumatoid arthritis. If the problem is excessive antigen, they tend to be deposited in the area of exposure as with the lung in the pneumonoconiosis.

CELL-MEDIATED, DELAYED-TYPE HYPERSENSITIVITY

Cell-mediated hypersensitivity is the primary cause of tissue damage in TB, contact dermatitis, acute and chronic transplant rejection, and in many fungal, viral, and parasitic infections.

The reaction requires antigen presentation and helper-T-cell sensitization to begin and then involves cytotoxic T cells, activated macrophages, K cells with their antibody-dependent cellular toxicity (ADCC) action, and NK cells.

IMMUNE DEFICIENCY

PRIMARY DEFICIENCIES

- Primary deficiencies are often genetic.
- They manifest as chronic or recurrent infections in infants over a few months of age because of the inability to replace passive immunity received from mother during pregnancy with active immunity.
- B-cell deficiency: low or absent gamma globulin resulting in infections with viruses such as rubella, which are normally neutralized by antibody, or bacteria such as *H. influenzae* that require opsonization to be phagocytized.
- T-cell deficiency: results in chronic or repeated infections due to viruses, yeasts/fungi such as *Candida*, and/or intracellular bacteria such as *M. tuberculosis*.
- Severe combined immunodeficiency: autosomal recessive or X-linked inherited disorder in which both T-cell and immunoglobulin production and function are deficient.
- Without successful bone-marrow transplant, death occurs before 1 year of age from opportunistic infection due to the same organisms as in AIDS (*Pneumocystis carinii*, *Candida*, *Pseudomonas*, cytomegalovirus, and herpes simplex virus).

SECONDARY DEFICIENCIES

- T-cell-mediated immune response decreases with increasing age.
- Immune deficiency occurs with severe malnutrition.
- Severe burns result in diminished ability to combat bacteria such as *H. influenzae* or *Staphylococcus* that require opsonization for phagocytosis.
- Diabetes results in reduced inflammatory and specific immune responses.
- Leukemias, lymphomas as well as infections such as cytomegalovirus, TB, and coccidiomycosis can suppress immune function.
- Iatrogenic deficiencies (related to medical treatment) occur with immunosuppressant drugs used to prevent graft rejection, chemotherapy or radiation used to treat cancer, use of drugs such as some anticonvulsants, tranquilizers, antimicrobials, analgesics, which are toxic to immune system components, surgery and anesthesia which can depress B-and T-cell function and cause lymphocyte deficiency for up to a month, stress, and corticosteroids.
- HIV infection (see Chapter 32).

RADIATION THERAPY

- Radiation therapy is used as a curative or palliative treatment for cancer alone or in combination with surgery and/or chemotherapy.
- The goal is to kill tumor cells without damaging normal cells; therefore, total radiation dose is divided and given in varying patterns to allow normal cells to recoup. However, there is always some damage to normal cells.
- Different body tissues have different levels of radiosensitivity (potential susceptibility to injury from ionizing radiation and time needed for damage to occur). Tissues that are highly proliferative are most affected by radiation. Thus, effects are first seen in bone marrow, skin, and GI tract.
- Hypoxic tissues are resistant to radiation.
- Radiosensitizers are drugs that enhance the effect of radiation; radioprotectors help protect normal cells from damage.
- Side effects of radiation primarily affect tissues at the site of therapy and may be acute (affect tissues with rapid cell division and occur within days) or late (due to blood vessel or connective tissue damage and occur after months or years, e.g., skin atrophy, fibrosis or ulceration, cataracts, and pulmonary fibrosis). Most common acute side effects are port-area skin reactions (erythema which increases over 2–3 weeks and then fades or progresses to dry then moist desquamation along with temporary alopecia), fatigue, and bone-marrow suppression (occurs with almost all ports with recovery time dependent on the size of port and dose of radiation).

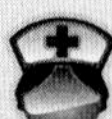

Practice Alert

Skin folds (intertriginous areas) such as axilla and groin are at high risk for skin reactions.

- Postradiation malignancies such as skin cancer, leukemia, non-Hodgkin's lymphoma, and sarcoma can develop.
- Monitoring for signs of bone-marrow depression (changes in laboratory values, infection, anemia, or bleeding) and for changes in weight at least weekly are critical nursing responsibilities.

INTERNAL RADIOTHERAPY (BRACHYTHERAPY)

- In internal radiotherapy, the radioactive source is placed in the body; the source may be sealed, for example, radioactive seeds inserted in prostate tumors, radioactive needles placed in breast tumors, or unsealed, for example, radioactive iodine (I 131) ingested/injected for thyroid tumors.
- Sealed radiation source may be inserted and removed at each treatment or afterloaded and left in place for duration of treatment.
- Afterloading: The container is placed in the body in the OR with its position confirmed by X-ray; client is placed in a private room; and radioactive substance is inserted. Exact positioning of the implant is essential to radiate tumor and prevent damage to normal tissue.
- Both sealed and unsealed sources require radiation precautions to protect others from exposure. Exposure risk of unsealed sources varies with the specific isotope used and its mode of excretion from the body; for example, I 131 is excreted from body fluids so there is exposure risk both from client and from contact with body discharges.

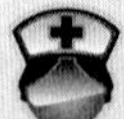

Practice Alert

- Time, distance, and shielding are the three essential elements in protection from hazardous radiation exposure. Minimize time with and maximize distance from clients with internal radiation sources.
- Remember a lead shield is not adequate protection against gamma rays.
- Follow guidelines from radiation safety officer carefully.
- Always wear dosimetry badge to measure radiation exposure.
- Rotate care of brachytherapy clients among the team of nurses.
- Never assign a pregnant nurse to care for a brachytherapy client.
- Trace doses of radiation used for diagnosis do not require special precautions.

EXTERNAL RADIOTHERAPY

- In external radiotherapy, the port (anatomic area that will receive the radiation) is marked in ink or tattoos.
- It is preoperatively used to decrease tumor size and eliminate stray cancer cells outside the operative area but

results in delayed healing of the parts of the surgical wound in the radiation-treated area.

- It is used postoperatively to eradicate any remaining tumor or subclinical disease.

Client teaching for self-care

Teach client to

- prevent irritation of skin over treated area: Cleanse area daily with mild soap and water (do not erase markings and take care to dry skin folds carefully); avoid irritating, rubbing clothes (cotton against skin is least irritating), use of perfumed soaps, ointments, powders, lotions, deodorants, heating pads, and hot or cold packs; use only an electric shaver; avoid scratching, vigorous rubbing or massage; also to avoid sun exposure when possible otherwise use sunscreen
- plan rest periods during the day and adequate sleep at night to combat fatigue
- eat a high-protein, high-CHO, and high-calorie diet and check weight weekly for loss
- take antiemetics and antidiarrheals as prescribed and eat a low-residue diet, for nausea and diarrhea associated with an abdominal port

For mucositis or xerostomia due to radiation involving the mouth or throat, teach as indicated under chemotherapy.

CHEMOTHERAPY

- Chemotherapy is used for the cure of cancer, long-term control of tumor growth, or for palliative shrinking of the tumor.
- Adjuvant chemotherapy (chemotherapy given along with either surgery or radiation) is designed to destroy any micrometastases.
- Chemotherapeutic agents that act on dividing cells are most effective when tumors are small and many cells are dividing; larger, slower growing tumors respond best to agents that act whether or not the cells are dividing.
- Mostly, chemotherapy involves a combination regimen because
  —different drugs attack tumor cells in different ways thereby increasing effectiveness,
  —risk of the tumor becoming resistant to therapy is decreased, and
  —different drugs produce toxicity in different organs and at different times after administration so larger amounts of chemotherapy can be given.
- Classifications of chemotherapeutic drugs include alkylating agents, antimetabolites, plant (vinca) alkaloids, antitumor antibiotics, and steroids.
- Doses of chemotherapy are usually based on body surface area (BSA), which is calculated using height and weight.
- Routes of administration are po, sc, IM, IV, topical, or direct instillation into bladder, peritoneum, CSF, or tumor bed, which allows high doses with less severe systemic effects. IV route often through a central VAD is most common.
- Side effects of chemotherapy, like those of radiotherapy, are seen first in tissues with rapid growth rates: bone marrow, GI epithelium, hair follicles, and the germinal epithelium of the testes. Fatigue and organ toxicities that are drug specific are also common. Table 33–2 discusses the side effects of chemotherapy.
- Some chemotherapy drugs are vesicants, i.e., cause severe tissue ulceration if they leak out of the vein into soft tissues

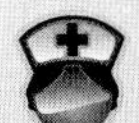

Practice Alert

Monitoring for IV infiltration when vesicant drugs are being administered is critical as is immediate treatment with appropriate antidotes and hot and cold applications to minimize tissue damage.

- Some chemotherapy drugs are associated with hypersensitivity reactions and specific precautions must be taken during administration.

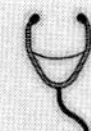

Assessment Alert

The most serious complication of bone-marrow suppression (specifically neutropenia) is infection, with the most common sites being oropharynx, lungs, urinary tract, and skin.

Table 33–2 Side Effects of Chemotherapy

Affected Tissue/Organ	Symptoms	Notes	Management
Bone-marrow suppression	Neutropenia (neutrophil count <1000/mm^3)	Each drug has a particular time at which maximum suppression occurs—for many drugs it is 7–10 d after drug administration	Implement regimen to maintain skin and mucous membrane integrity Avoid injections, rectal treatments, and other invasive procedures such as urinary catheterization Avoid medications that mask pain and other signs of infection Minimize exposure to sources of infection: Good hand washing by staff; restrict contact with persons with colds or other infection; avoid or thoroughly wash and cook fruits and vegetables; avoid obviously infected items such as litter boxes, and used tissues Monitor WBC and neutrophil count and for signs of infection Report stat fever over 101 F or other signs of infection Obtain bacterial and fungal cultures of body fluids before giving antibiotics Administer antibiotics and colony-stimulating factors as ordered
	Thromboctopenia (Platelets <50,000/mm^3)	May be mild such as bruising or a nosebleed or major hemorrhage into brain or GI tract	Minimize trauma by avoiding injections, rectal treatments, and other invasive procedures Avoid drugs which increase bleeding (ASA and NSAIDs) After venipuncture, apply pressure for 5 min to site Monitor platelet count Monitor for signs of bleeding Administer platelet Tx as ordered for count below 10,000/mm^3, for active bleeding or before invasive procedures Use soft toothbrush; avoid flossing and dental procedures Use only electric shaver Avoid activities that present risk of trauma
	Anemia	Signs of decreased tissue perfusion in any organ: fatigue, decreased endurance, headache, dizziness, tachycardia, and dyspnea	Administer EPO and/or Tx as ordered Design energy-conserving plan with client
GI tract	Stomatitis	Timing usually parallels bone-marrow suppression, i.e., 7–10 d after treatment	Remove and clean dentures or brush teeth with soft brush after eating and at bedtime, then rinse with salt and water or a mouthwash containing <6% alcohol Floss daily unless contraindicated

(continued on next page)

Table 33–2 *(continued from previous page)*

Affected Tissue/Organ	Symptoms	Notes	Management
			Do not wear dentures if they rub or are rough or if mouth is sore Lubricate lips and avoid irritants such as alcohol or tobacco Rinse every 2–4 hrs, increase fluid intake and use artificial saliva PRN for dry mouth Avoid spicy or acidic foods and use topical anesthetics and systemic analgesics PRN for sore mouth
	N&V	Typically peaks in first 12 hrs; may be followed by delayed nausea lasting 2–5 d Anticipatory N&V may also occur	Administer antiemetics Monitor fluid and electrolyte status
	Constipation and diarrhea	May be directly caused by drug but can be exacerbated by altered diet, opioid use, etc.	
Hair follicles	Alopecia	Amount of hair loss is dose and route-dependent; ranges from thinning of scalp hair to complete loss of all body hair; begins 2–3 wks after start of Rx; reversible with regrowth starting 1–2 mo after Rx and taking up to a year	
Ovaries/testes	Altered fertility: amenorrhea in young and menopause in older females; decreased sperm production and sperm and semen abnormalities in men	Most common with alkylating agents; fertility can be recovered but length and time for recovery depends on the drug and the dose; younger women more likely to recover than older	
Specific drug-related organ toxicities			Cryoprotectant drugs protect normal tissue and prevent some toxicities
Heart (cardiac cells)	EKG changes, heart failure over long term	Occurs with anthracycline agents	
Lungs	Pulmonary fibrosis	Occurs with bleomycin	
Liver	Hepatic toxicity	Occurs with high doses of many drugs	
Kidney	Nephrotoxicity	Occurs with cisplatin and high dose of methotrexate	
Urinary bladder	Hemorrhagic cystitis	Occurs with cyclophosphamide and ifosfamide	

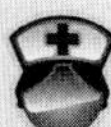

Practice Alert

Health care workers who handle chemotherapeutic drugs can be exposed to low doses and be at risk for their side effects including carcinogenicity and teratogenicity so following OSHA guidelines for safe handling of chemotherapeutic drugs is critical.

Most cytotoxic agents are metabolized or excreted within 48 hours although stool excretion can take a week.

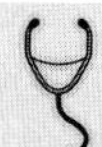

Assessment Alert

Neutropenic clients do not exhibit a normal inflammatory response. Mild localized tenderness and fever over 101 F may be the only signs of severe infection and represent a medical emergency.

Client teaching for self-care

- Clarify goal of chemotherapy: cure, palliation, and adjuvant therapy
- Reinforce planned protocol, i.e., treatment intervals and duration
- Teach client about expected side effects and supportive interventions as shown in Table 33–2

HEMODYNAMICS

The heart, large blood vessels, and the microcirculation (capillary circulation) interact to keep all body tissues perfused with blood. Effective perfusion requires good cardiac pumping ability, an adequate amount of blood to be pumped, and ability of blood vessels to constrict and to dilate to maintain blood pressure.

- Heart rate
  —Increased by sympathetic and decreased by parasympathetic nervous system stimulation.
  —Sustained rate of >180 bpm increases work of heart and decreases time of diastole so there is less time for ventricular filling.
  —Cardiac muscle receives oxygenated blood during diastole so at high heart rates the heart muscle becomes ischemic.
- Stroke volume
  —Volume of blood ejected by the ventricle with each heartbeat.
  —Normal: 60–70 ml.
- Cardiac output (CO)
  —Volume of blood pumped by the ventricle per minute. (Heart rate × stroke volume).
  —Normal: 4–6 l/min.
- Central venous pressure (CVP)
  —Pressure created by blood volume in the right side of the heart.
  —Normal: 2–4 mm Hg.
- Systemic vascular resistance (SVR)
  —Resistance in the arteries and the arterioles against which the left ventricle must pump. As SVR increases, CO decreases.
  —Normal: 900–1400 dynes/sec/cm^{-5}.
- Pulmonary vascular resistance
  —Resistance in the pulmonary arteries and the arterioles against which the right ventricle must pump.
  —Normal: 30–100 dynes/sec/cm^{-5}
- Preload
  —As the amount of blood filling the ventricle during diastole increases, the force of contraction increases up to a critical point after which effective contraction decreases.
  —Preload is a function of the volume of blood filling the ventricle and the ability of the ventricle to stretch (ventricular compliance).
  —Right ventricular preload is measured by CVP (normal range 2–4 mm Hg).

—Left ventricular preload volume pressure is measured as the pulmonary artery wedge pressure (PAWP) (normal range 5–12 mm Hg).

- Afterload
  —Tension in the ventricular wall during systole.
  —As afterload increases, work required for the heart to pump blood increases.
  —Afterload is increased by any factor that opposes the ejection of blood from the ventricle, e.g., aortic or pulmonary stenosis, septal hypertrophy, vasoconstriction, and increase in blood volume or viscosity.
- Contractility (contractile force of the heart or inotropy)
  —Inotropy is increased by sympathetic nervous system stimulation and by drugs such as digoxin, dopamine, and amrinone.
  —Inotropy is decreased by factors such as acidosis and hypoxia.
- Hemodynamic parameters which reflect these functions are
  —CVP,
  —pulmonary artery pressure (PAP), and
  —intra-arterial blood pressure.

CVP MEASUREMENT

- CVP is the pressure of the blood in the right atrium.
- It reflects right ventricular heart function and venous blood return.
- It indicates the heart's ability to manage fluid load.

Uses: CVP is a hemodynamic measure to manage a client's fluid volume status; it is used as a guide to the safe administration of intravenous fluid volume.

- Elevated CVP is indicative of hypervolemia: CHF, pulmonary edema, and cardiac tamponade.
- Decreased CVP is indicative of hypovolemia: dehydration and shock.

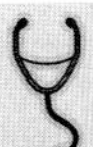

Assessment Alert

Normal range may be measured as 2–8 mm Hg *or* 5–10 cm of CVP of H_2O depending on the equipment used.

The zero point of the manometer or the transducer must be at the level of the right atrium (phlebostatic axis—fourth intercostal space midaxillary line)

Preparation: CVP catheter is inserted and connected to either a water manometer or a pressure-monitoring system.

Procedure: Procedure is generally done at the bedside. Equipment is prepared; insertion site is selected, shaved if necessary and cleansed with antiseptic solution; the physician inserts and threads a CVP catheter into the superior vena cava just above the right atrium.

Complications: Infection and air embolism.

Nursing Process Elements

- Provide client education concerning CVP monitoring
- Make sure the catheter is secure and a dry sterile occlusive dressing is in place
- Obtain portable chest X-ray to confirm placement
- Inspect site for signs of infection
- Perform dressing change per protocol
- Change lines per protocol
- Take CVP readings as ordered noting that trends are more important and accurate than individual readings
- Be sure to correctly zero prior to readings

PAP MEASUREMENT

- Pulmonary artery catheter is often referred to as Swan–Ganz catheter.
- It has four to five lumens to measure various cardiac pressures.
  —CVP or right atrial pressure
    - Reading is from the proximal lumen with normal CVP 0–5 mm Hg.
  —PAP
    - Normal mean pressure is 15 mm Hg.
  —PAWP
    - Balloon is inflated with 1 ml of air and becomes wedged in a pulmonary artery so that pressure of the left ventricle end diastolic pressure is obtained when the mitral valve is open, normal mean pressure is 10 mm Hg.
  —CO
    - Amount of blood pumped by the heart in 1 minute. Normal 4–8 lpm and is measured by thermodilution method where fluid is injected into the proximal lumen and the temperature change of the blood is recorded in the pulmonary artery by a thermistor and calculated by a computer.
  —It may also have pacing capabilities.

Uses: PAP measurement is used in hemodynamic monitoring to provide information about the efficiency of the right and left sides of the heart and evaluating a client's response to medical treatment.

Preparation: PAP catheter is a balloon-tipped catheter which is inserted through a large vein and then attached to a pressure-monitoring system (300 mm Hg heparinized pressure solution). It requires continuous ECG monitoring during insertion.

Procedure: Procedure is generally done at the bedside. Equipment is prepared; insertion site is selected, shaved if necessary and cleansed with antiseptic solution; the physician inserts and threads a PAP catheter into the superior vena cava → right atrium → right ventricle → pulmonary artery.

Complications: Infection, air embolism, thromboembolism, dysrhythmias, hemorrhage, pulmonary artery infarct, and pulmonary artery rupture.

Nursing Process Elements

- Provide client education concerning PAP monitoring
- Make sure the catheter is secure and a dry sterile occlusive dressing is in place
- Obtain portable chest X-ray to confirm placement
- Inspect site for signs of infection
- Perform dressing change per protocol using aseptic technique (every 48 hours is standard)
- Change lines per protocol (every 72 hours for line and 24 hours for IV solution is standard)
- Take PAP readings as ordered noting that trends are more important and accurate than individual readings
- Take readings between breaths to avoid effects of intrathoracic pressure
- Be sure balloon is completely deflated after PAWP is obtained
- Be sure that the catheter is correctly calibrated and zeroed prior to readings
- Keep pressure at 300 mm Hg at all times to ensure a continuous flow of flush solution to prevent clot formation and catheter occlusion
- Know procedures for immediate treatment if complications occur

INTRA-ARTERIAL BLOOD PRESSURE MEASUREMENT

- Intra-arterial blood pressure measurement refers to the continuous measurement of systolic, diastolic, and mean arterial blood (MAP) pressure.
- It provides continuous assessment of arterial perfusion to the major organs.
- MAP represents perfusion pressure throughout the cardiac cycle. Normal range 70–100 mm Hg

Uses: It is used to obtain direct and continuous BP monitoring when Kirchoff sounds are not heard, when client is hemodynamically unstable, when client is receiving potent vasoactive medications, and may also be used when frequent arterial blood gas measurements are required.

Preparation: Prepare client for procedure and gather materials including catheter, tubing, heparinized pressure solution, and monitor.

Procedure: Procedure is generally done at the bedside. Allen test is performed to determine that collateral circulation is adequate. Equipment is prepared; insertion artery site is selected and cleansed with antiseptic solution; the physician cannulates an artery and attaches the pressure-monitoring system.

Complications: Infection, air embolism, thromboembolism, and hemorrhage.

Nursing Process Elements

- Provide client education concerning intra-arterial BP monitoring
- Make sure the catheter is secure and a dry sterile occlusive dressing is in place
- Make sure site is visible
- Inspect site for signs of infection
- Assess peripheral perfusion by checking extremity for color, temperature, sensation, pulses, and movement
- Perform dressing change per protocol
- Change lines per protocol
- Monitor BP readings as ordered noting that trends are more important and accurate than individual readings
- Know procedures for immediate treatment if complications occur
- Compare monitor BP readings with manual readings per shift

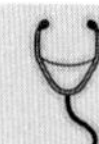

Assessment Alert

Intra-arterial BP readings may be 5–10 mm Hg higher than manual cuff BP readings.

WORKSHEET

FILL IN THE BLANKS

Fill in the blank spaces with the correct word or phrase to complete each statement.

1. The three most basic causes of cell injury are
   a. ______________________________
   b. ______________________________
   c. ______________________________
2. The five classic signs of infection are
   a. ______________________________
   b. ______________________________
   c. ______________________________
   d. ______________________________
   e. ______________________________
3. The two major components of the inflammatory response are
   a. ______________________________
   b. ______________________________
4. The three types of exudates are
   a. ______________________________
   b. ______________________________
   c. ______________________________
5. The four components of the healing process are
   a. ______________________________
   b. ______________________________
   c. ______________________________
   d. ______________________________
6. Collagen fibers in scar tissue are weak for ________ days.
7. The four most common sites of nosocomial infection are
   a. ______________________________
   b. ______________________________
   c. ______________________________
   d. ______________________________
8. Cancers arising in tissues derived from mesoderm such as muscles, bones, or connective tissue are called ________________.
9. The two distinct processes involved in carcinogenesis are
   a. ______________________________
   b. ______________________________
10. Another name for the contractile force of the heart is ____________________.

TRUE & FALSE QUESTIONS

Mark each of the following statements True or False. Correct all false statements in the space provided.

1. Calcification occurs only in necrotic tissue. ___ T ___ F
2. Chronic inflammation progressively destroys tissue and results in loss of function and scarring. ___ T ___ F
3. Once regeneration occurs, function is restored to damaged organs. ___ T ___ F
4. If a child cuts his hand on a piece of broken glass and has eight sutures to close the wound, healing will occur by second intention. ___ T ___ F
5. To facilitate healing of a wound across the middle knuckle of the index finger, the joint needs to be immobilized. ___ T ___ F
6. Signs of systemic infection include swollen lymph nodes, fever, and elevated ESR. ___ T ___ F
7. Total length of the cell cycle is the same for all cells; what differs is the length of time spent in each phase. ___ T ___ F
8. A characteristic of a benign tumor is that it is composed of cells that resemble the tissue of origin. ___ T ___ F
9. Malignant tumors cause systemic symptoms such as altered taste and weight loss. ___ T ___ F
10. The initial effect of an increase in heart rate is a decrease in cardiac output. ___ T ___ F

MATCHING QUESTIONS

Match the following:

1. ____ Adhesions	a. Type of nosocomial infection, which is the direct result of a diagnostic or therapeutic procedure
2. ____ Hypertrophy	b. Angioneogenesis
3. ____ Serous exudates	c. Ability of a microorganism to produce infection
4. ____ Dehiscence	d. Enlargement of cells and organs as a result of increased demand
5. ____ Apoptosis	e. Number of cells increased through cell division in response to demand
6. ____ Contracture	f. Fluid in blisters of a mild sunburn
7. ____ Suppurative exudate	g. Microorganism that causes infection only in a susceptible person

8. ______ Necrosis	h. Tissue death
9. ______ Granuloma	i. Process by which strains of microorganisms become resident flora in an area of the body
10. ______ Keloid	j. Tissue is disordered and cells vary in size and shape
11. ______ Hyperplasia	k. Shrinking of cells and organs as a result of decreased demand
12. ______ Phagocytosis	l. Lack of organ development
13. ______ Revascularization	m. Exaggerated contraction of maturing collagen, mostly affecting large wounds which results in distortion and limited mobility
14. ______ Colonization	n. Joining of serous membranes which normally move freely against each other due to organization of inflammatory exudates. Risk is greatest with trauma to abdominal organs, heart, and lungs
15. ______ Atrophy	o. Breaking open of a healing wound usually a result of pressure on the wound
16. ______ Opportunistic pathogen	p. Irregular masses of scar tissue protruding from the skin that result from overproduction of collagen
17. ______ Iatrogenic infection	q. Decreased number of cells as a result of self-destruction
18. ______ Virulence	r. Round masses of transformed macrophages surrounded by lymphocytes and fibroblasts
19. ______ Aplastic	s. Shortening of a muscle or scar tissue causing distortion or deformity
20. ______ Dysplasia	t. Ingestion of particles by cells
	u. Material that passes through vessels into adjacent tissues in inflammation

APPLICATION QUESTIONS

1. Of which process is gangrene an example?
   a. Coagulation necrosis
   b. Liquefaction necrosis
   c. Autolysis
   d. Phagocytosis
2. Which is the primary factor that determines the time interval that can elapse between removal of an organ from a donor and its transplantation into a recipient?
   a. Time an organ can survive ischemia
   b. Ability of the organ to withstand temperature change
   c. Amount of DNA present in the organ's cells
   d. Number of organelles in the organ's cells
3. Which factors can initiate an inflammatory response? (Select all that apply.)
   a. Heat or cold
   b. Trauma
   c. Infection
   d. Antigen–antibody-complex deposition
   e. Complement activation

(continued)

4. What type of diet should be encouraged for a client having radiation through an abdominal port who complains of nausea and vomiting? (Select all that apply.)
   a. High-protein
   b. High-carbohydrate
   c. High-fat
   d. High-residue
   e. High-calorie
   f. Low-protein
   g. Low-calorie
   h. Low-carbohydrate
   i. Low-residue
   j. Low-fat

5. When caring for a client having radiation therapy the nurse receives a report that the client's laboratory values are normal and there are no signs of anemia, infection, or bleeding. Which conclusion should the nurse draw from this information?
   a. Radiation has not yet reached a therapeutic level.
   b. The client is free of side effects of radiation.
   c. Nutritional status is normal.
   d. Bone-marrow suppression is not a problem.

6. The father of a 9-month-old boy just diagnosed with a primary immune deficiency says to the nurse "I don't understand it. Why did my son seem healthy until he was 6-months old and then start getting all these infections?" On which fact should the nurse's response be based?
   a. Under 6-months of age, most babies do not show signs of active infection.
   b. It takes about 6 months for babies to be exposed to enough pathogens for infection to readily occur.
   c. Until about 6 months, babies are protected from infection by immunity from their mothers.
   d. Before 6 months, babies are only susceptible to bacterial infections.

7. When assessing skin of a client having external radiation therapy, which fact should the nurse keep in mind?
   a. Skin damage is preceded by changes in oral mucous membranes.
   b. Most skin changes occur 4–8 weeks after the start of radiation.
   c. Skin areas with poor blood flow are at greatest risk for injury.
   d. Intertriginous areas are at particular risk for skin reactions.

8. How should the care of a client undergoing brachytherapy be assigned?
   a. To male nurses whenever possible
   b. On a rotating basis among nonpregnant nursing staff
   c. Consistently to the same nurses
   d. Never to a nurse with a history of cancer

9. A client having radiation therapy asks the nurse if his blood cells are going to be affected. Which fact should form the basis of the nurse's answer?
   a. Bone marrow and therefore blood cells is affected with almost all ports of radiation.
   b. If radiation is delivered to the hip or leg, no effect should occur.
   c. It depends on whether or not medications are being taken that sensitize blood cells to radiation.
   d. Speed and volume of blood to tissues of the port will determine the effect.

10. Which direction should be given to a client with a platelet count of 45,000 mm^3, a WBC count of 1250/mm^3, and an RBC count of 4.8 million/mm^3?
    a. Cook vegetables well.
    b. Use an electric razor.
    c. Rest at regular intervals.
    d. Increase vitamin B12 intake.

11. A client having chemotherapy for breast cancer reports a temperature of 101.4 F. How should the nurse interpret this fact?
    a. Sign of infection, which needs to be reported right away
    b. Side effect of chemotherapy, not requiring intervention
    c. Sign of infection, which needs monitoring and reporting if it persists for 48 hours
    d. Indicator of dehydration requiring client teaching regarding fluid intake

12. A client who had a dose of chemotherapy at 8 a.m. calls the clinic at 2:30 p.m. complaining of nausea and vomiting despite having taken the prescribed medication. She asks how much worse the nausea and vomiting is going to get. On which fact should the nurse's answer be based?
    a. Nausea and vomiting is totally unpredictable.
    b. Nausea and vomiting typically peak in the first 12 hours.
    c. Nausea and vomiting will ease on going to bed.
    d. Vomiting should cease in about 36 hours but nausea may persist for 7–10 days.

13. For which type of toxicity would the nurse plan to monitor a client who is being treated with cisplatin?
    a. Neurotoxicity
    b. Cardiotoxicity
    c. Nephrotoxicity
    d. Hepatotoxicity

14. Which class of chemotherapy drugs is most likely to affect fertility?
    a. Alkylating agents
    b. Antimetabolytes
    c. Cytotoxic antibiotics
    d. Mitotic inhibitors

15. Which information could be correctly included in the teaching plan for a client receiving chemotherapy?
    a. Scalp hair may be lost but body hair is unaffected.
    b. Hair loss usually occurs 6–8 weeks after chemotherapy starts.
    c. Regrowth usually starts 1–2 months after chemotherapy is completed.
    d. Hair regrowth can be expected to take 24–36 months.

16. Which comment about measuring pulmonary artery wedge pressure indicates a correct understanding of at least one aspect of the procedure?
    a. The pressure-monitoring system must be calibrated at least every 12 hours.
    b. Normal mean pressure is 15 mm Hg.
    c. The balloon must be completely deflated after each pressure measurement is obtained.
    d. The catheter is passed through the right heart and into the right pulmonary artery.

Think Smart/Test Smart

This question is looking for a correct statement because it asks which statement shows that the person making it correctly understands some aspect of the procedure. Thus, three distractors are going to be incorrect statements about the procedure and one is going to be correct and will be the answer.

17. Which statement is an appropriate practice guideline when CVP is being monitored?
    a. A pressure greater than 6 mm Hg must be reported immediately.
    b. A CVP of greater than 10 mm Hg indicates the need for immediate fluid.
    c. Overall trend is more important than any individual measure.
    d. A CVP of 1–3 mm Hg requires immediate intervention to prevent pulmonary edema.

18. Which statement made by a client receiving radiation therapy indicates a need for further teaching?
    a. "Today is my last treatment so by next week I will know if I am going to have any side effects from the radiation."
    b. "I'm tired of having blood drawn but I know I need it to check my bone marrow."
    c. "I need to check my skin for redness, especially in the skin folds."
    d. "I'm awfully fatigued all the time but I understand it is expected."

19. When caring for a client with a Swan–Ganz catheter, for which complications would the nurse monitor? (Select all that apply.)
    a. Heart failure
    b. Thromboembolism
    c. Hypervolemia
    d. Cardiac dysrhythmia
    e. Infection

20. A client who has received a biopsy report indicating dysplasia asks the nurse if this means she has cancer. Which is the most appropriate response?
    a. "Yes, it is cancer but an early form that is usually treatable."
    b. "It may be cancer. More tests have to be done and you will know in about 5 days."
    c. "No, it is not cancer but the tissue is abnormal and sometimes it becomes cancerous."
    d. "No, it is not cancer and it doesn't turn into cancer."

21. Which complication must the nurse be alert for when caring for a client on intra-arterial blood pressure monitoring?
    a. Ventricular tachycardia
    b. Myocardial infarct
    c. Pulmonary artery rupture
    d. Hemorrhage

(continued)

22. The spouse of a client who is to have intra-arterial blood pressure monitoring initiated, tells the nurse he heard someone say that an Allen test would be done and asks what it is for. Which fact should form the basis of the nurse's response?
   a. To make sure there is collateral circulation sufficient to keep tissue supplied with oxygenated blood.
   b. To check for abnormal clotting because of the risk of thromboembolism.
   c. To check if the volume of bloodflow is sufficient to provide an accurate measurement.
   d. To determine if the artery has a diameter great enough to allow passage of the catheter.
23. When measuring CVP, which is the reference point or the zero point of the manometer or the transducer?
   a. Fourth intercostal space at the left midclavicular line
   b. Fourth intercostal space at the left sternal border
   c. Sixth intercostal space at the right sternal border
   d. Sixth intercostal space at the left midclavicular line
24. A client having a Swan–Ganz catheter inserted asks how the MD will know when it is in the right place. What is the most accurate reply to the client's question?
   a. A chest X-ray shows the position.
   b. It is inserted under fluoroscopy so it can be seen on a television screen.
   c. The pressure in the artery changes depending on where the catheter is located.
   d. The distance from the point of entry to the heart is measured and the catheter is marked off in centimeters.
25. When preparing a client for insertion of a pulmonary artery catheter, the nurse's explanation of the procedure could include information based on which fact?
   a. Procedure is usually done in an operating room or treatment room.
   b. EKG is monitored continuously during insertion.
   c. Insertion is basically a risk-free procedure.
   d. Light, general anesthesia is used for client comfort.

ANSWERS & RATIONALES

ANSWERS FOR FILL IN THE BLANKS

Fill in the blank spaces with the correct word or phrase to complete each statement.

1. The three most basic causes of cell injury are
   a. deficiency
   b. intoxication/poisoning
   c. trauma/physical injury
2. The five classic signs of infection are
   a. redness
   b. heat
   c. pain
   d. swelling
   e. loss of function
3. The two major components of the inflammatory response are
   a. vascular
   b. cellular

4. The three types of exudates are
   a. serous
   b. purulent/suppurative
   c. hemorrhagic
5. The four components of the healing process are
   a. regeneration
   b. repair
   c. revascularization
   d. reepithelialization
6. Collagen fibers in scar tissue are very weak for 6–8 days.
7. The four most common sites of nosocomial infection are
   a. urinary tract
   b. respiratory tract
   c. bloodstream
   d. wounds
8. Cancers arising in tissues derived from mesoderm such as muscles, bones, or connective tissue are called sarcomas.
9. The two distinct processes involved in carcinogenesis are
   a. initiation
   b. promotion
10. Another name for the contractile force of the heart is inotropy.

TRUE & FALSE ANSWERS

Mark each of the following statements True or False. Correct all false statements in the space provided.

1. Calcification occurs only in necrotic tissue. *False*
   Deposits of calcium can occur in normal tissues as a result of marked hypercalcemia.
2. Chronic inflammation progressively destroys tissue and results in loss of function and scarring. *True*
3. Once regeneration occurs, function is restored to damaged organs. *False*
   Function is restored if the stroma is undamaged; if stroma is damaged then regeneration may be disorganized and some degree of functional loss results.
4. If a child cuts his hand on a piece of broken glass and has eight sutures to close the wound, healing will occur by second intention. *False*
   Healing is by first intention when the edges of the wound are approximated; it is second intention when the wound is not closed but is left to granulate in.
5. To facilitate healing of a wound across the middle knuckle of the index finger, the joint needs to be immobilized. *True*
6. Signs of systemic infection include swollen lymph nodes, fever, and elevated ESR. *True*

(continued)

7. Total length of the cell cycle is the same for all cells; what differs is the length of time spent in each phase. *False*
Total length of cell cycle varies with the type of cell ranging from 1 hour to 100 hours with the difference a result of time spent in G0 and G1.

8. A characteristic of a benign tumor is that it is composed of cells that resemble the tissue of origin. *True*

9. Malignant tumors cause systemic symptoms such as altered taste and weight loss. *True*

10. The initial effect of an increase in heart rate is a decrease in cardiac output. *False*
The initial effect is an increase in heart rate because cardiac output equals heart rate x stroke volume. When the heart rate reaches 180 bpm and is sustained there is less time for the ventricle to fill with blood so the stroke volume starts to decrease and ultimately the cardiac output decreases even though the rate is high.

MATCHING ANSWERS

Match the following:

1. _n_ Adhesions
2. _d_ Hypertrophy
3. _f_ Serous exudates
4. _o_ Dehiscence
5. _q_ Apoptosis
6. _s_ Contracture
7. _u_ Exudate
8. _h_ Necrosis
9. _r_ Granuloma
10. _p_ Keloid
11. _e_ Hyperplasia
12. _t_ Phagocytosis
13. _b_ Revascularization
14. _i_ Colonization

a. Type of nosocomial infection, which is the direct result of a diagnostic or therapeutic procedure
b. Angioneogenesis
c. Ability of a microorganism to produce infection
d. Enlargement of cells and organs as a result of increased demand
e. Number of cells increased through cell division in response to demand
f. Fluid in blisters of a mild sunburn
g. Microorganism that causes infection only in a susceptible person
h. Tissue death
i. Process by which strains of microorganisms become resident flora in an area of the body
j. Tissue is disordered and cells vary in size and shape
k. Shrinking of cells and organs as a result of decreased demand
l. Lack of organ development
m. Exaggerated contraction of maturing collagen, mostly affecting large wounds which results in distortion and limited mobility
n. Joining of serous membranes which normally move freely against each other due to organization of inflammatory exudates. Risk is greatest with trauma to abdominal organs, heart, and lungs

15. __k__ Atrophy	o. Breaking open of a healing wound usually a result of pressure on the wound
16. __g__ Opportunistic pathogen	p. Irregular masses of scar tissue protruding from the skin that result from overproduction of collagen
17. __a__ Iatrogenic infection	q. Decreased number of cells as a result of self-destruction
18. __c__ Virulence	r. Round masses of transformed macrophages surrounded by lymphocytes and fibroblasts
19. __l__ Aplastic	s. Shortening of a muscle or scar tissue causing distortion or deformity
20. __j__ Dysplasia	t. Ingestion of particles by cells
	u. Material that passes through vessels into adjacent tissues in inflammation

APPLICATION ANSWERS

1. Of which process is gangrene an example?
   a. Coagulation necrosis
   b. Liquefaction necrosis
   c. Autolysis
   d. Phagocytosis

Rationale
Correct answer: a.
Gangrene is an example of coagulation necrosis and is characterized by initial appearance of a firm area with the structure of normal tissue even though cells are dead; subsequently, the area is broken down and cleared by phagocytes. Gangrene is common when cells die due to anoxia or toxic injury except in the brain.
Liquefaction necrosis is characterized by an initial liquid area of dead cells. It is seen in death of nervous-system cells due to anoxia and in death of cells associated with bacterial infections.

2. Which is the primary factor that determines the time interval that can elapse between removal of an organ from a donor and its transplantation into a recipient?
   a. Time an organ can survive ischemia
   b. Ability of the organ to withstand temperature change
   c. Amount of DNA present in the organ's cells
   d. Number of organelles in the organ's cells

Rationale
Correct answer: a.
Oxygen, which is essential to cell survival, is brought to the tissues by the blood. Once an organ is removed from the donor its cells no longer have a source of oxygenated blood until it is implanted in the recipient. Different types of cells/tissues can withstand ischemia for different lengths of time. Hence, how long the organ can survive until implanted depends on this ability of the cells to withstand ischemia.

3. Which factors can initiate an inflammatory response? (Select all that apply.)
   a. Heat or cold
   b. Trauma
   c. Infection
   d. Antigen–antibody-complex deposition
   e. Complement activation

Rationale
Correct answers: a, b, c, and d.
Inflammation is a nonspecific response that occurs when there is damage to skin or mucous membranes, which serve as the body's first line of defense against infection. Anything that can damage these tissues can cause inflammation. Thus, factors such as prolonged exposure to the sun, surgery, exposure to irritating chemicals, and accidental cuts and scrapes are all initiators of the inflammatory response. The inflammatory response is nonspecific because it occurs as a result of many different kinds of damage and is the same regardless of the specific initiating factor.

(continued)

4. What type of diet should be encouraged for a client having radiation through an abdominal port who complains of nausea and vomiting? (Select all that apply.)
   a. High-protein
   b. High-carbohydrate
   c. High-fat
   d. High-residue
   e. High-calorie
   f. Low-protein
   g. Low-calorie
   h. Low-carbohydrate
   i. Low-residue
   j. Low-fat

Rationale

Correct answers: a, b, and e.

Clients having radiation therapy need a high-protein, high-carbohydrate, and high-calorie diet. Radiation causes tissue damage so extra protein is needed for tissue repair. Carbohydrates and calories are needed to provide the energy for tissue repair and to combat the fatigue associated with radiation therapy. Fat is high in calories but is harder to digest; neither a low-fat nor a high-fat diet is recommended. Amount of residue is unrelated.

5. When caring for a client having radiation therapy the nurse receives a report that the client's laboratory values are normal and there are no signs of anemia, infection, or bleeding. Which conclusion should the nurse draw from this information?
   a. Radiation has not yet reached a therapeutic level.
   b. The client is free of side effects of radiation.
   c. Nutritional status is normal.
   d. Bone-marrow suppression is not a problem.

Rationale

Correct answer: d.

Some effect on bone marrow occurs with almost all radiation therapy regardless of port. Bone-marrow suppression becomes a significant problem when RBC and WBC counts and platelet count drop below critical levels. This drop is seen in laboratory values and can result in the development of anemia, infection, or bleeding. Therefore, normal laboratory values and the absence of signs/symptoms of anemia, infection, and bleeding indicate that bone-marrow suppression is not a problem at this time.

6. The father of a 9-month-old boy just diagnosed with a primary immune deficiency says to the nurse "I don't understand it. Why did my son seem healthy until he was 6-months old and then start getting all these infections?" On which fact should the nurse's response be based?
   a. Under 6 months of age, most babies do not show signs of active infection.
   b. It takes about 6 months for babies to be exposed to enough pathogens for infection to readily occur.
   c. Until about 6 months, babies are protected from infection by immunity from their mothers.
   d. Before 6 months, babies are only susceptible to bacterial infections.

Rationale

Correct answer: c.

In utero, fetuses are protected against infection by passive immunity received from the mother via the placenta. This passive protection against pathogens that the mother has immunity to lasts for approximately 6 months at which time the infant becomes dependent on his or her own immune system for protection against infection. Therefore, it is not until the passive immunity has "worn off" that immunodeficiency in the infant manifests itself in chronic or recurrent infections. Infants develop signs of infection. Infection can occur at any time; it can even be present at birth. The cause of infection can be any type of microorganism.

7. When assessing skin of a client having external radiation therapy, which fact should the nurse keep in mind?
   a. Skin damage is preceded by changes in oral mucous membranes.
   b. Most skin changes occur 4–8 weeks after the start of radiation.
   c. Skin areas with poor blood flow are at greatest risk for injury.
   d. Intertriginous areas are at particular risk for skin reactions.

Rationale

Correct answer: d.

Skin fold areas are at particular risk for developing a reaction to radiation therapy.

It is important to keep these areas clean, dry, and free of irritation to help decrease the risk. Changes in oral mucous membranes do not always occur with radiation therapy; it depends on the port. This is different from chemotherapy, which is administered systemically. Acute skin reactions consist of erythema which increases over 2–3 weeks and then either fades or progresses to dry or moist desquamation.

Areas of poor bloodflow are less well-oxygenated and hypoxic tissues are resistant to radiation not at greater risk for injury.

8. How should the care of a client undergoing brachytherapy be assigned?
   a. To male nurses whenever possible
   b. On a rotating basis among nonpregnant nursing staff
   c. Consistently to the same nurses
   d. Never to a nurse with a history of cancer

Rationale

Correct answer: b.

To limit exposure to specific individuals, care of clients undergoing brachytherapy should be rotated among staff members with the exception of those who are pregnant because of the risk of damage to the developing fetus. Male gender or cancer history are not considered influencing factors. Assigning the same nurses would support consistency and efficiency of care but these benefits do not outweigh the risk of exposure.

9. A client having radiation therapy asks the nurse if his blood cells are going to be affected. Which fact should form the basis of the nurse's answer?
   a. Bone marrow and therefore blood cells are affected with almost all ports of radiation.
   b. If radiation is delivered to the hip or leg, no effect should occur.
   c. It depends on whether or not medications are being taken that sensitize blood cells to radiation.
   d. Speed and volume of blood to tissues of the port will determine the effect.

Rationale

Correct answer: a.

Radiation therapy exerts its greatest effect on well-oxygenated, actively dividing cells. As a result, bone-marrow cells are almost always affected. The hip and long bones of the leg contain large amounts of bone marrow so effects on the blood from radiation to these areas do occur. The effect on the blood occurs because the active cells in the bone marrow are affected, not because of any sensitizing drug.

10. Which direction should be given to a client with a platelet count of 45,000 mm^3, a WBC count of $1250/mm^3$, and an RBC count of 4.8 $million/mm^3$?
   a. Cook vegetables well.
   b. Use an electric razor.
   c. Rest at regular intervals.
   d. Increase vitamin B12 intake.

Rationale

Correct answer: b.

A platelet count of 45,000 mm^3 is significantly below the normal of $150{,}000–400{,}000/mm^3$ and so the client is at risk for bleeding. A basic bleeding precaution is to use an electric razor to avoid cutting the skin. The WBC and RBC counts are within normal range so do not require precautions. Cooking vegetables well is a direction given to neutropenic clients. Rest at regular intervals is needed by clients with anemia and other sources of fatigue. Increased vitamin B12 intake is needed by clients with pernicious anemia.

11. A client having chemotherapy for breast cancer reports a temperature of 101.4 F. How should the nurse interpret this fact?
   a. Sign of infection, which needs to be reported right away
   b. Side effect of chemotherapy, not requiring intervention
   c. Sign of infection, which needs monitoring and reporting if it persists for 48 hours
   d. Indicator of dehydration requiring client teaching regarding fluid intake

Rationale

Correct answer: a.

Any temperature over 101 F is considered a sign of infection and needs to be reported right away. Clients having radiation therapy are immunosuppressed because of the effect of the radiation on the bone marrow and so infection poses a particular risk for this population.

12. A client who had a dose of chemotherapy at 8 a.m. calls the clinic at 2:30 p.m. complaining of nausea and vomiting despite having taken the prescribed medication. She asks how much worse the nausea and vomiting is going to get. On which fact should the nurse's answer be based?
   a. Nausea and vomiting is totally unpredictable.
   b. Nausea and vomiting typically peak in the first 12 hours.
   c. Nausea and vomiting will ease on going to bed.
   d. Vomiting should cease in about 36 hours but nausea may persist for 7–10 days.

Rationale

Correct answer: b.

Nausea and vomiting typically peak in the first 12 hours so in this case the nausea and vomiting should begin to subside after 8 p.m. The degree of nausea and vomiting can vary from person to person and with different types of chemotherapy but broad patterns are evident; it is not totally unpredictable. Going to bed does not ease nausea and vomiting and its absolute duration is not known.

13. For which type of toxicity would the nurse plan to monitor a client who is being treated with cisplatin?
   a. Neurotoxicity
   b. Cardiotoxicity
   c. Nephrotoxicity
   d. Hepatotoxicity

(continued)

Rationale

Correct answer: c.

Cisplatin is associated with nephrotoxicity and as a result, the nurse must monitor for signs of renal tubule damage. Intake and output must be monitored. The client must be well-hydrated before administration of cisplatin and encouraged to maintain a fluid intake of 2–3 l daily for the duration of therapy. Cisplatin can also cause ototoxicity (deafness) and should be monitored for tinnitus.

14. Which class of chemotherapy drugs is most likely to affect fertility?
    a. Alkylating agents
    b. Antimetabolytes
    c. Cytotoxic antibiotics
    d. Mitotic inhibitors

Rationale

Correct answer: a.

Alkylating agents are the type of chemotherapeutic agents that most commonly affect the ovaries and testes resulting in changes in fertility. Amenorrhea is common in young females and induced menopause common in older females. Decreased sperm production as well as sperm and semen abnormalities occur in men. In some cases, fertility returns after treatment but this varies with the age of the client and the specific drug and dose of drug received.

15. Which information could be correctly included in the teaching plan for a client receiving chemotherapy?
    a. Scalp hair may be lost but body hair is unaffected.
    b. Hair loss usually occurs 6–8 weeks after chemotherapy starts.
    c. Regrowth usually starts 1–2 months after chemotherapy is completed.
    d. Hair regrowth can be expected to take 24–36 months.

Rationale

Correct answer: c.

Regrowth of hair usually starts 1–2 months after chemotherapy is completed. Both scalp and body hair may be lost and loss usually starts 2–3 weeks after treatment starts. Regrowth takes about a year.

16. Which comment about measuring pulmonary artery wedge pressure indicates a correct understanding of at least one aspect of the procedure?
    a. The pressure-monitoring system must be calibrated at least every 12 hours.
    b. Normal mean pressure is 15 mm Hg.
    c. The balloon must be completely deflated after each pressure measurement is obtained.
    d. The catheter is passed through the right heart and into the right pulmonary artery.

Think Smart/Test Smart

This question is looking for a correct statement because it asks which statement shows that the person making it correctly understands some aspect of the procedure. Thus, three distractors are going to be incorrect statements about the procedure and one is going to be correct and will be the answer.

Rationale

Correct answer: c.

The balloon must be completely deflated after each pressure measurement is obtained. This is correct. The other statements are incorrect because calibration should be checked before each reading; normal mean pressure is 10 mm Hg not 15; and the catheter passes through the left ventricle into the left pulmonary artery because it provides a measure of left ventricle end diastolic pressure, which is increased in left ventricular failure and pericardial tamponade and decreased in hypovolemia.

17. Which statement is an appropriate practice guideline when CVP is being monitored?
    a. A pressure greater than 6 mm Hg must be reported immediately.
    b. A CVP of greater than 10 mm Hg indicates the need for immediate fluid.
    c. Overall trend is more important than any individual measure.
    d. A CVP of 1–3 mm Hg requires immediate intervention to prevent pulmonary edema.

Rationale

Correct answer: c.

Trend in CVP change is more significant than any individual measurement. Normal range of CVP is 0–8 mm Hg or 5–10 cm H_2O depending on equipment used; so, a pressure of 6 mm Hg is within normal range and would not need to be reported immediately. A CVP 10 mm Hg is the upper limit of normal and does not indicate need for immediate fluid; elevated CVP is associated with hypervolemia not hypovolemia. Risk of pulmonary edema is indicated by an elevated CVP.

18. Which statement made by a client receiving radiation therapy indicates a need for further teaching?
    a. "Today is my last treatment so by next week I will know if I am going to have any side effects from the radiation."
    b. "I'm tired of having blood drawn but I know I need it to check my bone marrow."
    c. "I need to check my skin for redness, especially in the skin folds."
    d. "I'm awfully fatigued all the time but I understand it is expected."

Rationale
Correct answer: a.
There are late as well as immediate effects of radiation therapy. Late effects are due to blood vessel or connective tissue damage and occur months or years after therapy. Examples of late effects include skin atrophy, fibrosis or ulceration, pulmonary fibrosis, and cataracts.

19. When caring for a client with a Swan–Ganz catheter, for which complications would the nurse monitor? (Select all that apply.)
    a. Heart failure
    b. Thromboembolism
    c. Hypervolemia
    d. Cardiac dysrhythmia
    e. Infection

Rationale
Correct answers: b, d, and e.
Thromboembolism, cardiac dysrhythmia, and infection are risks associated with a Swan–Ganz catheter. Thromboembolism is a risk because the catheter is a foreign object in the circulatory system that interferes with bloodflow. Cardiac dysrhythmia is a risk because the catheter is threaded through the heart. Infection is a risk because the catheter enters through the skin and thus provides a potential source of entry for bacteria into normally sterile areas of the body.

20. A client who has received a biopsy report indicating dysplasia asks the nurse if this means she has cancer. Which is the most appropriate response?
    a. "Yes, it is cancer but an early form that is usually treatable."
    b. "It may be cancer. More tests have to be done and you will know in about 5 days."
    c. "No, it is not cancer but the tissue is abnormal and sometimes it becomes cancerous."
    d. "No, it is not cancer and it doesn't turn into cancer."

Rationale
Correct answer: c.
Dysplastic tissue is characterized by disorder and cells that vary in size and shape. It results from severe and prolonged irritation and often precedes neoplasia. Some forms are known as precancerous lesions.

21. Which complication must the nurse be alert for when caring for a client on intra-arterial blood pressure monitoring?
    a. Ventricular tachycardia
    b. Myocardial infarct
    c. Pulmonary artery rupture
    d. Hemorrhage

Rationale
Correct answer: d.
Hemorrhage is a potential complication because the catheter is inserted directly into a pulsating artery. Other complications are infection, air embolism, and throboembolism. The arterial line called an art line or A line does not pass through the heart so dysrhythmias are not a major risk nor do they enter or affect the pulmonary artery so pulmonary artery rupture is not a concern. Occurrence of MI is unrelated.

22. The spouse of a client who is to have intra-arterial blood pressure monitoring initiated, tells the nurse he heard someone say that an Allen test would be done and asks what it is for. Which fact should form the basis of the nurse's response?
    a. To make sure there is collateral circulation sufficient to keep tissue supplied with oxygenated blood.
    b. To check for abnormal clotting because of the risk of thromboembolism.
    c. To check if the volume of bloodflow is sufficient to provide an accurate measurement.
    d. To determine if the artery has a diameter great enough to allow passage of the catheter.

Rationale
Correct answer: a.
An Allen test is done to ascertain that inserting a catheter into one of the large arteries of an extremity will not result in a decrease in oxygenated blood to the part such that tissue damage occurs. When performing the Allen test on an upper extremity, both the radial and ulna arteries are compressed until the pulses are obliterated while the client is making a fist. The client is then asked to open the fist and pressure is released on one of the arteries and the palm is observed for flushing. This procedure is then repeated for the other artery.

(continued)

23. When measuring CVP, which is the reference point or the zero point of the manometer or the transducer?
    a. Fourth intercostal space at the left midclavicular line
    b. Fourth intercostal space at the left sternal border
    c. Sixth intercostal space at the right sternal border
    d. Sixth intercostal space at the left midclavicular line

Rationale

Correct answer: a.

The reference level for the transducer is the right atrium, whose filling pressure is measured by CVP. The right atrium is located below the fourth intercostal space at the left midclavicular line.

24. A client having a Swan–Ganz catheter inserted asks how the MD will know when it is in the right place. What is the most accurate reply to the client's question?
    a. A chest X-ray shows the position.
    b. It is inserted under fluoroscopy so it can be seen on a television screen.
    c. The pressure in the artery changes depending on where the catheter is located.
    d. The distance from the point of entry to the heart is measured and the catheter is marked off in centimeters.

Rationale

Correct answer: a.

A chest X-ray is done to confirm the position of a Swan–Ganz catheter once it is inserted. It is inserted usually as a bedside procedure; it is not done under fluoroscopy. Pressure in the arterial system does change in different locations but this is not how placement is confirmed nor is it confirmed by the length of catheter inserted. No IV fluid is run into a central line until placement is confirmed by X-ray.

25. When preparing a client for insertion of a pulmonary artery catheter, the nurse's explanation of the procedure could include information based on which fact?
    a. Procedure is usually done in an operating room or treatment room.
    b. EKG is monitored continuously during insertion.
    c. Insertion is basically a risk-free procedure.
    d. Light, general anesthesia is used for client comfort.

Rationale

Correct answer: b.

EKG is monitored continuously due to the risk of the catheter triggering a dysrhythmia as it passes through the right ventricle. The procedure is typically done at the bedside and general anesthesia is not needed. However, the procedure is not without risk. Air embolism, thromboembolism, pulmonary artery rupture or infarct, dysrhythmia, and infection can all occur.

Part III

TAKING THE TEST

CHAPTER 34

Practice Test for NCLEX-RN®

HEALTH PROMOTION AND MAINTENANCE

Human Sexuality

Counsel client/family/significant others on sexuality issues

1. A client who has experienced a myocardial infarction is being discharged from the hospital. The client questions when he can resume sexual activity with his spouse. The nurse's best response is:
   A. sex is no longer possible after your surgery.
   B. you must avoid foreplay but sex is acceptable as long as it is of a short duration.
   C. sex can be resumed when you can climb stairs without becoming short of breath.
   D. masturbation is the only allowable form of sexual expression after the surgery.

The answer is C. Sex can be resumed when the client can climb two flights of stairs without becoming short of breath or the client can walk more than 2 miles without shortness of breath.

A is incorrect—Sex is possible after a myocardial infarction. B is incorrect—Foreplay is encouraged to slowly prepare the body for the changes in heart rate and respiratory rate that accompany sex. D is incorrect—Masturbation is acceptable after a myocardial infarction but it is not the only form of sexual expression allowed.

SAFE AND EFFECTIVE CARE ENVIRONMENT

Safety and Infection Control

Disaster Planning

Identify nursing roles in disaster planning

2. What is the most important nursing role in disaster planning?
   A. Knowing the policy for disasters in the facility.
   B. Maintaining contact with community resources.
   C. Making a list of the most frequent contacts in the hospital.
   D. Attending meetings that discuss the potential for disasters in the community.

The answer is A. Knowing the policy for disasters in the facility is the most important role for the nurse. This allows the nurse to function within the policies of the hospital, which aids in maintaining patient and staff safety.

B is incorrect—Maintaining contact with community resources will benefit the nurse in a disaster situation, but is not the most important role. C is incorrect—Making a list of frequent contacts is helpful but not the most important nursing role. D is incorrect—Attending meetings on the disasters that can occur in the community will not prepare the nurse for how to handle the disaster in the facility.

SAFE AND EFFECTIVE CARE ENVIRONMENT

Safety and Infection Control

Medical and Surgical Asepsis

Evaluate whether aseptic technique is performed correctly

3. A nurse is working with a physician on the insertion of a central line. What action performed by the physician requires the nurse to stop the procedure due to a breach in asepsis?
   A. The kit is opened toward the physician last.
   B. The physician drops his or her gloved hands below the level of the chest.
   C. The physician touches two sterile hands together.
   D. The physician turns his or her back to the sterile field.

The answer is D. A person who is working in a sterile field should not turn his or her back to the sterile field or it is considered contaminated.

A is incorrect—A sterile kit is opened toward the outside first and toward the individual last to avoid contamination of the sterile contents. B is incorrect—The sterile field is from the chest to below the level of the sterile field. C is incorrect—A person wearing sterile gloves is allowed to touch two sterile gloved hands together without causing contamination to the field.

HEALTH PROMOTION AND MAINTENANCE

Developmental Stages and Transitions

Identify expected physical, cognitive, psychosocial, and moral stages of development

4. Which verbal complaint during the assessment of a 55-year-old female client is considered abnormal and requires further investigation?
   A. Absence of menstrual cycle
   B. Thinning of hair
   C. Periods of sweating and feeling warm
   D. Lumps in axilla area

The answer is D. Lumps in the axilla area could be lymph nodes, which could be a sign of cancer and needs further attention.

A is incorrect—The loss of menses is normal at the age of 55. B is incorrect—The thinning of hair is secondary to a drop in estrogen levels and is considered normal in the 55-year-old woman. C is incorrect—Periods of sweating and feeling warm are a response to the body's hormonal changes.

PSYCHOSOCIAL INTEGRITY

Coping Mechanisms

Assess client response to illness (rationalization, hopefulness, anger)

5. A client receives a diagnosis of cancer after a biopsy of a suspicious lymph node. The client states, "You must have made a mistake, I want a second opinion." Which stage of grief is the client experiencing?
   A. Denial
   B. Anger
   C. Bargaining
   D. Despair

The answer is A. The client is denying that the diagnosis is correct and desires a second opinion. This is a normal response and the client should be allowed to work through it with support from staff.

B is incorrect—The client is not yet angry but may encounter this response as time progresses. The client who is angry will blame others or himself as to why the health crisis occurred. C is incorrect—The client will begin to bargain with God or others whom he or she feels holds the key to healing. D is incorrect—The client will exhibit signs of depression in despair and will become disorganized with daily activities.

PHYSIOLOGICAL INTEGRITY

Basic Care and Comfort

Elimination

Perform irrigations

6. A nurse is performing continuous bladder irrigation at 1 L/h. Which assessment is the priority?
   A. The amount of fluid being returned.
   B. The size of the indwelling catheter.
   C. The client's knowledge level of the procedure.
   D. The percentage of formalin ordered for irrigation.

The answer is A. The amount of fluid being returned is priority since a decrease in output without a decrease in the input may indicate clot formation or catheter malfunction and needs to be addressed immediately.

B is incorrect—The size of the catheter is important but not priority in bladder irrigation. C is incorrect—The client should have his knowledge level assessed prior to the beginning of the procedure. D is incorrect—Formalin is used in the operating room under anesthesia due to the pain it causes and the need to prevent ureteral reflux.

SAFE AND EFFECTIVE CARE ENVIRONMENT

Safety and Infection Control

Standard/Transmission-Based/Other Precautions

Educate client/family/staff on infection control measures

7. A nurse is discharging a client who has been undergoing chemotherapy. When discussing at home care, the priority instruction should be to:
   A. avoid public places.
   B. include fresh fruits and vegetables in your diet.
   C. limit visitors in the home.
   D. wash your hands often.

The answer is D. Hand washing is the number one method of preventing infection and should be taught to all clients who are immunosuppressed.

A is incorrect—While avoiding public places is important and should be taught, it is not the priority teaching. B is incorrect—While fresh fruits and vegetables will aid in including vitamin C and other essential nutrients in the diet, this is not the priority. C is incorrect—Limiting visitors is important but not the priority.

HEALTH PROMOTION AND MAINTENANCE

Self-Care

Assess and intervene in client performance of instrumental activities of daily living

8. When planning the care of a client with rheumatoid arthritis, which plan would be best to assist with activities of daily living?
   A. Teach the client methods of energy conservation.
   B. Provide the client with a shower chair.
   C. Encourage family members to take over challenging activities.
   D. Provide the client with large handled instruments for eating.

The answer is A. The client should learn which activities are the most tiresome and limit the activities to conserve energy. The client with rheumatoid arthritis needs rest to limit increased inflammation in joints.

B is incorrect—The client can benefit with a shower chair but it is not the best plan to assist with activities of daily living. C is incorrect—The client needs to be able to perform the activities of daily living and delegate the activities that he or she is unable to perform. The nurse should not encourage family members to take over these activities. D is incorrect—The client does need instruments for eating but it is not the best plan to assist with activities of daily living.

PSYCHOSOCIAL INTEGRITY

Sensory/Perceptual Alterations

Evaluate client with altered ability to communicate effectively and intervene to promote successful adaptation

9. A client has undergone a total laryngectomy due to cancer. The nurse should plan on assisting the client with communicating by:
   A. providing an interpreter.
   B. providing a sheet explaining sign language.
   C. providing a tablet and pencil.
   D. talking to the client's face, accentuating words through lip movement.

The answer is C. The client should be given a tablet and pencil for communication postop.

A is incorrect—An interpreter is not needed unless the client does not speak English. B is incorrect—The client should be allowed to communicate through the written word unless he requests a sheet about sign language. D is incorrect—The client should not be expected to read lips to communicate with the nurse due to the possibility of miscommunication.

PHYSIOLOGICAL INTEGRITY

Basic Care and Comfort

Potential for Complications of Diagnostic Tests/Treatments/Procedures

Apply knowledge of nursing procedures and psychomotor skills when caring for a client with potential for complications

10. A client is 24 hours postop from gastric bypass surgery. Which of the following nursing actions is best in preventing thrombus formation?
   A. The application of sequential compression devices.
   B. Ambulating the client.
   C. Administering salicylate (Aspirin).
   D. Massaging of lower extremities.

The answer is B. The best method of preventing thrombus formation is ambulation. This will prevent a deep vein thrombosis as well as a pulmonary embolism.

A is incorrect—Sequential compression devices are beneficial in preventing thrombus formation but the best method is ambulation. C is incorrect—Aspirin is known for decreasing platelet aggregation and reduction in inflammation. It is not the best method of prevention of thrombus formation. D is incorrect—Massaging extremities is not appropriate in the postop client. Massaging of extremities may dislodge clots that have formed.

PHYSIOLOGICAL INTEGRITY

Reduction of Risk Potential

Monitoring Conscious Sedation

Assist with preparing client for conscious sedation

11. Prior to administering conscious sedation the nurse must first:
   A. verify informed consent.
   B. perform ABGs.
   C. assess vital signs.
   D. place high-flow oxygen on the client.

The answer is A. Prior to initiating conscious sedation, the nurse must ensure informed consent has been obtained and is on the chart.

B is incorrect—ABGs are not performed on a client before conscious sedation. C is incorrect—Vital signs are taken prior to medication administration but the first action is to verify consent has been obtained. D is incorrect—The client is not routinely placed on high-flow oxygen prior to conscious sedation. The client has a loss of protective reflexes but will breathe and the assessment of the client's oxygen saturation should occur.

PHYSIOLOGICAL INTEGRITY

Reduction of Risk Potential

System-Specific Assessment

Perform focused assessment or reassessment

12. A client presents to the ED complaining of acute low back pain, which is unrelieved with over the counter pain medications. The client is pacing the room, diaphoretic and grimacing. Which assessment data is most indicative of renal calculi?
    A. Hematuria
    B. Hypertension
    C. Vomiting
    D. Groin pain

The answer is A. A client with renal calculi will have hematuria or numerous red blood cells in the urine upon examination.

B is incorrect—Hypertension is not an indicative sign of renal calculi. Hypertension is common in a client who is experiencing severe pain. C is incorrect—While the client with renal calculi may experience vomiting, this is a side effect of the pain and not an indicative sign. D is incorrect—Some clients experience pain in the groin with renal calculi while some only experience unilateral flank pain making this not an indicative sign.

PHYSIOLOGICAL INTEGRITY

Reduction of Risk Potential

Vital Signs

Apply knowledge needed to perform related nursing procedures and psychomotor skills when assessing vital signs

13. The nurse will plan to avoid performing which nursing actions on the left arm of a client with an arteriovenous fistula?
    A. Blood pressure monitoring
    B. Oxygen saturation monitoring
    C. Blood glucose monitoring
    D. Assessment of capillary refill

The answer is A. A client with a arteriovenous fistula for hemodialysis should not have a blood pressure taken in that area to prevent damage and thrombosis formation inside the fistula.

B is incorrect—Oxygen saturation monitoring is acceptable in the site where a fistula is placed. C is incorrect—Blood glucose monitoring is appropriate in the affected arm as long as dialysis is not in progress. D is incorrect—Assessment of capillary refill is possible and safe for the client with an arteriovenous fistula.

PHYSIOLOGICAL INTEGRITY

Physiological Adaptation

Hemodynamics

Identify cardiac rhythm strip abnormalities

14. What is the most appropriate action for a rapidly occurring wide QRS complex with no discernable p-waves?
    A. Shock the client with 200 J
    B. Perform chest compressions
    C. Administer oxygen
    D. Take a manual blood pressure

The answer is C. The client has a rhythm known as ventricular tachycardia and needs to have oxygen applied to meet the standards of ABC.

A is incorrect—The client will not require a shock of the rhythm. B is incorrect—Chest compressions should not be initiated until it is determined if a pulse is present. D is incorrect—A blood pressure is measured after a pulse is obtained.

PHYSIOLOGICAL INTEGRITY

Physiological Adaptation

Hemodynamics

Identify cardiac rhythm strip abnormalities

15. The nurse is assessing his or her patients at the beginning of the shift. One of the client's exhibits a rhythm that displays p waves occurring regularly, a p–r interval of 0.20 and a QRS complex for every p wave measuring <0.12 with a rate of 70 and the t wave is upright. The nurse would document this rhythm as:
    A. normal sinus rhythm
    B. sinus bradycardia
    C. first-degree AV block
    D. second-degree AV block type I

The answer is A. The rhythm is regular since the rate is regular with a p–r interval and QRS complex measures within normal limits and the rate is above 60 and below 100.

B is incorrect—The rhythm is not below 60 beats per minute. . C is incorrect—The p–r interval is not elongated making this a normal sinus rhythm. D is incorrect—The relationship between the p wave and the QRS is consistently occurring.

PHYSIOLOGICAL INTEGRITY

Physiological Adaptation

Medical Emergencies

Perform emergency care procedures

16. When responding to a code in the hospital, the nurse finds a client who is being bagged with high flow oxygen by a fellow nurse. The client is pulseless and

CPR was begun less than 1 minute ago; there is no doctor on scene. Which action is next?

A. Reassess for a pulse

B. Attach the echocardiogram electrodes to the client

C. Begin a fluid bolus of normal saline

D. Ask another nurse for a history of the client

The answer is B. If CPR is in progress, the staff that arrives on scene should attach the electrodes to the client to prevent interruption of CPR.

A is incorrect—Reassessment for a pulse occurs after two full minutes of CPR. C is incorrect—Normal saline boluses must be ordered by the physician in the event the client has a history of heart failure. D is incorrect—A history regarding the client can occur after the electrodes are attached and the physician takes over the code.

PHYSIOLOGICAL INTEGRITY

Physiological Adaptation

Alterations in Body Systems

Provide postoperative care

17. A client is in the recovery room following a carotid endarterectomy. Place the following assessments in priority order

___ neurological status

___ signs of hemorrhage

___ intracranial pressure

___ blood pressure

The nurse's first priority is to assess the area for signs of hemorrhaging. This is most important since hemorrhage indicates that the brain is not receiving much needed oxygen and a stroke could occur as a result. Blood loss will affect the blood pressure and could cause the client to rapidly deteriorate. The second priority is the client's blood pressure. This is important since fluctuations are common during the first 24 hours postprocedure. The blood pressure should be monitored for hypertensive emergencies and hypotension, which will lead to poor perfusion of vital organs. The client's neurological status is the third assessment to monitor for changes consistent with a stroke. The last assessment is the intracranial pressure. The first three assessments will help identify if there is an increase in the intracranial pressure.

SAFE AND EFFECTIVE CARE ENVIRONMENT

Safety and Infection Control

Error Prevention

Ensure proper identification of client when providing care

18. Which of the following is the best method of identifying an infant before providing care?

A. Verify the information on the armband with the chart.

B. Ask the mom if the armband information is correct.

C. Ask the client if the information on the armband is correct.

D. Ask the previous nurse the client's name and date of birth.

The answer is B. Verifying the information on the armband with the mom will ensure that the correct armband was placed on the correct client before treatment is rendered.

A is incorrect—While verifying the chart against the band does demonstrate that the order for the client matches the client's armband, it does not ensure that the correct client is wearing the correct armband. Not verifying the information with a family member could still lead to a treatment error. C is incorrect—An infant will not be able to speak and so this is not an appropriate method. D is incorrect—Each nurse providing care should verify the correct client each time that care is provided during a shift.

SAFE AND EFFECTIVE CARE ENVIRONMENT

Management of Care

Ethical Practices

Intervene to promote ethical practice

19. A client returns from surgery with a diagnosis of cancer. The physician informs the staff to avoid telling the client the diagnosis. Upon awakening the client asks if he has cancer. Which response by the nurse is best?

A. I will call the physician and have him speak with you.

B. I do not know the results of the test.

C. You need to ask your family if they know the results.

D. The surgeon found what he feels is cancer; he will speak with you later.

The answer is A. Calling the physician is the best answer to this ethical dilemma. The physician is responsible for informing the client of the diagnosis; questions will be asked that the nurse may not be able to answer. By calling the physician, the nurse is not compromising fidelity and/or veracity.

B is incorrect—This is a violation of veracity, which is the principle that a nurse will not knowingly lie to a client. C is incorrect—The family is not responsible for informing a client of the results of a surgery performed. Informing a family member may fall into a HIPPA violation if the client does not want the family to know the results. D is incorrect—Informing the client of the diagnosis is a violation of fidelity. Fidelity is when a health care provider must maintain a professional loyalty to those in the profession, which in this case is the physician.

SAFE AND EFFECTIVE CARE ENVIRONMENT

Management of Care

Advocacy

Act as a client advocate

20. A client presents to the emergency department complaining of pain. The physician refuses to prescribe narcotic pain medication after stating the client is drug seeking. Which action by the nurse would be most appropriate?
    A. Report the physician to nursing administration for unethical behavior.
    B. Ask the physician why he or she believes the client is drug seeking.
    C. Discuss with the physician the client's chief complaint and ask if another type of pain reliever can be ordered.
    D. Go to the charge nurse, tell her of the physician's actions and ask if another physician can assess the client.

The answer is C. The nurse is responsible for acting as a client advocate. If the nurse feels that the physician is not addressing the client's pain due to a fear of narcotic addiction, the nurse is responsible for discussing alternative methods of pain relief with the physician.

A is incorrect—It does not address the needs of the client. B is incorrect—It only questions the physician and does not allow for a solution to the client's needs. D is incorrect—It does not address the issue that is with the physician and is not cost-effective to have another physician see the client.

SAFE AND EFFECTIVE CARE ENVIRONMENT

Management of Care

Confidentiality/Information Security

Maintain client confidentiality/privacy

21. You are working in an intensive care unit when an individual approaches you to ask about the unresponsive client in the bed you are assigned to. Before giving out information regarding the client you should first:
    A. verify that the individual is a family member by asking for the name of the client.
    B. ask the individual about his or her relationship to the client.
    C. ask the individual what is the personal identification number for the client.
    D. ask to see a driver's license and compare it to the information listed on the chart as the next of kin.

The answer is C. According to HIPPA laws, a person requesting information on a client must present the personal identification number before information can be distributed. In this case, the client is unresponsive; therefore, the nurse must ensure that a HIPPA violation does not occur.

A is incorrect—Knowing the name of the individual does not authorize information to be distributed. B is incorrect—Regardless of the relationship of the individual to the client, information cannot be distributed without the PIN. D is incorrect—It does not follow the policy for identification and distribution of medical information.

SAFE AND EFFECTIVE CARE ENVIRONMENT

Management of Care

Referrals

Assess the need to refer clients for assistance with actual or potential problems

22. While developing the clinical pathway of four clients, which client will need a referral to speech therapy based on the nurse's assessment?
    A. A client who experienced a fractured hip.
    B. A client who underwent a laryngectomy.
    C. A client who underwent a cholecystectomy.
    D. A client who was admitted for congestive heart failure.

The answer is B. A client who underwent a laryngectomy may require therapy to regain voice function or consume food.

A is incorrect—A client with a fractured hip will not require speech therapy. C is incorrect—A client who underwent a cholecystectomy will not require speech therapy. D is incorrect—A client with congestive heart failure will not require speech therapy.

SAFE AND EFFECTIVE CARE ENVIRONMENT

Safety and Infection Control

Safe Use of Equipment

Remove malfunctioning equipment from client care area and report the problem to appropriate personnel

23. While performing a morning check on the crash cart and defibrillator, the nurse notices the defibrillator does not charge and discharge as expected. Which action by the nurse is most appropriate?
    A. Place a repair tag on the equipment for biomedical services to pick up.
    B. Notify the charge nurse and page biomedical services to check the equipment.

C. Notify the house supervisor and request a temporary cart and defibrillator.
D. Ask the nursing assistant to take the cart to the biomedical department and ask for an immediate repair.

The answer is C. If a defibrillator is found to be nonfunctioning, then the nursing supervisor needs to replace the equipment immediately to cover the area in the event a code occurs.

A is incorrect—Placing a tag on the equipment does not resolve the problem, which leaves the clients on the floor vulnerable if cardiac arrest occurs. B is incorrect—Paging biomedical services is not a resolution to the need for a new defibrillator. D is incorrect—Although asking for an immediate repair is possible, it may not be repaired. The need to replace the defibrillator is immediate and a replacement is needed while repairs are being completed.

HEALTH PROMOTION AND MAINTENANCE

Health Screening

Perform targeted screening exams

24. A school nurse should schedule which type of screening exam for all 12-year-olds enrolled in the school?
    A. Scoliosis
    B. Diabetes
    C. Hypertension
    D. Hearing

The answer is A. Scoliosis screening occurs when a child reaches the age of puberty and should be conducted in the school setting with referrals made as needed.

B is incorrect—Diabetes is not a screening exam that needs to be performed in the school setting. C is incorrect—Hypertension screenings are not needed in the school setting. D is incorrect—Hearing exams are performed before school and if a child complains of difficulty hearing in class.

PSYCHOSOCIAL INTEGRITY

End-of-Life Care

Assist client/family/significant others in resolution of end-of-life issues

25. During the initial meeting with a client who has been referred for palliative care for a terminal illness, what is the primary nursing goal?
    A. To determine the client's religious preference.
    B. To determine the client's goals for the care to be provided.
    C. To form a trusting relationship with the client.
    D. To form a list of support systems that the client can use.

The answer is C. The primary goal of the nurse during the first encounter with a client who is in need of palliative care is to form a trusting relationship. The trusting relationship is the bridge to begin planning care that will focus on the level of care he or she desires and to ensure that the end of life is met with the client having a sense of control.

A is incorrect—The client's religious preference is important but is not the goal of the initial meeting. B is incorrect—The nurse will determine the client's goals for care after a trusting relationship has been formed with the client. D is incorrect—A list of support systems for the client will be formed after an analysis is performed of the client's goals, current financial situation, family members, physical abilities, religious preferences, and psychosocial status.

PSYCHOSOCIAL INTEGRITY

Unexpected Body Image Changes

Assess client/family/significant other's reactions to a change in body image

26. Which statement made by a client indicates that acceptance of a new colostomy has not occurred?
    A. "My husband will never want to be intimate with me again."
    B. "I will experiment with various pouches to see which one controls odor the best."
    C. "I plan on beginning elimination training for my colostomy as soon as the doctor says it is okay."
    D. "I will teach my spouse how to work with the colostomy in the event I ever need assistance."

The answer is A. The client is feeling despair that her spouse will not accept the changes she has undergone and will not desire her in a way he once did. She has not accepted the colostomy and assumes her spouse has not either.

B is incorrect—The client has accepted the colostomy and is ready to work with it so that it fits into her life. C is incorrect—The client has accepted the colostomy and is open to working with it to fit her needs. D is incorrect—The client has accepted the colostomy and is ready to teach others how to work with it as she does.

PHYSIOLOGICAL INTEGRITY

Basic Care and Comfort

Nutrition and Oral Hydration

Monitor client's hydration status

27. Which of the following is the best indicator of a negative hydration status in a client who weighed 200 pounds on admission and has been vomiting for 3 days after being diagnosed with diabetic ketoacidosis?
    A. Daily weight of 170 pounds on day 3.
    B. Serum glucose 100 mg/dL.

C. Ketones negative in urine.
D. Potassium level 4.0 mEq/L.

The answer is A. The client who is dehydrated will have a decrease in daily weights. This is a reflection of a negative fluid volume status.

B is incorrect—The serum glucose will rise in a client who is dehydrated due to insulin deficiency and glycogen breakdown to glucose of which cannot be eliminated by the body. C is incorrect—Ketones are positive due to free-floating fatty acids. The ketones are not eliminated due to low urine output and fluid volume deficit leading to ketones being in the urine. D is incorrect—As the client vomits and the potassium leaves the cell and goes to circulation, the level will rise; 4.0 mEq/L is considered a normal potassium level and therefore is an incorrect response.

PHYSIOLOGICAL INTEGRITY

Pharmacological and Parenteral Therapies

Central Venous Access Devices

Access implanted venous access devices

28. A client has a medi-port for chemotherapy administration. The nurse has an order to access the medi-port for a blood draw and the administration of normal saline at 125mL/hr. The nurse will plan on obtaining which of the following to access the device?
A. A 20-gauge 1.5-inch Huber needle
B. A 20-gauge 1.5-inch jelco
C. A butterfly needle
D. A needleless syringe system

The answer is A. A Huber needle is required to access a medi-port system so that damage will not occur to the structure of the system.

B is incorrect—A jelco is not the correct needle to access a medi-port. The use of a jelco would damage the implanted device and possibly the client. C is incorrect—A butterfly needle is small and used for lab collection only. It does not contain a catheter for fluid administration. D is incorrect—A needle is required to access the medi-port. A needleless system can be used after the medi-port is accessed by the appropriate needle.

PHYSIOLOGICAL INTEGRITY

Pharmacological and Parenteral Therapies

Total Parenteral Nutrition

Administer/maintain/discontinue total parenteral nutrition

29. Which site is the best for administering total parenteral nutrition to a client whose feeding contains greater than 10% glucose?
A. PEG tube
B. NG tube
C. Peripheral site
D. Central catheter site

The answer is D. The preferred site for the administration of parenteral nutrition is to use a central catheter site to prevent damage to the peripheral areas.

A is incorrect—Parenteral nutrition is administered intravenously not in a PEG tube site; tube feedings are reserved for PEG tube sites. B is incorrect—TPN is an intravenous form of feeding a client and an NG tube goes directly to the stomach, which requires tube feeding solutions. D is incorrect—Placing a high concentration of glucose in a peripheral site will irritate the vein and can cause damage to the client's surrounding tissues. TPN with greater than 10% glucose should use a central site.

PHYSIOLOGICAL INTEGRITY

Reduction of Risk Potential

Potential for Alterations in Body Systems

Monitor client output for changes from baseline

30. The client's output trend from a chest tube drainage system is as follows:

	0700	1500	2200
Day 1	600 mL	750 mL	648 mL
Day 2	500 mL	425 mL	400 mL
Day 3	400 mL	380 mL	400 mL
Day 4	500 mL	600 mL	700 mL

Based on the data trended, which initial action by the nurse would be best?
A. Report the trend to the physician.
B. Continue to monitor the client's drainage.
C. Review the chart to see what the acceptable parameters are.
D. Increase the suction on the chest tube.

The answer is C. On day 4 the output is similar to day 1, the nurse should verify with the chart what parameters are acceptable before consulting the physician.

A is incorrect—Before calling the physician, the nurse should verify the parameters with the chart to see what the physician considers acceptable. B is incorrect—Continuing to monitor the client comes after ensuring that the output is within expected limits. D is incorrect—The suction should never be increased unless a physician writes an order.

PHYSIOLOGICAL INTEGRITY

Physiological Adaptation

Fluid and Electrolyte Imbalances

Identify signs and symptoms of client fluid and/or electrolyte imbalance

31. A client's serum calcium level is 7 mg/dL. What would be the clinical manifestations of for this laboratory result?
    A. Abdominal cramps
    B. Depressed DTRs and dysrhythmias
    C. Lethargy and weakness
    D. Numbness and tingling in the extremities

The answer is D. Normal serum calcium range is 8.5–10.5 mg/dL and so the client has hypocalcemia. Symptoms of hypocalcemia include numbness and tingling in the extremities, carpopedal spasm, and ultimately tetany.

A, B, and C are incorrect—Lethargy and weakness as well as depressed deep tendon reflexes, anorexia, nausea, vomiting, constipation and dysrhythmias are symptoms of hypercalcemia. Abdominal cramping occurs with hyponatremia.

PHYSIOLOGICAL INTEGRITY

Pharmacological and Parenteral Therapies

Adverse Effects/Contraindications and Side Effects

Implement procedures to counteract adverse effects of medications and parental therapy

32. A client who takes digoxin (Lanoxin) at home has presented with a digoxin level of 4 ng/mL and a heart rate of 38. What is the priority nursing action?
    A. Set up the client for external pacing.
    B. Administer Atropine 1 mg IV.
    C. Administer Digibind 228 mg IV.
    D. Assess the client for visual changes and nausea/vomiting.

The answer is C. The therapeutic digoxin level is 0.5–2 ng/mL. The client who has digitalis toxicity will require a dose of Digibind, which binds to the digoxin in the serum and removes it from the circulating system.

A is incorrect—The client does not need external pacing for digoxin toxicity. B is incorrect—While Atropine will raise the heart rate, it will not remove digoxin from the serum, which is the cause of the bradycardia. D is incorrect—The client may have visual changes and nausea/vomiting but the priority nursing action is to remove the digoxin from the system. The nurse understands the client is has digoxin toxicity by the level in the serum and the client's heart rate.

PHYSIOLOGICAL INTEGRITY

Physiological Adaptation

Radiation Therapy

Implement interventions to address side/adverse effects of radiation therapy

33. What is the priority of care in a client that is undergoing external radiation therapy?
    A. Washing the markings off of the face.
    B. Maintaining a 6-ft distance.
    C. Grouping client care to minimize exposure to the radiation.
    D. Assessing the skin for burned areas.

The answer is D. The client should be assessed for areas that are burned so that treatment can occur to prevent further damage to the skin and underlying tissues. Fluid volume status should also be addressed due to the body's response to the burn.

A is incorrect—The markings placed on the body for radiation therapy should not be removed to ensure that alignment of the radiation can occur with preciseness. B is incorrect—Only with internal radiation should a distance be kept from the patient. C is incorrect—Grouping client care to minimize exposure to radiation is not necessary with external radiation.

PHYSIOLOGICAL INTEGRITY

Physiological Adaptation

Medical Emergencies

Apply knowledge of nursing procedures and psychomotor skills when caring for a client experiencing a medical emergency

34. A client presents to the emergency department after being involved in a vehicular accident. The client has obvious facial fractures and a head injury. The nurse should refrain from:
    A. placing a nasogastric tube.
    B. inserting a urinary catheter.
    C. cleaning the blood from the face.
    D. bagging the client with a bag valve mask and high flow oxygen.

The answer is A. With obvious facial fractures, the client should not receive a nasogastric tube through the nose.

B is incorrect—A urinary catheter is safe as long as there is not any blood at the meatus. C is incorrect—The nurse should clean blood from the face to see what injuries are present. D is incorrect—The client can be bagged with BVM until an artificial airway is placed by the physician.

SAFE AND EFFECTIVE CARE ENVIRONMENT

Safety and Infection Control

Standard/Transmission-Based/Other Precautions

Understand communicable disease and the modes of organism transmission

35. A client is admitted with active tuberculosis. Which form of isolation should the client be placed on?
    A. Contact
    B. Droplet
    C. Airborne
    D. Standard

The answer is C. Airborne isolation includes particles transmitted by droplet or airborne particles. By placing the client on airborne isolation, the client receives a room with negative airflow; mask are worn by staff while in the patient room and by the patient if out of the room for test.

A is incorrect—Contact isolation is for pathogens that are transmitted through direct or indirect contact with the client or items the client may have touched. B is incorrect—Droplet transmission is when the client coughs or the mucous membranes of the client are touched. Droplet transmission does not mean the client will need negative air pressure in his or her room since the particles are not suspended in the air as they are with airborne. D is incorrect—Standard is used for blood or body fluid pathogen transmission.

HEALTH PROMOTION AND MAINTENANCE

Family Systems

Assess impact of change on family system

36. Which statement made by a parent would indicate a need for immediate evaluation and counseling after the birth of the fifth child?
    A. "I just don't know how I will pay for college for all of the children."
    B. "I have thoughts of throwing the baby in a dumpster."
    C. "The four oldest siblings argue constantly over the remote."
    D. "I wish I made more money so my family would be happier."

The answer is B. The parent making the statement of the desire to throw the baby in the dumpster is indicative of a need for counseling. The parent could be experiencing depression or psychosis that needs intervention.

A is incorrect—Wondering how a parent will pay for college is a normal concern and does not pose an immediate threat to the parent or children. C is incorrect—A sibling arguing with another is normal and does not pose a threat to the children or parent. D is incorrect—A parent wishing he or she made more money is normal and does not pose an immediate threat.

HEALTH PROMOTION AND MAINTENANCE

Lifestyle Choices

Assess client lifestyle choices

37. Which statement made by a parent indicates that a child may need to be evaluated every year by a health care provider?
    A. "My children are home schooled to avoid societal influences."
    B. "I allow my children to attend private schools only."
    C. "We encourage our children to take a multivitamin at bedtime every night."
    D. "We don't allow our children to go outside alone."

The answer is A. The parents in this situation have chosen to teach the children at home to avoid societal influences. The children need a yearly screening to note for developmental delays and issues associated with a lack of social interaction with other children. The children are also at risk for being victims of abuse by not having outside observers to notice signs or symptoms of abuse leading for the need of the parents to participate in a yearly evaluation of the children by a health care professional.

B is incorrect—The parents have chosen to place their children in private schools, which still allows for health screenings by the school nurse and evaluations for signs of abuse. C is incorrect—Taking a multivitamin is not a reason for yearly visits to the physician. D is incorrect—By not allowing children to go outside alone, the children are being protected from external dangers; furthermore, this is not a reason for yearly visits by a health care provider.

PSYCHOSOCIAL INTEGRITY

Chemical and Other Dependencies

Assess client for drug-/alcohol-related dependencies, withdrawal, or toxicities

38. A client presents with a history of illegal use of prescription narcotics. Which assessment data is the earliest sign of withdrawal?
    A. BP 90/60, HR 100
    B. Anxiety, irritability
    C. Insomnia, diarrhea
    D. Nausea, vomiting

The answer is B. Anxiety and irritability is one of the first signs of opioid withdrawal with salivation, diaphoresis, and other symptoms following.

A is incorrect—The client presents with hypertension and tachycardia with an opioid withdrawal. C is incorrect—Insomnia does occur with opioid withdrawal but later in the cycle. Diarrhea is usually not seen as the client has a decrease in motility due to the opioid. D is incorrect—Nausea and vomiting occur late in the withdrawal process.

PSYCHOSOCIAL INTEGRITY

Grief and Loss

Assist client/family/significant others in coping with suffering grief, loss, dying, and bereavement

39. A client is nearing the end of his life. To assist the family to cope, the nurse should suggest that the family:
    A. tell the client good-bye.
    B. leave the client to die in peace.
    C. become visibly upset to expel all emotions.
    D. contact a local psychiatrist to discuss what has occurred.

The answer is A. The family will gain closure through telling the client good-bye. Gaining closure will help the family through the grieving and bereavement process.

B is incorrect—When the family leaves the client, they carry the fact that their family member died alone and this can harm the grieving process. C is incorrect—A family should respond to death in their own way; therefore, encouraging the family to become visibly upset is inappropriate. D is incorrect—The family should be provided with a list of support services to assist with grieving but a family should not be instructed to contact a psychiatrist by the nurse.

PSYCHOSOCIAL INTEGRITY

Stress Management

Implement measures to reduce environmental stressors

40. A client is being weaned from a patient controlled analgesic pump (PCA pump). Which nursing intervention would be best to assist in the control of pain?
    A. Provide small chatter in the background.
    B. Play classical music in the background.
    C. Darken the room and close the door.
    D. Teach the client to only call for pain meds when pain is a 10/10.

The answer is C. Dimming the lights and closing the client's door will lessen environmental stressors, which can precipitate pain.

A is incorrect—Chatter can be perceived as an added stress to the client. B is incorrect—While music in the background can assist in pain control, the client may find classical music annoying and not helpful. The client should be allowed his or her favorite music, if desired, during the period weaning. D is incorrect—The client should learn to call for pain medication before the pain is a 10/10 or pain management becomes more difficult.

PHYSIOLOGICAL INTEGRITY

Basic Care and Comfort

Nutrition and Oral Hydration

Monitor client hydration status

41. Based on the postsurgical client's 24-hour intake and output documentation, which data should be reported to the physician?

	Day 1		Day 2		Day 3		Day 4	
	Intake	**Output**	**Intake**	**Output**	**Intake**	**Output**	**Intake**	**Output**
A	2000	1000	1500	1250	1325	1300	1250	1300
B	2000	900	1800	1100	1750	1000	1500	1000
C	2000	1700	1700	1625	1575	1400	1300	1275
D	2000	1500	1500	1300	1400	1300	1425	1400

The answer is B. The client is not maintaining an appropriate fluid balance after surgery as expected and the chances of electrolyte imbalances and pulmonary edema are high. The physician should be notified so that pharmacological interventions can occur and a fluid restriction can be ordered.

A, C, and D represent a normal ratio of fluid intake to fluid lost and does not require notification of the physician.

PHYSIOLOGICAL INTEGRITY

Pharmacological and Parenteral Therapies

Blood and Blood Products

Check the client for appropriate venous access for red blood cell/blood product administration

42. Prior to administering a blood product, the nurse must ensure which of the following is present?
    A. A patent intravenous line
    B. Y-Site tubing
    C. An intravenous pump
    D. A 20 gauge or large intravenous line

The answer is D. A client must have a 20 gauge or larger intravenous line before blood products can be administered. If this is not present, a new IV must be initiated.

A is incorrect—While a patent line is important, the size of the line is the most important item a nurse must ensure is present before blood is administered. A 22-gauge line may be patent, but it is not sufficient for blood administration and a new site IV must be initiated. B is incorrect—Y-site tubing is important but not as important as the correct size intravenous line. C is incorrect—Blood should be administered on a pump, but it is not as important to ensure a pump is present as it is to ensure the proper size intravenous line is present.

PHYSIOLOGICAL INTEGRITY

Pharmacological and Parenteral Therapies

Medication Administration

Review pertinent data prior to medication administration

43. Prior to administration, a client starting an increased dose of clonidine (Catapress) should be assessed for which of the following
    A. Orthostatic hypotension
    B. Tachycardia
    C. Hyperglycemia
    D. Oliguria

The answer is A. A client who starts an increased dose of Catapress will experience orthostatic hypotension and so assessment for preexisting orthostatic hypotension is important and the physician can be notified for further orders.

B is incorrect—An adverse effect of Catapress is bradycardia not tachycardia and is not a contraindication to administering the medication. C is incorrect—Hyperglycemia is not a side effect of Catapress and is not a contraindication to administering the drug. D is incorrect—There is no contraindication to administering Catapress if oliguria is present.

PHYSIOLOGICAL INTEGRITY

Pharmacological and Parenteral Therapies

Total Parenteral Nutrition

Monitor client for side/adverse effects of TPN

44. For a client that is receiving total parenteral nutrition (TPN), which assessment data would be most indicative of infection within 48 hours of initiation of therapy?
    A. Confusion
    B. Diaphoresis
    C. Heart rate 120
    D. Temperature of 101°Fahrenheit.

The answer is D. Fever in an afebrile patient is indicative of sepsis in a client that is receiving TPN.

A is incorrect—Confusion is common in the first 24–48 hours of initiation of TPN. This is due to the shift of electrolytes from the plasma to the cell. B is incorrect—Diaphoresis is common with hypoglycemia associated with TPN. C is incorrect—While tachycardia accompanies a fever, it is not the most indicative sign of infection in the client.

PHYSIOLOGICAL INTEGRITY

Reduction of Risk Potential

Potential for Complications of Diagnostic Tests/Treatments/Procedures

Intervene to manage potential circulatory complications

45. Which finding in a client who has undergone repair of a radial fracture 12 hours ago would require immediate notification of the orthopedic surgeon?
    A. Pain at the incision site
    B. Edema of the affected arm
    C. Pain with passive movement of the fingers
    D. Fever

The answer is C. The client has compartment syndrome and one of the indicative signs is pain with passive movement of the fingers. This requires the physician to be notified immediately so that intervention can occur.

A is incorrect—Pain is common after a surgical repair of a fractured arm. B is incorrect—Edema is common after surgical repair due to the body's response to the injury and the beginning of repair. D is incorrect—Fever is a sign of infection and should be reported but it does not require the nurse to notify the orthopedic surgeon immediately.

PHYSIOLOGICAL INTEGRITY

Reduction of Risk Potential

System-Specific Assessment

Perform a risk assessment

46. A home health nurse is performing an admission assessment on a client who has been discharged from the hospital. Which finding on the risk for falls assessment must be resolved prior to the nurse leaving the home?
    A. Carpet in the home
    B. Throw rugs over hardwood floors
    C. Shower/tub combo with shower curtain
    D. Steps leading into the home

The answer is B. Throw rugs over hardwood floors are a common problem in homes of older clients and is an area where clients may fall. The nurse should remove the throw rugs prior to leaving the home and explain to the client her rationale.

A is incorrect—Carpet is not a falls risk. C is incorrect—While a tub/shower combo is not ideal and the client can fall getting into or out of the tub, the nurse cannot fix this before leaving and should request items that would assist the client to continue using the shower. D is incorrect—Although steps leading into the home present a fall risk, the nurse cannot modify these.

PHYSIOLOGICAL INTEGRITY

Physiological Adaptation

Alterations in Body Systems

Evaluate achievement of client treatment goals

47. A client with a history of COPD complains of increased shortness of breath and has wheezing noted upon auscultation. The client is administered a nebulizer treatment of Albuterol and Atrovent. Which evaluation would indicate a therapeutic response to this treatment?
    A. Increase in wheezing upon auscultation
    B. Pink frothy sputum
    C. Decrease in shortness of breath
    D. Decrease in heart rate

The answer is C. The client is complaining of shortness of breath, and therefore, a decrease would be considered a therapeutic response to the treatment.

A is incorrect—An increase in wheezing upon auscultation is not considered a therapeutic response to the breathing treatment. B is incorrect—Pink frothy sputum is indicative of pulmonary edema and is not a therapeutic response to the treatment. D is incorrect—A decrease in the heart rate is not a therapeutic response and indicates a complication since Albuterol and Atrovent are known to increase the client's heart rate.

PHYSIOLOGICAL INTEGRITY

Physiological Adaptation

Medical Emergencies

Apply knowledge of pathophysiology when caring for a client experiencing a medical emergency

48. A client presents to the emergency department after being ejected from an all terrain vehicle. The client received an opioid analgesic in route for control of pain associated with a lower leg injury. Which assessment data is most indicative of early increased intracranial pressure?
    A. Irritability
    B. Hypotension
    C. Pupils 2 mm
    D. Decreased respiratory rate

The answer is A. Irritability is the most indicative sign of increased intracranial pressure due to the changes the oxygen the brain receives due to compressed vessels. The absence of oxygen places the brain in a state of hypoxia, which causes irritability to occur.

B is incorrect—Hypertension is a sign of increased intracranial pressure due to the excited fibers, which control vasoconstriction. C is incorrect—Pupil dilation occurs due to increased intracranial pressure but in this case the pupils are constricted due to the administration of an opioid analgesic in the field. D is incorrect—Initially, the respiratory rate will be increased due to the body's response to hypoxia, as a late sign it will decrease.

PHYSIOLOGICAL INTEGRITY

Physiological Adaptation

Radiation Therapy

Apply knowledge of pathophysiology when discussing radiation therapy with client/family/significant others

49. A nurse is teaching a client about care of a wound after surgery, which will also be the site of radiation treatments. Discharge instructions should include:
    ___ How to care for the surgical site.
    ___ Signs and symptoms of delayed wound healing.
    ___ How often to report to outpatient for a treatment.
    ___ Signs and symptoms of anaphylactic reaction to radiation.
    ___ Signs of radiation toxicity.
    ___ Foods to avoid during therapy.

The discharge instructions should include how to care for the surgical site and the signs and symptoms of delayed wound healing since difficulties in wound healing are common in the client undergoing radiation therapy. Reporting to outpatient is important so that treatments stay on the scheduled path for the greatest benefits. Radiation toxicity is common and the signs and symptoms should be discussed with the client so that the individual can seek medical attention as needed. Foods to avoid are taught about due to the possibility of oral ulcerations and sores associated with radiation therapy.

Anaphylactic reactions are not a risk with radiation therapy.

PHYSIOLOGICAL INTEGRITY

Pharmacological and Parenteral Therapies

Blood and Blood Products

Administer blood products and evaluate the client response

50. A nurse has an order to administer packed red blood cells to a client. Prior to administration, the nurse should (check all that apply):
    ___ obtain consent
    ___ gather IV tubing with a filter
    ___ gather D5 ½ NS
    ___ prime the line with fluid
    ___ check the blood with either an RN or LPN

___ warm the blood to 100°F
___ assess the site for patency

Before administering blood, the nurse should obtain consent for blood administration, gather IV tubing ensuring a filter for blood administration is present, prime the line with fluid, and assess the site for patency.

The nurse should not use D5 ½ NS for blood administration. Only NS can be used for blood administration and only an RN can check blood with another RN. The blood should not be warmed unless orders are present to warm the blood to a specific temperature for rapid infusion. Warming of the blood will cause it to clot and can promote bacterial growth.

SAFE AND EFFECTIVE CARE ENVIRONMENT

Safety and Infection Control

Reporting of Incident/Event/Irregular Occurrence/Variance

Report error/event/occurrence per protocol

51. A nurse walks into a room after the bathroom call light is sounded and finds a client lying on the floor. The client states that he became dizzy and lost his balance after using the bathroom. Which documentation of the fall is most appropriate?
    A. "Client fell after standing-up from the toilet."
    B. "Client fell due to lowering in blood pressure upon standing."
    C. "Client found lying in floor, states 'I became dizzy and lost my balance after using the bathroom'."
    D. "Client experienced a vagal response and fell after using the bathroom."

The answer is C. The nurse should only document what she saw and what the client told her. Documentation other than what was stated and visualized is falsifying a document.

A is incorrect—This is a nursing assumption and is not legal. B is incorrect—This is not reporting what was seen or what the client told the nurse; therefore, it is inappropriate charting. D is incorrect—This is assuming the client experienced a vagal response and is not appropriate charting.

HEALTH PROMOTION AND MAINTENANCE

Ante-/Intra-/Postpartum and Newborn Care

Calculate expected delivery date

52. A client has her pregnancy confirmed by the nurse in a physician's office. The client wishes to know her expected date of delivery and the first day of her last menstrual period was July 4th. The nurse calculates the delivery date as:
    A. April 10th
    B. April 11th
    C. April 1st
    D. April 4th

The answer is B. The client's expected date of delivery is April 11th. This is calculated by subtracting 3 months from the month the client had her last menstrual period and adding 7 days to the date of the last menstrual period.

A, C, and D are incorrect using this method.

PHYSIOLOGICAL INTEGRITY

Reduction of Risk Potential

System-Specific Assessment

Perform focused assessment or reassessment

53. List in order from first to fourth the assessment technique used for a client who is complaining of abdominal pain.
    A. Inspection
    B. Palpation
    C. Auscultation
    D. Percussion

Inspection is the first step for an assessment of the gastrointestinal system. The second step is auscultation so that sounds can be heard since manipulation of the abdominal wall may alter sounds. The third step is to percuss for tympani or dullness and the last step is to palpate the abdomen for pain, tenderness, or other abnormalities.

PHYSIOLOGICAL INTEGRITY

Reduction of Risk Potential

Laboratory Values

Obtain specimens other than blood for diagnostic testing

54. A nurse has an order for a wound culture to be taken via aspiration; prior to aspirating the wound bed, the nurse should:
    A. massage the wound bed.
    B. irrigate the wound bed with normal saline.
    C. clean the wound bed edges with normal saline.
    D. dry exudate from the wound bed with sterile gauze.

The answer is B. The wound bed should be irrigated first with normal saline to remove exudate, which allows for fresh exudate from the wound bed to surface.

A is incorrect—The wound is massaged after the old exudate and saline irrigant is removed from the wound bed.

C is incorrect—Wound edges are not required to be cleaned when aspirating for a culture. D is incorrect—Exudate is removed from the wound bed with sterile gauze after saline irrigant is placed in the wound.

SAFE AND EFFECTIVE CARE ENVIRONMENT

Management of Care

Continuity of Care

Perform procedures necessary for admitting, transferring, or discharging a client

55. Prior to transferring a client from the medical surgical floor to the intensive care unit, the nurse should first:
    A. obtain a signed consent from the client for transfer.
    B. notify the nurse manager.
    C. obtain an accepting physician.
    D. phone a report to the nurse in the ICU who will receive the client.

The answer is D. The nurse must transfer care of the client to another nurse and this is performed in a patient report.

A is incorrect—A client does not need to sign consent if a transfer is within the same facility. B is incorrect—A nurse manager is not needed in a transfer as long as there is a physician order and a bed is available in the receiving unit. C is incorrect—The client's primary physician is responsible for following the client within the facility, and if a transfer of care to another physician is required, it is the responsibility of the physician to obtain an accepting physician.

SAFE AND EFFECTIVE CARE ENVIRONMENT

Management of Care

Staff Education

Assess purpose of staff education activities

56. A nurse understands that the primary rationale behind attending an in-service for newly acquired unit specific equipment is to:
    A. aid in medicaid reimbursement for the hospital.
    B. gain continuing education credits for licensure.
    C. meet JCAHO requirements for staff education of hospital equipment.
    D. maintain patient safety by understanding the proper use of hospital equipment.

The answer is D. The nurse possesses the responsibility to remain current on all equipment that is used in a specific area of employment so he or she can assist in maintaining patient safety. Being unfamiliar with equipment can lead to litigation if he or she is negligent and causes client harm.

A is incorrect—Medicaid does not require nurses to attend in-services before reimbursement for client care is awarded. B is incorrect—While gaining continuing education credits are possible with some in-services, those that deal specifically with equipment use are not governed by the licensure board therefore are not applicable for continuing education credits. C is incorrect—JCAHO requires that staff is educated regarding equipment used in the facility but the primary purpose of attending an in-service on equipment use is to maintain patient safety.

HEALTH PROMOTION AND MAINTENANCE

Aging Process

Provide care that meets the special needs of the preschool client ages 1 month to 4 years

57. When performing a routine assessment on a 1-year-old client, which data should be collected first?
    A. Rectal temperature
    B. Heart rate
    C. Respirations
    D. Blood pressure

The answer is C. Respirations should be counted first before the client becomes upset with the assessment process. Changes in respiratory rate will often occur before other signs and symptoms are present in a child.

A is incorrect—The rectal temperature should be performed last since it will upset the child. B is incorrect—The heart rate should be assessed after the respiratory rate since it requires a stethoscope and will alter the respiratory rate if the client becomes upset. D is incorrect—The blood pressure is not performed on the 1-year-old client unless there is a cause of concern such as altered level of consciousness, depressed or bulging fontanels, or signs and symptoms of dehydration. In this scenario, the assessment is routine.

HEALTH PROMOTION AND MAINTENANCE

Health and Wellness

Evaluate client/family/significant other understanding of health promotion behaviors/activities

58. A client in the doctor's office for a routine check-up demonstrates an understanding of health promotion behaviors and activities when he says that he will: (check all that apply)
    ___ walk at least twice a week.
    ___ avoid excessive caffeine.

___ cut down to one pack of cigarettes a day.
___ eat a vegetable at every meal.
___ take medication exactly as prescribed.
___ have blood pressure checked regularly.

The client voicing that he will walk at least twice a week, avoid excessive caffeine, eat a vegetable at every meal, take medication as prescribed and have blood pressure monitored frequently demonstrates an understanding of health promotion behaviors and activities.

The client stating he will cut down to one pack of cigarettes a day shows he does not realize the necessity of quitting smoking to improve health and further education is needed.

PSYCHOSOCIAL INTEGRITY

Abuse/Neglect

Identify risk factors for domestic, child and/or elder abuse/neglect, and sexual abuse

59. Which clients are at a high risk for sexual abuse? (Select all that apply.)
    ___ An 8-year-old boy who lives with both parents.
    ___ A 6-year-old girl living in foster care.
    ___ A 21-year-old female living in a college dorm.
    ___ An 88-year-old client living in a nursing home.
    ___ An 18-year-old male living in an apartment in a new town.

The answers are the 6-year-old girl living in foster care and the 21-year-old female living in a college dorm. Females are at a higher risk for sexual abuse than any other group. Sexual abuse for this group can consist of molestation of the 6-year-old girl or rape of either the 6- or 21-year-old.

Incorrect—The 8-year-old is at a low risk because he is male and lives with both parents making it a stable environment. The 88-year-old client living in a nursing home is at a low risk of being sexually abused due to age and facility. An 18-year-old male is at a low risk of being sexually abused even though he lives in a new town.

PSYCHOSOCIAL INTEGRITY

Psychopathology

Identify signs and symptoms of impaired cognition

60. A client's family is concerned about recent changes in their family member's behavior and is afraid that he is developing Alzheimer's disease. Which signs and symptoms reported by the family is associated with Alzheimer's disease? (Check all that apply.)
    ___ Memory loss
    ___ Seizures
    ___ Syncope
    ___ Personality changes
    ___ Anorexia
    ___ Poor judgment

The answers are memory loss, personality changes, anorexia, and poor judgment. All of these are signs and/or symptoms of Alzheimer's disease and require reporting to the physician for follow up.

Seizures is incorrect—they are not associated with the disease. Syncope is not associated with Alzheimer's unless a pre- or coexisting cardiac problem exists.

PHYSIOLOGICAL INTEGRITY

Basic Care and Comfort

Complementary and Alternative Therapies

Evaluate client/family/significant other outcomes of alternative and/or complementary therapy practices

61. A cancer client has been attending yoga to aid in relaxation and mind healing. Which evaluation would indicate a therapeutic response to this alternative therapy?
    A. The client claims to be "cancer free."
    B. The client has decided death will occur and is ready to "pass on."
    C. The client states she has found inner strength and has accepted the diagnosis.
    D. The client has decided to stop treatment and allow the body to heal itself.

The answer is C. The cancer patient will often turn to alternative therapies to assist in the treatment process. Yoga has proven to be a method of relaxation and allows for reflection and finding peace within one's self. The client who has a successful response to yoga will find the peace within and learn how to relax and channel thoughts until peace is achieved.

A is incorrect—The client has a false sense of being cancer free and this has proven to be a negative result of an alternative therapy. B is incorrect—The client has made the decision that the end will occur and this can leave the client with a negative outlook on the future and impede healing. D is incorrect—The client has a false assurance of the reality of yoga and the expectations of ones self. The client needs counseling on the benefits of yoga and the expected outcomes.

PHYSIOLOGICAL INTEGRITY

Pharmacological and Parenteral Therapies

Adverse Effects/Contraindications and Side Effects

Assess client for actual or potential side effects and adverse effects of medications

62. A client is being discharged home with a prescription for warfarin (Coumadin). Discharge instructions include:
    A. avoid Tylenol while taking Coumadin.
    B. avoid ginseng while taking Coumadin.

C. avoid clopidogrel (Plavix) while taking Coumadin.
D. avoid clonidine (Catapress) while taking Coumadin.

The answer is B. A client who takes Coumadin should avoid taking herbal supplements that contain ginseng due to the risk of increased risk of blood thinning beyond desired effects.

A is incorrect—Tylenol is acceptable to take while on Coumadin therapy unless hepatic function is impaired. C is incorrect—Plavix is a common drug used to prevent platelet aggregation and is compatible for use with Coumadin therapy. D is incorrect—Catapress is commonly used for hypertension and is compatible with Coumadin therapy.

PHYSIOLOGICAL INTEGRITY

Pharmacological and Parenteral Therapies

Pharmacological Interactions

Provide client/family/significant others with information on known pharmacological interactions of medication prescriptions

63. A client is prescribed theophylline (Theo-24) for COPD. Discharge instructions should include the interaction of which of the following:
    A. Nicotine transdermal patches
    B. fosinopril (Monopril)
    C. Advair Diskus 250/50
    D. clopidogrel (Plavix)

The answer is A. Nicotine is contraindicated with the use of theophylline because of the stimulant effects and may cause tachycardia.

B is incorrect—Monopril is an ACE inhibitor and does not carry any interactions with theophylline. C is incorrect—Advair is a nonsteroidal bronchodilator and is safe to be used concurrently with theophylline. D is incorrect—Plavix is a platelet aggregate and is safe to be used with theophylline.

PHYSIOLOGICAL INTEGRITY

Reduction of Risk Potential

Vital Signs

Intervene when client vital signs are abnormal

64. The vital signs on a client are as follows:
    - B/P 178/120
    - P 112
    - R 28
    - O_2Sat 98%
    - T 99.0

    The client is complaining of a headache and blurred vision. Which medication from the client's MAR should the nurse administer?
    A. Metoprolol (Toprol XL) 100 mg p.o.
    B. Clonidine (Catapress) 0.3 mg p.o.
    C. Metoprolol (Lopressor) 5 mg IV
    D. Tylenol 650 mg p.o.

The answer is C. The client meets criteria for a hypertensive crisis. Lopressor is to be given intravenously. This is the best drug to give from the client's MAR. Lopressor will lower the blood pressure and heart rate.

A is incorrect—The Toprol XL will also lower blood pressure and heart rate, but it is taken by mouth and will take 30 minutes to act. In hypertensive emergency, intravenous antihypertensives are given followed by oral dosing. B is incorrect—The client has an increased heart rate as well as increased blood pressure, the drug of choice would be an antihypertensive agent that will work on both areas. The Catapress is used for hypertensive emergencies but it does not have a labeled use for lowering the heart rate and the oral dose will take longer to show results. D is incorrect—The client does have a low-grade fever and a headache, but the headache will resolve with a resolution in the blood pressure.

PSYCHOSOCIAL INTEGRITY

Abuse/Neglect

Assess client risk for abuse/neglect

65. Which client is at the highest risk for neglect?
    A. Infant of a 30-year-old woman who is single.
    B. Infant of a 14-year-old girl who lives with her parents.
    C. 95-year-old client living in an assisted living facility.
    D. 79-year-old client living at home with her 41-year-old daughter.

The answer is B. Statistically, a child of a teenager is at the highest risk for neglect. The mother and father live with the teenager but in most situations, the teenager is still responsible for the care of the infant. A teenager generally does not have the coping skills and knowledge to care for an infant.

A is incorrect—The mother is an adult and the infant is less likely to be neglected. C is incorrect—A client in an assisted living facility is able to provide care with some assistance by other personnel lessening the chances of neglect. D is incorrect—The client living with her daughter is at a low risk with the daughter still young enough to provide adequate care.

PHYSIOLOGICAL INTEGRITY

Physiological Adaptation

Alterations in Body Systems

Perform peritoneal dialysis

66. A nurse is performing peritoneal dialysis and instills 2 L of dialysate into the peritoneal cavity. After 30 minutes has elapsed, the client returns only 1 L of solution. The nurse should:

A. have the client roll from side to side.

B. gather a syringe and pull fluid from the peritoneal cavity.

C. apply warm compresses to the abdomen.

D. stop the process and call the physician.

The answer is A. The client should move from side to side in the bed so that drainage can occur.

B is incorrect—A syringe should not be used to pull dialysate from the cavity. C is incorrect—Warm compresses on the abdomen will not help removing the solution from the peritoneal cavity. D is incorrect—The physician should not be notified unless moving the client is unsuccessful in removing the fluid.

PHYSIOLOGICAL INTEGRITY

Pharmacological and Parenteral Therapies

Medication Administration

Review pertinent data prior to medication administration

67. A client has vancomycin (Vancocin) ordered every 12 hours. The client has one IV access and it currently has dopamine (Intropin) infusing to maintain blood pressure. Prior to the administration of the vancomycin (Vancocin) the nurse should:

A. obtain another IV access.

B. check for patency of the existing IV site.

C. discontinue the Dopamine.

D. check for compatibility of Dopamine and Vancomycin.

The answer is D. Before obtaining another IV site, the nurse should check for compatibility of the Dopamine and the Vancomycin. If compatibility is not assured, then another IV site should be obtained.

A is incorrect—The nurse should check for compatibility first. B is incorrect—The patency of the IV line should be unquestionable if a medication is infusing in it currently. C is incorrect—Dopamine cannot be discontinued for the length of time it will take for Vancomycin to infuse.

PHYSIOLOGICAL INTEGRITY

Physiological Adaptation

Illness Management

Teach client about managing illness

68. A client is being discharged after receiving the diagnosis of human immunodeficiency virus (HIV). Priority teaching at the time of discharge is:

A. how to prevent the spread of infection to others.

B. when to take medications.

C. what foods to avoid.

D. when to follow up with physician.

The answer is A. Preventing the spread of the disease is the most important fact to teach the client prior to discharge from the hospital. This is most important with a new diagnosis of HIV.

B is incorrect—Although when to take medications is important, the nurse should first ensure that the client knows how to prevent the spread. C is incorrect—With a new diagnosis there are not any food restrictions. D is incorrect—When to follow up with the physician is important but not the most important fact to teach to the client before discharge.

SAFE AND EFFECTIVE CARE ENVIRONMENT

Management of Care

Client Rights

Recognize the client's right to refuse treatment/procedures

69. A client who is scheduled to undergo chemotherapy today states, "I do not wish to undergo my treatment today." Which action by the nurse is most appropriate?

A. Discuss with the client the need to follow the prescribed treatment regime.

B. Ask the client as to what has occurred to make him or her not want today's treatment.

C. Notify the physician that the client has refused a treatment.

D. Notify the chemotherapy nurse that the client has refused today's treatment.

The answer is B. The nurse needs to recognize that the client has the right to refuse treatment but he or she should also determine what has occurred to make the client refuse treatment so that an intervention can occur if needed.

A is incorrect—It discounts the client's feelings. C and D are incorrect—Although they recognize the client has refused treatment neither choice addresses the client and his or her current state of mind.

SAFE AND EFFECTIVE CARE ENVIRONMENT

Management of Care

Information Technology

Use information technology to enhance the care provided to a client

70. A 14-year-old client has been diagnosed with diabetes and needs diabetes education at the time of discharge. Which method of instruction would be best for this client?

A. A book that discusses diabetes, including how to administer medications.

B. Interactive computer software that discusses diabetes management.

C. A diabetes educator discussing diabetes management in a group environment.
D. A pamphlet that contains pictures on diabetes management.

The answer is B. A teenage would benefit most from computer software since teenagers are accustomed to a computer and learn best when they can interact with the information being given.

A is incorrect—A teenager is less likely to read a book discussing diabetes and thus leading to incomplete information. C is incorrect—Because of the nature of the illness and the psychological changes that a teenager goes through, a teenager often will not participate in a group discussion about diabetes management and therefore will not learn. D is incorrect—A pamphlet is not best for a teenager since they are active learners.

SAFE AND EFFECTIVE CARE ENVIRONMENT

Safety and Infection Control

Home Safety

Educate client/family on home safety issues

71. Which of the following should be included in the discharge teaching for a family who is in the pediatrician's office for a 2-year-old well baby check-up?
    A. Cover all outlets in the home.
    B. Place pots and pans on the front of the stove while cooking.
    C. Avoid leaving the child for more than 1 minute while in the tub.
    D. Remove all pets while the child is in the home.

The answer is A. A 2-year-old child is ambulatory and possess the motor skills to place objects in the electrical outlets which could potentially cause an electrical shock. The parents need to cover all outlets to prevent this from occurring.

B is incorrect—The parents should not place pots and pans on the front of the stove. They should be placed on the back. C is incorrect—A child should never be left alone in the tub. D is incorrect—Pets are not required to be removed from the home unless the child has an allergy to pets or other risks are associated.

SAFE AND EFFECTIVE CARE ENVIRONMENT

Safety and Infection Control

Emergency Response Plan

Implement emergency response plans

72. A nurse would expect the internal disaster plan to be enacted if which event occurs?
    A. Plane crash
    B. Infant abduction
    C. Fire in a client's room
    D. Explosion at a local plant

The answer is C. A fire in a client's room is an internal disaster and the plan should be enacted by administrative staff.

A is incorrect—A plane crash is an external disaster and requires an external disaster plan to be enacted. B is incorrect—An infant abduction carries a separate plan of action by the hospital and is not considered an internal disaster. D is incorrect—An explosion at a local plant is an external disaster and requires the external disaster plan to be enacted.

HEALTH PROMOTION AND MAINTENANCE

Expected Body Image Changes

Assess occurrence of expected body image changes

73. A client is in the hospital after experiencing a burn to the face. Which statement made by the client demonstrates an acceptance of the change in her appearance?
    A. "I will make sure to avoid going outside during the day."
    B. "I am ready to look into the mirror."
    C. "I can put a scarf over my face so no one will notice."
    D. "Going to a salon is worthless; a new hairstyle won't fix my deformity."

The answer is B. This statement made by the client demonstrates an acceptance of the changes that occurred as a result of the burn. The client is ready to see her face after the event, which is the first step to healing.

A is incorrect—This demonstrates that the client continues to have a disturbed body image. C is incorrect—Wearing a scarf is a sign that the client has not accepted the changes that have occurred. D is incorrect—The client continues with a disturbed body image and has yet to accept the changes that have occurred. The client needs continued support and counseling.

SAFE AND EFFECTIVE CARE ENVIRONMENT

Safety and Infection Control

Reporting of Incident/Event/Irregular Occurrence/Variance

Identify need/situation where reporting of incident/event/irregular occurrence/variance is appropriate

74. The nurse should fill out an incident report for which occurrence?

A. A client is found lying on the floor of his room.
B. An "as needed" medication is given for a complaint of pain.
C. Calling a physician for an illegible order.
D. A medication is held due to a decreased blood pressure.

The answer is A. A client found lying in the floor is considered an unexpected event and requires an incident report to be completed.

B is incorrect—A medication given for the complaint of pain is an expected occurrence and an incident report is not needed. C is incorrect—Calling a physician for an illegible order is preventing an error and does not require an incident report. D is incorrect—Holding a medication due to a low blood pressure is a valid nursing judgment and does not require an incident report.

PSYCHOSOCIAL INTEGRITY

Crisis Intervention

Assess the need for, initiate, and maintain suicide precautions

75. A client presents to the emergency department and states that he wants to kill himself. Which action by the nurse is the priority?
A. Removal of client's clothing.
B. Placement of client in room with camera.
C. Search of client for weapons.
D. Pad the side rails of the bed.

The answer is B. The first action by the nurse is to place the client in a room with a camera. The client will need to be monitored at all times and this is the best method.

A is incorrect—The client will need to remove clothing that could be used to assist with a suicide but this needs to be done in a room with a camera so that the staff can make sure the client is not harming self while alone. C is incorrect—The client's clothing will be searched for a weapon upon removal and the search of clothing is performed by security staff. D is incorrect—The side rails do not need to be padded for a suicidal client. The padding of side rails is reserved for the client experiencing seizures.

PSYCHOSOCIAL INTEGRITY

Therapeutic Communications

Use therapeutic communication techniques to provide support to client and/or family

76. A pediatric client is scheduled for a bone marrow biopsy. The mother begins to sob stating, "I am a horrible mother for letting this happen to my little girl." The nurse's best response is:
A. to leave the mother alone to cry.
B. to ask "Is there anyone I can call for you?"
C. to call the physician and request a sedative for the mother.
D. to state "You are not responsible for your child being ill; you have placed your child in the best environment for what she needs."

The answer is D. The mother needs hope for the situation at hand and needs to be reminded that this is not her fault and that she is doing what is best for her child.

A is incorrect—Leaving the mom will only worsen the situation. B is incorrect—The mother needs support at the moment. Calling other family is helpful but does not address the current situation. C is incorrect—The physician will not be able to prescribe a sedative for the mother. The mother must be of sound mind to make decisions for her child if needed and a sedative would impair her mental state.

PHYSIOLOGICAL INTEGRITY

Basic Care and Comfort

Personal Hygiene

Assist the client in the performance of activities of daily living

77. Which of the following should a nurse perform every day to ensure the client's activities of daily living have been met?
A. Set the client in a chair with the supplies needed to bathe.
B. Administer medications on time.
C. Place a consult for occupational therapy.
D. Perform wound care.

The answer is A. The client needs to bathe every day, and to assist the client the nurse should set him or her in a chair and allow time for bathing.

B is incorrect—Administering meds is not ensuring that activities of daily living have been met. C is incorrect—Placing the consult does not ensure that activities of daily living have been met. D is incorrect—Wound care is not part of the client's activities of daily living.

PHYSIOLOGICAL INTEGRITY

Pharmacological and Parenteral Therapies

Expected Effects/Outcomes

Evaluate and document client response to medication

78. Which of the following is a sign that IV ondansetron (Zofran) was therapeutic?
A. The client has a bowel movement within 6 hours.
B. The client no longer complains of a headache.

C. The client's abdominal pain is relieved.
D. The client no longer complains of nausea.

The answer is D. Zofran is an antiemetic and is used for nausea and vomiting associated with chemotherapy and surgery.

A is incorrect—Zofran, as with all antiemetics, has the tendency to cause constipation. B is incorrect—Zofran does not contain any pain-relieving properties. C is incorrect—Zofran does not contain any pain-relieving properties.

PHYSIOLOGICAL INTEGRITY

Reduction of Risk Potential

Diagnostic Tests

Evaluate the results of diagnostic testing and intervene as needed

79. The technician reports to the nurse that the client has 2 mm ST segment elevation in lead II and III on a 12-lead electrocardiogram. What is the priority nursing intervention?
    A. Assess the client
    B. Repeat the test
    C. Administer Oxygen 2L NC
    D. Phone the physician

The answer is A. When a nurse is presented with a suspicious test result, the nurse must first assess the patient for signs and symptoms of distress, as in this case, a suspected myocardial infarction. This allows the nurse to intervene as needed.

B is incorrect—The test may be repeated after an assessment of the client. C is incorrect—The nurse must first assess the client before performing any nursing action. D is incorrect—The physician is phoned after the nurse assesses the client and any actions are taken that are deemed necessary.

PHYSIOLOGICAL INTEGRITY

Reduction of Risk Potential

System-Specific Assessment

Identify factors that result in delayed wound healing

80. A nurse is assessing four of her assigned clients. Which client is at the highest risk for delayed wound healing?
    A. 18-year-old admitted after right knee arthroscopy.
    B. 34-year-old diabetic admitted for hernia repair.
    C. 64-year-old with peripheral vascular disease that underwent a toe amputation.
    D. 78-year-old with congestive heart failure admitted for a thoracentesis.

The answer is C. The 64-year-old client with peripheral vascular disease is at the highest risk for delayed wound healing. The client has vascular deficiency already as evidenced by the toe amputation. The body's ability to transport oxygen-rich blood and nutrients to the area is compromised and the client is likely to have difficulty healing from the procedure due to the already compromised state.

A is incorrect—The 18-year-old is not likely to have difficulty healing from the procedure. B is incorrect—While 34-year-old diabetic client will have difficulty with wound healing, the 64-year-old client with peripheral vascular disease is at the highest risk due to evidence of an already compromised system. D is incorrect—The 78-year-old client with congestive heart failure has a cardiac pump problem and will have decreased blood supply; although, for this question, C is the best answer.

PHYSIOLOGICAL INTEGRITY

Reduction of Risk Potential

Therapeutic Procedures

Educate client and family about home management of care

81. A client is being discharged with a CPAP machine for a diagnosis of sleep apnea. Which of the following should be included in the discharge instructions?
    A. Clean the face mask with bleach solution.
    B. Stop using the machine if noise precipitates insomnia.
    C. Place the mask securely on the face.
    D. Redness to the face where the mask is placed is normal.

The answer is C. The mask should fit securely on the face to prevent air leaking around the mask and causing eye irritation and maintain desired outcome.

A is incorrect—The bleach solution will harm the client's skin; the mask should be cleaned with vinegar and water solution. B is incorrect—The CPAP should be worn as directed by the physician and if the noise is causing insomnia, the physician should be notified. D is incorrect—Redness to the face may indicate an allergic reaction to the mask and should be reported to the physician.

PHYSIOLOGICAL INTEGRITY

Physiological Adaptation

Alterations in Body Systems

Perform or assist with dressing change

82. A nurse has an order to perform central line care. Which action by the nurse will be best in removing bacteria from the catheter insertion site?
    A. Allowing the chlora-prep to dry on the site.
    B. Scrubbing the insertion site for 2 minutes with chlora-prep.

C. Wearing a mask during the procedure.
D. Placing a medicated disk (bio-patch) around the insertion site.

The answer is B. Scrubbing the site with chlora-prep will be best nursing action in removing bacteria from the site of the catheter and prevent infection.

A is incorrect—The chlora-prep can dry on the site after it is scrubbed. C is incorrect—Wearing a mask is beneficial in preventing the introduction of new bacteria, but is not the best action when removing bacteria from the catheter insertion site. D is incorrect—Placing a bio-patch on the site will prevent growth of bacteria but it is not the best action in removing bacteria from the site.

PHYSIOLOGICAL INTEGRITY

Physiological Adaptation

Fluid and Electrolytes

Implement interventions to restore client fluid and/or electrolyte balance

83. A client has a magnesium level of 1.4 mg/dL. The nurse administers magnesium oxide at 1300 and will plan on ordering a redraw of the magnesium level at:
A. 1500
B. 1600
C. 1700
D. 2100

The answer is C. Magnesium has an onset of action in 3 hours of administration. The blood redraw is performed in 4 hours from administration to see if a desired response occurred.

A and B are incorrect—These time frames are not long enough from administration to onset for levels to increase. D is incorrect—This time frame is too long from the time of administration to know if desired outcomes occurred.

PHYSIOLOGICAL INTEGRITY

Physiological Adaptation

Hemodynamics

Apply knowledge of pathophysiology to interventions in response to the client's abnormal hemodynamics

84. Which client will not exhibit the expected assessment findings in response to septic shock?
A. A client with a previous myocardial infarction.
B. A client who is taking a beta blocker for hypertension.
C. A client who performs peritoneal dialysis.
D. A client with diabetes.

The answer is B. A client taking a beta blocker will not exhibit the heart rate change associated with septic shock and the blood pressures will remain at a lower level.

A is incorrect—A client with a myocardial infarction will exhibit the anticipated response. C is incorrect—A client who performs peritoneal dialysis will have the findings expected with septic shock. D is incorrect—While the client with diabetes will have an alteration such as an increase in blood pressure, the individual will exhibit the findings associated with septic shock.

PHYSIOLOGICAL INTEGRITY

Physiological Adaptation

Medical Emergencies

Provide emergency care for wound disruption

85. List in order the steps the nurse will take if faced with a wound dehiscence
___ Notify the physician
___ Cover the wound with sterile saline soaked gauze
___ Lay the client in low Fowlers and bend the client's knees
___ Instruct the client to splint the abdomen if needing to cough

The client should first lie down initially to prevent further strain on the incision site. Next, the nurse applies saline soaked sterile gauze to the area to keep the area moist. The nurse should then instruct the client on splinting during coughing in the event he or she needs to cough while the physician is being notified.

PHYSIOLOGICAL INTEGRITY

Physiological Adaptation

Unexpected Response to Therapies

Assess client for unexpected adverse response to therapy

86. A client is on the ventilator due to a diagnosis of acute respiratory distress syndrome (ARDS). Which assessment finding is most indicative of a complication?
A. Diminished breath sounds on auscultation
B. Deviation of the trachea
C. Weight gain
D. Decreased urine output

The answer is B. A deviated trachea is indicative of a tension pneumothorax associated with noncompliant lungs (as with ARDS) being ventilated at a higher pressure than the lung can tolerate. This requires immediate intervention by the physician.

A is incorrect—Diminished breath sounds are common in the client with ARDS due to decrease lung compliance and collapsed alveoli. C is incorrect—While weight gain may occur in ARDS, it is not the most indicative sign of a complication. D is incorrect—Although decreased urinary output is a problem and needs to be addressed, it is not the most indicative sign of a complication.

PHYSIOLOGICAL INTEGRITY

Reduction of Risk Potential

Potential for Complications of Diagnostic Tests/Treatments/Procedures

Implement measures to manage/prevent/lessen possible complications of the client condition and/or procedure

87. A client with a history of congestive heart failure who has gained 3 pounds in 1 day should be placed on:
    A. 1800 calorie ADA diet
    B. calorie count
    C. fluid restriction
    D. potassium restriction

The answer is C. The client who has gained more than 2 pounds in 1 day and has a history of congestive heart failure should be placed on a fluid restriction to keep the client from exacerbating his or her condition.

A is incorrect—The 1800 calorie ADA diet is for a diabetic and will not be beneficial in this situation of volume overload. B is incorrect—The client should not count calories but count liquid intake in volume. D is incorrect—A potassium restriction is not needed unless lab values indicate a high potassium level.

PHYSIOLOGICAL INTEGRITY

Physiological Adaptation

Illness Management

Administer oxygen therapy and evaluate response

88. A nurse is assessing the vital signs of a client and notices that the oxygen level is 91% on room air. The client complains of a headache and wheezing is noted upon auscultation. Which nursing intervention would be best?
    A. Ask the client to sit in high Fowlers.
    B. Ask the client to cough and reassess.
    C. Apply 2 L of oxygen per nasal cannula.
    D. Offer a pain medication for the headache.

The answer is C. The client has a low oxygen saturation level, is wheezing, and has a headache. The headache could be attributed to the low oxygen saturation level and so the nurse should place oxygen on the client to see if symptoms improve. The wheezing should be addressed with a bronchodilator.

A is incorrect—Making the client sit in high Fowlers will not resolve the situation of a low oxygen level. B is incorrect—Asking the client to cough is used when rhonchi is auscultated; wheezing is due to a narrowing of the airway. D is incorrect—Pain medication will worsen the oxygen saturation level.

SAFE AND EFFECTIVE CARE ENVIRONMENT

Safety and Infection Control

Medical Surgical Asepsis

Assess client environment area for sources of infection

89. In the room of a client who has sustained a burn, which of the following would be the greatest potential source of infection?
    A. Fresh flowers
    B. Fresh fruit
    C. Helium filled latex balloons
    D. Staff

The answer is D. Staff is the greatest source of infection for clients with a burn. For this reason, isolation is ordered for most clients who have sustained a burn.

A is incorrect—Fresh flowers produce toxins as they die; they are also a source of infection and should be limited in the rooms of client's with a burn. B is incorrect—Fresh fruit that is to be eaten is safe in the room of a client as long as it has not begun to rot. C is incorrect—Helium filled latex balloons are safe as long as the client does not have a latex allergy.

SAFE AND EFFECTIVE CARE ENVIRONMENT

Management of Care

Informed Consent

Ensure that client has given informed consent for treatment

90. A client is scheduled for a colonoscopy to be performed this morning. Prior to preparing the client for the procedure, the nurse must first:
    A. ensure that the client has an advance directive in the chart.
    B. assess the client's level of understanding about the procedure.
    C. verify that consent for the procedure has been signed by the client.
    D. verify that the client has not eaten since midnight.

The answer is C. Prior to preparing the client for the procedure, the nurse must ensure a signed consent is on the chart. The signing of the consent is the responsibility of the physician who will be performing the surgical procedure.

A is incorrect—An advanced directive is desired but not essential in the chart of a client who is going for a colonoscopy. B is incorrect—The client's level of understanding regarding the procedure is required prior to consent being signed. The signed consent establishes that the client understands the procedure that the physician will perform. D is incorrect—Verification that the client has remained NPO is less of a priority than verification that consent is on the chart prior to prepping the client for the procedure.

HEALTH PROMOTION AND MAINTENANCE

Ante/Intra/Postpartum and Newborn Care

Assess client for symptoms of postpartum complications

91. Which assessment data would be most indicative of a uterine infection in the postpartum client who underwent a vaginal delivery?
    A. Dark brown discharge from the vagina.
    B. Pain at the site of the episiotomy.
    C. Cramping in the lower abdomen.
    D. Foul smelling vaginal discharge.

The answer is D. Foul smelling discharge is indicative of an infection in the postpartum client and requires intervention.

A is incorrect—Dark brown discharge is old blood that is being expelled through the vagina and is normal. B is incorrect—Pain at the site of the episiotomy is normal until healed. C is incorrect—Cramping in the lower abdomen occurs as the uterus returns to its pre-pregnancy state.

HEALTH PROMOTION AND MAINTENANCE

Principles of Teaching/Learning

Assess readiness to learn, learning preferences, and barriers to learning

92. Which evaluation would be most indicative of readiness to begin self-wound care?
    A. The client does not wish to see the wound.
    B. The client no longer needs pain medication before wound care.
    C. The client watches the nurse perform care of the wound.
    D. The client begins to ask questions about the care of the wound.

The answer is D. When the client begins to ask questions about the care of the wound he or she has taken an interest in the procedure, which demonstrates a readiness to learn.

A is incorrect—If the client is unwilling to visualize the wound then he or she is not ready to care for the wound. B is incorrect—The client may no longer require pain medication before wound care but that does not show a readiness to learn how to care for the wound. C is incorrect—The client may begin to watch the care of the wound prior to being ready to take over the care. Watching the wound care is the first step but is not most indicative of a readiness to begin self-care.

PHYSIOLOGICAL INTEGRITY

Basic Care and Comfort

Mobility/Immobility

Maintain client skin integrity

93. Which of the following is the best method for preventing skin breakdown in an immobile client?
    A. Use of an alternating mattress.
    B. Turning every 2 hours.
    C. Keeping wrinkles out of sheets.
    D. Elevating heels off of the bed.

The answer is B. The best method of preventing skin breakdown is to turn the client every 2 hours.

A is incorrect—Even though a client uses an alternating mattress, a staff member must still turn the client every 2 hours. C is incorrect—The client will benefit from removal of wrinkles that may be in the sheets but it is not the best method of preventing skin breakdown. D is incorrect—While elevating the feet will prevent shearing, it is not the best method of preventing skin breakdown for an immobile client.

PHYSIOLOGICAL INTEGRITY

Pharmacological and Parenteral Therapies

Blood and Blood Products

Identify the client according to facility/agency policy prior to administration of red blood cells/blood products

94. Which of the following is the first action a nurse must take prior to initiating blood administration?
    A. Check the chart for the physician's order.
    B. Ask the client to sign consent for blood.
    C. Order a type and cross from the lab.
    D. Check the chart for the hematocrit and hemoglobin level.

The answer is C. Prior to blood administration, the nurse must be sure an order is on the chart signed by the physician. Without an order, the nurse cannot proceed with the process.

B is incorrect—The client should not sign consent unless an order is present on the chart. For the options given, ensuring an order is on the chart is the best answer. C is incorrect—The physician must write an order for a type and cross to be performed on the client. D is incorrect—After a physician's order is received, the nurse is responsible for checking the client's level before having a consent signed by the client.

PHYSIOLOGICAL INTEGRITY

Pharmacological and Parenteral Therapies

Pharmacological Pain Management

Evaluate and document client use and response to pain medications

95. The assessment of a client complaining of pain is documented as:
    - RR 24
    - BP 140/90
    - HR 100
    - grimacing, guarding

    Demerol 50 mg IM was administered 30 minutes prior to the pain reassessment. Which findings would best indicate a therapeutic response to the medication?
    A. RR 20
    B. HR 95
    C. BP 138/88
    D. Patient resting with eyes closed

The answer is D. The client is resting now, which shows a resolution from the grimacing and guarding the client was demonstrating before pharmacological intervention.

A is incorrect—The respiratory rate is not the best indicator of pain resolution. B is incorrect—The heart rate has only decreased by 5 bpm, which is not a significant indicator of pain relief. C is incorrect—The blood pressure has not decreased enough to demonstrate pain relief and is not the best indicator of pain relief.

PHYSIOLOGICAL INTEGRITY

Physiological Adaptation

Hemodynamics

Identify cardiac rhythm strip abnormalities

96. The nurse attaches an unresponsive client to the monitor. What is the rhythm the nurse sees on the monitor?
    A. Asystole
    B. Ventricular fibrillation
    C. Ventricular tachycardia
    D. Torsades De Pointes

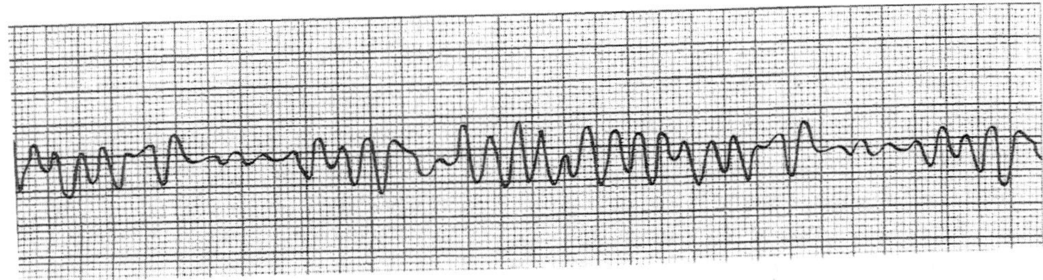

The answer is B. The rhythm is ventricular fibrillation. There are irregular ventricular contractions due to the absence of depolarization in the heart.

A is incorrect—With asystole, there is an absence of impulses to cause ventricular contractions. C is incorrect—Ventricular tachycardia exist with an increased and irregular ventricular rate. D is incorrect—Torsades De Pointes is due to prolonged repolarization and will progress to VF if left untreated.

PHYSIOLOGICAL INTEGRITY

Physiological Adaptation

Medical Emergencies

Apply knowledge of pathophysiology when caring for a client experiencing a medical emergency

97. A client is brought to the emergency department after working outdoors. The temperature is 99°F with a heat index of 102. The nurses assess for which of the following knowing it is the most indicative sign of a heat stroke?
    A. Agitation, confusion
    B. Nausea, headache
    C. Shedding of clothes, unable to move
    D. Syncope, neck stiffness

The answer is A. Agitation and confusion are the first signs of a heat stroke due to the body's response to the vasoconstriction and subsequent cerebral hypoxia associated with the body attempting to conserve fluid loss from sweating.

B is incorrect—Nausea and headache are common with heat exhaustion. C is incorrect—The shedding of clothes and inability to move is found with hypothermia. D is incorrect—Syncope and neck stiffness are not associated with heat stroke, but are associated with meningitis.

PHYSIOLOGICAL INTEGRITY

Reduction of Risk Potential

Potential for Complications of Diagnostic Tests/Treatments/Procedures

Implement measures to manage/prevent/lessen possible complications of client condition and/or procedure

98. A client is being admitted to the floor from the emergency department with possible seizures. Before the client arrives to the floor, the nurse should plan on:

A. padding the rails of the bed.
B. placing a bed alarm on the bed.
C. placing restraints at the bed side.
D. placing the crash cart at the bedside.

The answer is A. The rails of the bed should be padded to prevent injury if the client has a seizure while in the bed.

B is incorrect—Placing a bed alarm on the bed will not be beneficial in protecting the client if he or she has a seizure. C is incorrect—Restraints are not used on a client who might have a seizure. D is incorrect—There is no need for the crash cart to be at the bedside for a client with possible seizures.

PHYSIOLOGICAL INTEGRITY

Physiological Adaptation

Alterations in Body Systems

Counsel/teach client, family, or significant others about managing client health problems

99. The nurse is teaching the client and the family regarding peritoneal dialysis, which will be performed at home. The priority discharge instruction is:
A. signs and symptoms of peritoneal infection.
B. how to care for and clean the catheter.
C. how to take a blood pressure and heart rate.
D. how long the procedure should take.

The answer is B. How to care for and clean the catheter is priority teaching for the client. Prevention of infection is a high priority for clients who are performing peritoneal dialysis at home.

A is incorrect—Signs and symptoms of peritoneal infection are important and the client should be taught to report these to the physician. C is incorrect—How to take a blood pressure and heart rate is important but not necessary before every at-home treatment unless the client has complaints. D is incorrect—How long a procedure should take is important but it is better to teach the client about how to measure input to output to know that the treatment was successful.

PSYCHOSOCIAL INTEGRITY

Family Dynamics

Assist client/family/significant others to integrate new members into family structure

100. A mother states that her 3-year-old potty trained child has begun to urinate in his pants after the new baby was brought home from the hospital. Which response by the nurse is best?
A. "Children often regress when new members are introduced; continue to remind him to go to the rest room every hour."
B. "Punish him before this becomes a pattern."
C. "Children often regress at this age; it is normal and will improve with time."
D. "Talk to your child about what is occurring and then show him he is still important by spending an hour of one-on-one time with him every day while someone watches the baby."

The answer is D. The most important thing is to let the parents know it is okay to talk about what is occurring with their child and assist the family with a plan to help the child feel loved and still an important member of the family.

A is incorrect—This does explain to the family what is occurring but reminding the child to go to the restroom does not show the child that he or she is still a valuable member of the family. B is incorrect—Regression is a normal response to a new family member and punishment does not validate normalcy. C is incorrect—This will not resolve without intervention by the parents. Waiting for change to occur without action by the parents will only lead to more problems.

PHYSIOLOGICAL INTEGRITY

Reduction of Risk Potential

Laboratory Values

Provide client with information about the purpose and procedure of prescribed laboratory tests

101. A client presents to the ED with chest pain. The nurse draws blood during the initiation of an intravenous line for a triponin and CPK. The client asks what this test is for. The best response by the nurse is:
A. "the triponin looks for a heart attack."
B. "the triponin will verify what the EKG shows."
C. "the triponin is the cardiac marker test that shows cardiac injury."
D. "the triponin shows muscle damage."

The answer is C. The triponin is the only test that is explicitly for cardiac muscle ischemia making this the correct option.

A is incorrect—Although the client can have muscle ischemia from lack of blood supply, it is not the only indicator of a heart attack. B is incorrect—While the EKG and the triponin are used as indicators of muscle ischemia, this test is not used to verify another test. D is incorrect—The triponin is specifically a cardiac marker test. The CPK is the test that shows muscle damage.

PHYSIOLOGICAL INTEGRITY

Pharmacological and Parenteral Therapies

Dosage Calculation

Perform calculations needed for medication administration

102. A client has ordered Cardizem 250 mg in 250 mL to run at 10 mg/h. To deliver the ordered dose, the infusion pump should be set at:
A. 8 mL/h
B. 10 mL/h

C. 5 mL/h
D. 1 mL/h

The answer is B. The concentration of drug is a 1:1 ratio. The infusion pump should be set to 10 mL/h.

A, C, and D are incorrect—These choices would be under dosing the client.

PHYSIOLOGICAL INTEGRITY

Basic Care and Comfort

Assistive Devices

Assess client for actual/potential difficulty with communication and speech/vision/hearing problems

103. Which of the following drugs requires regular hearing exams with prolonged use?
A. Streptomycin
B. Ciprofloxacin (Cipro)
C. Hydromorphone (Dilaudid)
D. Isoniazid (INH)

The answer is A. The client who receives an aminoglycoside such as streptomycin requires auditory exams routinely to assess for hearing loss due to the drugs ototoxic affects.

B is incorrect—Cipro does not require routine exams of any sensory functions. C is incorrect—Dilaudid causes CNS depression, which leads to changes in respiratory rate and blood pressure and does not require routine auditory exams. D is incorrect—INH requires routine liver enzyme studies due to the possibility of liver toxicity with use.

SAFE AND EFFECTIVE CARE ENVIRONMENT

Management of Care

Resource Management

Plan safe, cost-effective care for the client

104. Which action by the nurse would be the safest and most cost-effective when administering daily medications?
A. Administer all morning meds at the same time regardless of time scheduled.
B. Date and time all IV tubing on piggybacks and continuous infusions.
C. Use only one medicine cup per client when administering meds in a 24-hour period.
D. Use Betadine versus alcohol swabs when cleaning sites for injections.

The answer is B. Dating and timing all tubing for intravenous medications and fluids eliminates the need to change tubing each shift. Tubing is acceptable for continuous use 24 hours after being attached to a bag and the client.

A is incorrect—Medications are scheduled by the pharmacy and should be followed. Administering medications as scheduled can prevent poor absorption and alterations in the client's physiologic status. C is incorrect—Using one medicine cup per day is unsanitary and should be avoided. D is incorrect—Betadine can damage the cells of the skin; using Betadine is not recommended for routine injections.

SAFE AND EFFECTIVE CARE ENVIRONMENT

Management of Care

Advance Directives

Provide client or family with information about advance directives

105. While admitting a client to the unit, the nurse asks the client if he or she has a living will. The client questions the nurse as to what a living will is. The nurse's best response is:
A. "A living will lets the family know your wishes if you go into cardiac arrest."
B. "A living will is a legal document that explains your wishes for health care depending on the severity of your illness."
C. "A living will is a written order by the physician."
D. "A living will allows you to name someone to make decisions for you."

The answer is B. A living will is an advance directive that states the wishes of a client in the event he or she is critically or terminally ill.

A is incorrect—A living will states more than the wishes of a client if he or she is in cardiac arrest. A living will not only informs the family of the client's wishes but also the health care team. C is incorrect—"Do not resuscitate" is the order written by the physician and placed in the chart after the wishes are made known by the client in an advance directive. D is incorrect—A living will does not allow the client to name an individual to make decisions for him or her, a durable power of attorney allows an appointed individual to make decisions for the client anytime he or she is unable to do so.

SAFE AND EFFECTIVE CARE ENVIRONMENT

Management of Care

Collaborate with Interdisciplinary Team

Identify significant information to report to other disciplines

106. A nurse enters a client's room to administer ferrous sulfate 324 mg. When the nurse checks the MAR against the medication, he or she notices that the dosage on

the package indicates ferrous sulfate 300 mg. Which action would be the most appropriate?

A. Notify the pharmacist of the dosage error and request the correct dosage.

B. Administer the medication since milligrams to be administered is lower than the ordered dose making it safe.

C. Hold the medication until the physician can be notified.

D. Ask the nurse who cared for the client yesterday what he or she administered to the client.

The answer is A. The nurse should phone the pharmacist first to request the correct dosage for the client before it is administered.

B is incorrect—Administering a medication that is under or over the ordered dose is a medication error unless an order is written for the dose being administered. C is incorrect—The pharmacy is responsible for dispensing medication and needs to be notified of the error. D is incorrect—The nurse should take responsibility for today and clarify the dosage with the pharmacy.

SAFE AND EFFECTIVE CARE ENVIRONMENT

Management of Care

Legal Rights and Responsibilities

Report unsafe practice of health care personnel to internal/external entities

107. A nurse walks by the room of a client and sees a licensed practical nurse beginning the administration of blood. Which action by the nurse would be most appropriate?

A. Confront the licensed practical nurse as to what is occurring.

B. Check the chart of the client to see if blood was ordered.

C. Report what was seen to the charge nurse.

D. Phone the board of nursing to report unsafe practice.

The answer is C. If a nurse suspects unsafe practice, it is imperative he or she follows the chain of command and report the nurse to the charge nurse. The charge nurse is responsible for confronting the nurse and continuing to report the nurse through the chain of command to the appropriate individuals.

A is incorrect—It is policy of most institutions to report unsafe practice to the nurse in charge of the unit. B is incorrect—Regardless of the order, it is not in the scope of practice of an LPN to administer blood. D is incorrect—The nursing administration is responsible for reporting a nurse for unsafe practice.

SAFE AND EFFECTIVE CARE ENVIRONMENT

Management of Care

Supervision

Evaluate effectiveness of staff member's time management skills

108. Which assessment by the charge nurse is most indicative that a staff member is demonstrating difficulty with time management of daily assignments?

A. Performing 3 minute assessments on all clients.

B. Being unable to leave the unit by the end of shift.

C. Administering medications as scheduled.

D. Not meeting the standards of client care during the shift.

The answer is D. Not meeting the standards of care is a sign that a nurse has difficulty with time management. Nurses are required to multitask to complete all assignments but meeting the standards of care is essential and should never be compromised.

A is incorrect—A 3-minute assessment is acceptable on a client that is not a new admission. It addresses the system-specific assessment and an overview of all other systems. B is incorrect—Being unable to leave the unit when the day is complete is not the highest indicator that a nurse has poor time management skills. Not meeting the standards of care ranks higher. C is incorrect—Administering medications on time demonstrates that a nurse does have the correct priorities for time management.

SAFE AND EFFECTIVE CARE ENVIRONMENT

Safety and Infection Control

Security Plan

Participate in maintaining the institution's security plan

109. The hospitals policy regarding infant abductions is below:

Hospital Policy Regarding Infant Abductions: Code Pink

1. If an infant is found to be missing or is reported missing by staff, phone the hospital operator immediately and a code pink will be called over the intercom system.
2. All staff should stand by elevators, doors leading to the outside, and stairwells in their department.
3. Anyone carrying a large bag, backpack, wearing a heavy coat or appears to be pregnant should be followed and a description of the person should be noted.
4. Phone security and follow the person.
5. Avoid confronting the individual, wait on security.

A nurse is working in a hospital and as she is exiting the elevator on the main floor a code pink is called over the intercom. Which action by the nurse is most appropriate?
A. Stand outside the elevator until an all clear is called.
B. Return to the assigned floor to stand outside the stairwell.
C. Leave the elevator and go to a stairwell and stand.
D. Begin stopping all staff and visitors and ask them to open bags and coats.

The answer is A. If a code pink is called, according to the policy the staff is to stand by any port of exit. In this case, the nurse should stand outside of the elevator so that it is attended during a possible abduction.

B is incorrect—Returning to the assigned floor does not follow the policy and leaves the elevator as a possible exit site for the abductor. C is incorrect—The elevator is a portal of exit as is the stairwell and so the one the staff member is at should be manned. D is incorrect—According to the policy, staff should not confront anyone suspected of being the abductor, but follow the possible abductor and phone security.

HEALTH PROMOTION AND MAINTENANCE

Health Promotion Programs

Instruct client on ways to promote health

110. A male should be instructed on using which method when performing a routine testicular self-examination?
A. Perform before taking a shower.
B. Perform every 3 months.
C. Roll the testicle between the thumb and fingers.
D. Pinch the epididymis until sensation is loss in the penis and release.

The answer is C. The client should be instructed to roll the testicle between the thumb and fingers to monitor for abnormalities.

A is incorrect—The test should be performed after taking a shower so that the scrotum is relaxed. B is incorrect—Self-exams should be performed every month to monitor for changes so they can be caught early. D is incorrect—The epididymis should not be pinched due to the potential for damage to the structure.

SAFE AND EFFECTIVE CARE ENVIRONMENT

Safety and Infection Control

Handling Hazardous and Infectious Materials

Identify biohazardous, flammable, and infectious materials

111. Which of the following should be placed in a biohazardous bag?
A. Foley urine bag of a client with CHF.
B. Used intravenous medication bag of a client suffering from dehydration.
C. Soiled diaper of a client with *Clostridium difficile*.
D. Syringe used to flush a central line.

The answer is C. Clostridium difficile is highly contagious and the stool of this client should be placed in a biohazardous bag for proper disposal.

A is incorrect—A client's Foley bag should be emptied in the toilet prior to throwing the bag in the trash can which removes waste into the appropriate facility. B is incorrect—A used intravenous bag can be thrown into the trash can in a client's room as long as a name is not on the bag. If a name is on the bag, the label should be removed and the bag can be placed in the trash receptacle. D is incorrect—A syringe used to flush a central line should be placed in a sharps receptacle and not into a biohazardous bag.

PSYCHOSOCIAL INTEGRITY

Mental Health Concepts

Explore why the client is refusing/not following the treatment plan (e.g., nonadherence)

112. A client with end stage renal disease (ESRD) tells the transporter that he is not going down for his dialysis treatment today. The nurse should
A. tell the client that it is okay and he can go tomorrow.
B. notify the physician.
C. ask the client if he is frustrated with the process of dialysis.
D. tell the client he will need to sign an "Against Medical Advice" form.

The answer is C. The most common reason for nonadherence to treatment regimens is a frustration with the procedure and the aspects of the disease process. Acknowledging that the client may be unhappy with the demands of the disease and the loss of control over life will help the nurse and client devise a plan to meet the treatment regimen that benefits both parties.

A is incorrect—The client needs to go to dialysis every scheduled day, telling him it is okay to miss a treatment will enable him to refuse every treatment and does not determine why he refused. B is incorrect—Notifying the physician does not explore why the client refused today's treatment. D is incorrect—Having the client to sign an AMA form does not explore why the client refused today's treatment.

PSYCHOSOCIAL INTEGRITY

Support Systems

Promote independence of client/family/significant others

113. Which of the following would promote independence in the client who recently underwent a below-the-knee amputation?

A. Teach range of motion exercises.
B. Provide the client with a wheelchair.
C. Instruct the client on proper wound care.
D. Provide analgesics for pain relief.

The answer is B. The client has the disability of limited mobility after an amputation. Providing the client with a wheelchair will enable him or her to move around in the environment and continue with independent activities.

A is incorrect—While a range of motion exercises prevent contractures and prepare the stump for prosthesis, it is not the best method of promoting independence initially. C is incorrect—Instructing the client on wound care promotes readiness to care for self, but does not promote independence overall. D is incorrect—Analgesics do not promote independence for the client.

PHYSIOLOGICAL INTEGRITY

Basic Care and Comfort

Palliative/Comfort Care

Assess client's symptoms related to end of life

114. Which of the following would a nurse find in her assessment of a client that is nearing the end of life? (Check all that apply.)
___ Decrease in time spent sleeping
___ Loss of appetite
___ Alteration in mental status
___ Generalized weakness
___ Periods of apnea
___ Seizures

The answers are loss of appetite, alteration in mental status, generalized weakness, and periods of apnea. These are consistent with the findings a nurse might see in his or her assessment of someone nearing the end of life. The loss of appetite is due to the decrease in metabolism that the body undergoes at death. Generalized weakness and an alteration in mental status is due to the changes in metabolism as well. Periods of apnea occur and are called Cheyne-Stokes; panting respirations will accompany the periods of apnea in some cases.

Incorrect answers are decrease in time spent sleeping and seizures. The client will often have an increase in time sleeping and seizures are uncommon.

PHYSIOLOGICAL INTEGRITY

Pharmacological and Parenteral Therapies

Medication Administration

Review pertinent data prior to medication administration

115. The morning assessment of a client reveals this data:
- BP 90/60
- HR 110
- RR 20
- Temp 98.9

The nurse should hold which of the following drugs:
A. levothyroxine (Synthroid)
B. carvedilol (Coreg)
C. gabapentin (Neurontin)
D. pioglitazone (Actos)

The answer is A. The nurse should hold the dose of Levothroid if the client has a resting pulse of greater than 100 bpm. This is a sign of hyperthyroidism and a dose will only compound the problem.

B is incorrect—While the blood pressure is borderline, it is within normal limits. Coreg is a beta blocker and is needed to lower the heart rate. C is incorrect—Neurontin is a drug used for nerve pain and there are no contraindications to administration based on vital signs. D is incorrect—Actos is used to serum glucose levels and does not carry a contraindication based on vital signs.

PHYSIOLOGICAL INTEGRITY

Pharmacological and Parenteral Therapies

Total Parenteral Nutrition

Provide client/family/significant others with information on TPN

116. A family is taking a client home that will be receiving total parenteral nutrition (TPN). The family should be instructed on:
A. how to perform glucose monitoring.
B. how to change the intravenous dressing every 24 hours.
C. how to dilute the TPN solution.
D. how to turn off the infusion pump.

The answer is A. The client receiving total parenteral nutrition requires frequent monitoring of glucose levels. The client's family will need to learn how to assess the client's glucose level and what action to take depending on the outcome.

B is incorrect—The dressing is changed every 48–72 hours unless contamination is suspected. Changing more often than needed is not cost-effective and opens the site to the possibility of contamination. C is incorrect—The TPN solution should not be diluted. The solution should be administered in its prepared form. D is incorrect—The infusion should never be stopped or changed abruptly to allow time for the body to change its metabolic needs.

PHYSIOLOGICAL INTEGRITY

Reduction of Risk Potential

Potential for Alterations in Body Systems

Identify client potential for aspiration

117. Which client is at the highest risk for aspiration pneumonia?

A. A client who has a nasogastric tube to low suction and an endotracheal tube in place.

B. A client who has a PEG tube feeding and is lying at 20 degrees

C. A client who has recently undergone surgery and is eating clear liquid diet.

D. A client who has returned from esophageal dilatation and is ready for discharge.

The answer is B. A client who has a PEG tube should not lie below 30 degrees to prevent aspiration of gastric contents.

A is incorrect—A client with an endotracheal tube has a protected airway and aspiration is not a worry. C is incorrect—A client on a clear liquid diet has an intact gag reflex and aspiration is a low risk. D is incorrect—A client who has undergone an esophageal dilatation and is ready for discharge is at a low risk for aspiration.

PHYSIOLOGICAL INTEGRITY

Reduction of Risk Potential

Potential for Complications from Surgical Procedures and Health Alterations

Apply knowledge of pathophysiology to monitoring for complications

118. A client has returned to the floor following a transverse loop colostomy. Which assessment finding would be indicative of a complication?
   A. Hypoactive bowel sounds
   B. A dusky color to the stoma
   C. Liquid stool measuring 900 mL
   D. Scant bleeding at the stoma site

The answer is B. A dusky colored stoma reveals that necrosis is occurring to the bowel that has been brought to the surface. The physician needs to be notified of this finding.

A is incorrect—Hypoactive bowel sounds are expected following a colostomy and are no cause for concern postoperatively. C is incorrect—Liquid stool is a normal finding following a colostomy. The bowel will need time to begin reabsorbing water from the GI track before stool will be more formed. D is incorrect—Scant bleeding is normal following a colostomy and is due to a rich blood supply from the GI track.

PHYSIOLOGICAL INTEGRITY

Reduction of Risk Potential

System-Specific Assessment

Assess client for signs of hypoglycemia or hyperglycemia

119. A nurse is performing the morning assessment on a client that has a diagnosis of diabetes mellitus controlled by diet. Which assessment finding requires notification of the physician?
   A. Urine output of 1000 cc in 2 hours
   B. BP 140/90
   C. Heart rate 100
   D. Temp 99.9°F

The answer is A. Polyuria is indicative of hyperglycemia and requires the physician to be notified so that orders can be written for fluid replacement and insulin administration if needed.

B is incorrect—This is borderline hypertension, but does not require notification of the physician. A reassessment of the blood pressure should occur. C is incorrect—Mild tachycardia is not a reason to consult the physician. The tachycardia may be secondary to the polyuria and may resolve when the condition improves. D is incorrect—This is a mildly elevated temperature and does not require notification of the physician.

PHYSIOLOGICAL INTEGRITY

Reduction of Risk Potential

Therapeutic Procedures

Provide pre- and/or postoperative education

120. Prior to a client undergoing a pinning of the right hip, the client should be instructed on:
   A. how to use the client controlled analgesic pump.
   B. when he can expect to eat a meal.
   C. how soon after surgery discharge is possible.
   D. how to care for the surgical wound.

The answer is A. The client should be instructed on how to use the client controlled analgesic pump prior to surgery to ensure understanding has occurred.

B is incorrect—When the client can eat is not something the nurse must prepare the client for prior to a surgical procedure. C is incorrect—Discharge is based on the individual's progress and the physician is responsible for writing the order and discussing a time frame for discharge with the client. D is incorrect—How to care for the wound occurs after the surgery when the client feels he or she is ready to take over the care.

PSYCHOSOCIAL INTEGRITY

Family Dynamics

Assess parental techniques related to discipline

121. A school nurse is evaluating families during an open house at a school. Which assessment indicates

abnormal discipline techniques and requires intervention?

A. A mother telling her child she will place her in "time out" once they are at home.

B. A mother yelling at her child to "behave" during a walk down the hall.

C. A mother stating "When we get home, I will beat you with a belt."

D. A mother stating "You need to learn to control your behavior or you will go straight to bed when we are home."

The answer is C. The mother is threatening the child with physical harm, which is a sign of abuse and should be acted on by the school nurse. Not reporting abuse or suspected abuse places the child in danger.

A is incorrect. Placing a child in "time out" is an appropriate method of discipline. B is incorrect—Asking a child to "behave" is a normal form of parental discipline. D is incorrect—Threatening a child with going to bed does not place the child in physical harm and is an appropriate form of parental discipline.

PHYSIOLOGICAL INTEGRITY

Physiological Adaptation

Radiation Therapy

Implement interventions to address side/adverse effects of radiation therapy

122. A client has experienced mucositis while undergoing radiation therapy. Which nursing action will be best to assist the client's nutritional intake?

A. Offer the client foods with enhanced taste.

B. Offering a commercially prepared mouth rinse.

C. Offer the client bland, soft foods such as puddings, shake.

D. Administer oral antibiotics to the client to swish daily.

The answer is C. The client should avoid spicy or hard foods if mucositis occurs. By offering the client foods that are bland and soft, he or she will be more likely to continue eating and maintain a nutritional intake sufficient for the body's needs.

A is incorrect—Offering foods with enhanced taste is equivalent to offering foods with spices. These foods may irritate or worsen the condition. B is incorrect—Most mouthwashes contain alcohol, which can worsen the mucositis. The client should rinse with water and hydrogen peroxide. D is incorrect—Oral antibiotics will not be beneficial in assisting the client with his or her nutritional intake when mucositis is present.

PHYSIOLOGICAL INTEGRITY

Physiological Adaptation

Hemodynamics

Connect and maintain pacing devices

123. Place an X where the nurse will place the pads for pacing on a client who is in a third-degree heart block with a rate of 38.

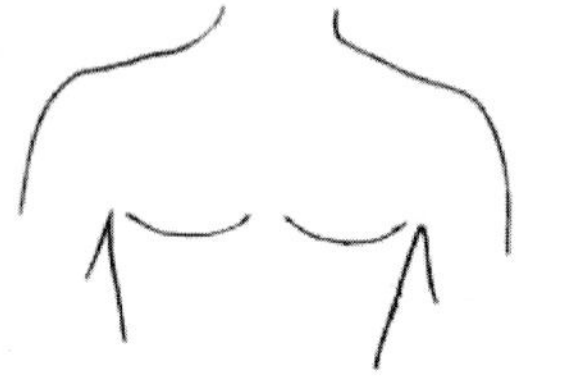

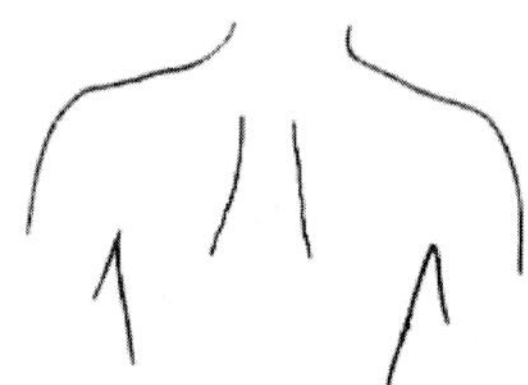

The pads should be placed on the anterior chest wall and the back for external, noninvasive transcutaneous pacing.

PHYSIOLOGICAL INTEGRITY

Reduction of Risk Potential

System-Specific Assessment

Perform focused assessment or reassessment

124. A client is admitted for pneumonia. Which assessment finding is most indicative of a potential complication?

A. Skin that appears dry

B. Clear sputum

C. Asymmetric fremitus

D. Bronchiovesicular breath sounds

The answer is C. Asymmetric fremitus is a significant finding. Fremitus is the vibration felt upon palpation in pneumonia. If this is asymmetrical, it means that the side with fremitus may have a tumor or the side without fremitus may be indicative of a pneumothorax. Decreased fremitus occurs when there is excess air in the lung space.

A is incorrect—Skin can appear dry and still be considered normal. B is incorrect—Clear sputum is a normal finding. D is incorrect—Bronchiovesicular breath sounds are the normal sounds heard upon auscultation of the lung fields.

HEALTH PROMOTION AND MAINTENANCE

Immunizations

Identify precautions and contraindications to immunizations

125. The MMR (measles, mumps, rubella) vaccine should be held if the client has a history of

A. anaphylactic reaction to eggs.
B. HIV.
C. rotavirus.
D. tuberculosis.

The answer is A. A client with a history of an anaphylactic reaction to eggs should not receive the MMR vaccine.

B is incorrect—A history of HIV is not a contraindication to the MMR vaccine. C is incorrect—The rotavirus is not a contraindication to receiving the MMR vaccine. D is incorrect—A client with tuberculosis or a positive PPD skin test can still receive the MMR vaccine.

HEALTH PROMOTION AND MAINTENANCE

Disease Prevention

Inform client/family/significant others of actions to maintain health and prevent disease

126. While preparing a client for discharge, which of the following should be included in the discharge instructions for a client who received stents during a heart catheterization?
A. Eat foods high in fat
B. Exercise daily
C. Limit fruits and vegetables
D. Increase intake of garlic

The answer is B. A client with new stents should exercise daily to maintain proper blood flow and improve overall health.

A is incorrect—Eating foods high in fat should be avoided after stent placement to prevent occlusion due to plague accumulation. C is incorrect—A client who has undergone stents needs a diet of fruits and vegetables for heart health. D is incorrect—Garlic should be avoided and may interact with postprocedure prescription medications administered at home.

SAFE AND EFFECTIVE CARE ENVIRONMENT

Management of Care

Case Management

Plan individualized care for client based on need

127. A client is being discharged from the hospital after experiencing a myocardial infarction. The client desires to have home health care scheduled to make biweekly visits. Which finding in the discharge needs assessment indicates that home health care will not be beneficial?
A. The client does not have a home telephone.
B. The client does not have a wheelchair ramp to get into the home.
C. The client is unable to drive.
D. The client does not have family in town to check on him daily.

The answer is A. If the client does not have a home telephone, he or she will not have the ability to call 911 for an emergency or a method for the home health care agency to contact the client, which is a requirement for admission into home health care services.

B is incorrect—The question does not state that there is a need for a wheelchair ramp. C is incorrect—In order for a client to receive home health care, he or she is considered homebound and the inability to drive is irrelevant. D is incorrect—Not having family in town does not indicate that home health care will not be beneficial.

SAFE AND EFFECTIVE CARE ENVIRONMENT

Management of Care

Consultation

Initiate consultations

128. Which of the following clients would benefit from the social services department consultation for help with prescription medications? (Check all that apply.)
___ A disabled veteran who uses the veterans' hospital facilities.
___ A homeless client with HIV.
___ A elderly client who has Medicare.
___ A child who does not have health insurance.
___ A client who is employed but is without health insurance.
___ A teenager who is currently enrolled on his parents' health insurance.

The homeless client, the child, and the client who is employed all are without health insurance and would benefit from social services for assistance with payment for prescription medications. These clients are the best choice for the answer since they are without any governmental or private assistance.

The veterans' hospital will assist the client who is a veteran, Medicare has prescription cards that are dependent upon the need of the client, and the teenager who is on his parent's health insurance will have coverage for medications.

SAFE AND EFFECTIVE CARE ENVIRONMENT

Safety and Infection Control

Ergonomic Principles

Review necessary modifications with client to reduce stress on specific muscle or skeletal groups

129. An elderly client is going home after hip replacement surgery. Which discharge instructions are most appropriate for this client?
   - A. Turn kneecap toward body while standing still to maintain balance.
   - B. Avoid crossing legs while sitting in a chair.
   - C. Keep the operative leg behind you when bending.
   - D. Use a long handled grabber to reach.
   - E. Avoid using an elevated toilet seat.
   - F. Keep a pillow between legs while sleeping.

The answers are B, C, D, and F. These activities will allow the client to avoid flexion greater than 90 degrees, adduction of the hip and internal rotation of the hip, which can cause the prosthesis to become dislocated.

A and E are incorrect answers—The client should not cause adduction by placing the kneecap inward toward the operative side to maintain balance. If balance is in question, an alternative assistive device should be used. Avoiding an elevated toilet seat is incorrect since it is recommended that clients use an elevated toilet seat to ease with standing and help to avoid dislocation of the prosthesis while standing and sitting.

PHYSIOLOGICAL INTEGRITY

Basic Care and Comfort

Nonpharmacological Comfort Interventions

Provide therapies for comfort and treatment of inflammation and swelling

130. A client has undergone repair of a fractured femur. Which nonpharmacological therapy is best for reducing swelling?
   - A. Application of heat.
   - B. Application of compression bandages.
   - C. Elevation of affected leg.
   - D. Acupuncture therapy.

The answer is C. Elevation of the leg will decrease swelling and subsequent pain in the leg.

A is incorrect—Heat is used to reduce muscle spasms and not for the reduction of swelling. Ice is used for the reduction of swelling. B is incorrect—Compression bandages are used to prevent deep vein thrombosis and do not provide relief from swelling. D is incorrect—Acupuncture therapy is an alternative therapy for pain relief but does not aid in the reduction of swelling.

PHYSIOLOGICAL INTEGRITY

Pharmacological and Parenteral Therapies

Adverse Effects/Contraindications and Side Effects

Identify symptoms/evidence of an allergic reaction

131. A client has an order for an intravenous injection of sodium ferric gluconate complex (Ferrlecit). Which nursing action would be best in monitoring for allergic reaction to the medication?
   - A. Administer the dose in twice the recommended time frame.
   - B. Perform an iron reaction scan prior to administration.
   - C. Administer 10 gtts/min for a 10 minute test dose.
   - D. Assess the client for allergy to eggs and wheat.

The answer is C. A test dose of 10 drops/minute for 10 minutes is best to monitor for allergic reaction to the iron-containing product.

A is incorrect—Administering a dose faster than the recommended time frame is not safe nursing practice and can lead to undesired effects. B is incorrect—There is no such scan as an iron reaction scan. D is incorrect—While a client taking iron supplements should avoid using eggs or whole grain breads an hour after the administration of iron-containing medications, there is no evidence of a correlation between these items and reactions to iron medications.

SAFE AND EFFECTIVE CARE ENVIRONMENT

Management of Care

Establishing Priorities

Assess/triage client(s) to prioritize the order of care delivery

132. Which client should be assessed first upon receiving report?
   - A. A 70-year-old postop client with hip replacement who has a new onset of A-fib.
   - B. A 54-year-old client admitted 2 hours ago with chest pain, which is relieved by ketorlac (Toradol) while in the ED.
   - C. A 69-year-old client scheduled for discharge today after being treated for a pulmonary embolism.
   - D. A 75-year-old client admitted 2 days ago for a myocardial infarction who has been transferred from CCU during the night shift.

The answer is A. The client who has a rhythm change is a priority to assess for symptoms associated with atrial fibrillation, such as shortness of breath and/or chest pain. This client is already at a high risk for thrombosis due to the nature of the surgical procedure.

B is incorrect—A client whose pain was relieved by an antiinflammatory is lower priority than option A. C is incorrect—A client who is scheduled to be discharged receives the last assessment of all four. This client is considered stable if discharge was ordered by the physician. D is incorrect—A client who is transferred from CCU is considered stable and requires assessment after the client described in option A.

HEALTH PROMOTION AND MAINTENANCE

Growth and Development

Compare client psychosocial/behavioral/physical development to norm for age/developmental stage of client

133. Which of the following is an abnormal finding in the growth and development assessment of a 6-month-old client?
    A. Imitates sounds
    B. Bears weight on hands while prone
    C. Holds bottle
    D. Pulls self to standing position

The answer is D. A child does not pull self to standing position until the ninth month. A 6-month-old child will bear most of weight if held in standing position by an adult.

A is incorrect—A 6-month-old child will babble sounds such as ma and hi. B is incorrect—A child of this age can bear weight on hands while prone and will lift chest and upper abdomen. C is incorrect—A child of this age can hold a bottle without assistance.

PSYCHOSOCIAL INTEGRITY

Behavioral Interventions

Orient client to reality

134. A client presents to the emergency department stating that he is an FBI agent and is there to secure the building. Which technique will be best in caring for this client?
    A. Following with the story and allow the client to continue with the delusion.
    B. Medicate the client till sedation occurs.
    C. Tell the client that he is in a hospital and he does not work for the FBI.
    D. Ask the client if he has used drugs in the last 24 hours.

The answer is C. The client needs to be oriented to reality to begin the process of treating the delusion.

A is incorrect—The nurse should not follow with the story, this only feeds the delusion and does not allow for interventions to begin. B is incorrect—The client does not need sedation until an assessment can be performed to see if the client is a danger to self or others and what other manifestations are associated with the current delusion. D is incorrect—The client is delusional and will not be able to tell the nurse what occurred in the last 24 hours.

Psychosocial Integrity

Situational Role Changes

Evaluate whether client/family/significant others have successfully adapted to situational role changes

135. Which statement made by a client's wife indicates that she has not accepted her husband's acute condition?
    A. "I will call a gardener to take over the yard until my husband recovers."
    B. "I know my husband will recover faster than expected and be ready to go back to work."
    C. "I will look into how we can modify our schedule so someone can always be by his side in the hospital."
    D. "I have planned on having someone at home to help me when we are discharged."

The answer is B. The wife has not accepted her husband's illness and the change in her role in the family as the support person and the caregiver.

A is incorrect—The wife realizes her husband is ill and will not be able to continue strenuous labor at the home. C is incorrect—The wife understands her role change as the caregiver and is ready to change as needed. D is incorrect—The wife understands her husband's illness and the need to gather support personnel to assist where needed.

PSYCHOSOCIAL INTEGRITY

Therapeutic Environment

Make client room assignments that promote the therapeutic milieu

136. When planning to provide a therapeutic environment for a client, the appropriate room assignment for a client who has recently been diagnosed with breast cancer is
    A. a room with a client who has renal cell carcinoma.
    B. a room with a client who has bone cancer.
    C. a room with a client who recently underwent a mastectomy.
    D. a room with a client who is scheduled for a lobectomy.

The answer is C. The client who has been diagnosed with breast cancer will be able to relate to the client who has undergone a mastectomy providing for a therapeutic environment.

A is incorrect—The client who has renal cell carcinoma is not a therapeutic choice for the client since the cancers differ and the treatments will differ as well. B is incorrect—The client with bone cancer is in chronic pain; therefore, sharing a room with a client is not a therapeutic environment for either. D is incorrect—A client who is undergoing a lobectomy is not a therapeutic choice for the client who has breast cancer due to the difference in the type of cancer and the treatments.

PHYSIOLOGICAL INTEGRITY

Pharmacological and Parenteral Therapies

Medication Administration

Administer and document medications given by common routes

137. Which of the following forms of insulin can be given intravenously?
   A. Novolin 70/30
   B. Novalog
   C. Lantus
   D. Novolin-R

The answer is D. Regular insulin is a short-acting insulin and is the only insulin approved to be given intravenously.

A is incorrect—Novolin 70/30 is a combination of 70% NPH and 30% regular insulin and therefore contains a short and intermediate acting form of insulin and is only approved to be administered subcutaneously. B is incorrect—Novalog is a rapid-acting insulin and is only administered subcutaneously. C is incorrect—Lantus is a long-acting insulin and is not approved to be given intravenously, only subcutaneously.

PHYSIOLOGICAL INTEGRITY

Reduction of Risk Potential

Laboratory Values

Know laboratory values for ABGs, BUN, cholesterol, glucose, hematocrit, hemoglobin, hemoglobin A1C, platelets, potassium, RBC, sodium, urine-specific gravity, and WBC

138. The respiratory therapist draws ABGs and shows them to the nurse. Which state is the client currently in based on the values:
   - pH: 7.39
   - CO_2: 40
   - HCO_3: 23
   - PaO_2: 90

   A. Metabolic acidosis
   B. Respiratory acidosis
   C. Respiratory alkalosis
   D. Homeostasis

The answer is D. The client's values are within normal limits and the client has compensated and is a state of homeostasis.

A is incorrect—For a client to be in a state of metabolic acidosis the pH less than 7.35 and the HCO_3 less than 22. B is incorrect—The client would need a pH less than 7.34 and a CO_2 greater than 45 to be in a state of respiratory acidosis. C is incorrect—The client would need a pH greater than 7.45 and CO_2 less than 45.

PHYSIOLOGICAL INTEGRITY

Reduction of Risk Potential

Potential for Complications of Diagnostic Tests/Treatments/Procedures

Intervene to manage potential circulatory complications

139. A client is found lying on the floor after a fall out of the bed. On assessment, the left foot appears shorter than the right and externally rotated. Palpation of the affected leg reveals a cold extremity with no palpable pulse at the doralis pedis or the posterior tibial. What is the priority nursing action?
   A. Palpate for a popiteal pulse
   B. Call the physician
   C. Try to realign the injured leg
   D. Elevate the injured leg and reassess

The answer is B. When an injury has caused disruption of the neurovascular system to the point that pulses are lost, the physician must be notified immediately so that action can be taken to prevent the tissue in the affected extremity from becoming necrotic.

A is incorrect—Palpating for a popiteal pulse would show whether the injury was severe enough to cause vascular compromise. Regardless if a pulse is present or not at the popiteal site, the area distal is without adequate blood supply and the physician needs to be notified immediately. C is incorrect—An injured leg should not be realigned by the nurse to prevent further injury. D is incorrect—The leg should not be elevated to prevent further injury to the vascular system.

PHYSIOLOGICAL INTEGRITY

Physiological Adaptation

Alterations in Body Systems

Monitor and maintain the client on a ventilator

140. A client is placed on the ventilator and has positive end-expiratory pressure (PEEP) added. Which assessment data will be most indicative of a potential complication?
   A. Tachycardia
   B. Wheezes

C. Hypotension
D. Hypertension

The answer is C. Hypotension is a sign of a complication. Hypotension can be related to a decreased venous return or a pneumothorax. Assessments should follow that determine the cause of hypotension.

A is incorrect—Tachycardia is due to the body's response to the illness and is not necessarily indicative of a complication. B is incorrect—Wheezing is due to bronchial constriction and is common with intubation. D is incorrect—Hypertension is due to the physiological response to the stress the client is under.

PHYSIOLOGICAL INTEGRITY

Physiological Adaptation

Fluid and Electrolytes

Implement interventions to restore client fluid and/or electrolyte balance

141. A client has a sodium level of 153. The nurse consults the physician and is given orders for dietary restrictions. The nurse should instruct the client to avoid which foods?
A. Cheese
B. Squash
C. Tomatoes
D. Apples

The answer is A. Cheese is considered to be high in sodium and should be restricted for the client who has a high sodium level.

B, C, and D are incorrect—These items are fresh foods and are not considered to be high in sodium.

PHYSIOLOGICAL INTEGRITY

Physiological Adaptation

Hemodynamics

Assess the client for decreased cardiac output

142. A client with congestive heart failure has been coughing up pink frothy sputum and exhibiting shortness of breath. The client's assessment 1 hour ago revealed:
- BP 80/40
- HR 90
- rhonchi upon auscultation
- oxygen saturation 90%
- normal sinus rhythm

Which assessment finding shows a worsening in the client's condition and a decrease in the client's cardiac output?
A. Premature ventricular contractions
B. HR 99
C. Wheezing upon auscultation
D. Oxygen saturation of 89%

The answer is A. Premature ventricular contractions are a direct result of cardiac muscle hypoxia, which is secondary to the pulmonary edema. PVCs do not allow for the diffusion of gasses to occur across the alveolar capillary membrane. All of this is directly proportional to the decrease in the cardiac output, which has caused blood to back up into the lungs.

B is incorrect—The heart rate change is due to the body trying to compensate for the state of hypoxia that exist by pumping faster in an attempt to supply dying cells with oxygen. C is incorrect—Wheezing does not indicate a worsening in the cardiac output. D is incorrect—The hypoxia is still present and is not the best indicator of a worsening in the client's condition.

PHYSIOLOGICAL INTEGRITY

Physiological Adaptation

Medical Emergencies

Monitor and maintain a client on the ventilator

143. A client on the ventilator becomes agitated and restless. Which action by the nurse is best?
A. Check the cuff pressure on the tube.
B. Remove the ventilator and bag the patient.
C. Assess for breath sounds.
D. Restrain the client to prevent tube dislodgement.

The answer is C. The client should be assessed for breath sounds to see if ventilation is occurring. Agitation is often due to hypoxia and lack of adequate ventilation would be seen with absent breath sounds.

A is incorrect—Checking the cuff pressure will not assist in determining the source of agitation. B is incorrect—Bagging the client will not be beneficial if the tube is not in the lungs. D is incorrect—Restraining the client will prevent tube dislodgement but it is not the best method to determine the cause of the agitation.

PHYSIOLOGICAL INTEGRITY

Physiological Adaptation

Unexpected Response to Therapies

Assess the client for unexpected adverse response to therapy

144. Which of the following are preventable adverse outcomes to the placement of a urinary catheter?
___ Infection
___ Urethral damage

___ Ureter damage
___ necrosis of the meatus
___ Vaginal tearing

A client who has an indwelling urinary catheter may develop infection from nonmaintenance of sterile technique, urethral damage if the balloon is placed in the urethra, and necrosis of the meatus due to shearing of the catheter on the meatus. All these are preventable by appropriate nursing actions such as maintenance of sterile technique and meticulous perineal care, ensuring the balloon is in the bladder before inflation, and applying a lubricant to the meatus to lessen shearing.

Ureter damage should not occur since the tube does go above the structure of the bladder. Vaginal tearing should not occur since the catheter is placed in the bladder and not the vaginal area.

PSYCHOSOCIAL INTEGRITY

Psychopathology

Identify signs and symptoms of impaired cognition

145. An elderly client is brought to the emergency department after being found trying to enter a home. The paramedics state that the client says she is 25 years old and lives in the home. The client is barefoot and has feces- and urine-stained clothes. The first nursing action is to:
    A. provide the client with a change of clothes.
    B. assess the client for bruising/injuries.
    C. reassure the client that she is safe and in a hospital.
    D. ask the client her name and date of birth.

The answer is C. The client should be assured that she is safe and of her location. Then the physical assessment can continue.

A is incorrect—The client can undergo a change of clothes after trust is formed. B is incorrect—The client's physical exam will show any bruising or injuries after the client is assured of her safety. D is incorrect—The client will not give the correct date of birth due to her current confused state.

PHYSIOLOGICAL INTEGRITY

Reduction of Risk Potential

Vital Signs

Evaluate invasive monitoring data

146. A client has a ventriculostomy after suffering a traumatic brain injury. The monitor is measuring the intracranial pressure at 30 mm Hg. Which nursing action is best for this client?
    A. Raise the head of bed to 30 degrees.
    B. Assess the client for peripheral edema.
    C. Dim the lights and place the bed at 15 degrees.
    D. Suction the client.

The answer is C. The client should have minimal stimuli and the bed should not be at a height that will cause increased pressure. This will help to lower the intracranial pressure and prevent it from rising.

A is incorrect—Raising the bed to semi Fowlers will cause the pressure to rise. B is incorrect—The client has increased pressure in the cranial vault. Assessment for peripheral is not a priority action for this situation. D is incorrect—Suctioning the client will increase the pressure, which can lead to ischemia of the brain.

SAFE AND EFFECTIVE CARE ENVIRONMENT

Management of Care

Informed Consent

Identify appropriate person to provide informed consent for client

147. An unidentified client is brought to the emergency department after being found on the side of the road with multiple stab wounds and an obvious head injury. After a series of radiological test, it is found that the client has a lacerated liver, brain injury, and needs immediate surgery. Which of the following would be best in obtaining consent for the surgical procedure?
    A. The client should be placed in state custody and consent obtained from the appropriate personnel.
    B. The physician should consider this implied consent and should follow the hospital policy for the situation.
    C. The nurse should sign consent for the client as the client advocate.
    D. The facility should wait to see if the client wakes up to give consent.

The answer is B. The hospital policy should be followed in this situation. In implied consent, the law recognizes that client in need of life saving measures will be provided with those measures unless documents can be provided that states otherwise. In this situation, the client is unidentified and needs surgery to save his life.

A is incorrect—To place a client in state custody, the state must go through a judge. In this case, there is not enough time for that to occur and this action would place the client's life in jeopardy. C is incorrect—The nurse cannot sign consent for a client. D is incorrect—The client may not wake up to give consent and while waiting on this to occur, the client's condition could decline.

HEALTH PROMOTION AND MAINTENANCE

Health Screening

Perform health history/health and risk assessment

148. When performing the health history of a pediatric client in for a well baby visit, the nurse should determine if which of the following is present?
   ___ Immunizations are up to date
   ___ Smoking in the home
   ___ History of cardiac disorders
   ___ History of Asthma
   ___ Eating habits
   ___ Toileting concerns

The nurse should assess for immunizations, smoking in the home, eating habits, and any toileting concerns to understand if the client is receiving the care needed and if there are concerns that may not be verbalized by the mom without a direct question.

A history of cardiac disorders or asthma should be questioned on a routine visit only if assessment findings indicate a concern.

PHYSIOLOGICAL INTEGRITY

Physiological Adaptation

Medical Emergencies

Perform emergency care procedures

149. A client is found in the room holding his hands to his throat and his lips are turning blue. Which action by the nurse is most appropriate?
   A. Lying the client on the floor and administering abdominal thrust.
   B. Ask the client to cough.
   C. Placing both fists around the abdomen above the umbilicus and administering abdominal thrust.
   D. Attempting a blind finger sweep.

The answer is C. The nurse should perform the Heimlich maneuver. The client is demonstrating the universal sign for choking and is obviously lacking oxygen.

A is incorrect—The client should not be lowered to the floor unless he or she is unconscious. B is incorrect—The client will not be able to cough at this point. D is incorrect—A blind finger sweep is not recommended since it can push the food further into the throat.

PHYSIOLOGICAL INTEGRITY

Pharmacological and Parenteral Therapies

Expected Effects/Outcomes

Notify primary health care provider of side effects, adverse effects, and contraindications of medications and parenteral therapy

150. A client is taking digoxin (Lanoxin) for atrial fibrillation and cardiomegally. Which assessment finding requires the nurse to notify the physician of a potential adverse effect?
   A. Abdominal pain and nausea
   B. Rhythm change to normal sinus rhythm
   C. Heart rate of 62
   D. Weight gain of ½ pound

The answer is A. Abdominal pain and nausea are the first signs of digoxin toxicity in the elderly and should be reported so that the physician can order a digoxin level desired.

B is incorrect—A rhythm change is not an adverse effect. The client continues to need the digoxin to treat the cardiomegally. C is incorrect—The heart rate is within normal limits for the drug to be administered. D is incorrect—A 1/2 pound weight gain is not an adverse effect. Monitoring of I&O should continue.

PHYSIOLOGICAL INTEGRITY

Physiological Adaptation

Illness Management

Interpret client data that needs to be reported immediately

151. Which of the following should be reported to the physician immediately?
   A. Monitor showing a sinus rhythm with a premature ventricular contractions (PVC) occurring every 10th beat.
   B. Sodium level 130 mEq/L.
   C. Potassium level of 5.9 mEq/L.
   D. Oxygen saturation level of 90% on room air.

The answer is C. The nurse should phone the physician to receive orders for treatment of the high potassium level, which can cause cardiac arrhythmias if untreated.

A is incorrect—This is considered sinus rhythm with occasional PVCs and is considered a normal finding. B is incorrect—This sodium level is lower than the normal range of 135–145 mEq/L, but is not low enough to bear reporting to the physician immediately. Lower than 127 mEq/L is considered critical. D is incorrect—The oxygen saturation level should not be reported unless it remains low after oxygen is applied. This finding requires a nursing intervention before phoning the physician.

PHYSIOLOGICAL INTEGRITY

Reduction of Risk Potential

Potential for Complications of Diagnostic Tests/Treatments/Procedures

Assess the client for an abnormal response following a diagnostic test/procedure

152. A client has just undergone a computerized tomography (CT) of the abdomen with oral contrast. Which assessment finding is indicative of an abnormal response to the exam?
    A. Feeling of fullness in the abdomen
    B. Redness of the face, generalized itching
    C. Increase in urination
    D. Nausea, diarrhea

The answer is B. The client who has undergone a CT of abdomen has been exposed to oral contrast. Those who are allergic to oral contrast will experience redness to the face, generalized itching, and other signs of a systemic reaction. This requires intervention by a physician order.

A is incorrect—Feeling of fullness is common after a CT where oral contrast was used. C is incorrect—The client will have an increase in urination following the ingestion of oral contrast for a CT. D is incorrect—The oral contrast contains a laxative and it is common for the client to become nauseated and experience diarrhea until the contrast has been passed through the system.

PHYSIOLOGICAL INTEGRITY

Physiological Adaptation

Unexpected Response to Therapies

Assess the client for unexpected adverse response to therapy

153. After placing a nasogastric tube into the right nare of a client, which assessment finding is indicative of an adverse response to this therapy?
    A. Epistaxis
    B. Vomiting
    C. Feeling of fullness in the throat
    D. Sore throat

The answer is A. Epistaxis is an adverse response to the placement of a nasogastric tube and measures should be implemented to stop the bleeding.

B is incorrect—The nasogastric tube will cause the client to vomit due to the irritation of the gag reflex. C is incorrect—The client will feel fullness in the throat until the body becomes accustomed to the tube. D is incorrect—A sore throat is common after a nasogastric tube is placed due to the irritation during insertion.

PHYSIOLOGICAL INTEGRITY

Physiological Adaptation

Radiation Therapy

Assess the client for signs and symptoms of adverse effects of radiation therapy

154. Which assessment finding requires immediate nursing intervention in a client who is receiving radiation therapy for esophageal cancer?
    A. Alopecia
    B. Skin ulceration
    C. Hearing loss
    D. Difficult swallowing

The answer is D. The nurse should take action regarding the client's difficulty swallowing. If there is damage to the esophagus then subsequent damage to the trachea could be occurring, which will compromise the client's airway.

A is incorrect—Alopecia is the loss of hair and is inevitable for the client undergoing radiation therapy. B is incorrect—Skin ulcerations are common with radiation therapy and require wound care to prevent infection. C is incorrect—Hearing loss is common with radiation to the neck and while precautions can be taken to lessen the effects, damage will likely occur.

PHYSIOLOGICAL INTEGRITY

Physiological Adaptation

Infectious Disease

Evaluate client response to treatment for an infectious disease

155. Which evaluation would indicate a therapeutic response to treatment for tuberculosis?
    A. A negative sputum culture after 3 months of therapy.
    B. Absence of symptoms.
    C. Decrease in cavities on an x-ray.
    D. Completion of medication therapy.

The answer is A. If cultures convert to negative within 3 months of therapy, the treatment is considered a success.

B is incorrect—Symptoms may disappear even if the bacteria are active. C is incorrect—Cavities on the x-ray are not a determinant for a therapeutic response to treatment. D is incorrect—Completion of medicinal therapy is not a therapeutic response to the treatment since the bacteria can still be active.

PHYSIOLOGICAL INTEGRITY

Physiological Adaptation

Hemodynamics

Monitor and maintain arterial lines

156. A nurse is assessing the arterial line via an intra-arterial catheter in a client in the ICU. Which assessment finding is most indicative of a potential complication?
   A. Cool extremities bilaterally
   B. Low blood pressure reading
   C. Capillary refill <2 seconds on affected arm
   D. Low mean arterial pressure

The answer is C. The capillary refill of less than 2 seconds is a sign that a thrombus may have formed and blood flow via the ulnar artery and the microcirculation is compromised.

A is incorrect—Cool extremities bilaterally are not the most indicative finding in a potential complication. B is incorrect—A low blood pressure reading is not a sign of a complication since the arterial line is used for monitoring the client's blood pressure. D is incorrect—A low mean arterial pressure is a direct reflection of the client's blood pressure and does not indicate a complication with the line itself.

PHYSIOLOGICAL INTEGRITY

Physiological Adaptation

Alterations in Body Systems

Provide suctioning via endotracheal or tracheostomy tube

157. Prior to suctioning a client who has an endotracheal tube, the nurse must first:
   A. hyperoxygenate the client.
   B. place saline in the endotracheal tube.
   C. ask the client to cough.
   D. deflate the cuff on the endotracheal tube.

The answer is A. Prior to suctioning a client with an artificial airway such as an endotracheal tube, the nurse must provide adequate oxygen to the client.

B is incorrect—While placing saline down the tube may loosen secretions, it is not what the nurse must first do prior to suctioning the client. C is incorrect—A client with an endotracheal tube should not cough to prevent tube dislodgement. D is incorrect—The endotracheal tube cuff is only deflated when moving of the tube is necessary.

PHYSIOLOGICAL INTEGRITY

Reduction of Risk Potential

Therapeutic Procedures

Monitor effective functioning of therapeutic devices

158. When performing an assessment on a client with a chest tube and an attached drainage system, which assessment finding is indicative of a complication?
   A. Continuous bubbling in the suction chamber.
   B. Yellow fluid accumulating in the drainage chamber.
   C. Suction in the off position.
   D. Vigorous bubbling in the water seal chamber.

The answer is D. Vigorous bubbling in the water seal chamber is indicative of a leak. The nurse must determine where the leak is and fix the problem before the lung is compromised.

A is incorrect—The suction chamber should have continuous bubbling if suction is connected. B is incorrect—Yellow fluid is serous and is normal with a chest tube drainage system. C is incorrect—Suction may or may not be connected to the drainage system depending on the client needs based on the physician's assessment.

SAFE AND EFFECTIVE CARE ENVIRONMENT

Management of Care

Concepts of Management

Supervise care provided by others

159. A member of the nursing team approaches you to complain that an unlicensed assistive personnel is not performing accuchecks on patients as assigned. Which action is most appropriate?
   A. Confront the unlicensed assistive personnel about the neglect in her role.
   B. Ask the nurse why he or she could not perform the accucheck on the patient.
   C. Ask the unlicensed assistive personnel if there is something preventing her from completing her assignment.
   D. Report the unlicensed assistive personnel to the nurse manager of the unit for a verbal reprimand.

The answer is C. Asking the unlicensed assistive personnel if there is something preventing her from completing her assignment gives the individual an opportunity to verbalize what is occurring that has delayed client care and follows the chain of conflict resolution.

A is incorrect—Confronting an individual will cause increased tension and does not resolve the conflict. B is incorrect—The licensed personnel is being asked to perform the duty of an unlicensed personnel therefore negating the delegation of duty. D is incorrect—This response does not follow the chain of conflict resolution and does not provide the unlicensed assistive personnel the opportunity to explain her actions.

SAFE AND EFFECTIVE CARE ENVIRONMENT

Management of Care

Delegation

Ensure appropriate education, skills, and experience of personnel performing delegated task

160. Match the appropriate personnel to the task that is within the scope of practice. (Choices may be used more than once.)
    ___ Insert a Foley catheter.
    ___ Perform an admission assessment.
    ___ Perform postprocedure vital signs.
    ___ Administer one unit of packed red blood cells.
    ___ Perform a morning assessment.
    A. Registered Nurse
    B. Licensed Practical Nurse
    C. Unlicensed Nursing Assistant

B *Insert a Foley catheter*: It is within the scope of practice for a LPN to insert an indwelling catheter.

A *Perform an admission assessment*: Only a registered nurse can perform an admission assessment.

C *Perform postprocedure vital signs*: It is within the scope of practice for unlicensed personnel to perform postprocedure vital signs as long as a licensed personnel is reviewing the data obtained and the unlicensed personnel has gone through the verification process in conjunction with the rules of the hospital.

A *Administer one unit of packed red blood cells*: Only a registered nurse can administer blood products.

B *Perform a morning assessment*: A LPN can perform a morning assessment on a client who has undergone an assessment by a RN upon admission to the area.

SAFE AND EFFECTIVE CARE ENVIRONMENT

Management of Care

Performance Improvement (Quality Improvement)

Define performance improvement/assurance activities

161. Which of the following is an example of quality assurance that meets the standards of JCAHO?
    A. Gathering a second opinion before administering as needed pain medications.
    B. Use of clinical pathways by all health care team members.
    C. Avoid admitting clients that have chronic conditions.
    D. Performing tests that are covered by insurance and avoiding those that are not.

The answer is B. The use of clinical pathways has replaced nursing care plans. Clinical pathways enable the staff to monitor for a progression of prescribed client care among all health care disciplines, which is a component of quality assurance.

A is incorrect—A client should receive pain medication based on his or her rating on the pain scale. Gathering a second opinion before medication is administered delays care and is not cost-effective and does not meet the standards. C is incorrect—Clients with chronic conditions may need to be admitted making this not an effective method of quality assurance. D is incorrect—Avoiding tests that are not covered by insurance may lessen overall cost, but is not meeting the standards of care a client deserves.

SAFE AND EFFECTIVE CARE ENVIRONMENT

Safety and Infection Control

Accident Prevention

Identify deficits that may impede client safety

162. Which finding in an admission assessment is most indicative of a potential falls risk?
    A. Hearing deficit
    B. Numbness in the left foot
    C. Confusion
    D. Unsteady gait

The answer is D. A client with an unsteady gait is at the highest risk for a fall due to an inability to correct a potential fall or brace during a fall.

A is incorrect—A loss of hearing is not the highest risk. A client who cannot hear can still maintain a steady gait while ambulating in a room. B is incorrect—Numbness in one foot does not place the client at the highest risk for falls risk, often a client will compensate with the normal extremity. C is incorrect—A confused client can possess a steady gait therefore not placing this client at the highest risk.

SAFE AND EFFECTIVE CARE ENVIRONMENT

Safety and Infection Control

Injury Prevention

Question prescriptions for treatments that may contribute to an accident or injury

163. Which discharge prescription should be questioned for a client who has peripheral neuropathy due to diabetes?

A. A prescription for shoes to be purchased at a health care supply store.
B. A prescription to follow up with diabetic services for routine foot care.
C. A prescription for a heating pad to be used on the lower extremities twice a day.
D. A prescription for TED hose to be used on the lower extremities unless bathing.

The answer is C. An order for a heating pad should be questioned because a client with diabetic neuropathy should not use a heating pad since he or she will be unable to feel if burning to the skin is occurring. A is incorrect—A prescription for shoes at a health care supply store is appropriate for the diabetic client. B is incorrect—The client with peripheral neuropathy due to diabetes should follow up with diabetic services for routine foot care such as nail cutting and inspections for ulcerations. D is incorrect—TED hose are useful to prevent deep vein thrombosis and swelling that may occur with peripheral neuropathy and diabetes.

SAFE AND EFFECTIVE CARE ENVIRONMENT

Safety and Infection Control

Use of Restraints/Safety Devices

Monitor client responses to restraints

164. Which assessment is priority for a client who is being placed in restraints due to confusion and agitation?
A. Toiletry needs
B. Hydrations needs
C. Circulation in restrained extremities
D. Client's knowledge of restraint purpose

The answer is C. Monitoring the extremities for adequate circulation is most important to prevent damage to underlying structures. Assessments of the area where the restraint is placed should be performed every 2 hours or per hospital policy.

A is incorrect—Toiletry needs are important while a client is in restraints but this is not the priority assessment. B is incorrect—Hydration needs are assessed every 2 hours but this is not the priority. D is incorrect—A client who is confused and agitated will not understand why he or she is being restrained.

HEALTH PROMOTION AND MAINTENANCE

Family Planning

Assess client need/desire for contraception

165. Which statement made by a client indicates a need for counseling regarding contraceptive devices?
A. "I plan on abstaining from sex until I am married."
B. "My boyfriend and I use condoms for protection."
C. "I have been having sex, but my boyfriend pulls out."
D. "It is against my religion to use birth control."

The answer is C. The client is using the withdrawal method, which is has a high failure rate. The client needs information regarding contraceptive devices to prevent pregnancy.

A is incorrect—The client does not have a plan to participate in sexual activity. The client should be reminded to contact her health care provider if her intentions change. B is incorrect—The client currently has a form of contraception in use. D is incorrect—The client is citing a religious restriction on the use of birth control; therefore, counseling is not needed.

HEALTH PROMOTION AND MAINTENANCE

High-Risk Behaviors

Assist client/family/significant others to identify behaviors/risks that may impact health

166. A client is being discharged after an admission for a sodium of 127 and recent weight loss. The family voices a concern that the client may be suffering from anorexia. At the time of discharge, the family will be instructed to monitor the client for which sign of the disorder?
A. Increase in menstrual cycles per month.
B. Pushing food around plate without taking bites.
C. Lack of desire to exercise.
D. Heat intolerance.

The answer is B. The client with anorexia nervosa will push food around on the plate and put bites of food to the face without eating the bite.

A is incorrect—A client with anorexia nervosa will experience amenorrhea due to loss of weight. C is incorrect—In anorexia nervosa, a client will exercise excessively and may not attend events/school to exercise. D is incorrect—With anorexia nervosa the client is intolerant of cold.

HEALTH PROMOTION AND MAINTENANCE

Techniques of Physical Assessment

Choose physical assessment equipment and technique appropriate for the client

167. Which equipment will be most important when performing the physical assessment of a client with a deep vein thrombosis (DVT) of the left leg?
A. Tape measure
B. Doppler

C. Tongue depressor

D. Penlight

The answer is B. When a client has a DVT, a Doppler is needed to assess for pulses in the affected extremity to ensure blood flow is occurring in the extremity at one of two pedal pulse areas.

A is incorrect—A tape measure is used to document the size of the leg compared to the unaffected leg, but it is not as important as the Doppler, which will assess for adequate blood flow to the affected foot. C is incorrect—A tongue depressor is not needed when assessing the client who has a DVT. D is incorrect—A penlight is needed to assess papillary response when performing a physical assessment, but is not the most important piece of equipment for this client.

PSYCHOSOCIAL INTEGRITY

Cultural Diversity

Incorporate client cultural practice and beliefs when planning and providing care

168. A client of Asian descent has been admitted to the surgical floor. Which of the following should the nurse consider when building the client care map for pain management?
   A. Consult an acupuncturist.
   B. Offer a narcotic every 4 hours.
   C. Offer daily medications only in the morning.
   D. Have a rabbi visit the client daily for prayer.

The answer is A. The Asian American culture uses acupuncture as a form of oriental medicine, which is based on an energy system that when used balances the yin and yang and promotes balance in the life and thus pain relief.

B is incorrect—This Asian American culture uses narcotics as a last form of pain relief, and the primary form of pain relief is acupuncture and herbs. C is incorrect—The Asian American culture does not have a preference on when medications are offered making this a nonjustified choice. D is incorrect—The Asian American culture uses a temple healer for religious needs and this is not a significant choice for care mapping of pain management.

PSYCHOSOCIAL INTEGRITY

Religious and Spiritual Influences on Health

Assess and plan interventions that meet client emotional and spiritual needs

169. A client who practises Catholicism will be undergoing a hip repair. Which nursing plan will be best to prevent tension between the patient and nurse and meet hospital policies and procedures?
   A. Allow the client to wear his medicine bundle into the operating room.
   B. Remove the client's traditional headpiece before leaving for the operating room.
   C. Inform the client that you will take his rosary and give it to his wife.
   D. Inform the client that all spiritual pieces need to be surrendered to security until after surgery.

The answer is C. The nurse should take the client's rosary and allow a trusted family member to hold it while he is in surgery. A rosary is sacred to the catholic religion and the nurse must treat is respectfully.

A is incorrect—Medicine bundles are worn by Native Americans. B is incorrect—Traditional headpieces are worn by Islamic Muslim women and they are not to be removed in public leaving the patient to remove it once in the holding room and giving it to a family member. D is incorrect—Spiritual pieces are not surrendered to security unless the client requests.

PHYSIOLOGICAL INTEGRITY

Basic Care and Comfort

Elimination

Insert/remove nasogastric, urethral catheter, or other tubes

170. A nurse is inserting a nasogastric tube when resistance is met. The nurse should:
   A. continue to push the tube into the nose.
   B. ask the client to swallow.
   C. pull out the tube and try the other side.
   D. check for correct placement with 30 cc of air.

The answer is C. If resistance is met during the insertion of a nasogastric tube, the nurse should remove the tube and try the other nostril to prevent damage to the nasal mucosa and internal structures.

A is incorrect—The nurse should avoid continuing to push the tube into the nose to prevent injury. B is incorrect—Asking the client to swallow will not prevent injury to the client. D is incorrect—The tube has met resistance and when it is inserted in the stomach, this does not occur; therefore, checking for placement is invalid.

PHYSIOLOGICAL INTEGRITY

Basic Care and Comfort

Nutrition and Oral Hydration

Assess client's ability to eat

171. A client has returned from having a procedure that required conscious sedation. Prior to offering food the nurse should:
   A. assess for the return of the gag reflex.
   B. administer morning medications missed due to NPO status.
   C. order a warm tray for the client.

D. view the chart to see the time the last dose of a medication was given for sedation.

The answer is A. Prior to offering food, the client should be evaluated to see if the gag reflex has returned. Without a gag reflex, the client should not eat due to the potential for aspiration.

B is incorrect—The client may need to eat before being offered meds. The client must also have an intact gag reflex before meds can be offered. C is incorrect—The client will need a warm tray but only after the client has been assessed to see if eating can occur without the risk of aspiration. D is incorrect—Regardless of the last dose of medication, the nurse is responsible for assessing to see if the gag reflex is intact before offering food.

PHYSIOLOGICAL INTEGRITY

Basic Care and Comfort

Rest and Sleep

Schedule client care activities to promote adequate rest

172. A burn client is recovering and needs periods of rest to aid in healing. Which plan would be best to promote rest periods for the client?
   A. Group activities such as physical assessment, bath, linen change, and morning meds together.
   B. Administer a sleeping aid every night from the "as needed" medication list.
   C. Schedule the client to go to occupational therapy and physical therapy consecutively.
   D. Place a sign on the door to limit visitors.

The answer is A. The best method for promoting rest is to group client care so that there are periods of time for the client to rest without interruption.

B is incorrect—The client may not need a sleeping aid at night when activities can be altered to assist with rest during the day. C is incorrect—Sending the client to both areas for therapy consecutively will place the client at a disadvantage. A client who has experienced a burn will need to rest between sessions due to an increased use of energy for healing. The client will not benefit from therapy sessions if he or she is too tired to participate. D is incorrect—Placing a sign on the door will help to warn visitors that the client is resting but it is not the best method of promoting rest.

PHYSIOLOGICAL INTEGRITY

Pharmacological and Parenteral Therapies

Blood and Blood Products

Administer blood products and evaluate client responses

173. A client who is experiencing an acute hemolytic transfusion reaction will exhibit what symptom?
   A. Hypertension
   B. Back pain
   C. Bradycardia
   D. Hyperglycemia

The answer is B. The symptoms of an acute hemolytic transfusion reaction are due to the breakdown of the red cell antibodies and cell destruction, which manifest as pain and an increase in body temperature.

A is incorrect—Hypotension occurs with an acute hemolytic transfusion reaction. C is incorrect—Tachycardia is common with an acute hemolytic transfusion reaction due to the body's response to the stress, increase in temperature, and hypotension. D is incorrect—Hyperglycemia does not occur in a hemolytic reaction.

PHYSIOLOGICAL INTEGRITY

Pharmacological and Parenteral Therapies

Pharmacological Agents/Actions

Identify a contraindication to the administration of a prescribed or over-the-counter medication to a client

174. During an admission assessment a client states an allergy to Motrin. Which drug order should be questioned?
   A. ketorlac (Toradol) 60 mg IM every 8 hours × 2 doses for pain.
   B. Tylenol 650 mg p.o. every 4 hours as need for pain.
   C. Morphine 2–4 mg IV every 4 hours as needed for pain.
   D. orphenadrine (Norflex) 100 mg p.o. BID prn pain.

The answer is A. Toradol is an antiinflammatory and is in the same classification as Motrin. A cross sensitivity may exist so it is best to avoid using Toradol for client's with an allergy.

B is incorrect—Tylenol is a non-opioid analgesic and Motrin is a nonsteroidal antiinflammatory. There is no evidence of cross sensitivity leaving this to be a safe drug for mild pain relief. C is incorrect—Morpine is an opioid analgesic and does not fall into the same category as Motrin. D is incorrect—Norflex is a muscle relaxant and is not contraindicated in the client with an allergy to Motrin.

PHYSIOLOGICAL INTEGRITY

Physiological Adaptation

Alterations in Body Systems

Provide wound care

175. A nurse caring for a client with a burn has an order to apply a silver sulfadiazine (Silvadene) dressing to the area. Which plan would be best to prevent infection of the wound during cleaning?
   A. Avoid applying Silvadene to areas that are not burned.
   B. Cleaning the area with Betadine.
   C. Using an irrigation system for cleaning.
   D. Wearing a mask, gown, and sterile gloves during care.

The answer is D. The nurse's goal for wound care is to prevent infection and promote revitalization of the tissue. The nurse should place a barrier between her and the client to prevent infection.

A is incorrect—Applying Silvadene to areas that are not burned will cause redness to the surrounding skin. B is incorrect—Betadine is avoided in burns since it can cause damage to the cells and will dry out the tissue. C is incorrect—While an irrigation system is best for removal of debris found in the wound bed, it is not the best plan for preventing infection.

PHYSIOLOGICAL INTEGRITY

Pharmacological and Parenteral Therapies

Expected Effects/Outcomes

Use clinical decision making/critical thinking when addressing expected effects/outcomes of medications

176. A client is complaining of tightness in her throat and arm pain. The nurse assesses the client and administers nitroglycerine 0.4 mg sublingual. After 4 minutes, the client claims no relief was felt. The nurse should:
    A. administer another dose and reassess in 5 minutes.
    B. check the client's blood pressure.
    C. administer Maalox from the "as needed" order list.
    D. notify the physician.

The answer is B. The client has no relief from the initial dose of nitroglycerine but with its potent vasodilatation, the nurse should assess the client's blood pressure before administering the second dose. If hypotension exist, the next dose should be held and other actions taken.

A is incorrect—The client's blood pressure should be assessed after every dose of nitroglycerine to assess for hypotension. C is incorrect—The nurse could attempt the use of Maalox to see if relief occurs but the blood pressure should be assessed prior to the administration of any other medications. D is incorrect—The physician should be notified after the nurse exhausts the protocol.

PHYSIOLOGICAL INTEGRITY

Physiological Adaptation

Medical Emergencies

Evaluate and document client response to emergency interventions

177. A client in respiratory distress is intubated by the physician. Which evaluation by the nurse best indicates the intubation was successful?
    A. Decrease in anxiety
    B. Lowering of blood pressure
    C. Increase in heart rate
    D. Bilateral breath sounds

The answer is D. Bilateral breath sounds are the best indicator of a successful intubation.

A is incorrect—While anxiety is an indicator of hypoxia, the resolution of anxiety is not the best indicator of a successful intubation. B is incorrect—Lowering of a client's blood pressure is not an indicator of a successful intubation. C is incorrect—An increase in the heart rate is not an indicator of a successful intubation.

PHYSIOLOGICAL INTEGRITY

Reduction of Risk Potential

Diagnostic Tests

Perform an electrocardiogram test

178. Place a client in lead II using a 5-lead monitor.

    An "X" should be placed at:

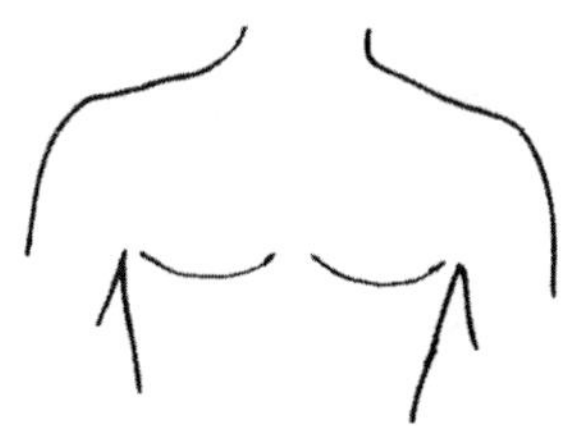

RA (white lead) is placed below the right clavicle where the arm and torso meet. The LA is placed below the left clavicle where the arm and torso meet. The LL is red and is placed on lower abdomen where the leg and torso meet. The RL is placed at the lower right abdomen and the C lead is placed at the fourth intercostal space, right sternal border.

PHYSIOLOGICAL INTEGRITY

Reduction of Risk Potential

Potential for Complications of Diagnostic Tests/Treatments/Procedures

Monitor client for signs of bleeding

179. A client has recently undergone a cardiac catheterization. Which assessment is the best to monitor for post-procedure bleeding?
    A. Assessing the insertion site.
    B. Assessing the area directly posterior to the insertion site.
    C. Assessment of vital signs.
    D. Assessment of neurological status.

The answer is A. Assessment of the insertion site is best when monitoring for postoperative bleeding. This site will be the first source of clot dislodgement and hemorrhage.

B is incorrect—The area posterior to the insertion site is secondary on the areas to assess for bleeding. This is usually noted if vital signs change. C is incorrect—Although vital signs are an appropriate assessment for the procedure that was performed, the first area to be assessed is the insertion site. D is incorrect—The neurological status will not be the best assessment for postprocedure bleeding.

PHYSIOLOGICAL INTEGRITY

Reduction of Risk Potential

Vital Signs

Apply knowledge needed to perform related nursing procedures and psychomotor skills when assessing vital signs

180. A nurse takes the blood pressure with an electronic blood pressure machine and receives a reading of 80/54. A review of the chart indicates this is uncharacteristic of the client's usual reading. The nurse should perform which action next?
    A. Retake the blood pressure using the electronic machine.
    B. Auscultate the blood pressure using a manual cuff.
    C. Phone the physician for orders.
    D. Leave the client and reassess in 30 minutes.

The answer is B. The nurse should assess the blood pressure using a manual cuff and stethoscope prior to taking any further action.

A is incorrect—The machine could be reading inappropriately. The nurse should perform option B. C is incorrect—The physician should not be notified until a manual pressure is taken. D is incorrect—The client should not be left for 30 minutes.

PHYSIOLOGICAL INTEGRITY

Physiological Adaptation

Fluid and Electrolytes

Apply knowledge of pathophysiology when caring for client with fluid and electrolyte imbalances

181. A nurse is assigned to four clients. Which client is at an increased risk for developing fluid volume deficit?
    A. A client who is in renal failure.
    B. A client receiving normal saline at 125 mL/h.
    C. A client who has an NG tube to low continuous suction.
    D. A client who has diarrhea related to *Clostridium difficile*.

The answer is D. The client with *Clostridium difficile* is at an increased risk for fluid volume deficit due to the loss of fluid via the GI tract.

A is incorrect—The client in renal failure is at an increased risk of fluid volume excess. B is incorrect—The client receiving normal saline is at a risk for fluid volume excess. C is incorrect—A client with an NG tube to low suction is not at as high a risk as the client with diarrhea.

PHYSIOLOGICAL INTEGRITY

Physiological Adaptation

Illness Management

Perform gastric lavage

182. A nurse has an order to perform a gastric lavage on a client who has overdosed on Tylenol. After the lavage tube is inserted in the nose, the nurse should:
    A. place tap water in the stomach and begin pulling out gastric contents.
    B. verify placement of the tube in the stomach using 60 cc of air.
    C. tape to tube in place.
    D. verify placement of the tube in the stomach using 30 cc of normal saline.

The answer is B. Prior to instilling anything in the stomach of a client who is undergoing gastric lavage, the nurse must make sure the tube is in the correct place by auscultation for air.

A is incorrect—While tap water can be used for lavage where the tap water will be pulled from the stomach, the nurse must assure the tube is in the stomach prior to performing the lavage. C is incorrect—The tube should not be taped in place until placement is verified. D is incorrect—Verification of the placement should be performed using air and not normal saline.

PHYSIOLOGICAL INTEGRITY

Physiological Adaptation

Fluid and Electrolyte Imbalances

Apply knowledge of pathophysiology when caring for client with fluid and electrolyte imbalances

183. A client is in a state of respiratory acidosis. The nurse understands that which of the following is a potential cause of the current acidotic state?
    A. Morphine (M.S. Contin)
    B. Vomiting
    C. Diarrhea
    D. Over the counter antacids

The answer is A. Morphine will place a client in a state of respiratory acidosis by lowering the respiratory drive, which causes the client to retain carbon dioxide.

B is incorrect—Vomiting will place a client in a state of metabolic alkalosis due to the loss of acid through the GI track. C is incorrect—Diarrhea will place the client in a state of metabolic acidosis by removing the bicarbonate from the GI track. D is incorrect—Antacids cause a build up on bicarbonate and will place the client in a state of alkalosis.

HEALTH PROMOTION AND MAINTENANCE

Ante/Intra/Postpartum and Newborn Care

Provide newborn care

184. An 8-pound infant is delivered via vaginal delivery. After the cord is cut and handed to the nurse, the nurse should first assess the baby's:
   A. respiratory effort
   B. Apgar score
   C. vital signs
   D. blood sugar

The answer is A. The respiratory effort should be assessed and assisted as needed.

B is incorrect—The Apgar score is second in the assessment. C is incorrect—Vital signs are assessed after the respiratory effort and Apgar score. D is incorrect—Unless mom was a diabetic, the baby does not require a blood sugar check.

SAFE AND EFFECTIVE CARE ENVIRONMENT

Management of Care

Concepts of Management

Apply principles of conflict resolution as needed when working with health care staff

185. Two staff nurses on the nursing unit disagree on how to involve a client's family in the client's care. Nurse A feels that only the husband needs to be included in the planning of the client's care as he will be the primary care giver when she is discharged home. Nurse B feels that both her husband and her son need to be involved as they are both very close to the client and both will have a role in her care once she is discharged. As the nurse leader you must decide how you will manage the conflict.
   A. Ignore the situation: if it isn't acknowledged it will go away.
   B. Do nothing and allow the two staff nurses to work out a mutually agreed upon decision.
   C. Make a decision for the staff nurses, as it is not appropriate for the client to be in the middle of the conflict.
   D. Sit down with the two staff nurses and allow them to express their points of view, encouraging both to consider the positive and negative aspects of their views.

The answer is D. By sitting with both nurses, each has a chance to consider the other's opinion. This will help the nurses to settle conflicts in the future.

Ignoring the situation and doing nothing will not resolve the problem. Decisions made by the authority will not resolve future problems and may lead to resentment on the nurses' part.

PHYSIOLOGICAL INTEGRITY

Physiological Adaptation

Alterations in Body Systems

Provide postoperative care

186. A client has been brought to the floor by the PACU nurse after having a cholecystectomy. When performing the postop assessment, which finding would be most indicative of a complication?
   A. Nausea, vomiting
   B. Abdominal pain
   C. Shoulder pain
   D. Rigid abdomen

The answer is D. A rigid abdomen is a sign of internal bleeding and requires immediate intervention.

A is incorrect—Nausea and vomiting are common after abdominal surgery and are not a complication. B is incorrect—Pain is common after surgery and is not a complication unless other symptoms of hemorrhage are present. C is incorrect—Shoulder pain is due to the gas that is placed in the abdomen for the surgeon to see the organs inside the abdominal cavity.

PHYSIOLOGICAL INTEGRITY

Reduction of Risk Potential

Potential for Complications of Diagnostic Tests/Treatments/Procedures

Position client to prevent complication following tests/treatments/procedures

187. A client who has undergone a spinal tap should be placed in what position after the procedure?
   A. Prone
   B. Supine
   C. Semi-Fowlers
   D. Side lying

The answer is B. A client who has undergone a spinal tap should be placed in the supine position for 2 hours after the procedure.

A is incorrect—The client should not be placed prone after the procedure to prevent airway compromise. C is incorrect—The client should remain supine. Semi-Fowlers would likely place pressure on the insertion site and cause bleeding. D is incorrect—While the client may be placed in the side-lying position during the procedure, after the procedure the client should be supine. Side-lying carries the possibility of placing pressure onto the insertion site.

PHYSIOLOGICAL INTEGRITY

Physiological Adaptation

Fluid and Electrolytes

Identify signs and symptoms of client fluid and/or electrolyte imbalance

188. A nurse will expect which assessment findings when caring for a client with a potassium level of 2.9?
   A. Irregular pulse
   B. Orthostatic hypertension
   C. Seizures
   D. Deep tendon hyperreflexia

The answer is A. An irregular pulse is found in the client with a low potassium level due to the effects on cardiac muscle activity.

B is incorrect—Hypokalemia will cause orthostatic hypotension not hypertension. C is incorrect—There are alterations in neuromuscular excitability leading to muscle weakness and flaccidness. D is incorrect—Hyporeflexia is common in hypokalemia due to alterations in neuromuscular excitability.

PHYSIOLOGICAL INTEGRITY

Physiological Adaptation

Alterations in Body Systems

Monitor wounds for signs and symptoms of infection

189. A nurse is caring for a surgical wound which is 3 days old. Which assessment data is most indicative of a wound infection?
   A. Increased white blood cell count
   B. Separated wound edges
   C. Purulent drainage
   D. Edema at the site

The answer is C. Purulent drainage is an indication of a wound infection due to the body's response to the bacteria that has invaded the wound.

A is incorrect—While an elevated white blood cell count is indicative of the activation of the body's immune response system, it does not mean the source of infection is the wound itself. B is incorrect—Wound edges may separate without infection being present. A client can strain and dislodge sutures or sutures can be dislodged if enough stress is placed on the operative area. D is incorrect—Edema is expected initially due to the body's response to invasion of skin integrity.

PSYCHOSOCIAL INTEGRITY

Abuse/Neglect

Provide a safe environment for an abused/neglected client

190. A client presents to the emergency department after her husband physically assaulted her during a fight. She states she feels as though he will come to the hospital to find her and she does not want to see him. Which nursing intervention will be best to protect this client from her husband?
   A. Notify security
   B. Place the client as "confidential"
   C. Notify the police department of the assault
   D. Place the client in a room separate from the emergency department

The answer is B. Placing the client as confidential places a restriction on employees of the hospital so they cannot tell any visitors that the client is at the hospital. This is best since the husband may try to search for his spouse and/or lie to security about who he is.

A is incorrect—Notifying security is not the best intervention for this client as evidenced by the rationale provided for answer A. C is incorrect—While the police should be notified on all assaults, it is not the best choice for protecting the client at the hospital. D is incorrect—Placing the client away from the emergency department is not an appropriate choice. If the client is away from the department, she is too far for the nurse to monitor and the husband may be able to find her.

PHYSIOLOGICAL INTEGRITY

Physiological Adaptation

Alterations in Body Systems

Remove sutures or staples

191. An order has been written to remove the staples, which were placed in a client's left hip during surgery. Prior to removing the staples, the nurse should first:
   A. assess the site for infection.
   B. determine the number of staples from the operative note.
   C. soak the site with normal saline.
   D. clean the site with hydrogen peroxide.

The answer is B. Prior to removing sutures from a wound, the nurse needs to determine how many staples were placed during surgery to make sure the same number of staples is removed as were placed.

A is incorrect—Assessing the site is part of the process but not the first step. C is incorrect—The site is soaked if excess dry blood is around the area or the staples are embedded into the wound bed but this is not the first step. D is incorrect—Hydrogen peroxide can be used as needed if the wound has dried exudate or the staples are embedded in the skin, but this is not the first step.

PHYSIOLOGICAL INTEGRITY

Physiological Adaptation

Infectious Disease

Recognize signs and symptoms of infectious diseases

192. A client presents to the emergency department complaining of cough, fever, and night sweats. Which nursing intervention would have the highest priority?
    A. Provide the client with a sputum cup.
    B. Place a mask on the client.
    C. Move the client to a private room in the treatment bay.
    D. Provide the client with a tissue to cover the mouth when he or she coughs.

The answer is B. The client exhibits signs of tuberculosis and should be placed on isolation via a mask until he or she can be placed in a room in the treatment bay to prevent spread to those in the surrounding area.

A is incorrect—The client can be given a sputum cup after isolation measures are taken to protect those in the area. C is incorrect—The client does need to be moved after begin given a mask to wear. D is incorrect—The client should wear a mask or airway coverage at all times versus only when coughing.

PHYSIOLOGICAL INTEGRITY

Reduction of Risk Potential

System-Specific Assessment

Perform focused assessment or reassessment

193. A nurse is assisting a physician with the intubation of a client. Which assessment is the priority after the intubation is complete?
    A. Oxygen saturation level
    B. Heart rate
    C. Breath sounds bilaterally
    D. Rise and fall of the chest

The answer is C. The breath sounds are the priority for a client who has just been intubated. If breath sounds are present, then the intubation was successful and the lungs are being ventilated.

A is incorrect—The oxygen saturation level is not the best indicator of successful intubation immediately after the procedure is complete. The oxygen level will improve as the lungs are ventilated and diffusion of gases occurs. B is incorrect—While the heart rate is important, the first assessment after intubation should be breath sounds in both lungs. The heart rate will respond to the physiological status of the body. Initially, the heart rate will be high while the heart is trying to pump blood to meet the oxygen needs of the body. It will return to a more normal state as oxygen rich blood is available. D is incorrect—The rise and fall of the chest is important, but the nurse must hear breath sounds bilaterally to ensure the intubation was successful and the lungs are being ventilated.

PHYSIOLOGICAL INTEGRITY

Physiological Adaptation

Hemodynamics

Identify cardiac rhythm strip abnormalities

194. A client on the unit was complaining of chest pain when he became unresponsive. The nurse attaches the monitor and sees the following rhythm. Which action by the nurse is most important?
    A. Begin chest compressions
    B. Palpate for a pulse
    C. Check to see if the leads are attached properly
    D. Assess for breathing

The answer is D. The first step in CPR is to assess for breathlessness and begin rescue breathing for the client. If breathing is present, assess for lead placement; if the client is not breathing, begin CPR.

A is incorrect—Chest compressions begin after airway, breathing, and pulses are assessed. B is incorrect—Palpation

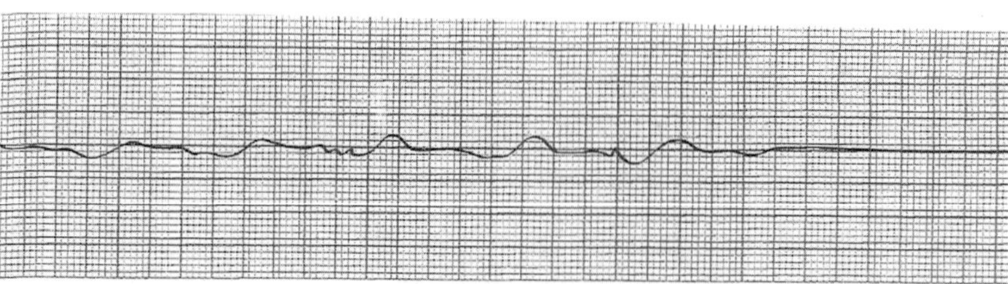

for pulses occurs after airway and breathing are assessed. C is incorrect—Lead placement is assessed after airway and breathing is assessed.

PHYSIOLOGICAL INTEGRITY

Physiological Adaptation

Illness Management

Teach client about managing illness

195. A client with a diagnosis of chronic obstructive pulmonary disease (COPD) is being discharged from the hospital. Which of the following is appropriate patient teaching before discharge?
   A. "Make sure to use a humidifier in your room while you sleep."
   B. "Apply powder to all crevices to prevent yeast while taking oral steroids."
   C. "Turn the oxygen up to no more than 6 L if you are short of breath."
   D. "Use your inhalers every day as directed even if symptoms are not present."

The answer is D. The client needs to use the inhalers every day regardless of symptoms to keep condition controlled and lessen the frequency of exacerbations.

A is incorrect—A humidifier is not necessary in the room of a client with COPD and can be a source of infection. B is incorrect—Powder can be an irritant to the client with COPD and cause an exacerbation of the disease. C is incorrect—The client with COPD should not use oxygen at greater than 2 L per nasal cannula.

PHYSIOLOGICAL INTEGRITY

Physiological Adaptation

Hemodynamics

Monitor and maintain arterial lines

196. A nurse is working with a client who has an arterial line for direct blood pressure monitoring. What is the first action the nurse should take when performing an assessment of the system?
   A. Ensure the transducer is at the phlebostatic axis.
   B. Zero out the system.
   C. Flush the system with normal saline.
   D. Administer a bolus of normal saline into the line.

The answer is A. The transducer should be placed at the phlebostatic axis, which is at the junction of the fourth intercostal space and the midchest area. If the transducer is placed above the axis, the monitor will give a low reading; if it is too low, the reading will be high.

B is incorrect—The transducer must be at the phlebostatic axis before zeroing occurs. C is incorrect—The system allows for blood draws but does not allow for fluid infusion. D is incorrect—The system has a Heparin solution which is used to keep the area from clotting; with that known other fluids such as normal saline are not to be instilled into the line as a flush or bolus.

PHYSIOLOGICAL INTEGRITY

Pharmacological and Parenteral Therapies

Expected Effects/Outcomes

Use clinical decision making/critical thinking when addressing expected effects/outcomes of medications

197. A nurse is reviewing a client's chart and notices the potassium level is 6.0; the nurse plans on administering which drug from protocol?
   A. Sodium polystyrene sulfonate (Kayexalate) 30 grams retention enema × 1 dose.
   B. 1 L normal saline with 20 mEq potassium chloride IV over 2 hours.
   C. Normal saline 1 L IV over 10 hours.
   D. phosphate/biphosphate (Phospho-Soda) 48 grams by mouth × 1 dose.

The answer is A. Kayexalate binds with the potassium and removes it from the body via the GI track. This drug carries less of a risk of hypovolemia than other preparations.

B is incorrect—This is adding potassium to the client, which will potentiate the problem. C is incorrect—Normal saline will not remove the potassium. Attempting to flush the system with normal saline places the client at risk for fluid overload. D is incorrect—Phospho-Soda inhibits absorption of fluids and electrolytes in the small intestine through an increase in peristalsis. This drug can potentially place a client in a state of hypovolemia and is not preferred for potassium reduction.

PHYSIOLOGICAL INTEGRITY

Reduction of Risk Potential

Vital Signs

Evaluate invasive monitoring data

198. A nurse is caring for a client who has a pulmonary artery catheter. Which assessment finding should be reported to the physician immediately?

A. Increase in capillary wedge pressure to 15 mm Hg.
B. Central venous pressure of 2 mm Hg.
C. Right ventricular pressure of 20 mm Hg systolic.
D. Cardiac output of 4 L/min.

The answer is A. The normal wedge pressure is from 8 to 12 mm Hg and anything above that indicates increased pressures in the left side of the heart, which are indicative of left sided heart failure and should be reported to the physician immediately.

B is incorrect—The normal central venous pressure is 2–6 mm Hg and indicates the volume status of the client. This reading will rise with volume overload. C is incorrect—The normal right ventricular pressure is 20–30 mm Hg and indicates the right ventricular function and volume. D is incorrect—The normal cardiac output is 4–8 L/min and is found by multiplying the stroke volume by the heart rate. This value is a direct reflection of the adequacy of cardiac function.

PHYSIOLOGICAL INTEGRITY

Physiological Adaptation

Pathophysiology

Identify client status based on pathophysiology

199. The nurse has received report on a client who has just been admitted for an acute myocardial infarction. The nurse's assessment findings are:
   - BP 90/66
   - HR 100
   - RR 16
   - skin cool to touch
   - A&O × 3 with mild anxiety
   - Urine output 40 mL/h

   The nurse understands that this assessment data is indicative of:
   A. class I cardiogenic shock
   B. class I hypovolemic shock
   C. class II septic shock
   D. class II neurogenic shock

The answer is A. In mild cardiogenic shock, the body responds to hypoperfusion by the heart through the activation of the Renin-Angiotensin system, which causes vasoconstriction. The heart rate increases to meet the demand of the body and the blood pressure is within normal limits during compensation. The antidiuretic hormone is secreted in response and urine output is decreased due to an increased resistance in the vascular system. Respirations will increase to provide oxygen to the critical organs. The cool skin is the response of the body shunting blood to the critical organs and the anxiety is due to the body's response to the shock and developing metabolic acidosis.

PHYSIOLOGICAL INTEGRITY

Elimination

Insert/remove nasogastric, urethral catheter, or other tubes

200. List in order the steps a nurse would follow prior to inserting a nasogastric tube:
   ___ Idenfy the client
   ___ Explain the procedure to the client
   ___ Wash hands
   ___ Gather supplies
   ___ Measure for tube placement
   ___ Assess the client
   ___ Turn suction to desired level
   ___ Sit client in high Fowlers

The nurse should first identify the client and then explain the procedure to gather a verbal acceptance. At that point, a system-specific assessment should be performed to ensure the client has no underlying complications that need immediate attention. Next the nurse gathers his or her supplies, washes hands, and then measures for tube placement. The suction is then set for the ordered level and finally the client is placed in high Fowlers.

MANAGEMENT OF CARE

Safety and Infection Control

Error Prevention

Verify appropriateness and/or accuracy of a treatment order

201. A client who has been in a car wreck resulting in head trauma and chest contusion is complaining of headache, chest pain radiating down his left arm, and difficulty breathing. The nurse receives the following orders from the physician. Which of the orders would the nurse question?
   A. Start an IV at a keep open rate.
   B. Raise the head of the bed 45 degrees.
   C. Start oxygen at 4 L per minute as ordered.
   D. Medicate with Nitrostat (Nitroglycerine) sublingual every 5 minutes × 3 for chest pain

The answer is D. Nitroglycerine is a vasodilator and may increase intracranial pressure.

The other actions would all be inappropriate.

HEALTH PROMOTION AND MAINTENANCE

Techniques of Physical Assessment

Perform comprehensive health assessment

202. Which cranial nerve is being tested when the nurse asks the client to shrug his/her shoulders and resist pressure to put them down?
    A. One (olfactory)
    B. Eleven (spinal accessory)
    C. Five (trigeminal)
    D. Seven (facial)

The answer is B. Cranial nerve eleven (spinal accessory) is tested by asking the client to shrug the shoulders and resist pressure to put them down because this cranial nerve controls muscular strength of the trapezius and sternocleidomastoid muscles.

A is incorrect—Cranial nerve one (olfactory nerve) is responsible for the sense of smell. It is tested by occluding each of the client's nostrils one at a time, holding a substance such as coffee or vanilla with a familiar aroma under the other nostril, and asking the client to identify the smell. The test is repeated with a different aromatic substance to determine if the client can differentiate smells.

C is incorrect—Cranial nerve five (trigeminal nerve) has both motor and sensory components. It is responsible for sensation in the face, scalp, oral and nasal mucous membranes, and the cornea and allows chewing movements of the jaw. Its three-part sensory division is tested by touching the forehead, cheek, and chin on each side with a wisp of cotton and asking the client whose eyes are closed to identify the type of touch and its location. Next the cornea of each eye is lightly touched with a wisp of cotton brought in from the side and the eye observed for the normal blink response. The motor function of cranial nerve five is tested by asking the client to clench the teeth and keep them clenched while the examiner pushes down on the chin to try and separate the jaws.

D is incorrect—Cranial nerve seven (facial nerve) is responsible for taste on the front two thirds of the tongue and for movement of the face including the ability to close the eyes and move the lips for speech. To test taste, an applicator dipped in a sugar, salt, or lemon solution is placed on the tongue and the client is asked what is tasted. Motor function of cranial nerve seven is tested by asking the client to smile, frown, grimace, show the upper and lower teeth, keep the eyes closed while the examiner tries to open them and puff out the cheeks. The examiner observes for symmetry and movement and presses the puffed out cheeks in to check if air is expelled equally from both sides.

PHYSIOLOGICAL INTEGRITY

Pharmacological and Parenteral Therapies

Medication Administration

Evaluate appropriateness/accuracy of medication order for client

203. A client is admitted with a diagnosis of cholecystitis. One of the admitting orders is for morphine PRN for pain. Why would the nurse question this order?
    A. Morphine is constipating.
    B. Morphine can cause nausea and vomiting.
    C. Morphine promotes biliary stone formation.
    D. Morphine causes spasm of the bile ducts.

The answer is D. Morphine is contraindicated for clients with cholecystitis because of the risk of precipitating duct spasm.

A, B, and C are incorrect—Morphine, which is an opioid, does cause constipation and also can cause nausea and vomiting but these are not the reason it is not used for clients with cholecystitis. Morphine is not documented as a factor in the formation of biliary stones.

HEALTH PROMOTION AND MAINTENANCE

Techniques of Physical Assessment

Perform comprehensive health assessment

204. Which would be a normal finding when percussing the left 10th intercostal space at the anterior axillary line?
    A. Tympany over the gastric air bubble
    B. Dullness over the spleen
    C. Resonance over the lungs
    D. Flatness over bone

The answer is B. Dullness over the spleen.

A, C, and D are incorrect. At the tenth intercostal space one is percussing over the spleen not over the gastric air bubble, lungs, or bone.

PHYSIOLOGICAL INTEGRITY

Reduction of Risk Potential

Diagnostic Tests

Obtain specimens other than blood for diagnostic testing

205. A diabetic client is admitted with a foul smelling, draining leg wound and a wound culture is ordered. When should the nurse plan to obtain the culture?
    A. Before any antiinfectives are administered.

B. When the blood sugar is within normal range.
C. Within 12 hours of a dose of a broad spectrum antibiotic.
D. After 48 hours of antimicrobial therapy

The answer is A. The culture needs to be obtained before any antiinfectives are given because antiinfectives will alter the microbial population. Blood sugar is unrelated to the timing of the culture.

PHYSIOLOGICAL INTEGRITY

Basic Care and Comfort

Elimination

206. The nurse is planning care for a client who requires a Sarita lift or the assistance of two people for transfer or ambulation. Which likely would be the best time to schedule having the client taken to the bathroom?
A. On awakening in the morning.
B. After breakfast.
C. Following mid-morning medications.
D. At bedtime after a warm drink.

The answer is B. The gastrocolic reflex is most active after breakfast so this is the time that the client is most likely to have a bowel movement. It is important to utilize the reflex because the client is somewhat immobilized and therefore prone to constipation. Warm fluids can stimulate the reflex but it is still most active in the morning.

PSYCHOSOCIAL INTEGRITY

Behavioral Interventions

Assess client appearance, mood, and psychomotor behavior and identify/respond to inappropriate/abnormal behavior

207. Which is an appropriate nursing intervention for a newly admitted client diagnosed with schizophrenia?
A. Avoid offering choices to the client.
B. Use touch to calm and reassure the client.
C. Keep explanations of care and activities to a minimum.
D. Spend time with the client even if there is no response.

The answer is D. The nurse should spend time with the client even if the client cannot respond. Being with the client is an indication of caring and is a form of human interaction. Initially, the client should not be offered choices; with treatment the client is gradually assisted in making decisions. Maintenance of ego boundaries is important when caring for the schizophrenic client and touching the client should be avoided. Explanations are an important part of the care of the schizophrenic client and everything that is being done should be explained to help create trust.

PHYSIOLOGICAL INTEGRITY

Physiological Adaptation

Illness Management

Teach client about managing illness

208. Which instruction would the nurse give when teaching a client pursed lip breathing?
A. Take a slow breath in through your mouth.
B. Breathe out through your mouth puffing out your cheeks.
C. Use your abdominal muscles to help exhale as deeply as possible.
D. Use this breathing technique before any strenuous activity.

The answer is C. Abdominal muscles should be used to help force as much air out as possible during each exhalation. All other instructions are incorrect. When teaching pursed lip breathing the client is instructed to breathe in through the nose with the mouth closed and then to purse the lips as if to whistle and exhale slowly (exhalation should be double the time of inspiration) through the mouth without puffing the cheeks using the abdominal muscles to maximize exhalation of air. Pursed lip breathing should be used during not before physical activity.

PHYSIOLOGICAL INTEGRITY

Physiological Adaptation

Illness management

209. Which statement made by a client with cirrhosis indicates the need for further clarification on self-care?
A. "I will not get any injections unless my doctor specifically approves."
B. "I will use an electric razor."
C. "I will take two acetaminophen tabs every 4 hours if I have pain."
D. "I will avoid exposure to people with colds or other infections."

The answer is C. Acetaminophen is hepatotoxic and contraindicated in cirrhosis so if the client says that he or she is going to take acetaminophen then further instruction is self-care is required.

A, B, and D are incorrect—Avoiding unnecessary injections and using an electric razor are appropriate because of the risk of bleeding due to impaired clotting. Avoiding exposure to infection is appropriate because of decreased immune function.

HEALTH PROMOTION AND MAINTENANCE

Techniques of Physical Assessment

Perform comprehensive health assessment

210. When assessing the heart, the nurse palpates for heaves over the tricuspid area which would be an abnormal finding. Which lettered block on the accompanying diagram marks the location where the nurse would place the ball of the hand to palpate over the tricuspid area. Write the letter of the block on the line provided.

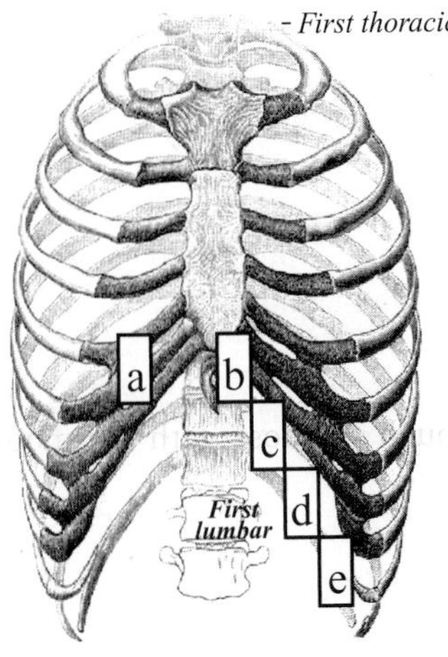

The answer is D.

PHYSIOLOGICAL INTEGRITY

Pharmacological and Parenteral Therapies

Medication Administration

Use the six "rights" when administering client medications

211. A client's order for pain medication reads "Codeine 15 sc q4h PRN for pain." Which aspect of this order should the nurse question?
A. Frequency
B. Route
C. Dose
D. None

The answer is C. The dose is incomplete and therefore needs to be questioned. No unit of dosage is specified and the nurse cannot assume mg or any other unit was intended. Route and frequency are specified. This is an as needed order and the reason for the need is also specified as required.

HEALTH PROMOTION AND MAINTENANCE

Techniques of Physical Assessment

Perform comprehensive health assessment

212. When assessing the knee, which types of motion must be present to a normal degree for the nurse to document full range of motion? (Mark all that apply.)
___ A. Supination
___ B. Flexion
___ C. Pronation
___ D. Hyperextension
___ E. Internal rotation
___ F. External rotation
___ G. Abduction
___ H. Adduction

The answers are B, D, E, and F. Normal range of motion in the knee is flexion, hyperextension, and internal and external rotation. Normal flexion is the ability to fully bend the knee so the calf touches the thigh. Hyperextension is the ability to extend the knee beyond the normal point of extension. Internal rotation is the ability to rotate the knee and lower leg toward the midline. External rotation is the ability to rotate the knee and lower leg laterally.

PHYSIOLOGICAL INTEGRITY

Physiological Adaptation

Fluid and Electrolyte Imbalances

Evaluate the client response to interventions to correct fluid and electrolyte imbalance

213. Which assessment finding indicates that a young adult client admitted with dehydration has been successfully rehydrated?
A. Urine output of 40 Ml/h.
B. Skin "tents" when pinched.
C. Urine-specific gravity of 1.031.
D. Apical pulse of 120 and blood pressure of 90/40.

The answer is A. Urinary output of 40 mL/h or more indicates adequate hydration and glomerular filtration rate.

B is incorrect—Tenting of the skin is indicative of dehydration, although care must be taken particularly with the elderly to check for tenting in areas such as around the top of the sternum because tenting can occur when the skin of the forearm or hand is pinched due to normal age changes and therefore does not always indicate dehydration. C is incorrect—Urine-specific gravity of 1.031 is indicative of concentrated urine, which would be seen when hydration is inadequate. D is incorrect—An apical pulse of 120 is abnormally rapid and a blood pressure of 90/40 is low. These findings are consistent with dehydration.

HEALTH PROMOTION AND MAINTENANCE

Techniques of Physical Assessment

Perform comprehensive health assessment

214. When assessing the heart, the nurse auscultates for abnormal heart sounds over the mitral area. Which lettered block on the accompanying diagram marks the location where the nurse would place the diaphragm of the stethoscope to auscultate the mitral area? Write the Letter of the block on the line provided.

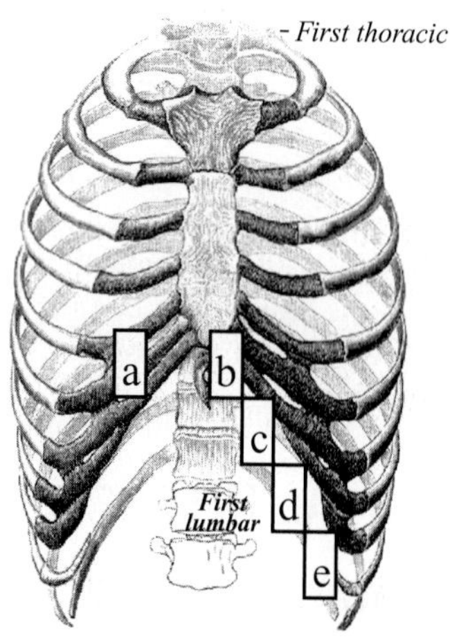

The answer is E.

PHYSIOLOGICAL INTEGRITY

Physiological Adaptation

Illness Management

Apply knowledge of client pathophysiology to illness management

215. When assessing a client with cholecystitis, a report of which type of pain would the nurse interpret as consistent with the diagnosis?
   A. Dull, aching upper right abdominal pain.
   B. Sharp, crampy periumbilical pain.
   C. Sharp pain in the back under the shoulder blade.
   D. Dull upper abdominal and right shoulder pain.

The answer is C. Cholecystitis causes right upper quadrant pain referred to the back under the shoulder blade.

A is incorrect—Liver cancer causes dull, aching pain in the right abdomen. B is incorrect—Crampy, sharp periumbilical pain is characteristic of a variety of intestinal disorders including food poisoning. D is incorrect—An enlarged spleen can press on the diaphragm and stimulate the phrenic nerve resulting in referred shoulder pain but this is pain on the left side not the right.

HEALTH PROMOTION AND MAINTENANCE

Techniques of Physical Assessment

Perform comprehensive health assessment

216. When assessing a client's hands, the nurse notes clubbing of the fingers. The nurse recognizes that clubbing is a sign of:
   A. respiratory disease
   B. cardiomegaly
   C. diabetes
   D. rheumatoid arthritis

The answer is A. Clubbing of the fingers occurs secondary to low oxygen tension leading to an increased hemoglobin and hematocrit. The other answers are incorrect.

PHYSIOLOGICAL INTEGRITY

Pharmacological and Parenteral Therapies

Expected Effects/Outcomes

Use clinical decision making/critical thinking when addressing expected effects/outcomes of medications

217. Which is the priority assessment when caring for a client taking a calcium channel blocker medication?
   A. Weight
   B. Breathing
   C. Blood pressure
   D. Urinary output

The answer is C. Calcium channel blockers cause coronary and peripheral vasodilation, which can lead to drop in blood pressure. There are no effects on weight, breathing, or urinary output requiring priority assessment.

HEALTH PROMOTION AND MAINTENANCE

Techniques of Physical Assessment

Perform comprehensive health assessment

218. Which lung sound if auscultated over point E in the diagram would be evaluated by the nurse as a normal assessment finding?

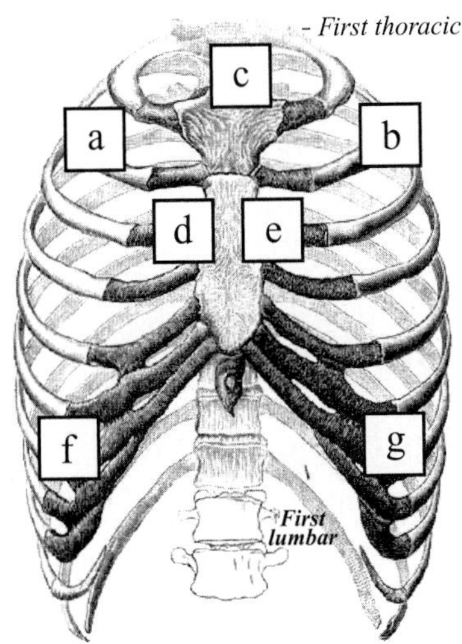

A. Bronchovesicular
B. Crackle
C. Gurgle
D. Sibilant
E. Tracheal
F. Vesicular
G. Wheeze

The answer is A. Bronchovesicular sounds are normally heard over the areas where the right and left bronchi branch. Anteriorly this is at the first and second intercostal spaces and posteriorly between the scapulae so this includes point B. Bronchovesicular sounds are of medium intensity and pitch with the inspiratory and expiratory phases equal.

PHYSIOLOGICAL INTEGRITY

Physiological Adaptation

Illness Management

Implement interventions to manage the client recovering from an illness

219. Which intervention would be inappropriate in the emergent care of a client with a dislocation?
A. Putting joint through passive range of motion
B. Splinting the joint in the dislocated position
C. Applying ice to the joint
D. Providing tactile stimulation distal to the affected joint

Option A is the inappropriate intervention. The joint is not moved through a ROM; so this option is incorrect.

Other interventions are correct actions—The joint would be splinted in the dislocated position until controlled reduction is possible. Cold is applied initially to reduce swelling. Tactile stimulation distal to the affected joint serves no purpose.

SAFE AND EFFECTIVE CARE ENVIRONMENT

Management of Care

Establishing Priorities

Assess/triage the client to prioritize the order of care delivery

220. The nurse is planning care for a client newly admitted for rectal bleeding. What is the priority order in which the nurse should plan to carry out the following nursing care activities? (Arrange the options in priority order. All options must be used.)
A. Start an intravenous.
B. Observe the client's level of anxiety.
C. Continue to monitor the client for rectal bleeding.
D. Teach the client self-care in preparation for the discharge.
E. Assess the client's skin, blood pressure, heart rate, and urine output.
F. Teach the client about the upcoming diagnostic tests that the doctor has ordered over the next couple of days.

Correct order of priorities: E, A, B, C, F, and D. Physical needs precede psychological needs. Client teaching would be the last priority in this situation.

PHYSIOLOGICAL INTEGRITY

Reduction of Risk Potential

Potential for Complications of Diagnostic Tests/Treatments/Procedures

Implement measures to manage/prevent/lessen possible complications of client condition and/or procedure

221. When caring for a client with a long intestinal tube attached to suction, the nurse would ensure that the suction does not exceed how many mm Hg? (Record your answer using a whole number.)

The answer is 25. Suction higher than 25 mm Hg can damage the intestinal mucosa.

HEALTH PROMOTION AND MAINTENANCE

Techniques of Physical Assessment

Perform comprehensive health assessment

222. The nurse asks a client what the client would do if she/he found a stamped and addressed envelope on the street.

The client says she/he would put it in a mailbox. What conclusion should the nurse draw from this exchange?
A. Judgment is intact
B. Short-term memory is intact
C. Mathematical abilities are intact
D. Abstract thinking is intact

The answer is A. Judgment is intact. This scenario requires the patient to exercise judgment before reacting.

B, C, and D are incorrect—The question and answer exchange does not address short-term memory, mathematical ability, or abstract thinking.

PHYSIOLOGICAL INTEGRITY

Pharmacological and Parenteral Therapies

Medication Administration

Educate the client/family about medications

223. A 19-year-old college student is diagnosed with a strep throat and penicillin is prescribed. Which question should the nurse ask the girl when giving her the prescription?
A. Do you drink milk?
B. Are you allergic to shellfish?
C. Do you take birth control pills?
D. Have you ever had vaginitis?

The answer is C. Penicillin can interfere with the action of oral contraceptives so if they are being used for birth control, the client needs to be advised to use an additional method while taking the medication. The other questions are not relevant to taking penicillin.

PHYSIOLOGICAL INTEGRITY

Reduction of Risk Potential

System-Specific Assessment

Perform focused assessment or reassessment

224. When monitoring abdominal girth, which guideline should the nurse follow?
A. Measure at the same time each day.
B. Measure before breakfast each morning.
C. Have the client empty the bladder before measuring.
D. Measure at the same location each time.

The answer is D. In order for the measurements to be comparable and therefore provide accurate information on the development of ascites, the girth of the abdomen must be measured at the same location each time. Usually the umbilicus is the location of choice but records of the measurements need to specify the location.

A, B, and C are incorrect—Time of day, breakfast, or a full bladder do not have the same potential for affecting the measurement as does location of the measurement on the abdomen.

PHYSIOLOGICAL INTEGRITY

Pharmacological and Parenteral Therapies

Adverse Effects/Contraindications and Side Effects

Assess the client for actual or potential side effects and adverse effects of medications

225. A client comes to the clinic complaining of unexplained black and blue areas and red tinged urine. Which type of medication is it most important to find out if the client is taking?
A. Urinary antiseptic
B. Systemic glucocorticoid
C. Antianemic
D. Anticoagulant

The answer is D. Unexplained black and blue areas and hematuria are signs of bleeding associated with excessive doses of anticoagulants. Because of the potential harmful effects of abnormal bleeding, checking for use of anticoagulants is the most important.

HEALTH PROMOTION AND MAINTENANCE

Techniques of Physical Assessment

Perform comprehensive health assessment

226. When assessing the hip, which types of motion must be present to a normal degree for the nurse to document full range of motion? (Mark all that apply.)
___ A. Supination
___ B. Flexion
___ C. Pronation
___ D. Extension
___ E. Internal rotation
___ F. External rotation
___ G. Abduction
___ H. Adduction

The answers are B, D, E, F, G, and H. The hip is a ball and socket joint as is the shoulder and this type of joint provides for the most movement. Types of movement possible are flexion, extension, adduction (movement toward the midline of the body), abduction (movement away from the midline of the body), and internal and external rotation.

PHYSIOLOGICAL INTEGRITY

Physiological Adaptation

Pathophysiology

227. Which are risk factors for cancer of the liver? Mark all that apply.
   A. ___ Hepatitis A
   B. ___ Cirrhosis
   C. ___ History of gastric cancer
   D. ___ Alcohol abuse
   E. ___ Portal hypertension
   F. ___ Exposure to environmental toxins
   G. ___ Smoking
   H. ___ Hepatitis C

The answers are B, D, F, G and H. Cirrhosis, alcohol abuse, exposure to chemicals and toxins, smoking, and hepatitis C are identified as risk factors for liver cancer. Liver cancer occurs more often among males and heredity seems to play a role in its occurrence.

A, C, and E are incorrect—Hepatitis A and a history of gastric cancer are unrelated to the development of liver cancer. Portal hypertension occurs with cirrhosis and can accompany liver cancer and other diseases. It is a result of rather than a cause of liver cancer.

PHYSIOLOGICAL INTEGRITY

Reduction of Risk Potential

Diagnostic Tests

Evaluate the results of diagnostic testing and intervene as needed

228. Which results of a CBC (complete blood count) with differential should the nurse interpret as indicating the client has a viral infection?
   A. WBC 8,500; lymphocytes 45%
   B. WBC 25,000; band neutrophils 20%
   C. WBC 15,000; segmented neutrophils 50%
   D. WBC 20,000; segmented neutrophils 58%

The answer is A. With a viral infection the WBC is normal with elevated lymphocytes.

B is incorrect—This indicates a severe bacterial infection because the total white blood cell count is above normal and the band neutrophils are elevated because the body is trying to fight the infection so quickly that the neutrophils are being released into the circulation before they are mature cells. C is incorrect—This indicates a bacterial infection, but not a severe one because the WBC count is above normal but the segs are normal. D is incorrect—This again indicates a bacterial infection, but not a severe one because although the WBC count is elevated, the segs are still within normal limits.

HEALTH PROMOTION AND MAINTENANCE

Immunizations

Assess the client/family/significant other knowledge of immunization schedules

229. Which statement made by a client at an immunization clinic indicates an understanding about the hepatitis B vaccine?
   A. "I have to come back in six months to a year for the booster dose."
   B. "I won't have maximum protection until after the third dose of the vaccine."
   C. "I'll be able to eat shellfish without worry once I get all these injections."
   D. "I regret I won't be able to give blood anymore after I get these injections."

The answer is B. Three doses of vaccine are needed for maximum protection.

A is incorrect—It is hepatitis A vaccine that requires a booster dose in 6–12 months after the initial dose is given. C is incorrect—Hepatitis A, not hepatitis B, can be contracted from eating contaminated shellfish. D is incorrect—Receiving hepatitis B vaccine does not prevent blood donation.

PHYSIOLOGICAL INTEGRITY

Physiological Adaptation

Illness Management

Apply knowledge of pathophysiology to illness management

230. Which would be an expected finding when assessing a client with gout?
   A. Rash over the nose and cheeks.
   B. Joint stiffness for 1–2 hours on arising.
   C. Reddened edematous joints.
   D. Intolerance of vegetable protein.

The answer is C. Reddened erythematous joints are signs of gout.

A is incorrect—Rash over the nose and cheeks is a symptom of SLE. B is incorrect—Joint stiffness for more than 1 hour on arising in the morning is characteristic of rheumatoid arthritis. D is incorrect—Intolerance to vegetable program is unrelated to a musculoskeletal disorder.

PHYSIOLOGICAL INTEGRITY

Pharmacological and Parenteral Therapies

Medication Administration

Review pertinent data prior to medication administration

231. Because of the risk of a toxic drug reaction, monitoring laboratory reports for hypokalemia would be a part of the plan of care for a client receiving which medication?
   A. Hydrodiuril
   B. Motrin
   C. Lovastatin
   D. Digoxin

The answer is D. Hypokalemia can precipitate a toxic reaction to digoxin.

A, B, and C are incorrect—Hypokalemia does not precipitate a toxic reaction to Hydrodiuril, Motrin, or Lovastatin.

HEALTH PROMOTION AND MAINTENANCE

Techniques of Physical Assessment

Perform comprehensive health assessment

232. In which group of clients would the nurse expect to find a positive plantar reflex with an up going first toe and the others fanning out?
   A. The elderly
   B. Adolescents
   C. Infants
   D. School aged children

The answer is C. Infants. The plantar or Babinski reflex in infants is positive, i.e., first toe goes up and toes fan.

A, B, and D are incorrect—In all other age groups, the first toe curls and the rest of the toes move downward.

PHYSIOLOGICAL INTEGRITY

Pharmacological and Parenteral Therapies

Medication Administration

Educate the client/families about medication

233. Which instruction should the nurse give to an elderly patient about the proper storage of medications?
   A. Keep medications in their original containers.
   B. Store in a bathroom cabinet out of the reach of children
   C. Keep in a brightly lit area to better read labels.
   D. Avoid storing in dry, cool locations.

The answer is A. Medications should always be kept in their original, properly labeled containers to decrease the risk of taking the wrong drug, or of taking the right drug but in the wrong amount, by the wrong route, or at the wrong time.

B is incorrect—Medications should be stored out of the reach of children but not in the bathroom cabinet where exposure to moisture can occur. C is incorrect—Drugs should be stored out of the light and away from heat and so a dark, cool location is needed. D is incorrect—It is important to pour pills from their containers in good lighting so that labels can be read accurately but bottles of medication should not be stored in bright light.

PSYCHOSOCIAL INTEGRITY

Behavioral Interventions

Assess client appearance, mood, and psychomotor behavior and identify/respond to inappropriate/abnormal behavior

234. Which is a priority goal for a client with borderline personality disorder?
   A. Acceptance of group therapy.
   B. Elimination of bizarre fantasies.
   C. Development of social relationships
   D. Decrease of actual and intended self-destructive behavior

The answer is D. Clients with borderline personality disorder make recurrent threats or gestures of self mutilation or suicide or actually attempt to mutilate or kill themselves. As a result a priority nursing intervention is to support efforts to decrease the actual behaviors as well as the client's intent to perform them. Group therapy can assist the client with borderline personality disorder in developing awareness of how one's behavior affects others.

PHYSIOLOGIC INTEGRITY

Reduction of Risk Potential

Potential for Complications of Diagnostic Tests/Treatments/Procedures

Implement measures to manage/prevent/lessen possible complications of the client condition and/or procedure

235. When caring for a client with pancreatitis, the nurse monitors the nasogastric tube attached to suction for proper functioning. It is important that proper functioning be maintained:

A. To prevent backup of secretions to the liver.
B. To protect the intestine from gastric secretions.
C. To allow for monitoring of gastric pH.
D. To protect the gastric lining from pancreatic enzymes.

The answer is B. The N/G tube serves to remove acidic gastric contents so these do not enter and damage the intestine. This is a risk because alkaline pancreatic secretions are not available to neutralize them.

A, C, and D are incorrect—Gastric secretions do not back up to the liver, gastric pH is not measured as part of the management of pancreatitis, and pancreatic enzymes back flowing to the stomach is not a problem.

HEALTH PROMOTION AND MAINTENANCE

Techniques of Physical Assessment

Perform comprehensive health assessment

236. When assessing the elbow, which types of motion must be present to a normal degree for the nurse to document full range of motion? (Mark all that apply.)
___ A. Supination
___ B. Flexion
___ C. Pronation
___ D. Extension
___ E. Rotation
___ F. Tilting

The answers are A, B, C, and D. As a hinge joint the basic movement possible in the elbow is flexion and extension. In addition checking ROM of the elbow joint includes pronation and supination. To assess pronation the nurse asks the client to hold each arm straight out and turn the palm upward toward the ceiling. To assess supination, the arms are held out straight and the palms turned downward toward the floor.

PHYSIOLOGICAL INTEGRITY

Pharmacological and Parenteral Therapies

Medication Administration

Administer and document medications given by common routes

237. What instruction would be most effective in helping a client relax the rectal sphincter in preparation for administration of a rectal suppository?
A. "Turn on your left side and flex your knees."
B. "Bear down as though for a bowel movement."
C. "Take a deep breath exhaling through the mouth."
D. "Think of something that you find soothing."

The answer is C. Taking a deep breath and exhaling through the mouth helps relax the rectal sphincter. Turning on the left side and flexing the knees is a desirable position for inserting the suppository. Bearing down as though for a bowel movement would act to eject the suppository. Thinking of something soothing may help the client relax but is not specific to the rectal sphincter.

PHYSIOLOGICAL INTEGRITY

Reduction of Risk Potential

Diagnostic Tests

Evaluate the results of diagnostic testing and intervene as needed

238. A nurse is reading a PPD test that he or she administered to a healthy 50-year-old grade school teacher. Which of the following measurements would the nurse interpret as a "positive" reading for this individual?
A. 10 mm of erythema
B. 5 mm of induration
C. 10 mm of induration
D. 15 mm of induration

The answer is C. With the exception of the immunocompromised, clients with risk factors such as teachers, health care workers, and people living in crowded areas, 10 mm and above of induration is considered positive.

A is incorrect—Erythema is not considered as positive. B is incorrect—5 mm of induration is positive if the person is immunocompromised. D is incorrect—15 mm of induration is positive for persons with no known risk factors.

PHYSIOLOGICAL INTEGRITY

Physiological Adaptation

Illness Management

Apply knowledge of pathophysiology to illness management

239. Which would be an expected finding when assessing a client with lupus erythematosis?
A. Rash over the nose and cheeks.
B. Joint stiffness for 1–2 hours on arising.
C. Reddened edematous joints.
D. Intolerance to milk sugar.

The answer is A. Rash over the nose and cheeks is a symptom of SLE, which is an autoimmune disease.

B is incorrect—Joint stiffness for more than 1 hour on arising in the morning is characteristic of rheumatoid arthritis. C is incorrect—Reddened erythematous joints are a sign of gout. Intolerance to milk sugar or lactose intolerance is unrelated to lupus erythematosis.

HEALTH PROMOTION AND MAINTENANCE

Techniques of Physical Assessment

Perform comprehensive health assessment

240. When assessing the ankle, which types of motion must be present to a normal degree for the nurse to document full range of motion? (Mark all that apply.)
___ A. Supination
___ B. Dorsiflexion
___ C. Pronation
___ D. Hyperextension
___ E. Eversion
___ F. Plantar flexion
___ G. Abduction
___ H. Adduction
___ I. Inversion

The answers are B, E, F, G, H, and I. Movements that are part of the normal range of motion for the ankles are dorsiflexion (foot bent upward with toes pointing at head), plantar flexion (foot pointed downward, abduction, adduction, and eversion (movement of the sole of the foot outward), and inversion (movement of the sole of the foot inward. Supination and pronation are movements of the elbow. Hyperextension is a movement of the shoulder, elbow, and knee.

PHYSIOLOGICAL INTEGRITY

Reduction in Risk Potential

Vital Signs

Apply knowledge needed to perform related nursing procedures and psychomotor skills when assessing vital signs

241. When delegating blood pressure measurement to an unlicensed assistant, the nurse cautions that correct technique must be used to avoid obtaining false low pressures. Which is one of the directions the nurse would give to prevent a false low pressure reading?
A. Take the blood pressure on an extremity positioned below heart level.
B. Use a cuff whose width is 40% of the diameter of the extremity.
C. Wrap the cuff loosely around the extremity.
D. Apply the cuff unevenly to the extremity.

The answer is B. The width of the cuff should be 40% of the diameter of the arm; use of a cuff that is too wide can cause false low blood pressure readings and use of a cuff that is too narrow can result in false high readings.

A is incorrect—Taking the blood pressure on an extremity positioned below heart level can result in a false low reading; it does not prevent it. The extremity needs to be supported and at heart level. C is incorrect—Wrapping the cuff too loosely on the extremity results in a false high reading not a false low reading. D is incorrect— If the cuff is wrapped unevenly around the extremity, the result can be a false high, not a false low, pressure reading.

HEALTH PROMOTION AND MAINTENANCE

Techniques of Physical Assessment

Perform comprehensive health assessment

242. When assessing the heart, the nurse auscultates for both aortic and pulmonic murmurs over Erb's point. Which lettered block on the accompanying diagram marks the location where the nurse would place the diaphragm of the stethoscope to auscultate over Erb's point? Write the letter of the block on the line provided.

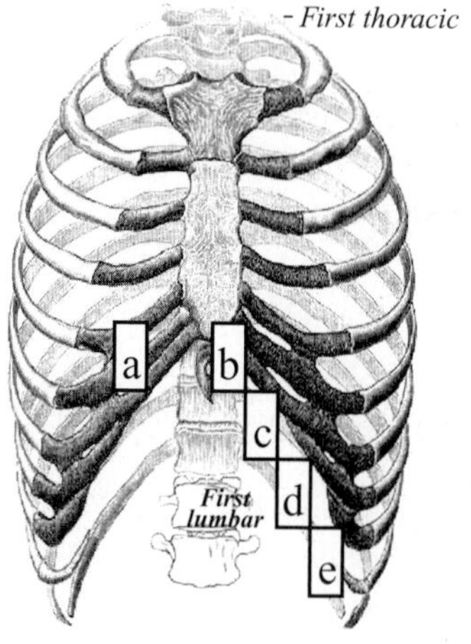

The answer is C.

PHYSIOLOGICAL INTEGRITY

Reduction of Risk Potential

Diagnostic Tests

Perform diagnostic testing

243. When instructing a client on obtaining a stool specimen for an FOBT, the nurse tells the client not to take aspirin or NSAIDs for how many days prior to collecting the specimen?
Record your answer using a whole number.

The answer is 2 days. FOBT is a screening test for colon cancer, a sign of which is occult blood in the stool. Aspirin and NSAIDS can cause GI irritation and bleeding and thus can result in a positive FOBT.

PHYSIOLOGICAL INTEGRITY

Pharmacological and Parenteral Therapies

Medication Administration

Administer and document medications given by parenteral routes

244. In which situation would the nurse need to administer an injection using Z-track technique?
   A. The client is malnourished with muscle wasting.
   B. The medication is thick and requires a large gauge needle.
   C. The medication is very irritating.
   D. The client's platelet count is 200,000 or more.

The answer is C. The Z-track method is designed to prevent backflow of medication through the needle track and into the surrounding tissues. It is used when medications are very irritating and can cause tissue damage.

A, B, and D are incorrect—Administration using a Z-track technique is not determined by the size of the client, the thickness of the medication, or the client's platelet count.

HEALTH PROMOTION AND MAINTENANCE

Techniques of Physical Assessment

Perform comprehensive health assessment

245. Which lung sound if auscultated over point F in the diagram would be evaluated by the nurse as a normal assessment finding?

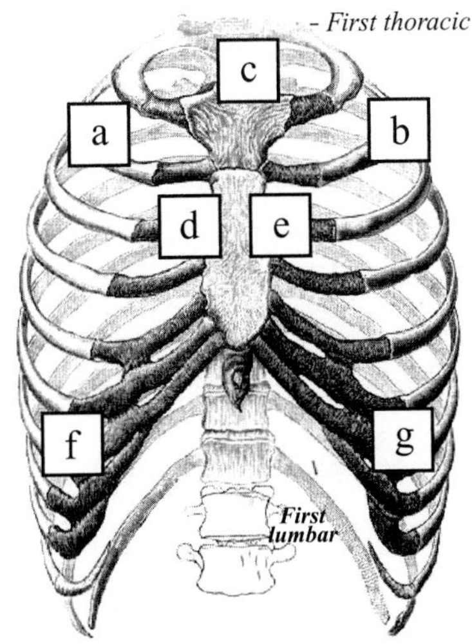

   A. Bronchovesicular
   B. Crackle
   C. Gurgle
   D. Sibilant
   E. Tracheal
   F. Vesicular
   G. Wheeze

The answer is F. Vesicular sounds are normally heard over alveolar lung tissue, which is the majority of both lungs including point B. Vesicular sounds are soft in intensity and low in pitch. The inspiratory phase is longer than the expiratory phase.

PHYSIOLOGICAL INTEGRITY

Reduction of Risk Potential

Laboratory Values

Provide the client with information about the purpose and procedure of prescribed laboratory tests

246. A client receives a report that his PSA level is 9 ng/mL and asks the nurse what this means. The nurse will base the response on the knowledge that:
   A. This result is within normal range and no follow up is required.
   B. This result is below the normal range and repeat testing is needed.
   C. This result is slightly elevated and may reflect problems such as urinary tract infection and benign prostatic hypertrophy as well as prostate cancer; follow up is needed.
   D. This result is above normal and indicative of prostate cancer; treatment is needed.

The answer is C. The normal PSA is less than 4 ng/mL but can be elevated into the hundreds with metastatic prostate cancer. Elevations can occur as a result of BPH, cirrhosis, prostatitis, urinary tract infection, and urinary retention. False elevated levels can occur after urinary catheterization, cystoscopy, transrectal ultrasound, or prostate biopsy.

PHYSIOLOGIC INTEGRITY

Reduction of Risk Potential

Laboratory Values

Recognizes deviations from normal

247. A pregnant woman is seen in the prenatal clinic. The following lab values are received during this visit. Which lab value requires further investigation?
   A. Positive HCG
   B. High alpha fetoprotein
   C. Low hemoglobin and hematocrit
   D. Urine negative for protein and glucose

The answer is B. High alpha fetoprotein is seen in conjunction with fetal abnormalities, such as spina bifida and Down's syndrome and should be investigated further.

A is incorrect—Positive HCG means she is pregnant. C is incorrect—During pregnancy, the volume portion of blood increases at a faster rate than the cellular portion producing a pseudoanemia. D is incorrect—Negative urine protein and glucose is normal.

PHYSIOLOGICAL INTEGRITY

Reduction of Risk Potential

Diagnostic Tests

Evaluate the results of diagnostic testing and intervene as needed

248. Because of the risk of spontaneous bleeding, the nurse would institute bleeding precautions for a client whose laboratory report documents a platelet count below ___ $/mm^3$. Record your answer using a whole number.

The answer is 20,000. Spontaneous bleeding can occur with a platelet count of less than 20,000/mm^3. Therefore bleeding precautions are required:

- Test all urine and stool for blood.
- No rectal treatments (temperatures, suppositories, enemas, etc.).
- No IM injections.
- Put firm pressure on all venipuncture sites for 5 minutes and on arterial puncture sites for 10 minutes.

PHYSIOLOGICAL INTEGRITY

Physiological Adaptation

Illness Management

Teach the client about managing illness

249. Which topic would be included in the teaching plan for a client with gout?
   A. Need to decrease dietary intake of foods high in purine.
   B. Importance of restricting caffeine in the daily diet.
   C. Necessity of limiting fluid intake.
   D. Benefits of decreasing intake of dairy products.

The answer is A. Clients with gout need to limit intake of high purine foods such as scallops, sadines, gravies, and cream sauces.

B is incorrect—Caffeine does not need to be restricted. C is incorrect—Fluid intake should be increased to aid renal filtration of uric acid from the blood; it should not be restricted. D is incorrect—Dairy products do not have to be decreased.

HEALTH PROMOTION AND MAINTENANCE

Techniques of Physical Assessment

Perform comprehensive health assessment

250. Which lung sound if auscultated over point D in the diagram would be evaluated by the nurse as a normal assessment finding?

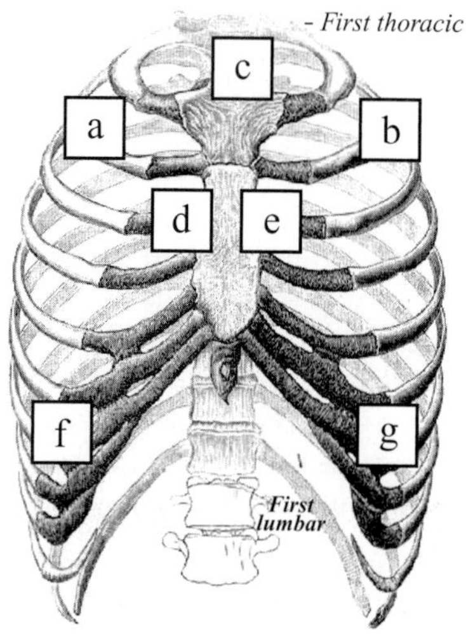

   A. Bronchovesicular
   B. Crackle
   C. Gurgle
   D. Sibilant
   E. Tracheal
   F. Vesicular
   G. Wheeze

The answer is A. Bronchovesicular sounds are normally heard over the areas where the right and left bronchi branch. Anteriorly this is at the first and second intercostal spaces and posteriorly between the scapulae so this includes point B. Bronchovesicular sounds are of medium intensity and pitch with the inspiratory and expiratory phases equal.

PHYSIOLOGICAL INTEGRITY

Pharmacological and Parenteral Therapies

Adverse Effects/Contraindications and Side Effects

Assess the client for actual or potential side effects and adverse effects of medications

251. When caring for a client on antibiotic therapy, monitoring for which type of common complication is an important component of the plan of care?
   A. Electrolyte imbalance
   B. Suprainfection

C. Liver failure

D. Abnormal bleeding

The answer is B. Suprainfection is a common complication of antibiotic therapy because as organisms susceptible to the prescribed antibiotic are eliminated, other nonsusceptible organisms can overgrow. This results in a second infection caused by an organism different from the one causing the infection for which the antibiotic was prescribed. Common examples of suprainfection are monilial vaginal infections and diarrhea.

SAFE AND EFFECTIVE CARE ENVIRONMENT

Management of Care

Delegation

Utilize five "rights" of delegations (right task, right circumstances, right person, right direction or communication, and right supervision or feedback)

252. When delegating blood pressure measurement to an unlicensed assistant, the nurse cautions that correct technique must be used to avoid obtaining false high blood pressures. Which errors in technique should be identified as the potential causes of false high blood pressures? Mark all that apply.

A. ___ Use of an unsupported limb to take the blood pressure

B. ___ Use of a cuff that is too wide.

C. ___ Immediate reinflation of the cuff

D. ___ Too rapid deflation of the cuff

E. ___ Uneven application of the cuff

The answers are A, C, and E. Taking the blood pressure on an unsupported extremity, reinflation of the cuff without waiting 1–2 minutes, and applying the cuff unevenly to the arm all can cause a false high blood pressure.

B and D are incorrect—Use of a cuff that is too wide or deflating the cuff too rapidly can cause false low blood pressures.

PHYSIOLOGICAL INTEGRITY

Pharmacological and Parenteral Therapies

Adverse Effects/Contraindications and Side Effects

Educate client/family about medications

253. Which statement made by a client who has been given instructions on taking NSAIDs for joint pain indicates the need for further teaching?

A. "I have to take these pills with food and a full glass of liquid."

B. "I can't have beer or other alcoholic drinks while taking these pills."

C. "I need to be on the alert for any signs of abnormal bleeding."

D. "I can take other over the counter drugs with these as long as I don't take more than the prescribed dose."

The answer is D. NSAIDS cannot be mixed with any over the counter drugs; safe use of other drugs varies with what they are and how they work. NSAIDS should not be mixed with any other NSAIDS. This statement indicates that the client has not understood all the information necessary for safe use of the prescribed NSAID. Therefore the client is in need of further teaching. Other responses are correct. NSAIDS should be taken with food and a full glass of fluid because of their irritating effects on the gastric mucosa; alcoholic beverages also should be avoided. Because aspirin and ibuprofen, which are classic examples of the two types of NSAIDS (a salicylate and a prostaglandin synthetase inhibitor respectively) affect platelet function and can cause GI bleeding, a client needs to observe for and report any signs of bleeding.

PHYSIOLOGIC INTEGRITY

Reduction of Risk Potential

Laboratory Values

Recognizes deviations from normal

254. A child is admitted to the hospital with a diagnosis of "rule out meningitis." A spinal tap is performed in the emergency room. It will take 24–48 hours before a culture is grown. Which finding in the spinal fluid indicates a probable bacterial meningitis?

A. Elevated protein

B. Decreased glucose

C. Elevated WBC count

D. Cloudy in appearance

The answer is B. The bacteria feed on the glucose lowering that level.

A, C, and D are incorrect—Elevated protein is usually indicative of a slowing or obstruction of the CSF, and elevated WBCs and cloudy appearance are seen in both types of meningitis.

HEALTH PROMOTION AND MAINTENANCE

Techniques of Physical Assessment

Choose physical assessment equipment and technique appropriate for the client

255. When assessing deep tendon reflexes, when does the nurse use the pointed end of the reflex hammer? Mark all that apply. The nurse uses the pointed end of the reflex hammer to check

A. ___ brachioradialis reflex
B. ___ biceps reflex
C. ___ triceps reflex
D. ___ patellar reflex
E. ___ Achilles reflex
F. ___ cremasteric reflex

The answers are A, B, and C. The brachioradialis reflex located in the forearm above the radial styloid process of the wrist, the biceps reflex located in front of the elbow, and the triceps reflex located just above the elbow on the back of the arm are all checked using the pointed end of the reflex hammer.

D, E, and F are incorrect—The patellar and Achilles reflexes located at the front of the knee and the back of the heel respectively are tested using the broad end of the reflex hammer. The cremasteric reflex is a superficial reflex, which causes elevation of one side of the testicle in response to stroking the thigh on that side. The handle of the reflex hammer is used to stroke the thigh.

PHYSIOLOGICAL INTEGRITY

Reduction of Risk Potential

Laboratory Values

Provide the client with information about the purpose and procedure of prescribed laboratory tests

256. Which instruction should the nurse give to a client who is to be scheduled for blood work, which includes measures of cholesterol?
   A. Do not drink alcohol for at least 24 hours before the test.
   B. Fast for 8 hours before the test.
   C. Drink at least 4 large glasses of water the evening before the test.
   D. Avoid fatty foods for 2 days before the test.

The answer is A. Alcohol should be avoided before the test.

B, C, and D are incorrect—Fasting is necessary for 9–12 hours before the test. There is no requirement regarding fluid intake or avoidance of fatty foods.

PHYSIOLOGICAL INTEGRITY

Reduction of Risk Potential

Potential for Complications of Diagnostic Tests/Treatments/Procedures

Apply knowledge of nursing procedures and psychomotor skills when caring for a client with potential for complications

257. A 72-year-old client is scheduled for a CT scan with contrast media. Prior to the test, the nurse checks to ascertain that which laboratory tests have been done?
   Mark all that apply.
   A. ___ Urinalysis
   B. ___ Fasting blood sugar
   C. ___ BUN
   D. ___ Aspartate aminotransferase (AST)
   E. ___ Alanine aminotransferase (ALT)
   F. ___ Creatinine

The answers are C and F. BUN and creatinine are tests of kidney function. Because contrast media is excreted through the kidneys, clients undergoing CT scans using contrast media need adequate kidney function. Because older clients are at risk for decreased renal function, those over age 60 have BUN and creatinine assessed prior to a test using contrast media.

Abnormal urinalysis, blood sugar (FBS), or liver function tests (AST, ALT) do not typically prevent a patient from having a CT scan.

PHYSIOLOGICAL INTEGRITY

Physiological Adaptation

Illness Management

Teach client about managing illness

258. Which instructions should be given to the client with gout?
   (Mark all that apply.)
   A. "Do not drink red wine or other alcohol."
   B. "Drink a lot of nonalcoholic fluids."
   C. "Decrease intake of foods high in purine."
   D. "Increase intake of foods high in calcium."
   E. "Reduce intake of salt."

The answers are A, B, and C. Clients with gout need to limit intake of high purine foods such as scallops, sadines, gravies, and cream sauces. Alcohol especially red wine should be avoided. Fluid intake should be increased to aid renal filtration of uric acid from the blood.

D and E are incorrect—Calcium does not need to be increased and salt does not need to be restricted.

PSYCHOSOCIAL INTEGRITY

Psychopathology

Provide client and family with information about acute and chronic mental illness

259. The nurse is speaking to a group of family members of clients with Alzheimer's disease. Which behaviors would the nurse identify as characteristic of Stage 2 Alzheimer's disease?

A. Progressive impairment primarily of short term memory
B. Difficulties with house keeping and cooking
C. Agitated movements and speech
D. Confabulation
E. Expressions of concern over loss of mental capacity

The answers are A, B, and D. Stage 2 of Alzheimer's disease is the stage of confusion. In this stage there is a progressive loss of memory with short term memory being most impaired. There is difficulty with the Instrumental Activities of Daily Living including house cleaning and cooking. Confabulation and stereotyped speech word usage occurs to cover up for memory loss. Agitation is a characteristic of stage 3 Alzheimer's disease which is ambulatory dementia. Expressions or awareness of the problem and concerns over mental abilities occur in Stage 1 which is the Stage of forgetfulness.

PHYSIOLOGIC INTEGRITY

Reduction of Risk Potential

Potential for Complications of Diagnostic Tests/ Treatments/Procedures

Implement measures to manage/prevent/lessen possible complications of client condition and/or procedure

260. When preparing to care for a client returning from surgery after a left lower extremity amputation, which piece of equipment is most critical to obtain for the bedside?
A. Traction set up
B. Alternating pressure mattress
C. Tourniquet
D. Wire cutters

The answer is C. If hemorrhage occurs, a tourniquet must be immediately applied and therefore is kept at the bedside.

A is incorrect—Traction is used for a variety of orthopedic conditions including fractures and low back pain. B is incorrect—An alternating pressure mattress is used to prevent or manage skin breakdown. D is incorrect—Wire cutters are needed at the bedside of clients who have wired jaws.

HEALTH PROMOTION AND MAINTENANCE

Ante-/Intra-/Postpartum and Newborn Care

Provide newborn care

261. A newborn is admitted to the newborn nursery. Initial assessment findings are axillary, temperature 97°F, pulse 128, and respirations 33. Based on these findings, the nurse would delay which normal admission activity?
A. Bath newborn and shampoo hair.
B. Complete a head to toe assessment.
C. Feed the infant 1 ounce or less of glucose water.
D. Place in an overbed warmer for easy observation.

The answer is A. Bathing a newborn with a low temperature will further lower the infant's temperature and put the infant in cold stress. All other responses are correct.

PHYSIOLOGICAL INTEGRITY

Basic Care and Comfort

Nutrition and Oral Hydration

Evaluate and monitor client height and weight

262. A 2-month-old infant was admitted for poor weight gain and frequent vomiting. The child is diagnosed with gastroesophageal reflux. Nursing interventions are implemented to reduce the vomiting. The nurse will know the interventions have been successful when:
A. urine output increases.
B. the infant is discharged home.
C. the child shows daily weight gain.
D. the mother says she is comfortable feeding her infant.

The answer is C. Weight gain is the best indication that sufficient food is being retained.

A is incorrect—Urine output may or may not increase. B is incorrect—Discharge home does not indicate the problem is totally solved. D is incorrect—This is a physical problem for the child, not the mother.

PHYSIOLOGICAL INTEGRITY

Physiological Adaptation

Alterations in Body Systems

Promote client wound healing

263. A client has been admitted to the hospital unit for stasis venous ulcers. Nursing care for this client would include:
A. doing Burger-Allen exercises.
B. providing bedrest with legs in a dependent position.
C. placing a foot board on the bed.
D. placing the client in a high fowlers position.

The answer is C. This keeps pressure off of the ulcer.

A is incorrect—Burger-Allen Exercises are done for Buerger's disease. B is incorrect—Keeping legs in a dependent position increases edema. D is incorrect—High Fowlers position increases pressure and kinking on the vascular system.

HEALTH PROMOTION AND MAINTENANCE

Techniques of Physical Assessment

Perform comprehensive health assessment

264. Which lung sound if auscultated over point G in the diagram would be evaluated by the nurse as a normal assessment finding?

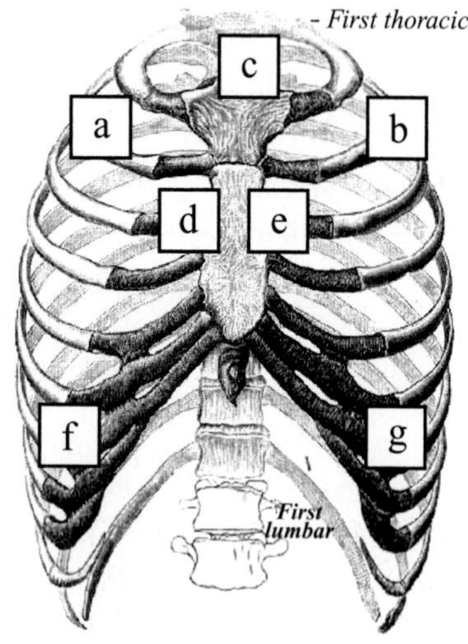

A. Bronchovesicular
B. Crackle
C. Gurgle
D. Sibilant
E. Tracheal
F. Vesicular
G. Wheeze

The answer is F. Vesicular sounds are normally heard over alveolar lung tissue, which is the majority of both lungs including point B. Vesicular sounds are soft in intensity and low in pitch. The inspiratory phase is longer than the expiratory phase.

PHYSIOLOGICAL INTEGRITY

Pharmacological and Parenteral Therapies

Expected effects/outcomes

265. Which class of drug is given to prevent heart failure in the first 24 hours after a myocardial infarction (MI)?
A. Calcium channel blocker
B. ACE inhibitor
C. Beta blocker
D. Digitalis derivative

The answer is B. Ace inhibitors prevent conversion of angiotensin I to angiotensin II.

A is incorrect—Calcium channel blockers cause coronary and peripheral vasoconstriction. C is incorrect—Beta blockers reduce heart rate and contractility. D is incorrect—Digitalis slows the heart and increases the force of contraction.

PHYSIOLOGICAL INTEGRITY

Pharmacological and Parenteral Therapies

Adverse Effects/Contraindications and Side Effects

Implement procedures to counteract adverse effects of medications and parenteral therapy

266. A client who is in the cardiac care unit complains of mediastinal chest pain, dyspnea, and anxiety. The nurse gives the client a nitroglycerine tablet sublingual. The client now complains of being dizzy. Which of the following nursing interventions should the nurse do first?
A. Get a 12 lead ECG.
B. Raise the side rails on the bed.
C. Open the D5W IV to 100 cc per hour.
D. Take the client's vital sign including pulse oximetry.

The answer is B. Safety is the priority.

Option C would not be correct because it is not an isotonic solution and would not help to maintain circulating volume. Option A would be done but would not be the priority. Option D is not indicated as a priority.

PHYSIOLOGICAL INTEGRITY

Pharmacological and Parenteral Therapies

Pharmacological Agents/Actions

Use clinical decision making/critical thinking when addressing actions of prescribed pharmacological agents on clients

267. A client with atrial fibrillation is receiving warfarin (Coumadin) 5 mg each day. His INR today is 1.8. What is the expected decision regarding change in medication dosage?
A. His INR is too low. His warfarin dose needs to be increased.
B. His INR is too high. His warfarin dose needs to be decreased.
C. His INR is too high. His warfarin dose needs to be increased.
D. His INR is within desired range. No change is warfarin dose is needed.

The answer is A. Target INR for clients with afib is 2.0–3.0. This client's INR is below this range so it would be expected that the dose of warfarin would be increased.

B and C are incorrect—The client's INR is not too low or high. D is incorrect—The INR is not within desired range.

SAFE AND EFFECTIVE CARE ENVIRONMENTS

Safety and Infection Control

Ergonomic Principles

Use ergonomic principles when providing care

268. While assisting a client to perform activities of daily living, how can the nurse best enhance his/her balance?
    A. By spreading his/her feet a comfortable distance.
    B. By stretching the thoracic cavity by taking deep breaths.
    C. By performing the activity(ies) to the level the client can tolerate without experiencing adverse effects.
    D. By exerting pressure against a solid object.

The answer is A. By spreading his/her feet a comfortable distance. Balance is achieved when there is a low center of gravity over a wide stable base of support.

B, C, and D are incorrect—Stretching the thorax will have no effect on balance; maintaining equilibrium responds to various head movements. Activity tolerance is performed to the level the individual can tolerate the activity, but this does not impact the nurse's balance. Isometric exercises involves exerting pressure against a solid object.

PHYSIOLOGICAL INTEGRITY

Physiological Adaptation

Illness Management

Plan nursing care based on assessment findings

269. A 4-year-old child was diagnosed with hydrocephaly shortly after birth and had a ventricular-peritoneal shunt inserted. The child has started vomiting and complaining of headaches in the morning but is well the rest of the day. Which problem would the nurse suspect?
    A. Meningitis
    B. Gastroenteritis
    C. Malfunctioning shunt
    D. The development of a brain tumor

The answer is C. The symptoms are those of increased intracranial pressure. Early morning vomiting and headaches are common. While the child is asleep at night, blood increases the intracranial contents causing symptoms. The other responses would not be early morning only symptoms.

PHYSIOLOGIC INTEGRITY

Reduction of Risk Potential

Potential for Complications from Surgical Procedures and Health Alterations

Apply knowledge of pathophysiology to monitoring for complications

270. Your patient is an 80-year-old female who is 4 hours postoperative from a right total hip replacement and is experiencing urinary retention. What is the most likely cause of this problem?
    A. Decreased renal blood flow
    B. Decreased bladder muscle tone
    C. Urethral edema
    D. Benign prostatic hypertrophy.

The answer is B. Decreased bladder tone will result in urinary retention.

A is incorrect—Decreased renal blood flow is incorrect because this would result in decreased production of urine (anuria or oliguria) not urinary retention, which refers to the inability to empty urine from the bladder. C is incorrect—Urethral edema is unlikely because the surgery does not involve manipulation of the urethra or any adjacent tissues. D is incorrect—Benign prostatic hypertrophy is incorrect because the patient is female.

HEALTH PROMOTION AND MAINTENANCE

Techniques of Physical Assessment

Perform comprehensive health assessment

271. Which lung sound if auscultated over point C in the diagram would be evaluated by the nurse as a normal assessment finding?

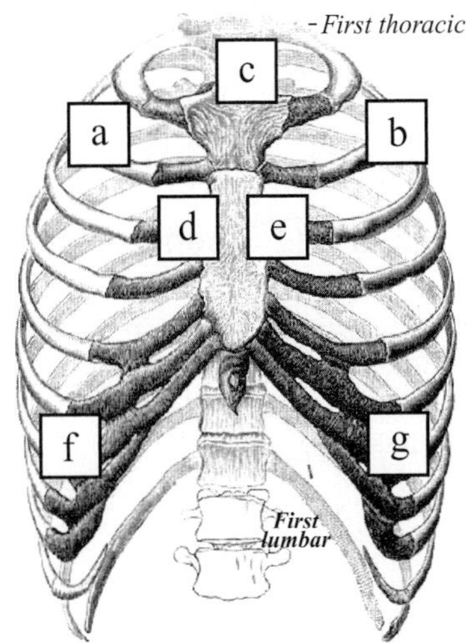

A. Bronchovesicular
B. Crackle
C. Gurgle
D. Sibilant
E. Tracheal
F. Vesicular
G. Wheeze

The answer is E. Tracheal sounds are normally heard over the trachea, which lies below point B. Tracheal sounds are very loud and high pitched rather like the sound made by blowing through the cardboard tube found at the center of a roll of paper towels. The expiratory phase is longer than the inspiratory phase.

PHYSIOLOGICAL INTEGRITY

Physiological Adaptation

Illness Management

Implement interventions to manage the client recovering from an illness

272. Which interventions would appropriately be included in the care plan of a client experiencing an acute episode of rheumatoid arthritis? (Mark all that apply.)
A. ___ Keep affected joints splinted for rest.
B. ___ Apply ice packs to affected joints.
C. ___ Maintain affected joints in a neutral, functional position.
D. ___ Assist the client to weight bear on affected joints for at least 15 minutes tid.
E. ___ Use heat to relieve pain.

The answers are A, B, and C. Ice helps reduce inflammation and relieve pain during acute episodes; heat is used to relax muscles and relieve pain at other times. During acute episodes affected joints are splinted for rest, are not exercised, are used to bear weight nor placed in a hyperextended position.

PHYSIOLOGICAL INTEGRITY

Pharmacological and Parenteral Therapies

273. A client is receiving vancomycin intravenously when the nurse notices the client's neck and face becoming red. The immediate response by the nurse should be to:
A. notify the physician
B. stop the infusion
C. administer benadryl
D. do nothing since this is a common reaction to vancomycin

The answer is B. The nurse would stop the infusion, then notify the physician who would order Benadryl. Once Benadryl has been administered and the flushing disappears, the antibiotic can be restarted, but at a slower rate. This reaction is called Red Man's syndrome and can be fatal if appropriate interventions do not occur.

PHYSIOLOGICAL INTEGRITY

Pharmacological and Parenteral Therapies

Indentify Pharmacological interactions

Educate the client/family about medications

274. Instructions given to a client taking which medication would include the need to keep the amount of green leafy vegetables eaten steady from day to day?
A. Heparin
B. Warfarin sodium
C. Lovastatin
D. Digoxin

The answer is B. Warfarin sodium exerts its anticoagulant effect through interference with the use of vitamin K for clotting. Green leafy vegetables are a major dietary source of vitamin K. If a person varies the amounts of green leafy vegetables in the diet significantly, the dosage of warfarin will be incorrect—either too much or too little depending on whether the client has increased or decreased intake of the green leafy vegetables. For correct dosage of warfarin amounts of vitamin K need to be stable and so dietary intake needs to be stable.

A, C, and D are incorrect—Green leafy vegetables do not impact the effect of heparin, lovastatin, or digoxin.

PSYCHOSOCIAL INTEGRITY

Behavioral Interventions

Assess client appearance, mood, and psychomotor behavior and identify/respond to inappropriate/abnormal behavior.

275. Which is a priority nursing intervention for a client with borderline personality disorder?
A. Encourage acceptance of intensive therapy.
B. Eliminate bizarre fantasies.
C. Facilitate social relationships
D. Promote verbalization of feelings about self.

The answer is D. Promoting verbalization of feelings about self is important in an attempt to gain insight for clients with borderline personality disorder. These clients have a poor and unstable self image and sense of self. They have overwhelming feelings of aloneness, emptiness and rage which is often manifested as self abusive behavior such as head banging, skin scratching, substance abuse, and suicide gestures and attempts. Relationships are typically unstable.

Clients with borderline personality disorder are dependent and needy and tend to seek help readily. Bizarre fantasies are not a prominent component of this disorder and facilitation of social relationships is not a priority need.

PHYSIOLOGICAL INTEGRITY

Pharmacological and Parenteral Therapies

Pharmacological Agents/Actions

Identify a contradiction to the administration of a prescribed or over-the-counter preparation to the client

276. You are reviewing the medications taken by a client who is going to be scheduled for surgery. You note that one baby aspirin is taken each day. When asked if the medications listed are all that he takes, the client says "Oh, I also take two garlic pills because I heard garlic was good for me." What should the nurse instruct the patient to do?
    A. Continue to take all of your medication including the garlic pill.
    B. Discontinue taking the garlic pill and continue all other medication.
    C. Discontinue taking the baby aspirin and continue all other medication.
    D. Discontinue taking both the baby aspirin and garlic pill now

The answer is D. Both the garlic pill and aspirin inhibit platelet aggregation and prolong bleeding.

A, B, and C are incorrect because the client is only told to stop either taking the garlic or aspirin.

HEALTH PROMOTION AND MAINTENANCE

Growth and Development

Assist client/family to identify/participate in activities fitting his/her age, preference, physical capacity, and psychosocial/behavior/physical development

277. The parents bring their 2-month-old to the clinic for a well baby check-up. The mother asks how they should start the baby on solid foods. Which information should be included in the nurse's response?
    A. It is too early to start solid foods.
    B. Rice cereal will be the first food added to the diet.
    C. Start with baby desserts as the baby will not spit that out.
    D. The solids can be put in the bottle with the milk in the beginning.

The answer is B.

A is incorrect—The parents did not ask when to start solids but how to start solids. C is incorrect—Desserts are not necessary and promote a "sweet tooth." D is incorrect—If the infant should need to take medication, it will be from a spoon and this new skill will not be learned if the solids are put in the bottle.

PHYSIOLOGICAL INTEGRITY

Pharmacological and Parenteral Therapies

Medication Administration

Instruct the client on medication self-administration procedures

278. Which client statement indicates understanding of the correct use of nitroglycerine paste?
    A. "I will decide on a convenient site for the medicine and use it consistently."
    B. "I will make sure I have medicine on 24 hours per day."
    C. "I will wipe the skin with alcohol before I put the paste on."
    D. "I will make sure to keep enough paste on hand because it is dangerous to just stop it."

The answer is D. Use of nitroglycerine paste is tapered off at the direction of the prescriber; it is not abruptly stopped.

A is incorrect—Sites need to be rotated to avoid skin irritation. B is incorrect—The medication is not used 24 hours per day; there needs to be a period each day when the medication is not used. This is typically 8 hours out of every 24. C is incorrect—Skin should not be shaved nor should alcohol be applied prior to application of the paste because of irritation and possible breaks in the skin, which allows for increased absorption of medication.

HEALTH PROMOTION AND MAINTENANCE

Techniques of Physical Assessment

Perform comprehensive health assessment

279. Which cranial nerve is being tested when the nurse asks the client to smile, frown, grimace, show the upper and lower teeth, keep the eyes closed while the examiner tries to open them and puff out the cheeks?
    A. One (olfactory)
    B. Five (trigeminal)
    C. Seven (facial)
    D. Eleven (spinal accessory)

The answer is C. Cranial nerve seven (facial nerve) is responsible for taste on the front two thirds of the tongue and for movement of the face including the ability to close the eyes and move the lips for speech. Motor function of cranial nerve seven is tested by asking the client to smile, frown, grimace, show the upper and lower teeth, keep the eyes closed, while the examiner tries to open them and puff out the cheeks. The examiner observes for symmetry and movement and presses the puffed out cheeks in to check if air is expelled equally from both sides. To test taste, an applicator dipped in a sugar, salt, or lemon solution is placed on the tongue and the client is asked what is tasted.

A is incorrect—Cranial nerve one (olfactory nerve) is responsible for the sense of smell. It is tested by occluding each of the client's nostrils one at a time, holding a substance such as coffee or vanilla with a familiar aroma under the other nostril, and asking the client to identify the smell. The test is repeated with a different aromatic substance to determine if the client can differentiate smells.

B is incorrect—Cranial nerve five (trigeminal nerve) has both motor and sensory components. It is responsible for sensation in the face, scalp, oral and nasal mucous membranes, and the cornea and allows chewing movements of the jaw. Its three-part sensory division is tested by touching the forehead, cheek, and chin on each side with a wisp of cotton and asking the client whose eyes are closed to identify the type of touch and its location. Next the cornea of each is lightly touched with a wisp of cotton brought in from the side and the eye observed for the normal blink response. The motor function of cranial nerve five is tested by asking the client to clench the teeth and keep them clenched while the examiner pushes down on the chin to try and separate the jaws.

D is incorrect—Cranial nerve eleven (spinal accessory) is tested by asking the client to shrug the shoulders and resist pressure to put them down because this cranial nerve controls muscular strength of the trapezius and sternocleidomastoid muscles.

PHYSIOLOGICAL INTEGRITY

Physiological Adaptation

Infectious Disease

Recognize signs and symptoms of infectious diseases

280. The nurse is assessing an infant in the newborn nursery. Which finding requires intervention?
    A. Milia on the nose
    B. Breasts are heavily engorged.
    C. Erythema toxicum on the trunk
    D. White adherent patches on the tongue

The answer is D. White patches are a sign of a candida infection called thrush. This must be reported to the physician so that a fungicide can be ordered.

A, B, and C are normal findings. Milia are white epidermal cysts that disappear on their own. Breast engorgement is normal and due to maternal hormones. Erythema toxicum or newborn rash is common and requires no intervention.

PHYSIOLOGICAL INTEGRITY

Reduction in Risk Potential

Laboratory Values

Recognize deviations from normal for values of WBC

281. How should the nurse interpret a laboratory report of "WBC 15,000; segmented neutrophils 50%"?
    A. Severe bacterial infection
    B. Low- to moderate-grade bacterial infection
    C. Viral infection
    D. No infection

The answer is B. WBC count is elevated but segs are normal. This indicates nonsevere bacterial infection. Severe infection is indicated by an elevated WBC with elevated band neutrophils. Viral infection is indicated by a normal WBC and elevated lymphocytes. No infection is indicated by a normal WBC with normal segs.

HEALTH PROMOTION AND MAINTENANCE

Techniques of Physical Assessment

Perform comprehensive health assessment

282. The nurse checks radial deviation as a part of the range of motion assessment of which joint (s) ?
    A. Cervical spine
    B. Elbow
    C. Wrist
    D. Ankle

The answer is C. Radial deviation occurs at the wrist and allows the hand to be pointed toward the side with the thumb and the radial artery. Other movements of the wrist are ulnar deviation in which the hand is pointed toward the side with the fifth or little finger and the ulnar artery.

PHYSIOLOGICAL INTEGRITY

Physiological Adaptation

Infectious Diseases

Apply knowledge of client pathophysiology when managing infectious disease

283. Which assessment findings would the nurse expect when caring for a client in the preicteric phase of hepatitis? Mark all that apply.
    A. ___ Anorexia
    B. ___ Scleral jaundice

C. ___ Fatigue
D. ___ Liver tenderness
E. ___ Headache
F. ___ Weight loss
G. ___ Vomiting

The answers are A, C, and E. Anorexia, headache, and fatigue are symptoms of the preicteric phase of hepatitis. Any jaundice, liver tenderness and weight loss are characteristic of the icteric phase. In the posticteric phase, the client begins to improve and anorexia lessens and jaundice begins to disappear.

PHYSIOLOGICAL INTEGRITY

Reduction of Risk Potential

Diagnostic Tests

Evaluate the results of diagnostic testing and intervene as needed

284. The nurse would interpret a PaO_2 value of less than how many mmHg as indicating hypoxemia? Record your answer using a whole number.

The answer is 70.

PHYSIOLOGICAL INTEGRITY

Physiological Adaptation

Illness Management

Teach the client about managing illness

285. Which statement made by a client who has a fractured hip indicates the need for additional teaching about required activity restrictions?
A. "I can't fully extend my leg at the hip for one month."
B. "I won't be able to cross my knees for up to 8 weeks."
C. "I can't put weight on the affected leg until my doctor says to."
D. "I can flex my hip but not more than 90 degrees for up to 2 months.

The answer is A. There is no restriction on extending the leg so if the client says she is not allowed to fully extend her leg for a month it means that she has misunderstood her self-care instructions.

B is incorrect—Adduction past the midline must be avoided for up to 2 months so the knees cannot be crossed for 2 months. C is incorrect—Weight bearing is restricted and doctor's orders regarding extent of restriction need to be followed. D is incorrect—Hip flexion of more than 90 degrees must be avoided for up to 2 months.

HEALTH PROMOTION AND MAINTENANCE

Growth and Development

Identify and report deviations from expected growth and development

286. When assessing the anterior fontanel, the nurse would interpret it as an abnormal finding requiring follow up if it was not closed in a child of which age?
A. Six months
B. Nine months
C. One year
D. Two years

The answer is D. It would be an abnormal finding if the anterior fontanel was not closed by age 2 years. The posterior fontanel is smaller and closes earlier.

PHYSIOLOGICAL INTEGRITY

Pharmacological and Parenteral Therapies

Medication Administration

Use the six "rights" when administering client medications

287. A 0.7-mL oral dose of liquid medication is ordered for an infant. In which device should the nurse measure the dose for administration?
A. 2 mL syringe
B. Tuberculin syringe
C. Infant teaspoon
D. Medicine cup

The answer is B. A tuberculin syringe allows accurate measurement of tenths of millimeters and so a dose of seven tenths of a milliliter can be obtained.

A, C, and D are incorrect—A 2-mL syringe is marked off in two tenths of a milliliter increments and so seven tenths cannot be accurately measured and for an infant very small extra amounts of drug have the potential to cause serious effects. Neither an infant teaspoon nor a medicine cup allow accurate measurement of tenths of millimeters.

PHYSIOLOGIC INTEGRITY

Reduction of Risk Potential

Potential for Complications of Diagnostic Tests/Treatments/Procedures

Implement measures to manage/prevent/lessen possible complications of client condition and/or procedure

288. Which postoperative exercise is best used to prevent deep vein thrombosis in postoperative clients?

A. Deep knee bends
B. Straight leg lifts
C. Side leg lifts
D. Forward lunges

The answer is B. Straight leg lifts exercise the muscle similar to walking to maintain normal blood flow to and from the lower extremity.

A, C, and D are incorrect. These exercises cannot normally be performed immediately following surgical procedures and require movement that may not be appropriate for all clients.

SAFE AND EFFECTIVE ENVIRONMENT

Management of Care

Establishing Priorities

Assess/triage the client to prioritize the order of care delivery

289. The nurse obtains the following vital signs on a client who has just been admitted to the unit. BP 162/84, pulse 100 and irregular, respirations 16, and pulse oximetry 88%. Which would be the immediate nursing intervention?
A. Place the client on cardiac telemetry.
B. Call the physician to report the vital signs.
C. Start a saline lock for IV medication access.
D. Start oxygen at 2–4 L per minute per nasal cannula per protocol.

The answer is D. The client's oxygen level is very low. All other interventions would be done later.

PHYSIOLOGICAL INTEGRITY

Physiological Adaptation

Illness Management

Teach the client about managing illness

290. Which statement made by the mother of a child with muscular dystrophy indicates a need for further teaching about the disease?
A. "I cannot believe that my son inherited this terrible disease."
B. "I'm going to try to see that my son has the best life possible even though it will be short."
C. "If intellectual impairment was not always a part of the disease, it would be easier to deal with."
D. "It will be very hard watching as the muscle wasting and loss of function occur."

Option C indicates a misunderstanding. Intellectual impairment occurs with a few forms of MD but not with all so the mother believing that intellectual impairment is always a part of the disease indicates a misunderstanding and therefore further teaching is needed.

The other statements are correct—Muscular dystrophy is an inherited disorder, with a shortened life expectancy. Muscle wasting, weakness, and loss of function are characteristic of muscular dystrophy.

HEALTH PROMOTION AND MAINTENANCE

Techniques of Physical Assessment

Perform comprehensive health assessment

291. When assessing the temporomandibular joint, where does the nurse palpate as the client is asked to clench the teeth and move the jaw?
A. In front of the ear
B. Behind the mastoid process
C. Just beneath the occipital lymph nodes
D. Over the insertion of the sternocleidomastoid muscle

The answer is A. The nurse palpates in front of the ear as the client clenches his/her teeth and moves the jaw. The temporomandibular joint is the junction of the temporal and mandibular bones in front of each ear and allows movement of the jaw.

PHYSIOLOGICAL INTEGRITY

Reduction of Risk Potential

Illness Management

Interpret client data that needs to be reported immediately

292. Which symptom reported in the health history of a 45-year-old man should be interpreted by the nurse as requiring immediate follow-up evaluation for possible upper GI bleeding?
A. Black, tarry stools
B. Loose, frothy stool
C. Flat, ribbon-shaped stool
D. Mahogany colored, formed stool

The answer is A. Black, tarry stools are indicative of blood from the upper GI tract, which has been in the GI tract long enough to be completely digested.

B is incorrect—Loose, frothy stool is indicative of high fat content and is associated with malabsorptive disorders. C is incorrect—Flat, ribbon shaped stool is consistent with a tumor, which alters the shape of the left colon and prevents formation and passage of normally formed stool. D is incorrect—Mahogany colored stool is a symptom of right-sided cancer of the colon. It results from the mixing of blood from the tumor with the stool and its exposure to digestive tract secretions as it progresses through the remaining colon.

PHYSIOLOGICAL INTEGRITY

Reduction in Risk Potential

Vital Signs

Assess vital signs

293. A client is assessed for orthostatic hypotension with blood pressure and pulse taken lying and standing after 3 minutes in the supine position and then after standing for 1 minute. Which sets of blood pressure measurements is indicative of orthostatic hypotension? Mark all that apply.
A. Supine 188/92; standing 164/78
B. Supine 148/84; standing 116/52
C. Supine 132/84; standing 102/50
D. Supine 114/72; standing 90/56

The answers are B and C. A drop of 30 mm Hg or more is indicative of orthostatic hypotension.

PHYSIOLOGIC INTEGRITY

Reduction of Risk Potential

Potential for Complications of Diagnostic Tests/ Treatments/Procedures

Implement measures to manage/prevent/lessen possible complications of client condition and/or procedure

294. Which direction given to a postoperative client will best promote comfort during coughing and deep breathing?
A. Listen to music
B. Practice imagery
C. Watch TV during the exercise
D. Splint the incision with a pillow

The answer is D. Splinting the incisional area prevents stress on the injured area and thereby reduces pain associated with coughing and deep breathing.

A, B, and C are incorrect—Listening to music, practising imagery, and watching TV are good distractors but do not address the actual prevention/limitation of pain that occurs with deep breathing and a forceful cough.

HEALTH PROMOTION AND MAINTENANCE

Techniques of Physical Assessment

Perform comprehensive health assessment

295. What is being assessed when the client is approached from the back and the nurse puts his or her hands on either side of the trachea pushing one side medially while asking the patient to swallow?
A. Patency of the trachea
B. Size and regularity of the thyroid gland
C. Size and movement of the pineal body
D. Elasticity of the cricoid cartilage

The answer is B. The size and regularity of the thyroid gland.

PHYSIOLOGICAL INTEGRITY

Pharmacological and Parenteral Therapies

Medication Administration

Administer and document medications given by common routes

296. When using an oral syringe to administer medications, where should the tip of the syringe be placed?
A. Between the cheek and the gums half way back in the mouth.
B. In the hollow of the mouth under the tongue.
C. One third of the way back on top of the tongue.
D. In the lower back corner of the mouth.

The answer is A. Placing the medication between the cheek and the gums half way back in the mouth helps prevent choking, medication running out of the mouth, or medication being spit out of the mouth. In the other locations these problems are more likely.

PHYSIOLOGICAL INTEGRITY

Physiological Adaptation

Illness Management

Teach the client about managing illness

297. Which statement made by a client indicates a need for further teaching about systemic lupus erythematosis?
A. Exposure to sunlight can exacerbate the disease.
B. Exacerbations are most likely to occur in the spring and summer.
C. Pulmonary function tests are needed annually because of frequent lung involvement.
D. Blood pressure needs monitoring because of the risk of hypertension.

Option C indicates a need for further teaching. Pleuritis can be a symptom of the disease, but monitoring with annual pulmonary function tests is not part of the medical routine. The client stating that pulmonary function tests are needed annually is incorrect and therefore indicates that self-care instructions have been misunderstood and more teaching is needed.

The other statements regarding the disease are correct—Sunlight can exacerbate the disease and exacerbations occur most often in the spring or summer. Clients with systemic lupus erythematosis are at risk for hypertension and therefore blood pressure monitoring is needed.

PHYSIOLOGICAL INTEGRITY

Reduction of Risk Potential

Potential for Complications of Diagnostic Tests/Treatments/Procedures

Implement measures to manage/prevent/lessen possible complications of the client condition and/or procedure

298. The charge nurse is observing another nurse who is inserting a nasogastric tube in a preterm infant. The charge nurse observes the following activities. Which action would the charge nurse correct?
The nurse
A. checks placement by aspirating stomach contents.
B. lubricates the tip of the tube with a water-soluble lubricant.
C. measures the length to be inserted from the tip of the nose to the ear to the sternum.
D. checks placement by inserting 5 mL air while listening over the stomach for the gurgle.

The answer is D. 5 mL of air would be an extremely large amount for the size of the infant. This volume is not necessary to check placement; 1 mL or less will provide adequate air for testing. All other activities are correct.

PHYSIOLOGICAL INTEGRITY

Reduction in Risk Potential

Laboratory Values

Recognize deviations from normal for values of WBC

299. Which results of a CBC (complete blood count) with differential should the nurse interpret as indicating the client has a severe bacterial infection?
A. WBC 8,500; lymphocytes 45%
B. WBC 15,000; segmented neutrophils 50%
C. WBC 25,000; band neutrophils 20%
D. WBC 20,000; segmented neutrophils 58%

The answer is C. With a severe bacterial infection, the total white blood cell count would be above normal. Band neutrophils would be elevated because the body is trying to quickly fight the infection; in fact, so quickly that the neutrophils are being released into the circulation before they are mature cells.

A is incorrect—The WBC count is normal with elevated lymphocytes, indicating viral infection. B is incorrect—WBC count is above normal but segs are normal, thus indicating the infection is not severe. D is incorrect—Although the WBC count is elevated, the segs are still within normal limits, again indicating the infection is not severe.

HEALTH PROMOTION AND MAINTENANCE

Techniques of Physical Assessment

Perform comprehensive health assessment

300. The nurse checks inversion as a part of the range of motion assessment of which joint(s)?
A. Lumbar spine
B. Knee
C. wrist
D. ankle

The answer is D. Movements that are part of the normal range of motion for the ankles are dorsiflexion (foot bent upward with toes pointing at head), plantar flexion (foot pointed downward, abduction, adduction, and eversion (movement of the sole of the foot outward) and inversion (movement of the sole of the foot inward)). Flexion, hyperextension, abduction, and adduction are movements of the knee. Movements at the wrist are flexion, extension, radial deviation, and ulnar deviation.

PHYSIOLOGICAL INTEGRITY

Basic Care and Comfort

Nutrition and Oral Hydration

Evaluate impact of disease/illness on nutritional status of the client

301. What symptom reported in the health history of a underweight teenager indicates the need for careful assessment of nutritional status?
A. Black, tarry stools
B. Loose, frothy stool
C. Flat, ribbon-shaped stool
D. Mahogany colored, formed stool

The answer is B. Loose, frothy stool is indicative of steatorrhea or fat in the stool. Large amounts of fat are expelled in the stool as a result of a variety of malabsorption syndromes. Therefore a report of this symptom would cause the nurse to carefully assess for other signs of malnutrition.

A is incorrect—Black, tarry stools are indicative of blood from the upper GI tract, which has been in the GI tract long enough to be completely digested. C is incorrect—Flat, ribbon shaped stool is consistent with a tumor, which alters the shape of the left colon and prevents formation and passage of normally formed stool. D is incorrect—Mahogany colored stool is a symptom of right-sided cancer of the colon. It results from the mixing of blood from the tumor with the stool and its exposure to digestive tract secretions as it progresses through the remaining colon.

PSYCHOSOCIAL INTEGRITY

Family Dynamics

Assess parental techniques related to discipline

302. The mother of a preschool child tells the child, "If you don't behave, I'll have the nurse give you a shot." The best nurse's response would be to:
   A. ignore the comment as it is obviously not true.
   B. reply, "Oh yes, you better be good while you are here."
   C. wait until the mother leaves the room and then tell the child that this was incorrect.
   D. reply, "Oh, no, I only give shots when the doctor thinks it will make you better."

The answer is D. This response provides the child with information about the nursing function and will reduce fear of the nurses.

A is incorrect—Ignoring the comment does not resolve any problem. B is incorrect—provides incorrect information. C is incorrect—would not help the mother to understand that her comment will make the child afraid of nurses.

PHYSIOLOGICAL INTEGRITY

Pharmacological and Parenteral Therapies

Medication Administration

Instruct the client on medication self-administration procedures

303. Which instruction should the nurse give a client for whom a vaginal cream has been prescribed?
   A. Lie on your left side for about 5 minutes.
   B. Remain supine with hips elevated for 5–10 minutes.
   C. Remove excess medication with soap and water in 15 minutes.
   D. Urinate and wipe front to back in 15–30 minutes.

The answer is B. Remaining supine with hips elevated for 5–10 minutes keeps the medication in place in the vagina where it is needed to exert its effect. If the client stands up immediately, the medication can slide down and out of the vagina.

A, C, and D are incorrect—Clients should lie on the left side following a rectal treatment such as an enema. Instructions regarding washing or urinating are not critical to the self-administration of the medication.

PHYSIOLOGICAL INTEGRITY

Pharmacological and Parenteral Therapies

Expected effects/outcomes

304. Which medication is given preoperatively to decrease gastric and pharyngeal secretions?
   A. Glycopyrrolate (Robinul)
   B. Pentobarbitol sodium
   C. Hydroxyzine hydrochloride (Vistaril)
   D. Lorazepam (Ativan)

The answer is A.

B, C, and D are incorrect— Pentobarbitol sodium is used as an induction agent for anesthesia, hydroxyzine hydrochloride is used to decrease anxiety, and lorazepam is used to provide sedation and impair memory of the perioperative events.

HEALTH PROMOTION AND MAINTENANCE

Developmental Stages and Transitions

Provide education on age-specific growth and development to clients and family

305. An 11-year-old girl is upset. She states her friends are buying bras and their breasts are much larger than hers. She is worried because only one of her breasts is developing and asks the school nurse what is wrong with her. How should the nurse respond? (Mark all that apply.)
   ___ A. Suggest an appointment with an endocrinologist
   ___ B. Explain that development is unique to each individual
   ___ C. Suggest she watch her progress by looking at the Tanner stages of development
   ___ D. Reassure that asymmetrical development is not unusual
   ___ E. Ask her to return weekly so her progress can be monitored

The answers are B, C, and D. Explaining that development is unique to each individual, suggesting she use the Tanner stages of development to watch her progress, and reassuring that asymmetrical development is not unusual are all appropriate responses.

A and E are incorrect—There is no information given to suggest an endocrine consult is needed and asking her to return for weekly monitoring is unnecessary and communicates the idea of a problem.

PHYSIOLOGICAL INTEGRITY

Pharmacological and Parenteral Therapies

Medication Administration

Review pertinent data prior to medication administration

306. For which of the following medications should a patient undergo therapeutic drug monitoring?
   A. Penicillin (antibiotic)
   B. Propranolol (beta-blocker)
   C. Furosemide (diuretic)
   D. Lithium (mood stabilizer)

The answer is D. There is a narrow margin of safety between therapeutic drug effect and drug toxicity with lithium.

A, B, and C are incorrect—There is a wide margin of safety with penicillin, propranolol, and furosemide and so therapeutic drug monitoring is not needed.

PHYSIOLOGICAL INTEGRITY

Physiological Adaptation

Illness Management

Implement interventions to manage the client recovering from an illness

307. Which intervention is inappropriate as part of the emergent treatment of a simple long bone fracture?
   A. Application of cold
   B. Elevating the limb
   C. Splinting above and below the fracture
   D. Application of a pressure bandage

Option D is the inappropriate intervention. A pressure bandage would not be used for a simple fracture.

Other interventions are correct actions—Cold is applied immediately and the limb is elevated not lowered to limit edema. Above and below the fracture is stabilized to prevent movement of the bone segments and further damage.

HEALTH PROMOTION AND MAINTENANCE

Techniques of Physical Assessment

Perform comprehensive health assessment

308. The nurse checks adduction as a part of the range of motion assessment of which joints? Mark all that apply.
   A. ___ Lumbar spine
   B. ___ Knee
   C. ___ Wrist
   D. ___ Ankle
   E. ___ Finger
   F. ___ Toe
   G. ___ Shoulder
   H. ___ Elbow

The answers are D, E, F, and G. The ankle, fingers, toes, and shoulders can all be adducted and abducted. Adduction is movement toward the midline of the body and abduction is away from the midline. When the ankle is adducted, the foot is turned inward toward the other foot; when the ankle is abducted, the foot is turned out to the side away from the other foot. When fingers and toes are adducted they are brought close together; when they are abducted, they are spread apart. When the shoulder is adducted the arm is brought across the body to the opposite side; when abducted the arm is extended out to the side away from the body. Remember ad means to or toward: you send a letter to an address. Ab means away from as when a student is absent or away from class.

PHYSIOLOGICAL INTEGRITY

Pharmacological and Parenteral Therapies

Medication Administration

Instruct the client on medication self-administration procedures

309. Which client statement indicates understanding of the procedure for using a steroid inhaler?
   A. "I will rinse my mouth out with water after using the inhaler."
   B. "I will take 5 to 6 slow deep breaths after each puff on the inhaler."
   C. "I will use my bronchodilator immediately after my steroid inhaler."
   D. "I will blow my nose forcefully after I finish with the inhaler."

The answer is A. Steroid residual in the mouth can lead to Candida overgrowth and infection. Rinsing the mouth out with water after using the inhaler removes residual steroid and can prevent this problem.

B is incorrect—Deep breaths do not have to be taken after using the inhaler. C is incorrect—Bronchodilator inhalers are always used first to open the lung passages so that other medications such as the steroids can get deep into the lung for maximum effect. D is incorrect— Blowing the nose forcefully has no role in the use of a steroid inhaler.

SAFE AND EFFECTIVE CARE ENVIRONMENTS

Safety and Infection Control

Medical and Surgical Asepsis

Use appropriate supplies to maintain asepsis

310. When getting a drainage set for an indwelling catheter, the nurse notices that the bag containing the set is not

entirely sealed at one end. Which is the appropriate action for the nurse to take?

A. Use it but notify purchasing about the condition of the bag.

B. Dispose of it and get another.

C. Use it only if the drainage system appears untouched.

D. Check with the nurse manager on agency policy.

The answer is B. If the protective packaging is not sealed then the equipment is not sterile and it cannot be used. This applies regardless of its appearance. Notifying purchasing or whomever is responsible for equipment can help with quality control. It is not necessary to check on agency policy regarding its use because use of contaminated sterile items places the client at risk for infection and so the decision to not use falls within the scope of ethical, professional decision making of the individual nurse.

PSYCHOSOCIAL INTEGRITY

Behavioral Interventions

Assess client appearance, mood, and psychomotor behavior and identify/respond to inappropriate/abnormal behavior

311. Which is an appropriate nursing intervention for a client diagnosed with schizophrenia?

A. Maintain a slightly higher level of environmental stimuli than usual.

B. Prevent the client from lapsing into periods of silence of longer than 5 minutes.

C. Tell the client if you do not understand what is being communicated.

D. Be warm with a show of positive emotion when interacting with the client.

The answer is C. The nurse should tell the client in a simple, direct manner that he or she is not being understood. Excessive environmental stimuli should be avoided; stimuli should not be increased. Clients may be silent and the nurse should accept this and sit with the client even during periods of silence if necessary. The client should be approached in a neutral manner as it is less threatening to the client than an overly warm approach.

PHYSIOLOGICAL INTEGRITY

Reduction of Risk Potential

Illness Management

Interpret client data that needs to be reported immediately

312. What symptom reported in the health history of a 64-year-old man should be interpreted by the nurse as requiring immediate follow-up evaluation for possible left colon cancer?

A. Black, tarry stools

B. Loose, frothy stool

C. Flat, ribbon-shaped stool

D. Mahogany colored, formed stool

The answer is C. Flat, ribbon shaped stool is consistent with a tumor, which alters the shape of the left colon and prevents formation and passage of normally formed stool.

A is incorrect—Black, tarry stools are indicative of blood from the upper GI tract, which has been in the GI tract long enough to be completely digested. B is incorrect—Loose, frothy stool is indicative of steatorrhea or fat in the stool. Large amounts of fat are expelled in the stool as a result of a variety of malabsorption syndromes. D is incorrect—Mahogany colored stool is a symptom of right-sided cancer of the colon. It results from the mixing of blood from the tumor with the stool and its exposure to digestive tract secretions as it progresses through the remaining colon.

HEALTH PROMOTION AND MAINTENANCE

Techniques of Physical Assessment

Perform comprehensive health assessment

313. When assessing the heart, the nurse palpates for pulsation over the aortic area which would be an abnormal finding. Which lettered block on the accompanying diagram marks the location where the nurse would place his or her finger tips to palpate over the aortic area. Write the letter of the block on the line provided.

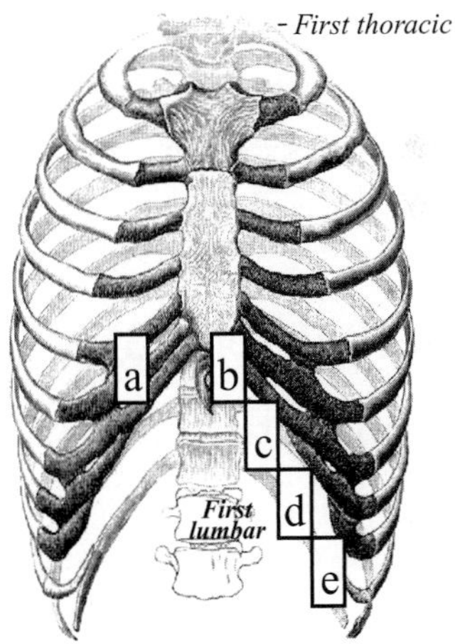

The answer is A.

PHYSIOLOGIC INTEGRITY

Reduction of Risk Potential

Therapeutic Procedures

Assess client response to recovery from local, regional, or general anesthesia

314. An elderly postoperative client has a history of chronic obstructive pulmonary disease. Based on this history,

the nurse is especially concerned with monitoring the client for which problem?
A. Aspiration
B. Delirium
C. Decreased gas exchange
D. Positioning difficulty

The answer is C. Decreased gas exchange is a particular risk with a history of COPD.

A is incorrect—Aspiration would be associated with the age related changes of the gastrointestinal system. B is incorrect—Delirium is associated with the age-related changes of the neurological system. D is incorrect—Positioning difficulty is associated with age related changes of the musculoskseletal system.

HEALTH PROMOTION AND MAINTENANCE

Techniques of Physical Assessment

Choose physical assessment equipment and technique appropriate for the client

315. Which criterion should the nurse use when selecting the proper size cuff to use when assessing the blood pressure of an 8-month-old infant?
The cuff will
A. say infant on the cuff
B. wrap around the arm twice
C. cover 1/4 of the upper extremity.
D. cover 80% of the length of the extremity section

The answer is D. The cuff should cover 80% of the extremity section, if the upper arm is the site, the cuff should cover 80% of the distance from the elbow to the acromian process. Another way to determine size is the bladder should cover 40% of the circumference of the extremity. All other responses are incorrect.

PHYSIOLOGICAL INTEGRITY

Physiological Adaptation

Illness Management

Apply knowledge of client pathophysiology to illness management

316. When assessing a client in the emergency room, which finding should be interpreted as a major indicator of acute pancreatitis?
A. Positive Cullen's sign.
B. Postprandial elevated serum amylase.
C. Decreased pancreatic secretion with secretin stimulation.
D. Midepigastric pain worsened by fasting.

The answer is A. A positive Cullen's sign (cyanosis of the periumbilical skin due to subcutaneous intraperitoneal hemorrhage) is symptomatic of acute disease. Reduced volume of pancreatic secretions on a secretin stimulation test is the most diagnostic measure of chronic disease. Elevated serum amylase is found with both acute and chronic disease. LUQ pain radiating to the back, not mid epigastric pain, is characteristic of acute disease.

PHYSIOLOGICAL INTEGRITY

Basic Care and Comfort

Nutrition and Oral Hydration

Provide/maintain special diets based on the client diagnosis/nutritional needs and cultural considerations

317. Which is the basic type of diet that the nurse would obtain for a client with celiac disease?
A. Fat free
B. Gluten free
C. Lactose free
D. Low sodium

The answer is B. Clients with celiac disease are unable to break down gluten, which is a protein. These clients are treated with a gluten-free diet. This diet excludes products containing wheat, rye, oats and barley since these grains contain gluten.

HEALTH PROMOTION AND MAINTENANCE

Techniques of Physical Assessment

Perform comprehensive health assessment

318. When assessing the heart, the nurse palpates for thrills over the pulmonic area which would be an abnormal finding. Which lettered block on the accompanying diagram marks the location where the nurse would place the ball of the hand to palpate over the pulmonic area. Write the Letter of the block on the line provided.

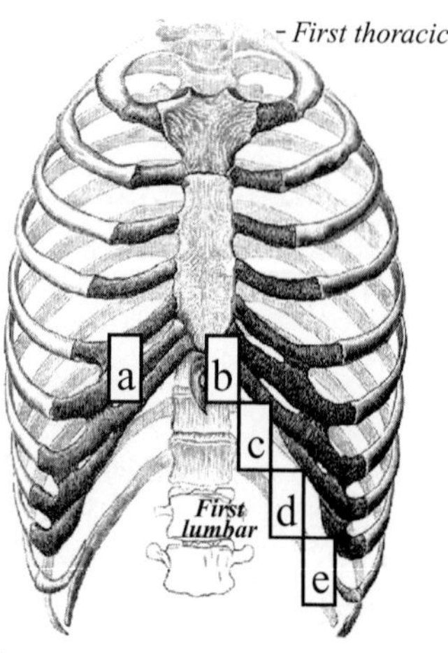

The answer is B.

PHYSIOLOGICAL INTEGRITY

Pharmacological and Parenteral Therapies

Pharmacological Agents and Actions

Apply knowledge of pathophysiology when addressing the pharmacological agents/actions of client prescriptions

319. During discharge teaching, a client asks the nurse how the prescribed antacids relieve heart burn. The nurse's response should be based on the knowledge that antacids work by
A. decreasing the secretion of gastric acid.
B. coating the stomach lining.
C. thickening the mucus secreted by the stomach wall.
D. neutralizing the acid present in the stomach.

The answer is D. Antacids are alkaline and they relieve heartburn by neutralizing the acid in the stomach.

PHYSIOLOGICAL INTEGRITY

Pharmacological and Parenteral Therapies

Pharmacological Agents/Actions

Identify a contraindication to the administration of a prescribed or over-the-counter medication to the client

320. On admission to the emergency room, a client with a traumatic lower extremity amputation is given an opioid for pain. Which herbal medication if taken by the client prior to the accident will prolong the sedative effects of the opioid?
A. Echinacea augustifolia
B. Hypericum perforatum (St. John's Wort)
C. Piper methysticum (Kava-kava)
D. Valeriana officinalis (Valerian)

The answer is B. Hypericum perforatum (St. John's Wort) prolongs the sedative effects of opioids. It also prolongs the sedative effects of anesthesia.

A, C, and D are incorrect—Echinacea augustifolia increases the effectiveness of corticosteroids. Piper methysticum (Kava-kava) potentiates central nervous system depressants, anesthetics, and corticosteroids. Valerian only prolongs the sedative effects of anesthesia.

PHYSIOLOGICAL INTEGRITY

Reduction of Risk Potential

System-Specific Assessment

Assess client for abnormal neurological status

321. The nurse is assessing for diminished deep tendon reflexes in a client with increasing intracranial pressure. Which location on the accompanying diagram would the nurse strike with the reflex hammer to check the biceps reflex?

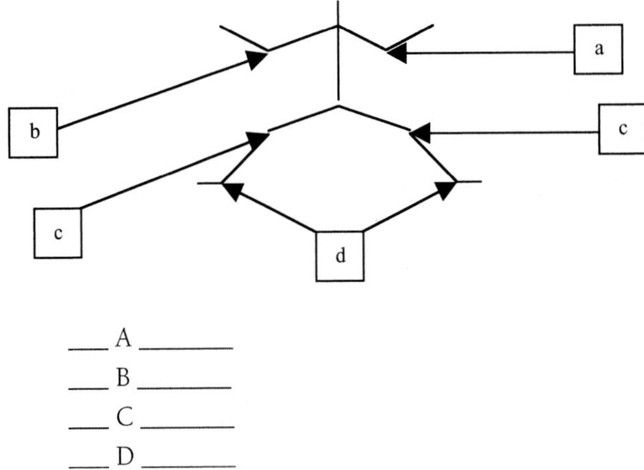

___ A ______
___ B ______
___ C ______
___ D ______

The answer is A. To check the biceps reflex, the examiner's thumb is placed over the biceps tendon located in the antecubital space. The thumb is struck with the pointed end of the reflex hammer. The forearm should flex in response.

Location B denotes the triceps reflex; location C denotes the patellar or knee jerk reflex; location D denotes the Achilles reflex.

HEALTH PROMOTION AND MAINTENANCE

Techniques of Physical Assessment

Perform comprehensive health assessment

322. Which cranial nerve is the nurse assessing when the client's gag reflex is checked?
A. Five (trigeminal)
B. Six (abducens)
C. Nine (glossopharyngeal)
D. Twelve (hypoglossal)

The answer is C. The glossopharyngeal nerve is responsible for the pharyngeal gag reflex as well as for movement of the phonation muscles of the pharynx. It is also responsible for taste on the posterior third of the tongue and sensation from the ear drum and ear canal. The gag reflex is tested by touching the posterior pharyngeal wall with a tongue blade and observing for gagging.

A is incorrect—Cranial nerve five (trigeminal nerve) has both motor and sensory components. It is responsible for sensation in the face, scalp, oral and nasal mucous membranes, and the cornea and allows chewing movements of the jaw. Its three-part sensory division is tested by touching the forehead, cheek, and chin on each side with a wisp of cotton and asking the client whose eyes are closed to identify the type of touch and its location. Next the cornea of each is lightly touched with a wisp of cotton brought in from the side and the eye observed for the normal blink response. The motor function of cranial nerve five is tested by asking the client to clench the teeth and keep them clenched while the examiner pushes down on the chin to try and separate the jaws.

B is incorrect—Cranial nerve six (abducens nerve) is responsible for lateral eye movement.

D is incorrect—Cranial nerve twelve (hypoglossal nerve) is responsible for tongue movement. It is tested by asking the client to stick out the tongue and later having the client say "late date night."

PHYSIOLOGICAL INTEGRITY

Reduction of Risk Potential

Potential for Complications from Surgical Procedures and Health Alterations

Apply knowledge of pathophysiology to monitoring for complications

323. After a difficult delivery, a newborn develops a large cephalohematoma. The nurse will monitor this infant for:
   A. infection
   B. brain damage
   C. hyperbilirubinemia
   D. congestive heart failure

The answer is C. Cephalohematoma is bleeding into the periosteum of the bone. When blood escapes the vascular system, it is broken down. When red blood cells are broken down, bilirubin is released. The immature liver is unable to handle large amounts of bilirubin and jaundice is the result. The nurse will need to monitor the child so early interventions can be instituted to prevent complications from high levels of bilirubin in the blood.

A, B, and D are incorrect—The hematoma is on the outside of the skull and will cause no brain damage. There is no risk of infection or congestive heart failure from this condition.

PHYSIOLOGICAL INTEGRITY

Reduction of Risk Potential

System-specific assessments

324. Which assessment finding should the nurse interpret as abnormal when admitting an infant to the newborn nursery?
   A. Pulse 142
   B. Respirations 38
   C. Head circumference: 29 cm
   D. Chest circumference: 34 cm

The answer is C. Head circumference should exceed the chest circumference and could indicate microcephaly. The other assessment findings are normal.

HEALTH PROMOTION AND MAINTENANCE

Techniques of Physical Assessment

325. When assessing the scrotum of a 64-year-old client, what would be a normal difference as compared to the scrotum of a 24-year-old client?
   The scrotum of the 64-year-old would be
   A. longer
   B. more pendulous
   C. less flexible
   D. more firm

The answer is B. The scrotum becomes more pendulous with age. It does not become longer, less flexible, or more firm.

PHYSIOLOGICAL INTEGRITY

Reduction of Risk Potential

System-Specific Assessment

Assess client for abnormal neurological status

326. The nurse is assessing for diminished deep tendon reflexes in a client with hypothyroidism. Which location on the accompanying diagram would the nurse strike with the reflex hammer to check the triceps reflex?

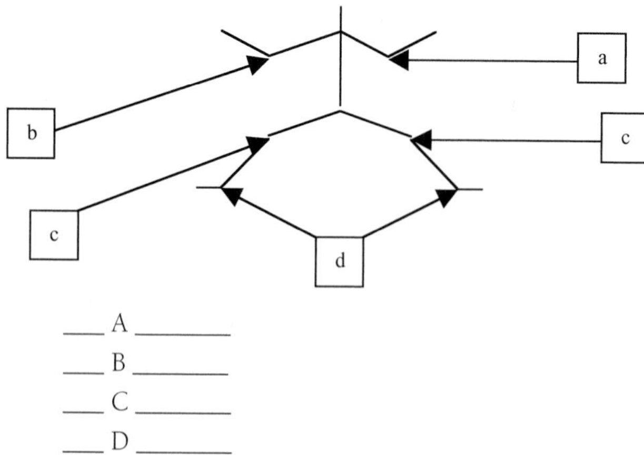

___ A ________
___ B ________
___ C ________
___ D ________

The answer is B. To check the triceps reflex, the client's arm is positioned with the elbow bent and the arm and the forearm and hand relaxed and down. The triceps tendon located just above the elbow on the back of the arm is struck with the pointed end of the reflex hammer. The forearm should extend in response.

Location A denotes the biceps reflex; location C denotes the patellar or knee jerk reflex; location D denotes the Achilles reflex.

PHYSIOLOGIC INTEGRITY

Reduction of Risk Potential

Therapeutic Procedures

Assess client response to recovery from local, regional, or general anesthesia

327. Which of the following is a common postoperative cause of airway obstruction?
    A. Difficult intubation
    B. Facial edema
    C. Po_2 greater than 60 mm Hg
    D. Tongue blocking the airway

The answer is D. The tongue blocking the airway is a risk in the postoperative client who has had general anesthesia.

A is incorrect—Difficult intubation is not a common cause of airway obstruction in postoperative clients; it is most often associated with age-related respiratory system changes in the elderly. B is incorrect—Facial edema does not necessarily cause a blocked airway. C is incorrect—A Po_2 greater than 60 mm Hg is not associated with respiratory difficulty.

PHYSIOLOGICAL INTEGRITY

Reduction of Risk Potential

Therapeutic Procedures

Educate the client and family about treatments and procedures

328. A client having surgery for glaucoma asks the nurse how the doctor will know if the surgery is successful. Which would be an appropriate response for the nurse to make?
    A. IOP will decrease.
    B. Ability to read small print will improve.
    C Pupil will remain permanently dilated.
    D. Peripheral vision will increase.

The answer is A. The reason surgery is done for glaucoma is to lower intraocular pressure because increased IOP causes progressive loss of vision. Surgery is done when medication is ineffective.

B is incorrect—Damage done by increased IOP is permanent therefore ability to read will not improve. C is incorrect—The pupil is not affected by the surgery so contraction and dilation occur normally. D is incorrect—Glaucoma causes loss of peripheral vision before loss of central vision and this loss is irreversible.

HEALTH PROMOTION AND MAINTENANCE

Techniques of Physical Assessment

Perform comprehensive health assessment

329. Which lung sound is auscultated over point A in the diagram would be evaluated by the nurse as a normal assessment finding?

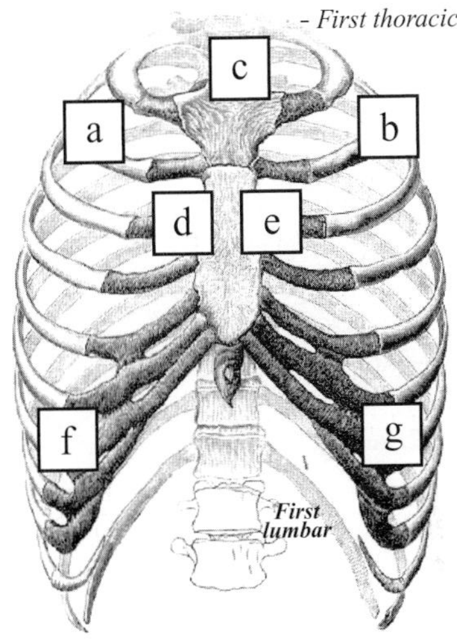

    A. Bronchovesicular
    B. Crackle
    C. Gurgle
    D. Sibilant
    E. Tracheal
    F. Vesicular
    G. Wheeze

The answer is F. Vesicular sounds are normally heard over alveolar lung tissue, which is the majority of both lungs including point A. Vesicular sounds are soft in intensity and low in pitch. The inspiratory phase is longer than the expiratory phase.

PHYSIOLOGICAL INTEGRITY

Physiological Adaptation

Alterations in body systems

330. Six hours after birth, an infant is found to have an axillary temperature of 97°F. The child is placed in an overbed warmer. When the nurse tells the mother that the infant will not be able to leave the nursery at the next feeding, the mother asks why this low temperature is a concern. The nurse explains that low body temperature in the newborn can cause which effects? (Select all that apply.)

A. Hypoglycemia
B. Metabolic acidosis
C. Respiratory distress
D. Hyperbilirubinemia
E. Caput Succedaneum

The answers are A, B, C, and D. Heat loss causes the body to try to produce heat which causes the respiratory rate to rise and can lead to respiratory distress. Metabolic acidosis occurs from the anaerobic burning of fats for energy. Hypoglycemia occurs because the body has burned the glucose to produce heat. All of the stress taxes the liver which is unable to convert the indirect bilirubin to direct bilirubin causing hyperbilirubinemia.

Caput is a swelling of the presenting part and not related to cold stress.

PSYCHOSOCIAL INTEGRITY

Behavioral Interventions

Assess client appearance, mood and psychomotor behavior and identify/respond to inappropriate/abnormal behavior

331. Which is a priority nursing intervention for a client with narcissistic personality disorder?
   A. Encourage acceptance of intensive therapy.
   B. Eliminate bizarre fantasies.
   C. Minimize potential for self harm.
   D. Promote verbalization of feelings about self.

The answer is D. Clients with narcissistic personality disorder are self-centered, independent, not easily intimidated, quite aggressive individuals who lack the ability to be empathetic and hence have difficulties with establishing and maintaining interpersonal relationships. They put forth a sense of grandiosity but underneath have low self esteem, and feel insecure and inadequate. These clients need to be helped to view themselves differently and verbalization of feelings about self is a first step toward this goal. Other responses do not apply to the client with a narcissistic personality disorder.

PHYSIOLOGICAL INTEGRITY

Reduction of Risk Potential

Potential for complications from surgical procedures and health alterations

332. A child is being discharged 18 hours after a tonsillectomy and adenoidectomy. Discharge instructions for the parents would include:
   A. Give the child aspirin for pain
   B. Use a straw to encourage drinking
   C. Offer a soft diet without spicy or acidic foods.
   D. Encourage the child to clear throat and cough frequently to remove secretions

The answer is C. A soft diet is maintained to prevent injury to the surgical area.

A, B, and D are incorrect—Aspirin would increase bleeding and would not be desirable. Drinking through a straw and throat clearing increases pressure and could dislodge a forming clot and cause hemorrhage.

HEALTH PROMOTION AND MAINTENANCE

Techniques of Physical Assessment

Perform comprehensive health assessment

333. Which direction would the nurse give to a client when assessing function of cranial nerve twelve (hypoglossal)?
   A. "Holding your head straight, move only your eyes to look first to the right and then to the left."
   B. "Clench your jaw as tightly shut as you can."
   C. "Stick out your tongue."
   D. "Raise your eyebrows."

The answer is C. Cranial nerve twelve (hypoglossal nerve) is responsible for tongue movement. It is tested by asking the client to stick out the tongue and later having the client say "late date night."

A, B, and D are incorrect—Cranial nerve six (abducens) is responsible for lateral eye movement. Clenching the teeth and keeping the jaw shut while the examiner pushes down on the chin to try and separate the jaws is a test of cranial nerve five (trigeminal nerve). Raising eyebrows along with smiling, frowning, and showing the upper and lower teeth are tests of the motor division of cranial nerve seven (facial nerve).

HEALTH PROMOTION AND MAINTENANCE

Techniques of Physical Assessment

Perform comprehensive health assessment

334. The nurse would assess a client's short-term memory by asking the client:
   A. his/her birth date
   B. to count backwards from 100 to 7
   C. to repeat the phrase "no ifs ands or buts"
   D. about current events

The answer is D. Asking about current events assesses short-term memory.

A is incorrect—Asking about birth date assesses long-term memory. B is incorrect—asking the client to count backwards from 100 by 7s assesses mathematical calculation. C is incorrect—Asking the client to repeat the phrase "no ifs ands or buts" assesses speech.

PHYSIOLOGICAL INTEGRITY

Physiological Adaptation

Illness management

335. When teaching a type II diabetic client about preventing hypoglycemic episodes, which information is appropriate for the nurse to include?
   A. Delaying a meal for as little as 15 minutes can significantly increase the risk of hypoglycemia.
   B. With the onset of menses, insulin requirement may decrease.
   C. Prolonged exercise can precipitate a hypoglycemic episode.
   D. Five grams of CHO raise blood sugar about 30 mg/dL.

The answer is B. With the onset of menses progesterone drops and this may cause a decrease in the need for insulin and so the risk of hypoglycemia is increased.

A, C, and D are incorrect—Delaying a meal for more than a half hour increases the risk of hypoglycemia. Exercise is associated with a drop in blood glucose levels in clients with type I diabetes. Prolonged exercise in these clients can cause increased rate of glucose uptake and use by cells for several hours after the exercise is complete. Thus blood glucose needs to be monitored and CHO supplements taken during exercise. Five grams of CHO raise blood sugar about 20 mg/dL not 30 mg/dL.

SAFE AND EFFECTIVE CARE ENVIRONMENTS

Safety and Infection Control

Ergonomic Principles

Use ergonomic principles when providing care

336. The nurse considers which of the following aspects when performing a client's activity and exercise assessment. Select all that apply:
   A. ___ body alignment and posture
   B. ___ routine exercised patterns
   C. ___ the body's response to activity and exercise
   D. ___ impact of activity and exercise on overall health

The answers are A, B, C, and D. All four aspects are components that necessary to consider to determine a correct nursing diagnosis. Assessment of activity tolerance, physical fitness, body alignment, and mobility are defining characteristics necessary to make a nursing diagnosis.

PHYSIOLOGICAL INTEGRITY

Pharmacological and Parenteral Therapies

Dosage Calculations

Perform calculations needed for medication administration

337. The drug book states that a therapeutic dose for a medication is 50–75 mg per kg of body weight per day. The child weighs 33 pounds and is to receive the medication 4 times a day. What would be the maximum amount of drug the child should receive per dose? Record your answer is a whole number carried out to two decimal places. _____ mg per dose

Answer: 281.25 mg per dose; 33 pounds divided by 2.2 pounds per kilogram = 15 (the child's weight in kilograms); 15 times 75 = 1125 mg per day divided by 4 doses equals 281.25 mg.

PHYSIOLOGICAL INTEGRITY

Reduction of Risk Potential

System-Specific Assessment

Assess client for abnormal neurological status

338. The nurse is assessing for hyperreflexia in a client with preeclampsia. Which location on the accompanying diagram would the nurse strike with the reflex hammer to check the patellar reflex?

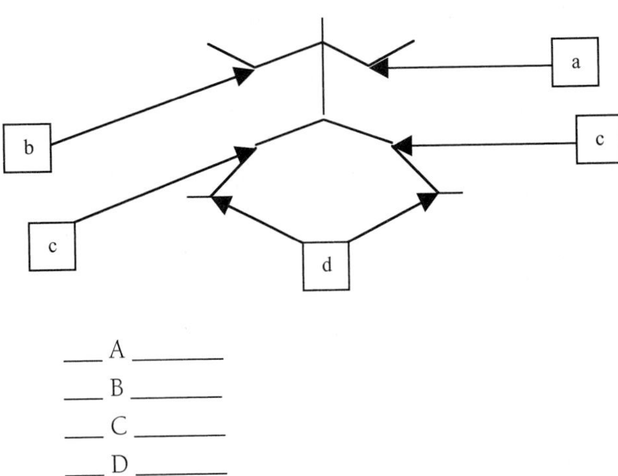

___ A ______
___ B ______
___ C ______
___ D ______

The answer is C. To check the patellar reflex, the client sits with legs dangling. The patellar tendon located just below the patella on the front of the knee is struck with the wide end of the reflex hammer. The lower leg should extend in response. If the client cannot dangle, the knee may be supported by the examiner's nondominant hand in a flexed position while the reflex is checked.

Location A denotes the biceps reflex; location B denotes the triceps reflex; location D denotes the Achilles reflex.

HEALTH PROMOTION AND MAINTENANCE

Health Promotion Programs

Plan and/or, Participate in the Education of Individuals in the Community

Provide the client information about health screening tests

339. A 24-year-old unmarried woman has never had a mammogram. The client states that she has heard that the exam is painful and she is afraid to have one. The nurse's response should be:
    A. "Why don't you have the test once and if it is too painful don't do it again?"
    B. "No, the mammogram is not painful. Whoever told you this was lying to you."
    C. "Yes, it is uncomfortable but it only lasts a few seconds. And the test is so important."
    D. "Since you are not married, it is okay to delay the test until you become sexually active."

The answer is C. Honesty is important when responding to the client. This response will assist the client in seeking health promotion activities.

A is incorrect as if she decides it was too uncomfortable, the nurse has given permission to not follow national guidelines. B and D are incorrect information.

MANAGEMENT OF CARE

Safety and Infection Control

Standard/Transmission-Based/Other Precautions

Apply knowledge of the client pathophysiology to interventions related to standard/transmission based/other precautions

340. A child is being treated for bacterial meningitis. Nursing interventions would include:
    A. forcing fluids.
    B. positioning in Trendelenburg position.
    C. maintaining a brightly lit room to observe for seizures.
    D. maintaining respiratory isolation for 24–48 hours after antibiotics are started.

The answer is D. Although the organism may be a common one (*H. influenzae* or *pneumococci*), other children on the unit must be protected from the infection. Isolation is maintained for at least 24 hours after antibiotics are started.

A is incorrect—Forcing fluids would not be advisable as cerebral edema is a concern. B is incorrect—The child should be positioned in semi-Fowler's position for comfort. C is incorrect—The child has photophobia; so a brightly lit room would not be appropriate.

PHYSIOLOGICAL INTEGRITY

Reduction of Risk Potential

System-Specific Assessment

Perform focused assessment or reassessment

341. Which is a step in the assessment of jugular venous pressure?
    A. Assist the client to a right side lying position.
    B. Raise the head of the bed 10–15 degrees.
    C. Shine a light across the client's neck.
    D. Measure the horizontal distance from the sternal angle to the meniscus of the internal jugular vein.

The answer is C. A light is shone tangentally across the client's neck to highlight the pulsations of the jugular vein. All other steps listed are incorrect. The client is placed in a supine position. The head of the bed is raised 30–45 degrees. The meniscus which is the highest point at which the pulsation of the internal jugular vein can be seen is identified. The sternal angle is located and a centimeter ruler is used to measure the vertical distance from the sternal angle to the meniscus. The number of centimeters, normally not more than 4, equals the jugular venous pressure.

PHYSIOLOGICAL INTEGRITY

Pharmacological and Parenteral Therapies

Parenteral/intravenous therapies

342. A client's parenteral antibiotic therapy has been completed. The physician writes orders to discontinue to IV line and discharge the client home. Which is a step the nurse will take when discontinuing the intravenous line?
    A. Leave the IV site open to the air.
    B. Use sterile gloves for catheter removal.
    C. Remove the catheter and apply an occlusive dressing.
    D. Use alcohol to prevent infection of the site during removal.

The answer is C. An occlusive dressing is recommended following catheter removal. The site should not be left open to the air. Clean gloves, not sterile gloves, are necessary for nurse protection. Alcohol will increase the bleeding at the site. A dry sterile dressing will be applied to the site.

PHYSIOLOGICAL INTEGRITY

Reduction in Risk Potential

Vital Signs

Assess vital signs

343. A client is assessed for orthostatic hypotension with blood pressure and pulse taken lying and standing after 3 minutes in the supine position and then after standing for 1 minute. Which sets of pulse rates is indicative of orthostatic hypotension? Mark all that apply.
   A. Supine 96 beats per minute; standing 54 beats per minute
   B. Supine 88 beats per minute; standing 62 beats per minute
   C. Supine 84 beats per minute; standing 70 beats per minute
   D. Supine 80 beats per minute; standing 50 beats per minute

The answer is A. A drop of 40 beats per minute or more in pulse rate is indicative of orthostatic hypotension.

HEALTH PROMOTION AND MAINTENANCE

Health Promotion Programs

Instruct the client on ways to promote health

344. A female client is being taught self-breast exam. Which information should the nurse include in the instructions?
   A. The nipple area should be avoided in palpating the breast.
   B. Breast exams are best performed immediately prior to menses.
   C. Self-breast exams are performed in the upright and supine positions.
   D. Should a lump be found, make an appointment for a professional examination if it hasn't disappeared in a month.

The answer is C. Supine and upright positions are used while palpating the breast.

A is incorrect—The entire breast including the nipple region should be palpated. B is incorrect—The best time for self-breast exam is immediately after their menstrual period as the hormonal influence will be at the minimal. D is incorrect—If a lump is found, a medical appointment should be made immediately.

PHYSIOLOGICAL INTEGRITY

Pharmacological and Parenteral Therapies

Applies knowledge of intravenous therapy to the care of client

345. A child is admitted to the hospital with gastroenteritis. The physician orders $D_5$1/4 NS with 20 mEq KCL per 1000 ml to be administered at a rate of 50 ml per hour. The appropriate nursing action for this order would be to
   A. delay adding the KCL until the child has voided.
   B. ask why the physician didn't include other electrolytes.
   C. question the physician why a hypertonic solution was ordered.
   D. monitor the child for fluid volume overload because of the fast rate.

The answer is A. Potassium would not be added until the child has voided. Hyperkalemia would occur if kidney function was impaired resulting in cardiac dysfunction.

The other responses are incorrect. Fluid replacement is the main concern in gastroenteritis, the fluid is hypotonic and the rate is not excessive.

PHYSIOLOGICAL INTEGRITY

Basic Care and Comfort

Mobility/Immobility

Apply knowledge of nursing procedures and psychomotor skills when providing care to clients with immobility

346. Mr. Clark, a 77-year-old, was admitted with a CVA 3 days ago. This is the first time you have been assigned to care for the gentleman. You carry out an assessment of Mr. Clark's mobility level and ability to participate in activities of daily living. You identify a nursing diagnosis of *Impaired Mobility related to Hemiplegia and Weakness*. Select all the nursing interventions that would be appropriate for the nursing diagnosis.
   A. ___ Change Mr. Clark's position every 2 hours, maintaining sound body alignment.
   B. ___ Use appropriate supportive devices to assist in maintaining correct positioning.
   C. ___ Teach client and his family correct positioning.
   D. ___ Prepare Mr. Clark for bed based on his usual bedtime patterns prior to the stroke.

The answers are A, B, and C. Correct positioning prevents contractures and maintains proper body alignment; support devices aid in maintaining correct body alignment; teaching involves the family in Mr. Clark's care from the beginning.

D is incorrect—Bedtime patterns are not related to nursing diagnosis of impaired mobility.

SAFE AND EFFECTIVE CARE ENVIRONMENTS

Safety and Infection Control

Ergonomic Principles

Use ergonomic principles when providing care

347. Identify the position depicted in the picture.

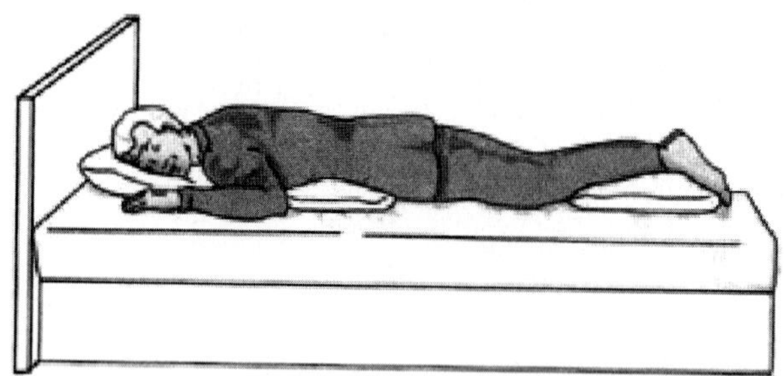

A. Sims' position
B. Supine position
C. Prone position
D. Fowlers position

The *answer is C.* In the prone position, the client has her/his head turned to the side when lying on the abdomen. The shoulders, head, and neck are in an erect position, the arms are in alignment with the shoulder girdle, the hips are extended.

A is incorrect—Sims' position is a position halfway between the lateral and prone positions where the lower arm is placed behind the client and the upper arm is flexed; both legs are flexed in front of the client. B is incorrect—Supine position is a position in which the client lies on his/her back with head and shoulders slightly elevated on a pillow. D is incorrect—Fowlers position is a semisitting position with the head of the bed elevated 45–60°.

PHYSIOLOGICAL INTEGRITY

Physiological Adaptation

Illness management

348. When teaching a client with type I diabetes, which factors would the nurse identify as increasing the risk of hypoglycemic episodes? Mark all that apply.
A. ___ End of menses
B. ___ Change in injection site
C. ___ Use of a new bottle of insulin
D. ___ Delaying a meal for 30 minutes

The answers are B, C, and D. Some individuals experience hypoglycemia as a result of an increased rate of absorption of insulin when the site of injection is changed. Hypoglycemia can occur when a new bottle of insulin is used if the old bottle had lost some of its potency. Delaying a meal for more than 30 minutes can also result in hypoglycemia because of deficient food intake.

Onset of menses with the associated drop in progesterone can increase the risk of hypoglycemia; the end of menses does not.

PHYSIOLOGICAL INTEGRITY

Physiological Adaptation

Pathophysiology

Uses assessment findings to plan nursing care

349. A nurse is working in the labor and delivery unit. The nurse assesses all the laboring clients and notes that one has a small baby in breech position, one has a large baby who is engaged, one has an average sized infant in a transverse lie, and the last has an average sized infant with a floating head. Which client will the nurse definitely have to prepare for a cesarean delivery? The client with the
A. small baby in breech position
B. large baby who is engaged
C. average sized infant in transverse lie
D. average sized infant with a floating head

The answer is C. A transverse lie is a shoulder presentation and cannot be delivered in this position. All of the other infants could be delivered vaginally.

HEALTH PROMOTION AND MAINTENANCE

Techniques of Physical Assessment

Perform comprehensive health assessment

350. Which parameters would the nurse assess as part of a complete neurological assessment? (Mark all that apply.)
___ A. Deep tendon reflexes
___ B. Shape of the head
___ C. Cranial nerves
___ D. Sensory perception
___ E. Coordination
___ F. Skin
___ G. Heart

The answers are A, C, D, and E. The other areas are not part of the neurological examination.

PHYSIOLOGICAL INTEGRITY

Reduction risk potential

Provide Pre- or Postoperative Education

351. A 4-year-old child has just returned from surgery for a tonsillectomy. Instructions that the nurse should give the parents would include:
   A. encourage the child to cough frequently.
   B. have the child drink through a straw to promote hydration.
   C. aviod red liquids in the postoperative period.
   D. aspirin is available for pain relief.

The answer is C. Red liquids are avoided to prevent confusion over bleeding in vomitus or stool.

A is incorrect—Coughing can cause the loss of a clot, leading to hemorrhage. B is incorrect—Drinking through a straw may cause the loss of the clot and lead to hemorrhage. D is incorrect—Aspirin inhibits clotting.

PHYSIOLOGICAL INTEGRITY

Basic Care and Comfort

Nutrition and oral hydration

352. A postpartum woman comes to the lactation clinic 2 weeks after birth. The woman states that she doesn't seem to produce enough milk for her infant. Which statement by the woman indicates a possible source of the lactation problem?
   A. "My breasts are not the least bit sore."
   B. "I am always hungry and just eat and eat."
   C. "I make sure I drink 500 ml of fluid every day."
   D. "The baby latches on and nurses for 20 minutes on each breast every 2 to 3 hours."

The answer is C. A minimal fluid intake is 1000 ml a day. Most breast feeding moms exceed this fluid intake as thirst is common.

A, B, and D are incorrect—The fact that the breasts are not sore is a positive finding. A breast feeding mother needs to increase her caloric intake by about 500 calories per day, which this woman seems to be doing. The infant is nursing for sufficient time.

PHYSIOLOGICAL INTEGRITY

Physiological Adaptation

Hemodynamics

353. A woman has delivered an infant by cesarean section. Which factors place this woman at risk for thromboembolic disease? (Select all that apply.)
   A. Due to the surgical procedure, the client will be less active.
   B. The platelet count is elevated as the body prepared for delivery.
   C. The pregnant woman's blood volume decreases in later pregnancy.
   D. Venous stasis in the lower extremities is common in late pregnancy.
   E. The fetus produces platelets which cross the placenta into the maternal circulation.

The answers are A, B, and D. Stasis of blood due to pressure of the term uterus and elevated platelet count in late pregnancy places all postpartum women at risk for thrombus. The cesarean client has the added burden of decreased mobility. The pregnant woman's blood volume increases not decreases. The fetal blood components do not readily cross the placenta.

HEALTH PROMOTION AND MAINTENANCE

Techniques of Physical Assessment

Perform comprehensive health assessment

354. Which lung sound if auscultated over point B in the diagram would be evaluated by the nurse as a normal assessment finding?

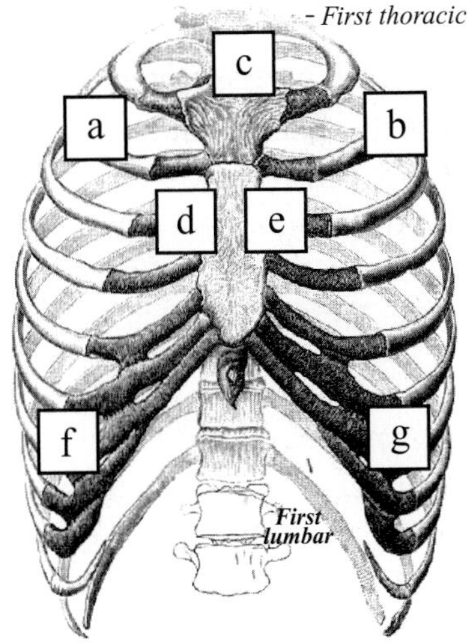

   A. Bronchovesicular
   B. Crackle
   C. Gurgle
   D. Sibilant
   E. Tracheal
   F. Vesicular
   G. Wheeze

The answer is F. Vesicular sounds are normally heard over alveolar lung tissue, which is the majority of both lungs including point B. Vesicular sounds are soft in intensity and low in pitch. The inspiratory phase is longer than the expiratory phase.

PHYSIOLOGICAL INTEGRITY

Physiological Adaptation

Medical emergencies

355. While being fed, a newly admitted infant with tetralogy of Fallot suddenly becomes very cyanotic and shows severe cardiac distress. Physician orders have not been written. Which action should the nurse take?
    A. Administer oxygen
    B. Administer morphine sulfate
    C. Place the child in knee chest position
    D. Place the child in high fowler's position

The answer is C. The child is displaying a "Tet" or hypercyanotic spell. Placing the child in knee chest reduces the blood return from the lower extremities and allows better recovery of the heart. High Fowler's position does not as effectively trap blood in the lower extremities and decrease venous return to the heart. The other responses are not appropriate as independent nursing actions.

HEALTH PROMOTION AND MAINTENANCE

Techniques of Physical Assessment

Choose physical assessment equipment and technique appropriate for the client

356. When assessing deep tendon reflexes, when does the nurse use the wide end of the reflex hammer? Mark all that apply.
    The nurse uses the wide end of the reflex hammer to check
    A. ___ brachioradialis reflex
    B. ___ biceps reflex
    C. ___ triceps reflex
    D. ___ patellar reflex
    E. ___ Achilles reflex
    F. ___ cremasteric reflex

The answers are D and E. The patellar and Achilles reflexes located at the front of the knee and the back of the heel respectively are tested using the broad end of the reflex hammer.

A, B, C, and F are incorrect—The brachioradialis reflex located in the forearm above the radial styloid process of the wrist, the biceps reflex located in front of the elbow, and the triceps reflex located just above the elbow on the back of the arm are all checked using the pointed end of the reflex hammer. The cremasteric reflex is a superficial reflex, which causes elevation of one side of the testicle in response to stroking the thigh on that side. The handle of the reflex hammer is used to stroke the thigh.

SAFE AND EFFECTIVE CARE ENVIRONMENTS

Safety and Infection Control

Standard/Transmission-Based/Other Precautions

Apply principles of infection control

357. Which type of precautions would be used when caring for a client with hepatitis A?
    A. Standard precautions
    B. Airborne precautions
    C. Droplet precautions
    D. Contact precautions

The answer is A. Standard precautions are used to decrease the risk of transmission from bloodborne pathogens and moist body substances. Moist body substances include blood, urine, feces, sputum, saliva, wound drainage, and all aspirated fluids. Because hepatitis A is spread by the fecal oral route, standard precautions are appropriate.

B is incorrect—Airborne precautions are used when the mode of spread of an organism is by small particle droplets borne on air currents. Airborne precautions require a private room with negative airflow and adequate filtration; those entering the room wear a mask and if the client leaves the room, a mask is worn. C is incorrect—Droplet precautions are used when the mechanism of transmission is by large droplets spread by coughing, sneezing, or talking. Droplet precautions require a private room or a room shared with someone infected with the same organism. Those entering the room and coming within 3 feet of the client need to wear a mask and the client wears a mask if taken out of the room. D is incorrect—Contact precautions are used when organisms causing serious disease are easily transmitted through direct contact. Contact precautions require a private room or a room shared with someone infected with the same organism. Gloves are worn at all times and gowns and protective barriers are used if direct contact is required.

PHYSIOLOGICAL INTEGRITY

Basic Care and Comfort

Nutrition and oral hydration

358. A young female adult client is admitted for anorexia nervosa. The client's weight has reached a precarious level and hospitalization was deemed necessary for the

client's physical well being. Which is the priority nursing intervention?
A. Obtaining daily weights
B. Referring for psychological counseling
C. Administering total parenteral nutrition
D. Reinforcing a positive body image

The answer is C. Because the client's weight loss has reached a critical level, it is important that nutritional support be begun immediately. The other interventions are not the priority interventions.

PSYCHOSOCIAL INTEGRITY

Psychopathology

Provide client and family with information about acute and chronic mental illness

359. The daughter of a woman who has just been admitted to an Alzheimer's care unit because of stage 3 symptoms of ambulatory dementia, asks the nurse what changes she should expect in her mother as the disease continues to progress. The nurse explains that stage 4 is endstage disease and identifies which symptoms that the client will likely manifest?
A. Does not recognize family members
B. Does not walk
C. Engages in minimal purposeful activity
D. May yell or scream spontaneously
E. Is incontinent
F. Does not recognize self in the mirror

The answers are A, B, C, D, E, and F. Endstage Alzheimer's Disease is characterized by inability to recognize family members, inability to recognize self in a mirror, incontinence and possibly seizures, inability to walk, little purposeful activity, spontaneous yelling or screaming often interspersed in periods of muteness, forgetting how to eat, swallow or chew, weight loss, and problems associated with immobility such as pressure ulcers, contractures, UTIs, and pneumonia.

PHYSIOLOGICAL INTEGRITY

Reduction of Risk Potential

Laboratory values

360. A child is admitted to the pediatric unit with acute glomerulonephritis. The unit secretary receives a phoned lab report from the laboratory. Which result should the nurse question?
A. Urine protein 3+
B. Urine RBCs 4+
C. Urine color: Smokey gray
D. Urine-specific gravity 1.003

The answer is D. Protein and RBCs are expected findings in the urine. The urine will be very concentrated. All of these facts will cause the urine-specific gravity to be high, not low. The color is smoky gray or "cola" colored.

PHYSIOLOGICAL INTEGRITY

Pharmacological and Parenteral Therapies

Medication Administration

Educate the client/family about medications

361. A pregnant woman has been found to be very anemic. Because she can't take pills, liquid iron supplements have been ordered. Which direction would the nurse give the client about taking the liquid iron preparation?
A. Take the iron with milk
B. Drink the iron through a straw
C. Take the iron on an empty stomach
D. Take the iron at the same time every day

The answer is B. Iron stains the teeth so should be taken in a manner to bypass the teeth.

A is incorrect—Milk will prevent iron absorption—iron should be taken with juice for the best absorption. C is incorrect—Iron can be irritating to the stomach. D is incorrect—It doesn't matter what time of day the iron is taken.

HEALTH PROMOTION AND MAINTENANCE

Techniques of Physical Assessment

Perform a comprehensive health assessment

362. What is the nurse assessing when, with the client's eyes closed, the nurse traces the number 3 on the palm of the client's hand with a capped pen and asks the client to identify what was traced?
A. Two-point discrimination
B. Stereognosis
C. Graphesthesia
D. Light touch

The answer is C. This is the procedure for assessing graphesthesia.

Two-point discrimination involves touching the skin simultaneously with two sterile needles at closer and closer distances to each other until the client perceives only one touch. Stereognosis is asking the client to identify a familiar object such as a key when it is placed in the client's hand with the client's eyes closed. Light touch is tested by stroking an area of the client's skin with a wisp of cotton.

PHYSIOLOGICAL INTEGRITY

Physiological Adaptation

Pathophysiology

363. An infant's crib is placed next to the window allowing the infant to lose heat to a cooler solid surface not in contact with the infant's skin. This type of heat loss is termed
A. radiation
B. convection
C. conduction
D. evaporation

The answer is A. This type of heat loss occurs by radiation. Convection is the loss of heat into the cooler room temperature. Conduction is the loss of body heat to a solid surface in direct contact with the body. Evaporation is the loss of heat when moisture on the skin is converted to a vapor.

SAFE AND EFFECTIVE CARE ENVIRONMENTS

Safety and Infection Control

Ergonomic Principles

Use ergonomic principles when providing care

364. Which activity requires an individual carrying out the activity to use the most energy:
A. Rolling
B. Pivoting
C. Lifting
D. Turning

The answer is C. Lifting a person or object requires going against the force of gravity.

A, B, and D are incorrect—Rolling, pivoting, and turning a client use a limited amount of energy compared to lifting a client. Moving an object along a level surface requires less energy than moving an object against the force of gravity.

PHYSIOLOGICAL INTEGRITY

Reduction of Risk Potential

Potential for alterations in body systems

365. The client has pulse oximetry ordered to monitor oxygen saturation. The nurse applies the monitoring probe to the right index finger and receives a reading of 91%. The nurse should
A. notify the physician.
B. encourage the client to take a deep breath.
C. check the oxygen level on each of the other fingers.
D. check the monitor site for skin breakdown from the probe.

The answer is A. The test is used to titrate levels of oxygen. This value is low. Taking a single deep breath will not resolve the problem. There is no reason to check the oxygen level of the other fingers, this is not a test of circulation to the hands. Although the probe uses heat to read the oxygen level, skin breakdown is not common in adults.

HEALTH PROMOTION AND MAINTENANCE

Techniques of Physical Assessment

Choose physical assessment equipment and technique appropriate for the client

366. Which equipment does the nurse need to perform a Rinne test on a client?
A. Reflex hammer
B. Pneumatic otoscope
C. Tuning fork
D. Snellen chart

The answer is C. The Rinne test utilizes a tuning fork to compare bone conduction and air conduction of sound. The base of a lightly vibrating tuning fork is placed on the mastoid process and the client is directed to state when the tone is no longer heard. When the client reports no longer hearing the tone the tuning fork is moved so the tines are in front of the opening to the suditory canal. The client is asked if sound is heard and if so to report when it stops. Normally, the client hears the sound for as long as the sound was heard with the base of the tuning fork on the mastoid bone. This means that air conduction is normally twice as long as bone conduction. If air conduction is found to be equal to or shorter than bone conduction, the client has a conductive hearing loss. If air conduction is longer, but not twice as long as bone conduction, sensorineural hearing loss is indicated.

A is incorrect—A reflex hammer is used to check reflexes. B is incorrect—A pneumatic otoscope is used to check for motion of the tympanic membrane. D is incorrect—A Snellen chart is used to test distance vision.

PHYSIOLOGICAL INTEGRITY

Reduction of Risk Potential

System-Specific Assessment

Assess the client for abnormal neurological status

367. The nurse is assessing for diminished deep tendon reflexes in a client with increasing intracranial pressure. Which location on the accompanying diagram

would the nurse strike with the reflex hammer to check the achilles reflex?

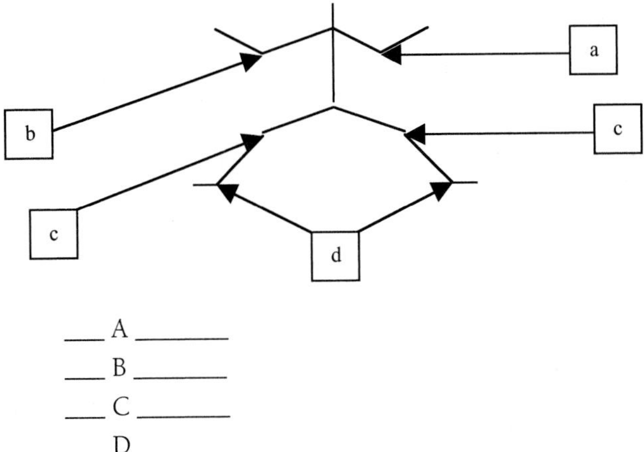

___ A _______
___ B _______
___ C _______
___ D _______

The answer is D. To check the Achilles reflex, the knee is flexed, the foot is dorsiflexed and held by the examiner, and the leg is externally rotated to allow easy access to the back of the heel. The Achilles tendon is struck with the wide end of the reflex hammer. The examiner should feel plantar flexion in the foot in response.

Location A denotes the biceps reflex; location B denotes the triceps reflex; location C denotes the patellar reflex.

PHYSIOLOGICAL INTEGRITY

Pharmacological and Parenteral Therapies

Pharmacological interactions

368. A client with known heart disease is being treated with digoxin and lasix. The client is admitted to the hospital for lethargy and shortness of breath. The admission labs show a potassium level of 2.9. The nurse would suspect
A. renal failure
B. digoxin toxicity
C. a respiratory infection.
D. decreased chloride levels

The answer is B. Low potassium levels can result from Lasix administration but would increase the action of the digoxin causing digoxin toxicity. The other responses are incorrect.

HEALTH PROMOTION AND MAINTENANCE

Growth and Development

Identify and report deviations from expected growth and development

369. When assessing a 5-month-old child, which finding would the nurse interpret as representing normal growth and development?
A. Presence of the tonic neck reflex
B. Presence of the crawling reflex
C. Presence of the dance reflex
D. Presence of the rooting reflex

The answer is A. The tonic neck reflex disappears between 4 and 6 months of age and so if it was still present at 5 months it would not be interpreted as an abnormal finding.

B, C, and D are incorrect—The crawling and dance reflexes disappear between 1 and 2 months of age. The rooting and sucking reflexes disappear at 3–4 months of age.

PHYSIOLOGICAL INTEGRITY

Reduction of Risk Potential

Laboratory values

370. An adult client with SIADH is on restricted fluids to return serum sodium to normal. A serum sodium level within which range would indicate that this client management goal was achieved?
A. 105–115 mEq/L
B. 118–125 mEq/L
C. 135–145 mEq/L
D. 148–158 mEq/L

The answer is C. The normal range of serum sodium is 135–145 mEq/L. Below 135 mEq/L is hyponatremia and above 145 mEq/L is hypernatremia. With SIADH serum sodium level is low as a result of dilution by retained fluid because of the inappropriate secretion of antidiuretic hormone which prevents diuresis.

SAFE AND EFFECTIVE CARE ENVIRONMENTS

Safety and Infection Control

Ergonomic Principles

Use ergonomic principles when providing care

371. When moving a client from the bed to a stretcher the nurse needs to consider utilizing a:
A. draw or pull sheet
B. pillow
C. footboard
D. trapeze bar

The answer is A. A draw or pull sheet will provide friction which will lead to less force needed to move the client.

Pillows are used in positioning clients. Footboards are used to prevent foot drop. Trapeze bar is used when the client can assist in pulling him/herself up in bed.

PHYSIOLOGICAL INTEGRITY

Physiological Adaptation

Pathophysiology

372. A newborn is being admitted to the newborn nursery. The father has accompanied the infant to the nursery. During the admission process, the nurse prepares to administer vitamin K intramuscularly. The father asks why his baby needs the vitamin K. Which response by the nurse would be most appropriate?
   A. "We give this to all babies born by cesarean section."
   B. "Babies can't take fruits and juices which are the main source of vitamin K in the diet."
   C. "Your baby will not have anything by mouth for the next 12 hours so he will be unable to get any vitamin K from his diet."
   D. "Newborns have sterile intestines. You and I get vitamin K from bacteria that live in our intestines."

The answer is D. The main source of vitamin K is from the intestinal flora and from the ingestion of fats.

A is incorrect because it is also given to infants born by vaginal delivery. Vitamin K is found in fats, not fruits. The infant will not be NPO.

PHYSIOLOGICAL INTEGRITY

Physiological Adaptation

Pathophysiology

373. A premature male infant is admitted to the high risk nursery. On the admission assessment, the nurse notes there are no testes in the scrotum. In relation to this finding, the nurse would
   A. document the finding.
   B. monitor urine output.
   C. prepare the parents for immediate orchiopexy.
   D. evaluate the child for low set ears.

The answer is A. Undescended testes are a common finding in the preterm infant and do not warrant further investigation at this time. Orchiopexy may be scheduled prior to the child starting school, but the testes may descend on their own. Low set ears are associated with renal abnormalities. Undescended testes are a sign of immaturity not renal abnormalities.

PSYCHOSOCIAL INTEGRITY

Therapeutic Communications

Develop and maintain therapeutic relationships with client/family/significant others

374. Upon return from a group meeting a client is visibly upset. When the nurse notes this fact and asks if the client would like to talk about it, the client replies "I'll tell you what happened but you can't tell anyone I told you." Which is the most appropriate response for the nurse to make?
   A. "I will respect your confidentiality."
   B. "I cannot make that promise."
   C. "As long as it doesn't involve another client, I won't say anything."
   D. "I won't write it in your record but I may need to tell someone."

The answer is B. "I cannot make that promise." This is the appropriate response because promising to keep information secret may be appropriate in a social relationship but is inappropriate in a therapeutic relationship. It is also an honest, direct answer to the client.

PHYSIOLOGICAL INTEGRITY

Reduction of Risk Potential

Potential for Complications from Surgical Procedures and Health Alterations

Applies knowledge of pathophysiology to selected assessment findings

375. A client is known to have hyperthyroidism with symptoms including recent weight loss, diarrhea and mild exophthalmos. The client is seen in the emergency room with a high temperature, tachycardia and hypertension. Tremors are noted in the hands. Which problem should the nurse suspect based on these assessment findings?
   A. Goiter
   B. Urinary tract infection
   C. Thyrotoxic Crisis (thyroid storm)
   D. Overdose of Synthroid (Levothyroxine sodium)

The answer is C. Thyroid storm is the sudden oversecretion of thyroid hormone and can be life threatening. Goiter is an enlargement of the thyroid gland secondary to decreased thyroid production. A urinary tract infection would cause hyperthermia but not the other symptoms. The client with hyperthyroidism would not be on medication for hypothyroidism (Synthroid).

PHYSIOLOGICAL INTEGRITY

Pharmacological and Parenteral Therapies

Expected effects/outcomes

376. A newly diagnosed asthma client calls the clinic nurse to ask which medication is taken routinely to prevent an asthma attack. Which medication is the one that would be taken prophylactically?
   A. Cromolyn sodium (Intal)
   B. Inhalant glucocorticoids such as flunisolide (Aerobid)

C. Short-acting bronchodilator such as albuterol (Preventil)
D. Long-acting bronchodilator such as salmeterol (Serevent)

The answer is A. Cromolyn sodium is a mast cell stabilizer and is used to prevent an asthmatic attack.

Glucocorticoids are anti-inflammatories used to reduce inflammation and airway constriction. Oral glucocorticoids may be administered for severe asthmatics as a prophylactic, the accumulated side effects are very problematic. Short-acting bronchodilators would be used prn for exercise induced asthma. Long-acting bronchodilators are used to obtain control of asthmatic attacks.

HEALTH PROMOTION AND MAINTENANCE

Techniques of Physical Assessment

Perform a comprehensive health assessment

377. What would you ask the client to do as you assess respiratory excursion?
A. "Take two or three rapid breaths."
B. "Say 99."
C. "Take a deep breath."
D. "Cough."

The answer is C. Respiratory excursion refers to the symmetry and degree of chest expansion upon taking a deep breath. Posteriorly excursion is measured by placing the palms of the hands with fingers spread wide and thumbs facing each other on either side of the spinal column with a skinfold pushed up between them. The client is then asked to exhale and then to take a deep breath and hold it. The examiner notes the amount of increased distance between his or her thumbs when the deep breath is taken. This increase in distance represents the amount of chest expansion or excursion. Normally the thumbs will separate by 1 ¼ to 2 inches.

PHYSIOLOGICAL INTEGRITY

Physiological Adaptation

Medical Emergencies

Perform emergency care procedures

378. A 59-year-old male was admitted to your unit following removal of a tumor on the sigmoid colon with a diverting colostomy. On the third postoperative day, the client's wife asks that you look at the dressing because it is all wet. Upon removal of the dressing you observe bowel protruding out of the abdomen through a dehisced incision. What is the priority nursing action?
A. Notify the surgeon
B. Reassure the client that he will be fine
C. Apply sterile, normal saline soaked gauze to the bowel and cover with a second sterile dressing
D. Gently push the bowel back into the abdominal cavity and apply an abdominal binder

The answer is C. Sterile gauze soaked with normal saline should be applied to the bowel to prevent drying and then covered with a secondary sterile dressing to prevent contamination.

A is incorrect—The nurse's priority action is to preserve the bowel; then the surgeon is notified. B is incorrect—Although the nurse does want to assure the client that this problem will be corrected immediately, it is not the priority action. D is incorrect—Pushing loops of bowel back into the abdominal cavity could result in injury to the bowel.

PHYSIOLOGICAL INTEGRITY

Pharmacological and Parenteral Therapies

Adverse effects/contraindications

379. A known drug addict arrived in the labor unit at 8 cm dilated. The client managed the contractions and the infant was delivered within 1 hour of the mother's admission. For which conditions would the infant be monitored? (Select all that apply.)
A. ___ Hyperbilirubinemia
B. ___ Congenital anomalies
C. ___ Narcotic depression immediately after birth
D. ___ Narcotic withdrawal within a few hours of delivery

The answers are B, C, and D. Many drug abusers will wait to the last minute to arrive at the labor unit and will have used recreational drugs immediately before admission. Therefore, the infant could be depressed at birth but then will develop withdrawal within a short period of time. Congenital anomalies are associated with some recreational drugs. The infant will probably not have problems with hyperbilirubinemia as the narcotic exposure in utero seems to mature the liver and infants born to substance abuses seem to have fewer problems with bilirubin than other infants.

SAFE AND EFFECTIVE CARE ENVIRONMENTS

Safety and Infection Control

Ergonomic Principles

Use ergonomic principles when providing care

380. A client needs help in transferring from his bed to a chair. He is 6 feet 2 inches tall, weighs approximately 250 lbs,

has weakness on his left side, and has been on prolonged bed rest. Which factors should the nurse consider prior to implementing the transfer? Select all that apply.

A. ___ Determine the need for assistance from other personnel

B. ___ Determine the client's activity tolerance

C. ___ Assess muscle strength in the client's legs and upper arms

D. ___ Assess the amount of instruction the nurse will need to provide the client's

The answers are A, B, C, and D. Clients require various levels of assistance; the nurse needs to recognize her/his strengths and limitations; a safe transfer is the first priority. Determining a client's activity tolerance will aid in determining the client's ability to assist in the transfer. Clients that have been immobile for a period of time may have decreased muscle strength, tone, and mass. This will effect his/her ability to bear weight and raise the body. By explaining the transfer procedure the client will be involved and maybe able to help in the transfer.

HEALTH PROMOTION AND MAINTENANCE

Growth and Development

Identify and report deviations from expected growth and development

381. When assessing a 6-month-old child, which finding should the nurse interpret as a sign of possible developmental delay?
 The child
 A. is not attempting to pull up to a standing position.
 B. does not turn toward a person who is speaking.
 C. does not imitate speech.
 D. does not respond to infant games like peek-a-boo.

The answer is B. At 6 months of age an infant should turn toward a person who is speaking. If the infant does not do this, the possibility of developmental delay or other disability exists.

A, C, and D are incorrect—At 1 year a child should have begun to pull up to a standing position; begun to imitate a variety of speech sounds; and begun to respond to games like peek-a-boo and pat-a-cake.

PHYSIOLOGICAL INTEGRITY

Physiological Adaptation

Alterations in body system

382. A pregnant woman at 39 weeks gestation tells the nurse "I started feeling like I can breathe better two days ago, but now I noticed I have to void a lot." How should the nurse would suspect interpret this information?
 A. Lightening has most likely occurred.
 B. Quickening has occurred.
 C. Labor has begun.
 D. A urinary tract infection has developed.

The answers is A. As the uterus descends into the pelvis in preparation for labor, the client will be able to breathe easier but will now have pressure on the bladder causing urinary frequency.

Quickening is feeling fetal movement. The client gives no indication of contractions although the body is preparing for labor. A urinary tract infection would cause frequent urination but not easier breathing.

PHYSIOLOGICAL INTEGRITY

Pharmacological and Parenteral Therapies

Adverse effects/contraindications and side effects

383. An 80-year-old man comes to the clinic complaining of erectile dysfunction. Which question is most important for the nurse to ask?
 A. How often do you usually have intercourse?
 B. What medications do you take?
 C. When was the last time you had your prostate examined?
 D. Do you have any problems urinating?

The answer is B. As clients age, the likelihood that they take medications increases. Many of the medications taken by the older population have erectile dysfunction as a side effect, including antihypertensives. In many cases the problem can be eliminated by changing the medication. The other questions, although they might be asked, do not most directly impact the problem.

PSYCHOSOCIAL INTEGRITY

Behavioral Interventions

Assist client with achieving and maintaining self-control of behavior

384. Which statement accurately describes a "no suicide" contract?
 A. The contract provides a boundary.
 B. The contract takes the responsibility for control away from the client.
 C. The contract serves to reinforce to the client that life is valuable.
 D. The contract must be written to be effective.

The answer is A. A "no suicide" contract is a way of providing boundaries. Contracts help place control in the domain of the client; they don't remove control. Contracts assure the client that someone is concerned enough about them to provide boundaries but do not directly reinforce that life is valuable. Verbal "no suicide" contracts have been proven effective.

PHYSIOLOGICAL INTEGRITY

Basic Care and Comfort

Nutrition and oral hydration

385. The husband of an elderly client tells the clinic nurse that the doctor has diagnosed his wife who has been increasingly confused, with anemia caused by a vitamin deficiency. The husband asks which vitamin could be causing the problem. Which vitamin deficiency would the nurse suspect is the cause of the problem?
   A. A
   B. B_{12}
   C. C
   D. D

The answer is B. Vitamin B_{12} deficiency is associated with anemia and mental confusion. This vitamin deficiency is common in the elderly. The other vitamins are not associated with these symptoms.

PHYSIOLOGICAL INTEGRITY

Physiological Adaptation

Alterations in body systems

386. A client was diagnosed with a hiatal hernia. Discharge teaching was provided and the client was discharged home. The client returns to clinic a week later to complain that the symptoms have not improved. The nurse questions the client on activities and notes that the client eats small frequent feedings; eats at least one hour before going to bed; has switched from coffee to tea to reduce caffeine ingestion; and has begun a smoking cessation program with moderate success.
   Which activity should the nurse counsel the client to change?
   A. Eats small frequent feedings.
   B. Eats at least one hour before going to bed.
   C. Has switched from coffee to tea to reduce caffeine ingestion.
   D. Has begun a smoking cessation program with moderate success.

The answer is C. Both coffee and tea are to be avoided as they increase stomach acidity. All the other activities are appropriate for a client with a hiatal hernia.

SAFE AND EFFECTIVE CARE ENVIRONMENTS

Safety and Infection Control

Ergonomic Principles

Use ergonomic principles when providing care

387. Prior to discharge, a client still experiencing some weakness on his left side has axillary crutches ordered for him. Which is the correct crutch gait for the nurse to teach this client?
   A. four-point gait
   B. three-point gait
   C. two-point gait
   D. swing through gait

The answer is B. The three-point gait requires the weight to be borne on both crutches and then on the uninvolved leg or side. Since this client still has some left sided weakness this would be the gait of choice.

The four-point gait requires weight bearing on both legs. The two-point gait requires at least partial weight bearing on each foot. The swing through gait is used by an individual wearing braces which assist in supporting the person's weight.

PHYSIOLOGICAL INTEGRITY

Physiological Adaptation

Pathophysiology

388. An obese 34-year-old black man with a high stress job is seen for primary hypertension. His diet is high in fried foods and sodium. The client asks why he developed this problem. Which are the risk factors for hypertension that this man has? (Select all that apply.)
   A. ___ Age
   B. ___ Race
   C. ___ Obesity
   D. ___ Fat Intake
   E. ___ High Stress
   F. ___ Sodium Intake

The answers are B, C, E, and F. Hypertension is more common in blacks. Obesity and high sodium intake have been associated with high blood pressure. Stress is associated with hypertension. This gentleman is young, the risk of hypertension increases with age. Although fat intake is related to obesity, fat intake alone has not been associated with hypertension.

PHYSIOLOGICAL INTEGRITY

Reduction of Risk Potential

Potential for Alteration in Body Systems

Compare current client data with baseline client data

389. A 63-year-old female, with a history of lymphoma treated with chemotherapy, is admitted for repair of a fractured right tibia. Postoperatively her white blood cell count is 4 mm^3 and temperature is 98.6°F. She is complaining of not feeling well and being chilled. Which is the priority nursing action?
   A. Compare the postoperative lab value and temperature to the preoperative data.
   B. Ask the client what her WBC and temperature has been in the past.
   C. Notify the physician of the change.
   D. Do nothing, these are normal values.

The answer is A. With a known history of cancer treated with chemotherapy the client has a low white blood cell count and a value close to normal is indicative of an infection.

B is incorrect—The client may not know what their lab values or temperatures typically have been. C is incorrect—The answer does not provide information that should be shared with the physician. D is incorrect—Doing nothing may result in a negative event for the patient.

HEALTH PROMOTION AND MAINTENANCE

Developmental Stages and Transitions

Identify expected physical, cognitive, psychosocial and moral stages of development

390. The nurse is observing a 9-month-old infant to see how the child is developing cognitively. Which behavior indicates object permanence has developed?
   The infant
   A. has found his hands
   B. reaches for a toy out of his reach
   C. cries when mother leaves the room
   D. puts a block into his mouth while playing

The answer is C. A child who cries when mother leaves the room is aware that mother exists outside his vision so object permanence has developed. None of the other activities indicate the child is aware of objects when not in his or her vision.

PHYSIOLOGICAL INTEGRITY

Pharmacological and Parenteral Therapies

Pharmacological agents/actions

391. The nurse caring for a client on digoxin checks the client's electrolyte reports because of the risk of toxicity precipitated by hypokalemia. To avoid this risk, the client's serum potassium level should be equal to or above how many milliequivalents per liter?
   Write your answer as a whole number carried to one decimal place. __________ mEq/L.

The answer is 3.5 mEq/L. The normal range of serum potassium is 3.5-5.0 mEq/L.

PSYCHOSOCIAL INTEGRITY

Behavioral Interventions

Assess client appearance, mood and psychomotor behavior and identify/respond to inappropriate/abnormal behavior

392. Which is a priority goal for a client with obsessive compulsive personality disorder?
   A. Acceptance of group therapy.
   B. Elimination of bizarre fantasies.
   C. Development of social relationships
   D. Decrease of maladaptive behaviors

The answer is D. Clients with obsessive compulsive personality disorder are rigid and preoccupied with issues of control and power. They fear losing control and utilize different maladaptive behaviors in an effort to control anxiety. Primary goals of therapy are to reduce anxiety, improve self esteem and understand and decrease maladaptive behaviors.

PHYSIOLOGICAL INTEGRITY

Basic Care and Comfort

Nutrition and oral hydration

393. The physician instructs a client to eat a low residue diet. Which foods would the nurse instruct the client to reduce or avoid? (Select all that apply.)
   A. ___ Eggs
   B. ___ Bananas
   C. ___ Strong cheeses
   D. ___ Lean tender meats
   E. ___ Whole grain cereals
   F. ___ Dried beans and beans

The answers are C, E, and F. These foods contain significant residue. The other foods are considered low residue.

HEALTH PROMOTION AND MAINTENANCE

Health Screening

Apply knowledge of pathophysiology to health screening

394. A 68-year-old client participating in a community skin screening tells the nurse about a raised "spot" on

his upper, outer arm, which has enlarged and changed color. Inspection discloses an irregular border and variegated color. What is the priority nursing response?

A. Caution the client to avoid sun exposure.
B. Advise the client to see a dermatologist as soon as possible.
C. Suggest use of a topical OTC antibiotic ointment to prevent infection.
D. Instruct to wash with a mild soap and avoid irritation.

The answer is B. See a dermatologist as soon as possible. A skin lesion that has an irregular border, inconsistent color, and is enlarging may be a serious condition such as melanoma. It is wise for the patient to see a specialist soon.

PHYSIOLOGICAL INTEGRITY

Pharmacological and Parenteral Therapies

Medication administration

395. A 10-year-old child is diagnosed in the pediatric clinic with conjunctivitis (pink eye) and an antibiotic eye ointment is ordered. Which instruction is appropriate for the nurse to give the mother in regard to the administration of the eye ointment?

A. Place the ointment directly on the pupil
B. Have the child apply the ointment by himself
C. Ask the child to close his eyes and spread the ointment on the lids
D. Pull the lower lid down and place the ointment into this "sack"

The answer is D. The lower lid is pulled down to form a sack and the ointment is spread into the sack from the inner corner to the outer corner.

The ointment should not be placed directly on the pupil. The child will be unable to instill the ointment by himself. The ointment should be placed into the subconjunctival sac not on the outer lids.

HEALTH PROMOTION AND MAINTENANCE

Growth and Development

Identify and report deviations from expected growth and development

396. When assessing a 12-month-old child, observation of which behavior is indicative of normal developmental progression?

A. Feeds self with a spoon
B. Smiles and babbles
C. Says two or three words such as mama, dada, and bye bye.
D. Arches the back and raises the head when lying on abdomen.

The answer is C. Saying two or three words is a developmental milestone that should be achieved by 1 year of age.

A is incorrect—Feeding self with a spoon is not expected until 18 months. B is incorrect—Smiling and babbling should be present by 6 months of age and so is not an indicator of normal development at the 1-year level. D is incorrect—Arching the back and raising the head when lying prone also is expected by the age of 6 months.

PHYSIOLOGICAL INTEGRITY

Pharmacological and Parenteral Therapies

Blood and blood products

397. A client is to receive a transfusion of packed cells. Prior to administering the unit, which steps will the nurse take? (Select all that apply.)

A. ___ Take vital signs
B. ___ Start an IV of D_5W
C. ___ Check that the blood types match
D. ___ Check the client's arm band for match to the unit of blood
E. ___ Double check the client's name and packed cells unit for match

The answers are A, C, D, and E. All are correct except B. The IV should be started with normal saline. Dextrose in the line will cause the cells to clot.

SAFE AND EFFECTIVE CARE ENVIRONMENTS

Safety and Infection Control

Standard/Transmission-Based/Other Precautions

Apply principles of infection control

398. Which type of precautions would be used when caring for a client with hepatitis B?

A. Standard precautions
B. Airborne precautions
C. Droplet precautions
D. Contact precautions

The answer is A. Standard precautions are used to decrease the risk of transmission from bloodborne pathogens and moist body substances. Moist body substances include blood, urine, feces, sputum, saliva, wound drainage, and all aspirated fluids. Because hepatitis B is spread by blood and blood products, standard precautions are appropriate.

B is incorrect—Airborne precautions are used when the mode of spread of an organism is by small particle droplets borne on air currents. Airborne precautions require a private room with negative airflow and adequate filtration; those entering the room wear a mask and if the client leaves the room, a mask is worn. C is incorrect—Droplet precautions are used when the mechanism of transmission is by large droplets spread by coughing, sneezing, or talking. Droplet precautions require a private room or a room shared with someone infected with the same organism. Those entering the room and coming within 3 feet of the client need to wear a mask and the client wears a mask if taken out of the room. D is incorrect—Contact precautions are used when organisms causing serious disease are easily transmitted through direct contact. Contact precautions require a private room or a room shared with someone infected with the same organism. Gloves are worn at all times and gowns and protective barriers are used if direct contact is required.

PHYSIOLOGICAL INTEGRITY

Pharmacological and Parenteral Therapies

Medication Administration

Administers parenteral medication in a safe and effective manner

399. The physician has ordered a medication to be given by IV push method. Which is an appropriate nursing action?
   A. Refuse to push the medication.
   B. Push the medication over 1 full minute.
   C. Push the medication over 5 full minutes.
   D. Determine the rate of infusion for this particular medication.

The answer is D. Each medication has an individual rate of infusion allowed for IV bolusing (pushing).

PHYSIOLOGICAL INTEGRITY

Reduction of Risk Potential

Potential for complications from surgical procedures and health alterations

400. During the third trimester of her pregnancy, a client develops mild PIH (pregnancy induced hypertension). Which instruction would be included in the teaching planned for this client?
   A. Avoid all sodium containing foods.
   B. Rest in bed during the mid-afternoon.
   C. When recumbent, always lay in the supine position.
   D. Notify the physician at the next prenatal visit if headaches or visual disturbances occur.

The answer is B. Rest is beneficial to reduce hypertension. Rest should be in the lateral position to prevent vena cava syndrome.

Sodium is a necessary nutrient so eliminating all sodium would be incorrect. If headaches or visual disturbances occur, the physician should be notified immediately as they may indicate worsening of the client's condition.

HEALTH PROMOTION AND MAINTENANCE

Growth and Development

Identify and report deviations from expected growth and development

401. When assessing a 3-month-old infant, which finding indicates the need for further evaluation?
   A. Infant reacts to sudden noise.
   B. Infant does not vocalize sounds.
   C. Infant does not reach for toys.
   D. Infant raises head without arching the back when in a prone position.

The answer is B. By 3 months of age, an infant should be vocalizing sounds and so the absence of this behavior indicates possible developmental delay or other disability and requires further evaluation.

A, C, and D are incorrect—It is normal for a 3-month-old infant to react to sudden noises and so no further investigation is required. Infants are not expected to reach for toys as a developmental marker until 6 months of age. It is normal for a 3-month-old to raise the head without arching the back when in a prone position; arching of the back is not expected until 6 months of age.

PHYSIOLOGICAL INTEGRITY

System Specific Assessment

Perform Focused Assessment or Reassessment (Respiratory)

Identify alterations

402. A client has COPD and a barrel chest. Which finding would the nurse expect when assessing the chest?
   A. Paradoxical chest movement
   B. Presence of a friction rub
   C. Decreased respiratory excursion
   D. Absent breath sounds

The answer is C. Respiratory excursion is decreased in the client with emphysema because a barrel chest develops as a result of air trapping in the alveoli and the accompanying lung hyperinflation and flattening of the diaphragm.

A, B, and D are incorrect—Paradoxical chest movement exists when an unaffected area of the chest wall rises on inspiration and the affected area falls and the reverse occurs during expiration. This is seen with flail chest not with emphysema. Friction rubs are associated with pleural inflammation secondary to problems such as pleuritis, tuberculosis, and pneumonia.

PHYSIOLOGICAL INTEGRITY

Reduction of Risk Potential

Laboratory values

403. A client has blood drawn for an electrolyte profile. The venipuncture was difficult and the blood aspiration was slow. The findings included the following: sodium 150 mEq/L, potassium 6.1 mEq/L, chloride 101 mEq/L, and CO_2 25 mEq/L. Which conclusion could the nurse draw from this information?
    A. The client is doing well as all values are normal.
    B. The sodium is low so the client may have heat stroke.
    C. The CO_2 is elevated so there may be a respiratory problem.
    D. The potassium is high, the specimen may have been hemolyzed.

The answer is D. The potassium is very high but all other values are normal. Because of the problems with the blood draw, the specimen could have been hemolyzed. Hemolysis results in the release of intracellular potassium and hence can cause hyperkalemia in the specimen. All other values are within normal limits.

HEALTH PROMOTION AND MAINTENANCE

Provide education on age specific growth and development to the client and families

404. A toddler is shopping with mother. The toddler grabs a toy off the shelf. When mother replaces the toy on the shelf, the toddler cries and falls on the floor. Which is the best response by the mother?
    A. Buy him the toy
    B. Spank his hands and tell him no
    C. Explain to the child why he can't have the toy.
    D. Remove the child from the area and divert attention to something else

The answer is D. The child is expressing his frustration. The goal of the parent is to allow the child to regain control without a loss of self-esteem. Removing and distracting him will allow him to regain self control.

Buying him the toy will not help him learn to deal with frustrations. Spanking his hand does not help with self-esteem. The child doesn't have the vocabulary for long explanations and frustration will continue as long as the desired object is in sight.

SAFE AND EFFECTIVE CARE ENVIRONMENTS

Safety and Infection Control

Ergonomic Principles

Use ergonomic principles when providing care

405. The nurse is reinforcing the correct way for a client to descend stairs using crutches. In which order would the nurse instruct the client to proceed with the listed steps?
    A. Places crutches on the next stair, transfers weight to the crutches, moves affected side (leg) forward
    B. Moves unaffected side (leg) forward
    C. Transfers body weight to the unaffected side (leg)

The answer is C, then A, and then B. The client transfers body weight to the unaffected side (leg) then places the crutches on the next stair. Next the client transfers weight to the crutches and moves the affected side (leg) forward. Finally the client moves unaffected side (leg) forward.

This order enables balance to be maintained and allows the client to more safely go down the stairs.

PHYSIOLOGICAL INTEGRITY

Pharmacological and Parenteral Therapies

Adverse effects/contraindications and side effects

406. A client is receiving a chemotherapy agent that is known to be irritating to the bladder wall. Which nursing action would best reduce irritation?
    A. Encourage the client to drink milk
    B. Restrict fluids to decrease urine volume
    C. Administer the once daily drug at bedtime
    D. Have the client void every two hours while awake

The answer is D. Having the client void frequently reduces the time the medication sits in the bladder. The nurse would also force fluids to dilute the medication and on once daily meds, give it early in the morning so the client can void frequently. Milk would have no effect on bladder irritation.

PSYCHOSOCIAL INTEGRITY

Psychopathology

Recognize signs and symptoms of impaired cognition

407. A client with schizophrenia says "raining turkeys" to himself and to others as he walks around the unit and

performs various activities. Which would be a correct label for the nurse to use when documenting this behavior?
A. word salad
B. clang association
C. neologism
D. verbigeration

The answer is D. Verbigeration is the purposeless repetition of words or phrases. Word salad refers to the meaningless connection of words and phrases. Clang association refers to repeating words and phrases which sound alike but are otherwise unconnected. A neologism is a new word coined by the client and with meaning only to the client.

PHYSIOLOGICAL INTEGRITY

Pharmacological and Parenteral Therapies

Total parenteral nutrition

408. A client has an order for total parenteral nutrition to run at 95 ml/hour. The TPN is infusing into a central line. While transferring the client to a stretcher to go to x-ray, the central line is accidentally pulled out. Which is the immediate nursing action?
A. Give the client sugar laced orange juice by mouth.
B. Start a peripheral line with D5W running at 95 ml/hour.
C. Start a peripheral line and administer the TPN at 95 ml/hour.
D. Notify the physician and wait for the central line to be restarted.

The answer is B. The client's body is accustomed to receiving a strong sugar solution at that rate so sudden stopping would cause hypoglycemia. TPN cannot be given by peripheral line. Sugar laced orange juice would not meet the need for continuous glucose infusion until the central line could be replaced.

PHYSIOLOGICAL INTEGRITY

Reduction of Risk Potential

Therapeutic procedures

409. A client has been severely burned in a house fire and admitted to the burn unit. After emergency stabilization, one of the primary nursing goals is to prevent contractures. Which nursing intervention supports achievement of this goal?
A. Administration of albumin
B. Promoting the intake of protein foods.
C. Application of splints to immobilize body parts
D. Treating the burns with the open method and not wrapping the burned injury.

The answer is C. Whereas all of the interventions may be used in the treatment of burns, the one intervention associated with prevention of contractions is the application of splints. In addition to splinting, ROM exercises are important in maintaining joint function.

HEALTH PROMOTION AND MAINTENANCE

Immunizations

410. An infant received her first immunization on schedule but is now past due for both the second and third immunization of the series. The nurse should
A. give the infant the second and third immunization during this visit.
B. start the immunizations over, giving the infant the first of the series.
C. give the second immunization and schedule the infant for a return visit for the third immunization.
D. give a double dose of the second immunization and then give the third immunization one month later.

The answer is C. Although there is an abnormal space between the first and second immunization, the nurse will give the second and schedule the third immunization for later. There is no need to restart the immunization. Two immunizations should not be given at the same time.

PHYSIOLOGICAL INTEGRITY

Physiological Adaptation

Pathophysiology

411. A teenager is admitted to the hospital with a diagnosis of osteomyelitis. An IV is started for administration of parenteral antibiotics. The teenager complains about hospitalization and asks the nurse: "Why can't I just be given some pills to take like my friend that had the abscess?" The nurse's response would be based on the knowledge that osteomyelitis:
A. Lacks an effective oral antibiotic.
B. Can cause pathologic fractures so the child must be hospitalized.
C. Is caused by a different organism than the one that causes abscesses.
D. Requires parenteral antibiotics to reach bone levels of the drug high enough to be effective.

The answer is D. Blood supply to the bones is less than to the skin. Parenteral antibiotics provide the best blood levels. The organism may or may not be the same as the other child had. Although pathologic fractures can occur from osteomyelitis, bedrest prevents the fracture not hospitalization.

PHYSIOLOGICAL INTEGRITY

Reduction of Risk Potential

Potential for complications from surgical procedures and health alterations

412. A child has a tonsillectomy. On return to the floor, the child is positioned prone until fully awake. Instructions given to the parents should include: (Select all that apply.)
   A. Avoid red liquids
   B. Use a straw to make drinking easier
   C. Cold liquids like popsicles will feel good.
   D. Give milk and non-acidic liquids to soothe the throat
   E. As soon as the child wakes up, start the child drinking

The answers are A, C, and E. Red liquids could be confused with blood in vomitus or stool. Cold liquids will reduce pain and promote blood clotting. Pushing orals fluids will keep the throat moist and reduce discomfort. A straw requires suction which could dislodge the clot that has formed in the throat. Milk thickens secretions requiring more throat clearing which is discouraged.

PHYSIOLOGICAL INTEGRITY

Reduction of Risk Potential

Potential for complications from surgical procedures and health alterations

413. A client with polycystic kidney disease needs a kidney transplant. Which action will the physician take prior to another family member being considered as a suitable donor?
   A. Discuss with the client feelings about the donor.
   B. Instruct the client to take over the counter drugs for pain
   C. Screen the family member for evidence of polycystic kidney disease
   D. Stop dialysis treatment so that the client's kidney function can be adequately evaluated

The answer is C. Polycystic kidney disease is inherited as an autosomal dominant disorder. Any family member should be screened for kidney disease before consideration as a donor. Until a donor is found, there is no need to discus the client's feelings about the donor. Medications are avoided because of the injury to the kidneys. If the client was on dialysis, the kidney function is known so stopping would be unnecessary and unhealthy.

SAFE AND EFFECTIVE CARE ENVIRONMENTS

Safety and Infection Control

Safe Use of Equipment

Ensure appropriate and safe use of equipment in performing client care procedures and treatments

414. Which are safety measures that the nurse needs to keep in mind when transporting a client in a wheelchair? Select all that apply.
   A. Lock the wheels before the client transfers from bed to wheelchair
   B. Push the wheelchair in a forward direction when getting on an elevator
   C. Be sure the footplates are in the down/lower position as the client gets into the wheelchair
   D. Position the client well back in the seat

The answers are A and D. The wheelchair's wheels always need to be locked before transferring a client into the wheelchair to prevent the wheelchair from moving and the client falling. Ensuring the client is sitting fully in the wheelchair will prevent the wheelchair from being off balance and possibly tipping forward.

PHYSIOLOGICAL INTEGRITY

Pharmacological and Parenteral Therapies

Pharmacological agents/actions

415. Due to an allergy to cats, a client has had several allergy attacks after visiting a family member. The physician has prescribed an antihistamine to reduce the symptoms. The client asks the nurse when would be the best time to take the antihistamine. The nurse's response is based on the knowledge that antihistamines
   A. transfer the allergic response to a mast cell.
   B. destroy the allergen that caused the symptoms
   C. block histamine from attaching to receptor sites.
   D. destroy histamine, the cause of allergic symptoms.

The answer is C. Antihistamines compete with histamine for the receptor sites. Once histamine is attached to the receptor site, an anti-histamine will not work. The best time to take the antihistamine would be before going to the house with cats.

PHYSIOLOGICAL INTEGRITY

Reduction of Risk Potential

Therapeutic procedures

416. Due to injuries in a car accident, a client has a tracheostomy. Which is a step in providing tracheostomy care?

A. Put on clean gloves in preparation for the procedure.
B. Advance the suction catheter while applying suction.
C. Insert the suction catheter as deep into the airway as possible and begin suctioning.
D. Rotate the suction catheter while applying intermittent suction during withdrawal.

The answer is D. Rotating the catheter cleans all surfaces of the trach. Intermittent suction prevents the client from becoming hypoxic. The procedure is sterile so sterile gloves are worn. Suction is never applied while inserting the catheter. The suction catheter is inserted fully and then withdrawn slightly before suctioning begins.

HEALTH PROMOTION AND MAINTENANCE

Human Sexuality

417. A woman is talking to her best friend who is a nurse. The woman knows that she does not carry the gene for sickle cell anemia. She tells the nurse she is going to marry a man who has the disease. She asks whether her future children will be affected with sickle cell anemia. The nurse's best response would be
A. no, but they will all be carriers for the disease.
B. one in four of your children will have the disease
C. none of your children will have the disease but 50% will be carriers.
D. there is no way to determine the possible outcome for your future children.

The answer is A. Sickle cell anemia is an autosomal recessive disorder, which means the child must receive an affected gene from each parent. Since she does not carry the affected gene, none of the children will be affected. However, since the both of the husband's genes are affected, the children will all receive one copy of the affected gene meaning they will be carriers. The other responses are incorrect.

PHYSIOLOGICAL INTEGRITY

Reduction in Risk Potential

Potential for complications of diagnostic tests/treatments/procedures

418. An infant was diagnosed with hydrocephalus shortly after birth and a ventriculo-peritoneal shunt was inserted. Three years later, the child is readmitted to the hospital with a malfunctioning shunt. Which assessment findings would the nurse interpret as expected based on the problem?
A. Vomiting and headache
B. Temperature and bradycardia
C. Abdominal pain and electrolyte imbalance
D. Bulging fontanels and increasing head circumference

The answer is A. Early symptoms of a malfunctioning shunt (and of hydrocephalus) are vomiting and headache, especially in the early morning. A younger child might have bulging fontanels and increasing head circumferences but this child is over 3 and fontanels should have closed.

PHYSIOLOGICAL INTEGRITY

Reduction of Risk Potential

Potential for alteration in body systems

419. There are several clients currently in the burn unit with extensive burns. Which client would be at greatest risk for infection in the burn?
The client who:
A. has skin grafts completely covering all burn surfaces.
B. is being discharged home with follow-up physical therapy.
C. is being treated with the open method (no dressings) of burn treatment.
D. is being treated with the closed method (dressings covering) of burn treatment.

The answer is C. The client whose burns are open to the air would be most likely to develop an infection. Dressed burns and grafted burns have coverings which will reduce the likelihood of infection. The client who is being discharged for follow-up physical therapy has burns that are well on the way to healing.

HEALTH PROMOTION AND MAINTENANCE

Techniques of Physical Assessment

Perform a comprehensive health assessment

420. Which question should the nurse ask the parent of a 7-month-old infant to obtain the most meaningful information about the child's development?
A. Can she sit up by herself?
B. Does she make cooing sounds?
C. Does she turn over?
D. Can she transfer a spoon hand to hand?

The answer is A. By seven months, the infant should be able to sit without support. The other options are appropriate for younger children.

PHYSIOLOGICAL INTEGRITY

Pharmacological and Parenteral Therapies

Medication administration

421. A 10-month-old infant needs an immunization. Which is the best site for the intramuscular injection?
   A. Deltoid
   B. Gluteal
   C. Dorsogluteal
   D. Vastus lateralis

The answer is D. This muscle is the best choice until the child is walking well.

The deltoid is never used on young children. The gluteal and dorsagluteal both refer to the same site and should not be used in children under 2.

SAFE AND EFFECTIVE CARE ENVIRONMENT

Safety and Infection Control

Injury Prevention

Protect the client from injury

422. After admission to the hospital unit, a 5-year-old child is diagnosed with a brain tumor involving the cerebellum. While providing care in the preoperative period, which would be the primary nursing intervention?
   A. Protect the child from falls
   B. Monitor the child for seizures
   C. Measure the head circumference daily
   D. Maintain the child's temperature within the normal range

The answer is A. Pathology in the cerebellum leads to ataxia which places the child at risk for falls.

B, C, and D are incorrect—Seizures are a late symptom in brain tumors so would not be expected here. The child's sutures have closed at 5 years of age so head circumference will not change. The temperature is not likely to be affected.

PHYSIOLOGICAL INTEGRITY

Reduction of Risk Potential

Therapeutic procedures

423. An elderly client is going to have a feeding tube permanently placed. The physician is debating placing a PEG gastrostomy tube or a jejunostomy tube. Which fact about the client suggests that a jejunostomy tube is the best option?
   A. The client's caloric needs are high.
   B. The client has a tendency to vomit.
   C. The client's family will be caring for the feeding tube.
   D. The client is mentally confused and may pull on a tube.

The answer is B. Vomiting would decrease with a jejunostomy tube as the feeding will be placed in the duodenum rather than in the stomach. The other statements would have no bearing on the decision.

HEALTH PROMOTION AND MAINTENANCE

Self-Care

424. A client has recently been diagnosed with a mild case of emphysema and has been instructed in self care at home. On a return visit to the clinic, the client makes the following statements. Which statement indicates the need for further client education?
   A. "I quit the gym since I shouldn't exercise."
   B. "I told my family they could no longer smoke in my house."
   C. "I have increased the water I drink by two extra glasses per day."
   D. "I had a room air conditioner put into my home so that I can stay indoors when the pollution level is high."

The answer is A. Moderate exercise can be beneficial to help keep the airways open and clean. All other statements were correct information and do not indicate need for further intervention.

PHYSIOLOGICAL INTEGRITY

Reduction of Risk Potential

Laboratory values

425. A nurse is working with several pediatric renal clients. The nurse notes similarities between the labs of the pediatric clients with nephrotic syndrome and those with acute glomerulonephritis. Which lab findings would be similar?
   A. Urine positive for protein
   B. Serum albumin decreased
   C. Elevated serum triglyceride levels
   D. Urine positive for red blood cells.

The answer is A. In nephrotic syndrome, albumin is lost while in acute glomerulonephritis, red blood cells are lost in the urine. Both are proteins and would give a positive proteinuria level. In nephrotic syndrome, the serum albumin is decreased and serum triglyceride levels are elevated. RBCs are in the urine for acute glomerulonephtirits.

PHYSIOLOGICAL INTEGRITY

Basic Care and Comfort

Nutrition and oral hydration

426. A child is found to be allergic to milk. To ensure adequate calcium intake, which foods would the nurse recommend be included in the child's diet?
   A. Coffee and tea
   B. Pork and ground beef
   C. Fruits such as apples and pears
   D. Green leafy vegetables such as collard greens and spinach

The answer is D. Greens and spinach are good sources of calcium. The other foods are not sources of calcium.

HEALTH PROMOTION AND MAINTENANCE

Growth and Development

427. Many high schools organize programs to discourage teenagers from driving drunk, e.g., a fatal car accident involving popular students is staged in a place where students will see it. On which developmental fact is the effectiveness of these programs postulated? Teenagers
   A. view death as a result of an accident.
   B. view death as a temporary separation.
   C. think death only occurs to the elderly and the sick.
   D. recognize that death is universal but usually do not see themselves as susceptible.

The answer is D. Teenagers can conceptionally view death as an adult does, but often do not think it can happen to them or their friends. These programs help them to understand the reality that driving and drinking can be fatal to everyone. The other views of death are those of younger children.

PHYSIOLOGICAL INTEGRITY

Pharmacological and Parenteral Therapies

Medication administration

428. Which is a step in the procedure for applying a transdermal patch for medication administration?
   A. Wear sterile gloves when handling the patch.
   B. Apply the patch to clean, dry, and un-inflamed skin.
   C. Wipe the skin with alcohol and Betadine before applying the patch.
   D. Rub the patch firmly after application to insure solid contact with skin.

The answer is B. Applying to clean dry and un-inflamed skin provides the best medication absorption.

Clean gloves should be worn, not sterile. The alcohol and Betadine are not used because they could affect medication absorption. Always follow manufacturer recommendations for application including rubbing the patch after application.

PHYSIOLOGICAL INTEGRITY

Reduction in Risk Potential

Diagnostic tests

429. A client admitted for a workup to rule out multiple sclerosis has an evoked response test. The client asks what this test will evaluate. Which is the correct reply? The test will evaluate:
   A. radiation uptake by the brain.
   B. the size of the brain for atrophy.
   C. the amount of protein in the cerebrospinal fluid.
   D. the length of time it takes for the nerve cell to conduct an impulse.

The answer is D. The evoked response test stimulates one nerve and evaluates how long it takes that message to travel to the brain. The stimuli can be visual, auditory or somatosensory. Radiation uptake would be a scan, a CT will evaluate atrophy of the brain. The amount of protein in the CSF is evaluated by a lumbar puncture.

PSYCHOSOCIAL INTEGRITY

Grief and Loss

430. A terminally ill client tells the nurse "If I can only live to see my grandchild born." The nurse recognizes this is an example of
   A. disbelief
   B. bargaining
   C. depression
   D. acceptance

The answer is B. Bargaining is the "If this, then that" response.

The disbelief response is "No, not me" and doctor shopping looking for a more acceptable diagnosis. In depression, the client accepts that death is inevitable and is saddened about all that they are losing. Acceptance is when the client is at peace with the terminal illness.

PHYSIOLOGICAL INTEGRITY

Reduction of Risk Potential

Potential for complications of diagnostic test/treatments/procedures

431. A client with a history of severe allergic reactions, is to be allergy tested. Which type of allergy test requires the most careful monitoring for a severe reaction?
   A. A RAST test
   B. Skin patch testing
   C. An eosinophil count
   D. Intracutaneous skin testing

The answer is D. This test provides the risk of the greatest exposure to potential allergens. Skin patch testing also involves exposure to potential allergens, but since the allergen is not injected, there is less risk of a systemic reaction. RAST test and eosinophil counts involve no risk of an allergic reaction.

PHYSIOLOGICAL INTEGRITY

Physiological Adaptation

Illness management

432. A client develops Bell's Palsy affecting the right side of their face. Which would be an important nursing intervention?
   A. Instill artificial tears into the right eye.
   B. Reinforce that appearance doesn't matter.
   C. Provide a clear liquid diet to prevent choking.
   D. Apply skin care products to the right side of the face from scalp to jaw line.

The answer is A. Because of the palsy, the client will be unable to blink on the right side. This will cause the right eye to dry out so artificial tears will keep the eye moist and promote comfort. Telling someone appearance doesn't matter doesn't affect how the client feels about appearance. Chewing and swallowing are only minimally affected so clear liquids are not appropriate. The skin on the affected side remains intact so skin care products are not required.

HEALTH PROMOTION AND MAINTENANCE

Self-Care

433. A diabetic client is being taught foot care. Which information will the nurse include in the teaching? (Select all that apply.)
   A. ___ Do not wear sandals or open toed shoes
   B. ___ Rubber/plastic shoes are best for your feet.
   C. ___ Use a mirror to inspect the soles and back of the foot daily
   D. ___ Buy your shoes in the late afternoon when your feet are their largest.
   E. ___ Cut your toenails first thing in the morning when they are the softest.

The answers are A, C, and D. Sandals and open toed shoes increase the risk of injury to the feet. A mirror will allow the inspection of hard to see areas. Your feet are their largest in late afternoon, so that is the best time to shop for shoes.

Natural fibers should as leather and canvas allow perspiration to escape and are better than rubber and plastic. Toenails should be cut after a bath when they are the softest.

PHYSIOLOGICAL INTEGRITY

Physiological Adaptation

Illness management

434. A client is seen in the emergency room for severe pain secondary to renal calculi. Following the administration of pain medication, the client is sent home and instructed to filter all urine for stones. Which other instructions will the nurse give the client? (Select all that apply.)
   A. ___ Limit milk intake
   B. ___ Rest in the lateral sims position
   C. ___ Void every two hours while awake
   D. ___ Increase intake of meat, eggs and cranberries
   E. ___ Increase fluid intake to 2 to 3 liters of fluid per day.

The answers are A, D, and E. In some clients, milk intake increases the calcium levels which are a component of some renal calculi. In addition, milk increases the alkalinity of the urine which can be a factor contributing to renal calculi. Meat, eggs, and cranberries produce acidic urine which reduces renal calculi. Fluid intake will help to reduce calculi. Resting in the lateral Sim's position and voiding every two hours will not reduce renal calculi.

PHYSIOLOGICAL INTEGRITY

Reduction in Risk Potential

Therapeutic procedures

435. A client with nutritional deficiencies has a jejunostomy tube placed for enteral feedings. The physician orders the client to receive 2400 ml of feeding per day. Which is an appropriate nursing action?
   A. Divide the feeding into 3 parts and feed at meal times.
   B. Feed the client an equal amount every two hours around the clock.

C. Place the feeding on a pump and feed continuously around the clock.
D. Divide the feeding into 6 feedings and feed every 4 hours around the clock.

The answer is C. Jejunostomy feedings should be continuous. Gastrostomy feedings can be bolused.

PSYCHOSOCIAL INTEGRITY

Mental Health Concepts

436. A client has been ordered by the court into a facility which specializes in the treatment of substance abuse. Group meetings are an integral part of the program. On the third day of treatment, the client says "I am not going to group this morning." In responding to the client, which fact must the nurse consider?
A. The client may be required to be in the facility but he has the right to informed consent in regard to participation in treatment.
B. The client can be physically escorted to the meeting room but cannot be made to enter.
C. The client can be coerced into attending the meeting as long as no physical force is used.
D. The client can elect not to attend 20% of treatment activities without any repercussions.

The answer is A. Because a client is involuntarily admitted to a facility does not mean that his right to informed choice is forfeited.

PHYSIOLOGICAL INTEGRITY

Pharmacological and Parenteral Therapies

Adverse effects/contraindications/side effects

437. The client has been on antibiotics for 10 days. When talking to the clinic nurse, the client mentions that diarrhea has become bothersome. Which would be an appropriate action for the nurse to suggest?
A. Decrease water intake
B. Add yogurt to the diet.
C. Increase milk in the diet.
D. Inform the physician at the next clinic visit

The answer is B. Antibiotics eliminate the normal flora of the intestines. Decreasing water intake will worsen the problem with dehydration. Adding yogurt to the diet will help replace the normal flora. Milk would not benefit the client. Putting off intervening until the next clinic visit is not appropriate.

PHYSIOLOGICAL INTEGRITY

Pharmacological and Parenteral Therapies

Parenteral/intravenous therapies

438. A client is receiving erythromycin by peripheral IV. On the third dose, the client complains of pain at the IV insertion site. The nurse checks the insertion site but the site is benign. Which action is appropriate for the nurse take to decrease the risk of phlebitis?
A. Give the infusion faster to reduce vein exposure.
B. Give the medication orally instead of intravenously.
C. Give the client the pain medication that has been ordered prn.
D. Call the pharmacist and ask for the medication to be diluted.

The answer is D. Diluting the concentration of the drug will reduce the irritation to the vein. The other responses will not improve the developing phlebitis.

HEALTH PROMOTION AND MAINTENANCE

Family Planning

439. A woman has just delivered her fourth baby in 5 years. She states she doesn't want to become pregnant again immediately. Which is the birth control option that would offer the best protection for this client in the first 6 weeks post partum?
A. Diaphragm
B. Breast feeding
C. Intrauterine device (IUD)
D. Natural family planning (Rhythm)

The answer is C. An IUD may be inserted soon after childbirth as it does not affect involution. A diaphragm needs to be fitted to the cervix. During involution, the cervical shape could change thus altering the fit of the diaphragm so it no longer provides protection. Breast feeding is not a method of contraception. Natural family planning can be used, but since many women ovulate before menstruation returns, it may not be successful in the immediate postpartal period.

PSYCHOSOCIAL INTEGRITY

Coping Mechanisms

440. A toddler has been hospitalized for several days. The mother visits irregularly. Although the toddler cried a lot at first, the child now seems to have settled in and is happy and playful. Which type of reaction is the child displaying?

A. Despair
B. Denial
C. Protest
D. Bargaining

The answer is B. Protest, despair, and denial are the three stages of toddler hospitalization reaction. Denial is a symptom of a severe psychological reaction. In despair, the child mourns the loss of the mother. In protest, the toddler is angry, and screams and kicks. Bargaining is not a component of toddler hospitalization reaction.

PHYSIOLOGICAL INTEGRITY

Physiological Adaptation

Illness management

441. A child is admitted with marked edema and frothy urine. Lab tests showed proteinuria and decreased serum albumin and globulin. Which is an appropriate diet for this child?
A. Low protein, high calorie
B. High protein, no added salt
C. High calorie, low sodium
D. High protein, low calorie

The answer is B. Nephrotic syndrome is the idiopathic loss of protein in the urine. With the loss of protein, there is a loss of osmotic pressure and fluid escapes from the vessels into the tissues. Replacement of protein is key to reducing edema. Sodium promotes fluid retention, however low sodium diets are not tasty. In children, low sodium diets are avoided if possible so no added salt would be the right choice.

HEALTH PROMOTION AND MAINTENANCE

Growth and Development

442. The mother tells the nurse that her older children have been trading money with her 3-year-old. The older children offer the toddler their pennies for her dimes. The nurse recognizes that the toddler has not developed:
A. Egocentrism
B. Conservation
C. Object permanence
D. Cognitive dysfunction

The answer is B. Conservation is the ability to deal with a number of different aspects at the same time. At this time, the toddler can only see that the penny is bigger than the dime and cannot understand that the dime has more value. This is a skill learned in the school-age period. Egocentrism is the inability to put themselves in others' place. Object permanence is the realization that objects exist even when the child cannot see the object.

PHYSIOLOGICAL INTEGRITY

Reduction of Risk Potential

Laboratory Test

Calculates an absolute neutrophil count

443. A client has a white blood cell count of $6000/mm^3$. The differential reports 47% of these are neutrophils (segs) and 5% are bands. What is the absolute neutrophil count?
A. 2520
B. 2820
C. 3120
D. 3420

The answer is C. ANC = segs + bands × white blood cell count. .47 + .05 = .52 × 6000 = 3120.

PHYSIOLOGICAL INTEGRITY

Reduction of Risk Potential

Diagnostic tests

444. A pregnant woman at term comes to the labor unit saying her membranes have ruptured. Which characteristic of the client's vaginal secretions would confirm that the membranes had ruptured? The vaginal secretions:
A. Are positive for glucose
B. Contain red blood cells
C. Turn nitrazine paper a reddish orange
D. Appear fern like under the microscope when dried on a slide.

The answer is D. Amniotic fluid present in the vagina indicates the membranes have ruptured. When dried amniotic fluid is examined under a microscope, a crystalline fern pattern may be observed.

When vaginal secretions are tested with nitrazine paper, the color change would be blue green if the membranes have ruptured as amniotic fluid is alkaline. The presence of glucose gives no indication of the status of the membranes. Red blood cells would be positive even before the membranes ruptures.

PSYCHOSOCIAL INTEGRITY

Therapeutic Communications

Use therapeutic communication techniques to provide support to the client and/or family

445. A client is scheduled for a surgical procedure under local anesthesia. Which is an appropriate nursing

intervention when preparing the client for the surgery?

A. Reassure the client that a nurse will stay with him.

B. Explain to the client what will be felt, seen, and heard.

C. Tell the client not to worry as the physician has done it many times before.

D. Explain what the nurse and the surgeon will be doing during the procedure.

The answer is B. Preparations for any procedure should be in terms of what the client will feel, see and hear.

Choice A does not prepare the patient for what will happen. C is not a reassurance. D explains the procedures in terms of what happens to the nurse and doctor, not the client.

PHYSIOLOGICAL INTEGRITY

Physiological Adaptation

Illness management

446. A client is suspected of having renal calculi. Which is the classic assessment finding indicative of this problem?

A. Oliguria

B. RBCs in the urine

C. Frothy appearing urine

D. Acute severe flank pain on one side

The answer is D. Pain is the chief symptom although blood may be noted especially in bladder calculi. The volume of urine does not change so oliguria is not a symptom. Frothy appearing urine is seen in the individual with albumin in the urine.

PHYSIOLOGICAL INTEGRITY

Pharmacological and Parenteral Therapies

Adverse effects/contraindications

447. An elderly client returned from surgery this am. Since surgery, the client has become increasingly confused. The nurse reviews the client chart and notes the following:

- The biopsy from surgery was positive for cancer.
- The wound dressing had a small amount of serosanguineous drainage.
- An NG tube to suction was in place during the first 6 hours post surgery.
- Meperidine HCL (Demerol) has been given every 4 hours for pain.

Which of these findings could account for the increasing mental confusion?

A. The biopsy from surgery was positive for cancer.

B. The wound dressing had a small amount of serosanquinous drainage.

C. An NG tube to suction was in place during the first 6 hours postsurgery.

D. Meperidine HCL (Demerol) has been given every 4 hours for pain.

The answer is D. Meperidine is broken down in the body and releases by-products that are difficult for the elderly client to excrete. These by-products build up in the body with repeated doses causing mental confusion. None of the other findings would be associated with mental confusion.

HEALTH PROMOTION AND MAINTENANCE

Ante-/Intra-/Postpartum and Newborn Care

448. When admitted for labor, the client had been excited and talkative. Now, two hours later, the client appears serious and does not participate in "chit-chat." How should the nurse interpret this behavior? The client is:

A. worn out from laboring.

B. in the active phase of labor.

C. dissatisfied with the nursing care.

D. displaying concern for the fetus' well-being.

The answer is B. Clients in early (latent) labor are excited and talkative. As they proceed into active labor, their demeanor becomes serious and they are less talkative. There is no evidence that any other of the statements are true.

PHYSIOLOGICAL INTEGRITY

Physiological Adaptation

Illness Management

Instructs the client on measures to promote health

449. A client is admitted for pneumonia. The nurse instructs the client to change positions every two hours. The client asks the nurse why this is important. The nurse explains that turning:

A. prevents Actelectasis of the lungs.

B. promotes drainage from the lung lobes by gravity.

C. changes the portion of the lung that is splinted by the bed.

D. keeps uninvolved portions of the lungs from becoming infected.

The answer is C. The bed splints the chest and limits the ability of the lung to expand. Turning changes the portion of the lung that is splinted promoting better oxygenation. The other responses are incorrect.

PHYSIOLOGICAL INTEGRITY

Physiological Adaptation

Illness management

450. A child has just been diagnosed with asthma. The nurse has taught the mother how to "allergy proof" the home. Which statement by the parent indicates a need for additional teaching?
   A. "I will remove all stuffed toys from my child's bedroom."
   B. "Out of season clothes will be stored away from my child's room."
   C. "I will enclose my child's mattress and box springs with plastic coverings."
   D. "I will put wall-to-wall carpeting in my child's room to reduce exposure to chemicals."

The answer is D. Wall to wall carpeting will hold dust and increase allergy exposure. A better option is hard wood floors which can be mopped on a daily basis. The other options are correct.

PHYSIOLOGICAL INTEGRITY

Physiological Adaptation

Infectious disease

451. The client has been diagnosed with syphilis and begins treatment with intramuscular penicillin G. Within 24 hours of this first injection, the client returns to the clinic complaining of joint pain and fever. On assessment, the nurse notes tachycardia and hypotension. How should the nurse interpret these signs and symptoms?
   A. A worsening of the syphilis
   B. An allergic reaction to the penicillin
   C. Cellular debris from the destruction of the spirochetes.
   D. Anxiety due to the diagnosis of a sexually transmitted disease

The answer is C. The symptoms describe Jarisch-Herxheimer reaction, indication that a large amount of spirochetes have been killed by the penicillin. The client would be treated symptomatically; the penicillin would not be stopped. Symptoms will abate in another 12 hours.

HEALTH PROMOTION AND MAINTENANCE

Growth and Development

452. During a well child visit, a mother tells the nurse she will be bringing her toddler to a play group for the first time and asks what the child's reaction is likely to be. As part of her response, which type of play does the nurse describe as characteristic of toddlers?
   A. Solitary
   B. Cooperatively with several toddlers
   C. Interactively in groups of no more than 3
   D. Beside another toddler but not with the other toddler

The answer is C. Parallel play in which a toddler plays beside but not with another toddler is the type of play characteristic of the age group. Infants play alone, called solitary play. Cooperative play is organized and seen in older children. Toddlers do not interact with other children well because of their egocentricity.

PHYSIOLOGICAL INTEGRITY

Physiological Adaptation

Illness management

453. A child is admitted to the hospital for Kwashiorkor, protein malnourishment. Which physical finding would be expected on the admission assessment?
   A. Eczema
   B. Edematous
   C. Height below normal range
   D. Weight below normal range

The answer is B. Protein provides the osmotic property of the blood and without protein, liquid escapes into the tissues. The child may be overweight if there were adequate carbohydrates in the diet.

PHYSIOLOGICAL INTEGRITY

Reduction of Risk Potential

Laboratory values

454. An adult client is scheduled for a tonsillectomy. Several labs are ordered pre-operatively. Which lab test is most significant prior to this surgery?
   A. CBC
   B. PTT
   C. Urinalysis
   D. WBC with differential

The answer is B. The surgery includes a significant risk for hemorrhage; so the client's ability to clot should be carefully evaluated prior to the surgical procedure. CBC is important but not the most important. Urinalysis is usually not significant. WBC with differential probably would be ordered as tonsillectomies are not done when there is infection present.

PHYSIOLOGICAL INTEGRITY

Physiological Adaptation

Infectious diseases

455. Several members of a family have been diagnosed with pinworms. In addition to treating the family with medications, which is an important instruction for the nurse to give the family?
A. Cook all meats well.
B. Never go barefoot outside
C. Wash all vegetables before eating
D. Wash all clothes and bed linens in hot soapy water.

The answer is D. Pinworms are spread from person to person and have no dirt cycle. The primary source of contamination is the clothing. Cooking meats reduces the risk tapeworms. Walking barefoot can lead to hookworm. Washing all vegetables reduces the risk of roundworms.

HEALTH PROMOTION AND MAINTENANCE

Techniques of Physical Assessment

Perform comprehensive health assessment

456. What is the nurse assessing when with the client's eyes closed, the nurse moves the client's toes up or down one by one and asks the client to say in which direction each was moved?
A. Two-point discrimination
B. Stereognosis
C. Position sense
D. Light touch

The answer is C. This procedure is a test of position sense.

A, B, and D are incorrect—Two-point discrimination involves touching the skin simultaneously with two sterile needles at closer and closer distances to each other until the client perceives only one touch. Stereognosis is asking the client to identify a familiar object such as a key when it is placed in the client's hand with the client's eyes closed. Light touch is tested by stroking an area of the client's skin with a wisp of cotton.

PHYSIOLOGICAL INTEGRITY

Pharmacological and Parenteral Therapies

Medication Administration

Administer and document medications given by common routes

457. A 2-year-old client with otitis media is to receive ear drops. To properly administer the ear drops, the nurse pulls the pinna:
A. Up and back
B. Up and forward
C. Down and back
D. Down and forward

The answer is C. The pinna of the ear is pulled down and back for children under three and up and back for children over three.

PHYSIOLOGICAL INTEGRITY

Reduction of Risk Potential

Potential for complications from surgical procedures and health alterations

458. A 1-week-old infant has surgery to repair a cleft lip. Which is the priority concern when the child returns from the recovery room?
A. Feeding method
B. Maintaining airway
C. Preventing scarring of the lip
D. Preventing incisional infection

The answer is B. Immediately after surgery, the concern is airway. Because of surgery to the nares and the fact that newborns are obligant nasal breathers, swelling could occlude the nares. Feeding method will be a concern because sucking will interfere with the integrity of the suture line. Preventing scarring and infection are also concerns but not immediately on return to the floor.

SAFE AND EFFECTIVE CARE ENVIRONMENT

Safety and Infection Control

Standard/transmission-based/other precautions

459. A client with cancer is being treated with chemotherapy. The client becomes neutropenic. To prevent infection, the nurse implements the following: (select all that apply)
A. Place the client in contact isolation
B. Eliminate fresh flowers from the client's room
C. Serve the client only cooked fruits and vegetables
D. Use a soft toothbrush to prevent the gums from bleeding
E. Allow only close family members (spouses and children) to visit

The answers are B and C. Fresh flowers may spread mold. Only cooked vegetables and fruits are allowed to be sure all organisms have been destroyed.

A, D, and E are incorrect—The client will be in protective isolation, not contact. Bleeding gums is thrombocytopenia. Visitors are acceptable as long as they are not sick. The client will avoid crowds and children who might be infected.

PHYSIOLOGICAL INTEGRITY

Reduction of Risk Potential

Therapeutic procedures

460. Following an automobile accident, the client is admitted to the hospital unit with a fractured femur. The client is placed in skeletal traction. Which is an appropriate nursing action?
  A. Restrict fluid
  B. Turn side to side every two hours
  C. Perform Range of Motion exercises on the affected hip
  D. Give sterile pin care using Betadine and sterile dressing

The answer is D. Skeletal traction involves a pin being inserted through the bone as a component of the traction. Since there is a loss of skin integrity at the site of the bone pinning, this site is at risk for infection. Therefore, pin care is an important part of the nursing care.

PHYSIOLOGICAL INTEGRITY

Pharmacological and Parenteral Therapies

Parenteral/intravenous therapies

461. The nurse is attempting to start a peripheral intravenous infusion line on a client with small veins. The nurse has made one attempt without success. The nurse states the veins aren't palpable with gloves on. Which action should the nurse take?
  A. Start the IV line without gloves.
  B. Wear a glove on the dominant hand only.
  C. Wear two gloves that the pointer finger of one glove has been removed for palpation
  D. Locate the vein without gloves and mark the site then put on gloves

The answer is D. For all procedures where blood exposure could occur, gloves are required. Removal of one finger has the same consequence as removing the whole glove and is not acceptable.

HEALTH PROMOTION AND MAINTENANCE

Techniques of Physical Assessment

462. The nurse is doing a complete physical assessment on a young child. Which is the most appropriate order of assessment for the nurse to use?
  A. Heart and lungs sounds first
  B. Percussion before auscultation
  C. Organized in a head to toe manner
  D. Invasive procedures first to get them over.

The answer is A. Listen to heart and lungs sounds first. Once an infant starts crying, it will be more difficult to hear these.

Auscultation is before percussion. Organized is appropriate but because of the child's developmental stage, it is not head to toe. Invasive should be performed last as children tend to be less cooperative after invasive procedures.

PHYSIOLOGICAL INTEGRITY

Reduction of Risk Potential

Therapeutic procedures

463. A baby has been diagnosed with developmental dysplasia of the hips and a Pavlik harness is applied. The Pavlik harness is a type of splint that abducts and flexes the hips while still allowing leg movement. The harness can be removed and reapplied by the parents. Instructions to include for the family caring for an infant in this type of harness would include:
  A. increase fluid intake to promote urine output.
  B. keep the harness on the child at least 23 hours a day.
  C. take the harness off at night if the baby is uncomfortable.
  D. the baby will need a high protein diet to allow hip repair.

The answer is B. When harnesses and splints can be applied and removed by the parents, there is a tendency for parents to remove them if the child complains.

C will result in insufficient treatment. A is not appropriate as this condition is not related to urinary function. D is incorrect as this is not a protein deficiency.

PSYCHOSOCIAL INTEGRITY

Psychopathology

Recognize signs of acute and chronic mental illness

464. A man brings his mother to the clinic and says she has been diagnosed with Alzheimer's disease but her behavior has changed drastically and he is concerned about what has happened. On obtaining the history, the nurse learns the client had been disoriented in terms of time and place, had loss of memory, and had difficulty with banking, housecleaning and other activities of daily living but has now become agitated and combative; doesn't bathe or groom; and rarely speaks. Which conclusion does the nurse draw from this information?
  A. The client has entered stage 2 of Alzheimer's disease.
  B. The client has passed from stage 2 to stage 3 of Alzheimer's disease.

C. The client has endstage disease.

D. The client has a secondary disease process going on.

The answer is B. The client's past symptoms of disorientation, memory loss and difficulty with instrumental activities of daily living are all characteristic of stage 2 Alzheimer's disease. The client's new symptoms of agitation, combativeness, lack of bathing and grooming, and rarely speaking are all symptoms of stage 3 Alzheimer's disease.

PHYSIOLOGICAL INTEGRITY

Physiological Adaptation

Illness management

465. During the initial assessment process, a client tells the nurse that he is lactose intolerant. When the nurse questions the client about the lactose intolerance, the nurse would expect the client to describe symptoms including (select all that apply).

A. ___ Rashes

B. ___ Flatus

C. ___ Constipation

D. ___ Black furry tongue

E. ___ Abdominal cramping

The answers are B and E. In addition to these symptoms, the other major symptom is diarrhea which can be explosive. Rashes are associated with allergic responses, not lactose intolerance. Black furry tongue is usually do to the overgrowth of organisms not susceptible to antibiotics and not associated with lactose intolerance.

PHYSIOLOGICAL INTEGRITY

Pharmacological and Parenteral Therapies

Adverse Effects/Contraindications

Implement procedures to counteract adverse effects of medications and parenteral therapy

466. A cancer client is receiving chemotherapy known to cause stomatitis. Which nursing action would be appropriate in an effort to reduce or prevent the development of stomatitis?

A. Ask the physician for a prophylactic antibiotic

B. Provide a firm toothbrush to enhance oral cleaning

C. Encourage the use of mouthwash containing alcohol

D. Instruct the client to rinse their mouth with water every two hours

The answer is D. Research has shown that simply rinsing the mouth with water on a frequent basis can reduce stomatitis in chemotherapy clients. A firm toothbrush could damage the oral mucous membranes. Alcohol is drying and would damage the mucous membranes. Antibiotics would be inappropriate.

SAFE AND EFFECTIVE CARE ENVIRONMENTS

Safety and Infection Control

Standard/Transmission-Based/Other Precautions

Apply principles of infection control

467. Which type of precautions would be used when caring for a client with *C. difficile*?

A. Standard precautions

B. Airborne precautions

C. Droplet precautions

D. Contact precautions

The answer is D. Contact precautions are used when organisms causing serious disease are easily transmitted through direct contact. This includes all multidrug resistant strains of organisms such as *C. difficile*, shigella, and impetigo. Contact precautions require a private room or a room shared with someone infected with the same organism. Gloves are worn at all times and gowns and protective barriers are used if direct contact is required.

A is incorrect—Standard precautions are used to decrease the risk of transmission from bloodborne pathogens and moist body substances. Moist body substances include blood, urine, feces, sputum, saliva, wound drainage, and all aspirated fluids. B is incorrect—Airborne precautions are used when the mode of spread of an organism is by small particle droplets borne on air currents. Airborne precautions require a private room with negative airflow and adequate filtration; those entering the room wear a mask and if the client leaves the room, a mask is worn. C is incorrect—Droplet precautions are used when the mechanism of transmission is by large droplets spread by coughing, sneezing, or talking. Droplet precautions require a private room or a room shared with someone infected with the same organism. Those entering the room and coming within 3 feet of the client need to wear a mask and the client wears a mask if taken out of the room.

PHYSIOLOGICAL INTEGRITY

Physiological Adaptation

Illness Management

Apply knowledge of client pathophysiology to illness management

468. A client presents to the emergency room in sickle cell crisis. The priority nursing intervention for this client to break the sickling cycle would be to:

A. administer oxygen as ordered.

B. teach sources of iron and folic acid in the diet.

C. draw blood for a hemoglobin and hematocrit value.

D. explain to the client the need to seek treatment as soon as a crisis begins.

The answer is A. The crisis is caused by a decrease in oxygen in the blood. Activities designed to reduce sickling would include administration of oxygen, fluids including intravenous fluids, promoting rest and providing pain relief.

All other activities would be inappropriate to break the sickling cycle.

HEALTH PROMOTION AND MAINTENANCE

Ante-/Intra-/Postpartum and Newborn Care

469. A pregnant woman is in early labor. After performing Leopold's maneuvers, the nurse determines that the infant is probably a right occiput posterior presentation. Where would the nurse check fetal heart tones?
   A. Through the mother's back.
   B. At the umbilicus on the left side.
   C. Below the umbilicus on the right side.
   D. Above the umbilicus on the right side.

The answer is C. The infant would be a vertex presentation on the right side making the fetal heart tones heard best below the umbilicus on the right. FHTs are never assessed through the maternal back. FHTs heard at the umbilicus are due to a transverse lie. Breech presentations put the FHTs above the umbilicus.

PHYSIOLOGICAL INTEGRITY

Reduction of Risk potential

Diagnostic tests

470. The client's history indicates several allergic diseases including eczema and asthma as a child and hay fever as an adult. Which laboratory findings support this history?
   A. Moderate anemia
   B. Elevated eosinophil count
   C. Elevated C reactive protein
   D. Alkaline Phosphatase decreased

The answer is B. Eosinophils are a type of WBC and are elevated in persons with allergies and worm infestations. The other responses are not related to allergic reactions.

PHYSIOLOGICAL INTEGRITY

Pharmacological and Parenteral Therapy

Medication Administration

Educate client/family about medications

471. A client was admitted to the burn unit after suffering extensive partial and full thickness burns in a house fire. At 24 hours postadmission, the physician orders albumin for the client. The family asks why the client is receiving albumin. The nurse's response would be based on the knowledge that albumin is a:
   A. blood product that will help restore circulating RBCs.
   B. hypertonic solution that will help restore plasma volume.
   C. source of clotting factors that will control wound bleeding.
   D. source of antibodies to help the client fight infection secondary to the loss of skin.

The answer is B. Following a burn injury, the blood vessels become permeable and fluid and protein is lost into the tissues. Administering a hypertonic solution will cause the fluid to return from the tissues and maintain circulating volume. Although albumin is a blood product, it does not contain red blood cells. Wound bleeding is not a problem this late in the injury. Albumin is not given to fight infection.

PSYCHOSOCIAL INTEGRITY

Behavioral Interventions

Assess client appearance, mood, and psychomotor behavior and identify/respond to inappropriate/abnormal behavior

472. Which is a priority nursing intervention for a client with paranoid personality disorder?
   A. Encourage acceptance of intensive therapy.
   B. Eliminate bizarre fantasies.
   C. Promote social relationships
   D. Minimize potential for aggression

The answer is D. Clients with a paranoid personality disorder is suspicious and hypervigilant with irritable, agitated moods. They can interpret all behavior as threatening and react in an aggressive manner. Therefore minimizing the potential for aggressive behavior is a priority nursing intervention. Clients with paranoid personality disorders are not good candidates for intensive therapy, especially group therapy, because it can heighten their suspiciousness and escalate the risk of aggressive response. Promotion of social relationships is a priority intervention for clients with schizoid personality disorder. Bizarre fantasies are characteristic of schizotypal personality disorder.

PHYSIOLOGICAL INTEGRITY

Reduction of Risk potential

Laboratory values

473. A preterm infant has significant respiratory distress due to the immaturity of the lungs. When arterial blood gases results are received, the nurse would expect to see which abnormality?
   A. Respiratory alkalosis

B. The pH is lower than normal
C. The oxygen saturation is 94%
D. The carbon dioxide pressure (PCO_2) is normal.

The answer is B. A lower pH is acidosis and an infant breathing poorly would have respiratory acidosis. An oxygen saturation of 94% is normal. The carbon dioxide pressure would not be normal.

PHYSIOLOGICAL INTEGRITY

Reduction of Risk Potential

Therapeutic procedures

474. A client had polio as a child and now wears a leg brace. A pressure sore has formed under the leg brace. Instructions for this client should include:
   A. wear the brace only 6 hours per day.
   B. do not wear the brace until the skin has healed.
   C. apply a dressing over the sore to protect it from the brace.
   D. cover the wound with petroleum prior to putting on the brace.

The answer is B. The brace should not be worn until the sore is healed as the brace is the most likely cause of the injury.

Wearing the brace 6 hours a day will further damage the skin. A dressing under a brace that is already rubbing on the skin will only make the pressure sore worse. Petroleum will not protect this wound if the brace is worn.

PSYCHOSOCIAL INTEGRITY

Therapeutic Communications

Uses therapeutic communications skills in providing care to the client

475. A 36-year-old woman has had a hysterectomy for fibroid disease. Prior to surgery, the woman stated her family was complete and she would be glad to not have to deal with her periods anymore. Two days after surgery, the nurse finds the woman crying. Which would be an appropriate response by the nurse?
   A. "I know what you are going through, I was upset after my hysterectomy too."
   B. "You shouldn't cry. Just think, no more periods, no more cramps, no more birth control."
   C. "I know that you thought you wouldn't be sad about the hysterectomy but it still bothers you, doesn't it?"
   D. "Other clients have told me that they were surprised about their feelings of loss even though they didn't want more children. Is that what you are feeling?"

The answer is D. This statement allows the client to recognize her feelings are common and seeks verification on the cause of the sadness.

A is incorrect—Usually it is best to avoid personal experiences when talking to clients about their feelings. Option B denies the validity of the client's sadness. Option C seeks clarification but does not let the client know that her feelings are common.

PHYSIOLOGICAL INTEGRITY

Pharmacological and Parenteral Therapies

Total Parenteral Nutrition

Provide client/family/significant others with information on TPN

476. When the family notices that the Total Parenteral Nutrition the surgical client is receiving contains insulin, they question the nurse about why insulin has been added to the bag. The nurse explains that the client:
   A. is a diabetic and needs the exogenous insulin.
   B. is underweight and the insulin will help with weight gain.
   C. is a pseudodiabetic due to the sugar content of the solution.
   D. needs the insulin because of ileus secondary to the surgical procedure.

The answer is C. TPN has a very high sugar content which stresses the client's pancreas. There is no evidence the client is diabetic or is underweight. Ileus does not affect the pancreas.

HEALTH PROMOTION AND MAINTENANCE

Techniques of Physical Assessment

Perform comprehensive health assessment

477. Which cranial nerve is the nurse assessing when the nurse the client's blink reflex is checked?
   A. One (olfactory)
   B. Five (trigeminal)
   C. Seven (facial)
   D. Eleven (spinal accessory)

The answer is B. The motor component of cranial nerve five (trigeminal nerve) controls the blink reflex, which is tested by bringing a wisp of cotton in from the side to touch the cornea of each eye.

A is incorrect—Cranial nerve one (olfactory nerve) is responsible for the sense of smell. It is tested by occluding each of the client's nostrils one at a time, holding a substance such as coffee or vanilla with a familiar aroma under the other nostril, and asking the client to identify the smell. The test is repeated with a different aromatic substance to determine if the client can differentiate smells.

C is incorrect—Cranial nerve seven (facial nerve) is responsible for taste on the front two thirds of the tongue and for movement of the face including the ability to close the eyes and move the lips for speech. Motor function of cranial nerve seven is tested by asking the client to smile, frown, grimace, show the upper and lower teeth, keep the eyes closed, while the examiner tries to open them and puff out the cheeks. The examiner observes for symmetry and movement and presses the puffed out cheeks in to check if air is expelled equally from both sides. To test taste, an applicator dipped in a sugar, salt, or lemon solution is placed on the tongue and the client is asked what is tasted.

D is incorrect—Cranial nerve eleven (spinal accessory) is tested by asking the client to shrug the shoulders and resist pressure to put them down because this cranial nerve controls muscular strength of the trapezius and sternocleidomastoid muscles.

PHYSIOLOGICAL INTEGRITY

Physiological Adaptation

Pathophysiology

478. A client has been admitted with a possible bowel obstruction. The nurse completes a head to toe assessment. Which finding should the nurse interpret as inconsistent with a bowel obstruction?
   A. Vital signs normal
   B. Vomitus has a fecal odor
   C. Complains of colicky pain
   D. Loud rumbling bowel sounds

The answer is D. Bowel sounds in early obstruction are often high pitched and tinkling above the obstruction. Bowel sounds will be absent in late obstruction. Vital signs may remain within the normal range in early obstruction and progress to shock as the obstruction continues. The pain is often colicky and the vomitus may have a fecal odor.

PHYSIOLOGICAL INTEGRITY

Reduction of Risk Potential

Therapeutic procedures

479. A client's care giver is performing tracheostomy care. Which action by the care giver would the nurse correct? The care giver
   A. Used half strength hydrogen peroxide to clean the inner cannula.
   B. Held the tracheostomy tube in place while changing the ties.
   C. Rinsed the inner cannula with sterile normal saline after cleaning.
   D. Used commercial tracheostomy dressing material to eliminate the need for cutting gauze

The answer is C. To prevent accidental decannulation, the soiled ties are not removed until the new ties have been put in place. Half strength hydrogen peroxide is used to clean the inner cannula and sterile saline is used to rinse it. Commercial tracheostomy dressings may be used for ease of application if desired.

SAFE AND EFFECTIVE CARE ENVIRONMENT

Safety and Infection Control

Standard/transmission-based/other precautions

480. A pregnant woman at term has an outbreak of genital herpes. She asks the nurse how this will affect her labor and delivery. Which response would be correct?
   A. "You will probably have a cesarean delivery."
   B. "The baby will require antibiotics after delivery."
   C. "You will be placed on antibiotics when you go into labor."
   D. "You will need antibiotics in the postpartum period to prevent a uterine infection."

The answer is A. With an outbreak of genital herpes, the baby is usually delivered by cesarean section to decrease the infant exposure. Herpes is a virus; so antibiotics will not be effective against this organism.

PHYSIOLOGICAL INTEGRITY

Reduction of Risk Potential

Potential for alteration in body systems

481. A child has been diagnosed with Wilms Tumor. Prior to surgery, a sign is placed over the child's bed that states: "Do Not Palpate Abdomen." The mother asks why that sign was placed over the bed. The nurse's response will be based on the knowledge that palpating the abdomen:
   A. would be painful for the child.
   B. can increase the child's anxiety.
   C. may affect the blood supply to the kidney.
   D. could release cancer cells that will migrate to other areas.

The answer is D. Wilms Tumor is encapsulated until relatively late in the disease. Palpating the abdomen may cause a seeding of tumor cells to other tissues by way of the blood and should be avoided except as absolutely necessary for diagnosis. Palpating the abdomen is not usually painful and should not cause anxiety. The blood supply to the kidney will not be affected except through cancer cell seeding.

PHYSIOLOGICAL INTEGRITY

Physiological Adaptation

Fluid and Electrolyte Imbalances

Identify signs and symptoms of client fluid and/or electrolyte balance

482. A child is admitted to the hospital unit for gastroenteritis and dehydration. Which laboratory values does the nurse interpret as indicative of dehydration? Select all that apply.
A. ___ Elevated WBC
B. ___ Elevated Hemoglobin
C. ___ Elevated Hematocrit
D. ___ Decreased urine-specific gravity.
E. ___ Elevated lymphocytes in the WBC differential

The answers are B and C. Both hemoglobin and hematocrit are comparisons of solids to liquids. If the amount of solids stays constant but the volume decreases, the Hgb and Hct would be elevated. Elevated WBC indicates infection, while the elevated lymphocytes indicate a viral infection. A decreased urine-specific gravity would be a more dilute urine and not associated with dehydration.

HEALTH PROMOTION AND MAINTENANCE

Ante-/Intra-/Postpartum and Newborn Care

483. A client is 12 weeks pregnant. During her regular prenatal visit, the following findings are noted:
- Leukorrhea is present
- Complains of urinary frequency
- Uterus is lower in the pelvis than 12 weeks gestation
- Has symptoms of PIH (pregnancy induce hypertension)

Which finding is suggestive of a hydatiform mole?
A. Leukorrhea is present
B. Complains of urinary frequency
C. Uterus is lower in the pelvis than 12 weeks gestation
D. Has symptoms of PIH (pregnancy induced hypertension)

The answer is D. PIH is rare in the first trimester except in the case of a hydatiform mole. Urinary frequency and leucorrhoea are normal in pregnancy. In molar pregnancies, the uterus is larger than anticipated.

PHYSIOLOGICAL INTEGRITY

Physiological Adaptation

Pathophysiology

484. A client has been diagnosed with pre-invasive cervical cancer. When assessing the client, what type of symptomology would the nurse expect?
A. Pain
B. Anorexia
C. Bleeding
D. None

The answer is D. There are usually no symptoms of preinvasive cervical cancer.

PHYSIOLOGICAL INTEGRITY

Pharmacological and Parenteral Therapies

Adverse effects/contraindications and side effects implement procedures to counteract adverse effects of medications and parenteral therapy

485. A toddler is seen in the emergency room after taking a number of codeine tablets belonging to a grandparent. Which antidote does the nurse expect the child to receive?
A. Glucagon
B. Naloxone
C. Vitamin K
D. Sodium Bicarbonate

The answer is B. Naloxone (narcan) is an antidote for narcotics such as codeine.

The other answers are incorrect.

SAFE AND EFFECTIVE ENVIRONMENT

Management of Care

Establishing Priorities

Apply knowledge of pathophysiology when establishing priorities for interventions with multiple clients

486. A nurse on the postpartum unit receives report on his or her assigned clients. Which client should the nurse assess first?
A. Primipara with problems breastfeeding.
B. Fresh delivery complaining of severe perineal pain.

C. Multipara, 48 hours postpartum, with elevated blood pressure.
D. Client who received spinal anesthesia for delivery and is complaining of a headache.

The answer is B. The severe perineal pain could be a labial hematoma. The other clients present no immediate concern.

PHYSIOLOGICAL INTEGRITY

Physiological Adaptation

Applies knowledge of bloodborne pathogens to the care of the client

487. A nurse has been diagnosed with hepatitis C. The source of the hepatitis C is not known. Which factor may have contributed to the nurse becoming infected?
A. Having a tattoo
B. Used oral street drugs during the teen years.
C. Failure to complete the Hepatitis Vaccine Series
D. Frequently eats vegetables straight from the garden

The answer is A. There is a major concern that tattoos may be a source of the hepatitis C if the tattoo artist does not use new or properly sterilized needles.

Oral drugs would not be a source of hepatitis C, injectibles would be. The hepatitis vaccine series protects against hepatitis B. It offers no protection for hepatitis C. Hepatitis C is a bloodborne pathogen. Hepatitis A comes from contaminated food and water.

PHYSIOLOGICAL INTEGRITY

Pharmacological and Parenteral Therapies

Total parenteral nutrition

488. A client is receiving total parenteral nutrition. In recognition of a common complication of TPN, the nurse will monitor the client for:
A. Dehydration
B. Renal failure
C. Cerebral edema
D. Pulmonary hypertension

The answer is A. TPN is a hypertonic solution which can lead to diuresis. The other complications are not associated with TPN.

PSYCHOSOCIAL INTEGRITY

Behavioral Interventions

Assess client appearance, mood and psychomotor behavior and identify/respond to inappropriate/abnormal behavior

489. Which behaviors exhibited by a client alert the nurse to the need to take measures to protect self and others against an aggressive outburst? Mark all that apply.
A. ___ fist clenching
B. ___ finger snapping
C. ___ foot tapping
D. ___ pacing
E. ___ shouting
F. ___ glaring

The answers are A, D, E, and F. Fist clenching, pacing, shouting, glaring along with jaw clenching are all common signs of markedly increased agitation and indicate that the risk of aggressive behavior is real and immediate. Foot tapping and finger snapping often occur unrelated to risk of aggression and if related generally indicate a lower level of agitation.

PHYSIOLOGICAL INTEGRITY

Basic Care and Comfort

Palliative/Comfort Care

Assess, intervene, and educate client/family/significant others about pain management

490. A client had a vulvectomy yesterday. On initial assessment, the nurse notes the client is dosing while sitting up in bed in Fowler's position. When she awakens, the client states she is uncomfortable. Which is the priority nursing action?
A. Call the physician
B. Change the client's position to Semi-Fowler's.
C. Give more pain medication
D. Explain it is normal to be uncomfortable after a surgical procedure

The answer is B. Lowering the head of the bed will reduce the pressure and tension on the incision and reduce the client's pain.

PHYSIOLOGICAL INTEGRITY

Physiological Adaptability

Illness Management

Apply knowledge of client pathology to illness management

491. A newborn has been transferred to the pediatric hospital from the birth hospital with a large myleomeningocele. On admission to the pediatric hospital, in which position will the nurse place the infant?
A. Prone
B. Supine
C. In semi-Fowler's
D. In trendelenburg

The answer is A. The myleomeningocele is extremely fragile prior to surgical removal. The infant is positioned prone to prevent pressure on the sac. The other responses are incorrect.

HEALTH PROMOTION AND MAINTENANCE

Ante-/Intra-/Postpartum and Newborn Care

492. The home economics class in a high school has a class on pregnancy as part of the family life curriculum. A nurse has been asked to present information about pregnancy to the class. The nurse tells the students that smoking during pregnancy can have a negative effect on the fetus. The nurse explains that mothers who smoke often give birth to:
    A. diabetic infants.
    B. low birth weight infants.
    C. large for gestational age babies.
    D. infants who grow up to be smokers.

The answer is B. Miscarriages, preterm birth, and low birth rate babies are associated with smoking during pregnancy. It is not associated with diabetic infants or large for gestational age babies. Seeing a parent smoke can be a influencing factor in the children smoking but the mother smoking during pregnancy does not encourage smoking by the infant when he or she grows up.

PHYSIOLOGICAL INTEGRITY

Reduction of Risk Potential

Potential for complications from surgical procedures and health alterations

493. An 18-month-old child has returned from cleft palate repair. The postoperative physician's orders include full liquid diet. Which would be the best feeding method for this child?
    A. Cup
    B. Straw
    C. Spoon
    D. Baby bottle

The answer is C. Anything that can be made into a liquid could be fed to the child. Drinking from a cup will prevent injury to the palate. Nothing rigid should be allowed in the mouth that could damage the palate repair. Sucking on a bottle or straw would also be inappropriate.

PSYCHOSOCIAL INTEGRITY

Coping Mechanisms

494. When the new baby comes home from the hospital, the older sibling, a toddler, begins wetting himself. The mother calls the clinic nurse to ask what is happening as the toddler was toilet trained over a year ago. Which is the most likely explanation for this problem? The client:
    A. May need more oral fluids.
    B. Has a urinary tract infection.
    C. Has regressed due to the stress of the new baby.
    D. Is mad at the mother for bringing home a new baby.

The answer is C. Regression is common when a child is psychologically stressed. There is no evidence of a need for increased fluids or a urinary tract infection. Even a toddler that is excited about a new sibling will feel stress when the family dynamics change.

PHYSIOLOGICAL INTEGRITY

Physiological Adaptation

Illness Management

Teach client about managing illness

495. Which statement made by a client with COPD after being taught about the use of pursed lip breathing indicates the need for additional instruction?
    A. "I will make sure to puff my cheeks out when I breathe out through my mouth."
    B. "I will set my lips for breathing out like I am going to whistle."
    C. "Breathing out should take me twice as long as breathing in."
    D. "I will never hold my breath when trying to lift something heavy."

The answer is A. Exhalation should be slow through pursed lips taking care not to let the checks puff out. All other statements accurately reflect instructions related to pursed lip breathing. Lips are set as if to whistle. Exhalation should be twice as long as inhalation. Pursed lip breathing should be used during any strenuous physical activity and the client should inhale before exerting and exhale during the activity. The breath should never be held.

PHYSIOLOGICAL INTEGRITY

Physiological Adaptation

Illness Management

Teach client about managing illness

496. The nurse has completed client teaching on activities to reduce the recurrence of kidney stones. Which statement by a client indicates the need for additional teaching?
    A. "I need to increase my intake of dried fruits and milk products."

B. "I should increase my intake of liquids to at least 2–3 liters per day."
C. "It is important that I drink extra water at bedtime to keep my urine dilute during the night."
D. "Cranberries, eggs and meats may help acidify my urine to reduce my kidney stones."

The answer is A. Dried fruits and milk products are high in calcium which is often associated with renal calculi so should be avoided. This statement indicates the need for additional teaching. Fluid intake, especially at night and acidifying the urine are all associated with reduced episodes of renal calculi.

PHYSIOLOGICAL INTEGRITY

Physiological Adaptation

Pathophysiology

497. Four days postoperatively, a client is noted to have thick yellow drainage on the operative dressing. The nurse would document this drainage as:
A. serous
B. purulent
C. sanguineous
D. serosanguineous

The answer is B. This drainage is purulent containing dead organisms and white blood cells. Serous is clear and watery; sanguineous is bloody; serosanguineous is pale, more watery but blood streaked.

HEALTH PROMOTION AND MAINTENANCE

Self-Care

498. Following a automobile accident, a client is treated for a head injury in the emergency room. After 12 hours of observation, the client is discharged. Which information should be given to the client/family in preparation for discharge?
A. Narcotic analgesics may be taken for headache
B. Memory of the car accident should return within the next 12 hours.
C. Vomiting may be a symptom of worsening neurologic status
D. The physician should be notified if the client is sleepy but easily aroused.

The answer is C. Vomiting could be a symptom of increased intracranial pressure. Narcotics would be avoided as they may mask increasing neurologic symptoms. Amnesia is common for the events surrounding the head injury. As long as the client is easily arousal, sleepiness is not a concern.

PHYSIOLOGICAL INTEGRITY

Reduction in Risk Potential

Vital signs

499. When delegating blood pressure measurement to an unlicensed assistant, the nurse cautions that correct technique must be used to avoid obtaining falsely high pressures. Which is one of the directions the nurse would give to prevent a falsely high pressure reading?
A. Take the blood pressure on an extremity positioned below heart level.
B. Use a cuff whose width is at least 60% of the diameter of the extremity.
C. If you have to inflate the cuff a second time, be sure to wait 1–2 minutes.
D. Apply the cuff loosely to the extremity.

The answer is C. Reinflating the cuff without a 1–2 minutes interval between inflations can result in a falsely high blood pressure reading. Therefore waiting the 1–2 minutes between inflations helps prevent a falsely high reading. Taking the blood pressure on an extremity positioned below heart level can result in a falsely low reading; the extremity needs to be supported and at heart level. The width of the cuff should be 40% of the diameter of the arm so a cuff that is at least 60% the diameter is too wide. Use of a cuff that is too wide can cause a falsely low blood pressure reading not a falsely high one. If the cuff is wrapped too loosely around the extremity the result can be a falsely high pressure reading so loose wrapping does not prevent a falsely high reading.

PHYSIOLOGICAL INTEGRITY

Pharmacological and Parenteral Therapies

Total parenteral nutrition

500. A client is receiving TPN. The bag of TPN arrives on the hospital unit with an ampule of multi-vitamins for the nurse to add. A new staff nurse asks why the pharmacy didn't add the vitamins before sending the bag to the floor. The experienced nurse will explain that:
A. The client may be allergic to the vitamins.
B. The vitamins are infused in the first 100 ml of the TPN bag.
C. The physician may change the order and leave out the vitamins.
D. Vitamins must be infused within 24 hours of being added to the bag.

The answer is D. The vitamins are stable only for 24 hours after being added to the TPN bag. The other responses are incorrect.

SAFE AND EFFECTIVE CARE ENVIRONMENTS

Safety and Infection Control

Standard/Transmission-Based/Other Precautions

Apply principles of infection control

501. Which type of precautions would be used when caring for a client with tuberculosis?
   A. Standard precautions
   B. Airborne precautions
   C. Droplet precautions
   D. Contact precautions

The answer is B. Airborne precautions are used when the mode of spread of an organism is by small particle droplets borne on air currents and tuberculosis is spread by this route. Airborne precautions require a private room with negative airflow and adequate filtration; those entering the room wear a mask and if the client leaves the room, a mask is worn.

A is incorrect—Standard precautions are used to decrease the risk of transmission from bloodborne pathogens and moist body substances. Moist body substances include blood, urine, feces, sputum, saliva, wound drainage, and all aspirated fluids. C is incorrect—Droplet precautions are used when the mechanism of transmission is by large droplets spread by coughing, sneezing, or talking. Droplet precautions require a private room or a room shared with someone infected with the same organism. Those entering the room and coming within 3 feet of the client need to wear a mask and the client wears a mask if taken out of the room. D is incorrect—Contact precautions are used when organisms causing serious disease are easily transmitted through direct contact. Contact precautions require a private room or a room shared with someone infected with the same organism. Gloves are worn at all times and gowns and protective barriers are used if direct contact is required.

PHYSIOLOGICAL INTEGRITY

Reduction in Risk Potential

Vital signs

502. A decrease in blood pressure of ____ mm Hg or more between the pressure taken after the client has been supine for 3 minutes and the pressure taken after the client arises and stands for a minute is indicative of orthostatic hypotension.

Answer is 30 mm Hg.

PHYSIOLOGICAL INTEGRITY

Reduction of Risk Potential

Therapeutic procedures

503. A wet to dry dressing has been ordered for an ulcer on the leg. Which is a step in the correct procedure for changing the dressing?
   A. Remove the soiled dressing dry.
   B. Apply the new dressing that has been wet with tap water.
   C. Moisten the soiled dressing with sterile water prior to removal.
   D. Moisten the soiled dressing with normal saline prior to removal.

The answer is A. A wet to dry dressing starts with sterile dressing wet with sterile water, sterile saline, or other prescribed liquid, placed over the wound and allowed to dry. Once dry, the soiled dressing is removed, taking with the dressing the adherent debris.

HEALTH PROMOTION AND MAINTENANCE

Ante-/Intra-/Postpartum and Newborn Care

504. A newborn is admitted to the nursery with a history of maternal diabetes that was poorly controlled during the pregnancy. The newborn's admission weight is over 9 pounds. The initial blood glucose level is within normal limits. Which is the priority nursing intervention for this infant?
   A. Initiate formula feedings.
   B. Encourage parental bonding.
   C. Avoid blood draws which could contribute to anemia
   D. Monitor the temperature because the infant is macrosomic.

The answer is A. Although the infant's blood glucose is normal now, the levels are expected to drop in the next two to three hours. Feeding protein foods (formula) will maintain blood glucose better than glucose water.

B, C, and D are incorrect—Parenteral bonding is not the priority intervention. Blood draws will be necessary to monitor glucose levels. The infant's temperature will need to be monitored but it is not the priority.

PHYSIOLOGICAL INTEGRITY

Reduction of Risk Potential

Potential for complications from surgical procedures and health alterations

505. The evening nurse is assessing a client who had a modified mastectomy earlier that morning. Which is a

fact that must be considered when planning nursing care?

A. The client will be depressed and asking for medication frequently
B. Blood pressures should not be performed on the arm of the operative side
C. The client will need to hold off doing arm exercises for 10 days
D. The client should not elevate involved extremity

The answer is B. Blood pressures should not be performed on the arm on the operative side to prevent venous congestion in the affected extremity. The other responses are incorrect.

PSYCHOSOCIAL INTEGRITY

Psychopathology

Recognize signs and symptoms of impaired cognition

506. A client with schizophrenia says "cat tree swim house sick jump pretty" when the nurse asks how he is feeling this morning. Which would be a correct label for the nurse to use when documenting this communication?
A. word salad
B. clang association
C. neologism
D. verbigeration

The answer is A. Word salad refers to the meaningless connection of words and phrases. Clang association refers to repeating words and phrases which sound alike but are otherwise unconnected. A neologism is a new word coined by the client and with meaning only to the client. Verbigeration is the purposeless repetition of words or phrases.

PHYSIOLOGICAL INTEGRITY

Pharmacological and Parenteral Therapies

Expected Effects/Outcomes

Evaluate and document client response to medication

507. A client on the burn unit is receiving IV albumin. Which parameter will the nurse monitor to determine the effectiveness of this treatment?
A. Weight
B. Pain
C. Wound healing
D. Hematocrit

The answer is A. With a burn injury, the integrity of the vessels is lost and fluid escapes into the tissues. Albumin is a hypertonic solution which draws fluids from the tissues to the plasma from where the kidneys can excrete it. Weight loss indicates fluid loss in this manner.

Albumin will not affect pain sensation. Albumin contains antibodies but does not promote wound healing directly and is not the reason for administering it. Albumin contains no red blood cells.

PHYSIOLOGICAL INTEGRITY

Physiological Adaptation

Teach client about managing illness

508. The nurse is working with the parents of a child newly diagnosed with hemophilia. Which topics should be included in teaching about home care of the child?
A. Providing extra iron in the child's diet
B. Oral administration of the missing factor
C. Avoiding sports activities as the child grows
D. Avoiding the use of aspirin for temperature elevations

The answer is D. Use of aspirin would decrease the clotting ability of the child's blood. The child does not need extra iron as the child is able to produce ample red blood cells. Factor is administered intravenously. The child would not avoid all sports. The nurse would provide guidance about sporting activities that would not put the child at risk for injury.

HEALTH PROMOTION AND MAINTENANCE

Immunizations

509. A child is in for a routine immunization. The child has recently received the following medications:
   - insulin
   - antibiotic
   - antihistamine
   - immunoglobulins (IVIG)

   Which would interfere with the effectiveness of the vaccination?
A. insulin
B. antibiotic
C. antihistamine
D. immunoglobulins (IVIG)

The answer is D. Immunoglobulins are antibodies. An immunization is a antigen designed to stimulate immunoglobulin production. If the immunoglobulins are already present, the antigen will be destroyed before antibodies are produced. The other responses would not have a significant effect on vaccination.

PHYSIOLOGICAL INTEGRITY

Basic Care and Comfort

Mobility/immobility

Maintain client skin integrity

510. At what inetrval should an elderly client be instructed to change position when up in her wheelchair during the day?
   A. Two (2) hours
   B. One (1) hour
   C. Thirty (30) minutes
   D. Fifteen (15) minutes

The answer is A. Frequent shifts of body weight are needed to maintain circulation and decrease the risk of a pressure ulcer. Repositioning is required every 2 hours.

A, B, and C are incorrect because more frequent body shifts while in a chair have been shown to be ineffective.

PHYSIOLOGICAL INTEGRITY

Physiological Adaptation

Alterations in body systems

511. A client has had a cesarean section. The client complains of postoperative discomfort due to abdominal distention. Which suggestion would reduce the client's discomfort?
   A. Walk to promote peristalsis
   B. Chew ice to facilitate peristalsis
   C. Lay flat in bed as much as possible
   D. Drink through a straw instead of sipping from a cup.

The answer is A. Walking promotes peristalsis. Drinking through a straw and chewing ice increases the amount of air the client swallows increasing the abdominal distention. Laying flat is not an appropriate intervention for abdominal distention.

PHYSIOLOGICAL INTEGRITY

Pharmacological and Parenteral Therapies

Blood and blood products

512. A hospitalized client receives a transfusion of whole blood. The client suddenly develops chest pain, fever and chills. The nurse suspects a hemolytic transfusion reaction. Which is the priority nursing intervention?
   A. Notify the physician.
   B. Flush the line with D_5NS.
   C. Stop the infusion and maintain the IV line with normal saline.
   D. Give the client the Benadryl (diphenhydramine) available as a prn order.

The answer is C. Hemolytic transfusion reactions are caused by a reaction from antibodies in the recipient blood reacting to the donor's blood protein. This can lead to serious consequences and may be fatal. Stopping the infusion is critical to reduce the source of the reaction. It is essential that the IV line be kept open for emergency access. The physician needs to be notified but it is not the priority action. Flushing the line with dextrose will cause the blood to clot. This is not an allergic reaction so Benadryl will not resolve the problem.

HEALTH PROMOTION AND MAINTENANCE

Ante-/Intra-/Postpartum and Newborn Care

513. A pregnant woman, whom the nurse notes has lordosis, asks why she has had bad back pain. Which factor explains the development of the lordosis and back pain and should serve as the basis of the nurse's response to the client's question?
   A. Maternal hormones
   B. The shifting center of gravity
   C. The loosening of the pelvic structure.
   D. Stasis of blood in the lower extremities

The answer is B. With the weight of the fetus shifting the center of gravity, the pregnant woman will develop lordosis and back pain.

Maternal hormones are present but not the cause of the back pain. The loosening pelvic structures affect the pregnant woman's balance and walk, not back pain. The pressure of the uterus will cause stasis of blood in the lower extremities but not back pain.

PHYSIOLOGICAL INTEGRITY

Physiologic Adaptation

Illness Management

Teach client about managing illness

514. Which actions might the nurse discuss with a client with multiple sclerosis who has recently had a number of exacerbations of the disease? (Select all that apply.)
   A. Joining a support group
   B. Avoiding the use of hot tubs.
   C. Preventing pregnancy
   D. Limiting fluid intake to 1250 ml per day
   E. Requesting a job transfer to a less stressful situation

The answers are A, B, and E. Support groups help support emotional coping mechanisms. The MS client is encouraged to avoid heat and cold situations as they have been implicated in exacerbations. A job transfer may allow the client to continue working. Pregnancy in general does not seem to affect the overall outcome of MS. Fluid intake is important to maintain body function and should not be limited.

PHYSIOLOGICAL INTEGRITY

Physiological Adaptation

Illness Management

Teach client about managing illness

515. A client with thrombocytopenia, secondary to leukemia, has developed epistaxis. Which instruction should the nurse give the client?
   A. Lie supine with the neck extended
   B. Sit upright, leaning slightly forward and apply heat.
   C. Blow the nose and then put lateral pressure on the nose
   D. Hold the nose while bending forward at the waist

The answer is D. This response provides pressure to halt the bleeding while preventing the blood from draining into the lungs. The other answers are incorrect. A would promote blood entering the respiratory system. Heat would increase bleeding. Blowing the nose will remove any clots which have formed and should be discouraged.

PSYCHOSOCIAL INTEGRITY

Psychopathology

Recognize signs and symptoms of acute and chronic mental illness

516. Which type of personality disorder does the nurse suspect when the client's history indicates an apparent lack of concern with others' opinions, a "loner", unfocused lifestyle without close friends, and a cold, aloof persona?
   A. paranoid
   B. schizoid
   C. antisocial
   D. borderline

The answer is B. Clients with schizoid personality disorder are detached from social relationships and demonstrate little emotional expression with other people. There appears to be no pleasure derived from interaction with other people. These individuals prefer solitary activities and can perform well when left alone.

Clients with paranoid personality disorder are suspicious of others believing that others are trying to exploit, deceive or harm them. They question the loyalty and trustworthiness of others; read hidden meanings into events; and bear grudges.

Clients with antisocial personality disorder are impulsive, risk takers who do not learn from experience, exploit others and ignore their rights; and lack guilt, honesty, fidelity and loyalty.

Clients with borderline personality disorder have a poor and unstable self image; are unable to maintain stable relationships; fear abandonment; engage in impulsive activities that are damaging to self such as substance abuse, binge eating and reckless sexual activity; repeatedly threaten or engage in self mutilating or suicidal behavior; experience a chronic sense of emptiness; and manifest inappropriate, intense, uncontrolled anger.

PHYSIOLOGICAL INTEGRITY

Pharmacological and Parenteral Therapies

Total Parenteral Nutrition

Monitor client for side/adverse effects of TPN

517. A client is receiving Total Parenteral Nutrition (TPN). Which is a common complication of TPN for which the nurse must monitor?
   A. Phlebitis
   B. Hypoglycemia
   C. Electrolyte Imbalance
   D. Fluid Volume Deficiency

The answer is D. The hypertonic fluid draws water from the tissues and can lead to fluid volume deficit. Hyperglycemia may be a problem, not hypoglycemia. The physician writes TPN orders based on the client's electrolyte balance TPN is always administered by central line so phlebitis would be a minimal risk.

PHYSIOLOGICAL INTEGRITY

Reduction of Risk Potential

Potential for Complications of Diagnostic Tests/Treatments/Procedures

Intervene to prevent potential neurological complications

518. A client has been casted for a fractured radius. The cast extends from the hand to above the elbow. The client complains of constant pain under the cast. The nurse completes a neurovascular check and notes swelling of the hand and loss of sensation to the little finger. Which is the priority nursing intervention?
   A. Elevate the arm
   B. Notify the physician
   C. Administer pain medication
   D. Reassure the client that these are common findings.

The answer is B. The client is demonstrating diminished circulation secondary to the cast which can lead to compartment syndrome. The cast may need bivalving. Elevating the arm is appropriate to reduce swelling but it is not the priority action at this time. Pain management may be appropriate but not the priority. These sensations are not normal but symptoms of compartment syndrome from a cast that is too tight.

PSYCHOSOCIAL INTEGRITY

Cultural Diversity

519. An ultra-orthodox Jewish client is 1 day postpartum. It is the Sabbath for this client. The client calls to the nurse and asks help in changing her peripad. The client asks the nurse to open the pad's packaging for her as this is considered work in her culture and not allowed on the Sabbath. Which is an appropriate nursing response?
   A. Ask the client if a family member couldn't open the package for her.
   B. Open several pads and leave them covered so that the client can use them as needed.
   C. Assign a male nurse to the client as she wouldn't ask him to open her peri packages.
   D. Tell the client that opening a peri pad package is not work and encourage her to do it for herself.

The answer is B. By opening several packages and leaving them within her reach, she will be able to perform self care without deviating from her religious beliefs.

The client's family would probably be of the same culture and therefore would not be willing to perform this task. A male nurse would make the ultraorthodox Jewish woman uncomfortable and not be culturally sensitive. Telling the client that this is not work does not consider her beliefs and feelings at all.

HEALTH PROMOTION AND MAINTENANCE

Immunizations

520. The clinic is running short of RSV Immune Globulin (the immunization for respiratory syncytival virus). Which child should have priority in receiving the vaccine?
   A. The 8-year-old with cystic fibrosis.
   B. The teenager who is sexually active.
   C. The 5-year-old with failure to thrive.
   D. The 6-month-old premie with a history of bronchial pulmonary dysplasia.

The answer is D. RSV is primarily a disease of infancy so preference would be given to children under 2 years of age.

PHYSIOLOGICAL INTEGRITY

Pharmacological and Parenteral Therapies

Medication Administration

Implement procedures to counteract adverse effects of medications

521. A client with leukemia is scheduled to get chemotherapy which includes vincristine. Which nursing action is appropriate?
   A. Insert the intravenous line in a vein in a joint area.
   B. Ensure that the intravenous is administered per pump.
   C. Administer the medication in a free flowing intravenous line.
   D. Always use an intravenous line that has been in place for several days.

The answer is C. Because it is so irritating to tissues, it is critical that extravasation of vincristine into tissue be prevented. A free flowing line means that the line is most likely in the vein. A pump will continue to pump IV fluids even after the line has extraversated. A fresh line is best to ensure its integrity and the joint areas should be avoided.

PHYSIOLOGICAL INTEGRITY

Basic Care and Comfort

Rest and sleep

522. A client informs the nurse that he is "unable to fall asleep at night and tends to walk around until he gets sleepy." Which suggestion can the nurse make to help the client to develop better sleep habits?
   A. Have an alcoholic drink prior to bedtime
   B. Exercise when unable to sleep
   C. Increase fluid intake prior to bedtime to maintain hydration
   D. Avoid stressful situations prior to bedtime
   E. Wear loose clothing to bed
   F. Avoid caffeinated beverages before bedtime

The answers are D, E, and F. Stress will deter the client from falling asleep so avoiding stressful situations prior to bedtime will promote sleep. Wearing loose clothing to bed and avoiding caffeinated beverages before bedtime will also facilitate sleep.

Alcohol, exercise, and increasing fluid intake before bed all interfere with sleep.

HEALTH PROMOTION AND MAINTENANCE

Ante-/Intra-/Postpartum and Newborn Care

523. Which comment made by a teenager who is attending a health class on pregnancy indicates the need for clarification of information?

A. "I didn't realize that smoking during pregnancy could cause a miscarriage."
B. "I didn't realize that smoking during pregnancy could cause the baby to have high blood pressure as an adult."
C. "I didn't realize that smoking during pregnancy could result in a large baby and a difficult birth."
D. "I didn't realize that smoking during pregnancy is associated with asthma as the child grows older.

The answer is A. Miscarriages, preterm birth and low birth weight babies are associated with smoking during pregnancy. It is not known to be associated with adult hypertension nor with childhood asthma.

PHYSIOLOGICAL INTEGRITY

Physiological Adaptation

Illness Management

Teach client about managing illness

524. Following a long history of vomiting, a child is diagnosed with GERD, Gastric esophageal reflux disease. Instructions are given to the parents for conservative management to reduce the reflux. Following the parent teaching, the nurse will recognize the need for additional information when the parent states:
A. "I will keep my child's weight at the recommended levels."
B. "My child should avoid caffeine, and spicy foods to reduce reflux."
C. "I will lay my child down in bed after meals to allow time for digestion."
D. "I will see that my child receives the antacid that his physician prescribed for him."

The answer is C. The child should not be placed flat in bed following feedings but should be maintained in a semi to high fowler's position to promote formula retention. Overweight children are more prone to GERD. Caffeine, chocolate and spicy foods seems to weaken the esophageal pressure and increase the reflux. The physician may order an H2 antagonist, a proton pump inhibitor or other drugs to promote stomach emptying.

PHYSIOLOGICAL INTEGRITY

Basic Care and Comfort

Assistive Devices

Evaluate correct use of assistive devices by staff/client/family

525. A client is recovering from a broken tibia and is walking on wooden crutches. Which observed client behavior requires nursing intervention?
A. The client props his foot up while sitting.
B. The cast is visibly dirty.
C. While standing, the client rests his body weight on the top of the crutches.
D. The client uses a swing through motion when walking with the crutches.

The answer is C. Resting the arm pits on the top of the crutches could damage nerves and circulation. A visibly dirty cast can be covered with adhesive tape for better appearances but this is not the priority intervention. It is appropriate to elevate the foot while sitting. A swing through motion is often used to prevent weight bearing on the casted leg.

HEALTH PROMOTION AND MAINTENANCE

Ante-/Intra-/Postpartum and Newborn Care

Provides safe nursing care to the pregnant client

526. A pregnant woman has developed diabetes during the pregnancy. After several attempts to control the diabetes with diet alone, the physician plans to place the woman on insulin. The woman asks the nurse why she can't take the "oral" insulins like her grandpa. The nurse's response is based on the knowledge that oral hypoglycemics:
A. May cross the placenta and be teratogenic
B. Contain too little insulin and would require multiple pills.
C. Will affect the fetal pancreas leading to infantile diabetes.
D. Contain too much insulin and would be dangerous to the fetus.

The answer is A. The full effect of the oral hypoglycemics on the fetus is not yet known. The oral hypoglycemics are not insulin but stimulate insulin production.

PHYSIOLOGICAL INTEGRITY

Reduction of Risk Potential

System-Specific Assessment

Perform focused assessment or reassessment

527. A newborn is suspected of having hydrocephalus. For which symptoms would the nursery nurse monitor the child? (Select all that apply.)
A. Sunset eyes
B. Depressed fontanels
C. Thin scalp and sparse hair
D. Increasing head circumference
E. Head circumference equal to chest circumference

The answers are A, C, and D. The fontanels would be bulging, not depressed. The head circumference is larger than the chest circumference at birth in normal children. In this child, the difference would be even greater.

PSYCHOSOCIAL INTEGRITY

Psychopathology

Recognize signs and symptoms of acute and chronic mental illness

528. When assessing a client newly admitted with a diagnosis of active phase schizophrenia, which are negative symptoms of schizophrenia which the nurse might find?
Mark all that apply.
A. ___ disorganized speech
B. ___ flat affect
C. ___ alogia
D. ___ impaired attention
E. ___ bizarre behavior
F. ___ avolition

The answers are B, C, D, and F. Flat affect, alogia, attention impairment, avolition along with anhedonia are all negative symptoms of schizophrenia.

Disorganized speech and bizarre or disorganized behavior are positive symptoms of schizophrenia.

PHYSIOLOGICAL INTEGRITY

Pharmacological and Parenteral Therapies

Adverse Effects/Contraindications and Side Effects

Implement procedures to counteract adverse effects of medications and parenteral therapy

529. A client is receiving Vancomycin HCL for an infection. Shortly after the nurse starts the intravenous infusion, the client appears flushed and complains of feeling hot. The nurse should:
A. slow the infusion.
B. stop the infusion and call the physician.
C. speed up the infusion as it seems to be making the client nervous.
D. recognize the client is having a drug interaction.

The answer is B. The client is showing symptoms of red man syndrome. The flushing is caused by a release of histamine causing vasodilatation. If untreated, the problem could be fatal. The physician will usually order Benadryl and order the vancomycin to be restarted at a slower rate.

PHYSIOLOGICAL INTEGRITY

Physiological Adaptation

Pathophysiology

Understand general principles of pathophysiology

530. The nurse is reviewing the laboratory report of a client who underwent a bone marrow biopsy. The finding that would most strongly support a diagnosis of acute leukemia is the existence of a large number of immature:
A. nucleated red blood cells
B. thrombocytes
C. reticulocytes
D. leukocytes

The answer is D. Leukocytes are immature WHCs. Thrombocytes are immature platelets and reticulocytes and nucleated red blood cells are immature red blood cells.

SAFE AND EFFECTIVE CARE ENVIRONMENT

Safety and Infection Control

Standard/Transmission Based/Other Precautions

Provides care to the child with an infectious disease

531. A child has been diagnosed with tubercule (tuberculosis) meningitis and is admitted to the hospital. The child should be placed on:
A. contact isolation.
B. droplet isolation.
C. respiratory isolation.
D. standard precautions.

The answer is D. These children are not considered contagious. Active, untreated respiratory tuberculosis is spread by droplets. The CDC recommends these individuals be placed in a negative flow (airflow) room with caregivers wearing masks and gowns.

HEALTH PROMOTION AND MAINTENANCE

Techniques of Physical Assessment

532. The nurse is performing a physical examination of a client's abdomen. In what order should the assessment be performed?
A. Inspection, palpation, auscultation
B. Palpation, auscultation, inspection
C. Inspection, auscultation, palpation
D. Auscultation, inspection, palpation

The answer is C. Inspection is always the first step. Palpation is always performed last because palpation of the abdomen may interfere with bowel sounds and could cause pain.

PHYSIOLOGICAL INTEGRITY

Reduction of Risk Potential

Potential for Complications of Diagnostic Tests/Treatments/Procedures

Provide nursing care that identifies potential complications

533. A client has been admitted to the hospital for a gastrointestinal procedure. The physician orders the following:
   - NPO at midnight
   - Clear liquids except those that are red
   - Multiple tap water enemas until clear
   - One dose of an oral antibiotic the morning of the procedure.

   Which order should the nurse question?
   A. NPO at midnight
   B. Clear liquids except those that are red
   C. Multiple tap water enemas until clear
   D. One dose of an oral antibiotic the morning of the procedure.

The answer is C. Multiple tap water enemas can lead to water intoxication. NPO at midnight is a common order preceding a treatment. Prophylactic antibiotics may be ordered. Clear liquids will maintain the cleanliness of the bowel—reds are avoided as it cannot be differentiated from blood in stool or vomitus.

PHYSIOLOGICAL INTEGRITY

Physiological Adaptation

Pathophysiology

534. Two clients are comparing symptoms while waiting in the endocrine clinic. One client has been diagnosed with diabetes insipidus while the other client has diabetes mellitus. The clients note that they have many similar symptoms. Which symptom would differentiate the two disorders?
   A. Polyuria
   B. Polydipsia
   C. Polyphagia
   D. Nocturnal voidings

The answer is C. Both clients will have excessive urination and thirst. Nighttime voiding would be common. Polyphagia, excessive hunger, would only be seen in the client with diabetes mellitus.

SAFE AND EFFECTIVE CARE ENVIRONMENT

Safety and Infection Control

Injury prevention

535. An elderly client is admitted to the hospital unit. On admission, the family tells the nurse that the client has fallen several times recently. The nurse evaluates the client and finds the client alert and without symptoms of ataxia. Which is an appropriate nursing action?
   A. Place the client on fall precautions
   B. Ask physical therapy to evaluate the client.
   C. Not place the client of fall precautions
   D. Question the family about what they did for the falls.

The answer is A. The nurse has been warned and therefore has a heightened legal liability to protect this client. The other responses are inappropriate.

PHYSIOLOGICAL INTEGRITY

Physiological Adaptation

Illness Management

Teach client about managing illness

536. A client has been diagnosed with fibrocystic breast disease. Which information should be included in the self care teaching for this client?
   A. Occasional nipple discharge is normal.
   B. If breast pain is not relieved after menses begins, the client should see her primary care provider.
   C. Breast pain due to inflammation and root stimulation begins before the luteal phase of the menstrual cycle.
   D. Diuretics are never used to relieve symptoms of fibrocystic breast disease.

The answer is B. If breast pain is not relieved after menses begins, the client should see her primary health care provider as inflammation and nerve root stimulation begin at 4–7 days into the luteal phase of the menstrual cycle and end with the beginning of menses.

PHYSIOLOGICAL INTEGRITY

Reduction of Risk Potential

Vital Signs

Apply knowledge needed to perform related nursing procedures and psychomotor skills when assessing vital signs

537. A nursing assistant reports to a staff nurse that the neonate assigned to her care is crying and has axillary

temperature of 90°F. Which is the appropriate action on the part of the staff nurse?
A. Call a code
B. Notify the physician
C. Retake the temperature
D. Place the infant in a warming unit

The answer is C. A temperature of 90 axillary is not compatible with life. When infants cry they also tend to wave their arms around which can interfere with obtaining an accurate axillary temperature. The temperature should be retaken.

PSYCHOSOCIAL INTEGRITY

Chemical and Other Dependencies

Assess client for drug/alcohol related dependencies, withdrawal, or toxicities

538. A client comes to the clinic saying he is withdrawing from heroin and needs help. Which assessment findings would support the client's statement?
A. Vomiting and decreased respirations
B. confusion and ataxia
C. muscle twitching and dilated pupils
D. impaired memory and seizure activity

The answer is C. Symptoms of withdrawal from heroin include muscle twitching and dilated pupils along with yawning, rhinorrhea, lacrimation, abdominal cramps, diaphoresis, irritability, restlessness, anxiety, agitation, sleep disturbance, body aches, muscle cramps, "goose flesh" sensations of hot or cold, nausea, diarrhea, anorexia, fever, hypertension, tachycardia, tachypnea, dysphoria, and craving.

Confusion, impaired memory and seizure activity occurs with withdrawal from alcohol, sedatives/hypnotics, and anxiolytic drugs. Vomiting and ataxia are associated with withdrawal from alcohol, sedatives/hypnotics, and anxiolytic drugs. Respirations are increased with withdrawal from alcohol, opiates, and sedatives/hypnotics, and anxiolytics.

PHYSIOLOGICAL INTEGRITY

Pharmacological and Parenteral Therapies

Blood and Blood Products

Administer blood products and evaluate client response

539. A client is to receive a blood transfusion. When will the nurse plan to take vital signs? (Select all that apply.)
A. Prior to starting the transfusion.
B. Every 15 minutes during the first hour of the transfusion.
C. Fifteen minutes after the transfusion is completed
D. At least twice during the transfusion.

The answers are A, B, and C. Changes in vital signs are early indications of reactions to the blood. Therefore baseline vital signs should be taken prior to starting the transfusion. Subsequently vital signs should be taken every 15 minutes during the first hour, periodically during the rest of the transfusion and then upon completion of the transfusion.

PHYSIOLOGICAL INTEGRITY

Pharmacological and Parenteral Therapies

Medication Administration

Use the six "rights" when administering client medications

540. The nurse is administering Cyanocobalamin (vitamin B_{12}) to a client with pernicious anemia, secondary to a gastrectomy. Which route should the nurse use to most effectively administer the vitamin?
A. topical route
B. enteral route
C. parenteral route
D. transdermal route

The answer is C. Cyanocobalamin is administered IM or SC. The other routes are incorrect.

SAFE AND EFFECTIVE CARE ENVIRONMENT

Management of Care

Delegation

Assure appropriate education, skills, and experience of personnel performing delegated task

541. There are three clients on the unit who are receiving chemotherapy. Which type of assignment of care is appropriate?
A. Care divided among two newly hired and one experienced registered nurses
B. Care divided among three experienced registered nurses
C. Care assigned to an experienced Licensed Practice Nurse
D. Care assigned to a chemotherapy certified pregnant nurse

The answer is B. Chemotherapy administration should be divided among a number of nurses rather than assigning all chemotherapy to one nurse to decrease the cytotoxic chemical exposure. Chemotherapy certified nurse would be the best option, but because the nurse is pregnant, she should protect her fetus by avoiding all exposure possible. The nurse administering chemotherapy does not have to be certified.

PHYSIOLOGICAL INTEGRITY

Basic Care and Comfort

Elimination

Assess and intervene with a client who has an alteration in elimination

542. Which intervention would be included in the plan of care for a client who is post operative from pelvic surgery?
   A. Administer stool softeners to prevent constipation
   B. Teach a low fat diet.
   C. Limit fluid intake to reduce bladder filling.
   D. Encourage pelvic tilt exercises.

The answer is A. Constipation will cause straining which will cause discomfort and pressure on the suture lines. There is no rationale for a low fat diet. Fluid intake is important to reduce urinary stasis. Pelvic tilt exercises are not appropriate at this time.

PSYCHOSOCIAL INTEGRITY

Family Dynamics

Assist the family in crisis and under stress to adapt and change

543. An elderly woman was diagnosed with Alzheimer's disease several years ago. Her confusion is increasing. During AM care, the woman tells the nurse about something that happened to her years ago. The husband, who overheard, immediately corrects the woman and explains the correct information to the nurse. The nurse would talk to the husband in private to encourage him to:
   A. continue to correct her stories to help her stay in touch with reality.
   B. discourage his wife from talking so that listeners will not be confused.
   C. allow her to tell stories as she remembers them to reduce risk of agitation.
   D. ignore all of the woman's rantings as everyone is aware of her confusion.

The answer is C. Clients with Alzheimer's are aware of their confusion and try to mask their loss of memory. That is why they spend so much time talking about the past. Eventually the past memories also become confused. Repeated corrections will increase the woman's agitation and may affect her self-esteem. In addition, it will not keep the woman in touch with reality. Discouraging the woman from talking will further isolate the woman from the world as will ignoring her.

HEALTH PROMOTION AND MAINTENANCE

Ante-/Intra-/Postpartum and Newborn Care

544. During the later part of her pregnancy, a woman was treated for pregnancy-induced hypertension. The woman delivered a healthy infant 6 hours ago. Why is close monitoring of this client during the first two postpartum days an important nursing action?
   The client
   A. will have problems bonding to her infant.
   B. could have heart damage from the hypertension.
   C. is at high risk for renal failure in the postpartal period.
   D. may become eclamptic for up to 48 hours after delivery.

The answer is D. Eclampsia or seizures could occur for up to 48 hours after delivery. The other responses are not correct.

PHYSIOLOGICAL INTEGRITY

Pharmacological and Parenteral Therapies

Adverse effects/contraindications/side effects

545. A woman is getting married and asks for birth control pills. Which assessment finding suggests that "the pill" may not be the best choice of birth control for this client because of the associated risk of heart disease?
   The client
   A. is a heavy smoker.
   B. is 22 years old.
   C. had an abortion as a teenager.
   D. has a sexually transmitted disease.

The answer is A. Smokers on oral contraceptives are significantly more at risk for the development of heart disease. This risk increases with age. The other findings are not significant risk factors.

PHYSIOLOGICAL INTEGRITY

Physiological Adaptation

Medical Emergencies

Perform emergency care procedures

546. A client receives a dose of penicillin and has an anaphylactic reaction. Which is the priority nursing intervention for this client?

A. Monitoring vital signs
B. Maintaining a patent airway
C. Assessing for adequate circulating blood volume
D. Treating symptoms of vascular overload

The answer is B. Maintaining a paten airway is essential for the maintenance of tissue oxygenation. Monitoring vital signs and assessing for adequate circulating blood volume are both assessments and will not provide any relief to the client. The client will have circulatory collapse.

SAFE AND EFFECTIVE CARE ENVIRONMENTS

Safety and Infection Control

Error Prevention

Verify appropriateness and/or accuracy of a treatment order

547. A newborn with a diaphragmatic hernia and respiratory distress is admitted to the pediatric unit. The admitting physician writes the following orders:
- Position in semi- to high Fowlers
- Position on affected side.
- Diet for age.
- NG tube to suction

Which order should the nurse question in the preoperative period?
A. Position in semi- to high Fowlers
B. Position on affected side.
C. Diet for age.
D. NG tube to suction

The answer is C. Feeding the infant would increase the contents in the GI tract. Since bowel material is in the chest, this would increase the contents of the chest further compressing the unaffected lung. Semi to high Fowlers would use gravity to decrease the contents of the chest which would help respirations. Position on the affected side so the unaffected lung has full expansion ability. NG tube to suction is used to decompress the gastric contents and is appropriate.

PHYSIOLOGICAL INTEGRITY

Pharmacological and Parenteral Therapies

Expected Effects/Outcomes

Evaluate and document client response to medication

548. A client is admitted with third degree burns. On the second day post burn, the physician orders the client to receive albumin. The nurse will know that the treatment was successful when the client:
A. loses weight
B. feels less pain
C. doesn't develop a burn infection
D. has an increased hemoglobin and hematocrit

The answer is A. With a burn injury, the integrity of the vessels is lost and fluid escapes into the tissues. Albumin is a hypertonic solution which draws fluids from the tissues to the plasma from where it can be excreted by the kidneys. Weight loss indicates fluid loss in this manner. Albumin will not affect pain sensation. Although albumin does contain antibodies, this is not the reason for administering it. Albumin contains no red blood cells.

PHYSIOLOGICAL INTEGRITY

Reduction of Risk Potential

Diagnostic Tests

Apply knowledge of related nursing procedures and psychomotor skills when caring for clients undergoing diagnostic testing

549. A woman 9 months pregnant is admitted for a Non-Stress Test. How will the nurse position the woman?
A. Prone
B. Supine
C. With legs elevated
D. With right hip tilted with a pad.

The answer is D. The client is positioned with a pad used to slightly elevate the right hip. This position will prevent vena cava syndrome, a side effect of lying supine. When in the supine position, the pregnant uterus lies on the inferior vena cava reducing blood flow to the heart. The other options are incorrect.

PHYSIOLOGICAL INTEGRITY

Pharmacological and Parenteral Therapies

Expected Effects/Outcomes

Use clinical decision making/critical thinking when addressing expected Effects/Outcomes of medications

550. A client is receiving levothyroxine (Synthroid) for hypothyroidism. Occurrence of which symptom would cause the nurse to suspect the dosage is too high?
A. Weight gain
B. Hypotension
C. Diarrhea
D. Round the clock sleepiness.

The answer is C. Symptoms of overdose would be those of hyperthyroidism. All the listed symptoms are those of hypothyroidism except for diarrhea.

SAFE AND EFFECTIVE CARE ENVIRONMENTS

Safety and Infection Control

Standard/Transmission-Based/Other Precautions

Apply principles of infection control

551. Which type of precautions would be used when caring for a client with *H. influenzae*?
   A. Standard precautions
   B. Airborne precautions
   C. Droplet precautions
   D. Contact precautions

The answer is C. Droplet precautions are used when the mechanism of transmission is by large droplets spread by coughing, sneezing, or talking. This is the mechanism of spread of *H. influenzae*.

A is incorrect—Standard precautions are used to decrease the risk of transmission from bloodborne pathogens and moist body substances. Moist body substances include blood, urine, feces, sputum, saliva, wound drainage, and all aspirated fluids. B is incorrect—Airborne precautions are used when the mode of spread of an organism is by small particle droplets borne on air currents. Airborne precautions require a private room with negative airflow and adequate filtration; those entering the room wear a mask and if the client leaves the room, a mask is worn. D is incorrect—Droplet precautions require a private room or a room shared with someone infected with the same organism. Those entering the room and coming within 3 feet of the client need to wear a mask and the client wears a mask if taken out of the room. Contact precautions are used when organisms causing serious disease are easily transmitted through direct contact. Contact precautions require a private room or a room shared with someone infected with the same organism. Gloves are worn at all times and gowns and protective barriers are used if direct contact is required.

PSYCHOSOCIAL INTEGRITY

Psychopathology

Assess client for alterations in mood, judgment, cognition, and reasoning as evidence of psychopathology

552. Which type of personality disorder presents a challenge to treatment because it is characterized by a charming manner often used to manipulate staff into agreeing with or granting client demands?
   A. dependent
   B. histrionic
   C. antisocial
   D. narcissistic

The answer is C. Clients with antisocial personality disorder are typically intelligent, charming, manipulative and with outstanding verbal and nonverbal communication skills. As a result, staff must be on guard against being inadvertently manipulated by these clients and must consistently set firm limits to avoid reinforcing the clients maladaptive behaviors.

PHYSIOLOGICAL INTEGRITY

Pharmacological and Parenteral Therapies

Pharmacological interactions

553. Which assessment findings would the home care nurse interpret as increasing a new client's risk for problems related to polypharmacy? (Select all that apply.)
   A. Uses several practitioners
   B. Currently being treated for several chronic conditions
   C. Has switched health care providers frequently
   D. Has a history of cataracts
   E. Currently is on an antibiotic for an acute UTI

The answers are A, B, and C. Using several physicians, and switching physicians both can lead to multiple conflicting prescriptions. Multiple chronic conditions will be treated with numerous medications. History of cataracts is not a significant factor in polypharmacy. Short term use of antibiotic for UTI is not a problem.

SAFE AND EFFECTIVE CARE ENVIRONMENT

Safety and Infection Control

Error prevention

554. A client is admitted with a draining wound. MRSA is suspected as the causative agent. The physician writes the following orders. Which order should the nurse question?
   A. Diet as tolerated
   B. Contact isolation
   C. D_5 1/4 NS at keep vein open
   D. Procaine Penicillin G 150,000 units every 4 hours IV

The answer is D. Procaine is an additive that is to slow the absorption of the medication from the muscle. Procaine is never administered intravenously. The intravenous form of penicillin is Aqueous penicillin.

PHYSIOLOGICAL INTEGRITY

Physiologic Adaptation

Pathophysiology

Identify client status based on pathophysiology

555. An infant in the newborn nursery has been cyanotic since birth. Which type of congenital problem could account for the cyanosis?

A. A left to right shunt
B. A right to left shunt
C. Congestive heart failure
D. Red blood cell deficiency

The answer is B. A right to left shunt is a cyanotic heart defect. A left to right shunt is acyanotic. The presence of cyanosis does not provide any information about congestive heart failure. A child with inadequate red blood cells would be hypoxic but not cyanotic as cyanosis is unoxygenated hemoglobin.

HEALTH PROMOTION AND MAINTENANCE

Techniques of Physical Assessment

Perform a comprehensive health assessment

556. What is the nurse assessing when, with the client's eyes closed, the nurse places a key in the client's hand and asks the client to identify what it is?
    A. Two-point discrimination
    B. Stereognosis
    C. Position sense
    D. Light touch

The answer is B. Stereognosis is asking the client to identify a familiar object such as a key when it is placed in the client's hand with the client's eyes closed.

A, C, and D are incorrect—Two-point discrimination involves touching the skin simultaneously with two sterile needles at closer and closer distances to each other until the client perceives only one touch. Position sense is tested by moving the client's toes up or down one by one and asking the client, whose eyes are closed, to say in which direction each was moved. Light touch is tested by stroking an area of the client's skin with a wisp of cotton.

PHYSIOLOGICAL INTEGRITY

Reduction of Risk Potential

Potential for Complications of Diagnostic Tests/Treatments/Procedures

Educate client and family about home management of care

557. The nurse is preparing a client with a full leg cast for discharge. Discharge instructions on cast care have been provided. Which statement by the client indicates the need for more information?
    A. "I will not get my cast wet."
    B. "I will contact my physician immediately if the cast breaks."
    C. "Keeping my toes still will reduce my pain."
    D. "I should put nothing into the cast."

The answer is C. The client would be encouraged to wiggle his toes. All other responses would be correct responses by the client.

PHYSIOLOGICAL INTEGRITY

Pharmacological and Parenteral Therapies

Central Venous Access Devices

Provide care for a client with a central venous access device

558. A client is admitted to the hospital unit with a PICC that was placed at another facility. Although the client has documentation indicating the PICC has been x-ray verified, there is no information about whether the catheter is valved or non-valved. Which is an appropriate nursing action?
    A. Flush the line with normal saline only.
    B. Do not flush the line.
    C. Ask the client what other nurses have done with the line.
    D. Flush the line with heparin flush solution per hospital protocol.

The answer is D. Flushing the line with heparin flush solution will not harm a valved catheter but failure to flush with heparin in a non-valved line will result in occlusion of the line.

HEALTH PROMOTION AND MAINTENANCE

Ante-/Intra-/Postpartum and Newborn Care

559. A client with known cardiac disease becomes pregnant. The nurses monitor the woman throughout her pregnancy. At what point during her pregnancy is the client at greatest risk of developing congestive heart failure?
    A. First trimester
    B. 20 weeks gestation
    C. As the woman approaches 30–32 weeks gestation
    D. As she goes into labor

The answer is C. The blood volume and workload for the heart reaches its maximum at 30–32 weeks. If the pregnant cardiac client makes it beyond this point, she will probably complete the pregnancy.

SAFE AND EFFECTIVE CARE ENVIRONMENT

Management of Care

Establishing Priorities

Assess/triage clients to prioritize the order of care delivery

560. The nurse is working in the emergency room. On what basis should the nurse determine the order that clients in the reception room should be seen?
    A. Triage
    B. Time of arrival
    C. Comprehensive assessment
    D. Age

The answer is A. Triage identifies the clients who need medical attention first. Order of arrival is not appropriate because it does not address immediacy of need for care. Comprehensive assessment takes substantial time and slows the organization of client interventions. Age is not appropriate because by itself it does not determine the severity of a problem or the immediacy of the need for care.

PHYSIOLOGICAL INTEGRITY

Pharmacological and Parenteral Therapies

Medication Administration

Educate client/family about medications

561. A client with sickle cell anemia has been treated with several blood transfusions. Now deferoxamine (Desferal) has been ordered and the client asks the nurse the purpose of this medication. Which is the correct answer for the nurse to give?
    The medication will:
    A. prevent the RBCs from sickling
    B. remove excessive iron from the body
    C. improve the longevity of the red blood cells.
    D. increase the oxygen carrying capacity of the blood.

The answer is B. When repeated blood transfusions are given, the RBCs will eventually be broken down. The body retains the iron from these donated cells leading to iron toxicity. All other responses are incorrect.

PHYSIOLOGICAL INTEGRITY

Physiological Adaptation

Medical Emergencies

Perform emergency care procedures

562. A nurse stops at the scene of a car accident and provides first aid to the victim who has a neck injury. Which is the most appropriate way to open the airway of this victim?
    A. jaw-thrust
    B. head lift
    C. neck thrust
    D. neck tilt.

The answer is A. A jaw thrust will prevent damage to the spinal cord that could occur with other methods of opening the airway.

HEALTH PROMOTION AND MAINTENANCE

Growth and Development

563. A 3-year-old child is scheduled for surgery. The nurse is explaining the procedure to the child. Which is the most appropriate statement for the nurse to make about the anesthesia?
    "The doctor will give you some special medicine that:
    A. "Will help you take a nap."
    B. "Will put you to sleep."
    C. "Make you unconscious."
    D. "Mommy wants you to have."

The answer is A. Children may be familiar with animals which have been "put to sleep" and never returned. Unconscious is a word that would not be in their vocabulary

Telling the child that mommy wants them to take the medicine does not explain what will happen.

PHYSIOLOGICAL INTEGRITY

Physiological Adaptation

Illness Management

Teach client about managing illness

564. Which statement made by a client with Multiple Sclerosis indicates that the nurse needs to clarify self care instructions with the client?
    A. "When I am tired, I lay down and rest."
    B. "When I feel stressed, I get in the hot tub."
    C. "I try to avoid conflicts with my husband."
    D. "I'm thinking of changing jobs to reduce stress."

The answer is B. Heat increases the risk of exacerbations in Multiple Sclerosis so hot tubs should be avoided. All the other statements will promote wellness in the client.

HEALTH PROMOTION AND MAINTENANCE

Immunizations

565. While administering the hepatitis vaccine to a group of medical students, the nurse is asked: "Is this going to

produce active or passive immunity?" Which is the correct response?

A. This is passive immunity because I am giving you the vaccine.

B. This is passive immunity because this shot contains the antibodies.

C. This is active immunity because you did not get it from your mother.

D. This is active immunity because your body must respond to the vaccine.

The answer is D. Most vaccinations contain toxins or attenuated organisms. Your body views the vaccine as an antigen and produces antibodies against it. That is what makes it active.

A, B, and C are incorrect—Vaccination produces active immunity. Antibodies received from the mother provides passive immunity.

PHYSIOLOGICAL INTEGRITY

Physiological Adaptation

Illness Management

Implement interventions to manage client recovering from an illness

566. A client is experiencing severe respiratory distress. The nurse would perform which of the following activities to promote gas exchange? Select all that apply

A. Sit the client up in bed

B. Support both arms on a pillow

C. Encourage the client to drink clear liquids

D. Keep the room temperature somewhat warmer than usual

The answers are A and B. Sitting the client up in bed with both arms supported on pillows allows for better lung expansion by reducing pressure from abdominal contents and removing the weight of the arms from the chest. The client would not be encouraged to drink because the severe respiratory distress could cause aspiration. Keeping the room warm would raise the client's basal metabolism rate increasing the body's requirement for oxygen and should be avoided. The room should be kept cool.

PHYSIOLOGICAL INTEGRITY

Pharmacological and Parenteral Therapies

Blood and blood products

567. An immunocompromised client is to receive a blood transfusion for anemia. Which type of blood product would the nurse expect the physician to order?

A. Platelets

B. Whole blood

C. Filtered packed cells

D. Irradiated packed cells

The answer is C. An immunocompromised client is at risk for graft versus host disease. Irradiated packed blood cells will reduce this risk. Whole blood is rarely administered as packed cells provide the needed cells without the volume.

SAFE AND EFFECTIVE CARE ENVIRONMENTS

Safety and Infection Control

Standard/Transmission-Based/Other Precautions

Understand communicable diseases and the modes of organism transmission

568. A college student has been admitted to the hospital unit with a diagnosis of meningococcal meningitis. The client should be placed in:

A. droplet isolation

B. airborne isolation

C. protective isolation

D. no isolation as universal precautions is sufficient

The answer is A. Meningococcal meningitis is spread by droplets and is the only meningitis form that is readily transmitted to others. Droplet transmission involves contact with a large particle in the conjunctivae or mucous membranes of the nose or mouth. Transmission by large particle requires close contact whereas airborne can be transmitted through the air. Protective isolation protects the client from others and is not appropriate.

PHYSIOLOGICAL INTEGRITY

Basic Care and Comfort

Palliative/comfort Care

Assess client for nonverbal signs of pain/discomfort

569. A client is seen in the emergency room following a fall at home. The client is known to have late stage Alzheimer's disease. A fractured hip is diagnosed and surgery is scheduled for the next morning. When asked, the client denies pain. Which symptoms would cause the nurse to suspect the client is in pain?

A. Client yells for her long deceased husband

B. Client's hands finger the sheets continuously.

C. Blood pressure is elevated from admission findings

D. Client reaches for the nurse's hand when the nurse approaches the client.

The answer is C. Elevation in blood pressure may indicate an increase in pain.

Clients with Alzheimer's disease often call for individuals from their past, finger sheets, and other material and want physical contact.

PHYSIOLOGICAL INTEGRITY

Physiological Adaptation

Pathophysiology

570. A newborn has been diagnosed with osteogenesis imperfecta. Which assessment findings would the nurse expect? Select all that apply.
   A. Blue sclera
   B. Simian crease
   C. Hyperbilirubinemia
   D. Multiple fractures apparent at birth
   E. Cephalohematoma developed within hours of birth

The answers are A and D. Blue sclerae and multiple fractures at birth are signs of osteogenesis imperfecta. Simian crease is a soft neurologic sign associated with Down's syndrome. Hyperbilirubinemia is not a symptom of osteogenesis imperfecta although it could result from bleeding injuries secondary to the broken bones. Cephalohematoma is not a symptom of osteogenesis imperfecta.

PHYSIOLOGICAL INTEGRITY

Reduction of Risk Potential

Diagnostic tests

571. Which is the most important question to ask a 36-year-old woman prior to having a bone scan?
   A. Do you have an allergy to seafood?
   B. Did you have anything to eat or drink after midnight?
   C. Are you claustrophobic?
   D. Are you pregnant?

The answer is D. With a bone scan, there is a risk of radiation exposure to the fetus.

A is incorrect—this question is asked of any client receiving an isotope. B is incorrect—the client does not have to be NPO for this diagnostic test. C is incorrect—not all CT or MRI machines are full enclosures.

PHYSIOLOGICAL INTEGRITY

Physiological Adaptation

Pathophysiology

572. A 68-year-old female is admitted with a chief complaint of low back pain. Spinal x-ray indicates that the client has intervertebral disc disease. When asked by the client's family, the nurse would explain the etiology of this disease as:
   A. caused by weakening of the bone due to loss of calcium from the bone.
   B. the degeneration of the spine due to dehydration of the intervertebral discs.
   C. caused by inflammation of the joints and surrounding tissues.
   D. the displacement and loss of contact of articulating surfaces.

The answer is B.

A is incorrect—Weakening of bone due to loss of calcium occurs with osteoporosis. C is incorrect—Inflammation of joints and surrounding tissue occurs with arthritis. D is incorrect—Displacement and loss of contact of articulating surfaces occurs with dislocation of a joint.

SAFE AND EFFECTIVE CARE ENVIRONMENT

Management of Care

Confidentiality/Information Security

Maintain client confidentiality/privacy

573. The nurse is working on the pediatric unit when a call is received from a school teacher asking about the condition of one of her students who is hospitalized on the unit. The nurse should:
   A. give only general information about the child.
   B. encourage the teacher to contact the child's parents.
   C. transfer the call to the hospital administrator.
   D. answer her questions if the nurse can verify that the person on the phone is the child's teacher.

The answer is B. No information can be given to the teacher. Only the guardians may receive information about the child.

PHYSIOLOGICAL INTEGRITY

Pharmacological and Parenteral Therapies

Adverse Effects/Contraindications and Side Effects

Assess client for actual or potential side effects and adverse effects of medications

574. Gentamicin is known to be nephrotoxic. The nurse administering gentamicin should independently evaluate the client's:
   A. BUN
   B. Urinary output
   C. Fluid intake
   D. Creatinine clearance

The answer is B. Urinary output provides information about renal functioning. BUN and Creatinine clearance also evaluate renal functioning but require a physician's order so may not be available for monitoring.

HEALTH PROMOTION AND MAINTENANCE

Ante-/Intra-/Postpartum and Newborn Care

Identifies deviations from normal in the newborn

575. After a difficult vaginal delivery, a newborn is admitted to the newborn nursery. During the assessment, it is noted that the baby's moro reflex does not include the right arm. Which problem would the nurse suspect?
    A. Brain damage
    B. Fractured radius
    C. Erb Duchenne palsy
    D. Cephalohematoma

The answer is C. Erb Duchenne Palsy usually is due to pulling the head away from the shoulder. The palsy, which may be permanent, prevents movement of the shoulder and upper arm. There is no evidence of brain damage. A fractured radius would not affect shoulder movement. Cephalohematoma is bleeding into the periosteum of the skull bone.

PHYSIOLOGICAL INTEGRITY

Pharmacological and Parenteral Therapies

Central Venous Access Devices

Provide care for client with a central venous access device

576. A client's PICC line will not flush. The nurse is unable to aspirate blood from the line. Which is an appropriate nursing action to restore patency?
    A. Instill heparin into the line
    B. Increase the pump pressure setting
    C. Use increased pressure to flush the line with saline.
    D. Contact the physician for orders for Activase (alteplase)

The answer is D. Activase is a thrombolytic which breaks down clots. Heparin prevents the formation of clots, it does not break down clots. Increased pressure may cause the clotted line to release an embolus into the client's circulation. Increasing the pump's pressure setting would not cause the clot to disintegrate.

PHYSIOLOGICAL INTEGRITY

Reduction of Risk Potential

577. A client has developed a pulmonary embolism. Which factors predispose a client to this problem? (Select all that apply.)
    A. Bradycardia
    B. Hypertension
    C. Hypercoagulability
    D. Fluid volume overload
    E. Venous stasis in the lower extremities

The answers are C and E. Hypercoagulability and venous stasis in the lower extremities predispose to development of a pulmonary embolism. The other options are unrelated to pulmonary embolism.

PHYSIOLOGICAL INTEGRITY

Physiological Adaptation

Illness Management

Apply knowledge of pathophysiology to illness management

578. A client is admitted to the hospital unit with a diagnosis of hemophilia A. The nurse reviews the client's lab report. Which lab result should the nurse interpret as unexpected and requiring further investigation?
    A. Low platelet count
    B. Low factor VIII values
    C. Prolonged bleeding time
    D. Prolonged partial thromboplastin time

The answer is A. The client with hemophilia A has insufficient levels of factor VIII which is a component of the clotting cascade. The platelet counts are normal. The other laboratory values would be prolonged due to the inadequacy of the clotting cascade.

SAFE AND EFFECTIVE CARE ENVIRONMENT

Safety and Infection Control

Home safety

579. A client is brought to the emergency room for acute lead poisoning. When determining the source of the lead poisoning, the nurse will question the client about which topic?
    A. Eating lead pencils
    B. Recent house painting
    C. Using homemade pottery or ceramic dishes.
    D. Eating unwashed vegetables from the garden.

The answer is C. Poorly fired pottery and ceramics may be improperly glazed allowing the lead to leak out of the clay. Lead pencils are made of carbon. Paint is now lead free. Unwashed vegetables do not contribute a risk of lead.

PHYSIOLOGICAL INTEGRITY

Reduction of Risk Potential

Potential for Complications of Diagnostic Tests/Treatments/Procedures

Provide nursing care that includes interventions designed to reduce post procedure complications

580. A client has returned to the cardiac unit following a cardiac catheterization performed through the left femoral artery. Which item is an appropriate part of the nursing care plan for this client?
   A. Out of bed as soon as awake from anesthesia
   B. Neurovascular check to the insertion site times two
   C. Pressure dressing and immobility for the insertion site
   D. Range of motion exercises to the left leg every two hours.

The answer is C. The site is kept immobile for up to 24 hours after cardiac catheterization to reduce the risk of a severe arterial bleed. Range of motion exercises would be contraindicated. The client would be on bedrest. Neurovascular checks should be performed at least hourly for the first 24 hours due to the risk of thrombosis.

PHYSIOLOGICAL INTEGRITY

Physiological Adaptation

Fluid and Electrolyte Imbalances

Identify signs and symptoms of client fluid and/or electrolyte imbalance

581. A client with multiple myeloma is beginning chemotherapy. The client's serum calcium level is 15 mg/dl. For which clinical manifestations related to this laboratory finding would the nurse assess?
   A. Abdominal cramps
   B. Confusion and anxiety
   C. Lethargy and weakness
   D. Muscle twitching

The answer is C. Normal serum calcium range is 8.5– 10.5 mg/dL so the client has hypercalcemia. Symptoms of hypercalcemia include lethargy and weakness as well as depressed deep tendon reflexes, anorexia, nausea, vomiting, constipation and dysrhythmias.

A, B, and D are incorrect—Abdominal cramping occurs with hyponatremia; confusion and anxiety occur with hypocalcemia; muscle twitching occurs with hyponatremia.

HEALTH PROMOTION AND MAINTENANCE

Ante-/Intra-/Postpartum and Newborn Care

582. The nurse is working on the postpartum unit and is assigned to four clients. Which of the four clients is most likely to suffer afterbirth pain based on their obstetrical history?
   A. Mother of twins
   B. Bottle feeding mother.
   C. Multipara with a premature infant
   D. Primipara with an average for gestational age infant

The answer is A. Factors which increase afterbirth pain include overdistended uterus such as in twins or large infants, breast feeding, and multiparas.

PHYSIOLOGICAL INTEGRITY

Reduction of Risk Potential

Therapeutic Procedures

Provide pre- and/or postoperative education

583. A client with a recent below the knee amputation of the left lower extremity is admitted to the rehabilitation unit and will be fitted with a prosthesis. Which is the priority self care instruction to be given to the client?
   A. Keep a diary of time and type of activity related to the use of the prosthesis.
   B. Assess skin integrity of the stump daily.
   C. Apply cold compresses to the residual extremity bid.
   D. Take analgesics if needed for phantom pain.

The answer is B. Preserving the integrity of the skin over the residual extremity is critical to use of the prosthesis and resumption of mobility. Thus the client is instructed to assess the skin at least daily so any problem is identified and treated early.

A is incorrect—a diary related to the use of the prosthesis is not a standard recommendation. C is incorrect—application of cold is not a standard part of residual extremity care. D is incorrect—although self-administration of analgesic may be required secondary to phantom limb pain it is not considered a priority in client education at this time.

PHYSIOLOGICAL INTEGRITY

Physiological Adaptation

Pathophysiology

584. A client arrives in the emergency room with a chief complaint of new onset stiff neck and muscle aches. A physical exam reveals erythema migrans on the right

upper arm. Which is the most likely cause of the client's signs and symptoms?
A. Gout
B. Lyme disease
C. Lupus erythematosis
D. Polymyositis

The answer is B. Lyme disease, caused by the spirochete Borrelia burgdorferi carried and transmitted by ticks, is characterized by erythema migrans or the "bull's eye" rash. Other symptoms of Stage I disease are muscle and joint pain and stiffness. Symptoms of gout are acute pain and inflammation of one or more small joints. Lupus erythematosis can affect virtually every body system. It can cause joint inflammation and myositis. It also can cause a rash but the rash is the dry, scaly, raised "butterfly" rash typically involving the cheeks and bridge of the nose resulting in the butterfly shape. The rash is not a bull's eye rash. Polymyositis is an inflammation of striated muscle causing symmetrical weakness and atrophy. It is not characterized by erythema migrans.

SAFE AND EFFECTIVE CARE ENVIRONMENTS

Management of Care

Principles of Management

Supervise care provided by others

585. The charge nurse is observing a newly hired nurse measure jugular venous pressure. Which action on the part of the new nurse requires correction by the charge nurse? The newly hired nurse
A. positions the client supine.
B. raises the head of the bed 30–45 degrees.
C. shines a light tangentally across the client's neck.
D. measures the vertical distance from the manubrium to the meniscus of the internal jugular vein.

The answer is D. The distance is measured vertically is from the sternal angle (angle of Louis) to the meniscus of the internal jugular vein. This distance which is measured in centimeters equals the jugular venous pressure which usually does not exceed 4 cm.

PSYCHOSOCIAL INTEGRITY

Chemical and Other Dependencies

Assess client for drug/alcohol related dependencies, withdrawal, or toxicities

586. When examining a two and a half year old, which assessment findings would the nurse interpret as consistent with fetal alcohol syndrome?
A. ___ strabismus
B. ___ Irritability
C. ___ Absence of teeth
D. ___ Hyperactivity
E. ___ Developmental delay

The answers are A, B, D, and E. Abnormalities associated with fetal alcohol syndrome which would be evident on assessing a two and one half year child include strabismus, myopia, irritability, hyperactivity, poor attention span, developmental delay and growth deficiency. Teeth are malformed not absent. Once in school, poor school performance is characteristic.

PHYSIOLOGICAL INTEGRITY

Basic Care and Comfort

Mobility/immobility

587. You are caring for a 40-year-old male who is on complete bed rest following a traumatic injury to his pelvis. The data collected during your morning assessment include elevated oral temperature (100°F), diminished lung sounds in right lower lobe and oxygen saturation of 90% on room air. The most likely cause of these findings:
A. hypostatic pneumonia
B. atelectasis
C. bronchitis
D. asthma

The answer is A. immobility results in respiratory complications which include pooling of respiratory secretions.

B is incorrect—atelectasis is a collapse of a single lobe or an entire lung. C is incorrect—bronchitis is the acute inflammation of airway passages. D is incorrect—asthma is not caused by immobility.

HEALTH PROMOTION AND MAINTENANCE

Developmental Stages and Transitions

Modify approaches to care in accordance with client's developmental stage

588. An 11-year-old boy is admitted to the hospital unit following a bicycle accident. A fractured femur is diagnosed and the child is placed in traction. The best room assignment for this child would be a room:
A. with other boys of the same age as roommates.
B. near the nurse's station so the child can be closely supervised.

C. away from other children so that the child can rest adequately.
D. with an alert adult roommate who can respond to the child's needs.

The answer is A. Boys of this age are usually active. This child has restricted activity and will be easily bored. The child will enjoy the company of the other children.

This child's condition is not a high risk condition so any room location on the unit would be acceptable. It is not the job of other clients to care for a client who is immobilized so option D would be incorrect.

PHYSIOLOGICAL INTEGRITY

Pharmacological and Parenteral Therapies

Adverse effects/contraindications

589. Which statement made by the parent of a 15-year-old girl receiving doxorubicin (Adriamycin) to treat leukemia indicates that information regarding side effects of the medication was understood?
A. "My daughter is lucky that the major side effects of her medication are headache and drowsiness; they could be a lot worse."
B. "It will be hard to see my daughter confused and hallucinating from the medication but at least these side effects won't last forever."
C. "I hope my daughter's heart isn't damaged from this medication; she is already going through so much that would just be awful for her."
D. "I worry about the effect of the medication on my daughter's kidneys but the important thing is to cure the cancer then we will deal with the rest."

The answer is C. heart damage is one of several side effects of doxorubicin (Adriamycin) so this statement indicates the client's parent understands this fact.

Answer A is incorrect—headache and drowsiness are side effects of methotrexate. Answer B is incorrect—hallucinations and confusion are side effects of ifsoamide (Ifex). Answer D is incorrect—kidney damage is a side effect of carboplatin (Paraplatin).

PHYSIOLOGICAL INTEGRITY

Reduction of Risk

Potential for complications of diagnostic Tests/Treatments/ Procedures

590. A client is admitted for an arthrogram of the right knee. Which is the most important information to obtain as part of the admission history?
A. Allergies to iodine, seafood, or local anesthetic
B. Current pain level to right knee
C. Previous experience with arthrogram
D. Time of last meal or fluid intake

The answer is A. it is important to know if the client has any of these allergies because a radiopaque dye, administered IV, is given to visualize the joint.

B and C are incorrect—Although collecting information related to pain and previous experience with an arthrogram should be included, it is not the most important information. D is incorrect—The client does not have to be NPO prior to this diagnostic test.

PSYCHOSOCIAL INTEGRITY

Therapeutic Communication

Use therapeutic communication techniques to provide support to client and/or family

591. A woman has recently been diagnosed with a terminal illness. Although her physical condition is stable at this time, the client seems depressed. Which approach by the nurse would be most effective in encouraging the client to talk about her feelings?
A. "You seem down today."
B. "Why are you feeling so depressed?"
C. "What can I do to make you feel better?"
D. "Would you like to talk to the hospital chaplain?"

The answer is A. The nurse has made a statement of his or her perceptions. The client can agree or deny these perceptions.

The client is never asked to explain feelings so asking why is a incorrect response. In option C, the nurse offers his or her self but this does not get at the client's feelings. Option D limits the conversation and is a way for the nurse to get out of an uncomfortable situation.

PHYSIOLOGICAL INTEGRITY

Pharmacological and Parenteral Therapies

Pharmacological agents/actions

592. A client is admitted to the hospital with a diagnosis of disseminated intravascular coagulation (DIC). The physician orders the client treated with heparin. A family member asks why heparin is being given to the client who is bleeding internally. The nurse's response is based on the knowledge that heparin:
A. increases the production of clotting factors.
B. preserves the platelets to prevent the client from bleeding out.

C. activates the clot disintegration process which breaks up the clots that have formed.
D. promotes neutralization of thrombin and prevents the conversion of fibrinogen to fibrin.

The answer is D. This action blocks the coagulation cascade at the common pathway and stops the intravascular coagulation disorder. The other responses do not accurately describe the effect of heparin.

PHYSIOLOGICAL INTEGRITY

Pharmacological and Parenteral Therapies

Medication Administration

Educate client/family about medications

593. A client is being placed on long-term corticosteroid therapy. Which information should be included as part of the client's discharge teaching?
A. Drink lots of water daily
B. Do not stop the medication suddenly
C. The medication may cause weight loss
D. It is critical not to not smoke while on corticosteroid therapy

The answer is B. Corticosteroids depress the body's natural production of corticosteroids. Sudden stopping of the medication could be fatal. The other responses are not correct.

PHYSIOLOGICAL INTEGRITY

Physiological Adaptation

Fluid and Electrolyte Imbalances

594. In caring for a client with a serum calcium level of 15 mg/dl, which instruction would be given to the client?
A. Increase the amount of calcium rich foods eaten each day
B. Incorporate fiber into the daily diet to decrease constipation
C. Avoid foods high in sodium content
D. Limit fluid intake of water

The answer is B. Normal serum calcium range is 8.5– 10.5 mg/dl so the client has hypercalcemia. Hypercalcemia can cause constipation.

A, C, and D are incorrect—Increasing calcium food consumption is indicated for hypocalcemia; a decrease in sodium intake is appropriate for hypernatremia; free water intake is indicated with hyponatremia.

SAFE AND EFFECTIVE CARE ENVIRONMENT

Safety and Infection Control

Standard/Transmission-Based/Other Precautions

Educate client/family/staff on infection control measures

595. A client goes to a clinic requesting to be tested for Acquired Immunodeficiency Syndrome (AIDS). The test was positive. Instructions to avoid spreading the infection will include:
A. Avoid sharing toothbrushes and razors
B. Do not share a bathroom with other individuals
C. Keep your dishes seperate
D. Keep fresh flowers and plants out of the home to reduce the accumulation of mold.

The answer is A. Body fluids can be spread by sharing toothbrushes and razors. Sharing a bathroom is acceptable. Others do not need to wear gloves during casual contact with the client.

PHYSIOLOGICAL INTEGRITY

Pharmacological and Parenteral Therapies

Medication Administration

Educate client/family about medications

596. A client with sickle cell anemia has been treated with several blood transfusions. Now Deferoxamine (Desferal) has been ordered and the client asks the nurse the purpose of this medication. Which is the correct answer for the nurse to give?
The medication will:
A. prevent the RBCs from sickling.
B. remove excessive iron from the body.
C. improve the longevity of the red blood cells.
D. increase the oxygen carrying capacity of the blood.

The answer is B. When repeated blood transfusions are given, the RBCs will eventually be broken down. The body retains the iron from these donated cells leading to iron toxicity. All other responses are incorrect.

PHYSIOLOGICAL INTEGRITY

Physiological Adaptation

Alterations in Body Systems

Provide postoperative care

597. A client has a cesarean section and delivers a healthy infant. Which of the following interventions are useful

in preventing pulmonary embolism in the postoperative mother?

A. Low salt diet and exercise

B. Compression stockings and leg exercises

C. Daily aspirin and daily breathing exercises

D. Low fat diet and rehabilitation therapy

The answer is B. Pulmonary emboli would result from thrombus formation. The pregnant woman is at greater risk for the development of thrombus. All surgical clients would also have this risk while bed ridden. Compression stockings and leg exercises would be most effective in preventing circulatory stasis.

PSYCHOSOCIAL INTEGRITY

Psychopathology

Assess client for alterations in mood, judgment, cognition, and reasoning as evidence of psychopathology

598. Nurses working with a client with which type of personality disorder must be particularly alert for splitting behavior?

A. Antisocial

B. Borderline

C. Narcissistic

D. Histrionic

The answer is B. Splitting is an unconscious mechanism characteristic of the client with an borderline personality disorder. The client is unable to accept imperfections in others and sees people as all good or all bad with the result that persons are set up against one another. For example, nurses may be good if they say only positive things to the client; nurses are bad if they provide negative feedback even when appropriate. Splitting is a coping behavior.

PHYSIOLOGICAL INTEGRITY

Basic Care and Comfort

Mobility/immobility

Provide nursing care that incorporates knowledge of the risks associated with immobility

599. A client has been bed ridden for several months due to the effects of Alzheimer's Disease. For which musculoskeletal problem is the client at risk?

A. Deep vein thrombosis

B. Osteoporosis

C. Avascular necrosis of hip

D. Embolism

The answer is B. prolonged bed rest result in loss of calcium leading to osteoporosis.

A is incorrect—this is a complication of the vascular system due to bed rest. C is incorrect—avascular necrosis is due to trauma and/or chronic steroid use. D is incorrect—an embolism is a cardiovascular complication from long term bed rest.

PHYSIOLOGICAL INTEGRITY

Physiological Adaptation

Pathophysiology

600. An elderly client develops disuse osteoporosis. The client's adult son asks why his parent has this disease. The nurse would explain that disuse osteoporosis occurs because of:

A. a decrease in calcium intake.

B. contractures to the lower extremities.

C. lack of stress to weight-bearing activity.

D. stiff and painful joints of the extremities.

The answer is C. calcium loss in the bones occurs due to lack of weight-bearing activity to the bones.

A is incorrect—a decrease in calcium content does not directly have an impact on disuse osteoporosis. B is incorrect—contractures of lower extremities can be the result of immobility. D is incorrect—immobility will eventually result in stiff and sore joints.

PHYSIOLOGICAL INTEGRITY

Pharmacological and Parenteral Therapies

Medication Administration

601. A 13-month-old child is to receive an oral medication. The child starts crying as soon as the nurse enters the room with the medication despite the fact that his mother is telling him a story. After checking the child's identification bracelet, how should the nurse proceed with administering the medication?

A. Blow gently across his face with a soft whistling sound to stop the crying.

B. Allow the mother to administer the medication.

C. Delay giving the medication until the child is calmer.

D. Hold the child on his or her lap in a semi-Fowler's position.

The answer is B. After the nurse checks the bracelet, the mother can be allowed to administer the medication while the nurse watches. The nurse would not blow across the child's face; microorganisms can be spread in this way. Medication must be given in a timely fashion to be effective. The child would be held upright to prevent choking.

HEALTH PROMOTION AND MAINTENANCE

Developmental Stages and Transitions

Assist the client to achieve an appropriate outcome

602. A mother asks the nurse when she should begin toilet training her toddler. Which is an appropriate response for the nurse to give?
An indication that a child is ready to begin toilet training is that the child
A. pulls on the diaper when it is wet.
B. has a BM at the same time every day.
C. doesn't want to lay down for diaper changes.
D. hides behind the living room chair when having a BM

The answer is D. This indicates the child is aware that he is about to have a BM, a necessary step in toilet training. A indicates the child is aware that he has eliminated, but does not show anticipation of the event. Having a BM at the same time every day makes toilet training easier for mother, but does not indicate readiness. Toddlers are so busy they often complain about the need to have diapers changed. It doesn't indicate readiness.

PHYSIOLOGICAL INTEGRITY

Pharmacological and Parenteral Therapies

Medication Administration

Use clinical decision making/critical thinking when calculating dosages

603. What is the maximum daily dose of acetaminophen in mg/Kg of body weight that can safely be given to children? Record your answer in a whole number.
_____ mg/Kg.

The answer is 90 mg/Kg. The maximum daily dose for adults is 4 gm.

PHYSIOLOGICAL INTEGRITY

Pharmacological and Parenteral Therapy

Expected effects/outcomes

604. The nurse is comparing laboratory results on admission with laboratory results following treatment of a client with DIC. Which change in laboratory values from admission indicates a positive response to therapy?
A. Decrease in platelet count
B. Increase in fibrinogen level
C. D-dimer assay increase
D. Decreased bleeding time

The answer is B. Heparin is used in the treatment of DIC. If therapy is effective, the heparin should stop the process of intravascular coagulation thereby allowing the fibrinogen level in the blood to increase. Platelet count would increase not decrease with effective therapy. D-dimer assay is a global marker of coagulation activation measuring a fibrin degradation product. Clotting time, not bleeding time, is a reliable indicator of effective therapy for DIC.

PSYCHOSOCIAL INTEGRITY

Therapeutic Communications

Use therapeutic communication techniques to provide support to client and/or family

605. A woman has given birth to a preterm infant. The infant is doing well in the high risk nursery. The woman states to the nurse: "I am so worried about my baby." The best response by the nurse would be:
A. "You're worried about your baby?"
B. "Don't be worried, your baby is doing fine."
C. "God will take care of your baby if it is meant to be."
D. "Babies born at the gestation of your baby usually do very well.'

The answer is A. It is reflective and encourages the mother to provide more information. The other responses are not therapeutic.

PHYSIOLOGICAL INTEGRITY

Pharmacological and Parenteral Therapies

Parenteral/Intravenous Therapy

Monitor and maintain infusion site(s) and rate(s)

606. The nurse is scheduled to administer 500 mg of ampicillin IV by secondary line. The drug is to be infused over 20 minutes. The ampicillin is in a 50 ml baggie of D5W. The IV drop factor for this IV is 15. How many drops per minute should the nurse regulate the IV to infuse at over the required 20 minutes?
A. 20 gtts/min
B. 30 gtts/min
C. 40 gtts/min
D. 60 gtts/min

The answer is B. 50 ml in 20 minutes or $2\frac{1}{2}$ ml per minute. Each ml contains 12 drops so 12 times $2\frac{1}{2} = 30$ gtts/min.

PHYSIOLOGICAL INTEGRITY

Physiological Adaptation

Medical emergencies

607. When performing the Heimlich maneuver on a pregnant or markedly obese client, the nurse should position her hands in which area? Mark the spot with the letter "X".

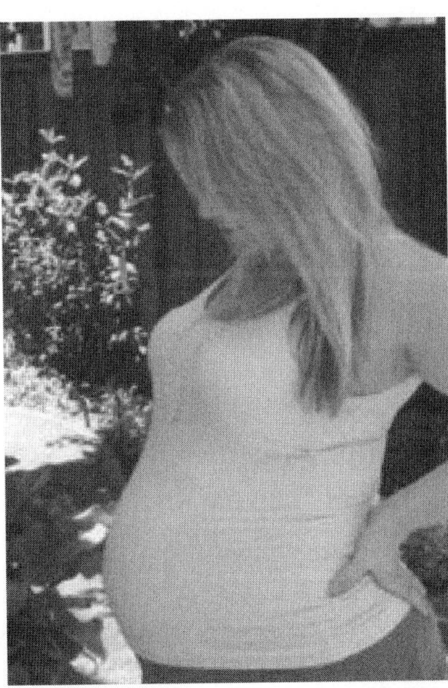

Correct response:

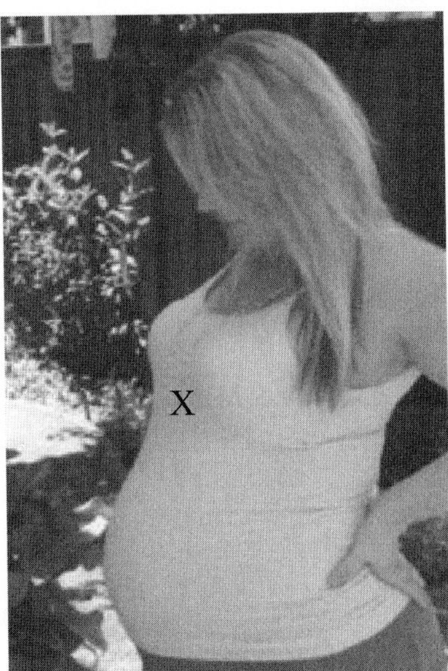

PHYSIOLOGICAL INTEGRITY

Physiological Adaptation

Fluid and Electrolyte Imbalances

Identify signs and symptoms of client fluid and/or electrolyte imbalance

608. A child has been admitted to the pediatric unit with gastroenteritis. Which laboratory finding indicates the child is dehydrated?
   A. Elevated reticulocyte count
   B. Elevated white blood cell counts
   C. Decreased urine-specific gravity
   D. Elevated hemoglobin and hematocrit

The answer is D. Since both hemoglobin and hematocrit are comparisons of solids to liquids, dehydration causes an increase in these values. The other responses do not indicate dehydration.

HEALTH PROMOTION AND MAINTENANCE

Techniques of Physical Assessment

Choose physical assessment equipment and technique appropriate for client

609. A client is transferred from the operating room to the postpartum unit following a cesarean section for fetal distress. When the nurse performs the postpartum assessment, the client complains of pain and asks the nurse not to palpate the fundus. Which is the appropriate nursing action?
   A. Ask a more experienced nurse to palpate the fundus.
   B. Palpate the fundus anyway while avoiding the incision area.
   C. Avoid palpating the fundus as long as the vital signs are stable.
   D. Explain the need for fundal palpation and then palpate the fundus from the side.

The answer is D. Fundal palpation is essential for the well-being of the client. Contraction of the fundus occludes open blood vessels and prevents excessive bleeding from the site of placental implantation. The client will be more cooperative if the client understands the rationale.

PHYSIOLOGICAL INTEGRITY

Reduction of Risk Potential

Potential for alterations in body systems

610. An 84-year-old female is brought to the E.R. presenting with confusion, restlessness and altered mental status. Which nursing action is appropriate?

A. Ask the client about the medications she is currently taking.
B. Give electrolyte replacing fluids.
C. Refer the client for a psychiatric evaluation.
D. Prepare for a physical exam including a chest x-ray, EKG, UA, and CBC.

The answer is D. Changes in mental status such as confusion and restlessness are typical signs of acute illness in older adults requiring physical exam and lab work to r/o UTI, MI, pneumonia.

PHYSIOLOGICAL INTEGRITY

Basic Care and Comfort

Mobility/immobility

611. An elderly client has been hospitalized for two weeks and develops the beginning of a pressure ulcer on the coccyx. The nurse recognizes that pressure ulcers in older adults are considered:
A. primary changes
B. secondary changes
C. normal changes
D. expected changes when hospitalized

The answer is B. Primary, normal, and expected changes are the same thing and pressure ulcers are not a normal sign, rather a pathological one.

SAFE AND EFFECTIVE CARE ENVIRONMENT

Safety and Infection Control

Accident Prevention

Identify and facilitate correct use of infant and child safety seats

612. The nurse is teaching a prenatal class on child safety. Where would the nurse instruct the expectant mothers to put their baby's car seat?
A. Front passenger seat
B. Middle of the back seat
C. Back seat behind the driver
D. Back seat behind the passenger

The answer is B. The middle of the back seat is the safest place for the infant car seat.

PHYSIOLOGICAL INTEGRITY

Reduction of Risk Potential

Potential for complications from surgical procedures and health alterations

613. A client had a left total knee replacement two days ago and is now having dyspnea and appears to be very apprehensive. Pulse rate is 110 and she is diaphoretic. Which problem does the nurse suspect?
A. Infection
B. Pneumonia
C. Fat embolus
D. Anaphylaxis

The answer is C. These are symptoms of a fat embolus which is a risk when the marrow cavities of long bones are opened due to accidental trauma or surgery.

A is incorrect—the symptoms listed are not indicators of infection, B is incorrect—Data collected does not include temperature. D is incorrect—information provided does not include drug history.

PSYCHOSOCIAL INTEGRITY

Psychopathology

Recognize signs and symptoms of impaired cognition

614. A client with schizophrenia says "skipping, whipping, tripping" over and over during his waking hours. Which would be a correct label for the nurse to use when documenting this communication?
A. word salad
B. clang association
C. neologism
D. echolalia

The answer is B. Clang association. Clang association refers to repeating words and phrases which sound alike but are otherwise unconnected. Word salad refers to the meaningless connection of words and phrases. A neologism is a new word coined by the client and with meaning only to the client. Echolalia is the repetition of words or phrases heard from another person.

PHYSIOLOGICAL INTEGRITY

Pharmacological and Parenteral Therapy

Pharmacological interactions

615. A client is on anticoagulant therapy following a pulmonary embolism. During the first visit to the client's

home, the home health nurse asks the client to take out all the medications that he has on hand. Which medication is a cause for concern when taken by a client on an anticoagulant?

A. Ferrous sulfate (Iron)
B. Acetylsalicylic acid (Aspirin)
C. Isoniazid (INH)
D. Phenytoin (Dilantin)

The answer is B. Aspirin can potentiate the effects of anticoagulants. Ferrous sulfate does not affect anticoagulants; it is used for RBC production. INH is an antitubercular product and does not affect clotting time. Phenytoin is an antiseizure med and does not affecting clotting time.

PHYSIOLOGICAL INTEGRITY

Pharmacological and Parenteral Therapies

Central Venous Access Devices

Access implanted venous access devices

616. While visiting the area from another state, a client presents to the emergency room with severe pain secondary to a kidney stone. The physician orders an IV line started with 125 ml per hour of D5 ¼ NS and morphine for pain. The client shows the nurse his chest where he states he has a Subcutaneous venous port and asks the nurse to start the IV there. Prior to starting an IV line in this port, the nurse would need to verify that the:

A. Brand of subcutaneous port.
B. Medications can be given by central line.
C. Port internal tip lies in the superior vena cava.
D. Intravenous fluids can be administered by central line.

The answer is C. Prior to administering anything through a central line, the location of the internal tip must be verified. Since this client is not known in the area, the tip location can be verified by x-ray if the client does not have a card documenting this information. Any medication and intravenous fluids that can be administered by peripheral line can be administered in a central line.

SAFE AND EFFECTIVE CARE ENVIRONMENT

Safety and Infection Control

Standard/Transmission Based/Other Precautions

Evaluate infection control precautions implemented by staff members

617. A client is on contact isolation due to a MSRA abscess. The charge nurse observes all of the following nursing activities. Which nursing activity fails to safely protect others from the client?

The nurse:

A. washes hands after removing gloves.
B. does not wear gloves when changing the bed.
C. does not wear a gown when checking the IV level.
D. covers the client with a sheet when being transported to x-ray.

The answer is B. The abscess could have drained onto the bedding. The nurse does not need to wear a gown unless contact with items in the room is expected. Hands should always be washed or disinfected after removing gloves. Covering the client with a sheet when out of the room will reduce exposure to others.

PHYSIOLOGICAL INTEGRITY

Physiological Adaptation

Alterations in Body Systems

618. The nurse is assessing an elderly client and notes the following findings. Which assessment findings would the nurse identify as a normal signs of aging? Mark all that apply.

A. Increase in diastolic blood pressure
B. Reduced lens elasticity
C. Reduced vital capacity
D. Decreased force of myocardial contraction

The answers are B, C, and D. Decreases in lens elasticity, vital capacity and force of myocardial contraction all occur normally with aging. Mild increase in systolic BP also occurs, however an increase in diastolic BP is pathological and requires monitoring.

PHYSIOLOGICAL INTEGRITY

Pharmacological and Parenteral Therapies

Adverse Effects/Contraindications

Provide nursing care that incorporates knowledge of adverse effects of selected pharmaceutical agents

619. A client presents to the emergency department, dehydrated and with metabolic acidosis. An overdose of which drug can result in these problems?

A. Digitalis
B. Aspirin
C. Insulin
D. Acetaminophen

The answer is B. Aspirin toxicity causes hyperventilation leading to respiratory alkalosis which leads to metabolic acidosis and dehydration. In digitalis toxicity, the major symptoms would be bradycardia. Insulin overdose would lead to hypoglycemia. Acetaminophen toxicity would result in symptoms of liver damage including AST and ALT elevations.

SAFE AND EFFECTIVE CARE ENVIRONMENT

Safety and Infection Control

Standard/Transmission-Based/Other Precautions

Apply principles of infection control

620. The charge nurse is orienting a new nurse to the mother baby unit. The charge nurse explains that gloves should be worn (select all that apply):
   A. when changing diapers.
   B. for the initial newborn bath.
   C. when changing the bag of IV fluids.
   D. while performing initial assessment on a newborn.
   E. when assisting the new mother to the bathroom for the first time after delivery.

The answers are A, B, D, and E. The nurse would be at risk for exposure to bloodborne pathogens during all these events. Newborns are covered with amniotic fluid and blood. Diaper changes might expose the nurse to body fluids. The first time the mother is out of bed, a large amount of blood usually escapes from the vagina. Combine that with the fact that many new mothers become weak or faint when first up, gloves at this time provide protection for the nurse.

PHYSIOLOGICAL INTEGRITY

Pharmacological and Parenteral Therapies

Central Venous Access Devices

Provide care for a client with a central venous access device

621. A client has had a PICC line for 2 weeks which is being used for intermittent infusion of an antibiotic. Between uses, the PICC line is heparinized and locked. The nurse is ready to administer the PM dose of antibiotic. The nurse flushes the line which flushes easily, but is unable to aspirate blood. The nurse should:
   A. administer the medication as planned.
   B. ask for x-ray verification of the PICC placement.
   C. discontinue this PICC line and insert a new PICC line.
   D. hold the dose until the physician sees the client in the AM.

The answer is A. PICC lines have a very small lumen and blood aspiration is often not possible after several weeks of use. The easy flush with no other complaints usually indicates that the PICC is intact. X-ray verification is used whenever the location of the tip is in question. Only specially trained nurses can insert PICC lines. Holding the dose until the next day would allow the client's blood level to drop and could allow the organism to become resistant.

PSYCHOSOCIAL INTEGRITY

Family Dynamics

Assist client/family/significant others to integrate new members into family structure

622. A young teenage girl has just given birth to a baby girl. She has decided to keep her baby. The nurses are concerned about bonding between mother and infant. To promote bonding, the nurse will:
   A. tell the mother her baby is beautiful.
   B. delay eye prophylaxis immediately after birth.
   C. leave the mother and baby alone to get acquainted.
   D. keep the lights in the room on bright so the mother can see her infant clearly.

The answer is B. Bonding is supported when the mother looks at her infant and the infant looks back. Delaying eye prophylaxis and lowering the lights in the room will promote the infant looking back.

The mother may be afraid to be alone with her infant. Telling the mother the baby is beautiful is not the best intervention to promote bonding.

PHYSIOLOGICAL INTEGRITY

Pharmacological and Parenteral Therapies

Total Parenteral Nutrition

Provide client/family/significant others with information on TPN

623. A 4-year-old child with cystic fibrosis has difficulty maintaining adequate nutrition and has had a subcutaneous venous port surgically implanted for home administration of total parenteral nutrition. The child receives the TPN for 8 hours each night and is disconnected from the IV line during the day. The home health nurse teaches the mother to:
   A. Calculate the drip rate since a pump will not be needed.
   B. Check the child's blood glucose every two hours during the night.
   C. Limit the child's intake during the day so the child will not become obese.

D. Start the TPN slow and taper up to the desired rate each night and then taper off each morning.

The answer is D. TPN is always tapered on and tapered off. Sudden onset will cause hyperglycemia, sudden stopping will cause hypoglycemia. An electronic infusion pump is always used with TPN. It is not necessary to check the child's glucose as often as every two hours. Limiting the child's daily intake would be inappropriate as the child is malnourished.

PHYSIOLOGICAL INTEGRITY

Physiological Adaptation

Pathophysiology

624. A 67-year-old female is returning to the medical clinic for a follow-up visit due to complaints of back pain, frequent fevers and weight loss. CBC and serum chemistry disclosed high serum calcium and protein levels and low levels of hemoglobin, red blood cells, platelets, and white blood cells. With which problem are these signs and symptoms consistent?
A. Anemia
B. Arthritis
C. Multiple myeloma
D. Systemic lupus erythematosis

The answer is C. Multiple myeloma is correct.

A is incorrect—there is only a decrease in hemoglobin and hematocrit with anemia. B is incorrect—these tests would not be performed to diagnose arthritis. D is incorrect—these tests are not performed to diagnose lupus erythematosis.

HEALTH PROMOTION AND MAINTENANCE

Principles of Teaching/Learning

Assess readiness to learn, learning preferences, and barriers to learning

625. A nurse is preparing to teach a newly diagnosed diabetic about the disease. Which is the initial step the nurse should take?
A. Identify the client's willingness to learn.
B. Find out what the client knows about the disease.
C. Determine the client's level of formal education.
D. Select written material available for the client's use.

The answer is B. The initial step is always to begin where the client is. All other responses may be helpful, but initially determining the client's current knowledge is most important.

PHYSIOLOGICAL INTEGRITY

Reduction of Risk Potential

System-Specific Assessment

Perform focused assessment

626. The nurse is checking Homan's sign on a client suspected of having a venous thrombosis. Which action should the nurse take?
A. Flex the client's hip and the knee
B. Flex the client's hip while extending the knee
C. Ask the client to point the toes while bending the knee
D. Push the client's foot forward toward the knee while maintaining the knee in extension

The answer is D. A positive Homan's sign is calf pain on dorsiflexing the foot while maintaining the knee in extension. If Homan's is positive, a venous thrombosis is suspected. The other responses do not describe the appropriate technique to assess for Homan's sign.

PHYSIOLOGICAL INTEGRITY

Reduction of Risk Potential

Therapeutic Procedures

Use precautions to prevent further injury when moving a client with a musculoskeletal position

627. A client has had spinal surgery and the physician has ordered the client to be "log-rolled." To be log rolled, the nurse will:
A. have the client turn slowly and stiffly.
B. use a draw sheet to maintain body alignment.
C. only position the client prone or supine to prevent spinal trauma.
D. ask for assistance from another nurse to maintain the body alignment.

The answer is D. Log rolling will require two nurses or more to maintain alignment of the spine and prevent trauma. The other actions are not the correct methods for log-rolling.

PSYCHOSOCIAL INTEGRITY

Psychopathology

Recognize signs of acute and chronic mental illness

628. The nurse would expect to encounter withdrawal and odd eccentric behaviors when caring for a group of clients with which cluster of personality disorders?
A. Paranoid, schizoid, schizotypal
B. Antisocial, borderline, histrionic, narcissistic

C. Avoidant, dependent, obsessive-compulsive

D. Passive-aggressive, masochistic

The answer is A. Withdrawal and odd, eccentric behaviors are characteristic of clients with paranoid, schizoid, and schizotypal personality disorder. Attention seeking and erratic behaviors are characteristic of clients with antisocial, borderline, histrionic and narcissistic personality disorders. Clients with avoidant, dependent or obsessive compulsive personality disorder are attempting to avoid or minimize anxiety or fear.

Clients with passive-aggressive or masochistic personality disorder are covertly aggressive against self or others.

PHYSIOLOGICAL INTEGRITY

Physiological Adaptation

Alterations in body systems

629. A woman is admitted to the emergency room with bleeding from a stab wound in the right chest area. Which assessment findings would the nurse interpret as indicating the initial phase of hypovolemic shock? Mark all that apply.

A. Increased hematocrit

B. Narrowed pulse pressure

C. Elevated heart rate

D. Oxygen saturation of less than 80%

E. Increased rate and depth of respiration

F. Absent superficial peripheral pulses

G. Slowed capillary refill

The answers are B, C, and G. Pulse pressure narrows because in the initial stage of hypovolemic shock the body attempts to compensate for the blood loss through vasoconstriction which decreases the size of the vascular bed. Vasoconstriction increases the diastolic blood pressure but not the systolic, thus the pulse pressure is decreased or narrowed before the systolic pressure drops from loss of volume. Heart rate also increases as part of the compensatory effort. The increased heart rate is an attempt to maintain cardiac output despite the fact that stroke volume is decreased. Capillary refill or the time taken for color to return to the nail bed after being pressed until it blanches is slow or even absent in shock.

Hematocrit and hemoglobin are decreased in shock caused by hemorrhage; they are increased in other types of hypovolemic shock. Oxygen saturation of less than 80% is not a sign of initial shock; it is a sign of later progressive shock. Increased respiratory rate is a sign of initial shock but depth does not increase until shock has progressed to the point that lactic acidosis is present. Superficial peripheral pulses may be difficult to locate and easily obliterated in initial shock but absent superficial peripheral pulses are a sign of later shock.

PHYSIOLOGICAL INTEGRITY

Reduction of Risk Potential

Therapeutic Procedures

Provide preoperative care

630. A child is scheduled for surgery. Which are nursing actions to be carried out prior to surgery? (Select all that apply.)

A. Check the child for loose teeth.

B. Remove finger nail polish from fingers and toes.

C. Have appropriate lab reports available on the chart.

D. Verify that the parents have signed an informed consent.

E. Check that the child has been NPO for a specified period of time.

The answers are A, B, C, D, and E. All responses are correct and should be included in the presurgery routine.

PHYSIOLOGICAL INTEGRITY

Physiological Adaptation

Alterations in Body System

631. A 44-year-old client is admitted to the emergency department with burns to the neck and face received from an explosion while working on a gas pipeline. During the nurse's initial assessment, highest priority should be given to:

A. Noting signs of increased intracranial pressure (ICP)

B. Monitoring hourly intake and output

C. Assessing changes in circumference of the neck

D. Replacing fluid loss since based on weight

The answer is C. Assessing circumference of the neck will identify increases in girth and potential restriction of the airway from edema. ICP not pertinent in the absence of head injury and would not replace maintenance of a patent airway as a priority. Monitoring I&O is important but not the initial priority. Replacing fluid is essential in burn therapy but not a priority over airway.

SAFE AND EFFECTIVE CARE ENVIRONMENTS

Safety and Infection Control

Standard/Transmission-Based/Other Precautions

Apply principles of infection control

632. Which precaution measures would be instituted when a client has a Mycoplasma pneumoniae infection? (Mark all that apply.)

A. ___ Client is placed in a private, negative airflow pressure room.
B. ___ Client is placed in a private room or with other clients with infection caused by the same organism.
C. ___ Use mask at all times while in the client's room.
D. ___ Use mask when working within 3 feet of the client
E. ___ Use gown and protective barriers when giving direct care.
F. ___ Mask on client if transported out of room.
G. ___ Use gloves at all times when caring for clients.
H. ___ Use gloves when there is risk of exposure to blood or body fluids.

The answers are B, D, F, and H. Mycoplasma pneumoniae is spread by droplet transmission. Transmission-based precautions for droplet transmission require a private room or a room shared with someone infected with the same organism. Those entering the room and coming within 3 feet of the client need to wear a mask and the client wears a mask if taken out of the room. Standard precautions, which involve wearing gloves whenever there is the risk of touching something wet that comes from the body surface or a body cavity, i.e., when there is the risk of contact with blood or body fluids, are used at all times for all clients.

PHYSIOLOGICAL INTEGRITY

Physiological Adaptation

Medical Emergencies

Perform emergency care procedures

633. A client comes into the Emergency Room with a heavily bleeding thigh wound. Which is the priority nursing action?
   A. Start oxygen
   B. Put pressure on the wound
   C. Establish an IV line
   D. Determine the cause of the wound

The answer is B. The first priority is to put pressure on the wound to stop the bleeding and prevent further blood loss which can lead to hypovolemic shock. Oxygen is given to aid maintenance of tissue oxygenation. An IV line is established for fluid replacement and the cause of the wound would be determined as a guide to management. However none of these is the first priority.

PHYSIOLOGICAL INTEGRITY

Pharmacological and Parenteral Therapies

Dosage calculations

634. Using the Parkland formula (4 ml of lactated ringer's solution/% TBSA burn/kg body weight/24 hours), the nurse would calculate fluid replacement for a 70-kg client with a 50% TBSA burn over 24 hours as
   A. 1400 ml
   B. 14,000 ml
   C. 6720 ml
   D. 700 ml

The answer is B. 14,000 ml is the correct number. 4 × 50 = 200 ml/kg. Client weighs 70 kilograms so 70 × 200 = 14000 ml.

SAFE AND EFFECTIVE CARE ENVIRONMENT

Management of Care

Informed Consent

Ensure that client has given informed consent for treatment

635. The physician has ordered IVIG (intravenous immunoglobulins) to be administered to a client on a monthly basis. Prior to starting this therapy, the nurse would make certain that the client:
   A. is aware of the importance of being NPO the morning of the infusion.
   B. has signed an informed consent for a blood product.
   C. understands that once started, the therapy cannot be stopped.
   D. recognizes that he or she will be contagious for 2 days after receiving the IVIG product.

The answer is B. IVIG are antibodies removed from the blood of blood donors. One dose of IVIG can contain antibodies from 60,000 individuals. All other statements are not correct.

PHYSIOLOGICAL INTEGRITY

Pharmacological and Parenteral Therapies

Medication Administration

Educate client and family about medications

636. Due to a severe asthma attack, a client has been on corticosteroids for more than 2 weeks. Which information should the nurse give the client about when the time comes to stop the medication?

A. Fluid intake will need to be limited.
B. The dose of medication will be tapered down slowly.
C. Extra calcium will be needed for a week to ten days.
D. Vitamin supplements will be needed to prevent bone loss.

The answer is B. Corticosteroids suppress the body's own production of corticosteroids by the adrenal gland. Sudden stopping of the medication could be fatal. The other responses are incorrect.

PSYCHOSOCIAL INTEGRITY

Psychopathology

Recognize signs and symptoms of acute and chronic mental illness

637. Which symptoms would the nurse expect to find when assessing a client in the prodromal stage of schizophrenia?
A. social isolation and withdrawal
B. impaired role function
C. Speech aberration
D. peculiar beliefs
E. markedly odd behavior

The answers are A, B, C, D, and E. Social isolation withdrawal, impaired role function, speech aberration, peculiar beliefs, and markedly odd behavior are all symptoms that can occur in the prodromal phase of schizophrenia. Speech disturbance may be manifested as vague or circumstantial speech, over elaborate speech, or poverty of speech and content. Other prodromal symptoms include unusual perceptual experience and marked lack of initiative, interests and energy. At least two of these symptoms persisting continuously for six months must occur for the diagnosis of prodromal schizophrenia to be made.

PHYSIOLOGICAL INTEGRITY

Physiological Adaptations

Fluid and electrolyte imbalances

638. A client arrives in the emergency department after having been burned with hot oil over the upper entire anterior chest and right leg. When the client is being triaged, which is the most important question for the nurse to ask?
A. "What time did the burn occur?"
B. "Have you had any pain meds since the burn?"
C. "How did you stop the burning process?"
D. "What caused this burn initially?"

The answer is A. The time the burn occurred will determine the amount of fluid replacement.

The other questions may be asked but none is more important than the time of the burn because fluid replacement is of critical importance and none of the other questions provide information needed to determine it. Pain assessment is important but fluid replacement is priority. Knowing how the burning process was stopped is not critical in fluid replacement. Option D is important but not priority.

PHYSIOLOGICAL INTEGRITY

Physiological Adaptation

Medical Emergencies

639. A visitor falls to the floor in front of the nursing station. Which assessment findings are indicative of sudden cardiac death?
A. Fixed, dilated pupils
B. Absent respirations
C. Absent pulses
D. Absent blood pressure
E. Loss of consciousness

The answers are B, C, D, and E. Absence of respirations, pulses and blood pressure along with loss of consciousness are signs of full cardiac arrest. Pupils become fixed but not necessarily dilated.

SAFE AND EFFECTIVE CARE ENVIRONMENT

Safety and Infection Control

Use of Restraints/Safety Devices

Comply with federal/state/institutional policy regarding the use of client restraints and/or safety devices

640. A 2-year-old child has had a cleft palate repair. Elbow restraints have been placed on the child's arms to prevent the child from damaging the suture line. How does the nurse manage the restraints?
The nurse
A. never removes the restraints.
B. removes both restraints at the same time every 2 hours.
C. removes the restraints one at a time when providing range of motion.

D. removes the restraints only when there is another adult present to prevent suture damage.

The answer is C. The restraints are removed every two hours, one at a time. At that time the underlying skin is evaluated and range of motion exercises are provided.

A is incorrect as the restraints need to be removed periodically. B is incorrect as the restraints would be removed one at a time. D is incorrect as the nurse does not need another adult to remove the restraints.

PHYSIOLOGICAL INTEGRITY

Physiological Adaptation

Alterations in Body Systems

Counsel/teach client/family/significant others about managing client health problem

641. A 3-month-old infant has been diagnosed as being at risk for sudden infant death and apnea monitors are being used in the home. Parent teaching will include:
    A. infant CPR.
    B. heimlich maneuver for infancy.
    C. postural drainage techniques.
    D. use of portable oxygen.

The answer is A. Unless the parents know infant CPR, they will be unable to respond if their child has an apneic period. The other responses are incorrect.

HEALTH PROMOTION AND MAINTENANCE

Growth and Development

642. A newborn infant has been diagnosed with Down's syndrome. The parents have been informed that the child will have mental retardation. The parents ask the nurse what they can expect of their child's development. The best response by the nurse would include the information that their child will:
    A. develop in an undeterminable pattern.
    B. never develop basic skills due to the mental retardation.
    C. develop in the same pattern as other children but at a slower rate.
    D. will follow the same developmental time frame as other children but will stop developing before the other children.

The answer is C. Mentally retarded children develop in the same order as other children—they will learn to sit before they stand, stand before they walk, etc. The other answers are incorrect.

PHYSIOLOGICAL INTEGRITY

Physiological Adaptation

Illness Management

Teach client about managing illness

643. A child has been diagnosed with scabies. In addition to washing the child with the prescribed medication, the nurse would instruct the mother to:
    A. wash all bed linens in hot soapy water.
    B. wash all fruits and vegetables before use.
    C. have the family's dog checked for evidence of infestation.
    D. discard all of the child's clothing and replace with new clothing.

The answer is A. All bed linens and clothing should be washed in hot soapy water to kill the itch mites. This itch mite is not acquired from food sources. The dog does not transmit the itch mite to humans. It is not necessary to discard all clothing.

PHYSIOLOGICAL INTEGRITY

Physiological Adaptation

Medical emergencies

644. An industrial nurse responds to an emergency in the plant where a worker is burned. Which is the correct sequence of nursing actions?
    A. Eliminate the source of the burn, ensure airway patency, observe for and treat associated injuries, treat burn shock.
    B. Eliminate the source of the burn, ensue airway patency, cool the burn wound, apply topical antibiotic cream.
    C. Ensure airway patency, insert a nasogastric tube, insert a bladder catheter, stare IV fluid infusion.
    D. Treat burn shock, ensure airway patency, start IV antibiotics and put the client in reverse isolation.

The answer is A. The appropriate sequence of nursing actions for clients with major burn injuries is to eliminate the source of the burn, ensure airway patency, assess for and treat associated injuries, and treat burn shock. Options B, C, and D may be appropriate during care of such a client, but response (A) represents the correct sequence for initial assessment.

PHYSIOLOGICAL INTEGRITY

Reduction of Risk Potential

Potential for complications from surgical procedures and health alterations

645. Why are clients who have had back surgery, such as a laminectomy or spinal fusion, turned by log rolling?
   A. Guard against wound dehiscence
   B. Prevent excess pressure on the operative site
   C. Maintain body alignment
   D. Protect against skin breakdown

The answer is C. In log rolling, the client is turned all at once with the back as straight as possible. This maintains proper body alignment and avoids disruption of the surgical site. Other answers are incorrect.

SAFE AND EFFECTIVE CARE ENVIRONMENT

Management of Care

Confidentiality/Information Security

Maintain client confidentiality/privacy

646. The nurse is working in the emergency department when a call is received from a police officer asking about the condition of one his colleagues who has been injured while on duty. Which is an appropriate nursing action?
   A. Give only general information about the client.
   B. Encourage the officer to contact a member of the client's family.
   C. Transfer the call to the hospital administrator.
   D. Answer his questions once the identity of the officer is confirmed.

The answer is B. Sharing of a client's health information is governed by the HIPPA regulations. No information can be given to a friend or coworker. Referring the officer to a family member does not guarantee that this person has or will share information but does not violate the privacy requirements.

PHYSIOLOGICAL INTEGRITY

Reduction of Risk Potential

Potential for complications from surgical procedures and health alterations

647. Your client has an external fixator to the right lower extremity to stabilize an open fracture of the tibia and fibia with extensive soft tissue damage. The client is complaining of a tingling sensation in the foot. Which is the priority nursing action in response to the client's new complaint?
   A. Administer pain medication
   B. Assess pain level using a pain scale
   C. Notify physician of client's status
   D. Perform neurovascular assessment

The answer is D. Prior to any of the other interventions, the nurse will need to do a full assessment of the status of the leg. The physician will need the additional information to determine the appropriate medical intervention.

PHYSIOLOGICAL INTEGRITY

Physiological Adaptation

Illness management

648. A client suffered blunt trauma to the chest in a motor vehicle accident (MVA) and is later diagnosed with adult respiratory distress syndrome (ARDS). The nurse is formulating a plan of care for this client and knows that the nursing goal with the highest priority should relate to which area?
   A. Improving nutritional status and decreasing protein wasting
   B. Administering diuretics and antibiotics to combat infection
   C. Maintaining oxygenation and eliminating underlying cause of ARDS
   D. Monitoring the client's blood pressure and $PaCO_2$ levels

The answer is C. Airway and oxygenation are always the first priority. Maintaining oxygenation takes the priority over monitoring blood pressure and ensuring good nutrition.

PSYCHOSOCIAL INTEGRITY

Psychopathology

Recognize signs of acute and chronic mental illness

649. The nurse would expect to encounter attention seeking and erratic behaviors when caring for a group of clients with which cluster of personality disorders?
   A. Paranoid, schizoid, schizotypal
   B. Antisocial, borderline, histrionic, narcissistic
   C. Avoidant, dependent, obsessive-compulsive
   D. Passive-aggressive, masochistic

The answer is B. Attention seeking and erratic behaviors are characteristic of clients with antisocial, borderline, histrionic and narcissistic personality disorders. Withdrawal and odd, eccentric behaviors are characteristic of clients with paranoid, schizoid, and schizotypal personality disorder. Clients with avoidant, dependent or obsessive compulsive personality disorder are attempting to avoid or minimize anxiety or fear.

Clients with passive-aggressive or masochistic personality disorder are covertly aggressive against self or others.

PHYSIOLOGICAL INTEGRITY

Physiological Adaptation

Illness management

650. The nurse is caring for a client with ARDS. To reduce oxygen consumption in this client, the nurse should provide
 A. ample time for rest and relaxation
 B. 100% oxygen per nasal cannula
 C. increased daily caloric intake
 D. 21% oxygen per mask as needed

The answer is A. It is the only response that considers and reduces oxygen consumption.

PHYSIOLOGICAL INTEGRITY

Physiological Adaptation

Medical Emergencies

651. A suicidal client has ingested a large amount of an unknown poison. The client has no signs of injury to the mouth but is difficult to arouse. Which would be the appropriate intervention for this client?
 A. Administer syrup of ipecac immediately
 B. Initiate gastric lavage after assessment
 C. Give milk or water orally to dilute gastric content
 D. Call the poison control center for an antidote

The answer is B. Gastric lavage would be instituted to remove the poison. Gastric lavage would not be used if signs of injury from a corrosive poison are present because the lavage tube might perforate the burned esophagus. Syrup of ipecac should not be given to induce vomiting with a difficult to arouse client because of the risk of aspiration. Giving oral fluids also is contraindicated because of the risk of aspiration. Since the poison is unknown, calling the Poison control center for an antidote is not possible.

HEALTH PROMOTION AND MAINTENANCE

Developmental Stages and Transitions

Identify expected physical, cognitive, psychosocial, and moral stages of development

652. The nurse is observing a group of preschoolers in a day care. The nurse recognizes that the child who is showing signs of a developing conscience is the child who:
 A. tattles on a classmate.
 B. stays close to the teacher.
 C. ignores other children's toys.
 D. carries a security object with them at all times.

The answer is A. When a child is developing a sense of conscience, they often tattle because of their recognition of right and incorrect in others. None of the other behaviors are related to the development of conscience.

PHYSIOLOGICAL INTEGRITY

Physiological Adaptation

Illness Management

Apply knowledge of pathophysiology to illness management

653. A newborn was diagnosed with osteogenesis imperfecta. When handling the infant, the nurse would:
 A. wear gloves to prevent contamination.
 B. maintain the infant in semi-fowler's position.
 C. restrain the infant to prevent trauma to the bones.
 D. use the palms of the hands to handle the infant's extremities.

The answer is D. Children with osteogenesis imperfecta have fragile bones and must be handled by the palms of the hands. None of the other responses are appropriate for this child.

HEALTH PROMOTION AND MAINTENANCE

Growth and Development

654. Which of the following principles of growth and development is being addressed when the nurse explains to the parent that the infant will develop control of the head before control of the torso and legs?
 A. Cephalocaudal
 B. Proximodistal

C. Mass to specific
D. Simple to complex

The answer is A. Cephalocaudal means head to tail and refers to the fact that development occurs from the head downward. Normal development simultaneously occurs from midline to periphery which is proximodistal. Mass to specific refers to differentiation. Simple to complex refers to operations in which simple precedes complex ones and is similar to mass to specific.

PSYCHOSOCIAL INTEGRITY

Therapeutic Communications

655. A 78-year-old male in the late stages of Alzheimer's disease is in an extended care facility. He complains to the nurse that he is tired and his neck is sore from working in the field all day. Which of the following is the best response from the nurse?
    A. "You know you don't work in the field anymore"
    B. "What type of motion caused the soreness"
    C. "You're 78-years-old, You've been here all day with me, you haven't worked in the field in years"
    D. "Would you like me to rub your neck and apply a warm compress?"

The answer is D. Validating the client's reality is the most appropriate intervention for later stages of Alzheimer's disease. He is not a candidate for reality orientation. The nurse is responding to what she can help with, his sore neck. The other answers are confrontational and close off communication.

PHYSIOLOGICAL INTEGRITY

Reduction of Risk Potential

Potential for complications from surgical procedures and health alterations

656. A client is transported to the emergency department following multiple traumatic fractures from a motor vehicle accident. Which assessment findings would be a priority for the nurse to report to the physician 6 hours after a spica body cast has been applied?
    A. Pedal pulses are equal but weak.
    B. The lower extremities are cool to touch.
    C. The client is complaining of itch under the cast.
    D. The client complains of pain with respirations

The answer is D. Pain with respirations could mean restricted lung expansion and compartment syndrome. This is the priority because it involves airway and oxygenation.

PHYSIOLOGICAL INTEGRITY

Basic Care and Comfort

Palliative/comfort care

657. The client in the burn unit is complaining of severe pain in the first 24 hours following the burn injury. Which of the following is the usual method of dealing with pain during this period?
    A. Liquid narcotics are given via the NG (nasogastric) tube as needed.
    B. Narcotics are administered via the intramuscular route into non-burned tissue.
    C. Intravenous narcotic agents are administered for pain as needed.
    D. No medications are given during this period because of respiratory depression.

The answer is C. The client will have IV access as a component of the resuscitation process. Intravenous administration allows for quick results of the narcotic. Narcotics administered through the NG or IM route would be slower in providing relief. Although respiratory depression would be monitored, narcotic pain relief would still be given.

PHYSIOLOGICAL INTEGRITY

Physiological Adaptation

Medical Emergencies

658. A client is seen in the emergency room following an industrial accident involving chemical burns. The nurse recognizes that the severity of a chemical burn depends on which factors?
    A. The mechanisms of action.
    B. Penetrating strength and concentration.
    C. The amount and duration of exposure.
    D. The age of the client
    E. The occupation of the client

The answers are A, B, C, and D. Factors related to the chemical itself, type of chemical, concentration, amount and duration of exposure, all affect the severity of the burn. The age of the skin affects how easily it is injured as well as healing ability. Age affects general condition of client. The occupation will have no effect.

PSYCHOSOCIAL INTEGRITY

Psychopathology

Recognize signs and symptoms of acute and chronic mental illness

659. When assessing a client newly admitted with a diagnosis of active phase schizophrenia, which are positive

symptoms at least one of which the nurse would expect to find?
Mark all that apply.
A. ___ disorganized speech
B. ___ flat affect
C. ___ delusion
D. ___ impaired attention
E. ___ bizarre behavior
F. ___ hallucination

The answers are A, C, E, and F. The positive signs of active phase schizophrenia are delusion, hallucination, disorganized speech, and bizarre or disorganized behavior. At least one of these positive signs must be present for at least one month for a diagnosis of active phase schizophrenia to be made. Flat affect and impaired attention are negative symptoms of schizophrenia.

PHYSIOLOGICAL INTEGRITY

Reduction of Risk Potential

Potential for complications from surgical procedures and health alterations

660. A client with burns on the face and neck is at risk for airway obstruction. Which of the following would be most indicative of a potential airway obstruction?
A. Singed nasal hairs
B. Neck and face pain
C. PaO_2 of 80 mm Hg
D. Coughing up large amounts of thick, white sputum

The answer is A. Singed nasal hairs indicate the client breathed in hot gases. This can lead to edema of the oral mucus membranes. Pain in these areas does not indicate airway problems. PaO_x of 80 is low normal. Thick white sputum would not indicate airway burns.

PHYSIOLOGICAL INTEGRITY

Physiological Adaptation

Pathophysiology

661. A client with a suspected pulmonary embolus is admitted to a medical unit from the emergency department. The client complains of shortness of breath and severe chest pain. Which other signs and symptoms would support the diagnosis of pulmonary embolism?
A. Low grade fever
B. Productive white sputum
C. 2 degree AV block
D. Frothy sputum
E. Tachycardia
F. Blood-tinged sputum

The answers are A, E, and F. Chest pain and dyspnea are cardinal signs and symptoms of pulmonary embolism. Clients may also have a low grade fever, tachycardia which is a compensatory mechanism for decreased oxygen supply, and blood tinged sputum. Productive white sputum is not suggestive of pulmonary embolism. Frothy sputum would indicate pulmonary edema.

PHYSIOLOGICAL INTEGRITY

Basic Care and Comfort

Nutrition and oral hydration

662. An older gentleman reports that he has needed to use more salt than usual to make his food taste good. He asks the nurse what this could mean. The nurse's response should be based on the knowledge that
A. the number of taste buds decreases with age.
B. older persons need more sodium to ensure good kidney function.
C. increased sodium is needed to compensate for lost fluids.
D. the client may be confused due to his advancing age.

The answer is A. The taste buds begin to atrophy at age 40 and after age 60 there is an insensitivity to taste qualities. There are also studies that indicate that there are changes in the salt threshold in some elderly individuals. The other options are incorrect.

HEALTH PROMOTION AND MAINTENANCE

Developmental Stages and Transitions

Identify common developmental patterns of a pediatric client

663. When observing a two year old in the hospital playroom, which type of play would the nurse interpret as representative of normal development?
A. Solitary
B. Parallel
C. Associative
D. Dramatic

The answer is B. Solitary play is seen in the infant, associative play is seen in a preschooler. A school age child may demonstrate dramatic play.

PHYSIOLOGICAL INTEGRITY

Physiological Adaptation

Medical emergencies

664. The client is admitted to the emergency room with massive bleeding and a gunshot wound to the chest in severe respiratory distress. Which nursing action has the highest priority when managing the emergency?
   A. Establish and maintain an open airway
   B. Start cardiopulmonary resuscitation
   C. Initiate oxygen therapy via nasal cannula
   D. Apply pressure to wound to control bleeding

The answer is A. Establish airway is the correct response. Without a patent airway, all other measures are not critical. CPR is not appropriate since the client is not pulseless. Oxygen therapy via nasal cannula is not appropriate for severe respiratory distress. Applying pressure to the wound to control bleeding is critical but does not take priority over establishing and maintaining an airway.

PHYSIOLOGICAL INTEGRITY

Pharmacological and Parenteral Therapies

Medication Administration

665. A client is being discharged home on anticoagulant therapy. Which instructions should the nurse include as part of discharge teaching? (Select all that apply.)
   A. ___ Avoid use of aspirin containing drugs while receiving Coumadin.
   B. ___ Do not keep fresh flowers in the home.
   C. ___ Report dark, tarry stools to primary health care provider.
   D. ___ Avoid brushing teeth to prevent bleeding gums.
   E. ___ Avoid inactivity for prolonged periods of sitting with legs crossed.
   F. ___ Change positions frequently while traveling; walk occasionally; exercise legs and ankles.
   G. ___ Continue anticoagulants for length of time ordered.

The answers are A, C, and G. Aspirin has an anticoagulant effect and as a result enhances the effect of Coumadin. Therefore it is contraindicated for clients taking Coumadin. Dark tarry stools need to be reported because bleeding is an adverse effect of anticoagulation and bleeding in the upper GI tract can present as dark, tarry stools as a result of the presence of blood which has been exposed to digestive secretions. It is important that clients for whom anticoagulants are prescribed follow the directions for taking the medications precisely; this includes taking the medication for the length of time ordered. Fresh flowers are not contraindicated for clients on Coumadin; they are contraindicated for clients who are immunocompromised. Brushing the teeth should be done regularly, not avoided. However, a soft bristled toothbrush should be used. Moving and avoiding inactivity are instructions that would be given to clients at risk for venous thrombosis.

PHYSIOLOGICAL INTEGRITY

Reduction of Risk Potential

Laboratory values

666. A client suffered deep partial-thickness and full-thickness burns over 40% of his body approximately 12 hours ago. Urine output is 22 ml/hour and the hematocrit is 50%. ABG values show pH, 7.32; paO_2, 95 mm Hg; $PaCo_2$, 35 mm Hg; and HCO_3-, 18 mEq/L. Based on this data, which conclusion can the nurse draw about the client's status?
   The client
   A. is hypovolemic from fluid shift and has metabolic acidosis.
   B. is in the early stages of heart failure caused by over hydration.
   C. is adequately hydrated, but in acute renal failure and respiratory acidosis
   D. has developed a polycythemia as the body attempts to compensate for metabolic acidosis and renal failure.

The answer is A. During the first 24 hours after a burn injury, fluid is lost from the intravascular space into the tissues causing hemoconcentration and diminished urine output.

There is no indication of over hydration. The client does not show symptoms of respiratory alkalosis. The condition is hemoconcentration not polycythemia.

PSYCHOSOCIAL INTEGRITY

Chemical and Other Dependencies

Assess client for drug/alcohol related dependencies, withdrawal, or toxicities

667. When examining a neonate on admission to the newborn nursery, which assessment findings would the nurse interpret as consistent with fetal alcohol syndrome? Mark all that apply.
   A. ___ Elongated palpebral fissures
   B. ___ Strawberry hemangioma
   C. ___ Thick upper lip
   D. ___ Cleft palate
   E. ___ Congenital hip dislocation

The answers are B, D, and E. Malformations associated with fetal alcohol syndrome which would be evident in the neonate include strawberry hemangioma, low set posteriorly rotated ears, cleft lip/cleft palate, pointy chin, thin upper lip, short palpebral fissures, microcephaly, joint dysfunction including congenital hip dislocation, abnormal palmar creases, thoracic cage abnormalities, atrial and ventricular septal defects.

PHYSIOLOGICAL INTEGRITY

Reduction of Risk Potential

Potential for alterations in body systems

668. The client is admitted to the emergency room for acetaminophen overdose. The nurse should prepare to
   A. place an intravenous catheter and administer 1000cc D5W intravenously.
   B. induce gastric emptying by inserting a nasogastric tube for lavage.
   C. give syrup of ipecac and follow with activated charcoal.
   D. insert a Foley catheter and start diuresis immediately.

The answer is C. Removal of the poison by inducing vomiting followed by preventing absorption is standard treatment for a non-caustic poisoning. Gavage would be unnecessary as a way to remove the poison. The other two options have nothing to do with poison removal.

HEALTH PROMOTION AND MAINTENANCE

Techniques of Physical Assessment

Choose physical assessment equipment and technique appropriate for the client

669. When examining a 3-year-old, which part of the health assessment should be done first?
   A. Abdominal palpation
   B. Otoscopic examination
   C. Oral examination
   D. Chest auscultation

The answer is D. Chest auscultation is the least intrusive part of the physical examination and should be done first to provide time for the child to adjust somewhat to being examined and to delay upsetting the child.

PHYSIOLOGICAL INTEGRITY

Physiological Adaptation

Pathophysiology

670. An 18-year-old client is brought to the emergency room for a hornet sting. Which symptoms suggest that the client is having an anaphylactic reaction?
   A. rhinorrhea
   B. wheezing
   C. local edema
   D. urticaria
   E. angioedema
   F. generalized pruritus

The answers are A, B, D, E, and F. Signs of anaphylaxis which is a hypersensitivity reaction, typically begin with feelings of apprehension and impending doom. Generalized pruritus, urticaria, and sometimes swelling of the eyes, lips, and tongue (angioedema) follow. Respiratory congestion, rhinorrhea, wheezing and dyspnea occur as a result of bronchoconstriction, mucosal edema and production of excess mucus. Laryngeal edema is associated with hoarseness and stridor. Full blown shock may ensue.

PSYCHOSOCIAL INTEGRITY

Therapeutic Environment

671. A new mother of a 1-month-old infant is concerned that she is spoiling the baby "because she carries her around the house in an infant sling against her chest." The nurse's best response would be:
   A. "You should not carry her in the sling except when you are going out and need to take her."
   B. "She should spend at least half of her waking time on a firm surface by herself."
   C. "Spoiling an infant is difficult; cuddling and holding are essential for normal development."
   D. "Carrying an infant in a sling is not advised because of potential problems with development of the spine."

The answer is C. Cuddling and holding along with meeting other basic needs builds trust and is essential for normal growth and development. The child can be carried in the infant sling at home as well as when the mother goes out. There is no set time the infant should be alone and on a flat surface. Use of a sling has not been shown to cause problems with the spine.

PHYSIOLOGICAL INTEGRITY

Reduction of Risk Potential

Potential for Complications of Diagnostic Tests/Treatments/Procedures

Provide nursing care in a safe and effective manner

672. The nurse would question an order for a mydriatic medication to be administered to a client with which disorder?
   A. Narrow angle glaucoma
   B. Drug overdose

C. Blunt force head injury

D. Suspected spinal cord injury

The answer is A. A mydriatic medication dilates the pupils. Pupil dilation is contraindicated with narrow angle glaucoma so an order for a mydriatic would be questioned because of its ability to cause harm. Pupil dilation does not have the potential for injury in relationship to the other disorders.

HEALTH PROMOTION AND MAINTENANCE

Expected Body Image Changes

673. During the routine well check up of an 18 month old, the mother asks the nurse about her son's protruding abdomen. Which fact should form the basis of the nurse's response?
   A. The abdomen protrudes as a result of increased food intake at this age
   B. Underdeveloped abdominal muscles are the reason for the protruding abdomen.
   C. A protruding abdomen indicates a possible abnormal curvature of the spine.
   D. A protruding abdomen is uncommon in toddlers and requires further assessment.

The answer is B. Undeveloped abdominal musculature gives the toddler the characteristic protruding abdomen.

A is incorrect because during toddlerhood food intake decreases. C is incorrect because, although it's normal, it doesn't provide the answer to the mother's question. D is incorrect as protruding abdomen is common in toddlers.

PHYSIOLOGICAL INTEGRITY

Reduction of Risk Potential

Potential for alterations in body systems

674. The client with which problem would be at greatest risk for developing a pulmonary artery thrombosis?
   A. Fluid volume overload
   B. Ventricular fibrillation
   C. Increased cardiac output
   D. Polycythemia

The answer is D. Polycythemia predisposes to stasis of blood as a result of increased viscosity secondary to the increased numbers of red blood cells. None of the other problems predispose to thrombosis.

PHYSIOLOGICAL INTEGRITY

Reduction of Risk Potential

Potential for Complications of Diagnostic Tests/Treatments/Procedures

675. A client presents to the emergency department with a foreign object in the eye. Which action should the nurse take?
   A. Remove the object after an x-ray is taken.
   B. Remove the object after notifying the ophthalmologist.
   C. Leave the object untouched while awaiting the ophthalmologist..
   D. Flush the eye with saline to dislodge the object.

The answer is C. The nurse would make no attempt to remove the foreign body until the client has been examined by an ophthalmologist.

HEALTH PROMOTION AND MAINTENANCE

Techniques of Physical Assessment

Choose physical assessment equipment and technique appropriate for the client

676. The nurse is admitting a 2-year-old child to the hospital unit for a minor surgical procedure. When examining the child, which approach is most appropriate?
   A. Have the parent wait in the next room
   B. Have the toddler sit on the parent's lap
   C. Allow the child to remain clothed.
   D. Keep equipment to be used out of sight

The answer is B. The child will be more cooperative if his or her parent holds the toddler on lap for the exam. Separating the child from the parent will most likely increase the child's distress and there is no reason to do so. It is not possible to perform an effective physical examination with clothing in place. The child should not only see but be allowed to handle equipment to decrease fear and anxiety.

PSYCHOSOCIAL INTEGRITY

Psychopathology

Recognize signs of acute and chronic mental illness

677. The nurse would expect to encounter clients who are covertly aggressive against self or others when working with a group diagnosed with which types of personality disorder?

A. Paranoid, schizoid, schizotypal
B. Antisocial, borderline, histrionic, narcissistic
C. Avoidant, dependent, obsessive-compulsive
D. Passive-aggressive, masochistic

The answer is D. Clients with passive-aggressive or masochistic personality disorder are covertly aggressive against self or others. Withdrawal and odd, eccentric behaviors are characteristic of clients with paranoid, schizoid, and schizotypal personality disorder. Attention seeking and erratic behaviors are characteristic of clients with antisocial, borderline, histrionic and narcissistic personality disorders. Clients with avoidant, dependent or obsessive compulsive personality disorder are attempting to avoid or minimize anxiety or fear.

PHYSIOLOGICAL INTEGRITY

Pharmacological and Parenteral Therapies

Adverse effects/contraindications

678. Which statement made by a client taking methotrexate for rheumatoid arthritis indicates that information regarding side effects of the medication was understood?
   A. "It's too bad medications have to have side effects but I guess I can deal with headache and nausea."
   B. "I don't know how my husband will cope if I become confused and hallucinate from this medication."
   C. "I already have a heart murmur; I am afraid that this medication will make it worse and I will end up needing heart surgery."
   D. "I know this medication is very likely to cause kidney damage but the symptoms of the rheumatoid arthritis are so bad that I have to take it anyway."

The answer is A. Side effects of methotrexate include headache and nausea and this statement indicates the client understands that fact. Heart damage is one of several side effects of doxorubicin (Adriamycin). Hallucinations and confusion are side effects of ifsoamide (Ifex). Kidney damage is a side effect of carboplatin (Paraplatin).

PHYSIOLOGICAL INTEGRITY

Physiological Adaptation

Medical Emergencies

679. While being helped out of bed to a chair, a client who is two days postoperative from abdominal surgery starts to cough forcefully and the surgical wound eviscerates. What is the priority nursing intervention?
   A. Cover the wound with a moist sterile dressing
   B. Start intravenous fluids and antibiotics
   C. Apply an abdominal binder
   D. Notify the physician.

The answer is A. The wound should be covered with a moist sterile dressing. Moisture prevents the wound from drying out and becoming necrotic prior to surgery. Wound evisceration is a surgical emergency and while one nurse is with the client and covering the wound, a second should be notifying the surgeon. If a client is at known risk for evisceration, sterile dressing and sterile saline should be available in the client's room. Intravenous fluids and antibiotics will be part of the client's care but are not the immediate priority. Abdominal binders are not appropriate and could cause damage to wound.

HEALTH PROMOTION AND MAINTENANCE

Developmental Stages and Transitions

680. A toddler is hospitalized for medical treatment. When the mother leaves, the child screams and cries for his mother. He refuses to be comforted and will not eat while mother is not present. The nurse interprets the child's behavior as indicative of which stage of toddler hospitalization reaction?
   A. Protest
   B. Despair
   C. Detachment
   D. Regression

The answer is A. Protest is a stage of anger at the separation from the parent. Despair is mourning the loss of the parent. The child would no longer display anger but would be saddened by the loss. Detachment is a stage where the toddler appears to be the "good client"—appears happy with the parent present.

PHYSIOLOGICAL INTEGRITY

Physiological Adaptation

Alterations in body systems

681. The client is diagnosed with a life-threatening condition characterized by inadequate blood flow to the tissues and cells of the body to meet metabolic demands. Nursing care should focus on:
   A. restoring circulating volume
   B. maintaining adequate IV access

C. monitoring intake and output
D. weighing daily
E. observing for fluid overload

The answers are A and B. These activities are designed to restore circulation while observing for complications of nursing interventions.

Responses C, D and E are assessment tools to evaluate the success of the interventions.

PHYSIOLOGICAL INTEGRITY

Basic Care and Comfort

Rest and sleep

682. Which information should the nurse include when teaching the parent of an 8-year-old child about bedtime schedules?
   A. The child's need for sleep is greater now than in adolescence.
   B. Minimum requirement for optimal growth and development is 10 hours of sleep a night.
   C. The child is often unaware of his own fatigue level.
   D. Nightmares and night tremors are common in this age group.

The answer is C. School-age children are often unaware of their own fatigue level. If allowed to stay awake they will be tired the next day.

Because of slowed growth rate, during the school-age period less sleep, not more, is required than in adolescence. Eight-year-old children do not require a minimum of 10 hours of sleep. Nightmares and night terrors are common in the preschool period.

PHYSIOLOGICAL INTEGRITY

Pharmacological and Parenteral Therapies

Medication administration

683. A client is requiring resuscitation secondary to a respiratory arrest. During the code, epinephrine is ordered. The most effective route of administration would be:
   A. Intravenously
   B. Endotracheally
   C. Intradermally
   D. Subcutaneously

The answer is B. The quickest and most effective route would be via endotracheal tube.

The IV route is slower but effective. Subcutaneous or intradermal administration is inappropriate.

HEALTH PROMOTION AND MAINTENANCE

Developmental Stages and Transitions

684. The nurse is discussing readiness for toileting with a child's parents. Which factor would the nurse identify as a contraindication to beginning toilet training at this time?
   A. The toddler wakes up dry from a nap
   B. The toddler stays dry for up to 3 hours
   C. The toddler wants to have a soiled diaper changed promptly.
   D. The toddler has a toilet adjacent to his bedroom in the family's brand new home.

The answer is D. Moving is a stressful and toilet training should not be initiated during stressful period.

Choices A, B, and C are all signs of readiness for toilet training.

PHYSIOLOGICAL INTEGRITY

Physiological Adaptation

Alterations in body systems

685. A child is admitted to the emergency room with multiple blunt trauma to the chest, and crushing wounds to the abdomen, and legs. Which are the priority nursing assessments?
   A. Level of consciousness and pupil size
   B. Abdominal contusions and other wounds
   C. Pain, respiratory rate, and blood pressure
   D. Quality of respirations and presence of pulses

The answer is D. These are top priorities in trauma management; basic life functions must be maintained or reestablished. Level of consciousness and pupil size are part of the assessment for head injury. Assessment for head injury and assessment for abdominal injury and pain follow appraisal of airway, breathing, and circulation.

PHYSIOLOGICAL INTEGRITY

Pharmacological and Parenteral Therapies

Adverse effects/contraindications

686. Which instructions would the nurse give to a client starting on Pentoxifylline (Trental)? Mark all that apply.
   A. ___ Take on an empty stomach
   B. ___ Report any unusual bleeding or bruising

C. ___ There may be toxic drug effects if taken with Theophylline

D. ___ Drug reduces red blood cell aggregation

The answers are B, C, and D. Pentoxifylline (Trental) should be taken with food to decrease GI symptoms. Information in all other answers should be included in client teaching regarding self administration of Pentoxifylline (Trental).

SAFE AND EFFECTIVE CARE ENVIRONMENTS

Safety and Infection Control

Standard/Transmission-Based/Other Precautions

Apply principles of infection control

687. Which precaution measures would be instituted when a client has tuberculosis? (Mark all that apply.)

A. ___ Client is placed in a private, negative airflow pressure room.

B. ___ Client is placed in a private room or with other clients with infection caused by the same organism.

C. ___ Use mask at all times while in the client's room.

D. ___ Use mask when working within 3 feet of the client.

E. ___ Use gown and protective barriers when giving direct care.

F. ___ Mask on client if transported out of room.

G. ___ Use gloves at all times when caring for clients.

H. ___ Use gloves when there is risk of exposure to blood or body fluids.

The answers are A, C, F, and H. Tuberculosis is spread in small particle droplets by airborne transmission. Airborne precautions require a private room with negative airflow and adequate filtration; those entering the room wear a mask and if the client leaves the room, a mask is worn. Standard precautions, which involve wearing gloves whenever there is the risk of touching something wet that comes from the body surface or a body cavity, i.e., when there is the risk of contact with blood or body fluids, are used at all times for all clients.

PHYSIOLOGICAL INTEGRITY

Physiological Adaptation

Alteration in body systems

688. A client is admitted to the emergency room with a diagnosis of acute respiratory distress syndrome. Which assessment findings would the nurse expect?

A. A systolic blood pressure greater than 170

B. Tenacious thick greenish yellow sputum

C. An altered level of consciousness

D. Slow abdominal breathing

The answer is C. Cognition and level of consciousness are reduced secondary to cerebral hypoxia which accompanies ARDS. Blood pressure may be reduced. Sputum is not tenacious, but may be frothy if pulmonary edema is present. Breathing will be rapid and shallow not slow and abdominal.

HEALTH PROMOTION AND MAINTENANCE

Growth and Development

689. After administering an IM injection to 3-year-old child the nurse puts an adhesive bandage on the site. The reason for applying the bandage is based on the fact that:

A. the child will "pick" at the injection site.

B. the bandage will relieve pain at the site.

C. the preschool child is afraid his "insides will fall out" and the bandage prevents "insides from leaking."

D. the bandage will remind the nurses that the child has received an injection recently.

The answer is C. Preschoolers want a bandage on any scrape or bruise to prevent their insides from leaking out. Most children will not pick at the site, bandages do not relieve pain, and nurses should not need a reminder that a child has received an injection.

PHYSIOLOGICAL INTEGRITY

Physiological Adaptation

Illness management

690. Which type of delivery system would the nurse use when administering oxygen to a client who has experienced a cardiac arrest?

A. A nasal cannula at 1 liter per minute.

B. A 100% non-rebreather mask.

C. A 28% venti-mask

D. A face mask at 4 liters per minute

The answer is B. A non-rebreather mask provides the highest concentration of oxygen available. All other choices would provide insufficient oxygen. With a simple face mask, the flow rate must be at least 5 liters per minute to flush the mask of carbon dioxide.

PSYCHOSOCIAL INTEGRITY

Family Dynamics

Assist client/family/significant others to integrate new members into family structure

691. A very young teenager has just given birth to a healthy infant. The nurse is concerned about bonding. To promote bonding, the nurse would:
   A. Encourage early parent–infant interaction and close body contact.
   B. Allow mother infant interaction only when a nurse can be present.
   C. Require the new mother to breastfeed the infant.
   D. Tell the new mother how bright and alert her baby is.

The answer is A. Studies have shown that immediately after birth is the best time for maternal infant bonding.

B, C, and D are incorrect because maternal-child contact would not be limited; the mother has the right to choose to breast feed or not; telling the mother her baby is bright and alert does not promote bonding.

PHYSIOLOGICAL INTEGRITY

Physiological Adaptation

Pathophysiology

692. A client with disseminated intravascular coagulation has a severe reaction to a unit of packed cells and develops a humoral immunity. The nurse knows that humoral immunity:
   A. Is produced by T-cell activity
   B. Involves immunoglobulins
   C. Occurs only in anaphylactic reactions
   D. Involves the thymus

The answer is B. Humoral immunity is mediated by B lymphocytes and is involved in an anaphylactic reaction. A is incorrect as it is B cell activity. Humoral immunity can also involve immunocomplex hypersensitivities. The thymus is not involved.

PHYSIOLOGICAL INTEGRITY

Physiological Adaptation

Pathophysiology

693. Which symptoms occurring in a 4-week-old male infant are consistent with a diagnosis of pyloric stenosis?
   A. Metabolic alkalosis
   B. Uninterested in feeding
   C. Vomiting bile stained fluid.
   D. 2 ounce weight loss over last 3 days.
   E. Peristalsis observed over the abdomen.

The answers are A, D, and E. A and D are related to the vomiting that occurs. Peristalsis may be visible on the abdomen as the stomach tries to push formula past the obstruction. The infant will be hungry, vomiting will not be bile stained.

PHYSIOLOGICAL INTEGRITY

Physiological Adaptation

Alterations in Body Systems

694. A client has been admitted to the hospital unit for stasis venous ulcers. Which nursing intervention would be included in the plan of care?
   A. Performing Burger-Allen Exercises
   B. Providing bedrest with legs in a dependent position
   C. Placing a foot board on the bed
   D. Placing the client in a high fowler's position

The answer is C. Use of a footboard keeps pressure off of the ulcer. Burger-Allen Exercises are done for Buerger's disease. Keeping legs in a dependent position increases edema. High Fowler's position increases pressure and kinking on the vascular system.

PSYCHOSOCIAL INTEGRITY

Sensory/Perceptual Alterations

Assess needs of clients with altered sensory perception

695. When planning care for a client with hallucinations, the nurse would consider that the client is most likely to harm self or others in which stage of the hallucinatory process?
   A. comforting
   B. condemning
   C. threatening
   D. controlling

The answer is D. Controlling. There are four stages in the hallucinatory process. In stage 1, the hallucination is familiar and comforting and anxiety level is mild. In stage 2, the hallucination is condemning; it is accusing and makes the person feel guilty and isolated. In stage 3, the hallucination is threatening and begins to rule all different aspects of behavior. In the fourth or controlling stage, anxiety has increased to the panic level and the individual is unable to control behavior. It is in this stage that the risk of harm to self or others is greatest.

PHYSIOLOGICAL INTEGRITY

Physiological Adaptation

Pathophysiology

696. A maternity client is seen for her regular checkup at 20 weeks gestation. On assessment, the nurse notes that the uterus is at the level of the xiphoid process. The nurse would suspect:
   A. Oligohydramnios
   B. Multiple Gestation
   C. Intrauterine growth retardation
   D. Fetal demise

The answer is B. At 20 weeks gestation, the fundus should be at the level of the umbilicus. This finding indicates the fundus is above the expected location. The only response that would cause the fundus to be higher than normal is B. All other conditions would lead to a fundus below the expected level.

HEALTH PROMOTION AND MAINTENANCE

Developmental Stages and Transitions

697. The parent of a 3-year-old child tells the nurse that she is worried because the child has irrational fears. "My child is afraid to go to bed, afraid of the neighbor's gentle Golden Retriever, every day there's a new fear" Which of the following is the best response from the nurse?
   A. "Preschool children have the most fears; try a night light to help going to bed and know that being afraid of large dogs is very common in this age group."
   B. "Your child should be growing out of these irrational fears by now, let's get her involved in some play and see what seems to be going on."
   C. "Don't make too much of it; just be patient; this phase will pass soon"
   D. "Going to bed is often a problem, let her fall asleep in your bed and then carry her back to her bed when she is sleeping"

The answer is A. The preschool years are the time when children have the most fears. Option A reassures the mother her child's behavior is normal and it gives the mother information that will help her deal with the child's fear.

PHYSIOLOGICAL INTEGRITY

Physiological Adaptation

Medical Emergencies

698. A 4-month-old infant puts a toy in their mouth and begins to choke. Which is the appropriate nursing action?
   A. Position infant head down and provide back blows.
   B. Elevate the infant's head and provide back blows.
   C. Position the fist below the navel, then using both fists perform four abdominal thrusts.
   D. Place one fist on the sternum and perform chest thrusts.

The answer is A. The infant is positioned head down and back blows are given. Back blows are used on the conscious infant. Trendelenburg position is used to assist with foreign body removal. The other responses are incorrect.

HEALTH PROMOTION AND MAINTENANCE

Developmental Stages and Transitions

699. Which suggestion could the school nurse make to the parents of a 10-year-old child who want to promote their child's psychosocial development?
   A. Encourage the child to start a collection of model cars, baseball cards, or other similar items.
   B. Meet the needs of the child in a consistent manner.
   C. Avoid disciplining the child during this difficult period.
   D. Reinforce that the child is a good person even if behavior is bad.

According to Erikson, the school age child's task is to develop industry vs. inferiority. A child's sense of industry is enhanced by building a collection. Being consistent helps meet the needs of the infant. Informing the child that he is a good person even if his behavior is bad is appropriate for a toddler. All children need discipline as they are uncomfortable when there are no rules.

PHYSIOLOGICAL INTEGRITY

Physiological Adaptation

Medical Emergencies

700. While providing nursing care, the client has a respiratory arrest. Which are the priority interventions for the resuscitation of this client?
   A. Intubating with an endotracheal tube
   B. Starting 100% oxygen
   C. Drawing serial arterial blood gases
   D. Checking the Glasgow coma scale
   E. Monitoring oxygen saturation level

The answers are A and B. Both of these actions would promote oxygenation.

C and D are assessment measures that would be done but they are not the priority. Response E is unrelated to a respiratory arrest.

PHYSIOLOGICAL INTEGRITY

Reduction of Risk Potential

Potential for complications from surgical procedures and health alterations

701. A client returns to the hospital unit following an appendectomy. Which finding on the postoperative admission assessment should be reported to the physician immediately?
   A. Oral temperature 99°F
   B. Pulse 98 and thready
   C. Complaints of nausea
   D. Absent bowel sounds

The answer is B. A pulse of 98 and thready is suggestive of hemorrhage. Oral temperature may be slightly elevated as a result of the procedure. Nausea is common in the post operative period. Absent bowel sounds are common in the immediate post operative period.

HEALTH PROMOTION AND MAINTENANCE

Aging Process

702. An 89-year-old man came to the clinic for his annual checkup. Which finding related to pulmonary function would the nurse expect?
   A. An increase in functional alveoli
   B. A reduction of residual volume
   C. A decrease in vital capacity
   D. Blood gases that show mild acidosis

The answer is C. A decrease in vital capacity because loss of elastic forces in the lung lead to an increase in residual volume, and a decrease in vital capacity.

PHYSIOLOGICAL INTEGRITY

Reduction of Risk Potential

Potential for complications of diagnostic tests/treatments/procedures

703. A client in the emergency department is intubated and connected to a mechanical ventilator. She becomes extremely anxious, and the pressure alarm sounds with each inspiration. Which is the priority nursing intervention?
   A. Increase the tidal volume
   B. Increase the oxygen concentration
   C. Disconnect the ventilator and manually ventilate the client using a ventilator bag for a few breaths.
   D. Administer the prescribed diazepam or morphine sulfate as needed.

The answer is C. This allows the nurse to assess for a mucus plug which would occlude the ET tube causing the increased pressure alarm. The other interventions would be inappropriate.

PHYSIOLOGICAL INTEGRITY

Physiological Adaptation

Hemodynamics

704. The nurse is teaching self care to a client who has been diagnosed with Raynaud's disease. Which instruction best meets the goal of maintaining optimal tissue perfusion?
   A. Inspect skin daily for breakdown
   B. Alleviate factors that increase pain
   C. Wear mittens when going out into the cold
   D. Elevate extremities when color changes occur due to vasoconstriction

The answer is C. Keeping the hand warm enhances vasodilation and tissue perfusion. Inspection of the skin is important to prevent complications but does not enhance vasodilation. Alleviating factors that increase pain promotes comfort and may help prevent further decreases in tissue perfusion but does not optimize it. Elevating extremities decreases circulation to the extremity.

PSYCHOSOCIAL INTEGRITY

Psychopathology

Recognize signs and symptoms of impaired cognition

705. The nurse says to a schizophrenic client "Swallow your pills, John." The client responds by saying "Swallow your pills John; swallow your pills John; swallow your pills John; swallow your pills John" Which would be a correct label for the nurse to use when documenting this communication?
   A. word salad
   B. clang association
   C. neologism
   D. echolalia

The answer is D. Echolalia. Echolalia is the repetition of words or phrases heard from another person. Word salad refers to the meaningless connection of words and phrases.

Clang association refers to repeating words and phrases which sound alike but are otherwise unconnected. A neologism is a new word coined by the client and with meaning only to the client.

PHYSIOLOGICAL INTEGRITY

Reduction of Risk Potential

Potential for complications from surgical procedures and health alterations

706. A teenager has been admitted to the hospital unit with a diagnosis of appendicitis. While awaiting the start of surgery, it becomes apparent that the appendix has ruptured. At this time, in what position will the nurse maintain the client?
   A. Prone
   B. High Fowlers
   C. Left side-lying
   D. Trendelenburg

The answer is B. High Fowlers position utilizes gravity to collect the infectious material in one area of the abdomen reducing the extent of peritonitis. The other responses would not be correct.

PHYSIOLOGICAL INTEGRITY

Physiological Adaptation

Pathophysiology

707. A client is admitted to the emergency room with a blood pressure of 72/42 mm HG and a diagnosis of septic shock. Which assessment finding would best confirm this diagnosis?
   A. Hot, dry skin with poor skin turgor
   B. ABG analysis revealing metabolic alkalosis
   C. Temperature of 105°F (40.6°C) and a pulse rate of 122 beats/minute
   D. Urine output of 30 ml/hour and central venous pressure of 8 cmH_2O

The answer is C. Septic shock is related to the presence of endotoxins or exotoxins released from bacteria. Symptoms include fever, tachycardia, increased respiratory rate and shock and coma. The other responses are not related to septic shock.

HEALTH PROMOTION AND MAINTENANCE

Developmental Stages and Transitions

Identify expected physical, cognitive, psychosocial, and moral stages of development

708. When planning care for a 4-year-old, the nurse considers the fact that the child does not yet comprehend which concepts?
   A. Alternative points of view
   B. Conservation
   C. Reversibility
   D. Object permanence

The answers are A, B, and C. A 4-year-old child is egocentric and doesn't understand another's view yet. Conservation, which is permanence of mass and volume, is not comprehended nor is the concept of reversibility i.e. if 2 + 3 = 5, then 5 − 3 = 2. Object permanence is mastered and understood in toddlerhood.

PHYSIOLOGICAL INTEGRITY

Physiological Adaptation

Hemodynamics

709. A client is experiencing septic shock and the attending physician wants to titrate medications to be regulated so that a mean arterial pressure (MAP) between 75 and 85 mmHg is maintained. When evaluating the response of the drug, which of the blood pressure readings meet the goal?
   A. 135/90
   B. 125/80
   C. 115/70
   D. 110/60

The answer is C. The formula for mean arterial pressure (MAP) is SBP +2 DBP divided by 3. The blood pressure with mean arterial pressure between 75 and 85 is 115/70 (MAP), (115 + 70 + 70 = 255/3 = 85) is 85.
A, B, and C are incorrect.

PHYSIOLOGICAL INTEGRITY

Physiological Adaptation

Illness management

710. A 24-year-old post partum client is transferred to the ICU after developing disseminated intravascular coagulation (DIC). The nurse develops a care plan in collaboration with the physician knowing that the care of a client with a bleeding(clotting disorder usually includes:
   A. Monitoring core body temperature
   B. Initiating heparin therapy
   C. Administering blood
   D. Restricting dairy products in the diet

The answer is B. Heparin is given because the abnormal clotting that occurs with DIC uses up available clotting factor. Heparin inhibits clotting and therefore allows clotting factor to be replenished. Monitoring core body temperature is not a priority with DIC. Blood is not administered because the problem is clotting, not bleeding. Dairy products are unrelated to DIC.

HEALTH PROMOTION AND MAINTENANCE

Aging Process

711. Which finding when reviewing the record of an elderly client would the nurse interpret as a normal occurrence with aging?
   A. Very concentrated urine
   B. Microscopic hematuria
   C. Occasional urinary incontinence
   D. Decreased glomerular filtration rate

The answer is D. Changes in the renal tubules cause a dramatic decrease in the glomerular filtration rate. Hematuria, either microscopic or gross, is always abnormal. Incontinence is also abnormal.

PHYSIOLOGICAL INTEGRITY

Physiological Adaptation

Illness management

712. After diagnosis of diverticulitis, a client has been taught about the appropriate dietary changes. Which statements by the client indicate that teaching was successful?
   A. "I will eat a low-fiber diet."
   B. "Milk will increase my episodes of diverticulitis."
   C. "Whole grains are better for me than refined grains."
   D. "Starches, fruits and vegetables will increase my flatus and diarrhea."

The answers are B and C. A diet to prevent constipation is recommended. Milk can be constipating so it can contribute to increase episodes of diverticulitis. Whole grains are better than refined grains because they provide more fiber. Option A is incorrect because a high fiber not a low fiber diet is needed to prevent constipation. Starches, fruits and vegetables are good sources of fiber so they decrease not increase symptoms.

PHYSIOLOGICAL INTEGRITY

Reduction of Risk Potential

Potential for Complications of Diagnostic Tests/Treatments/Procedures

713. A 20-year-old male suffered a broken jaw in an automobile accident. The jaw has been wired shut. The nurse will ensure that which of the following equipment will be available at the client's bedside for safety?
   A. Call light
   B. Wire cutters
   C. Clear liquids
   D. Paper and pencil

The answer is B. If the client should vomit, he could choke and aspirate. Wire cutters would need to be immediately available. The call light is appropriate for all clients. Clear liquids would not be a safety feature. Paper and pencil may aid communication but are not emergency supplies.

PSYCHOSOCIAL INTEGRITY

Chemical and Other Dependencies

Provide symptom management for clients experiencing withdrawal or toxicity

714. When planning care for a client withdrawing from cocaine, which is a critical nursing intervention?
   A. Monitor for seizures
   B. Protect from self harm
   C. Orient to time and place
   D. Monitor for hypotension

The answer is D. Protect from self harm. The client withdrawing from cocaine or another central nervous stimulant experiences severe dysphoria, anxiety, disturbed sleep and is at significant risk for suicide. Hence a priority nursing intervention is to prevent self harm. Seizures and confusion can occur with withdrawal from alcohol, sedatives/hypnotics, and anxiolytic drugs. Hypertension, not hypotension is a risk with cocaine withdrawal.

PHYSIOLOGICAL INTEGRITY

Physiological Adaptation

Medical emergencies

715. A client is brought into the emergency department complaining of severe back pain. He is diaphoretic, pale, tachycardic, and has absent pedal pulses. Which is the immediate nursing intervention?
   A. Start an IV with a 16 gauge catheter
   B. Get a stat back x-ray
   C. Prepare the client for insertion of hemodynamic monitoring
   D. Get a 12 lead ECG

The answer is A. The client is showing signs of shock and needs immediate vascular access. The other interventions could be done later.

PHYSIOLOGICAL INTEGRITY

Reduction of Risk Potential

Potential for complications from surgical procedures and health alterations

716. A 2-week-old infant has returned from surgery for repair of a unilateral cleft lip. The nurse instructs the mother to comfort the baby when the baby becomes upset and starts to cry. The mother asks why it is important that the baby not cry. The nurse's response would be based on the knowledge that crying:
   A. puts strain on the suture line.
   B. may prevent the infant from developing trust.
   C. causes the infant to swallow air and may cause vomiting.
   D. simulates coughing in the post operative infant.

The answer is A. A crying infant will open the mouth wide putting strain on the sutures in the upper lip. Although meeting the infant's needs in a timely fashion is important in the development of trust, it is not the correct response in this situation. Crying does cause the infant to swallow air, but that is not the primary reason for comforting the child. Crying stimulates coughing but is not appropriate for this child.

PSYCHOSOCIAL INTEGRITY

Coping Mechanisms

717. A 15-year-old boy was admitted to the pediatric unit following an injury to his leg. When told that the complicated fracture would require surgical repair and prevent a return to the football team for an unknown extended period of time, the boy throws an apple from the lunch tray at the nurse. Which type of coping behavior is the teenager exhibiting?
   A. Reaction formation
   B. Projection
   C. Denial
   D. Displacement

The answer is D. Displacement is shifting focus from an undesired object or feeling to a more acceptable object or feeling. Reaction formation is acting opposite to how one feels. Projection occurs when one attributes ones own unacceptable feelings to another. In denial one ignores unacceptable realities.

PHYSIOLOGICAL INTEGRITY

Reduction of Risk Potential

Diagnostic tests

718. A client is suspected of having osteoporosis. Which test will provide the best information regarding this problem?
   A. Serum calcium
   B. X-ray of pelvis
   C. CT scan of spine
   D. DEXA scan

The answer is D. Dual energy x-ray absorptiometry (DEXA) measures bone mineral density. It allows detection of early osteoporotic changes in the wrist, spine and/or hip. It is the best diagnostic tool available for osteoporosis. There are no laboratory tests that definitively diagnose primary osteoporosis. Serum calcium is one of a battery of laboratory tests used to rule out secondary osteoporosis or other metabolic disease. X-rays and CT scans do not provide an accurate picture of the mineral content in bone that denotes bone density and do not detect early bone changes.

HEALTH PROMOTION AND MAINTENANCE

Aging Process

719. Which assessment finding on a 78-year-old woman most likely reflects age-related decreased blood vessel elasticity and increased peripheral resistance?
   A. An irregular peripheral pulse
   B. An increase in blood pressure
   C. Night time confusion
   D. Wide QRS complexes on the ECG

The answer is B. Thickening of the blood vessels and less distensible arteries and veins cause impeded blood flow and increased vascular resistance, leading to hypertension.

PHYSIOLOGICAL INTEGRITY

Pharmacological and Parenteral Therapies

Medication administration

720. The nurse is pushing IV medications during a "code blue." Which is a critical step in the procedure?
   A. Check the orders with the chart
   B. Inspect the IV site for infiltration
   C. Evaluate the peripheral pulses
   D. Flush the line with dextrose between drugs

The answer is B. Inspecting the IV site for infiltration is critical because medication will not be effective if administered into the tissue rather than the blood stream. Orders are usually verbal during a code situation. Pulses are generally absent if in a code blue situation. Lines should be flushed with sodium chloride.

PSYCHOSOCIAL INTEGRITY

Therapeutic Communications

Develop and maintain therapeutic relationships with client/family/significant others

721. Which is an appropriate guideline for the nurse to utilize when communicating with an adolescent?
   A. Reassure that what he or she is going through is understood.
   B. Invite the parents to be present when talking with the adolescent.
   C. Ask meaning of expressions if not clearly understood as a result of teen culture.
   D. Share with the parents information received in their absence.

The answer is C. Understanding the meaning of the adolescent's expression will aid in understanding the communication and display interest in the adolescent's point of view.

A is incorrect as this statement will discourage further comments. B is incorrect as the adolescent may not be willing to talk in front of his parents. The child will feel betrayed if the nurse reports the conversation to the parents.

PHYSIOLOGICAL INTEGRITY

Reduction of Risk Potential

Laboratory values

722. A child is admitted to the hospital unit with a diagnosis of pyloric stenosis, On admission, the nurse would expect to see which electrolyte imbalance?
   A. Hypokalemia
   B. Hypernatremia
   C. Hyperchloremia
   D. Hypomagnesemia

The answer is A. Potassium is lost by vomiting. All other responses are incorrect.

PHYSIOLOGICAL INTEGRITY

Pharmacological and Parenteral Therapies

Expected effects/outcomes

723. A client is being treated for Gastroesophageal Reflux Disease (GERD). When the nurse administers famotidine (Pepcid) to the client, the client asks how this medication will help. The nurse's reply will be based on the knowledge that the medication will:
   A. Decrease gastric acidity reducing irritation to the esophagus.
   B. Relax the lower esophageal sphincter (LES) preventing further reflux.
   C. Increase intraabdominal pressure to maintain positive pressure in the esophagus.
   D. Decrease the intra-gastric pressure putting less strain on the lower esophageal sphincter (LES).

The answer is A. Symptoms of the disease are due to the regurgitation of stomach acids into the esophagus. By reducing the acidity of stomach contents, symptoms will be reduced.

The other responses are incorrect. The activity described in B and C would increase the symptoms.

HEALTH PROMOTION AND MAINTENANCE

Disease Prevention

724. Working on a geriatric unit, the nurse knows that the bed bound hospitalized older adult is at risk for pressure ulcers. Which factors seen in the unit's clients would increase the risk for pressure ulcers?
   A. Diminished sensory perception
   B. Dry fragile skin
   C. Decreased mobility
   D. Indwelling urinary catheter
   E. Decreased appetite since hospitalization
   F. Nursing assessment every shift

The answers are A, B, C, and E. Dry fragile skin increases the risk for skin breakdown. Diminished sensory perception diminishes the amount of normal shifting and movement, not allowing for the relief of pressure, increasing the risk for skin breakdown. This is true with decreased mobility as well. Incontinence, not an indwelling catheter would increase the risk of pressure ulcers. Nursing assessment and interventions including a turning and positioning schedule, bed bath and massage, ROM exercises, and providing appetizing nutritious foods with adequate protein that the client likes, is key to the prevention of pressure ulcers.

PHYSIOLOGICAL INTEGRITY

Physiological Adaptation

Alterations in Body System

725. In preparing a discharge teaching plan for a client diagnosed with thrombophlebitis and being treated with warfarin, which instructions would the nurse include?
   A. Eat a diet high in fiber and leafy green vegetables
   B. Start a progressive exercise program
   C. Drink at least eight glasses of fluid daily
   D. Do not use oral contraceptives

The answers are B, C, and D. The instruction to eat a diet high in leafy green vegetables would not be included because green leafy vegetables contain vitamin K, which can affect the needed dose of warfarin. All other instructions are appropriate and would be included in discharge plan.

PSYCHOSOCIAL INTEGRITY

Psychopathology

Recognize signs of acute and chronic mental illness

726. The nurse would expect to encounter clients who are attempting to avoid or minimize anxiety or fear when working with a group diagnosed with which types of personality disorder?
    A. Paranoid, schizoid, schizotypal
    B. Antisocial, borderline, histrionic, narcissistic
    C. Avoidant, dependent, obsessive-compulsive
    D. Passive-aggressive, masochistic

The answer is C. Clients with avoidant, dependent or obsessive compulsive personality disorder are attempting to avoid or minimize anxiety or fear. Withdrawal and odd, eccentric behaviors are characteristic of clients with paranoid, schizoid, and schizotypal personality disorder. Attention seeking and erratic behaviors are characteristic of clients with antisocial, borderline, histrionic and narcissistic personality disorders. Clients with passive-aggressive or masochistic personality disorder are covertly aggressive against self or others.

PHYSIOLOGICAL INTEGRITY

Physiological Adaptation

Pathophysiology

727. The nurse is caring for a client with Alzheimer's disease (AD), the most common form of dementia in older adults. Which factors are associated with AD? Select all that apply:
    A. Acute onset
    B. Impaired memory
    C. Confusion
    D. Difficulties with language
    E. Reversible organic disorder
    F. Amyloid plaques

The answers are B, C, D, and F. AD is a progressive, irreversible, organic disorder, characterized by confusion, disorientation, impaired memory and cognition. Personality changes are seen, and in later stages eventual dependency for all ADLs and IADLs. Amyloid plaques and neurofibrillary tangles are found in the brains of AD clients.

PHYSIOLOGICAL INTEGRITY

Pharmacological and Parenteral Therapies

Pharmacological agents/actions

728. A child has been admitted to the hospital unit for gastroenteritis. The child has been having diarrhea for 3 days and is moderately severely dehydrated. The stool cultures indicate a rotovirus as the cause of the diarrhea. The mother questions the nurse why her child isn't on antibiotics like the other children on the unit with GE. The nurse's response would be based on the knowledge that:
    A. antibiotics will make the diarrhea worse.
    B. the diarrhea has probably already run its course.
    C. antibiotics are not used for rotovirus gastroenteritis.
    D. the child is too dehydrated for antibiotics to be effective.

The answer is C. Antibiotics are used to treat bacterial infections not viral. Diarrhea is often a side effect of antibiotics but is not the correct response here. The other responses are incorrect.

HEALTH PROMOTION AND MAINTENANCE

Developmental Stages and Transitions

Recognize behaviors associated with psychosocial development

729. Which of the following behaviors indicates a 3 month old infant is developing a sense of trust?
    A. Eats and sleeps well
    B. Makes cooing noises
    C. Has developed object permanence
    D. Clings to mother and cries when she is not present

The answer is A. A sense of trust indicates trust in the world around them that basic needs will be met. Cooing noises occur because a child can hear himself. Object permanence is a component of Piaget's theory and not related to trust versus mistrust. Clinging to the mother occurs after object permanence develops in a much older infant.

PSYCHOSOCIAL INTEGRITY

Therapeutic Communications

Develop and maintain therapeutic relationships with client/family/significant others

730. A toddler is hospitalized for minor surgery. The parents are unable to stay with the child. The child reacts to the separation with a saddened expression, refusal to eat and continues to cry for momma. How should the nurse respond?

A. Encourage the child to forget mom and dad.

B. Hold the child and tell him mommy loves him and will come back.

C. Ignore his cries as they do not represent physical discomfort.

D. Avoid mentioning parents while holding and comforting the child.

The answer is B. This is the despair phase of toddler hospitalization reaction. The appropriate response is for the nurse to provide physical comfort and reinforce that the parents will return. The child's psychological needs can not be ignored. The child needs the parents for healthy development.

PHYSIOLOGICAL INTEGRITY

Reduction of Risk Potential

Therapeutic procedures

731. After an infant has a barium enema reduction of intussception, the nurse will know the reduction was successful when the infant:
   A. smiles at mother.
   B. passes a solid stool.
   C. falls asleep without medications.
   D. takes his regular amount of formula.

The answer is B. In addition to pain, the symptoms of intussception include passing a "currant jelly" stool followed by intestinal obstruction. Passing a solid stool would indicate the obstruction has cleared. The other responses do not address the pathology.

PHYSIOLOGICAL INTEGRITY

Physiological Adaptation

Medical Emergencies

732. A 22-year-old man has accidentally ingested about 200 ml of a lye-based liquid drain cleaner. Which treatment should the nurse be prepared to administer when the client arrives at the emergency department?
   A. A cathartic to promote elimination of the poisonous substance
   B. 30 ml of ipecac syrup followed by 240 ml of water to induce vomiting
   C. 150 ml of milk or water to dilute the ingested substance
   D. 75 g of activated charcoal to absorb the ingested chemical

The answer is C. The goal is to dilute the lye based product because it is caustic and tissue burn can result from contact with the agent. Diluting the product decreases the burn. Vomiting is contraindicated because the caustic product would come into contact with tissues of the esophagus, throat and mouth a second time and do more damage. Absorption of the chemical into the body is not the immediate concern so activated charcoal is not used.

HEALTH PROMOTION AND MAINTENANCE

Health and Wellness

733. A home health nurse sees many elderly clients and is concerned about their nutritional status. The nurse recognizes that the following factors contribute to the risk of malnutrition in older adults:
   A. Gastrointestinal changes including diminished saliva, decreased gastric acid and digestive enzyme secretions
   B. Chronic illness
   C. Poor dentition
   D. Inadequate financial resources
   E. Decline in functional ability
   F. Moving to an Assisted Living Facility

The answers are A, B, C, D, and E. Poor dentition, GI changes, and chronic illness result in inadequate intake, poor ingestion and digestion of food. The older adult may believe that limited resources will prevent them from purchasing nutritional foods and eat junk food instead. The nurse needs to educate regarding affordable nutritional foods and work as case manager and arrange for food stamps. Functional ability is the extent to which one is able to perform Activities of Daily Living (ADLs) & Instrumental Activities of Daily Living (IADLs). Decline in ADLs includes the ability to prepare meals; a decline in IADLs includes the ability to go food shopping. With functional limitations, the nurse as case manager can arrange for meals on wheels. Assisted living provides balanced meals that promotes good nutrition.

PHYSIOLOGICAL INTEGRITY

Pharmacological and Parenteral Therapies

Medication Administration

Use the "six rights" when administering client medications

734. A dose of intravenous acyclovir should be administered over what period of time? Record your answer as a whole number of minutes in the space provided.
   ____________minutes

Answer is 60 minutes.

Acyclovir is nephrotoxic. It is excreted primarily by glomerular filtration and tubular secretion. To decrease the risk of nephrotoxicity, the client must be well hydrated; the drug must be administered over a period of 60 minutes; and urinary output must be measured for two hours after the infusion. Output of less than 500 mL of urine per gram of acyclovir must be reported immediately.

PHYSIOLOGICAL INTEGRITY

Reduction of Risk Potential

Therapeutic Procedures

735. The nurse preparing a client for a cardiac catheterization and revascularization should include which information in the pre-op teaching.
   A. The client will be asleep during the procedure
   B. The client may experience a hot flash as the dye is injected
   C. There may be a sand bag placed over the cannulated site following the procedure
   D. The client will be on fluid restrictions until the gag reflex returns
   E. The client may experience chest pain when the balloon is inflated
   F. The client will experience a headache as the dye is injected

The answers are B, C, and E. The client is generally awake during the procedure and fluid intake is encouraged in order to assist the kidneys with excretion of the dye. Generally a client may experience a metallic taste in the mouth or a hot flash when the dye is injected.

PSYCHOSOCIAL INTEGRITY

Coping Mechanisms

Assess client response to illness

736. An 8-year-old child is hospitalized and undergoing diagnostic testing. Her parents can spend very little time with her because of the demands of work and four younger children at home. Nonetheless the child appears calm, does not complain, and seems unperturbed by all the stress. How would the nurse interpret this behavior?
   A. The child is mature for her age and is dealing well with hospitalization.
   B. A child of this age is not invested in health or family matters; peers are the concern and she will be receiving a lot of attention from them.
   C. The child is employing reaction formation which is a primary defense mechanism for her age.
   D. The child is coping by regressing.

The answer is C. The primary defense mechanism at this stage is reaction formation, which is acting brave, when really being quite frightened.

A, B, and D are incorrect—The child is interested in peers, but the rest of the comments are not true. Regression is seen in younger children and the symptoms of this child are not those of regression but are typical in reaction formation.

PHYSIOLOGICAL INTEGRITY

Pharmacological and Parenteral Therapies

Adverse effects/contraindications

737. The client is receiving Heparin IV at 1200 units/hour as part of the treatment regime for pulmonary embolism. The nurse notes that the urine has become bright red in color. The nurse would prepare to administer which of the following medications?
   A. Protamine Sulfate
   B. Aquamephyton (vitamin K)
   C. Warfarin (Coumadin)
   D. Acetylcysteine (Mucomyst)

The answer is A. The antidote for Heparin is protamine sulfate. Bright red urine suggests hematuria which is a potential adverse effect of anticoagulation. Aquamephyton is the antidote for Coumadin overdose and Acetylcysteine is the antidote for acetaminophen poisoning.

HEALTH PROMOTION AND MAINTENANCE

Developmental Stages and Transitions

Incorporate knowledge of theories of development in planning care for the client

738. A chronically ill adolescent has been hospitalized frequently for extended periods of time. Because of the severity of the illness and as a result of the hospitalization, the adolescent has been unable to develop a sense of who he is or what he will become. According to Erikson, these deficiencies will result in which of the following:
   A. role diffusion
   B. inferiority
   C. isolation
   D. stagnation

The answer is A. The adolescent is working on developing a sense of identity. Other answers are for other stages.

PHYSIOLOGICAL INTEGRITY

Pharmacological and Parenteral Therapies

Adverse effects/contraindications and side effects

739. A client who is in the Cardiac Care Unit complains of mediastinal chest pain, dyspnea, and anxiety. The nurse gives the client a nitroglycerine tablet sublingual. The client now complains of being dizzy. Which is the priority nursing intervention?
   A. Get a 12 lead ECG
   B. Raise the side rails on the bed
   C. Open the D5W IV to 100 cc per hour
   D. Take vital signs including pulse oximetry

The answer is B. Safety is the priority.

C would not be correct because it is not an isotonic solution and would not help to maintain circulating volume. A would be done but would not be the priority. D is not the priority.

HEALTH PROMOTION AND MAINTENANCE

Aging Process

740. Which of the following would the nurse identify as normative signs of aging, as opposed to pathologic signs?
   A. Increase in diastolic blood pressure
   B. Decrease in glomerular filtration rate
   C. Reduced lens elasticity
   D. Reduced vital capacity
   E. Dulled sense of taste
   F. Pressure ulcers

The answers are B, C, D, and E. A mild increase in systolic BP is expected, however an increase in diastolic BP is pathological. Normative changes in renal tubules cause a dramatic decrease in glomerular filtration rate. There is a normal decrease in lens elasticity. A normative decrease in chest wall compliance and atrophy of respiratory muscles contributes to reduced vital capacity. There is a normative dulled sense of taste, touch, and pain. Pressure ulcers are a pathological sign.

PHYSIOLOGICAL INTEGRITY

Reduction of Risk Potential

Potential for complications from surgical procedures and health alterations

741. Which is an indication of a successful outcome for a client who is recovering from an abdominal aortic aneurysm repair?
   A. Capillary refill of the toes >5 seconds
   B. Pulse Oximetry of the foot = 88%
   C. BP diastolic = 80 mm Hg.
   D. Urine output = 15 cc per hour

The answer is C. Diastolic blood pressure of 80 mm Hg.. High BP puts pressure on the surgical site. Capillary refill should be ≤3 seconds. Pulse oximetry should be ≥95%. Urine output should be ≥30 cc per hour.

PSYCHOSOCIAL INTEGRITY

Behavioral Interventions

Assist client with achieving and maintaining self-control of behavior

742. Which statement made by the parent of a suicidal client indicates the need for further explanation about a "no suicide" contract?
   A. The contract provides a boundary.
   B. The contract gives the client responsibility for control.
   C. These contract serve to reinforce to the client that life is valuable.
   D. Verbal as well as written contracts have been shown to be effective.

The answer is C. No suicide contracts do not directly reinforce that life is valuable. Therefore this is an incorrect statement and indicates that the parent needs further explanation.

All other statements about a no suicide contract are correct. A "no suicide" contract is a way of providing boundaries. Contracts help place control in the domian of the client. Both verbal and written "no suicide" contracts have proven effective.

PHYSIOLOGICAL INTEGRITY

Physiological Adaptation

Pathophysiology

743. Which symptoms identified during the assessment of a 4-week-old male infant are consistent with the diagnosis of pyloric stenosis?
   A. Metabolic alkalosis
   B. Lack of interest in feeding
   C. Vomiting bile stained fluid.
   D. 2 ounce weight loss over last 3 days.
   E. Peristalsis observed over the abdomen.

The answers are A, D, and E. Metabolic alkalosis, weight loss, and visible peristalsis are signs of pyloric obstruction. Metabolic alkalosis and weight loss result from vomiting that occurs with pyloric stenosis. A and D are related to the vomiting that occurs. Peristalsis may be visible on the abdomen as the stomach tries to push formula past the obstruction. The infant will be hungry, vomiting will not be bile stained.

HEALTH PROMOTION AND MAINTENANCE

Aging Process

744. When doing an intake assessment on the older adult, which factor should the nurse consider?

 The older adult
 A. responds with increased emotion to questions related to family history.
 B. often has diminished auditory acuity and may impede communication.
 C. is uncomfortable with the physical assessment because of multiple physical changes.
 D. has an increased response to pain requiring extreme caution with the physical assessment.

The answer is B. Diminished auditory acuity is common and communication is affected. Response to pain is decreased. Other responses are incorrect.

PHYSIOLOGICAL INTEGRITY

Basic Care and Comfort

Nutrition and oral hydration

745. A two week old infant has had several periods of apnea. After work-up, the physician diagnoses the infant with GERD and instructs the nurse to teach the mother feeding techniques to diminish reflux. The nurse will teach the mother to:
 A. avoid burping the baby to discourage reflux.
 B. keep the infant in an upright position after feeding.
 C. rock the baby during the feeding to keep him calm.
 D. place the baby prone after feeding to prevent aspiration if reflux occurs.

The answer is B. Upright position uses gravity to assist in formula retention. Burping would be more frequent in the GERD infant. Rocking will mix air with the formula making vomiting more likely. Prone position would put pressure on the abdomen and may increase vomiting.

HEALTH PROMOTION AND MAINTENANCE

Aging Process

746. The nurse knows the older adult has an increased risk for drug toxicity. Which of the following contributing factors increase the risk for drug toxicity?
 A. Impaired renal function
 B. Decrease in blood flow to the kidneys
 C. Polypharmacy
 D. Urinary incontinence
 E. Possibility of multiple chronic conditions requiring medications
 F. Using many physicians and lack of communication between physicians

The answers are A, B, C, E, and F. The decline in renal function in the older adult results in inefficient excretion of active drug, allowing toxic levels of drug to accumulate, placing the older adult at risk for drug toxicity. Polypharmacy is the concurrent use of many drugs, which is common in older adults as a result of: increased number of chronic conditions, using many physicians, changing physicians frequently, using more than one pharmacy, lack of information about over the counter medications, and assumption that once a drug is started it must be finished.

PHYSIOLOGICAL INTEGRITY

Pharmacological and Parenteral Therapies

Medication Administration

Instruct client on medication self-administration procedures

747. Which information/instruction would the nurse include when teaching the mother of child diagnosed with ADD about the proper use of the prescribed stimulant medication?
 A. Take the medication before a meal.
 B. If a dose is missed, take it as soon as remembered.
 C. Expect heavy sweating and heat intolerance as side effects of the medication.
 D. Follow up visits for lab tests or other monitoring are needed.

The answer is D. Follow up visits are critical so that the effects of the prescribed medication can be monitored. Monitoring may include laboratory studies, vital sign checks or EKGs. Stimulant medications should be taken after eating to avoid problems with appetite or indigestion. If a dose is missed, it is not "made up", the next dose is simply taken as scheduled. Side effects of stimulant medications are anorexia, nausea and vomiting, insomnia, tachycardia and chest pain, headache, and irritability, nervousness or confusion.

PSYCHOSOCIAL INTEGRITY

Behavioral Interventions

Assess client appearance, mood, and psychomotor behavior and identify/respond to inappropriate/abnormal behavior

748. An elderly client in an extended care facility hollers from her bed "Nurse, help me. They are throwing

dishes at me." Which is the best response on the part of the nurse?

A. "What kind of dishes is someone throwing at you?"

B. "Have a drink of water and by then it will be over."

C. "I don't see anyone throwing dishes but it must be scary for you; you are safe here."

D. "Why do you think anyone would want to throw dishes at you? You have never hurt anyone have you?

The answer is C. This response is empathetic; acknowledges the client's feeling; and offers reassurance. Responses A and D encourage the client to get more involved and add detail to the delusion and this is not therapeutic. Response B makes light of the client's experience and has an element of false reassurance.

PHYSIOLOGICAL INTEGRITY

Reduction of Risk Potential

Potential for complications of diagnostic tests/treatments/procedures

749. A client has just had an arthroscopy of the right knee for diagnostic evaluation of chronic knee pain. Which assessment finding has the highest priority for being reported to the surgeon?

A. Report of pain is 7 out of 10 on pain scale

B. Strength of right pedal pulse is decreased.

C. Capillary refill time is 3 seconds..

D. Pain is unrelieved by application of ice.

The answer is B. The decrease in pedal pulse could be indicative of obstruction to arterial flow to the foot.

A, C, and D are not correct because pain immediately following the arthroscopy is expected. Capillary refill time of three seconds is normal and indicates good blood flow through the capillaries. In older individuals, up to 5 seconds is considered normal.

PHYSIOLOGICAL INTEGRITY

Physiological Adaptation

Medical Emergencies

750. A 35-year old man is brought to the emergency department by EMS personnel after he was found sitting in the car in an enclosed garage with the motor running. He is unresponsive and hypotensive, and his skin is bright red. Which intervention would have the greatest priority?

A. Administration of oxygen

B. Placing the client in a prone position.

C. Administration of Narcan

D. Initiating CPR.

The answer is A. Being found in an enclosed space in a car with its motor running with symptoms of bright red skin and unresponsiveness is indicative of carbon monoxide poisoning. The immediate intervention is to remove the client from exposure to carbon monoxide and administer oxygen. Oxygenation is always the first priority. Placing the client in a prone position is inappropriate. Narcan is an opiate antagonist; it is not used in the treatment of carbon monoxide poisoning. The client does not need CPR because his heart is beating if he is hypotensive.

PHYSIOLOGICAL INTEGRITY

Physiological Adaptation

Unexpected response to therapies

751. The nurse is performing post operative assessments on a client who has had a femoral artery revascularization. Which is the most critical finding?

A. A quarter sized area of bright red drainage on the dressing

B. An apical pulse of 100 beats per minute

C. Complaint of numbness of the toes on the operative leg

D. An ankle-brachial index (ABI) of 1.0

The answer is C. Numbness is a symptom of arterial occlusion therefore it is the most critical finding as it can result in death of tissue. A quarter size area of bright red drainage on the dressing is not immediately critical; the nurse would circle the area and observe for continued bleeding. The apical pulse of 9 and the ABI pf 1.0 are both within normal range.

PSYCHOSOCIAL INTEGRITY

Abuse/Neglect

752. The home care nurse is providing an in-service on elder abuse to the home health aides that will be going out in the field. Which should be identified as potential signs of abuse? (Select all that apply.)

A. Bruises in various stages of healing

B. Malnutrition and dehydration

C. Poor personal hygiene, disheveled unkempt appearance

D. Burns and broken bones

The answers are A, B, C, and D. All responses are possible signs of abuse.

PHYSIOLOGICAL INTEGRITY

Physiological Adaptation

Pathophysiology

753. A nurse is a guest on a health related radio show. A listener calls in and asks what is the most common symptom of esophageal cancer. Which is the correct reply?
   A. Projectile vomiting.
   B. Progressive indigestion.
   C. Progressive dysphagia.
   D. Hoarseness progressing to loss of voice.

The answer is C. Progressive dysphagia is the most common symptom of esophageal cancer. It is insidious in onset and often the client simply eliminates foods from the diet which are difficult to swallow and so remains unaware of the problem until suddenly realizing that only liquids can be swallowed. Projectile vomiting is associated with increased intracranial pressure, not with cancer. Progressive indigestion is associated with GERD and hiatal hernia. Hoarseness and ultimately voice loss is associated with laryngeal cancer.

HEALTH PROMOTION AND MAINTENANCE

High Risk Behaviors

754. When teaching about accidental injury to adolescents, what does the nurse identify as the most common cause of injury?

Answer: Motor vehicle accidents.

The adolescent is prone to Motor Vehicle Accidents due to reckless driving and speeding to show off, driving under the influence of drugs or alcohol (doing drugs and alcohol to be part of the gang), and failure to use seatbelts because it isn't 'cool'.

PHYSIOLOGICAL INTEGRITY

Reduction of Risk Potential

Laboratory values

755. The nurse is reviewing laboratory findings for a client who has Congestive Heart Failure. Which laboratory value should be reported to the physician immediately?
   A. Cholesterol level of 240 mg/dl
   B. Digoxin level of 2.5ng/ml
   C. Troponin 1 level of 0.30 ng/ml
   D. Triglyceride level of 160 md/dl

The answer is B. Normal digoxin level is <2ng/ml and 2.5 ng/ml is a toxic level. Cholesterol level is slightly high but not critical. Troponin 1 level is normal. Triglyceride level is borderline high but not critical.

SAFE AND EFFECTIVE CARE ENVIRONMENT

Safety and Infection Control

Home safety

756. The home care nurse is concerned with reducing the risk of falling for an 86-year-old client. Which statement represents the most appropriate approach to the problem?
   A. "I understand that you are concerned about finances, however adequate non glare lighting is very important to keep you safe. Can I speak to your son about trying the new florescent bulbs that are much less expensive to use."
   B. "This house is not safe, it has years of accumulated clutter. Why don't you consider selling the house and move to a nursing home, where you will be safe and well fed."
   C. "The old rug in the dining room under the table will have to go, it's worn out anyway."
   D. "Never leave your room, when you are home alone, sit in the lounge chair or stay in bed, I'll set up a bed side commode for you."

The answer is A. When reading questions on communication listen to the tone of the response, abrupt, impolite, overly paternalistic responses can be eliminated. Responses with absolute terms such as all or never can be eliminated. Option A offers not only information needed but helps discover options within the client's means.

PHYSIOLOGICAL INTEGRITY

Physiological Adaptation

Pathophysiology

757. A nurse is speaking to a community group on the early detection of cancer. A member of the audience asks what is a symptom of cancer of the larynx. Which is the correct response for the nurse to give?
   A. Projectile vomiting.
   B. Progressive indigestion.
   C. Progressive dysphagia.
   D. Hoarseness progressing to loss of voice.

The answer is D. Hoarseness and ultimately voice loss is associated with laryngeal cancer.

Projectile vomiting is associated with increased intracranial pressure, not with cancer. Progressive indigestion is associated with GERD and hiatal hernia. Progressive dysphagia is the most common symptom of esophageal cancer.

HEALTH PROMOTION AND MAINTENANCE

Health Screening

Perform targeted screening examination

758. The nurse is performing health screening at the local junior high school for scoliosis. Which test should the nurse perform?
   A. Ask the child to stand on one foot to see if the pelvis shifts down.
   B. Have the child bend at the waist to see if there is a difference between the sides.
   C. Have the child twist at the waist from side to side to see if there is pain with the motion.
   D. Ask the child to stretch toward the ceiling first with the left, then with the right side to see if one hand reaches higher.

The answer is B. This test is called the Adam's Forward Bend Test. Children with scoliosis will have a prominence on one side or the other. The other responses are not tests for scoliosis.

PHYSIOLOGICAL INTEGRITY

Reduction of Risk Potential

Therapeutic Procedures

759. A registered nurse and an LPN are working as a team to provide care for a group of clients. Which action by the LPN requires the RN to intervene?
   A. The LPN raises the knee gatch on the bed of a client who has an intraaortic balloon pump in order to relieve pressure on the client's back.
   B. The LPN prepares to administer Lasix (furosimide) to a client whose potassium level is 4.2 mEq/L
   C. The LPN returns a client to bed after the client's heart rate increases from 72 to 96 beats per minute while ambulating in the hall
   D. The LPN brings breakfast to a client who is scheduled for an echocardiogram later in the morning.

The answer is A. The knee gatch should not be raised because it could cause the balloon catheter to be kinked off. All other actions are appropriate and do not require corrective intervention by the RN.

PHYSIOLOGICAL INTEGRITY

Physiological Adaptation

Pathophysiology

760. Which disorder places the client at risk for tissue necrosis and breakdown of bone structure with decalcification?
   A. Osteoarthritis
   B. Osteomyelitis
   C. Osteoporosis
   D. Osteogenesis

The answer is B.

A is incorrect—osteoarthritis or degenerative joint disease. C is incorrect—osteoporosis is a loss of bone density. D is incorrect—osteogenesis refers to the formation of bone in the body.

PHYSIOLOGICAL INTEGRITY

Reduction of Risk Potential

Potential for complications from surgical procedures and health alterations

761. A 5-year-old child has just returned from a tonsillectomy. The child's mother is at the bedside and caring for her child. Which observation made by the nurse while taking vital signs, requires nursing intervention?
   A. The child is lying supine.
   B. An ice collar is lying on the child's neck.
   C. The mother is offering the child ice chips from a spoon.
   D. The child is drooling and the mother is wiping the child's mouth with a wash rag.

The answer is A. The child should not be in a supine position because of the risk of aspirating blood if the surgical wound should ooze. Nursing intervention is required to reposition the child in a side lying position and to explain to the mother the importance of maintaining the child in this position. None of the other options indicate the need for nursing intervention.

HEALTH PROMOTION AND MAINTENANCE

Aging Process

762. Many body systems manifest deteriorative changes to a greater or lesser degree with aging. The expected, normal signs of aging are called —— changes.

Answer: Primary.

Primary changes are the expected normal changes associated with aging. An example of a primary change is decreased elasticity of the skin. Pathological or disease related changes are referred to as secondary changes.

PHYSIOLOGICAL INTEGRITY

Pharmacological and Parenteral Therapies

Adverse effects/contraindications

763. A client has rheumatoid arthritis and is receiving hydroxychloroquine (Plaquenil). Which instruction should be given to the client prior to discharge home?
   A. Take this medication on an empty stomach.
   B. Expect your urine to be greenish-yellow in color while taking this medication.
   C. Report a weight gain of more than 5 lbs. to your physician.
   D. Notify your physician if you experience any changes in vision.

The answer is D. because hydroxychloroquine can produce over time changes in vision due to ocular toxicity or retinopathy. These manifest as episodes of misty or foggy vision, "disappearing words" when reading, light flashes before the eyes, or seeing only half of the visual field. Hydroxychloroquine can be taken with meals to minimize gastrointestinal side effects. Hydroxychloroquine may discolor urine red or brown not green. Weight gain is not related to use of hydroxychloroquine.

PHYSIOLOGICAL INTEGRITY

Reduction of Risk Potential

Diagnostic tests

764. The CCU nurse notices that a client's T wave has become inverted. Which is the priority nursing intervention?
   A. Give the client nitroglycerine sublingual, 1 tablet every 5 minutes three times
   B. Start oxygen at 2–4 liters per minute via nasal cannula
   C. Check for T wave elevation in the V1 lead
   D. Check the client and verify lead placement

The answer is D. The leads may have gotten moved. It is priority to always check your client to verify that monitoring data is correct.

HEALTH PROMOTION AND MAINTENANCE

Health Screening

765. You are assessing an infant brought to the pediatric clinic. Which assessment finding would indicate that follow up is needed because of possible developmental dysplasia of the hip?
   A. Outward turning of both legs
   B. Limited range of motion in the hip joint
   C. Crying and other signs of pain on flexing the hips
   D. Asymmetrical thigh and buttock skin creases

The answer is D. Asymmetrical thigh and buttock skin creases are an obvious sign of developmental dysplasia of the hip.

A is incorrect—there is no outward turning of the legs. B is incorrect—there is no limited range of motion in the hip. C is incorrect—developmental hip dysplasia is not painful.

PHYSIOLOGICAL INTEGRITY

Physiological Adaptation

Pathophysiology

Identify client status based upon pathophysiology

766. Which interpretation should the nurse assign to assessment findings of delayed capillary refill, cyanosis and clubbing?
   A. Arterial oxygen levels are chronically low.
   B. Carbon dioxide levels in the blood are elevated.
   C. Compensatory polycythemia has developed.
   D. Vital capacity has progressively decreased over time.

The answer is A. Delayed capillary refill, cyanosis and clubbing are signs of chronically decreased arterial oxygen levels. Elevated carbon dioxide levels (hypercarbia) is not always associated with hypoxemia and does not cause these signs. Polycythemia is an increase in red blood cells which does occur as a compensatory effort in clients with chronic hypoxemia; it does not cause the signs. Changes in vital capacity which is the amount of gas that can be expired after a maximum inspiration do not cause delayed capillary refill, cyanosis or clubbing.

PHYSIOLOGICAL INTEGRITY

Reduction of Risk Potential

Potential for complications from surgical procedures and health alterations

767. On assessing a client who has had coronary artery bypass grafting the nurse finds: T 100.2°F; pulse 110 beats per minute; BP 96/60 mm Hg; Respirations 20 per minute; distended neck veins; muffled heart sounds. Based on this assessment data, which is the priority nursing action?
   A. Increase frequency of client monitoring.
   B. Ask the client about pain.
   C. Report findings immediately to the physician
   D. Call the lab to draw blood cultures

The answer is C. The client is displaying signs and symptoms of cardiac tamponade which is a medical emergency. Increased monitoring will occur but calling the physician is the priority. Pain may cause tachycardia but it wouldn't cause JVD. Lab cultures are usually not done until the temperature is 102°F or above.

PSYCHOSOCIAL INTEGRITY

Chemical and Other Dependencies

768. A client in a methadone program, is admitted with a broken pelvis following an automobile accident. Which fact should be considered when planning care for this client?
    A. The client is likely to be euphoric at intervals.
    B. Methadone should continue to be given while the client is in the hospital.
    C. The client will not need pain medication if he is receiving methadone.
    D. If methadone is stopped, delusions or hallucinations may ensue.

The answer is B. Methadone maintenance should be continued while the client is in the hospital if at all possible. Methadone does not cause euphoria so if it is continued, the client will not have intervals of euphoria. Methadone does not adequately relieve acute pain so it will not eliminate the need for pain medication; it can be used with success in the management of chronic pain. Delusions and hallucinations are not symptoms of withdrawal from methadone and other opiates; delusions and hallucinations are associated with withdrawal from alcohol, sedatives/hypnotics, and anxiolytics.

PHYSIOLOGICAL INTEGRITY

Pharmacological and Parenteral Therapies

Adverse effects/contraindications

769. Which is the most common side effect of salicylates and NSAIDs used in the management of the pain and swelling associated with rheumatoid arthritis?
    A. Anorexia
    B. Dizziness
    C. Gastrointestinal distress
    D. Weight loss

The answer is C. Long term use can result in irritation of the stomach lining.

Answers A, B, and D are incorrect because they are side effects for different classes of medication.

PHYSIOLOGICAL INTEGRITY

Pharmacological and Parenteral Therapies

Medication Administration

770. The nurse is providing discharge instructions for a client who has been diagnosed with stable angina and has a prescription for nitroglycerine sublingual tablets. Which statement by the client indicates that further teaching is needed?
    A. "I should keep my pills in the original container."
    B. "I need to replace my pills every month."
    C. "I should go to the hospital if the pain is not relieved after taking a nitroglycerine."
    D. "I should stop all activity and rest when having chest pain."

The answer is B. Pills should be replaced every 3–6 months.

A, C, and D are all correct.

HEALTH PROMOTION AND MAINTENANCE

Developmental Stages and Transitions

771. According to Piaget's theory of cognitive development which of the following cognitive developmental skills are mastered between the ages of 7 and 11 (school-age years)?
    A. Concrete thought
    B. Conservation
    C. Complex classification
    D. Abstract thinking
    E. Sees another's point of view

The answers are A, B, C, and E. The stage of concrete operations is between 7 and 11 years of age. Thought becomes logical, concrete, and based on tasks in the here and now. The school-age child masters conservation and complex classification and is also starting to understand that other's have a different point of view form their own. Abstract thinking and reflecting on theoretical matters begins in the preadolescent years.

PHYSIOLOGICAL INTEGRITY

Physiological Adaptation

Alterations in Body Systems

772. The nurse on the hospital unit receives a call from admitting stating a client with a question of an intestinal obstruction is being admitted. In preparing for

the arrival of the client, the nurse will gather equipment for:

A. Gastric lavage

B. Morphine drip

C. Gastric decompression

D. Soap suds enema

The answer is C. The client will be NPO in preparation for surgery and a NG tube will be inserted for gastric decompression. There is no reason to lavage the stomach. Morphine and other opioids are generally withheld until after the diagnosis is established. Soap suds enema are contraindicated.

SAFE AND EFFECTIVE CARE ENVIRONMENT

Management of Care

Establishing priorities

773. Which client being treated in the emergency room requires the most immediate intervention?

A. A client whose initial assessment disclosed elevated T waves and a serum potassium level of 6.1.

B. A client whose x-ray showed a fractured radius.

C. A client with a stab wound to the thigh covered with a bloody gauze pad.

D. A woman who is 30 weeks pregnant with abdominal pain.

The answer is A. An elevated T wave is suggestive of a cardiac problem and the potassium is dangerously elevated. Thus this client is in a potentially life threatening situation and requires rapid intervention. All of the other clients are in need of treatment for significant problems but none are in immediate danger.

PHYSIOLOGICAL INTEGRITY

Reduction of Risk Potential

System-specific assessment

774. Which assessment findings would the nurse expect when examining a client with chronic low arterial oxygen levels? Mark all that apply.

A. ___ cyanosis

B. ___ skin tenting

C. ___ positive Cullen's sign

D. ___ delayed capillary refill

E. ___ clubbing

F. ___ muffled heart sounds

The answers are A, D, and E. Delayed capillary refill, cyanosis and clubbing are signs of chronically decreased arterial oxygen levels. Skin tenting is an indicator of dehydration. A positive Cullen's sign is bluish discoloration around the umbilicus and is indicative of bleeding into the peritoneal cavity. Muffled heart sounds are not a sign of chronic low arterial oxygen levels.

HEALTH PROMOTION AND MAINTENANCE

Ante-/Intra-/Postpartum and Newborn Care

775. The nurse is doing the neurologic assessment of the newborn infant. Which would be normal findings?

A. ___ Sucking in response to touching infant's lips; strong and coordinated

B. ___ Blinking in response to light or touch

C. ___ Gag in response to stimulation of the posterior pharynx by food or tube

D. ___ Asymmetrical sporadic movement of the extremities

E. ___ Extremities extended when prone

F. ___ Minimal head lag when pulled to a sitting position

The answers are A, B, and C. Sucking, blinking, and gag reflexes are present at birth. Sucking reflex disappears at 3–4 months, blinking and gag reflexes persist for life. Movements are symmetrical, sporadic and involve all extremities. Extremities are flexed and knees are flexed under abdomen in the newborn. The neonate has minimal head control therefore there is significant head lag when pulled to a sitting position.

PHYSIOLOGICAL INTEGRITY

Physiological Adaptation

Fluid and electrolyte imbalance

776. A client has a CVP reading of 12mmHg. Which physical assessment finding is consistent with this measurement?

A. Increased JVD

B. 1+ peripheral pulses

C. Tachycardia

D. Crackles in the lung bases

The answer is A. Increased JVD is an indication of volume overload. Tachycardia, not bradycardia, is the physiologic response to decreased cardiac output. Crackles in the lung bases are indicative of pulmonary overload.

PHYSIOLOGICAL INTEGRITY

Reduction of Risk Potential

Potential for complications from surgical procedures and health alterations

777. The nurse teaches new parents about nutrition for the first year of life. What information does the nurse include in her teaching plan?
   A. Breast milk is a complete and healthful diet for first 6 months of life.
   B. Commercially prepared fortified infant formula is a good alternative if breast feeding is not desirable or feasible.
   C. No additional fluids are needed for first 4–6 months with breast or formula fed infant.
   D. In the second 6 months skim or regular cow's milk may be used depending on infant's weight pattern.
   E. Solid foods are started with cereals at 2 months, and then fruits, vegetables and meats are gradually introduced over next 4 months.
   F. Honey is not given for the first year because it is a source of botulism.

The answers are A, B, C, and F. Breast feeding and fortified commercially prepared infant formulas are the best and only sources of nutrition appropriate for the first 6 months of life and continue to be the primary source of nutrition in the second six months of life as well. Cows' milk, skim or regular, and imitation milks are not acceptable during the first year, as they are difficult to digest and lack the nutrients needed for growth. Solid foods are generally introduced at 5 to 6 months starting with cereals and progressing and gradually progressing to fruits, vegetables and meats. Honey is not given in the first year as it is associated with botulism.

PHYSIOLOGICAL INTEGRITY

Physiological Adaptation

Medical Emergencies

778. While shopping the nurse observes a school age child put something in his mouth and immediately begins coughing. Which would be an appropriate initial action for the nurse to take?
   A. Ask the child if he is choking.
   B. Place the child in reverse Trendelenburg position.
   C. Perform the Heimlich maneuver.
   D. Check pulse and respirations.

The answer is A. Asking for a response is a method of determining if the airway is obstructed and immediate emergency intervention is needed. If a person can speak the airway is not obstructed. Reverse Trendelburg position in which the client is supine with feet lower than the head would serve no purpose. A Heimlich maneuver is performed if a foreign body is occluding the upper airway. Checking pulse and respirations serves no purpose in the immediate situation.

PHYSIOLOGICAL INTEGRITY

Physiological Adaptation

Fluid and electrolyte imbalance

779. A client has a CVP reading of 12mm Hg. Which physician order for fluids would the nurse question?
   A. 5% Dextrose and Normal Saline IV at 100 cc hr
   B. Oral fluid restrictions of 1500 cc per 24 hours
   C. Normal Saline at 20 cc hr.
   D. Nitroglycerine IV drip at 5 mcg per minute

The answer is A. D_5NS is a hypertonic IV solution and would pull more fluid into the vascular system which is already overloaded. Fluid restrictions would help decrease fluid overload. Normal Saline at 20 cc/hr would only keep the vein open and would not add to overload. Nitroglycerine would cause vasodilation and decrease circulating volume.

SAFE AND EFFECTIVE CARE ENVIRONMENT

Management of Care

Establishing priorities

780. The nurse has just received report on assigned clients. Which client should the nurse see first?
   A. A 23-year-old admitted two hours ago with a gunshot wound; 3 cm area of dark drainage noted on the dressing.
   B. A 38-year-old with a collapsed lung due to an accident; no drainage noted in the previous 3 hours.
   C. A 47-year-old who had a stab wound to the abdomen one day ago; client complains of chills and fever.
   D. A 34-year-old with a mastectomy two days ago; 15 cc of serosanguineous fluid noted in the Hemovac drain. Complaining of pain in axilla.

The answer is C. Because the client is at risk for internal bleeding, infection, or peritonitis. This client should be assessed for further symptoms of infection.

The client in option A would not be first because there is apparently no active bleeding as indicated by the small amount of drainage on the dressing. The client in option B has no more than the expected amount and color of drainage. The client in option D has no unexpected signs or symptoms.

PHYSIOLOGICAL INTEGRITY

Physiological Adaptation

Alterations in Body Systems

781. Which problem associated with Hirschsprung's Disease in a newborn is the most critical?
   A. Respiratory distress.
   B. Abdominal distention.
   C. Vomits several feedings.
   D. Failure to pass meconium by 48 hours of life.

The answer is A. Respiratory distress can occur with Hirschsprung's disease as a result of abdominal distention. Because respiratory distress can be immediately life threatening it is the most critical problem associated with the disease. All of the other responses are symptoms of Hirschsprung's Disease but none are immediately life threatening.

SAFE AND EFFECTIVE CARE ENVIRONMENT

Safety and Infection Control

Disaster planning

782. As a nurse manager at the area medical center you have been asked to participate as a member of the team to develop the community's disaster preparedness plan. As you begin to think through the steps of a sound plan you identify the following key phases in a disaster management program:
   A. Preparedness, mitigation, response, recovery, and evaluation
   B. Planning, organizing, leading, controlling
   C. Assessment, analyzes planning, implementation, evaluation
   D. Prevention, warning, rehabilitation, reconstruction

The answer is A. There are five basic phases to a disaster management program, there may be some overlapping between the phases but each phase has a specific component relating to disaster management.

B lists the four concepts of the management process, C lists the components of the nursing process, and D is a listing of terms that are not related to each other.

PHYSIOLOGICAL INTEGRITY

Reduction of Risk Potential

Alterations in Body Systems

Evaluate achievement of client treatment goals

783. How would the nurse best evaluate the effectiveness of a client's oxygen therapy?
   Monitor change in
   A. Hematocrit
   B. Hemoglobin
   C. Arterial blood gases
   D. Pulmonary function tests

The answer is C. Oxygen is used to treat hypoxemia and hypoxia. The best measure of its effectiveness in reversing these conditions is ABG analysis.

PHYSIOLOGICAL INTEGRITY

Therapeutic Communications

Use therapeutic communication techniques to provide support to client and/or family

784. A client standing in the doorway to his room, screams at the nurse as she comes down the hall "How long am I supposed to wait for someone to straighten my bed? Do you know how much this room is costing me per day? I want my bed fixed and I want it done now." How should the nurse respond?
   A. Say "I don't think you need your bed straightened this minute. . ."
   B. Place a hand on the client's arm and lead him to a chair in his room.
   C. Ask the client if he really thinks this type of behavior will help him feel better.
   D. Acknowledge the distress and obtain more information about what the pateint needs.

The answers is D. Acknowledging a person's distress is therapeutic. Dismissing a person's feelings is nontherapeutic and interferes with establishing an effective nurse–client relationship. Obtaining more information about the situation allows for discussion of a solution.

A is incorrect—Disagreeing/arguing with the angry client can lead to escalation of angry behavior. B is incorrect—Touching an angry client or entering the client's personal space can also escalate anger. C is incorrect— it is patronizing and this type of response increases anger.

PHYSIOLOGICAL INTEGRITY

Physiological Adaptation

Hemodynamics

785. A client has a pulmonary artery pressure catheter inserted for hemodynamic monitoring. The client's cardiac output reading is 2 liters per minute. Which physical assessment finding is consistent with this measurement?
   A. Increased JVD
   B. 1+ peripheral pulses
   C. Bradycardia
   D. Crackles in the lung bases

The answer is B. 1+ peripheral pulses. The normal CO is 4–7 liters per minute so the client would display signs and symptoms of decreased cardiac output. Increased JVD is an indication of volume overload. Tachycardia, not bradycardia, is the physiologic response to decreased cardiac output. Crackles in the lung bases are indicative of pulmonary overload.

PHYSIOLOGICAL INTEGRITY

Physiological Adaptation

Fluid and electrolyte imbalances

786. A 4-week-old infant boy has been admitted to the pediatric unit with a diagnosis of "rule out pyloric stenosis." For signs of which electrolyte imbalance would the nurse monitor the infant?
   A. Hypokalemia
   B. Hypernatremia
   C. Metabolic acidosis
   D. Respiratory alkalosis

The answer is A. Vomiting causes the loss of potassium, hence hypokalemia would occur as well as metabolic alkalosis from the loss of stomach acids.

PHYSIOLOGICAL INTEGRITY

Pharmacological and Parenteral Therapies

Adverse effects/contraindications

787. A physician writes the following orders for a client being evaluated for a possible bowel obstruction. Which order would the nurse question?
   A. Intake and Output
   B. NG tube to suction
   C. IV, $D_5$1/4 NS at 125 ml/hr
   D. Morphine q 3 hours prn pain

The answer is D. Morphine suppresses peristalsis and would increase the bowel obstruction. Morphine and other opioid analgesics are usually withheld during the diagnostic period because of the effect on peristalsis and also because they can cause vomiting. Vomiting can complicate the diagnosis and determination of the plan of care because vomiting is also a sign of worsening bowel obstruction and of N/G tube obstruction.

HEALTH PROMOTION AND MAINTENANCE

Ante-/Intra-/Postpartum and Newborn Care

788. The nurse is assessing a newborn. A sudden noise causes the newborn infant to extend and then flex the arms and fingers. The nurse would document this as a positive:
   A. Moro reflex
   B. Gag reflex
   C. Babinski reflex
   D. Tonic neck reflex

The answer is A. The Moro reflex occurs in response to a sudden noise or movement. The infant extends arms and legs and then flexes them. The infant's hands form a C with the thumb and fingers.

PHYSIOLOGICAL INTEGRITY

Reduction of Risk Potential

Alterations in Body Systems

Evaluate achievement of client treatment goals

789. Which would be an expected effect of resistive breathing training in a client with COPD?
   A. Energy conservation
   B. Increased oxygen saturation
   C. Decreased hypercarbia
   D. Increased respiratory muscle strength

The answer is D. Resistive breathing training is used for clients with exercise induced dyspnea and may be done as part of a pulmonary rehabilitation program. In resistive breathing the client breathes against a set resistance with the goal of developing strength and endurance in the respiratory muscles. The goal of resistive breathing is not energy conservation, increased oxygen saturation, or decreased hypercarbia.

PSYCHOSOCIAL INTEGRITY

Therapeutic Communications

Use therapeutic communication techniques to provide support to client and/or family

790. The daughter of a nursing home client comes to the nurse's station and shouts angrily "My mother's condition is a disgrace–this place should be closed down and you all should lose your licenses." How should the nurse respond?
   A. Say "I was just into your mother and there is nothing disgraceful about her condition."
   B. Place a hand on the daughter's arm and lead her to a chair.
   C. Ask the daughter if she really thinks this is a proper way for an adult to behave.
   D. Acknowledge the distress and obtain more information about the problem.

The answer is D. Acknowledging a person's distress is therapeutic; dismissing a person's feelings is non-therapeutic and interferes with establishing an effective nurse-client relationship. Determining the immediate trigger of the daughter's anger allows the possibility of addressing the problem and opening the door to discussion of underlying issues.

Response A is inappropriate because it disagrees/argues with the angry daughter and this can lead to escalation of angry behavior. Similarly response B is incorrect because touching an angry client or entering the client's personal space can also escalate anger.

Response C is incorrect because it is patronizing and this type of response increases anger.

PHYSIOLOGICAL INTEGRITY

Physiological Adaptation

Pathophysiology

791. The parents of a child with Tetralogy of Fallot are very upset by the cyanotic "tet" spells and asks the nurse what causes them. Which fact should be the basis of the nurse's response?
   A. The aorta carries mixed deoxygenated and oxygenated blood into the systemic circulation.
   B. Low hemoglobin and circulating iron levels of the newborn cause low oxygen saturation.
   C. A left to right shunt increases blood return to the lungs.
   D. Increased heart rate causes a ventilation/perfusion mismatch when the child becomes stressed.

The answer is A. Increased right ventricular pressure creates right to left shunt. The hemoglobin and iron levels are not one of the factors associated with Tetralogy of Fallot. A left to right shunt involves an acyanotic defects. Ventilation/perfusion mismatch occurs in pulmonary embolisms.

PHYSIOLOGICAL INTEGRITY

Pharmacological and Parenteral Therapies

Expected effects/outcomes

792. The CCU nurse admits a client from ER who has been diagnosed with an evolving MI and has received thrombolytic therapy with T-PA, tissue plasminogen activator, and heparin. Which is an expected client outcome?
   A. ST elevation of 2 mm in two chest leads
   B. PTT level of 1.5–2.5 times the control
   C. An INR value of 2–3
   D. A cardiac ejection fraction of 30%

The answer is B. PTT level of 1.5–2.5 times the control is the therapeutic range during heparin therapy. ST elevation is an indication of cardiac tissue injury. INR is for warfarin (Coumadin) therapy. Normal cardiac ejection fraction is 60% or higher.

SAFE AND EFFECTIVE CARE ENVIRONMENT

Management of Care

Legal rights and responsibilities

793. A nurse is explaining to a client that she has the right to be treated in a certain manner, receive adequate information, and have her confidentiality maintained while hospitalized. The client asks what gives her these rights. Which document should the nurse refer to in responding to the client's question?
   A. Client Constitution
   B. Client Bill of Rights
   C. Client Medical Record
   D. Client Self-Determination Act

The answer is B. The Client Bill of Rights is a document published by the American Hospital Association to promote the rights of hospitalized clients.

Client Constitutions is not a document but is a form of law–constitutional law. The Medical Record is the record of the hospitalization includes medical tests, procedures and nursing documentation. The Client Self-Determination Act is a legal act that requires every competent adult be informed in writing upon admission to a health care institution about the client's rights to accept or refuse treatment.

PHYSIOLOGICAL INTEGRITY

Reduction of Risk Potential

Therapeutic Procedures

Provide nursing care of surgical clients

794. A client has just returned from surgery for colorectal cancer. In assessing the client, the nurse notes that the perineal dressing is soaked with bright red drainage. Which action should the nurse take?
   A. Reinforce the existing dressing.
   B. Change the dressing using sterile technique.
   C. Apply a pressure dressing using clean technique.
   D. Cover the existing dressing with waterproof material.

The answer is A. The first dressing following surgery is changed by the surgeon. The nurse would reinforce the dressing. If the drainage continues, the nurse would notify the surgeon. The other responses are incorrect.

PHYSIOLOGICAL INTEGRITY

Physiological Adaptation

Illness management

795. The mother of an 8-week-old infant is telling the pediatric nurse that her baby has colic and cries all the time. The mother is visibly tired and frustrated. In helping the mother to cope with an infant with colic, the nurse can remind the mother that colic usually disappears by the age of:
A. 3 months
B. 6 months
C. 9 months
D. 12 months

The answer is A. Colic is a short-term complaint and the infant usually outgrows it by 3 months of age.

PHYSIOLOGICAL INTEGRITY

Pharmacological and Parenteral Therapies

Pharmacological Agents/Actions

Use clinical decision making/critical thinking when addressing actions of prescribed pharmacological agents on clients

796. A client receiving chemotherapy for cancer also has epoetin alfa prescribed. The client's spouse asks what the epoetin alfa will do for the client. The nurse's response is based on the knowledge that the therapeutic goal of therapy with epoetin alfa for clients receiving chemotherapy for cancer is to:
A. Potentiate the chemotherapy drugs
B. Decrease the need for transfusions.
C. Bolster immune system activity
D. Protect against renal damage

The answer is B. Epoetin alfa is used to treat chemotherapy induced anemia and reduce the need for transfusions in clients with cancer who will receive chemotherapy for two months or more. It does not potentiate chemotherapeutic drugs. Like endogenous erythropoietin, It stimulates the production of red blood cells not immune system cells. Epoetin alfa is used to treat the anemia associated with chronic renal failure; it does not protect against kidney damage.

HEALTH PROMOTION AND MAINTENANCE

Disease Prevention

797. The nurse teaches new parents about infant dentition and care of the teeth. Which of the following will the nurse include in the teaching plan?
A. Beginning signs of tooth eruption are not seen before 10–11 months
B. A frozen teething ring may be used to reduce inflammation and relieve discomfort
C. Prevent dental carries by avoiding having infant fall asleep with bottle
D. Fluoride should not be supplemented in the first year
E. Infant Tylenol may be given with practitioners approval, for teething pain disrupting sleep and feeding
F. Teeth may be cleaned with damp cloth

The answers are B, C, E, and F. Beginning signs of tooth eruption are commonly seen by 5 or 6 months. In areas where water supply is not adequately fluorinated, supplemental fluoride begins at around 6 months. A frozen teething ring is used to reduce inflammation and manage pain. Infant Tylenol may be used for severe pain disrupting function with practitioners order. Teeth may be cleaned with a damp cloth.

PHYSIOLOGICAL INTEGRITY

Pharmacological and Parenteral Therapies

Medication Administration

Instruct client on medication self-administration procedures

798. The nurse is giving a client instructions on the use of an inhaled beta 2 agonist for mild symptoms associated with emphysema and chronic bronchitis. The nurse cautions that the maximum number of puffs to be taken in 24 hours is how many?
A. 12–16
B. 8–12
C. 6–10
D. 4–8

The answer is B. For mild symptoms 1–2 puffs of a beta 2 agonist can be taken every 2 to 6 hours PRN not to exceed 8 to 12 puffs in any 24 hour period.

HEALTH PROMOTION AND MAINTENANCE

Health and Wellness

799. The nurse is teaching parents of toddlers about nutritional needs, food preferences and expected appetite patterns. Which information would the nurse include in the teaching plan?
A. ___ Do not overwhelm the toddler with large portions.
B. ___ Serve stews with meat and vegetables in one bowl to maximize nutrition with minimal fuss.

C. ___ It is important to encourage eating because growth is increasing and appetite is decreasing.
D. ___ Toddlers are very concerned with the plate or cup used.
E. ___ Serve foods that are new and interesting to the toddler as often as possible.
F. ___ Substitute cow's milk if meat isn't eaten.

The answers are A and D. Toddlers are easily overwhelmed by large portions. Toddler's prefer single foods and often refuse mixtures such as stews. The toddler will even refuse foods that are touching each other. In toddlerhood growth slows, and appetite is diminished, with periods of physiologic anorexia. The toddler has a favorite cup, spoon, dish, and will often refuse a well-liked food because it's not served in the favorite dish. Repeat a set of nutritious foods often so they will be recognized by the toddler, and better received. Cow's milk is a poor source of iron and interferes with iron absorption leading to iron deficiency anemia if not curtailed.

SAFE AND EFFECTIVE CARE ENVIRONMENTS

Safety and Infection Control

Standard/Transmission-Based/Other Precautions

Apply principles of infection control

800. Which precaution measures would be instituted when a client has shigella? Mark all that apply.
A. ___ Client is placed in a private, negative airflow pressure room.
B. ___ Client is placed in a private room or with other clients with infection caused by the same organism.
C. ___ Use mask at all times while in the client's room.
D. ___ Use mask when working within 3 feet of the client.
E. ___ Use gown and protective barriers when giving direct care.
F. ___ Mask on client if transported out of room.
G. ___ Use gloves at all times when caring for clients.
H. ___ Use gloves when there is risk of exposure to blood or body fluids.

The answers are B, E, and G. Shigella is a serious disease that is easily transmitted through direct contact. Contact precautions require a private room or a room shared with someone infected with the same organism. Gloves are worn at all times and gowns and protective barriers are used if direct contact is required. Since gloves are worn at all times, the requirements of standard precautions, which involve wearing gloves whenever there is the risk of touching something wet that comes from the body surface or a body cavity, i.e., when there is the risk of contact with blood or body fluids, are met.

PHYSIOLOGICAL INTEGRITY

Physiological Adaptation

Pathophysiology

801. A client who has Rheumatic Fever is being admitted to your floor. Admitting has assigned the client to share a room with a client who is a fresh post-operative client. As the charge nurse, you would
A. arrange for the new client to be reassigned to a private room.
B. ask that the new client be assigned to a room with a non-surgical client.
C. admit the client to the room assigned.
D. move the postoperative client to a room with another postoperative client.

The answer is C. The client can be admitted to the room assigned because rheumatic fever is an autoimmune response to a streptococcal infection and is not contagious.

PHYSIOLOGICAL INTEGRITY

Reduction of Risk Potential

Laboratory values

802. A client is admitted for hemorrhagic gastritis of prolonged standing. The nurse reviews the lab results on this client. Which lab result would the nurse question?
A. Hematocrit 29
B. Hemoglobin 9.9
C. Guaiac negative
D. Reticulocyte count elevated

The answer is C. Guaiac evaluates blood in the stool which should be positive. The client with hemorrhagic gastritis would likely be anemic from chronic bleeding so low hemoglobin and hematocrit would be expected. An elevated reticulocyte count is the body's attempt to replace lost blood cells.

PHYSIOLOGICAL INTEGRITY

Pharmacological and Parenteral Therapies

Adverse Effects/Contraindications and Side Effects

Implement procedures to counteract adverse effects of medications and parenteral therapy

803. Guarding against suicide is a priority nursing intervention for which client?

A client who is withdrawing from
A. Methylphenidate (Ritalin)
B. Alprazolam (Xanax)

C. Propoxyphene (Darvon)
D. Butabarbital (Butisol)

The answer is A. Methylphenidate (Ritalin) is a central nervous system stimulant and like other CNS stimulants such as cocaine and the amphetamines, clients who are withdrawing from it are severely dysphoric, anxious and at risk for suicide. Suicide is not a withdrawal effect of any of the other drug options.

HEALTH PROMOTION AND MAINTENANCE

Growth and Development

804. When teaching new mothers about play and stimulation for the first 6 months, which of the following toys would be recommended?
A. Unbreakable mirror in a soft black and white frame
B. Large brightly colored balloon
C. 5" doll with removable clothing and shoes
D. Push-pull toy
E. Soft cuddly stuffed toy
F. Musical Mobile

The answers are A, E, and F. Balloons are a choking hazard. Push-pull toys will be useful later on when the child can manipulate the toy. With a 5' doll the removable shoes and possibly other accessories are too small and therefore a choking hazard. Mirrors, toys with contrasting colors, musical mobiles and soft stuffed toys are appropriate for the first 6 months.

PHYSIOLOGICAL INTEGRITY

Pharmacological and Parenteral Therapies

Medication Administration

Instruct client on medication self-administration procedures

805. Which directions should be given to a patient taking Fosamax?
Mark all that apply.
A. ___ Take with a full glass of water
B. ___ Take at bedtime
C. ___ Take on an empty stomach
D. ___ Avoid fatty foods.
E. ___ Avoid heavy lifting
F. ___ Do not lie down until after eating once the pill is taken.
G. ___ Do not eat for 30 minutes

The answers are A, C, F, and G. Fosamax should be swallowed, not chewed or sucked, with a full glass of water on an empty stomach after getting up for the day. After taking Fosamax, the client should not eat, drink, or take another medication for at least 30 minutes. Clients should not lie down once the pill is taken until 30 minutes has passed and they have eaten. Fosamax should not be taken at bed time or before getting up for a day. If a dose is missed, a tablet should be taken the morning after the client remembers and then the usual dosage schedule followed. Two tablets should not be taken on the same day.

SAFE AND EFFECTIVE CARE ENVIRONMENT

Safety and Infection Control

Disaster planning

806. During a disaster the director of the command post sends a nurse to the emergency department to assist in triaging causality victims as they arrive. Which is the priority concern of this nurse?
A. Meet the needs of the largest number of victims
B. Provide care to the most seriously injured
C. Record names of victims as they arrive
D. Place victims in zones according to their color coded tags

The answer is A. Triage is the process of prioritizing which clients are to be treated first during a disaster. Triage is based on making decisions that will do the greatest good for the greatest number. Treating the most seriously injured is describing "daily triage." The victim is expected to arrive at the hospital with a tag already filled out. Victims are evaluated and a color coded tag is applied for easy identification of the victims status.

PSYCHOSOCIAL INTEGRITY

Behavioral Interventions

Assess client appearance, mood, and psychomotor behavior and identify/respond to inappropriate/abnormal behavior

807. A client with delusions says to the nurse "The aliens are after me because they think I am going to take over their planet." Which is the most appropriate response for the nurse to make?
A. "I don't know anything about aliens. Do you feel afraid that people are trying to harm you?"
B. "Why would the aliens think you are going to take over their planet?"
C. "You are a good person; no one wants to kill you."
D. "What makes you think the aliens want to kill you?"

The answer is A. This is an empathetic response that acknowledges the client's feeling.

Responses B and D encourage the client to get more involved and add detail to the delusion and this is not therapeutic. Response C has an element of false reassurance and cliché as well as disagreement with the client's delusion. Disagreeing can result in a defensive reaction with the client sticking even more firmly to the delusion.

PHYSIOLOGICAL INTEGRITY

Physiological Adaptation

Illness management

808. After being diagnosed with diverticulitis, a client has been taught about the appropriate dietary changes. The nurse recognizes that additional teaching is needed when the client states:
   A. "I will follow a high-fiber diet."
   B. "Milk will decrease my episodes of diverticulitis."
   C. "Whole grains are better for me than refined grains."
   D. "Fruits and vegetables are good for me but not nuts and seeds."

The answer is B. A diet to prevent constipation is recommended. Milk can be constipating. A high fiber diet helps to prevent constipation. Whole grains are a good source of fiber. Fruits and vegetables are good sources of fiber but nuts and seeds should be avoided because of the risk of them getting trapped in a diverticulum and serving as a source of inflammation.

PHYSIOLOGICAL INTEGRITY

Physiological Adaptation

Pathophysiology

809. A client has recently been diagnosed with cancer of the tongue. Client teaching about oral cancer has been completed. Which comment by the client indicates the need for additional client teaching?
   A. "My type of cancer metastasizes quickly because of the rich lymph and blood supply in the area."
   B. "Like me, most clients don't have early symptoms of tongue cancer."
   C. "The doctor may need to do a neck resection to get to the lymph nodes there."
   D. "I never thought that smoking would get me, but they tell me that studies show a direct link between smoking and cancer of the tongue."

The answer is D. Smoking has been linked to all oral cancers except that of the tongue. All other responses are correct.

PHYSIOLOGICAL INTEGRITY

Basic Care and Comfort

Elimination

810. The nurse is teaching a group of pregnant clients about hemorrhoid prevention. Which risk factors would the nurse identify?
   A. Constipation
   B. Straining on elimination
   C. Sitting for prolonged periods
   D. Excessive roughage in the diet.
   E. Standing for prolonged periods

The answers are A, B, C, and E. Constipation and straining on elimination increases the pressure in the rectal area. Maintaining one position for an extended period will cause stasis of circulation. Roughage is encouraged to prevent constipation so is not a risk factor for hemorrhoids.

HEALTH PROMOTION AND MAINTENANCE

Growth and Development

811. The nurse teaches parents about fears in the preschool years. Which information does the nurse include in the teaching plan?
   A. Past fears of the toddlerhood years are gradually disappearing
   B. The preschool child is no longer bothered by imagined fears; fears are more realistic
   C. The preschool child is no longer afraid to go to bed as in the toddler years
   D. The preschool child finds large dogs and other animals frightening
   E. The preschool child is afraid of mutilation and pain
   F. Playing out fears with dolls that helped in toddlerhood is not effective for the pre-schooler.

The answers are D and E. The preschool child experiences a greater number of real and imagined fears than in any other time of childhood. The child is afraid of the dark, being alone at bedtime, large dogs, ghosts, thunderstorms, pain, and mutilation. Playing out fears with dolls is useful in alleviating fears as well as desensitization.

PHYSIOLOGICAL INTEGRITY

Pharmacological and Parenteral Therapies

Medication Administration

Instruct client on medication self-administration procedures

812. What is the primary reason why the nurse teaches a client to wear a glove or finger cot when applying topical acyclovir to a herpetic lesion?
   A. Prevent suprainfection
   B. Prevent autoinoculation
   C. Prevent overdose from excess absorption
   D. Prevent unnecessary staining of the skin

The answer is B. Herpes can spread by autoinoculation. Wearing a glove to apply medication to the lesions helps prevent this. Even when wearing a glove or finger cot, clients must also be taught the importance of hand washing before and after each application of medication. Use of a barrier also helps prevent possible bacterial contamination and suprainfection but is not the primary reason for teaching the use of a barrier rather than just hand washing alone.

PSYCHOSOCIAL INTEGRITY

Therapeutic Communications

Use therapeutic communication techniques to provide support to client and/or family

813. The nurse asks a client with Alzheimer's Disease "Do you want some orange juice?" The client responds "Wha....". What should be the nurse's response?
   A. "Do you want a glass of orange juice?"
   B. "Are you thirsty–do you want some juice?"
   C. "Have a nice cold glass of juice; it will taste good."
   D. "Do you want some orange juice?"

The answer is D. "Do you want some orange juice?" This is the same question the nurse asked first. When communicating with a client with Alzheimer's disease one guideline to be followed is repeat questions if needed but do not rephrase them because this would only further confuse the client. Other guidelines for communicating with the client with Alzheimer's disease are: use simple words and short sentences; ask only one question at a time; give only one direction at a time; speak slowly and clearly.

HEALTH PROMOTION AND MAINTENANCE

Developmental Stages and Transitions

814. The nurse teaches new parents about gross motor and fine motor development of the infant. What can the mother expect by 6 months?
   A. Head lag at 6 months
   B. Can usually roll from prone to supine and supine to prone
   C. Can transfer cube from one hand to the other hand
   D. Can pull self to stand
   E. Crude pincer grasp
   F. Palmer grasp with fingers encircling object

The answers are B, C, and F. Head lag at 6 months is an ominous sign and should be reported for follow up. The 6 month old can roll from the prone to supine and supine to prone position. With the new practice of placing infants on their backs for sleep, as opposed to the abdomen, because of SIDs, there is a noted delay in many infants in rolling from abdomen to back, but by 6 months infants have accomplished this task. The 6-month-old has a palmer grasp and is beginning to transfer a cube from one hand to the other. The infant pulls himself to stand, and develops a crude pincer grasp at 9 months.

PHYSIOLOGICAL INTEGRITY

Reduction of Risk Potential

Monitoring conscious sedation

815. The nurse is caring for a client who has received conscious sedation for elective cardioversion. Following the procedure the arterial blood gas results are as follows: pH 7.32; PaO_2 95mm Hg; $PaCO_2$ 62 mm Hg; HCO_3 19 meq/L; O_2 Sat 95%. Based on these values which action would the nurse take?
   A. Chart the values and continue assessing the client
   B. Start supplemental oxygen at 2 liter per minute via nasal cannula
   C. Have the client perform deep breathing exercises
   D. Have the client breathe into a paper bag

The answer is C. Deep breathing exercises will help the client blow off carbon dioxide and bring down the $PaCO_2$ level.

A is incorrect because the blood gas results are showing respiratory acidosis.

O_2 is not needed because the Os 2 level is within the normal range. Breathing into a paper bag is used when the client is experiencing respiratory alkalosis.

SAFE AND EFFECTIVE CARE ENVIRONMENT

Management of Care

Establishing priorities

816. The nurse assigned to a client being admitted for rectal bleeding, must establish priorities of care. In which order would the nurse carry out the following care activities?
   A. Start an intravenous
   B. Observe the client's level of anxiety
   C. Continue to monitor the client for rectal bleeding
   D. Teach the client self care in preparation for her discharge
   E. Assess the client's skin, blood pressure, heart rate, and urine output
   F. Teach the client about the diagnostic tests ordered during the next 48 hours

Record your answer by placing the letter of each activity in proper sequence in the space provided.

Correct order of priorities: E, A, B, C, F, D. Physical needs precede psychological needs. Client teaching would be the last priority in this situation.

PHYSIOLOGICAL INTEGRITY

Physiological Adaptation

Alterations in Body Systems

817. A 3-week-old infant has been diagnosed with Hirschsprung's Disease and has just returned from surgery with a double barreled colostomy. The mother cries when she sees the colostomy stoma and says: "My poor baby, to have to go through life with that thing on his abdomen." The nurse's response would be based on the knowledge that
    A. colostomy care is not as difficult as it may seem.
    B. the colostomy will not be permanent.
    C. the child will never have known anything but the colostomy.
    D. colostomy stomas are hidden easily under clothing.

The answer is B. A double barreled colostomy indicates the intention to reconnect the bowel at a later time so the mother's misconception needs to be addressed. All the other options are inappropriate as the basis of the nurse's response because the colostomy is not going to be permanent. Colostomy care during infancy is relatively simple as the child would not be continent anyway. Stomas can be hidden under clothing. The child would eventually know that he or she is different.

HEALTH PROMOTION AND MAINTENANCE

Developmental Stages and Transitions

818. The nurse is planning a class to promote effective parenting of toddlers. Which topics should the nurse plan to discuss?
    A. Negativism
    B. Ritualism
    C. Egocentrism
    D. Temper Tantrums
    E. Possessiveness
    F. Altruism

The answers are A, B, C, D, and E. These are all topics pertinent to toddler behavior. Negativism refers to strongly expressed emotions: 'no'. Ritualism is seen as the toddler having a favorite doll, favorite blanket and various rituals of behavior, especially at bedtime. Egocentrism refers to the fact that the toddlers can not comprehend that others think differently than they do. Temper Tantrums which are characteristic of toddlers are attention seeking and best dealt with by ignoring them. Possessiveness indicates the toddler's beginning awareness of ownership, as shown by the use of the word "mine." Altruism is not a characteristic of toddlerhood.

PHYSIOLOGICAL INTEGRITY

Pharmacological and Parenteral Therapies

Adverse Effects/Contraindications and Side Effects

Assess client for actual or potential side effects and adverse effects of medications

819. Which is the priority factor for the nurse to assess when a client is receiving IV acyclovir?
    A. mental status
    B. cardiac rhythm
    C. urinary output
    D. temperature

The answer is C. Monitoring urinary output is critical when acyclovir is given systemically because it is excreted primarily by glomerular filtration and tubular secretion and therefore can be nephrotoxic. To decrease the risk of nephrotoxicity, the client must be well hydrated; the drug must be administered over a period of 60 minutes; and urinary output must be measured for 2 hours after the infusion. Output of less than 500 mL of urine per gram of acyclovir must be reported immediately.

Confusion and hallucinations along with tremors and seizures are some of the serious adverse reactions to systemic acyclovir but they are uncommon. Cardiac rhythm is unaffected. Temperature may be monitored because of existing infection but not directly because of the acyclovir; it does not present an immediate threat so does not take priority over monitoring urinary output.

SAFE AND EFFECTIVE ENVIRONMENT

Management of Care

Establishing priorities

820. Vital signs on a client who has just been admitted to the unit are: BP 162/84, Pulse 100 and irregular, Respirations 16, and Pulse Oximetry 88%. Which would be the immediate nursing intervention?
    A. Place the client on cardiac telemetry
    B. Call the physician to report the vital signs
    C. Start a saline lock for IV medication access
    D. Start oxygen at 2–4 liters per minute per nasal cannula per protocol

The answer is D. The client's oxygen level is very low. All other interventions would be done later.

PHYSIOLOGICAL INTEGRITY

Pharmacological and Parenteral Therapies

Evaluate appropriateness/accuracy of medication order for client

821. A nurse would question an order for misoprostol to prevent gastric ulcers for which client?
   A. A client allergic to shellfish
   B. A pregnant client
   C. A client taking warfarin sodium
   D. A client with a history of hepatitis

The answer is B. Misoprostol is a synthetic form of prostaglandin E which is used to prevent NSAID-induced gastric ulcers in high risk clients. It is a pregnancy category X drug because of its abortifacient action and therefore the order would be questioned if the client is pregnant. Before beginning treatment with misoprostol women of childbearing age must have a negative serum pregnancy test within two weeks of start of treatment which should be on day 2 or 3 or menses. They must also be warned both orally and in writing that the drug causes uterine contractions and miscarriage and be able and willing to use an effective form of contraception.

HEALTH PROMOTION AND MAINTENANCE

Health Promotion Programs

822. The nurse teaches new parents about nutrition for the first year of life. What information does the nurse include in her teaching plan?
   A. Breast milk is a complete and healthful diet for the first 6 months of life.
   B. Commercially prepared fortified infant formula is a good alternative if breast feeding is not desirable or feasible.
   C. No additional fluids are needed for the first 4–6 months when the infant is breast or formula fed.
   D. In second 6 months skim or regular cow's milk used depending on infant's weight pattern.
   E. Solid foods starting with cereals at 2 months, and gradually introducing fruits, vegetables and meats over next 4 months.
   F. Honey is not given for the first year because it is a source of botulism.

The answers are A, B, C, and F. Breast feeding and fortified commercially prepared infant formulas are the best and only sources of nutrition appropriate for the first 6 months of life and continues to be the primary source of nutrition in the second 6 months of life as well. Cows' milk, skim or regular, and imitation milks are not acceptable during the first year, as they are difficult to digest and lack the nutrients needed for growth. Solid foods are generally introduced at 5–6 months starting with cereals with gradual introduction of fruits, vegetables and meats. Honey is not given in the first year as it is associated with botulism.

PHYSIOLOGICAL INTEGRITY

Physiological Adaptation

Hemodynamics

823. The nurse is caring for a client when the cardiac monitor shows that cardiac pattern has changed from a normal sinus rhythm. QRSs are now widened and bizarre at a rate of 160 beats per minute. The client begins complaining of being dizzy. Which is the nurse's immediate action?
   A. Call a code
   B. Administer a precordial thump
   C. Give Lidocaine 50–100 mG. IV push
   D. Assess the client's vital signs

The answer is D. The nurse needs to assess the client to determine cardiac perfusion and to be sure of what the monitor is showing. The nurse would not call a code because the client has not arrested. Precordial thump is only used with a witnessed arrest. Lidocaine would be the drug of choice if the client were in a sustained Ventricular Tachycardia and was symptomatic.

SAFE AND EFFECTIVE CARE ENVIRONMENT

Safety and Infection Control

Handling hazardous and infectious materials

824. The nurse is serving on a safety committee which is currently examining policies regarding the proper handling and storage of dangerous chemicals. Which guidelines would the nurse expect the policies to address?
   A. ___ Label the containers containing materials
   B. ___ Maintain an inventory list of the materials
   C. ___ Keep older products in the front, newer products in the back
   D. ___ Store chemicals on open shelves
   E. ___ Segregate chemicals alphabetically

The answers are A, B, and C. Containers containing hazardous chemicals need to be clearly labeled with the full chemical name. Current hazard waste inventory list is required to be maintained. Older chemicals need to be used before newer products.

Chemicals stored on open shelves could be accidentally knocked off the shelf. Chemicals also need to be stored based on compatibility and not necessarily alphabetically.

PHYSIOLOGICAL INTEGRITY

Physiological Adaptation

Alterations in Body Systems

825. A client has a permanent colostomy for colon cancer. The client is struggling to learn colostomy care. In frustration, the client throws the equipment and says, "It's not worth it. I might as well be dead." Which interpretation of this behavior should be the basis of the nurse's initial response to the client?
   A. The client has not developed an adult level of self control.
   B. The client does not want to learn.
   C. The approach to teaching is incorrect for this client.
   D. The client is having difficulty coping.

The answer is D. The most likely interpretation of this behavior and the one that should serve as the basis of the nurse's first response is that the client is displaying signs of inadequate coping with his life threatening disease and the need for a colostomy. It is possible that the client is lacking in self control or doesn't want to learn but these are not as likely as difficulty coping given the client's health problems. It is also possible that the approach to teaching is not ideal for this client and this may need to be addressed but it is not the most likely cause of the behavior.

HEALTH PROMOTION AND MAINTENANCE

Growth and Development

826. The nurse at a day care is observing pre-school children at play. Which types of play observed would the nurse evaluate as normal for a preschooler?
   A. Playing house and doing housekeeping chores.
   B. Jumping, running or climbing
   C. Riding a tricycle
   D. Having an "imaginary playmate"
   E. Playing dress up

The answers are A, B, C, D, and E. Imitative, imaginary and dramatic play are characteristic of the pre-school period. Playing house, dress up, and housekeeping chores are examples of imitative, imaginary and dramatic play. Imaginary playmates are a normal healthy and useful part of the preschoolers play. Parents can even set a place setting for a "friend," but can not allow the child to avoid responsibility by blaming "friend" for mess.

Activities for motor development should also be encouraged including: running, jumping, climbing and tricycle riding. Reading or watching an educational video are examples of mutual activities that can be enjoyed with a parent.

PHYSIOLOGICAL INTEGRITY

Reduction of Risk Potential

System-specific assessment

827. To calculate central venous pressure from the jugular venous pressure, how many centimeters are added to the JVP? Record your answer as a whole number in the space provided.

   ____

The answer is 4 cm. Four centimeters are added to the jugular venous pressure to obtain the central venous pressure.

PSYCHOSOCIAL INTEGRITY

Behavioral Interventions

Assess client appearance, mood, and psychomotor behavior and identify/respond to inappropriate/abnormal behavior

828. What is the most important reason for monitoring a client with a borderline personality disorder and depression for a sudden change in mood?
   A. Mood change can be the first indication that therapeutic gains are being made.
   B. Mood change can indicate a need for change in medication.
   C. Mood change can herald a decision to commit suicide.
   D. Mood change can signal the appropriate time to introduce group therapy.

The answer is C. A mood change can indicate a decision to commit suicide. Client safety is always the priority hence this is the most important reason for monitoring mood. Change in mood may indicate any of the other options but they are not the priority over protecting the client's life.

PHYSIOLOGICAL INTEGRITY

Reduction of Risk Potential

Potential for Complication of Diagnostic Tests/Treatments/Procedures

829. Following eye surgery, the client is told by the physician that care must be taken to avoid elevating intraocular pressure. Which activities would the nurse identify as those the client needs to avoid? Mark all that apply.

A. ___ Blowing the nose
B. ___ Straining at stool
C. ___ Wearing a tight collar
D. ___ Bending over at the waist
E. ___ Coughing
F. ___ Keeping the head down

The answers are all A, B, C, D, E, and F. All of these activities increase pressure within the eyeball as does sneezing, vomiting and sexual intercourse.

INDEX

D

E

R